药品监管法律制度系列研究

Compilation of FDA
GCP and GLP Warning Letters

美国FDA药物
临床试验与非临床研究
警告信汇编
（2008~2017）

国家食品药品监督管理总局食品药品审核查验中心
上海药品审评核查中心　组织编译

中国医药科技出版社

编委会

前言
Foreword

药物非临床研究和临床试验是药品研发过程中的关键环节，是研发者在资源和时间上投入最大的部分，其研究数据和结果是评价药物安全性、有效性的重要依据。2015年7月22日，国家食品药品监督管理总局发布《关于开展药物临床试验数据自查核查工作的公告》，启动了药物临床试验数据检查工作。从检查结果来看，近年来在我国开展的药物临床研究中存在不少问题，包括一定数量的数据不可靠及弄虚作假行为，较严重地影响了药物临床试验的质量，甚至直接影响到对上市药品安全性、有效性的客观评价。有鉴于此，国家食品药品监督管理总局正在加大药物临床试验现场检查监管力度，并将监管重点从对研究机构的资格认定检查向对临床试验项目的过程检查转变，以通过建立更为行之有效的监管机制，促进我国药物非临床研究和临床试验的健康发展，以进一步落实党中央“四个最严”的要求。

“他山之石，可以攻玉”。美国食品药品监督管理局（FDA）多年来实施的“生物研究监查项目”（Bioreseardn Monitoring Program，BIMO），基于风险和问题，对药物非临床研究（GLP）和临床试验（GCP）进行监督检查，为我国药物临床试验的监管提供了参考典范。该项目美国FDA已实施20多年，其目的：一是保护美国FDA监管的以药品注册为目的开展的临床试验和非临床研究中受试者及试验动物的权利和安全；二是核实用于支持药物上市申请的临床试验和非临床研究数据的准确性和可靠性；三是保证美国FDA监管的GCP和GLP研究的实施符合法规要求。该项目通过常规检查和有因检查的方式对提交美国FDA的新药或仿制药非临床研究及临床试验相关单位（包括伦理委员会、申办企业、研究者及生物样本检测实验室等）进行现场检查，以发现并评估试验过程的合规性和试验数据及结果的可靠性方面存在的问题，并根据问题的严重程度对相关方给予相应的处罚措施（包括警告信、限制或取消资格、拒绝接受数据、暂缓或终止临床研究、禁令等），甚至移送追究刑事责任。其中，发出警告信是最常见的一种行政处罚措施。在美国FDA给相关方的警告信中会详尽列出检查对象信息、检查发现的问题、违反的相关法规条款，以及对企业整改的要求等内容。由于警告信不仅寄送被检查的相关方，而且还在美国FDA网站的数据库中全文公布，供社会各界查询，因此对违规的被检查单位或相关人员构成了很大的威慑及警示作用。同时，这些警告信也成为各国监管机构、研究机构和企业了解美国FDA检查重点和发现问题的很好信息资源。

国家食品药品监督管理总局食品药品审核查验中心与上海药品审评核查

中心合作，对2008年以来美国FDA网站上公布的在BIMO现场检查中发现问题的药物非临床研究和临床试验警告信进行了收集、翻译、整理和分析，以通过系统研究美国FDA药物非临床研究和临床试验警告信案例，分析美国FDA在现场检查中发现的主要问题和缺陷情况，了解美国FDA相关检查的重点和模式，为探索我国基于风险的现场检查模式提供可借鉴的经验。展现在各位读者面前的本汇编就是该课题的主要成果之一。

该汇编收集了美国FDA官方自2008年1月至2017年12月期间由其药品评价与研究中心（CDER）和生物制品评价与研究中心（CBER）发布的药物GCP和GLP警告信共152封中译文和英文原文。为了方便读者参阅，该汇编将全部警告信分成药物GCP警告信，给伦理委员会、给申办者、给合同研究组织、给申办-研究者、给研究者以及药物GLP警告信六部分。各部分按照警告信的发布日期从近到远排列。正文后附专业术语及缩略语英汉对照表。在编译时，对原文中存在的部分姓名表示方式不一致、因保密需要使用的代码、用语不统一、序号不连贯等情况，基本按原文保留；对个别明显的拼写错误给予了更正。为了节省篇幅，中译文中每封警告信正文前后的通讯信息及格式化内容均予省略，需要的读者可参见原文。

该汇编可供我国各级药品监管机构、审评检查机构、药品研发企业及临床研究机构相关人员参考，是药物非临床研究与药物临床试验合规性检查不可多得的参考书。

参加本汇编翻译、审校工作的同志有上海药品审评核查中心、国家食品药品监督管理总局食品药品审核查验中心人员，以及部分来自业界的专业人士。这些同志在完成紧张的本职工作的同时，为本书的翻译和出版倾注了大量心血，同时也得到了所在单位和部门领导的大力支持，在此一并表示诚挚的感谢！

编译者

2018年1月

目 录
Contents

第一部分

药物 GCP 警告信

——给伦理委员会

FDA

第 1 封　给 Oeyama-Moto 癌症研究基金会伦理委员会的警告信

2016年4月7日

参考号：16-HFD-45-03-04

尊敬的Wada博士：

2015年8月11日至9月29日，Uttaniti Limchumroon先生、Greg K. Keshishyan先生和Quynh-Van Tran博士代表美国食品药品监督管理局（以下简称FDA）对贵伦理委员会（IRB）进行了现场检查，这封警告信特告知您现场检查中发现的违规情况。本次现场检查的目的是核实贵伦理委员会受试者的保护程序是否符合美国联邦法规（CFR）第21篇第50和第56部分的要求。这些法规均适用于FDA所监管产品的临床研究。

本次现场检查是FDA的生物研究监查项目的一部分，该项目通过设定的检查方法，对FDA所监管的相关研究的实施情况进行评估，以确认研究数据在科学上是有效和准确的，并帮助确保这些研究中受试者的权益、安全和福利得到了保护。

在现场检查结束时，Limchumroon和Keshishyan先生向伦理委员会委员Judy Fu Chuan Li女士出示了FDA 483表，即现场检查发现的问题，并与她进行了讨论。贵伦理委员会2015年10月8日提交的针对该FDA 483表的书面回复已收悉。

经对现场检查报告、该报告的附件，以及贵伦理委员会于2015年10月8日的书面回复进行审查，我们认为，贵伦理委员会未能遵循监管受试者保护的FDA法规。我们想强调以下几点：

1. IRB未能制定、维护和遵守管理IRB职能和运行的必要书面程序［21 CFR 56.108（a）、21 CFR 56.108（b）和21 CFR 56.115（a）（6）］

为了符合IRB法规要求，每个IRB必须制定、维护并遵守IRB职能与运行相关的书面程序。贵IRB未能遵循这一要求。具体来说，Oeyama-Moto癌症研究基金会IRB未能制定、维护和遵守FDA法规所要求的如下书面程序：

a. IRB关于进行初始审查和跟踪审查的书面程序，向研究者和机构报告IRB发现的问题和采取的措施的书面程序［21 CFR 56.108（a）（1）和21 CFR 56.115（a）（6）］。

b. 确定哪些项目需要进行超过每年一次的审查，哪些项目需要从研究者以外的来源确认自先前的IRB审查后材料没有发生变更的书面程序［21 CFR 56.108（a）（2）和21 CFR 56.115（a）（6）］。

c. 确保将研究活动中的变动及时向IRB报告的书面程序［21 CFR 56.108（a）（3）］。

d. 确保将任何非预期的、给受试者或他人带来风险的问题及时向IRB、适当的机构管理人员以及FDA报告的书面程序［21 CFR 56.108（b）（1）和21 CFR 56.115（a）（6）］。

e. 确保将任何严重的或持续不符合法规要求或IRB决定的情况及时向IRB、适当的机构管理人员以及FDA报告的书面程序［21 CFR 56.108（b）（2）和21 CFR 56.115（a）（6）］。

f. 确保将任何IRB批件的暂停或终止及时向IRB、适当的机构管理人员以及FDA报告的书面程序［21 CFR 56.108（b）（3）和21 CFR 56.115（a）（6）］。

贵IRB的书面回复不能充分地解决这一违规，因为回复引用了实施临床研究的书面程序，而不是21 CFR 56.108（a）、21 CFR 56.108（b）和21 CFR 56.115（a）（6）所要求的监管IRB职能和运行的书面程序。

请提交贵IRB计划采取的解决上述违规的任何纠正或预防措施。与这些纠正或预防措施一起，请提交一份IRB最终版本的书面程序或任何拟定中的程序草案的复印件，以及新的书面程序实施的计划时间表。此外，请提交对IRB员工和委员进行新的书面程序培训的说明，以及接受培训的人员和委员名单，或者计划培训的项目时间表。

IRB未能制定、维护和遵守必要的书面程序这一情况，引起对IRB确保受试者权益和福利的审查程序的关注。

2. IRB未能准备和保存足够的包括IRB会议记录的IRB活动记录［21 CFR 56.115（a）（2）］

IRB必须准备和保存IRB活动的足够记录，包括IRB会议的会议记录，其中应当用充分的细节来显示会议的出席情况，IRB采取的行动，关于这些行动的投票，包括赞成、反对和弃权的委员人数，要求对研究进行修改或不批准研究的依据，对有争议问题的讨论和处理的书面概要。贵IRB未能遵循这个要求，具体而言：

a. 2014年1月18日的会议记录显示，IRB“审查并通过了用于IND（b）（4）的（b）（4）临床试验方案”。但该记录没有包含对这项行动的投票情况，包括赞成、反对与弃权的委员人数。

针对上述2.a.项，我们承认贵IRB对FDA483表的书面回复提到，所有投票的IRB委员，都同意采取的行动。但是，该回复并不充分，因为没有任何为预防将来发生类似违规而采取的措施。

b. 2014年2月8日的会议记录显示，贵IRB批准“随机双臂研究，且以人道主义原因同意将低剂量组患者转至高剂量组继续接受治疗”。2014年4月18日的IRB会议记录显示那次会议上也采取了类似的行动。该记录没有包含对这项行动的投票情况，包括赞成、反对与弃权的委员人数。

c. 2014年5月28日和2014年8月28日的会议记录显示，IRB批准（b）（4）临床试验“在报纸上招募患者参与”。该记录没有包含对这项行动的投票情况，包括赞成、反对与弃权的委员人数。

我们确认上述2.b.项2.c.项的问题并未列入给贵IRB的FDA483表，因此，贵IRB对FDA483表的书面回复没有对这些违规进行说明。

请提交一份贵IRB为确保符合FDA法规和IRB书面程序而计划采取的措施的书面说明，因为这些措施与会议记录有关。回复应包含一份对IRB员工和委员进行培训的说明，以及接受培训的IRB人员和委员的名单，或者计划培训的项目时间表，以解决以上2.a.项到2.c.项描述的违规。

由于贵IRB未能在2014年1月18日、2月8日、4月18日、5月28日和8月28日的IRB会议记录投票的计票情况，导致我们无法确定作为（b）（4）临床研究的授权研究者医生的两位IRB委员（b）（4）和（b）（4）医生是否参加到对研究的IRB审查，除非是按照IRB的要求提供信息。

未能准备和保存关于IRB会议的充分记录，引起对贵IRB审查程序充分性的关注。而且，不充分的记录引起对贵IRB召开会议时委员数量是否达到法定人数的关注。

3. IRB未能以书面形式通知研究者和机构批准或不予批准被提议的研究的决定，或为保证IRB批准研究而要求的修改意见［21 CFR 56.109（e）］

IRB需要以书面形式通知研究者和机构对于提出的研究的批准或不批准的决定，或为确保IRB批准要求进行的修改。贵IRB未能遵循这一要求，具体而言：

a. IRB于2014年2月8日批准“随机双臂研究”和“人道主义原因同意将低剂量组患者转至高剂量组继续治疗”时，没有以书面形式通知研究者。与此类似，2014年4月18日贵IRB采取同样的行动时，也未以书面形式通知研究者。

b. IRB于2014年12月8日“停止从报纸广告招募患者参与该项临床研究”时，未以书面形式通知研究者。与此类似，2015年1月28日贵IRB采取同样的行动时，也未以书面形式通知研究者。

贵IRB对FDA483表的书面回复中提到，IRB理解为一张小“备忘便条”也可以算是书面通知。然后写到，“请见各每个会议记录的P.S.部分”。然而，现场检查期间提供的会议记录并未包括“P.S.部分”。

贵IRB的书面回复已收悉，但是我们不能对该回复进行知情评价，因为其并没有包括据称是作为IRB对以上3.a.项和3.b.项提到的研究活动的决定的书面通知的“备忘便条”的复印件。请提交IRB回复中引用的以上3.a.项和3.b.项反映的、书面告知研究者IRB决定的“备忘便条”的复印件。

如果贵IRB不能够提供上述要求的“备忘便条”复印件，请提交IRB为解决上述违规情况的发生计划采取的纠正或预防措施。与纠正或预防措施一起，请提交一份贵IRB书面程序的复印件，或任何拟定中的程序草案的复印件，以及实施任何新的书面程序的项目时间表。此外，请提供一份对IRB员工和委员进行新的书面程序培训的说明，以及接受培训的IRB员工和委员的名单，或者计划培训的项目时间表。

未能以书面形式通知研究者和机构批准或不予批准被提议的研究的决定，或为保证IRB批准研究而要求的修改意见，引起我们对贵IRB与研究者沟通的充分性的关注。

本警告信的目的并非是罗列贵IRB在审查和批准试验方案中存在的所有缺陷。确保实际操作和程序完全符合所有适用法规的要求是贵IRB的责任。

自收到这封信的15个工作日内，贵IRB应当书面告知本办公室为预防将来发生类似违规情况而采取的措施。如果不能充分、迅速地解释上述违规问题，可能导致我们在不再通知的情况下采取监管措施。如果您认为已符合FDA法规要求，请陈述理由，并提供所有支持资料，以供我们参考。

附：英文原文

Oeyama-Moto Cancer Research Foundation IRB

WARNING LETTER

APR 7, 2016

CERTIFIED MAIL
RETURN RECEIPT REQUESTED

Ref: 16-HFD-45-03-04

Masao Wada, M.D.
Chair
Oeyama-Moto Cancer Research Foundation IRB
3106 East Garvey Avenue South
West Covina, California 91791-2344

Dear Dr. Wada:

This Warning Letter informs you of objectionable conditions observed during the U.S. Food and Drug Administration (FDA) inspection of your Institutional Review Board (IRB) that was conducted between August 11and September 29, 2015,by Mr. Uttaniti Limchumroon, Mr. Greg K. Keshishyan, and Quynh-Van Tran, Pharm.D., representing FDA. The purpose of this inspection was to determine whether the IRB procedures for the protection of human subjects complied with Title 21 of the Code of Federal Regulations (CFR), parts 50 and 56. These regulations apply to clinical investigations of products regulated by FDA.

This inspection is a part of FDA's Bioresearch Monitoring Program, which includes inspections designed to evaluate the conduct of FDA-regulated research to ensure that the data are scientifically valid and accurate, and to help ensure that the rights, safety, and welfare of the human subjects of those studies have been protected.

At the conclusion of the inspection, Mr. Limchumroon and Mr. Keshishyan presented and discussed with IRB member Ms. Judy Fu Chuan Li the Form FDA 483,Inspectional Observations. We acknowledge receipt of the IRB's October 8, 2015,written response to the Form FDA 483.

From our review of the FDA Establishment Inspection Report, the documents submitted with that report,and the IRB's October 8, 2015,written response, we conclude that the IRB did not adhere to FDA regulations governing the protection of human subjects. We wish to emphasize the following:

1. The IRB failed to prepare, maintain, and follow required written procedures governing the functions and operations of the IRB [21 CFR 56.108(a), 21 CFR 56.108(b), and 21 CFR 56.115(a)(6)].

In order to fulfill the requirements of the IRB regulations, each IRB must prepare, maintain, and follow written procedures describing IRB functions and operations that are specified in the regulations. The IRB failed to adhere to this requirement. Specifically, the Oeyama-Moto Cancer Research Foundation IRB failed to prepare, maintain, and follow the written procedures below that are required by FDA regulations:

a. Written procedures for conducting the IRB's initial and continuing review of research and for reporting the IRB's findings and actions to the investigator and the institution [21 CFR 56.108(a)(1) and 21 CFR 56.115(a)(6)].

b. Written procedures for determining which projects require review more often than annually, and which projects need verification from sources other than the investigator that no material changes have occurred since the previous IRB review [21 CFR 56.108(a)(2) and 21 CFR 56.115(a)(6)].

c. Written procedures for ensuring prompt reporting to the IRB of changes in research activity [21 CFR 56.108(a)(3)].

d. Written procedures for ensuring prompt reporting to the IRB, appropriate institutional officials, and the FDA of any unanticipated problems involving risks to human subjects or others [21 CFR 56.108(b)(1) and 21 CFR 56.115(a)(6)].

e. Written procedures for ensuring prompt reporting to the IRB, appropriate institutional officials, and the FDA of any instance of serious or continuing noncompliance with these regulations or with the requirements or determinations of the IRB [21 CFR 56.108(b)(2) and 21 CFR 56.115(a)(6)].

f. Written procedures for ensuring prompt reporting to the IRB, appropriate institutional officials, and the FDA of any suspension or termination of IRB approval [21 CFR 56.108(b)(3) and 21 CFR 56.115(a)(6)].

The IRB's written response does not address this violation adequately because the response refers to written procedures for conducting the clinical investigation, rather than written procedures governing the functions and operations of the IRB, as required by 21 CFR 56.108(a), 21 CFR 56.108(b), and 21 CFR 56.115(a)(6).

Please submit any corrective or preventive actions the IRB plans to take to address the violation described above. With these corrective or preventive actions, please submit a copy of the IRB's finalized written procedures, or any draft procedures in development, and a projected timeline for the implementation of any new written procedures. In addition, please provide a description of any training provided to IRB staff and members on the new written procedures, and a list of staff and members trained, or a projected timeline of planned training.

Failure of the IRB to prepare, maintain, and follow required written procedures raises concerns about the adequacy of the IRB's review processes for ensuring protection of the rights and welfare of human research subjects.

2. The IRB failed to prepare and maintain adequate documentation of IRB activities, including minutes of IRB meetings [21 CFR 56.115(a)(2)].

The IRB is required to prepare and maintain adequate documentation of IRB activities, including the minutes of IRB meetings, which shall be in sufficient detail to show attendance at the meetings; actions taken by the IRB; the vote on these actions, including the number of members voting for, against, and abstaining; the basis for requiring changes in or disapproving research; and a written summary of the discussion of controverted issues and their resolution. The IRB failed to adhere to this requirement. Specifically:

a. Minutes of the January 18, 2014, IRB meeting indicate that the IRB "reviewed, agreed on the protocol for IND**(b)(4)**, in **(b)(4)** clinical trial." However, the minutes do not include documentation of a vote on this action, including the number of members voting for, against, and abstaining.

Regarding Item 2.a. above, we acknowledge that the IRB's written response to the Form FDA 483 indicates that all members of the IRB who voted, voted in favor of the action taken. However, the response is inadequate because it does not describe any actions taken to prevent similar violations in the future.

b. Minutes of the February 8, 2014, IRB meeting indicate that the IRB approved "of double arm study by coin toss, and agreed to transfer low dose group patients to high dose group for continuing treatment due to humanitarian reason." Minutes of the April 18, 2014, IRB meeting indicate that similar actions were taken during that meeting. The minutes do not include documentation of a vote on these actions, including the number of members voting for, against, and abstaining.

c. Minutes of the May 28, 2014, and August 28, 2014, IRB meetings indicate that the IRB approved "for newspaper soliciting of patients to participate" in the **(b)(4)** clinical trial. The minutes do not include documentation of a vote on this action, including the number of members voting for, against, and abstaining.

We acknowledge that Items 2.b. and 2.c. above were not included as observations on the Form FDA 483 that was issued to the IRB, and therefore, the IRB's written response to the Form FDA 483 did not address these violations.

Please submit a written description of the actions the IRB plans to take to ensure compliance with FDA regulations and the IRB's written procedures as they relate to meeting minutes. The response should include a description of any training provided to the IRB staff and members and a list of IRB staff and members trained, or a projected timeline of planned training, to address the violations described in Items 2.a. through 2.c. above.

Because of the IRB's failure to document vote counts in the minutes of IRB meetings held on January 18, February 8, April 18, May 28, and August 28, 2014, we are unable to determine if two IRB members, Dr. **(b)(4)**and Dr. **(b)(4)**, who are subinvestigators for the **(b)(4)** clinical study, participated in the IRB's review of the study in any way, other than to provide information requested by the IRB.

Failure to prepare and maintain adequate documentation of IRB meetings raises concerns about the adequacy of the IRB's review process. Furthermore, inadequate documentation raises concerns about whether the IRB members maintained a quorum for the duration of the IRB meetings.

3. The IRB failed to notify investigators and the institution in writing of its decision to approve or disapprove proposed research activities or of modifications required to secure IRB approval of the research activity [21 CFR 56.109(e)].

The IRB is required to notify investigators and the institution in writing of its decision to approve or disapprove proposed research, or of modifications required to secure IRB approval. The IRB failed to adhere to this requirement. Specifically:

a. The IRB did not notify the investigator in writing when it approved the "double arm study by coin toss" and "agreed to transfer low dose group patients to high dose group for continuing treatment due to humanitarian reason" on February 8, 2014. Similarly, the IRB did not notify the investigator in writing when it took the same action on April 18, 2014.

b. The IRB did not notify the investigator in writing when it "discontinued for newspaper soliciting advertizement [*sic*] of patients to participate in this clinical trial" on December 8, 2014. Similarly, the IRB did not notify the investigator in writing when it took the same action on January 28, 2015.

The IRB's written response to the Form FDA 483 notes the IRB's understanding that a small "memorandum note" would serve as written notification; then it states, "Please see P.S. segment of the meeting minutes of each meeting." However, the meeting minutes provided during the inspection do not contain a "P.S. segment."

We acknowledge the IRB's written response; however, we are unable to undertake an informed evaluation of the response, because it does not contain copies of the memoranda that reportedly served as written notification of the IRB's decisions regarding the research activities noted in Items 3.a. and 3.b. above. Please submit copies of the memoranda referred to in the IRB's response regarding written notification to investigators for the IRB's decisions reflected in Items 3.a. and 3.b. above.

If the IRB is unable to provide copies of the memoranda requested above, please submit any corrective or preventive actions the IRB plans to take to address the violation described above. With these corrective or preventive actions, please submit a copy of the IRB's written procedures, or any draft procedures in development, and a projected timeline for the implementation of any new written procedures. In addition, please provide a description of any training provided to IRB staff and members on the new written procedures, and a list of staff and members trained, or a projected timeline of planned training.

Failure to notify investigators in writing of IRB decisions to approve or disapprove proposed research activities, or of modifications required to secure IRB approval, raises concerns about the adequacy of the IRB's communications with investigators.

This letter is not intended to be an all-inclusive list of deficiencies for the protocols reviewed and approved by the IRB. It is the IRB's responsibility to ensure that its practices and procedures comply fully with all applicable regulations.

Within fifteen (15) working days of the IRB's receipt of this letter, the IRB should notify this office in writing of the actions that will be taken to prevent similar violations in the future. Failure to address the violations noted above adequately and promptly may result in regulatory action without further notice. If you believe you have complied with FDA regulations, include your reasoning and any supporting information for our consideration.

We recommend that the IRB visit the following FDA Web page for information on human subject protections that may assist the IRB in its efforts to come into compliance with FDA regulations:*http://www.fda.gov/ScienceResearch/SpecialTopics/RunningClinicalTrials/default.htm.*

We appreciate the cooperation shown to the FDA investigators during the inspection. If the IRB has any questions, please contact Constance Cullity, M.D., M.P.H., at 301-796-3397; FAX 301-847-8748. The IRB's written response and any pertinent documentation should be addressed to:

Constance Cullity, M.D., M.P.H.
Branch Chief
Good Clinical Practice Compliance Oversight Branch
Division of Clinical Compliance Evaluation
Office of Scientific Investigations
Office of Compliance
Center for Drug Evaluation and Research
Food and Drug Administration
Building 51, Room 5354
10903 New Hampshire Avenue
Silver Spring, MD 20993

Sincerely,

{See appended electronic signature page}

David Burrow, Pharm.D., J.D.
Acting Director
Office of Scientific Investigations
Office of Compliance
Center for Drug Evaluation and Research
Food and Drug Administration

第2封　给Pikeville医疗中心有限公司伦理委员会的警告信

2016年3月1日

参考号：16-HFD-45-02-03

尊敬的May先生：

2015年8月17日至8月21日，Richard W. Berning先生代表FDA对贵伦理委员会（IRB）进行了现场检查。这封警告信特告知您现场检查中发现的违规情况。本次现场检查的目的是核实贵伦理委员会受试者保护程序是否符合美国联邦法规（CFR）第21篇第50和第56部分的要求。这些法规适用于FDA所监管产品的临床研究。

本次现场检查是FDA的生物研究监查项目的一部分。该项目通过设定的检查方法，对FDA所监管的相关研究的实施情况进行评估，以确认研究数据在科学上是有效和准确的，并帮助确保这些研究中受试者的权益、安全和福利得到了保护。

在现场检查结束时，Berning先生向贵伦理委员会主席Holly H. Gallion博士出示了FDA483表，即现场检查发现的问题，并与其进行了讨论。您2015年9月14日对该FDA483表的书面回复已收悉。

经对现场检查报告、该报告的附件，以及您2015年9月14日的书面回复进行审查，我们认为，贵伦理委员会没有遵循适用的监管受试者保护的FDA法规。我们想强调以下几点：

1. IRB未能制定、维护和遵守管理IRB职能和运行的必要书面程序［21 CFR 56.108（a），21 CFR 56.108（b）与21 CFR 56.115（a）（6）］

为了满足IRB法规的要求，每个IRB必须制定、维护和遵守法规中规定的描述IRB职能与运行的书面程序。贵IRB未能遵循该项要求，具体而言：

Pikeville医疗中心有限公司IRB（PMC IRB）未能制定、维护和遵守FDA法规要求的以下书面程序。

a. IRB关于对研究进行初始审查和跟踪审查的书面程序，向研究者和机构报告IRB发现的问题和采取的措施的书面程序［21 CFR 56.108（a）（1）和21 CFR 56.115（a）（6）］。

b. 确定哪些项目需要进行超过每年一次的审查，哪些项目需要从研究者以外的来源确认自先前的IRB审查后材料没有发生变更的书面程序［21 CFR 56.108（a）（2）和21 CFR 56.115（a）（6）］。

c. 确保将任何非预期的、给受试者或他人带来风险的问题及时向IRB、适当的机构管理人员以及FDA报告的书面程序［21 CFR 56.108（b）（1）和21 CFR 56.115（a）（6）］。

d. 确保将任何严重的或持续不符合法规要求或IRB决定的情况及时向IRB、适当的机构管理人员以及FDA报告的书面程序［21 CFR 56.108（b）（2）和21 CFR 56.115（a）（6）］。

e. 确保将任何IRB批件的暂停或终止及时向IRB、适当的机构管理人员以及FDA报告的书面程序［21 CFR 56.108（b）（3）和21 CFR 56.115（a）（6）］。

我们确认您在2015年9月14日对FDA 483表的书面回复中声称PMC已决定将PMC IRB的管理转交给PMC董事会的一个委员会。您的回复还表示该委员会将负责报告所有供研究参考的建议，且最终的裁决由董事会来作出所有决定。我们确认您的书面回复中含有政策草案，您的书面回复声称这个新的委员会将制定新的政策，并应当在2015年12月得到批准和就位。但是，我们注意到政策终稿和针对新政策对PMC新IRB委员的培训计划没有与您的回复一并提交。

因为以下原因，我们不能对您的书面回复进行知情评价：

a. 我们无法确定是否新的委员会将一直行使PMC的IRB职责，还是只管理当前的PMC IRB。我们注意到您的回复指出，新委员会将负责报告所有供研究参考的建议，且最终的裁决由董事会来作出所有决定。在研究建议报告方面，PMC IRB与新委员会两者角色上的差异不明确。如果新委员会将一直行使IRB的职能，该委员会必须准备和保存一份IRB委员名单，标识姓名；获得学位；代表性能力；经验证明，如董事会证书、执照等足以描述每名委员对IRB审议能带来的主要预期贡献的指标，以及每名委员与机构之间的雇佣或其他关系［21 CFR 56.115（a）（5）］。

b. 回复中没有说明该委员会将在多长时间内管理PMC IRB，并负责报告所有供研究参考的研究建议。

c. 回复中没有描述针对新的书面程序，用来对IRB委员、员工和临床研究者进行培训和教育的过程。

请提交下列材料：

a. 若新的委员会将一直行使IRB的职能：一份当前委员会委员的名单，标识姓名；获得学位；代表性能力；经验证明，如董事会证书、执照等足以描述每名委员对IRB审议能带来的主要预期贡献的指标，以及每名委员与机构之间的雇佣或其他关系。

b. 一份在报告研究建议方面PMC IRB与新的委员会角色上的差异的说明。

c. 一份新委员会将会在多长时间内管理PMC IRB并负责报告所有研究建议的说明。

d. 一份此警告信第2页中1.a.项到1.e.项提出的要求的书面程序的终稿复印件。

e. 一份对IRB委员和员工就要求的书面程序进行培训的情况说明。

f. 一份已经接受过关于要求的书面程序的培训的IRB委员和委员名单，或者计划培训的项目时间表。

贵IRB未能制定、维护和遵守必要的书面程序，从而引起我们对贵IRB用于确保受试者的权益和福利的审查程序充分性的关注。

2. IRB未能准备和保存足够的包括IRB会议记录的IRB活动记录［21 CFR 56.115（a）（2）］

IRB必须准备和保存IRB活动的充分记录，包括IRB会议的会议记录，其中应当用充分的细节来显示会议的出席情况；IRB采取的行动；关于这些行动的投票，包括赞成、反对和弃权的委员人数，要求对研究进行修改或不批准研究的依据，对有争议问题的讨论和处理的书面概要。贵IRB未能遵循这个要求，具体而言：

九次IRB会议（2011年8月11日、9月8日、9月27日、12月1日；2012年1月24日、3月27日、8月28日、12月6日；2015年1月14日）的会议记录中，没有充分记录对IRB采取的行动的投票情况，包括赞成、反对与弃权的委员人数。

我们确认您的书面回复，称2015年6月后的会议记录将撰写充分的细节来显示对行动的投票情况，包括赞成、反对与弃权的委员人数。若执行得当，您的回复看来应能够预防将来类似违规再次发生。

未能准备和保存IRB活动包括会议记录的充分记录，引起对贵IRB审查程序充分性的关注。

3. IRB未能在大多数IRB委员出席，其中至少包括一位来自非科学领域的委员的召集会议上，对拟开展的研究进行审查［21 CFR 56.108（c）］

除非采用了快速审查程序，IRB只能在大多数IRB委员出席（即法定人数），其中至少包括一位来自非科学领域的委员的召集会议上，对拟开展的研究进行审查。贵IRB未能遵循该项要求，具体而言：

贵IRB在缺少大多数IRB委员出席的会议上，对FDA所监管的研究进行了审查。如果召集会议未达法定人数（例如，有利益冲突的委员离开、早退或因非科学领域委员缺席），除非重新达到法定人数，否则IRB不能采取下一步的行动或投票［21 CFR 56.108（c）］。此外，请注意当IRB委员有利益冲突时，那些委员必须全部回避投票环节，且不得参与审议，而不是当有利益冲突时仅仅放弃投票权［21 CFR 56.107（e）］。

a. 2012年1月24日，贵IRB在没有大多数IRB委员出席的情况下，对FDA所监管的研究进行了审查。2012年1月24日IRB会议的会议记录显示，贵IRB有10位委员。因此，IRB应当有至少6位投票委员（包括一位非科学领域委员）出席才能审查FDA所监管的研究。IRB会议记录显示，只有4位投票委员出席该会议。

b. 2011年9月8日，贵IRB在没有大多数IRB委员在场的情况下，对FDA所监管的研究进行了审查。当日

IRB会议的会议记录显示，贵IRB有9位委员。因此，IRB应当有至少5位投票委员（包括一位非科学领域委员）在场，才能审查FDA所监管的研究。IRB会议记录显示，只有4位投票委员出席该会议。

我们确认您的书面回复称，PMC董事会的新委员会将审查和采取政策管理召集会议的活动，也包括严格地列出参赛人数达到大多数才能采取行动的要求。我们也确认您的回复提出，这些政策将概述出席的要求，包括至少有一名非科学领域的委员出席。但是，由于以下原因，我们无法进行知情评价：

a. 正如上述第1项中提到的，我们无法判断新的委员会是将一直行使PMC的IRB职能，还是只管理现阶段的PMC IRB。我们注意到贵方在回复中提出，新委员会将审查和采取政策管理召集会议上的活动、行动的多数要求和参会要求。我们无法判断上述政策是为现阶段PMC IRB而制定，还是为新委员会（若该委员会行使IRB的职能）而制定的。

b. 该回复中未包括任何与所召集会议活动相关的书面程序终稿的复印件、行动的多数要求，或参会要求的复印件。

c. 贵回复中未包括任何针对书面程序对IRB委员与员工提供培训的说明；接受培训的员工与委员的名单，或计划培训的项目时间表。

请提交下列文件：

a. 一份作为PMC的IRB实体（即现阶段PMC IRB或PMC理事会组成的新委员会）需遵守的书面程序终稿复印件，以确保当IRB对拟开展的研究进行审核时，大多数IRB委员，包括至少一位来自非科学领域的委员均在场。

b. 一份对IRB委员与员工针对新的书面程序进行培训的说明。

c. 一份针对新书面程序的接受培训的IRB委员与员工的名单，或一份计划培训的项目时间表。

根据21 CFR 56.107（a），为了促进研究活动的完成与审查的充分性，要求IRB由不同背景的委员组成。IRB不能确立并维护IRB会议的法定参会人数，可能对研究活动的审核不充分而影响对研究受试者权益和福利的保护。

4. IRB未能以不低于一年一次的频次对研究进行跟踪审查［21 CFR 56.109（f）］

为了满足IRB法规的要求，要求IRB依据风险程度对研究进行适度频次的跟踪审查，但不得低于一年一次。贵IRB未能遵守该要求，具体表现为：

a. PMC IRB于2011年8月11日的IRB会议上，审查并批准了以下研究：

i.（b）（4），“（b）（4）”。

ii.（b）（4），“（b）（4）”。

对研究（b）（4）与（b）（4）的跟踪审查日期应为2012年8月11日。然而，直到2013年2月28日，贵方才对这两项研究进行跟踪审查。

b. PMC IRB于2012年1月24日的IRB会议上，审查并批准了试验方案（b）（4），“（b）（4）”。该研究的跟踪审查日期应为2013年1月24日。然而，直到2013年2月28日才进行了跟踪审查。

我们确认收到贵方于2015年9月14日的书面回复。该回复称PMC研究人员已在PMC IRB的审查下，审核了全部研究项目，并确认所有项目都是依照现行批件运行的。我们同样确认贵方回复中表明PMC的理事会组成的委员会将准备并采用新的符合FDA法规的政策，并确保所有与这些政策相关的研究活动合规，包括对研究的恰当的跟踪审查。然而，我们无法对该回复进行知情评价，原因如下：

a. 如上述第1.项中提到的，我们无法判断新委员会是将一直行使PMC的IRB职能，还是只管理现阶段的PMC IRB。我们注意到您在回复中提出，新委员会将准备并采纳符合FDA法规的新政策，包括对研究的恰当跟踪审查。我们无法判断上述政策是为现阶段PMC IRB而制定，还是为新委员会（若该委员会行使IRB的职能）而制定的。

b. 该回复中未包括任何与跟踪审查相关的书面程序终稿的复印件、针对书面程序对IRB委员与员工提供任何培训的说明及受训员工与委员的名单，或一份计划培训的项目时间表。

请提交以下材料：

a. 一份作为PMC的IRB实体（即现阶段PMC IRB或PMC董事会的新委员会）需遵守的书面程序终稿复印件。

b. 一份针对新的书面程序，对IRB委员与员工的培训说明。

c. 一份针对新的书面程序，IRB接受培训委员与员工的名单，或一份计划培训的项目时间表。

贵IRB未能以不低于一年一次的频次对研究进行跟踪审查，从而引发我们对贵IRB对此前已批准而正在进行的研究的监管充分性的关注。

如上所述，我们无法确认现阶段PMC IRB、新成立的委员会与PMC董事会的角色。请提交对这三个组织各自角色的书面说明。

本警告信的目的并非是罗列贵伦理委员会在审查和批准试验方案中存在的所有缺陷。确保实际操作和程序完全符合所有适用法规的要求是贵伦理委员会的责任。

自收到这封信的15个工作日内，贵伦理委员会应当书面告知本办公室为预防将来发生类似违规情况而采取的措施。如果不能充分、迅速地解释上述违规问题，可能导致我们在不再通知的情况下采取监管措施。如果贵方认为已符合FDA法规要求，请陈述理由，并提供所有支持资料，以供我们参考。

附：英文原文

Pikeville Medical Center Inc., Institutional Review Board

WARNING LETTER

MAR 1, 2016

CERTIFIED MAIL
RETURN RECEIPT REQUESTED

Ref: 16-HFD-45-02-03

Walter E. May
President and Chief Executive Officer
Pikeville Medical Center, Inc., IRB
911 Bypass Road
Pikeville, Kentucky 41501

Dear Mr. May:

This Warning Letter informs you of objectionable conditions observed during the U.S. Food and Drug Administration (FDA) inspection of your Institutional Review Board (IRB) that was conducted between August 17 and August 21, 2015,by Mr. Richard W. Berning, representing FDA. The purpose of this inspection was to determine whether the IRB procedures for the protection of human subjects complied with Title 21 of the Code of Federal Regulations (CFR), parts 50 and 56. These regulations apply to clinical investigations of products regulated by FDA.

This inspection is a part of FDA's Bioresearch Monitoring Program, which includes inspections designed to evaluate the conduct of FDA-regulated research to ensure that the data are scientifically valid and accurate, and to help ensure that the rights, safety, and welfare of the human subjects of those studies have been protected.

At the conclusion of the inspection, Mr. Berning presented and discussed with Holly H. Gallion, M.D, IRB

Chairperson, Form FDA 483, Inspectional Observations. We acknowledge receipt of your September 14, 2015, written response to the Form FDA 483.

From our review of the FDA Establishment Inspection Report, the documents submitted with that report, and your September 14, 2015, written response, we conclude that the IRB did not adhere to the applicable FDA regulations governing the protection of human subjects. We wish to emphasize the following:

1. The IRB failed to prepare, maintain, and follow required written procedures governing the functions and operations of the IRB [21 CFR 56.108(a), 21 CFR 56.108(b), and 21 CFR 56.115(a)(6)].

In order the fulfill the requirements of the IRB regulations, each IRB must prepare, maintain, and follow written procedures describing IRB functions and operations specified in the regulations. The IRB failed to adhere to this requirement. Specifically:

The Pikeville Medical Center, Inc., IRB (PMC IRB) failed to prepare, maintain, and follow the written procedures listed below that are required by FDA regulations.

a. Written procedures for conducting the IRB's initial and continuing review of research and for reporting the IRB's findings and actions to the investigator and the institution [21 CFR 56.108(a)(1) and 21 CFR 56.115(a)(6)]

b. Written procedures for determining which projects require review more often than annually, and which projects need verification from sources other than the investigator that no material changes have occurred since the previous IRB review [21 CFR 56.108(a)(2) and 21 CFR 56.115(a)(6)]

c. Written procedures for ensuring prompt reporting to the IRB, appropriate institutional officials, and the FDA of any unanticipated problems involving risks to human subjects or others [21 CFR 56.108(b)(1) and 21 CFR 56.115(a)(6)]

d. Written procedures for ensuring prompt reporting to the IRB, appropriate institutional officials, and the FDA of any instance of serious or continuing noncompliance with these regulations or with the requirements or determinations of the IRB [21 CFR 56.108(b)(2) and 21 CFR 56.115(a)(6)]

e. Written procedures for ensuring prompt reporting to the IRB, appropriate institutional officials, and the FDA of any suspension or termination of IRB approval [21 CFR 56.108(b)(3) and 21 CFR 56.115(a)(6)]

We acknowledge that your September 14, 2015, written response to the Form FDA 483 states that PMC has decided to transition governance of the PMC IRB to a committee of PMC's Board of Directors. Your response also states that this committee will be responsible for reporting all recommendations made in reference to research, with final authority resting in the Board of Directors to make all decisions. We also acknowledge that your written response contains draft policies, and that your written response states that this new committee will prepare new policies that should be approved and in place by November 2015. However, we note that the finalized policies and plan for training PMC's new IRB members on the new policies were not submitted with your response.

We are unable to perform an informed evaluation of your written response for the following reasons:

a. We are unable to determine if the new committee will function as PMC's IRB for any period of time, or if it will serve only to govern the current PMC IRB. We note that your response indicates that the new committee will be responsible for reporting all recommendations made in reference to research, with final authority resting in the Board of Directors to make all decisions. With respect to the reporting of research recommendations, any difference in roles between the PMC IRB and the new committee is unclear. If the new committee will function as an IRB for any period of time, the committee must prepare and maintain adequate documentation of a list of IRB members identified by name; earned degrees; representative capacity; indications of experience, such as board certifications, licenses, etc., sufficient to describe each member's chief anticipated contributions to IRB deliberations; and any employment or other relationship between each member and the institution [21 CFR 56.115(a)(5)].

b. The response does not indicate how long the committee will govern the PMC IRB and be responsible for reporting all research recommendations made in reference to research.

c. The response does not describe the process that will be used to train and educate IRB members, staff, and clinical investigators with respect to any new written procedures.

Please submit the following:

a. If the new committee will be serving as an IRB for any period of time: A current list of committee members identified by names, earned degrees, representative capacities, indications of experience sufficient to describe each member's chief anticipated contributions to IRB deliberations, and any employment or other relationship between each member and the institution

b. A description of any difference in roles between the PMC IRB and the new committee with respect to reporting research recommendations

c. An indication of how long the new committee will govern the PMC IRB and report all research recommendations

d. A finalized copy of the required written procedures identified in Items 1.a through 1.e on page 2 of this letter

e. A description of any training provided to IRB members and staff on the required written procedures

f. A list of IRB members and staff who have been trained on the required written procedures, or a projected timeline of planned training

Failure of the IRB to prepare, maintain, and follow required written procedures raises concerns about the adequacy of the IRB's review processes for ensuring the protection of the rights and welfare of human research subjects.

2. The IRB failed to prepare and maintain adequate documentation of IRB activities, including minutes of IRB meetings [21 CFR 56.115(a)(2)].

The IRB is required to prepare and maintain adequate documentation of IRB activities, including minutes of IRB meetings, which must be in sufficient detail to show attendance at the meetings; actions taken by the IRB; the vote on these actions, including the number of members voting for, against, and abstaining; the basis for requiring changes in or disapproving research; and a written summary of the discussion of controverted issues and their resolution. The IRB failed to adhere to this requirement. Specifically:

For nine IRB meetings (August 11, September 8, September 27, and December 1, 2011; January 24, March 27, August 28, and December 6, 2012; and January 14, 2015), the meeting minutes did not adequately document the vote on actions taken by the IRB, including the number of members voting for, against, and abstaining.

We acknowledge your written response that the minutes of meetings after June 2015 will be prepared in sufficient detail to show the vote of actions, including the number of members voting for, against, and abstaining. If properly carried out, your response appears adequate to prevent the recurrence of this violation in the future.

Failure to prepare and maintain adequate documentation of IRB activities, including IRB meeting minutes, raises concerns about the adequacy of the IRB's review process.

3. The IRB failed to review proposed research at convened meetings at which a majority of the members of the IRB are present, including at least one member whose primary concerns are in nonscientific areas [21 CFR 56.108(c)].

Except when an expedited review procedure is used, the IRB may review proposed research only at convened meetings at which a majority of the IRB members is present (that is, a quorum), including at least one member whose primary concerns are in nonscientific areas. The IRB failed to adhere to this requirement. Specifically:

The IRB reviewed FDA-regulated research at meetings where a majority of the IRB members was not present. If a quorum is lost during a convened meeting (for example, because those with conflicts are excused, because of early departures, or because of the absence of a nonscientist member), the IRB may not take further actions or votes unless the quorum can be restored [21 CFR 56.108(c)]. Further, please note that when IRB members have a conflict of interest, those members are required to recuse themselves from voting altogether and may not participate in deliberation, as opposed to simply abstaining from votes in which they have a conflict of interest [21 CFR 56.107(e)].

a. The IRB reviewed FDA-regulated research on January 24, 2012, without a majority of members present. Minutes of the January 24, 2012, IRB meeting indicate that the IRB had ten members. Therefore, at least six voting members (including a nonscientist) needed to be present for the IRB to review FDA-regulated research. IRB meeting minutes indicate that only four voting members of the IRB attended the meeting.

b. The IRB reviewed FDA-regulated research on September 8, 2011, without a majority of members present. Minutes of the September 8, 2011, IRB meeting indicate that the IRB had nine members. Therefore, at least five voting members (including a nonscientist) needed to be present for the IRB to review FDA-regulated research. IRB meeting minutes indicate that only four voting members of the IRB attended the meeting.

We acknowledge that your written response states that the new committee of PMC's Board of Directors will review and adopt policies governing activities at convened meetings, as well as strictly outlining the majority requirements for action. We also acknowledge that your response indicates that these policies will outline attendance requirements, including the presence of at least one member from a nonscientific area. However, we are unable to perform an informed evaluation of the response for the following reasons:

a. As noted in Item 1 above, we are unable to determine if the new committee will function as PMC's IRB for any period of time, or if it will serve only to govern the current PMC IRB. We note that your response indicates that the new committee will review and adopt policies related to activities at convened meetings, majority requirements for action, and attendance requirements. We are unable to determine if the policies mentioned above are intended for the current PMC IRB or for the new committee (if it is to function as an IRB).

b. The response does not contain a copy of any finalized written procedures related to activities at convened meetings, majority requirements for action, or attendance requirements.

c. The response does not contain a description of any training provided to the IRB members and staff on such written procedures; a list of IRB members and staff who have been trained; or a projected timeline of planned training.

Please submit the following:

a. A finalized copy of the written procedures to be followed by the entity that will serve as PMC's IRB (that is, either the current PMC IRB or the new committee of PMC's Board of Directors) to ensure that a majority of the IRB members, including at least one member whose primary concerns are in nonscientific areas, is present when the IRB reviews proposed research.

b. A description of any training provided to the IRB members and staff on the new written procedures

c. A list of IRB members and staff who have been trained on the new written procedures, or a projected timeline of planned training

Under 21 CFR 56.107(a), to promote complete and adequate review of research activities, the IRB is required to have members with varying backgrounds. Failure of the IRB to establish or maintain a quorum at IRB meetings may result in the inadequate review of research activities, which can impact the protection of the rights and welfare of human research subjects.

4. The IRB failed to conduct continuing review of research at intervals of not less than once per year [21 CFR 56.109(f)].

In order to fulfill the requirements of the IRB regulations, the IRB is required to conduct continuing review of research at intervals appropriate to the degree of risk, but not less than once per year. The IRB failed to adhere to this requirement. Specifically:

a. The PMC IRB reviewed and approved the following studies at the August 11, 2011, IRB meeting:

i. **(b)(4)**, "**(b)(4)**"

ii. **(b)(4)**, "**(b)(4)**"

Continuing review for Studies **(b)(4)** and **(b)(4)** was due by August 11, 2012. However, continuing review for both studies was not conducted until February 28, 2013.

b. The PMC IRB reviewed and approved Protocol **(b)(4)**, "**(b)(4)**," at the January 24, 2012, IRB meeting. Continuing review for this study was due by January 24, 2013. However, continuing review was not conducted until February 28, 2013.

We acknowledge that your September 14, 2015, written response states that PMC research staff has reviewed all research projects under the review of the PMC IRB and has determined that all projects are operating under current approval. We also acknowledge that your response indicates that the new committee of PMC's Board of Directors will prepare and adopt new policies consistent with FDA regulations and will ensure the compliance of all research activities related to those policies, including appropriate continuing review of research. However, we are unable to perform an informed evaluation of the response for the following reasons:

a. As noted in Item 1 above, we are unable to determine if the new committee will function as PMC's IRB for any period of time, or if it will serve only to govern the current PMC IRB. We note that your response indicates that the new committee will prepare and adopt new policies consistent with FDA regulations, including policies for appropriate continuing review of research. We are unable to determine if the policies mentioned above are intended for the current PMC IRB or for the new committee (if it is to function as an IRB).

b. The response does not contain a copy of any finalized written procedures related to continuing review, a description of any training provided to the IRB members and staff on such written procedures, and a list of IRB members and staff who have been trained or a projected timeline of planned training.

Please submit the following:

a. A finalized copy of the written procedures to be followed by the entity that will serve as PMC's IRB (that is, either the current PMC IRB or the new committee of PMC's Board of Directors)

b. A description of any training provided to the IRB members and staff on the new written procedures

c. A list of IRB members and staff who have been trained on the new written procedures, or a projected timeline of planned training

Failure of the IRB to conduct continuing review at intervals of not less than once per year raises concerns about the adequacy of the IRB's oversight of ongoing research that the IRB had previously approved.

As noted above, we are unable to determine the roles of the current PMC IRB, the new committee, and the PMC Board of Directors. Please submit a written description explaining the respective roles of the three entities.

This letter is not intended to be an all-inclusive list of deficiencies for the protocols reviewed and approved by the IRB. It is the IRB's responsibility to ensure that its practices and procedures comply fully with all applicable regulations.

Within fifteen (15) working days of your receipt of this letter, the IRB should notify this office in writing of the actions that have been taken to prevent similar violations in the future. Failure to adequately and promptly address the violations noted above may result in regulatory action without further notice. If you believe you have complied with FDA regulations, include your reasoning and any supporting information for our consideration.

We recommend that the IRB visit the following FDA Web page for information on human subject protections that may assist the IRB in its efforts to come into compliance with FDA regulations:

http://www.fda.gov/ScienceResearch/SpecialTopics/RunningClinicalTrials/default.htm

We appreciate the cooperation shown to the FDA Investigator during the inspection. If the IRB has any questions, please contact Constance Cullity, M.D., M.P.H., at 301-796-3397; FAX 301-847-8748. Your written response and any pertinent documentation should be addressed to:

Constance Cullity, M.D., M.P.H.
Branch Chief
Good Clinical Practice Compliance Oversight Branch
Division of Clinical Compliance Evaluation
Office of Scientific Investigations
Office of Compliance
Center for Drug Evaluation and Research
U.S. Food and Drug Administration
Building 51, Room 5354
10903 New Hampshire Avenue
Silver Spring, MD 20993

Sincerely,

{See appended electronic signature page}

David C. Burrow, Pharm.D., J.D.

Acting Director
Office of Scientific Investigations
Office of Compliance
Center for Drug Evaluation and Research
U.S. Food and Drug Administration

This is a representation of an electronic record that was signed electronically and this page is the manifestation of the electronic signature.

/S/

DAVID C BURROW
03/01/2016

第3封　给Jamaica医院医疗中心伦理委员会的警告信

2016年2月24日

参考号：16-HFD-45-02-02

尊敬的Mendelson博士：

2015年8月13日至8月20日，Tara K. Carmody女士代表FDA对贵伦理委员会（IRB）进行了现场检查。这封警告信特告知您现场检查中发现的违规情况。本次现场检查的目的是核实贵IRB受试者保护程序是否符合美国联邦法规（CFR）第21篇第50和56部分的要求。该法规适用于FDA所监管产品的临床研究。

本次现场检查是FDA的生物研究监查项目的一部分。该项目通过设定的检查方法，对FDA所监管的相关研究的实施情况进行评估，以确认研究数据在科学上是有效和准确的，并确保这些研究中受试者的权益、安全和福利得到了保护。

在现场检查结束时，Carmody女士向您出示了FDA483表，即现场检查发现的问题，并与您进行了讨论。您2015年9月1日对该FDA483表的书面回复已收悉。

经对现场检查报告、该报告的附件，以及您2015年9月1日的书面回复进行审查，我们认为，IRB没有遵循适用的监管受试者保护的FDA法规。我们想强调以下几点：

IRB未能准备和保存足够的包括IRB会议记录与IRB委员名单的IRB活动记录［21 CFR 56.115（a）（2）］

IRB必须准备和保存足够的IRB活动记录，包括 IRB会议记录，要有充分的细节来显示会议的出席情况；IRB采取的行动；对行动的投票情况，包括同意、反对和弃权票数；需要修正或不批准研究的依据；对争议问题进行讨论和解决的书面总结［21 CFR 56.115（a）（2）］。

- 一份IRB委员名单，标识姓名；获得学位；经验证明，例如认证、许可证等足以描述每名委员对IRB审议能带来的主要预期贡献的指标，以及每名委员与机构之间的雇佣或其他关系［21 CFR 56.115（a）（5）］。

贵IRB未能遵守这些要求，具体表现为：

a. 2013年1月7日至2015年7月6日期间召开的IRB会议，投票计数情况没有保持记录在会议记录中。会议记录显示，不是记录投票计数，而是代之以，例如“委员会认可并批准了该申请”等说明。检查中审查的28份会议记录中，9份记录的所有事项均没有任何投票计数的记录，19份记录只有某些事项有投票计数的记录。例如：

1. 2014年1月6日的会议记录表明，IRB会议未包括已经过审查和批准的FDA监管研究的投票计数记录。
2. 2014年2月3日的会议记录表明，IRB会议未包括已经过审查和批准的FDA监管研究的投票计数记录。
3. 2015年1月5日的会议记录表明，IRB会议未包括已经过审查和批准的FDA监管研究的投票计数记录。
4. 2015年3月9日的会议记录表明，IRB会议未包括已经过审查和批准的FDA监管研究的投票计数记录。
5. 2015年5月4日的会议记录表明，IRB会议未包括已经过审查和批准的FDA监管研究的投票计数记录。

我们确认您2015年9月1日的书面回复中包括了贵IRB修订的标准操作规程（SOPs）（2015年9月14 日版）复印件。这些修订后的SOPs与IRB之前的SOPs版本均表明对行动进行投票的情况，包括同意、反对与弃权的委员人数，都将记录于会议记录中。

请提交一份IRB拟采取的确保符合FDA法规，以及与会议记录有关的IRB书面程序的措施的说明。回复中应包括一份对IRB员工与委员的培训说明，和IRB已接受培训员工与委员的名单，或一份计划培训的项目时间表。

贵IRB未能准备和保存对IRB会议的充分记录，引起我们对贵IRB审查程序适宜性的关注。此外，还引起我们关注的是：贵IRB会议期间IRB委员能否达到法定人数，是否有IRB委员除了应IRB要求提供信息外，还参与了对自己研究项目的审查。

b. 2013～2015年，贵IRB未能按照21 CFR 56.115（a）（5）所要求的，准备和保存IRB委员名单。检查期间所提供的委员名单显示，委员变更没有对名单进行更新，因为会议记录和出席名单中的委员姓名与委员名单姓名有时不一致。具体而言：

1.（b）（6）未被列入任何委员名单中，但在2013年1月7日至2015年7月6日之间20次会议的会议记录中均被列为投票委员。

2.（b）（6）未被列入任何委员名单中，但在2013年举行的12次会议的会议记录中均被列为投票委员。

3.（b）（6）未被列入任何委员名单中，但在2013年9月9日、2013年10月7日、2013年12月2日、2014年2月3日和2014年3月10日的会议记录中均被列为投票委员。

4.（b）（6）未被列入任何委员名单中，但在2013年6月3日、2013年11月11日和2015年7月6日的会议记录中均被列为投票委员。

5.（b）（6）未被列入任何委员名单中，但在2014年12月1日的会议记录中被列为投票委员。

我们确认您在书面回复中表明，检查期间查到了一份委员名册模板，且新的名册在制定中。这份名册包括委员姓名、学历、职务、性别、是否隶属于机构，以及委员状态（委员或替补）；且下一步，委员名单将会持续更新，加入版本号与日期。若执行得当，该措施看来应能满足要求。

贵IRB未能准备和保存IRB委员的准确名单，引起我们对贵IRB委员结构的适宜性及其保障研究受试者权益与福利能力的关注。

本警告信的目的并非是罗列贵伦理委员会在审查和批准试验方案中存在的所有缺陷。确保Jamaica医院医学中心IRB的实际操作和程序完全符合所有适用法规的要求是您的职责。

自收到这封信的15个工作日内，您应当书面告知本办公室为预防将来发生类似违规情况而采取的措施。如果不能充分、迅速地解释上述违规问题，可能导致我们在不再通知的情况下采取监管措施。如果您认为已符合FDA法规要求，请陈述理由，并提供所有支持资料，以供我们参考。

附：英文原文

Jamaica Hospital Medical Center IRB

WARNING LETTER

FEB 24, 2016

CERTIFIED MAIL
RETURN RECEIPT REQUESTED

Ref: 16-HFD-45-02-02

Robert I. Mendelson, M.D., FACC, FACP Chairman
Jamaica Hospital Institutional Review Board
Jamaica Hospital Medical Center
8900 Van Wyck Expressway
Jamaica, New York 11418-2832

Dear Dr. Mendelson:

This Warning Letter informs you of objectionable conditions observed during the U.S. Food and Drug Administration (FDA) inspection of your Institutional Review Board (IRB) that was conducted between August 13 and August 20, 2015, by Ms. Tara K. Carmody, representing FDA. The purpose of this inspection was to determine whether the IRB procedures for the protection of human subjects complied with Title 21 of the Code of Federal Regulations (CFR), parts 50 and 56. These regulations apply to clinical investigations of products regulated by FDA.

This inspection is a part of FDA's Bioresearch Monitoring Program, which includes inspections designed to evaluate the conduct of FDA-regulated research to ensure that the data are scientifically valid and accurate, and to help ensure that the rights, safety, and welfare of the human subjects of those studies have been protected.

At the conclusion of the inspection, Ms. Carmody presented and discussed with you Form FDA 483, Inspectional Observations. We acknowledge receipt of the IRB's September 1, 2015, written response to the Form FDA 483.

From our review of the FDA Establishment Inspection Report, the documents submitted with that report, and your September 1, 2015, written response, we conclude that the IRB did not adhere to the applicable FDA regulations governing the protection of human subjects. We wish to emphasize the following:

The IRB failed to prepare and maintain adequate documentation of IRB activities, including minutes of IRB meetings and a list of IRB members [21 CFR 56.115(a)(2) and 21 CFR 56.115(a)(5)].

The IRB is required to prepare and maintain adequate documentation of IRB activities, including:

Minutes of IRB meetings, which must be in sufficient detail to show attendance at the meetings; actions taken by the IRB; the vote on these actions, including the number of members voting for, against, and abstaining; the basis for requiring changes in or disapproving research; and a written summary of the discussion of controverted issues and their resolution [21 CFR 56.115(a)(2)]

- A list of IRB members identified by name; earned degrees; representative capacity; indications of experience such as board certifications, licenses, etc., sufficient to describe each member's chief anticipated contributions to IRB deliberations; and any employment or other relationship between each member and the institution [21 CFR 56.115(a)(5)]

The IRB failed to adhere to these requirements. Specifically:

a. For IRB meetings held between January 7, 2013, and July 6, 2015, vote counts were not recorded in the meeting minutes consistently. Instead of recording vote counts, the minutes indicate, for example, "The committee acknowledged and approved the submission." Of the 28 sets of minutes reviewed during the inspection, 9 have no vote counts recorded for any items, and 19 have vote counts recorded for some items only. For example:

1. Minutes of the January 6, 2014, IRB meeting do not include documentation of vote counts for FDA-regulated research that was reviewed and approved.

2. Minutes of the February 3, 2014, IRB meeting do not include documentation of vote counts for FDA-regulated research that was reviewed and approved.

3. Minutes of the January 5, 2015, IRB meeting do not include documentation of vote counts for FDA-regulated research that was reviewed and approved.

4. Minutes of the March 9, 2015, IRB meeting do not include documentation of vote counts for FDA-regulated research that was reviewed and approved.

5. Minutes of the May 4, 2015, IRB meeting do not include documentation of vote counts for FDA-regulated research that was reviewed and approved.

We acknowledge that in your September 1, 2015, written response, you included a copy of the IRB's revised standard operating procedures (SOPs) (version date 14 September 2015). These SOPs and the previous version of the IRB's SOPs both indicate that the votes on actions, including the number of members voting for, against, and abstaining, will be recorded in meeting minutes.

Please submit a written description of the actions the IRB plans to take to ensure compliance with FDA regulations and the IRB's written procedures as they relate to meeting minutes. The response should include a description of any training provided to IRB staff and members and a list of IRB staff and members trained, or a projected timeline of planned training.

Failure to prepare and maintain adequate documentation of IRB meetings raises concerns about the adequacy of the IRB's review process. Furthermore, inadequate documentation raises concerns about whether the IRB members maintained a quorum for the duration of the IRB meetings, and whether any IRB member participated in the review of his or her own research, except to provide information requested by the IRB.

b. During the time period from 2013 to 2015, the IRB failed to prepare and maintain a list of IRB members, in accordance with 21 CFR 56.115(a)(5). Membership lists provided during the inspection indicate that the lists had not been updated as the membership changed, in that members' names listed in meeting minutes and on attendance sheets did not always match the names on membership lists. Specifically:

1. **(b)(6)** is not listed on any membership lists, but she is listed as a voting member in the minutes of 20 meetings held between January 7, 2013, and July 6, 2015.

2. **(b)(6)** is not listed on any membership lists, but he is listed as a voting member in the minutes of 12 meetings held in 2013.

3. **(b)(6)** is not listed on any membership lists, but she is listed as a voting member in the minutes of meetings held on September 9, 2013; October 7, 2013; December 2, 2013; February 3, 2014; March 10, 2014; and September 8, 2014.

4. **(b)(6)** is not listed on any membership lists, but he is listed as a voting member in the minutes of meetings held on June 3, 2013; November 11, 2013; and July 6, 2015.

5. **(b)(6)** is not listed on any membership lists, but he is listed as a voting member in the minutes of a meeting held on December 1, 2014.

We acknowledge your written response indicating that during the inspection, a membership roster template was obtained and a new roster was developed. The roster now includes each member's name, degree, occupation, gender, whether or not affiliated with the institution, and membership status (member or alternate); and that going forward, membership lists will be updated on a continuous basis and will include a version number and date. If properly carried out, this action appears to be adequate.

Failure to prepare and maintain an accurate list of IRB members raises concerns about the adequacy of the IRB's composition and its ability to safeguard the rights and welfare of research subjects.

This letter is not intended to be an all-inclusive list of deficiencies for the protocols reviewed and approved by the IRB. It is your responsibility to ensure that Jamaica Hospital Medical Center IRB's practices and procedures comply fully with all applicable regulations.

Within fifteen (15) working days of your receipt of this letter, you should notify this office in writing of the actions that will be taken to prevent similar violations in the future. Failure to adequately and promptly address the violations noted above may result in regulatory action without further notice. If you believe you have complied with FDA regulations, include your reasoning and any supporting information for our consideration.

We recommend that you visit the following FDA Web page for information on human subject protections that may assist you in bringing the IRB into compliance with FDA regulations:http://www.fda.gov/ScienceResearch/SpecialTopics/RunningClinicalTrials/default.htm.

We appreciate the cooperation shown to the FDA investigator during the inspection. If you have any questions, please contact Constance Cullity, M.D., M.P.H., at 301-796-3397; FAX 301-847- 8748. Your written response and any pertinent documentation should be addressed to:

Constance Cullity, M.D., M.P.H.
Branch Chief
Good Clinical Practice Compliance Oversight Branch
Division of Clinical Compliance Evaluation
Office of Scientific Investigations
Office of Compliance
Center for Drug Evaluation and Research
U.S. Food and Drug Administration
Building 51, Room 5354
10903 New Hampshire Avenue

Silver Spring, MD 20993

Sincerely,

{See appended electronic signature page}

David C. Burrow, Pharm.D., J.D.
Acting Director
Office of Scientific Investigations
Office of Compliance
Center for Drug Evaluation and Research
U.S. Food and Drug Administration

This is a representation of an electronic record that was signed electronically and this page is the manifestation of the electronic signature.

/S/

DAVID C BURROW
02/24/2016

第4封 给Monmouth医疗中心伦理委员会的警告信

2015年11月10日

参考号：16-HFD-45-11-01

尊敬的Jaeger博士：

2015年4月1日至4月20日，Denise M. Viscon女士代表FDA，对贵伦理委员会（IRB）进行了现场检查。这封警告信特告知您现场检查中发现的违规情况。本次现场检查的目的是核实贵IRB受试者保护程序是否符合美国联邦法规（CFR）第21篇第50和第56部分的要求。该法规适用于FDA所监管产品的临床研究。

本次现场检查是FDA的生物研究监查项目的一部分。该项目通过设定的检查方法，对FDA所监管的相关研究的实施情况进行评估，以确认研究数据在科学上是有效和准确的，并帮助确保这些研究中的受试者的权益、安全和福利得到了保护。

在现场检查结束时，Visco女士向您出示了FDA483表，即现场检查发现的问题，并与您进行了讨论。您2015年5月1日对该FDA483表的书面回复已收悉。

经对现场检查报告、该报告的附件，以及您2015年5月1日的书面回复进行审查，我们认为，IRB没有遵循监管受试者保护的FDA法规。我们想强调以下几点：

1. IRB未能在初始审查时，确定涉及儿童的研究需要依照21 CFR 50（D），临床试验中对儿童的额外保护措施［21 CFR 56.109（h）］

21 CFR 56.109（h）规定，当临床试验中的部分或全部受试者是儿童时，伦理委员会在初始审查时，必须确定临床试验符合21 CFR 50（D）（临床试验中对儿童的附加安全保护）。21 CFR 50.50规定，伦理委员会必须对临床试验进行审查，仅批准满足21 CFR 50.51（临床试验不会产生比最小风险更大的风险）、21 CFR 50.52（临床试验会产生比最小风险更大的风险，除非存在能够给个人受试者带来直接利益的希望）或者21 CFR 50.53（临床试验会产生比最小风险更大的风险，也不存在能够给个人受试者带来直接利益的希望，但是对于受试者的身体功能紊乱或病情可能产生普遍性的知识）标准的临床试验。

21 CFR 50（D）（临床试验中对儿童的额外保护措施）规定，伦理委员会对涉及儿童的临床试验必须作出某种类型的调查。此外，21 CFR 56.115规定，伦理委员会必须记录其活动情况，包括伦理委员会在会议期间采取的行动。

但是，在现场检查过程中，无论是在会议记录或者是其他任何审查的材料中，都没有记录表明伦理委员会在初始审查时进行必要的确认，下列临床试验涉及儿童受试者，需要依照21 CFR 50（D）：

a）IRB 研究（b）（4），“（b）（4）”；

b）IRB 研究（b）（4），“（b）（4）”。

在2015年5月1日的书面回复中，您提出伦理委员会将要实施以下的纠正或预防措施：

a）伦理委员会将在下一个财务季度内将试验方案（b）（4）（已于2014年2月停止入组）提上议事日程。

b）将会草拟伦理委员会会议补充表，来确定弱势的受试者的类型（如果有的话），以及风险的种类。

c）伦理委员会将按照需要，对政策进行审查和修改，使其中包含相关内容，在制定用于审查涉及儿童和其他弱势的受试者的临床试验的标准操作规程（SOP）时可以参考。

d）伦理委员会将按照需要，对用于儿科研究的伦理委员会检查表进行审查和修改。

我们承认您的书面回复中含有关于2015年4月13日伦理委员会对试验方案（b）（4）进行审查和对D部分作出决定的记录，但是我们无法对您的书面回复进行知情评价，因为您没有提供下列项目的文件：

a）伦理委员会对于试验方案（b）（4）D部分作出的决定；

b）伦理委员会会议补充表的定稿复印件；

c）用于评估儿科研究的伦理委员会检查表的定稿复印件；

d）已经修订过的相关SOP；

e）提供情况简述：对伦理委员会员工和委员进行的关于新SOP的培训，接受培训的员工和委员名单，或者进行计划培训的项目时间表。

请提交伦理委员会准备采取的纠正或预防措施，以确保所有正在进行的或将来进行的FDA监管下的儿科研究中儿科风险确认得以适当地完成，避免违规行为再次发生。请包括上面列出的a）~e）项。

研究中儿童的额外保护措施必须得到满足，未能确定这一点可能导致将这个弱势的群体置于不必要的风险中，可能导致儿童的父母（们）或监护人（们）对要进行的研究不能充分知情。

2. IRB未能在大多数IRB委员出席，其中至少包括一位来自非科学领域委员的召集会议上，对拟开展的研究进行审查［21 CFR 56.108（c）］

除了采用快速审查程序以外，伦理委员会仅在召集会议上对即将开展的研究进行审查，召集会议要求伦理委员会的委员多数出席（也就是说，法定人数），并且包括至少一位来自非科学领域的委员。伦理委员会未能遵照这个要求，具体表现在：

伦理委员会在多数委员未出席、某位出席的委员有利益冲突使达不到法定人数（下面会描述具体情况）的会议上审查FDA监管的研究。请注意：当伦理委员会在审查的研究中有委员存在利益冲突时，有利益冲突的委员不能够参与投票，该委员也不能够算到法定人数内。如果在召集会议上达不到法定人数（例如，因为有利益冲突的委员需要回避，因为委员提前离开或因为没有非科学领域委员参加会议），伦理委员会不得采取进一步行动或投票，除非可以重新达到法定人数［21 CFR 56.108（c）］。

a）2012年6月11日和2013年1月13日，在没有多数委员出席的情况下，伦理委员会审查了FDA监管的研究。在这些日期里有效的伦理委员会委员名册中，每一个名册上由10名主要委员组成，这意味着在会议中为评审FDA监管的研究至少需要6名有投票权的委员（其中包括1名非科学领域委员）出席。伦理委员会会议记录显示这些会议中每次只有5名有投票权的委员出席。

b）2012年1月17日，在会议缺少多数委员出席的情况下，伦理委员会审查并批准了IRB研究（b）（4），“（b）（4）”。会议记录显示，如果不是同时对研究（b）（4）进行审查和批准的话，伦理委员会出席委员符合法定人数要求的数量（10名委员中有6名出席，其中包括1名非科学领域委员）。

出席会议的6名伦理委员会委员中的（b）（6）医学博士，是研究（b）（4）的主要研究者。（b）（6）医生作为主要研究者，存在利益冲突，不应该计算在审查和批准这项研究的法定人数当中。但是，会议记录显示（b）（6）医生被算在法定人数当中。

伦理委员会不应该审查或批准研究（b）（4），因为伦理委员会并没有达到审查这项研究所需的法定人数。

c）2012年2月13日，在会议缺少多数委员出席的情况下，伦理委员会审查并批准了下列研究：

i. IRB 研究（b）（4），“（b）（4）”；

ii. IRB 研究（b）（4），“（b）（4）”。

会议记录显示如果不是上述两项研究同时进行审查和批准的话，伦理委员会出席委员符合法定人数要求的数量（10名委员中有6名出席，其中包括1名非科学领域委员）。出席会议的6名伦理委员会委员中的（b）（6）博士，是这些研究的主要研究者。（b）（6）博士作为主要研究者，存在利益冲突，不应该计算在审查和批准这些研究的法定人数当中。

然而，会议记录显示（b）（6）博士被算在法定人数当中。伦理委员会不应该审查或批准IRB 研究（b）（4）和（b）（4），因为伦理委员会并没有达到审查这些研究所需的法定人数。

在2015年5月1日的书面回复中，您指出伦理委员会将实施下列纠正或预防措施：

a）伦理委员会会议补充表将被完善用于在伦理委员会会议前和会议期间，记录投票情况和判别法定人数不足（如果有这种情况的话）。

b）伦理委员会将按照需要，对政策和程序进行审查和修改，使其中包含相关内容，在制定关于伦理委员会会议管理的标准操作规程（SOP）时可以参考。

我们收到了您的书面回复，但是我们不能对您的书面回复进行知情评价，因为您没有提供下列项目的文件：

a）伦理委员会会议补充表的定稿复印件；

b）已经修订过的任何相关的书面SOP；

c）提供情况简述：对伦理委员会员工和委员进行的关于新SOP的培训，接受培训的员工和委员名单，或者进行计划培训的项目时间表。

请提交伦理委员会准备采取的任何纠正或预防措施，以确保伦理委员会在对即将开展的研究进行审查时，多数委员出席并且其中包括至少一位来自非科学领域的委员。请包括上述a）~c）项。

21 CFR 56.107（a）规定，伦理委员会应当有不同专业背景的委员，以促进对研究活动进行全面和充分的审查。伦理委员会未能建立或保持法定人数可能会导致对研究活动的审查不够充分，这可能影响对受试者权益和福利的保护。

3. IRB未能准备和保存足够的包括IRB会议记录的IRB活动记录［21 CFR 56.115（a）（2）］

伦理委员会应当准备和保持关于伦理委员会活动情况的文件，包括伦理委员会会议记录，其中应该用足够的细节说明会议的出席情况、伦理委员会采取的措施、关于这些措施的投票情况（包括投票赞成、反对和弃权的委员数量）、要求研究进行必要改动或者不批准研究的依据、对有争议的问题的讨论和决议的书面总结。伦理委员会没有遵循这些要求，具体表现在：

伦理委员会2013年2月11日的会议记录显示：（b）（6）医生是3项FDA监管研究（b）（4）的主要研究者或授权研究者，他出席了会议并在会议期间投票批准了这些研究。但是，在伦理委员会对FDA483表的回复中，含有日期为2015年4月6日和4月30日的信函，（b）（6）医生在信件中声明他对这些研究投票弃权。

请注意没有任何伦理委员会可以让一名存在利益冲突的委员参加伦理委员会对该项研究的初始审查或跟踪审查，除非是为了让该委员提供伦理委员会需要的信息［21 CFR 56.107（e）］。因此如果委员在某项研究中存在利益冲突，伦理委员会在讨论针对该项研究所要采取的行动时，该名存在利益冲突的伦理委员会委员不能够参与评议和投票。

请提交伦理委员会准备采取的任何纠正或预防措施，以解决上述的违规行为。和纠正或预防措施一起，请提交伦理委员会书面SOP，或者任何在完善中的SOP草案的复印件，以及准备采用新SOP的项目时间表。此外，请提供简述：对伦理委员会员工和委员进行的关于新SOP的培训，接受培训的员工和委员名单，或者计划培训的项目时间表。

未能准备和保持关于伦理委员会活动情况的文件，包括伦理委员会会议记录，这引起对伦理委员会审查过程充分性的关注。

此外，我们注意到在上述的几次伦理委员会会议中，一名委员在对有利益冲突的研究进行审查时投票弃权。我们要注意，当存在利益冲突时，委员应当回避表决，不能参与评议，而不是简单的投弃权票［21 CFR 56.107（e）］。

本警告信的目的并非是罗列贵伦理委员会在审查和批准试验方案中存在的所有缺陷。确保Monmouth 医疗中心伦理委员会实际操作和程序完全符合所有适用法律和法规的要求是您的职责。

自收到这封信的15个工作日内，您应当书面告知本办公室为预防将来发生类似违规情况而已经采取的措施。如果不能充分、迅速地解释上述违规问题，可能导致我们在不再通知的情况下采取监管措施。

附：英文原文

Monmouth Medical Center IRB

WARNING LETTER

Nov 10, 2015

CERTIFIED MAIL
RETURN RECEIPT REQUESTED

Ref: 16-HFD-45-11-01

Joseph Jaeger, Dr.P.H.
Chief Academic Officer
Monmouth Medical Center
300 Second Avenue
Long Branch, New Jersey 07740

Dear Dr. Jaeger:

This Warning Letter informs you of objectionable conditions observed during the U.S. Food and Drug Administration (FDA) inspection of your Institutional Review Board (IRB) that was conducted between April 1 and April 20, 2015,by Ms. Denise M. Visco, representing FDA. The purpose of this inspection was to determine whether the IRB procedures for the protection of human subjects complied with Title 21 of the Code of Federal Regulations (CFR), parts 50 and 56. These regulations apply to clinical investigations of products regulated by FDA.

This inspection is a part of FDA's Bioresearch Monitoring Program, which includes inspections designed to evaluate the conduct of FDA-regulated research to ensure that the data are scientifically valid and accurate, and to help ensure that the rights, safety, and welfare of the human subjects of those studies have been protected.

At the conclusion of the inspection, Ms. Visco presented and discussed with you Form FDA 483, Inspectional Observations. We acknowledge receipt of your May 1, 2015, written response to the Form FDA 483.

From our review of the FDA Establishment Inspection Report, the documents submitted with that report, and the IRB's May 1, 2015, written response, we conclude that the IRB did not adhere to FDA regulations governing the protection of human subjects. We wish to emphasize the following:

1. The IRB failed to determine at the time of initial review that studies involving children are in compliance with 21 CFR part 50, subpart D, Additional Safeguards for Children in Clinical Investigations [21 CFR 56.109(h)].

Under 21 CFR 56.109(h), when some or all of the subjects in a clinical investigation are children, the IRB must determine that the clinical investigation is in compliance with 21 CFR part 50, subpart D (Additional Safeguards for Children in Clinical Investigations) at the time of the initial review of the research. Under 21 CFR 50.50, the IRB must review the clinical investigation and approve only those clinical investigations that satisfy the criteria described in 21 CFR 50.51 (clinical investigations not involving greater than minimal risk), 21 CFR 50.52 (clinical investigations involving greater than minimal risk but presenting the prospect of direct benefit to individual subjects), or 21 CFR 50.53 (clinical investigations involving greater than minimal risk and no prospect of direct benefit to individual subjects, but likely to yield generalizable knowledge about the subject's disorder or condition).

Under 21 CFR part 50, subpart D (Additional Safeguards for Children in Clinical Investigations), the IRB must make certain findings with respect to clinical investigations involving children. In addition, under 21 CFR 56.115, the IRB is required to document its activities, including actions taken during IRB meetings.

However, there is no documentation, either in the meeting minutes or in any other materials reviewed during the inspection, of the IRB's requisite determination at the time of the initial review that the following clinical investigations involving pediatric subjects were in compliance with subpart D:

a) IRB Study **(b)(4)**, "**(b)(4)**"

b) IRB Study **(b)(4)**, "**(b)(4)**"

In the May 1, 2015, written response, you indicate that the IRB will implement the following corrective or preventive actions:

a) The IRB will place Protocol **(b)(4)**, which was closed to enrollment in February 2014, on an IRB agenda within the next fiscal quarter.

b) An IRB meeting supplement form will be drafted to identify the type of vulnerable subjects, if any, and the risk category.

c) The IRB will review and revise, as needed, its policy to include a reference to a standard operating procedure (SOP) for reviewing research involving children and other vulnerable subjects.

d) The IRB will review and revise, as needed, an IRB checklist used for evaluating pediatric studies.

We acknowledge that your written response contains documentation of the IRB's review of Protocol **(b)(4)** and subpart D determination on April 13, 2015. However, we are unable to undertake an informed evaluation of your written response because you did not provide documentation for the following items:

a) The IRB's subpart D determination for Protocol **(b)(4)**

b) A finalized copy of the IRB meeting supplemental form

c) A finalized copy of the IRB checklist used for evaluating pediatric studies

d) Any relevant SOPs that have been revised

e) A description of any training provided to the IRB staff and members on the new SOPs, and a list of staff and members trained, or a projected timeline of planned training

Please submit any corrective or preventive actions the IRB plans to take to ensure that the pediatric risk determinations are appropriately completed for all ongoing and future FDA-regulated pediatric studies in order to avoid the recurrence of the violations. Please include items a) through e) listed above.

Failure to determine that the additional safeguards for children in research are met may expose this vulnerable population to unnecessary risks, and may result in the child's parent(s) or guardian(s) not being fully informed about the proposed research.

2. The IRB failed to review proposed research at convened meetings at which a majority of the members of the IRB are present, including at least one member whose primary concerns are in nonscientific areas [21 CFR 56.108(c)].

Except when an expedited review procedure is used, the IRB may review proposed research only at convened meetings at which a majority of the IRB members is present (that is, a quorum), including at least one member whose primary concerns are in nonscientific areas. The IRB failed to adhere to this requirement. Specifically:

The IRB reviewed FDA regulated research at meetings where a majority of the IRB members was not present, and at meetings where the quorum was lost when an IRB member in attendance had a conflict of interest, as described below. Please note that an IRB member with a conflict of interest may not vote or be counted toward the quorum when the IRB is reviewing research in which the member has a conflict. If a quorum is lost during a convened meeting (for example, because those with conflicts are excused, because of early departures, or because of the absence of a nonscientist member), the IRB may not take further actions or votes unless the quorum can be restored [21 CFR 56.108(c)].

a) The IRB reviewed FDA-regulated research on June 11, 2012, and January 13, 2014, without a majority of members present. The IRB membership rosters in effect on these dates consisted of ten primary members on each roster, meaning that at least six voting members needed to be present (including a nonscientist) in order to review FDA-regulated research at these meetings. IRB meeting minutes indicate that just five voting members of the IRB attended each of these meetings.

b) The IRB reviewed and approved IRB Study **(b)(4)**, "**(b)(4)**," at the January 17, 2012, IRB meeting without a majority of members present. The meeting minutes indicate that the IRB had the required membership present for quorum (six of the ten IRB members including a nonscientist) except for when Study **(b)(4)** was reviewed and approved.

(b)(6), M.D., who was one of the six IRB members present, was the principal investigator for Study **(b)(4)**. As the principal investigator, Dr. **(b)(6)** had a conflict of interest and should not have counted toward the quorum for review and approval of this study. However, the meeting minutes indicate that Dr. **(b)(6)** was counted toward the quorum.

The IRB should not have reviewed or approved Study **(b)(4)** because the IRB did not have a quorum available for review of this study.

c) The IRB reviewed and approved the following studies at the February 13, 2012, IRB meeting without a majority of members present:

i. IRB Study **(b)(4), "(b)(4)"**

ii. IRB Study **(b)(4), "(b)(4)"**

The meeting minutes indicate that the IRB had the required membership present for quorum (six of the ten members, including a nonscientist), except for when the two studies above were reviewed and approved. **(b)(6)**, M.D., who was one of the six IRB members present, was the principal investigator for these studies. As the principal investigator, Dr. **(b)(6)** had a conflict of interest and should not have been counted toward the quorum for review and approval of these studies. The meeting minutes indicate, however, that Dr. **(b)(6)** was counted toward the quorum. The IRB should not have reviewed or approved IRB Studies **(b)(4)** and **(b)(4)** because the IRB did not have a quorum present for review of these studies.

In your May 1, 2015, written response, you indicate that the IRB will implement the following corrective or preventive actions:

a) An IRB meeting supplement form will be developed for recording votes and identifying quorum deficiencies, if any, before and during an IRB meeting.

b) The IRB will review and revise, as needed, their policies and procedures to include a reference to an SOP regarding IRB meeting administration.

We acknowledge your written response; however, we are unable to undertake an informed evaluation of the written response because you did not provide documentation of the following items:

a) A finalized copy of the IRB meeting supplemental form

b) Any relevant written SOPs that have been revised

c) A description of any training provided to IRB staff and members on the new SOPs, and a list of staff and members trained, or a projected timeline of planned training

Please submit any corrective or preventive actions the IRB plans to take to ensure that a majority of the members of the IRB is present, including at least one member whose primary concerns are in nonscientific areas, when the IRB reviews proposed research. Please include items a) through c) listed above.

Under 21 CFR 56.107(a), the IRB is required to have members with varying backgrounds to promote complete and adequate review of research activities. Failure of the IRB to establish or maintain a quorum may result in an inadequate review of research activities, which can impact the protection of the rights and welfare of human research subjects.

3. The IRB failed to prepare and maintain adequate documentation of IRB activities, including minutes of IRB meetings [21 CFR 56.115(a)(2)].

The IRB is required to prepare and maintain adequate documentation of IRB activities, including minutes of IRB meetings, which shall be in sufficient detail to show attendance at the meetings; actions taken by the IRB; the vote on these actions, including the number of members voting for, against, and abstaining; the basis for requiring changes in or disapproving research; and a written summary of the discussion of controverted issues and their resolution. The IRB failed to adhere to this requirement. Specifically:

The minutes of the IRB's February 11, 2013, meeting indicate that Dr. **(b)(6)**, who was either a principal investigator or a subinvestigator for three FDA-regulated studies (**(b)(4)**, attended the meeting and voted to approve these studies during the meeting. However, in letters dated April 6 and April 30, 2015, which were included in the IRB's response to the Form FDA 483, Dr. **(b)(6)** stated he had abstained from voting on these studies.

Please note that no IRB may have a member participate in the IRB's initial or continuing review of research in which the member has a conflict of interest, except to provide information requested by the IRB [21 CFR 56.107(e)]. Therefore, an IRB member with a conflict of interest may not participate in deliberation or voting on IRB actions taken for research in which the member has a conflict of interest.

Please submit any corrective or preventive actions the IRB plans to take to address the violation described above. With these corrective or preventive actions, please submit a copy of the IRB's written SOPs, or any draft SOPs in development, and a projected timeline for the implementation of any new SOPs. In addition, please provide a description of any training provided to IRB staff and members on the new SOPs, and a list of staff and members trained, or a projected timeline of planned training.

Failure to prepare and maintain adequate documentation of IRB activities, including IRB meeting minutes, raises concerns about the adequacy of the IRB's review process.

In addition, we note that in several of the IRB meetings described above, a member of the IRB abstained from voting on a review of research in which that member had a conflict of interest. We note that members are required to recuse themselves from voting altogether, and may not participate in deliberation, as opposed to simply abstaining from votes in which they have a conflict of interest [21 CFR 56.107(e)].

This letter is not intended to be an all-inclusive list of deficiencies for the protocols reviewed and approved by the IRB. It is your responsibility to ensure that the Monmouth Medical Center IRB's practices and procedures comply fully with all applicable statutes and regulations.

Within fifteen (15) working days of your receipt of this letter, you should notify this office in writing of the actions you have taken to prevent similar violations in the future. Failure to address the violations noted above adequately and promptly may result in regulatory action without further notice.

We recommend that you visit the following FDA Web page for information on human subject protections that may assist you in bringing the IRB into compliance with FDA regulations: http://www.fda.gov/ScienceResearch/SpecialTopics/RunningClinicalTrials/default.htm.

We appreciate the cooperation shown to the FDA Investigator during the inspection. If you have any questions, please contact Constance Cullity, M.D., M.P.H., at 301-796-3397: FAX 301-847-8748. Your written response and any pertinent documentation should be addressed to:

Constance Cullity, M.D., M.P.H.
Branch Chief
Good Clinical Practice Compliance Oversight Branch
Division of Clinical Compliance Evaluation
Office of Scientific Investigations
Office of Compliance
Center for Drug Evaluation and Research
U.S. Food and Drug Administration
Building 51, Room 5354
10903 New Hampshire Avenue
Silver Spring, MD 20993

Sincerely,

{See appended electronic signature page}

David C. Burrow, Pharm.D., J.D.
Acting Director
Office of Scientific Investigations
Office of Compliance
Center for Drug Evaluation and Research
U.S. Food and Drug Administration

This is a representation of an electronic record that was signed electronically and this page is the manifestation of the electronic signature.

/S/

DAVID C BURROW
11/10/2015

第5封　给St. Vincent医院和健康护理中心的警告信

2013年11月27日

参考号：13-HFD-45-11-03

尊敬的Worden博士：

2013年8月12日至8月26日，Myra Casey女士代表FDA对St. Vincent医院和健康护理中心伦理委员会（SVHHCC IRB）进行了现场检查。这封警告信特告知您现场检查中发现的违规情况。该项检查的目的是核实贵伦理委员会受试者保护程序是否符合美国联邦法规（CFR）第21篇第50和56部分的内容。该法规适用于FDA所监管产品的临床研究。

本次现场检查是FDA的生物研究监查项目的一部分。该项目通过设定的检查方法，对FDA所监管的相关研究的实施情况进行评估，以确认研究数据在科学上是有效和准确的，并帮助确保这些研究中受试者的权益、安全和福利得到了保护。

在现场检查结束时，Casey女士向Academic Affairs and Research的代理执行主任Niceta C. Bradburn博士出示了FDA483表，即现场检查的发现，并进行了讨论。我们确认收到了伦理委员会于2013年9月11日对该FDA483表作出的书面回复。

经对现场检查报告、该报告的附件，以及伦理委员会提交的书面回复进行审查，我们认为，伦理委员会没有遵循适用的法律要求和监管受试者保护的FDA法规。我们想强调以下几点：

1. IRB未能在初始审查时确定涉及儿童的研究需要遵循21 CFR 50（D），临床试验中对儿童的额外保护措施［21 CFR 56.109（h）］

21 CFR 56.109（h）规定，当一项临床研究部分或全部受试者为儿童时，伦理委员会必须在初始审查时确认该研究遵循21 CFR 50（D），对临床研究中儿童受试者的额外保护。根据21 CFR 50.50规定，伦理委员会必须对临床试验进行审查，仅批准符合21 CFR 50.51（临床试验不会产生比最小风险更大的风险）、21 CFR 50.52（临床试验会产生比最小风险更大的风险，除非存在能够给个人受试者带来直接利益的希望）或者21 CFR 50.53（临床试验会产生比最小风险更大的风险，也不存在能够给个人受试者带来直接利益的希望，但是对于受试者的身体功能障碍或病情可能产生通用的知识）标准的临床试验。

为了确认涉及儿童的研究是否需要符合21 CFR 50（D）的标准，伦理委员会对这类研究作出某种类型的调查。除了需遵循21 CFR 56.115规定外，伦理委员会也必须将包括伦理委员会会议期间采取的行动等活动记录下来。我们调查发现，在审查并批准的31个在研的涉及儿童受试者的临床研究中，SVHHCC伦理委员会未能确认研究满足D部分的标准。

例如，2012年5月23日SVHHCC伦理委员会审查并批准了一项名为“（b）（4）”的儿科临床研究。但是，不管是在会议记录还是在任何其他伦理委员会材料中，都没有伦理委员会在初始审查时对临床研究符合D部分进行必要确认的记录。

贵伦理委员会的日期为2013年9月11日的书面回复承认上述所列违规行为，并包含了一份“涉及儿童研究的检查表”的复印件。这份检查表记录着，作为伦理委员会纠正措施计划的一部分，将对上述所提到的儿科临床研究及另两项［研究（b）（4）和（b）（4）］在FDA483表上提到的儿科临床研究进行D部分审查。贵伦理委员会的回复也声明，将对31项中剩余28项在研的儿科临床研究进行D部分审查。贵伦理委员会的回复是不充分的，因为没有提供其余28项在研儿科临床研究已完成D部分审查的书面保证。

未能确保对研究中儿童受试者的额外保护得到满足，可能将这个弱势群体暴露于不必要的风险中，可能导致儿童的父母或监护人不能对您开展的研究充分知情。

2. IRB未能满足委员的要求［21 CFR 56.107］

伦理委员会允许非委员投票。具体而言：

a. 2012年3月28日伦理委员会会议记录显示，姓名为（b）（6）的参会者参与了投票。根据伦理委员会名册，（b）（6）女士在会议召开时还不是伦理委员会委员。

b. 2011年6月29日伦理委员会会议记录显示，姓名为（b）（6）的参会者参与了投票。根据伦理委员会名册，（b）（6）女士在会议召开时还不是伦理委员会委员。

c. 2010年6月23日伦理会议记录显示，姓名为（b）（6）的参会者参与了投票。根据伦理委员会名册，（b）（6）女士在会议召开时还不是伦理委员会委员。

我们承认在2013年9月11日的书面回复中，贵伦理委员会声明已实施了数项纠正措施，包括重组IRB会议记录的考勤表格，也包括对伦理委员会委员开展SOP 403、“伦理委员会考勤监控”，SOP 404、“伦理委员会会议记录”，SOP 803、“伦理委员会委员增补”等内容的培训。如果能正确实施并执行，这项措施似乎足以预防将来类似违规的再次发生。请确保伦理委员会遵守SOP，包括满足委员要求并更新委员名册。

21 CFR 56.107中描述的伦理委员会委员要求准备就绪，以确保伦理委员会通过委员的经验、专业和多样性使伦理委员会有资格来保护受试者。允许非委员投票的行为引起我们对伦理委员会满足这一要求能力的关注。

本警告信的目的并非是罗列贵伦理委员会在审查和批准试验方案中存在的所有缺陷。确保SVHHCC伦理委员会的实际操作和程序完全符合所有适用法律和法规的要求是您的职责。

自收到这封信的15个工作日内，您应当书面告知本办公室为预防将来发生类似违规情况而采取的措施。您的书面回复中应当包括能显示出已经达到全面和充分整改所需要的文件。请包括每项将要完成的措施的预计完成日期。如果不能充分、迅速地解释上述违规问题，可能导致我们在不再通知的情况下采取监管措施。

附：英文原文

St. Vincent Hospital and Health Care

WARNING LETTER

NOV 27, 2013

CERTIFIED MAIL
RETURN RECEIPT REQUESTED

Ref: 13-HFD-45-11-03

Ian Worden, MHA, MBA, CPA
Interim Chief Executive Officer
St. Vincent Health
2001 West 86th Street
Indianapolis, IN 46260

Dear Mr. Worden:

This Warning Letter informs you of objectionable conditions observed during the U.S. Food and Drug Administration (FDA) inspection of St. Vincent Hospital and Health Care Center Institutional Review Board (SVHHCC IRB) that was conducted between August 12, 2013, and August 26, 2013, by Ms. Myra Casey, representing FDA. The purpose of this inspection was to determine whether the IRB procedures for the protection of human subjects complied with Title 21 of the Code of Federal Regulations (CFR), parts 50 and 56. These regulations apply to clinical investigations of products regulated by FDA.

This inspection is a part of FDA's Bioresearch Monitoring Program, which includes inspections designed to evaluate the conduct of FDA-regulated research to ensure that the data are scientifically valid and accurate, and to help ensure that the rights, safety, and welfare of the human subjects of those clinical investigations have been protected.

At the conclusion of the inspection, Ms. Casey presented the Interim Executive Director for Academic Affairs and Research, Dr. Niceta C. Bradburn, with a Form FDA 483, Inspectional Observations. We acknowledge receipt of the IRB's September 11, 2013, written response to the Form FDA 483.

From our review of the FDA establishment inspection report, the documents submitted with that report and the IRB's written response, we conclude that the IRB did not adhere to the applicable statutory requirements and FDA regulations governing the protection of human subjects. We wish to emphasize the following:

1. The IRB failed to determine at the time of initial review that clinical investigations involving children were in compliance with 21 CFR part 50, subpart D, Additional Safeguard for Children in Clinical Investigations [21 CFR 56.109(h)].

Under 21 CFR 56.109(h), when some or all of the subjects in a clinical investigation are children, the IRB must determine that the clinical investigation is in compliance with 21 CFR part 50, subpart D (Additional Safeguards for Children in Clinical Investigations) at the time of initial review. Under 21 CFR 50.50, an IRB must review the clinical investigation and approve only those clinical investigations that satisfy the criteria described in section 50.51 (clinical investigations not involving greater than minimal risk), section 50.52 (clinical investigations involving greater than minimal risk but presenting the prospect of direct benefit to individual subjects), or section 50.53 (clinical investigations involving greater than minimal risk and no prospect of direct benefit to individual subjects, but likely to yield generalizable knowledge about the subject's disorder or condition).

In order to determine if a clinical investigation involving children meets the criteria in 21 CFR part 50, subpart D, the IRB must make certain types of findings with respect to such investigations. In addition under 21 CFR 56.115, the IRB is required to document its activities, including actions taken during IRB meetings. Our inspection revealed that in its review and approval of 31 active clinical investigations involving pediatric subjects, SVHHCC IRB failed to determine that the clinical investigation satisfied the criteria of subpart D.

For example, on May 23, 2012, SVHHCC IRB reviewed and approved a pediatric clinical investigation titled "(b)(4)." However, there is no documentation, either in the meeting minutes or in any other IRB materials, of the IRB's requisite determination at the time of initial review that the clinical investigation was in compliance with subpart D.

Your IRB's written response dated September 11, 2013, acknowledges the violation listed above and includes a copy of a "Checklist for Research Involving Children." This checklist documents that, as a part of the IRB's corrective action plan, a subpart D review was performed for the above mentioned pediatric clinical investigation and for two other pediatric clinical investigations (Studies(b)(4) and (b)(4)) that were included in the Form FDA 483. Your IRB's response also states that the IRB will perform a subpart D review for the remaining 28 of 31 active pediatric clinical investigations. Your IRB's response is inadequate because it does not provide written assurance that a subpart D review has been completed for the remaining 28 active pediatric clinical investigations.

Failure to determine that the additional safeguards for children in research are met may expose this vulnerable population to unnecessary risks, and may result in the child's parent(s) or guardian(s) not being fully informed about the proposed research.

2. The IRB failed to fulfill membership requirements [21 CFR 56.107].

The IRB allowed nonmembers to vote on clinical investigations. Specifically:

a. IRB meeting minutes from March 28, 2012, show that an attendee identified as (b)(6) participated in voting. According to the IRB membership roster, Ms. (b)(6) was not a member of the IRB when this meeting was conducted.

b. IRB meeting minutes from June 29, 2011, show that an attendee identified as (b)(6) participated in voting. According to the IRB membership roster, Ms. (b)(6) was not a member of the IRB when this meeting was conducted.

c. IRB meeting minutes from June 23, 2010, show that an attendee identified as(b)(6) participated in voting. According to the IRB membership roster, Ms. (b)(6) was not a member of the IRB when this meeting was conducted.

We acknowledge your IRB's September 11, 2013, written response, stating that several corrective actions have been implemented. These include the restructuring of the attendance grid of IRB meeting minutes, as well as training for IRB members on Standard Operating Procedure (SOP) #403, "IRB Attendance Monitoring"; SOP #404, "IRB Meeting Minutes"; and SOP #803, "IRB Membership Addition." If properly implemented and executed, these procedures/actions appear adequate to prevent recurrence of similar violations in the future. Please ensure that the IRB is adhering to its SOPs, including fulfilling membership requirements and updating the membership roster.

IRB membership requirements described in 21 CFR 56.107 are in place to ensure that the IRB is qualified through its members' experience, expertise, and diversity to protect human subjects. Allowing nonmembers to vote calls into question the IRB's ability to fulfill this requirement.

This letter is not intended to be an all-inclusive list of deficiencies for the protocols reviewed and approved by the IRB. It is your responsibility to ensure that SVHHCC IRB's practices and procedures comply fully with all applicable statutes and regulations.

Within fifteen (15) business days of your receipt of this letter, you should notify this office in writing of the actions you have taken to prevent similar violations in the future. Your written response should include any documentation necessary to show that full and adequate correction will be achieved. Please include the projected completion dates for each action to be accomplished. Failure to explain the violations noted above adequately and promptly may result in regulatory action without further notice.

We recommend that you visit the following FDA Web page for information on human subject protection that may assist you in your efforts to bring the IRB into compliance with FDA
regulations: *http://www.fda.gov/ScienceResearch/SpecialTopics/RunningClinicalTrials/default.htm.*

We appreciate the cooperation shown to the FDA Investigator, Ms. Myra Casey, during the inspection. I you have any questions, please contact Catherine Parker, R.N., at 301-796-5553; FAX 301-847-8748. Your written response and any pertinent documentation should be addressed to:

Catherine Parker, R.N.
Team Lead, Human Subject Protection Branch
Office of Scientific Investigations
Office of Compliance
Center for Drug Evaluation and Research
Food and Drug Administration
Building 51, Room 5247 10903 New Hampshire Avenue
Silver Spring, MD 20993

Sincerely yours,

{See appended electronic signature page}
Thomas N. Moreno, M.S.
Acting Office Director
Office of Scientific Investigations
Office of Compliance
Center for Drug Evaluation and Research
Food and Drug Administration

Cc: Kyle DeFur, FACHE
President
St. Vincent Indianapolis Hospital
2001 West 86th Street
Indianapolis, IN 46260
Tina G. Noonan, MBA, CHRC
Director, Research & Regulatory Affairs
St. Vincent Research & Research Regulatory Affairs
8402 Harcourt Road, Suite 805
Indianapolis, IN 46260

第 6 封　给 BRI 伦理委员会的警告信

2013年9月23日

参考号：3377341

尊敬的Hazelwood博士：

2013年1月22日至2月7日，FDA对BRI伦理委员会（以下简称BRI IRB）进行了现场检查。这封警告信特告知您现场检查中发现的违规情况。本次现场检查的目的是核实IRB的操作和受试者保护程序是否符合美国联邦法规（CFR ）第21篇第50和56部分的内容。该法规适用于FDA所监管产品的临床研究，以帮助确保受试者在临床研究期间所受到的危害和风险得到最大的保护。

在现场检查结束时，检查员向您出示了FDA483表，即现场检查发现的问题，并与您进行了讨论。我们确认收到了伦理委员会于2013年2月28日对FDA483表作出的书面回复，以及2013年3月28日的增补回复。我们已经审查了报告、FDA483表以及伦理委员会的书面回复，伦理委员会的书面回复意见无法让人接受，具体解释如下：此封IRB限制信是书面告知您BRI伦理委员会未遵守（或违反了）美国联邦法规关于临床研究的相关法规，未履行21CFR 56所要求的伦理委员会职责。BRI伦理委员会应当向FDA药品评价与研究中心（CDER）、科学研究办公室（OSI）提交书面的改进计划，该计划由伦理委员会、研究机构分别或共同执行，以确保伦理委员会工作能符合FDA法规要求［21 CFR 56.120（a）］。本信件末尾列出了您需要发送改进计划的人员名单及地址。违规行为列举如下，每条违规所依据的CFR法规一并列出。

1. IRB未能遵守关于快速审查程序的FDA法规［21 CFR 56.110（b）］

根据快速审查程序，快速审查可由伦理委员会主席单独执行，或由主席指定一位或多位伦理委员会委员来执行。此外，对下列情形之一才可采用快速审查程序：①联邦注册登记簿目录上所列符合快速审查资格并经审评专家认为不超过最小风险的部分或全部研究；或者②对伦理委员会已批准的研究方案仅做较小修正。

我们的现场检查发现，BRI伦理委员会对单一受试者方案（SPPs）实施了不恰当的快速审查，此类受试者不符合入选标准却被批准在开放性临床研究中使用抗肿瘤治疗。根据本次检查记录以及伦理委员会副主席Gary L. Harvey先生在检查期间的声明，伦理委员会在下次会议审查之前先行给予SPP“临时批准”的批复，允许受试者接受抗肿瘤治疗。“临时批准”不被FDA认为是有效的伦理委员会行动。伦理委员会相关法规规定，研究必须经全体委员审查或在某些合适情形下快速审查批准。因为BRI伦理委员会在全体委员审查之前就授权研究者收到“临时批准”后给予受试者研究药物，所以看起来伦理委员会是使用“临时批准”的名称以快速审查方式批准了研究。

BRI伦理委员会未能遵循FDA有关快速审查程序的法规。特别是在不适用快速审查的情形下采用了快速审查方式。对患者接受抗肿瘤治疗的SPP的批准既不是对先前批准研究的微小变动，也不属于联邦登记注册通知所列符合快速审查资格的研究。因此，此类SPP必须在召集会议上由全体委员进行审查。

不恰当采用快速审查的例子包括，但不仅限于以下：

a. 2012年3月29日，BRI伦理委员会对受试者023115作出“临时批准”（经快速审查批准），而直到4个月后的2012年8月3日才进行了要求的全体委员审查。

b. 2012年5月2日，BRI伦理委员会对受试者023320作出“临时批准”（经快速审查批准），而直到3个月后的2012年8月3日才进行了要求的全体委员审查。

c. 2012年5月3日，BRI伦理委员会对受试者023410作出“临时批准”（经快速审查批准），而直到3个月后的2012年8月3日才进行了要求的全体委员审查。

2013年2月28日书面回复中的纠正措施声称，伦理委员会已对SPPs审查程序进行了修正，由至少3名伦理委员会委员加伦理委员会主席或副主席组成的小组进行审查，该小组将通过BRI伦理委员会建立的快速审批方法对“需FDA批准的”SPP申请进行审查和批准。经小组审查后，由伦理委员会主席或副主席将在“临时批准”批件上签字确认。这些“临时批准”将在下一次伦理委员会会议上进行宣读并记录在会议记录中。这个过程被描述在2013年3月28日（13版）题为：“紧急情况下对前瞻性伦理委员会批准进行豁免”的标准操作规程中，并提交在2013年3月28日的书面回复中。您的纠正措施是不可接受的。按照FDA法规规定，SPPs不适于进行快速审查。因此，您的对SPPs进行快速审查的纠正措施不符合FDA法规的要求。

我们注意到2013年3月28日书面回复中提交的SOP，似乎将21 CFR 56.104（c）中关于紧急使用试验样品的要求与21 CFR 56.110中关于快速审查的要求相混淆了。紧急情况下使用试验样品可豁免伦理委员会审查，但快速审查如其名称所示是伦理审查的加快程序。FDA认为这类SPPs不符合紧急使用试验样品情况。BRI伦理委员会于2012年3月29日、2012年5月2日及2012年5月3日收到过来自于FDA的邮件，FDA已在邮件中阐明“每一例豁免的受试者在治疗前必须经负责对这些研究进行审查的伦理委员会批准（21 CFR 56）。”因此，FDA认为这些SPPs（邮件中提到的“特别豁免”）需要审查和批准，BRI伦理委员会对此是知晓的。

根据21 USC 360bbb条例，FDA通过扩大可及性计划，使罹患严重或很快危及生命的疾病或状况且缺乏有效治疗手段的受试者能够使用研究药物进行治疗。个例患者方案（也称为单一患者方案）属于这个计划的范围。伦理委员会开展前瞻性审查和批准是扩大可及性的关键性监管要求，以保证给这些天然的弱势群体提供伦理上的监督。缺少在有大多数委员出席的召集会议上对SPPs进行前瞻性全部委员的审查和批准，引起对在BRI伦理委员会监督下进行治疗的患者的监护水平的关注。

请递交针对上述违规行为所采取的纠正和预防措施（CAPA）计划。请随该计划一起，递交书面程序或任何正在制定中的程序草案的复印件，以及实施新程序的时间表。请提供一份对伦理委员会委员进行或将要进行针对新程序的说明，接受培训的人员名单，或计划培训的项目时间表。

2. IRB在未确认符合以下标准的情况下批准了研究：受试者的风险最小化［21 CFR 56.111（a）（1）］；受试者的风险与预期的效益（如果存在），以及与预期可以获得的重要知识相比是合理的［21 CFR 56.111（a）（2）］

为批准一项研究，伦理委员会必须确认21 CFR 56.111中明确的所有要求都得到满足。具体而言，伦理委员会必须确认受试者风险最小化以及风险-预期效益比是合理的。伦理委员会通过审查充分的信息来评估对受试者的预期效益才作出这样的决定。

我们现场检查发现，BRI伦理委员会未能确保受试者风险最小化以及风险-预期效益比是合理的，因为在批准项目前未审核受试者病史及其他相关信息。此外，伦理委员会委员Gary L. Harvey，也是伦理委员会副主席，批准了大多数项目，他是社区（即非科学领域背景）委员，有工商管理硕士学位。根据2013年2月28日您书面回复时递交的伦理委员会人员名册，Harvey先生是提供水上康复服务的个体经营者，因此他并不具备必需的临床专业知识，以对给受试者带来的风险和与预期收益相关的合理性进行必需的知情评价。

例如：

a. 2012年6月21日，伦理委员会副主席Gary Harvey代表BRI伦理委员会批准受试者022056接受抗肿瘤治疗。但是，当时伦理委员会批准时仅有的文件是知情同意书（ICD）。ICD是提供给受试者的书面信息概要，许多研究者在获取潜在的受试者知情同意时，将知情同意书作为对试验方案口头解释的指南。但是，单独以此文件上内容对伦理委员会确定一项提议研究的可行性是不充分的。

在2013年2月28日递交的书面回复中，您声称伦理委员会副主席在作出批准决定前已审查了此例受试者的病史及体检资料。您的回复与2012年12月7日（伦理委员会已批准后）写给Burzynski诊所的信件内容相矛盾，写给诊所的信就是为了索取受试者022056的病史资料。

b. 2012年6月21日，伦理委员会副主席Gary Harvey代表BRI伦理委员会批准受试者023356接受抗肿瘤治疗。当时伦理委员会批准时仅有的文件是知情同意书（ICD）。如上所讨论的，单独以此文件上内容对伦理委员会确定一项提议研究的可行性是不充分的。

在2013年2月28日递交的书面回复中，您声称伦理委员会副主席在作出批准决定前已审核了这例受试者的病史及体检资料，您的回复与2012年12月7日（伦理已批准后）写给Burzynski诊所的信件内容相矛盾，写信就是为了索取受试者023356的病史资料。

c. 2012年6月21日，伦理委员会副主席Gary Harvey代表BRI伦理委员会批准受试者023520接受抗肿瘤治疗。但从现场检查期间审查的材料来看，伦理委员会批准时仅有的文件是ICD。如上所讨论的，单独以此文件上内容对伦理委员会确定一项提议研究的可行性是不充分的。

在2013年2月28日递交的书面回复中，您声称伦理委员会已审核了这例受试者详细的病史及体检资料，但您的回复没有包括任何证明材料（即病史和体检资料）。

d. 2011年6月28日，伦理委员会主席Carlton Hazelwood代表BRI伦理委员会批准受试者021237接受抗肿瘤治疗。但是审批表上清晰地记录着Hazelwood先生的手写批注，质疑为何入选卡氏评分50的患者："请阐明卡氏评分50的病史及体检资料——目前资料不清。"直到2011年8月2日，BRI伦理委员会才收到这例受试者更正的病史和体检资料。

在2013年2月28日递交的书面回复中，您声称"既然病史及体检资料已证明了该评分，伦理委员会觉得没有必要再去要求澄清了。"但您的回复与审批表上的手写批注相矛盾，在质疑卡氏评分50的情况下却仍进行批准。

2013年2月28日递交书面回复中的纠正措施，声称正在起草一份SOP，以确保对受试者的风险与预期效益比的合理性，该项SOP最迟于2013年4月1日定稿。2013年2月28日的书面回复中还包含两项SOP，但其中没有任何一项SOP是针对此违规行为制定的。

BRI伦理委员会不能符合批准SPPs的监管要求（即保证受试者风险的最小化和合理性），没有做到以下方面：①审核受试者医疗记录（病史及体检资料）；②在批准前，搞清楚任何有关受试者是否适于抗肿瘤治疗的突出问题（例如卡氏评分）。BRI伦理委员会没有对必要资料进行审查就作出批准，这种行为让人关注其对接受抗肿瘤治疗受试者的监护水平。

请递交针对上述违规行为所采取的CAPA计划。在CAPA计划中，请递交书面程序或任何正在制定中的规程的复印件，以及实施新规程的时间表。请提供一份对伦理委员会委员进行或将要进行针对新规程培训的说明，接受培训的人员名单，或计划培训的项目时间表。

3. IRB未能在初始审查时确定涉及儿童的研究需要遵循21 CFR 50（D），临床试验中对儿童的额外保护措施［21 CFR 56.109（h）］

这是自2010年现场检查的重复违规。

根据21 CFR 56.109（h）规定，当一项临床研究部分或全部受试者为儿童时，伦理委员会必须在初始审查时确认该研究遵循21 CFR 50（D）（对临床研究中儿童受试者的额外保护）。21 CFR 50.50规定，伦理委员会必须对临床研究进行审查，仅批准满足21 CFR 50.51（临床试验不会产生比最小风险更大的风险）、21 CFR 50.52（临床试验会产生比最小风险更大的风险，除非存在能够给个人受试者带来直接利益的希望）或者21 CFR 50.53（临床试验会产生比最小风险更大的风险，也不存在能够给个人受试者带来直接利益的希望，但是对于受试者的身体功能紊乱或病情可能产生通用的知识）标准的临床试验。

根据21 CFR 50（D）（对临床研究中儿童受试者的额外保护），伦理委员会必须对涉及儿童的临床研究作出某些调查。按照21 CFR 56.115的要求，伦理委员会需要将包括采取的行动等活动记录下来。我们现场检查发现，在经批准开展的涉及儿童受试者的临床研究中，BRI伦理委员未能充分地记录研究满足D部分的标准。特别是下列SPPs由伦理委员会审查并批准，但是伦理委员会记录未能详细说明伦理委员会已明确这些研究满足D部分的标准。

a. 2012年5月2日，BRI伦理委员会对受试者023320（5岁）作出"临时批准"接受抗肿瘤治疗，后续于

2012年8月3日再经全体委员批准，但没有文件，证明伦理委员会根据21 CFR 56.115的要求按照D部分的规定进行必要的确定。

b. 2012年5月3日，BRI伦理委员会对受试者023410（4岁）作出“临时批准”接受抗肿瘤治疗，后续于2012年8月3日再经全体委员批准，但没有文件证明伦理委员会根据21 CFR 56.115的要求按照D部分的规定进行了必要的确定。

c. 2012年3月29日，BRI伦理委员会对受试者023115（3岁）作出“临时批准”接受抗肿瘤治疗，后续于2012年8月3日再经全体委员批准，但没有文件证明伦理委员会根据21 CFR 56.115的要求按照D部分的规定进行了必要的确定。

2013年2月28日书面回复中，您声称已为潜在的绝症患者制定了儿科风险评估表，对涉及儿童研究审查的新程序包括以下内容：

- 要求临床研究者提供风险/效益评估；
- 依照法规规定的超过最小风险的定义作出所有风险程度确定；
- 伦理委员会将审查并确定是否赞同研究者的决定；
- 伦理委员会开展的风险/效益评判将记录于会议记录上。

此外，您声称伦理委员会在SOP中正式列明风险分级依据，此项工作将于2013年4月1日前完成。

2013年3月28日书面回复包括如下内容：SOP 13“紧急情况下豁免提前的伦理委员会批准，”SOP 35“涉及儿童的研究。”但是，您的回复是无法接受的，因为伦理委员会对涉及儿童作为受试者的SPPs审查，必须在召集会议上进行［21 CFR 56.108（c）］，而不能如SOP 13所述的使用快速审查程序。

未能确保对研究中儿童受试者的额外保护得到满足，可能使这个弱势群体暴露于不必要的风险中，也可能导致儿童的父母或监护人对拟开展研究不能充分知情。涉及儿童的SPP缺乏前瞻性伦理审批，BRI伦理委员会对接受治疗的儿童受试者的监护水平引起关注。

请递交针对上述违规行为所采取的CAPA计划。在CAPA计划中，请递交已定稿或任何正在制定中的程序的复印件，以及实施新程序的时间计划表。请提供一份对伦理委员会委员进行或将要进行针对新程序培训的说明，接受培训的人员名单，或计划培训的项目时间表。

4. IRB未能制定、维护和遵守管理IRB职能和运行的书面程序，并保存足够的记录［21 CFR 56.108（a），21 CFR 56.108（b）和21 CFR 56.115（a）（6）］

为达到FDA法规所要求的、对FDA所监管的研究进行审查的伦理委员会的要求，每个伦理委员会制定、维护和遵守法规中规定的说明IRB职能和运行的书面程序。贵伦理委员会没有遵守这些要求，遵守法规要求是为了保护受试者的权益。具体而言：

a. BRI 伦理委员会在作出“临时批准”时未能遵守操作规程。因为“SOP 4 向伦理委员会申请”下4.4“伦理委员会对申请进行审查”的 4.4.1“BRI 伦理委员会决定”中陈述：“BRI 伦理委员会将在召集会议上对伦理申请进行审核”。伦理委员会没有制定专门用于SPP审批的书面程序，即使用快速审查程序（指“临时批准”）。初始审查程序中没有任何有关可通过快速途径开展审核的条款内容，快速审查只在“SOP 5 对研究进行跟踪审查”中被提及。

b. BRI伦理委员会未制订就下列情况向伦理委员会、适当的机构人员和FDA确保进行快速报告的书面程序：①任何给受试者或他人带来风险的非预期事件；②任何严重或持续违反伦理规程、要求或伦理委员会决定的情况。

2013年2月28日书面回复中，对初始审查未遵循书面程序做了解释，您的解释是伦理委员会对“FDA预先已批准的情况”一直采用了快速审查程序。我们想强调一下，FDA确定21 CFR 312.305 和312.310的标准得到满足，与伦理委员会的审查和批准是截然不同完全独立的行动。伦理委员会必须作出自己的确定，并对FDA所监管的研究遵循21 CFR 50和56的要求。特别是，伦理委员会的纠正措施是无法接受的，因为看起来伦理委员会意图继续应用快速审查程序来批准SPPs。具体而言，您的回复中称：“我们立即启动的流程已在观察项1中做了描述，其中包括成立一个由至少3名伦理委员会委员加伦理委员会主席或副主席组成的小组，来审查和批准任何FDA批准的个例患者治疗申请”。如之前所述，根据FDA法规，SPPs不适用于快速审查程序，因此，您的对SPPs使用快速审查程序的纠正措施未能符合FDA法规要求。

2013年2月28日书面回复中，对未能起草将任何给受试者或他人带来风险的非预期问题及时报告给伦理委员会、适当的机构人员和FDA的书面程序进行了说明。您的解释是贵方将制定指南和规程，以保证研究者快速上报任何给受试者或他人带来风险的非预期问题，并提到了题为“给参与者和他人带来风险的非预期问题的上报”的SOP。您的纠正措施是不能接受的，因为SOP没有明确提供向FDA报告的流程。

2013年2月28日书面回复中，您对未能制定将任何严重或持续违反伦理规程、要求或伦理委员会决定的情况及时向伦理委员会、适当的机构人员和FDA报告的书面程序进行了解释。提到了题为“给参与者和他人带来风险的非预期问题的上报”的SOP。但此SOP显示仅伦理委员会的批件暂停或终止才需上报。这个SOP是不能接受的，因为其未能包含报告严重或持续不合规的程序。

书面程序是重要的，因为其描述了伦理委员会如何操作和履行主要职责。伦理委员会未能制定、维护和遵守书面程序可能会对受试者权益和福利产生不良影响，因为这可能导致违反现行以保护受试者权益和福利的法规（例如我们检查中发现的问题）。

请递交针对上述违规行为所采取的CAPA计划。在CAPA计划中，请递交已定稿或任何正在制定中的程序的复印件，以及实施任何新程序的时间表，并请提供针对伦理委员会委员已开展或拟开展培训的说明，接受培训的人员名单，或计划培训的项目时间表。

本警告信的目的并非是罗列存在的所有缺陷。确保遵循法律和相关法规的每一项要求是您的职责。

鉴于在既往3次现场检查中发现的缺陷问题持续存在，BRI伦理委员会未达到21 CFR 56的法规要求。我们无法确保其规程是否可充分保护受试者权益和福利。因此，立即采取如下措施：

（1）禁止BRI伦理委员会批准需遵循 21 CFR 50和56要求的新研究［21 CFR 56.103（a）和 56.120（b）（1）］；

（2）禁止需遵循 21 CFR 56 的在研项目入组新的受试者［21 CFR 56.120（b）（2）］；

（3）FDA暂停伦理委员会采用快速审查程序，以保护受试者权益或福利［21 CFR 56.110（d）］。

在FDA得到贵伦理委员会充分的改进措施证据并书面通知贵伦理委员会的纠正措施令人满意前，这些限制措施持续有效。您有责任将这些限制措施通知受影响的申办者及研究者（见 21 CFR 312.66）。在此期间，伦理委员会应当继续负责接收、处理给受试者或他人带来风险的非预期事件报告，在研项目的常规进展报告。限制措施禁止SPP项目或其他在研2、3期研究入组新的受试者，但对已入组的受试者来说，只要入组对其个人利益与安全处于最佳状况，限制措施对其就没有影响。

在收到本警告信的30个工作日内，您应当书面回复说明将要采取的或已经实施的使达到合规的纠正措施。

您的回复应当对上述每条不合规进行解释。如果您不认为贵伦理委员会违反了FDA的法规要求，请提供理由及任何支持文件供我们参考。如果您确信已经达到全面充分的纠正，应当提供包含确认您纠正措施的所有文件。对每项将要完成的措施，请包括预计完成日期。

与您的回复一起，请包含一份伦理委员会与每个受影响的申办者和临床研究者进行交流，告诉他们当前FDA施加的禁令的书面材料的复印件。此外，请提供遵循21 CFR 56并正被贵伦理委员会审查的所有研究的名单，列出所有受到上述禁令影响的研究。

附：英文原文

BRI Institutional Review Board

By Certified Mail – Return Receipt Requested

Carlton F. Hazelwood, Ph.D.
Chairman
BRI Institutional Review Board
9432 Katy Freeway, Suite 105
Houston, TX 77055

Dear Dr. Hazelwood:

This letter imposing restrictions (IRB Restrictions Letter) informs you of objectionable conditions observed during the U.S. Food and Drug Administration (FDA) inspection of the BRI Institutional Review Board (BRI IRB) that was conducted between January 22, 2013, and February 7, 2013. The purpose of this inspection was to determine whether the IRB's activities and procedures for the protection of human subjects comply with FDA regulations published in Title 21 of the Code of Federal Regulations (21 CFR), parts 50 and 56. These regulations govern clinical investigations of products regulated by FDA, and help ensure that human subjects are protected from undue hazard or risk during the course of clinical investigations.

At the conclusion of the inspection, a Form FDA 483, Inspectional Observations, was presented and discussed with you. We acknowledge receipt of the IRB's February 28, 2013, written response to the Form FDA 483, and a follow-up response dated March 28, 2013. We have reviewed the FDA inspection report, the Form FDA 483, and your responses. The IRB's written responses are unacceptable, as explained below. This IRB Restrictions Letter provides you with written notice describing BRI IRB's noncompliance with (violations of) applicable federal regulations governing the operation and responsibilities of IRBs under 21CFR part 56. The BRI IRB is required to respond in writing to FDA's Center for Drug Evaluation and Research (CDER), Office of Scientific Investigations (OSI) with a description of the corrective actions that will be taken by the IRB, the institution, or both, to achieve compliance with FDA regulations [21 CFR 56.120(a)]. The name and address of the person to whom you should submit your corrective action plan is provided at the end of the letter. A listing of the violations follows. The applicable provisions of the CFR are cited for each violation.

1. The IRB failed to follow FDA regulations regarding expedited review procedures [21 CFR 56.110(b)].

Under an expedited review procedure, the IRB's review may be carried out by the IRB chairperson or by one or more experienced reviewers designated by the IRB chairperson from among the members of the IRB. Further, the IRB may use the expedited review procedure to review either or both of the following: (1) some or all of the research appearing on the Federal Register list of categories of research eligible for expedited review and found by the reviewer(s) to involve no more than minimal risk; or (2) minor changes in previously approved research during the period for which approval is authorized.

Our inspection revealed that BRI IRB used expedited review inappropriately to approve Single Patient Protocols (SPPs) for patients who failed to meet enrollment criteria for open clinical investigations to receive antineoplaston therapy. Based on our review of records from the inspection, as well as statements made by Mr. Gary L. Harvey, IRB Vice-Chairman, during the inspection, the IRB would grant "provisional approval" before placing an SPP on the agenda for the next scheduled IRB meeting, and that upon granting this "provisional approval," the subject was able to receive treatment with antineoplastons. A "provisional approval" is not recognized by FDA as a valid IRB action. The IRB regulations provide for studies to be approved by either full board review or by expedited review when applicable. Because BRI IRB authorized the investigator to provide the investigational product to subjects after receiving "provisional approval" and prior to a full board review, it appears that BRI IRB uses the term "provisional approval" to mean approval via expedited review.

BRI IRB has failed to comply with the regulations for employing an expedited review procedure. Specifically, BRI IRB used expedited review to approve research that was not eligible for review under an expedited review procedure. Approval of an SPP for patients to receive antineoplaston therapy is not a minor change in previously approved research and is not a category of research eligible for expedited review as listed in the *Federal Register* notice.[1] Therefore, SPPs must be reviewed by a full board during a convened IRB meeting.

Examples of your inappropriate use of the expedited review procedure include, but are not limited, to the following:

a. On March 29, 2012, BRI IRB granted "provisional approval" (approval via expedited review) for Subject 023115. The requisite full board review did not occur until four months later, on August 3, 2012.

b. On May 2, 2012, BRI IRB granted "provisional approval" (approval via expedited review) for Subject 023320. The requisite full board review did not occur until three months later, on August 3, 2012.

c. On May 3, 2012, BRI IRB granted "provisional approval" (approval via expedited review) for Subject 023410. The requisite full board review did not occur until three months later, on August 3, 2012.

The corrective action in your February 28, 2013, written response states that the IRB has initiated a revised IRB approval process for SPPs, to include review by a subcommittee of at least three IRB members plus the IRB Chairman or Vice-Chairman, which will review and approve any "FDA-sanctioned" SPP requests through the expedited approval method established by BRI IRB. After review by the subcommittee, the IRB Chairman or Vice-Chairman will signoff on a "provisional approval." These "provisional approvals" will then be read into the record at a subsequent IRB meeting and documented in the meeting minutes. This process is described in your Standard Operating Procedure (SOP) titled, "Emergency Exemption from Prospective IRB Approval," dated March 28, 2013 (Version 13), which was submitted in your March 28, 2013, written response. Your corrective action is unacceptable. Under FDA regulations, SPPs are not eligible for review via the expedited review procedure. Therefore, your corrective action documenting an expedited review procedure for SPPs fails to comply with FDA's regulatory requirements.

We note that the SOP submitted with your March 28, 2013, response appears to confuse the requirements under 21 CFR 56.104(c) regarding emergency use of a test article, with the requirements under 21 CFR 56.110 for expedited review. Emergency use of a test article is exempt from IRB review, whereas expedited review, as its name suggests, is an expedited process for IRB review. FDA does not consider these SPPs to qualify as an emergency use of a test article. BRI IRB was in possession of e-mails from FDA to the clinical site, dated March 29, 2012; May 2, 2012; and May 3, 2012, stating that "each special exception patient must be approved, prior to treatment, by the IRB that is responsible for review of these clinical investigations (21 CFR part 56)." Thus, BRI IRB was aware that FDA considered these SPPs (referred to in the e-mails as "special exceptions") to require IRB review and approval.

FDA facilitates access to investigational drugs for treatment use for patients with serious or immediately life-threatening diseases or conditions who lack therapeutic alternatives through its expanded access program under 21 USC 360bbb. Individual patient protocols (also referred to as single patient protocols) are part of this program. Prospective IRB review and approval is a critical regulatory requirement for expanded access, in order to provide ethical oversight for this inherently vulnerable population. The absence of prospective full board IRB review and approval of SPPs at a convened meeting at which a majority of the members of the IRB are present [21 CFR 56.108(c)] raises concerns about the level of oversight given to patients whose treatments are overseen by BRI IRB.

Please submit a corrective and preventive action (CAPA) plan to address the violations cited above. With your CAPA plan, submit a copy of your written procedures, or any draft procedures in development, and a timeline for the implementation of any new procedures. Please provide a description of any training provided or to be provided to IRB members on the new procedures and a list of attendees, or a projected timeline of planned training.

---

1 "Conditions for IRB Use of Expedited Review," *Federal Register*, November 9, 1998 (Volume 63, Number 216).

2. The IRB approved research without determining that the following criteria were met: risks to subjects were minimized [21 CFR 56.111(a)(1)]; risks to subjects were reasonable in relation to anticipated benefits, if any, to subjects, and the importance of the knowledge that may be expected to result [21 CFR 56.111(a)(2)].

In order to approve research, an IRB must determine that all of the requirements as defined in 21 CFR 56.111 are satisfied. Specifically, an IRB must determine that risks to subjects are minimized and reasonable in relationship to the anticipated benefit. An IRB makes such a determination by reviewing sufficient information to assess anticipated benefits to subjects.

Our inspection revealed that BRI IRB failed to ensure that the risks to subjects were minimized and reasonable in relation to the anticipated benefits, because BRI IRB did not review the subjects' medical records and other pertinent information prior to granting approval. In addition, the IRB member who granted the majority of these approvals, IRB Vice-Chairman Gary L. Harvey, was a community (i.e., nonscientific) member of the IRB with a Master's degree in Business Administration. According to the IRB roster submitted with your February 28, 2013, written response, Mr. Harvey is self-employed in water rehabilitation services; therefore, he does not have the clinical expertise necessary to make the required informed evaluation of the risks to subjects and their reasonableness in relation to anticipated benefits.

For example:

a. On June 21, 2012, IRB Vice-Chairman Gary Harvey, on behalf of BRI IRB, granted approval for Subject 022056 to receive antineoplastons. However, the only document in the IRB's possession at the time of approval was the Informed Consent Document (ICD). The ICD is a written summary of the information that should be provided to the subject. Many clinical investigators use the consent document as a guide for the verbal explanation of the study when obtaining consent from a potential subject; however, it alone is insufficient information for an IRB to determine the approvability of a proposed protocol.

Your February 28, 2013, written response states that the IRB Vice-Chairman reviewed the history and physical exam for this subject prior to granting approval. Your response contradicts an IRB letter sent to the Burzynski Clinic on December 7, 2012 (after the IRB had already granted approval), requesting medical records for Subject 022056.

b. On June 21, 2012, Vice-Chairman Gary Harvey, on behalf of BRI IRB, granted approval for Subject 023356 to receive antineoplastons. However, the only document in the IRB's possession at the time of approval was the ICD. As discussed above, an ICD alone is insufficient information for an IRB to determine the approvability of a proposed protocol.

Your February 28, 2013, written response states that the IRB Vice-Chairman reviewed the history and physical exam for this subject prior to granting approval. Your response contradicts an IRB letter sent to the Burzynski Clinic on December 7, 2012 (after the IRB had already granted approval), requesting medical records for Subject 023356.

c. On June 21, 2012, Vice-Chairman Gary Harvey, on behalf of BRI IRB, granted approval for Subject 023520 to receive antineoplastons. However, it appears from the evidence reviewed during the inspection that the only document in the IRB's possession at the time of approval was the ICD. As discussed above, an ICD alone is insufficient information for an IRB to determine the approvability of a proposed protocol.

Your February 28, 2013, written response states that a detailed history and physical exam for this subject were reviewed by the IRB. However, your response fails to include any documentation (i.e., history and physical exam) to support your statement.

d. On July 28, 2011, Chairman Carlton Hazelwood, on behalf of BRI IRB, granted approval for Subject 021237 to receive antineoplastons. However, the approval form sought clarity as to why a Karnofsky score of 50 had been assigned, as evidenced by Dr. Hazelwood's handwritten comment: "Please clarify history and physical for assigning KPS 50 – not evident at present." BRI IRB did not receive a corrected medical history and physical exam for this subject until August 2, 2011.

Your February 28, 2013, written response states that "the IRB did not feel it necessary to clarify the rating, since the history and physical supported the rating." Your response, however, contradicts the handwritten comment on the approval form which questioned the Karnofsky score of 50, but still granted the approval.

The corrective action as described in your February 28, 2013, written response states that an SOP was being prepared to ensure that the risks to subjects are reasonable in relation to the anticipated benefits, and that it will be finalized no later than April 1, 2013. You included two SOPs in your March 28, 2013, written response, neither of which appears to address this violation.

BRI IRB cannot meet the regulatory requirements for approval of SPPs (i.e., ensuring that risks to subjects are minimized and reasonable) without (1) reviewing the subject's medical records (history and physical exam), and (2) clarifying any outstanding issues with respect to the suitability of treating the subject with antineoplastons (for example, the Karnofsky score) prior to granting IRB approval. BRI IRB's approval without reviewing necessary information raises concerns about the level of oversight given to patients who received antineoplaston therapy.

Please submit a CAPA plan to address the violations cited above. With your CAPA plan, submit a copy of your written procedures, or any draft procedures in development, and a timeline for the implementation of any new procedures. Please provide a description of any training provided or to be provided to IRB members on the new procedures and a list of attendees, or a projected timeline of planned training.

3. The IRB failed to determine at the time of initial review that studies involving children are in compliance with 21 CFR part 50, subpart D, Additional Safeguards for Children in Clinical Investigations [21 CFR 56.109(h)].

This is a repeat violation from our 2010 inspection.

Under 21 CFR 56.109(h), when some or all of the subjects in a study are children, the IRB must determine that the research study is in compliance with 21 CFR part 50, subpart D (Additional Safeguards for Children in Clinical Investigations) at the time of initial review. Under 21 CFR 50.50, an IRB must review the clinical investigation and approve only those clinical investigations that satisfy the criteria described in section 50.51 (clinical investigations not involving greater than minimal risk), section 50.52 (clinical investigations involving greater than minimal risk but presenting the prospect of direct benefit to individual subjects), or section 50.53 (clinical investigations involving greater than minimal risk and no prospect of direct benefit to individual subjects, but likely to yield generalizable knowledge about the subject's disorder or condition).

Under 21 CFR part 50, subpart D (Additional Safeguards for Children in Clinical Investigations), the IRB must make certain findings with respect to clinical investigations involving children. Under 21 CFR 56.115, the IRB is required to document its activities, including actions taken. Our inspection revealed that in its review and approval of research involving pediatric subjects, BRI IRB failed to document adequately that the research satisfied the criteria of subpart D. Specifically, the following SPPs were reviewed and approved by the IRB, but the IRB records fail to specify that the IRB had determined that the study satisfied the criteria under subpart D.

a. On May 2, 2012, BRI IRB granted "provisional approval" for Subject 023320 (5-year-old child) to receive antineoplastons, followed by a full board approval on August 3, 2012. There is no documentation, as required by 21 CFR 56.115, of the IRB's requisite determination under subpart D.

b. On May 3, 2012, BRI IRB granted "provisional approval" for Subject 023410 (4-year-old child) to receive antineoplastons, followed by a full board approval on August 3, 2012. There is no documentation, as required by 21 CFR 56.115, of the IRB's requisite determination under subpart D.

c. On March 29, 2012, BRI IRB granted provisional approval for Subject 023115 (3-year-old child) to receive antineoplastons, followed by a full board approval on August 3, 2012. There is no documentation, as required by 21 CFR 56.115, of the IRB's requisite determination under subpart D.

In your February 28, 2013, written response, you state that a pediatric risk assessment form for potentially terminally ill patients had been created, and that your new procedure for review of research involving children includes the following:

- The clinical investigator is asked to provide his/her risk/benefit assessment;
- All determinations about the degree of risk will be made in accordance with the regulatory definition of greater than minimal risk;
- The IRB will review and determine whether there is concurrence with the clinical investigator's determination; and
- The IRB's risk/benefit determination will be documented in the meeting minutes.

In addition, you stated that the IRB will formally specify the justification of risk in its SOPs, which will be completed by April 1, 2013.

Your written response dated March 28, 2013, includes the following: SOP #13, "Emergency Exemption from Prospective IRB Approval," and SOP #35, "Research Involving Children." Your responses, however, are unacceptable, because the IRB's review of SPPs involving children as subjects must be performed during a convened IRB meeting [21 CFR 56.108(c)] and not under an expedited review procedure, as described by your SOP #13.

Failure to determine that the additional safeguards for children in research are met may expose this vulnerable population to unnecessary risks and result in the child's parent(s) or guardian(s) not being fully informed about the proposed research. The absence of prospective IRB review and approval of SPPs involving children raises concerns about the level of oversight given to pediatric patients whose treatments are overseen by BRI IRB.

Please submit a CAPA plan to address the violations cited above. With your CAPA plan, submit a copy of your written procedures, or any draft procedures in development, and a timeline for the implementation of any new procedures. Please provide a description of any training provided or to be provided to IRB members on the new procedures and a list of attendees, or a projected timeline of planned training.

4. The IRB failed to prepare, maintain, and follow written procedures and maintain adequate documentation governing the functions and operations of the IRB [21 CFR 56.108(a), 21 CFR 56.108(b), and 21 CFR 56.115(a)(6)].

In order to fulfill the requirements of an IRB that reviews clinical investigations regulated by FDA, each IRB must prepare, maintain, and follow written procedures describing IRB functions and operations specified in the regulations. Your IRB failed to adhere to these requirements. Compliance with these requirements is intended to protect the rights and welfare of research subjects involved in such investigations. Specifically:

a. BRI IRB failed to follow its written procedures when it granted "provisional approvals," because the IRB's written procedures in "SOP 4 Application to the IRB," section 4.4, "IRB Review of Application," subsection 4.4.1, "BRI IRB Decision," state: "BRI IRB will consider the application at a convened meeting." The IRB had no written procedures for the process that it used to review and approve SPPs, i.e., using expedited review (which it refers to as "provisional approval"). The written procedures for conducting initial review do not contain any provision for conducting IRB review through an expedited mechanism. Expedited review is only discussed under "SOP 5 Continuing Review of Research."

b. BRI IRB failed to prepare written procedures for ensuring prompt reporting to the IRB, appropriate institutional officials, and the Food and Drug Administration of (1) any unanticipated problems involving risks to human subjects or others, and (2) any instance of serious or continuing noncompliance with these regulations or the requirements or determinations of the IRB.

In your February 28, 2013, written response addressing your failure to follow written procedures for conducting initial review of research, you explain that the IRB had been using the expedited review procedure "for cases that have been pre-approved by the FDA." We wish to emphasize that an FDA determination that the criteria in 21 CFR 312.305 and 312.310 are met is a distinct and completely separate action from IRB review and approval. The IRB must make its own determinations and comply with the regulations in 21 CFR parts 50 and 56 for FDA-regulated clinical investigations. Specifically, the IRB must ensure that all of the criteria specified in 21 CFR 56.111 have been met prior to IRB approval. Your corrective action is unacceptable, because it appears that the IRB intends to continue to use the expedited review procedure to approve SPPs. Specifically, your response states, "The procedure we have immediately initiated is described in Observation #1, which requires a sub-committee of at least 3 IRB members plus the IRB Chairman or Vice-Chairman to review and approve any FDA-sanctioned single patient protocol requests." As stated earlier, under FDA regulations, SPPs are not eligible for review via the expedited review procedure. Therefore, your corrective action documenting an expedited review procedure for SPPs fails to comply with FDA's regulatory requirements.

In your February 28, 2013, written response addressing your failure to prepare a written procedure for ensuring prompt reporting to the IRB, appropriate institutional officials, and FDA of any unanticipated problems involving risks to human subjects or others, you explain that you will institute guidelines and procedures to ensure that investigators promptly report any unanticipated problems involving risk to subjects or others, and referred to the SOP titled "Reporting of Unanticipated Problems Involving Risks to Participants and Others." Your corrective action is unacceptable, because the SOP does not explicitly provide a procedure for reporting to FDA.

In your February 28, 2013, written response addressing your failure to prepare a written procedure for ensuring prompt reporting to the IRB, appropriate institutional officials, and FDA of any instance of serious or continuing noncompliance with these regulations or the requirements or determinations of the IRB, you refer to the SOP titled "Reporting of Unanticipated Problems Involving Risks to Participants and Others." The SOP indicates only that the suspension or termination of IRB approval will be reported. This SOP is unacceptable, because it fails to include a procedure for reporting serious or continuing noncompliance.

Written procedures are important because they describe how an IRB operates and conducts its major functions. Failure of an IRB to prepare, maintain, and follow written procedures may have an adverse impact on the rights and welfare of research subjects, because it may lead to violations of regulations (such as those observed during our inspection) that were put in place to protect the rights and welfare of these subjects.

Please submit a CAPA plan to address the violations cited above. With your CAPA plan, submit a copy of your written procedures, or any draft procedures in development, and a timeline for the implementation of any new procedures. Please provide a description of any training provided or to be provided to IRB members on the new procedures and a list of attendees, or a projected timeline of planned training.

This letter is not intended to be an all-inclusive list of deficiencies. It is your responsibility to ensure adherence to each requirement of the law and relevant regulations.

Based on the continuing pattern of deficiencies found during the last three inspections, BRI IRB does not meet the requirements of 21 CFR part 56. We have no assurance that the IRB procedures are adequately protecting the rights and welfare of the human subjects involved in research. For this reason, and effective immediately:

(1) No new studies subject to the requirements of 21 CFR parts 50 and 56 are to be approved by BRI IRB [21 CFR 56.103(a) and 56.120(b)(1)];

(2) No new subjects are to be added to ongoing studies subject to 21 CFR part 56 [21 CFR 56.120(b)(2)]; and

(3) FDA is suspending the IRB's use of the expedited review procedure to protect the rights or welfare of subjects [21 CFR 56.110(d)].

These restrictions will remain in effect until such time as FDA has evidence of adequate corrective actions, and notifies you in writing that the IRB's corrective actions are satisfactory. You are responsible for notifying the affected sponsors and clinical investigators about these restrictions (see 21 CFR 312.66). These restrictions do not relieve the IRB of its responsibilities for receiving and reacting to reports of unanticipated problems involving risks to human subjects or others, and routine progress reports from ongoing studies. The restrictions state that no new subjects are to be enrolled in SPPs or in any active Phase 2 or 3 studies; however, this restriction would not affect any subjects already enrolled in ongoing SPPs or Phase 2 or 3 studies, as long as it is in the best interest and safety of individual subjects to remain enrolled.

Within 30 working days of receipt of this letter, you should respond in writing with a description of the corrective actions that will be taken or that have been implemented to achieve compliance with the regulations.

Your response should address each item of noncompliance listed above. If you do not believe your IRB is in violation of FDA requirements, include your reasoning and any supporting information for our consideration. If you assert that full and adequate correction has been achieved, you should include any documentation necessary that affirms your corrective actions. For each action to be accomplished, include the projected completion dates.

Include with your response a copy of the IRB's written communication to each of the affected sponsors and clinical investigators, notifying them of the current FDA-imposed restrictions. In addition, please provide a list of all studies being reviewed by your IRB that are subject to 21 CFR part 56, and list all studies that are affected by the above restrictions.

Your failure to adequately respond to this letter may result in further administrative actions, as authorized by 21 CFR 56.120 and 56.121.

Your written reply should be sent to:

Catherine Parker, R.N.

Team Lead, Human Subject Protection Branch

Office of Scientific Investigations
Office of Compliance
Center for Drug Evaluation and Research
Food and Drug Administration
Building 51, Room 5247 10903 New
Hampshire Avenue
Silver Spring, MD
20993

FDA's Center for Drug Evaluation and Research will carefully consider your written response. Additionally, your corrective actions will be verified during a future inspection.

Sincerely yours,

{See appended electronic signature page}

Thomas N. Moreno, M.S.
Acting Office Director
Office of Scientific Investigations
Office of Compliance
Center for Drug Evaluation and Research
Food and Drug Administration

第 7 封　给 Agnesian 健康护理中心伦理委员会的警告信

2013年3月25日

参考号：13-HFD-45-03-01

尊敬的Little博士：

2012年11月7日至11月13日，Denise L. Burosh女士代表FDA，对贵伦理委员会（IRB）进行了现场检查，这封警告信特告知您现场检查中发现的违规情况。本次现场检查的目的是核实贵伦理委员会受试者保护程序是否符合美国联邦法规（CFR）第21篇第50和56部分的要求。该法规适用于研究机构，如Agnesian健康护理中心进行FDA所监管产品的临床研究。这次检查结果显示Agnesian健康护理中心伦理委员会很大程度上未能遵循这些法规。

本次现场检查是FDA的生物研究监查项目的一部分。该项目通过设定的检查方法，对FDA所监管的相关研究的实施情况进行评估，以确认研究数据在科学上是有效和准确的，并帮助确保这些研究中受试者的权益、安全和福利得到了保护。

在现场检查结束时，Burosh女士向伦理委员会主席James P. Mugan先生出示了FDA483表，即现场检查发现的问题。贵伦理委员会2012年11月21日对该FDA483表的书面回复已收悉。

经对现场检查报告、该报告的附件，以及伦理委员会提交的书面回复进行审查，我们认为，伦理委员会没有遵循适用的法律要求和监管受试者保护的FDA法规。我们想强调以下几点：

1. IRB未能制定、维护和遵守管理IRB职能和运行的书面程序［21 CFR 56.108（a），21 CFR 56.108（b）和21 CFR56.115（a）（6）］

为满足伦理委员会相关法规的要求，每个伦理委员会都必须制定、维护和遵守书面程序，这些程序描述了法规规定的伦理委员会的职能和运行。

Agnesian健康护理中心伦理委员会提供了关于伦理委员会活动的、题为“方针与程序”的两份文件，第一份文件副标题为“伦理委员会”，生效期为2008年11月；第二份文件副标题为“临床试验筛查”，生效期为2012年9月17日。伦理委员会没有向FDA提供其他描述它的规程的文件。这两份文件并没有包含FDA法规所要求的所有书面程序。尤其是，贵伦理委员会未能创建或遵循用于以下方面的书面程序：

- 实施对研究的初始审查以及跟踪审查，并向研究者和机构报告审查的发现以及采取的行动；
- 确定哪些项目需要比每年一次更频繁地审查，哪些项目需要从研究者以外的来源进行验证，自上次伦理委员会审查以来没有发生材料的改变；
- 确保研究活动中的变动快速地向伦理委员会报告；
- 确保在伦理委员会已经给出批准意见期间，在已经批准的研究中的变更，未经伦理委员会的审查和批准不能启动，除非是需要消除对受试者明显的、直接的伤害。
- 确保快速向伦理委员会、适当的机构管理人员、FDA报告：
  - 给受试者或其他人带来风险的任何非预期的问题；
  - 任何严重或者持续性的不符合规定、要求或伦理委员会决定的情况；
  - 任何伦理委员会批准的暂停或终止。

详见FDA法规：21 CFR 56.108（a）（1~4）、（b）（1~3）。

伦理委员会于2012年11月21日对FDA483表的书面回复，并不反对FDA做出的“伦理委员会违反了21 CFR 56.108（a~b）、56.115（a）（6）”这一结论的有效性。回复称伦理委员会将修订书面程序来解决这些违规行为，并在30~60天内或在2013年1月17日前对所有的员工进行培训。请将这些新的书面程序提交给FDA。

2. IRB未能以书面形式通知研究者和机构批准或不予批准被提议的研究的决定，或为确保IRB批准研究而要求的修改意见［21 CFR 56.109（e）］

伦理委员会必须以书面形式通知研究者和机构批准或不予批准所申请的研究的决定，或者为确保伦理委员会批准而要求的修改意见。

对于所审查的研究项目作出的批准或不批准决定，贵伦理委员会未能提交与研究者进行的书面沟通。相反，FDA检查员被告知，临床研究者在会议期间被口头通知了伦理委员会的决定。伦理委员会并没有给临床研究者提供后续决定的书面通知或沟通。

对FDA检查员审计的这些试验，贵伦理委员会未能向她提交伦理委员会与癌症试验支持部门［CTSU，是国立肿瘤研究所（NCI）发起的一个组织，为癌症试验提供更大的便利］之间书面沟通的证据。实际上，与伦理委员会委员和员工的会谈表明，对于这些试验，贵伦理委员会的书面沟通仅限于证明表，这些表在他们针对某一试验采取行动时发给CTSU。

伦理委员会于2012年11月21日对FDA483表的书面回复，并不反对FDA作出的“伦理委员会违反了21 CFR 56.109（e）”这一结论的有效性。回复称伦理委员会将在60天内，或2013年1月17日前用新的书面程序来解决这些违规行为。请将这些新的书面程序提交给FDA。

3. IRB未能准备和保存足够的包括IRB会议记录的IRB活动记录［21 CFR 56.115（a）（2）］

伦理委员会应当准备和保存包括伦理委员会会议记录在内的、伦理委员会活动的足够文件记录，这些记录应当用足够的细节来说明会议的出席情况，伦理委员会采取的行动，关于这些行动的投票情况（包括投票赞成、反对、弃权的委员数量），要求对研究进行修改或不批准研究的理由，对有争议问题进行的讨论、解决措施的书面总结。贵伦理委员会未能遵循上述规定。

我们的现场检查表明，弃权委员的数量没有记录在伦理委员会会议记录里。例如，2012年8月21日的伦理委员会会议记录显示（b）（6）医生和（b）（6）医生向伦理委员会做批准增编和对不同研究项目年度更新的报告。这两名医生都是伦理委员会委员。会议记录显示了投票“同意”和“不同意”的委员数量，但是没有弃权的记录。为了充分记录伦理委员会所采取的行动，会议记录应当显示弃权的委员数量（如果没有，记录为“0”），因利益冲突没有投票的委员的数量也是如此。当存在利益冲突的研究正在被伦理委员会审查时，存在利益冲突的伦理委员会委员不能进行投票或者被计算在法定人数以内。

伦理委员会于2012年11月21日对FDA483表的书面回复，并不反对FDA作出的“伦理委员会违反了21 CFR 56.115（a）（2）”这一结论的有效性。回复称伦理委员会将在60天内，或2013年1月17日前用新的书面程序来解决这些违规行为。请将这些新的书面程序提交给FDA。

4. IRB未能确保IRB批准的知情同意书中包含知情同意的基本要素［21 CFR 56.109（b）］

按照21 CFR 50.25，伦理委员会必须要求在知情同意过程中提供给受试者的信息中包括基本的要素，这些要素是获得受试者的知情、理解和自愿同意所必需的。知情同意中这些最基本的部分决定了研究受试者至少得到以下信息：

- 本试验与研究有关的告示；
- 对所有可合理预见的风险或不适的描述；
- 对研究的结果、可合理预期获得的任何好处的描述；
- 对可能存在的、任何适当的替代程序或治疗的解释；
- 告知机密性被保持的程度；
- 对研究期间如果发生涉及超过最小风险的伤害，任何补偿和/或医学治疗的解释；
- 对问题进行解答以及发生研究相关的伤害时的联系人信息；

详见21CFR50.25（a）（1~7）。

我们的现场检查发现，伦理委员会未能确保批准的研究（b）（4），“（b）（4）”的知情同意书中包含

21CFR50.25（a）（2）所要求的、与合理的可以预见的风险或不适有关的足够信息。下面将讨论到，尽管在2012年8月21日的伦理委员会会议上，（b）（4）进行了通知，临床研究者进行了讨论，但是贵伦理委员会仍未能将4项少见但又是严重的风险吸收入研究试验方案（b）（4）补遗10中的知情同意文件（ICD）中。

2012年6月18日，（b）（4）通知伦理委员会，“附录I 模板，方案（b）（4）补遗10中知情同意文件”被发现有一处错误，（b）（4）信函中警告称，下列4种罕见但严重的风险被意外地从试验方案补遗10中知情同意文件的附录第8页中删除了：

- 心脏功能衰竭：心脏不能充分地泵血给身体供氧；
- 在心跳的“活跃”期（收缩期），心脏泵血功能下降；
- 堵塞或心脏血液供应减少导致的心脏病发作；
- 肺部血管的高血压；

（b）（4）在信中称，即将发布的补遗11将改正这些错误。但是，既然补遗11还没有发布，（b）（4）指示伦理委员会人员要确保在这段时间内，没有“在您的研究场所用于招募受试者的知情同意文件中加入这些风险”附录10不会被提供给研究受试者。

这封信并不认为是贵伦理委员会的唯一通知，补遗10中知情同意文件未能告知试验受试者研究中的四大风险。在一次伦理委员会会议上，临床研究者和（b）（6）医生解释说：“补遗10中知情同意文件被发现有一处错误”“删除的内容需要再加入到补遗10中的知情同意文件中”。

尽管有（b）（4）的指示、伦理委员会会议上坐在委员席位上的临床研究者的报告，但在同一次会议上，Agnesian健康护理中心伦理委员会还是批准了没有添加四大严重风险的研究试验方案（b）（4）补遗10。伦理委员会本不应批准已知有错误的知情同意文件，应指导临床研究者进行改正并重新提交知情同意文件，供伦理委员会做进一步审查。未能确保FDA要求的所有知情同意要素得到满足，使受试者不能获得研究的足够的信息来作出有效的知情同意。

伦理委员会于2012年11月21日对FDA483表的书面回复，并不反对FDA作出的“伦理委员会违反了21 CFR 50.25（a），56.109（b）”这一结论的有效性。回复称伦理委员会将在60天内或2013年1月17日前用新的书面程序来解决这些违规行为。请将这些新的书面程序提交给FDA。

5. IRB未能准备和保存足够的包括IRB会议记录的IRB活动记录［21 CFR 56.115（a）（1，4）］

伦理委员会应该准备和保存足够的伦理委员会活动的文件记录，包括但不限于研究者提交的进展报告复印件、伦理委员会与研究者之间所有通信的复印件。伦理委员会未能遵循这些要求。

对FDA审计的这些研究，贵审查委员会研究文件仅包括初始方案和知情同意文件、更新后的方案和知情同意文件、CTSU伦理委员会的证明表。从获得的证据来看，伦理委员会未能保存伦理委员会与临床研究者之间关于伦理委员会决定（如本警告信第2项所述）的任何书面沟通文件，未能保存这些研究的任何非预期问题或进展报告的文件记录。

此外，伦理委员会一直没有要求临床研究者向伦理委员会提交非预期的问题或进展报告。相反，伦理委员会一直是通过与CTSU的沟通来获取正在进行的研究情况。

按照法规要求保留的记录提供了重要证据，以确认伦理委员会所用的程序是否足以保护其审查的临床试验的受试者。

伦理委员会于2012年11月21日对FDA483表的书面回复，并不反对FDA作出的“伦理委员会违反了21 CFR 56.115（a）（1）和21 CFR 56.115（a）（4）”这一结论的有效性。回复称伦理委员会将在60天内或2013年1月17日前用新的书面程序来解决这些违规行为。请将这些新的书面程序提交给FDA。

如上所述，贵伦理委员会于2012年11月21日对FDA483表的书面回复，承认上面列出的每一条违规行为的有效性。回复中称伦理委员会将针对每一条违规行为起草新的规程，但是，回复中并没有提出将草稿或最终的规程提交给FDA。伦理委员会对FDA483表的书面回复并不足以解决这些违规，因为回复中并没有描述伦理委员会将用来针对新的规程对伦理委员会委员、员工和临床研究者进行培训和教育的流程。没有这些信息，FDA无法准确评估提出的纠正和预防措施的潜在能力，以防止将来这些违规行为或类似违规行为复发。

本警告信的目的并非是罗列贵伦理委员会在审查和批准试验方案时存在的所有缺陷。确保Agnesian健康护理中心伦理委员会的实际操作和程序完全符合所有适用法律和法规的要求是您的职责。

自收到这封信的15个工作日内，您应当书面告知本办公室为预防将来发生类似违规行为情况采取的措施。您的书面回复应当包括所有必要的文件，足以证明已经完成完全和充分的纠正措施。请明确每项措施的预计完成日期。如果不能对上述违规行为进行充分、迅速的解释，可能导致我们在不再通知的情况下采取监管措施。

附：英文原文

Agnesian Healthcare IRB

WARNING LETTER

Mar 25, 2013

CERTIFIED MAIL
RETURN RECEIPT REQUESTED

Ref.: 13-HFD-45-03-01

Mr. Steven Little
President and Chief Executive Officer
Agnesian Healthcare
430 East Division Street
Fond du Lac, WI 54935

Dear Mr. Little:

This Warning Letter informs you of unacceptable conditions observed during the U.S. Food and Drug Administration (FDA) inspection of your Institutional Review Board (IRB) that was conducted between November 7, 2012, and November 13, 2012, by Ms. Denise L. Burosh, representing FDA. The purpose of this inspection was to determine whether the IRB's procedures for the protection of human subjects complied with Title 21 of the Code of Federal Regulations (CFR), parts 50 and 56. These regulations apply to institutions that, like Agnesian Healthcare, conduct clinical investigations of products regulated by FDA. This inspection revealed that Agnesian Healthcare's IRB has substantially failed to follow these regulations.

This inspection is a part of FDA's Bioresearch Monitoring Program, which includes inspections designed to evaluate the conduct of FDA-regulated research to ensure that the data are scientifically valid and accurate, and to help ensure that the rights, safety, and welfare of the human subjects of those studies have been protected.

At the conclusion of the inspection, Ms. Burosh presented the IRB Chairman, Mr. James P. Mugan, with Form FDA 483, Inspectional Observations. We acknowledge receipt of the IRB's November 21, 2012, written response to the Form FDA 483. From our review of the FDA's establishment inspection report, the documents submitted with that report, and the IRB's written response, we conclude that the IRB did not adhere to the applicable statutory requirements and FDA regulations governing the protection of human subjects. We wish to emphasize the following:

1. The IRB failed to prepare, maintain, and follow required written procedures governing the functions and operations of the IRB [21 CFR 56.108(a), 21 CFR 56.108(b), and 21 CFR56.115(a)(6)].

In order to fulfill the requirements of the IRB regulations, each IRB must prepare, maintain, and follow written procedures describing IRB functions and operations specified in the regulations.

Agnesian Healthcare IRB provided two documents titled “Policy and Procedure” concerning the IRB’s activity to FDA. The first document is subtitled “Institutional Review Board” and has an effective date of November, 2008. The second document is subtitled “Clinical Trial Screening” and has an effective date of September 17, 2012. The IRB provided no other documents describing its procedures to FDA. These two documents do not contain all of the written procedures required under FDA’s regulations. Specifically, your IRB failed to create or follow written procedures for:

- Conducting its initial and continuing review of research and for reporting its findings and actions to the investigator and the institution;
- Determining which projects require review more often than annually and which projects need verification from sources other than the investigator that no material changes have occurred since previous IRB review;
- Ensuring prompt reporting to the IRB of changes in research activity;
- Ensuring that changes in approved research, during the period for which IRB approval has already been given, may not be initiated without IRB review and approval except where necessary to eliminate apparent immediate hazards to the human subjects; or
- Ensuring prompt reporting to the IRB, appropriate institutional officials, and the Food and Drug Administration of:
  - any unanticipated problems involving risks to human subjects or others;
  - any instance of serious or continuing noncompliance with these regulations or the requirements or determinations of the IRB; or
  - any suspension or termination of IRB approval.

See FDA’s regulations at 21 CFR 56.108(a)(1-4) and (b)(1-3).

The IRB’s written response to the Form FDA 483, dated November 21, 2012, does not object to the validity of FDA’s conclusion that it violated 21 CFR 56.108(a-b) and 56.115(a)(6). The response states that the IRB would revise written procedures to address these violations. and would train all staff within 30-60 days, or by January 17, 2013. Please provide these new written procedures to FDA.

2. The IRB failed to notify investigators and the institution in writing of its decision to approve or disapprove proposed research activities or of modifications required to secure IRB approval of the research activity [21 CFR 56.109(e)].

The IRB is required to notify investigators and the institution in writing of its decision to approve or disapprove proposed research, or of modifications required to secure IRB approval.

Your IRB failed to provide written communication to investigators of its decisions to approve or disapprove research studies reviewed by the IRB. The FDA investigator was told that, instead, clinical investigators were only verbally informed of IRB decisions during meetings. The IRB did not provide the clinical investigators with subsequent written notification or communication of that decision.

For the trials audited by the FDA investigator, your IRB failed to provide her with evidence of written communication between the IRB and any parties outside of the Cancer Trials Support Unit (CTSU), an organization sponsored by the National Cancer Institute (NCI) to provide greater access to cancer trials. In fact, interviews with IRB members and staff revealed that your IRB’s written communication regarding these trials was limited to the certification forms that the IRB sends to the CTSU whenever they take action with regard to a trial.

The IRB’s written response to the Form FDA 483, dated November 21, 2012, does not object to the validity of FDA’s conclusion that it violated 21 CFR 56.109(e). The response states that the IRB would have new written procedures to address this violation within 60 days, or by January 17, 2013. Please provide these new written procedures to FDA.

3. The IRB failed to prepare and maintain adequate documentation of IRB activities, including minutes of IRB meetings [21 CFR 56.115(a)(2)].

An IRB shall prepare and maintain adequate documentation of IRB activities, including minutes of IRB meetings, which shall be in sufficient detail to show attendance at the meetings, actions taken by the IRB, the vote on these actions, including the number of members voting for, against, and abstaining, the basis for requiring changes in or disapproving research, and a written summary of the discussion of controverted issues and their resolution. Your IRB failed to adhere to the abovestated regulations.

Our inspection revealed that the number of members abstaining is not recorded in the IRB's meeting minutes. For example, minutes of the August 21, 2012, IRB meeting indicate that Dr. (b)(6) and Dr. (b)(6) made presentations to the IRB for approval of addendums and annual renewal of various studies. Both of these physicians are IRB members. The minutes indicate the number of members voting "yes" and "no," but there is no documentation of abstentions. In order to adequately document actions taken by the IRB, the minutes should indicate the number of members abstaining (if none, document as "0"), as well as the number of members who did not vote due to a conflict of interest. IRB members with a conflict of interest may not vote or be counted towards quorum when research in which they have a conflict is being reviewed by the IRB.

The IRB's written response to the Form FDA 483, dated November 21, 2012, does not object to the validity of FDA's conclusion that it violated 21 CFR 56.115(a)(2). The response states that the IRB would have new written procedures to address this violation within 60 days, or by January 17, 2013. Please provide these new written procedures to FDA.

4. The IRB failed to ensure that basic elements of informed consent are included in the IRB-approved consent form [21 CFR 56.109(b)].

The IRB must require that information given to subjects during the informed consent process includes the fundamental elements necessary to obtain the informed, understanding, and voluntary consent of subjects in accordance with 21 CFR 50.25. These most basic components of informed consent dictate that study subjects receive at minimum:

- notice that the study involves research;
- a description of all reasonably foreseeable risks or discomforts;
- a description of any benefits that can be reasonably expected to accrue as a result of the research;
- an explanation of any appropriate alternative procedures or treatments that might be available;
- notice of the extent to which confidentiality will be maintained;
- an explanation of any compensation and/or medical treatments available if injury occurs during research involving more than minimal risk;and
- information on whom to contact both for answers to questions and in the event of a research-related injury.

See 21 CFR 50.25(a)(1-7).

Our inspection revealed that the IRB failed to ensure that the IRB-approved informed consent form for Study (b)(4), "(b)(4)," contained adequate information about reasonably foreseeable risks or discomforts as required by 21 CFR 50.25(a)(2). As discussed below, your IRB failed to incorporate four rare but serious risks into the informed consent document (ICD) in Addendum 10 of Study Protocol (b)(4), despite notification by the (b)(4) and discussion by the clinical investigator during the August 21, 2012, IRB meeting.

On June 18, 2012, (b)(4) informed the IRB that an error had been discovered in "Appendix I model informed consent document in Addendum 10 of protocol (b)(4)." [1] (b)(4) letter warned that the following four rare but serious risks had been accidentally deleted from page 8 of the appendix to the ICD in Addendum 10 to the protocol:

- Heart failure: inability of the heart to adequately pump blood to supply oxygen to the body;
- Decrease in heart's ability to pump blood during the 'active' phase of the heartbeat (systole);
- Heart attack caused by a blockage or decreased blood supply to the heart; and
- High blood pressure of the blood vessels in the lungs.

(b)(4) noted in the letter that the forthcoming Addendum 11 would correct the mistake. However, since Addendum 11 had not yet been issued, (b)(4) instructed IRB personnel to ensure that, in the meantime, Addendum 10 would not be provided to study subjects without "adding these risks to the informed consent document used to enroll patients at your site."

This letter did not constitute your IRB's only notification that the ICD in Addendum 10 failed to inform research subjects of four major risks of the research. During an IRB meeting, clinical investigator and IRB member Dr. (b)(6) "explained that an error was discovered in the informed consent for Addendum 10," and that the " deletions needed to be re-added to the consent for Addendum 10." [2]

Despite (b)(4)'s instruction and the presentation by a clinical investigator who sat on your IRB during an IRB meeting, during that same meeting, Agnesian Healthcare's IRB approved Addendum 10 for Study Protocol (b)(4) without adding the four serious risks. The IRB should have not approved an ICD known to contain an error and should have instructed the clinical investigator to correct and resubmit the ICD for further IRB review. Failure to ensure that all of the FDA-required elements of informed consent are met prevents human subjects from being provided with enough information about a study to give effective informed consent.

The IRB's written response to the Form FDA 483, dated November 21, 2012, does not object to the validity of FDA's conclusion that it violated 21 CFR 50.25(a) and 56.109(b). The response states that the IRB would have new written procedures to address these violations within 60 days, or by January 17, 2013. Please provide these new written procedures to FDA.

5. The IRB failed to prepare and maintain adequate documentation of IRB activities [21 CFR 56.115(a)(1) and (4)].

An IRB is required to prepare and maintain adequate documentation of IRB activities including, but not limited to, copies of progress reports submitted by investigators and copies of all correspondence between the IRB and the investigators. The IRB failed to adhere to this requirement.

For the studies audited by FDA, your IRB's study files only included the initial protocols and ICDs, updated protocols and ICDs, and Clinical Trial Support Unit (CTSU) IRB certification forms. From the evidence obtained, it appears that the IRB has failed to maintain any written communication between the IRB and clinical investigators of IRB decisions (as described under Item 2 of this letter) or any written documentation of any unanticipated problems or progress reports for these studies.

Additionally, the IRB has not been requiring clinical investigators to submit unanticipated problems or progress reports to the IRB. Rather, the IRB's process for receiving information with respect to ongoing research has been through communication with the CTSU. [3]

Maintaining records, as required under the regulations, provides significant evidence of whether the procedures utilized by the IRB are adequately protecting the human subjects of the clinical investigations that the IRB is reviewing.

The IRB's written response to the Form FDA 483, dated November 21, 2012, does not object to the validity of FDA's conclusion that it violated 21 CFR 56.115(a)(1) and 56.115(a)(4). The response states that the IRB would have new written procedures to address these violations within 60 days, or by January 17, 2013. Please provide these new written procedures to FDA.

As noted above, your IRB's written response to the Form FDA 483, dated November 21, 2012, acknowledges the validity of each of the violations listed above. The response states that the IRB will develop new written procedures to address each violation. However, the response does not indicate that the draft or final procedures will be provided to FDA. In addition, the IRB's written response to the Form FDA 483 is inadequate to address these violations because it does not describe any process that the IRB will use to train and educate IRB members, staff, and clinical investigators with respect to its new written procedures. Without this information, FDA cannot conduct a proper evaluation of the proposed corrective and preventive action's potential ability to prevent the recurrence of these or similar violations in the future.

This letter is not intended to be an all inclusive list of deficiencies for the protocols reviewed and approved by the IRB. It is your responsibility to ensure that Agnesian Healthcare IRB's practices and procedures comply fully with all applicable statutes and regulations.

Within fifteen (15) business days of your receipt of this letter, you should notify this office in writing of the actions you have taken to prevent similar violations in the future. Your written response should include any documentation necessary to show that full and adequate correction will be achieved. Please include the projected completion dates for each action to be accomplished. Failure to explain the violations noted above adequately and promptly may result in regulatory action without further notice.

We recommend that you visit the following FDA Web page for information on human subject protection that may assist you in your efforts to bring the IRB into compliance with FDA regulations:

http://www.fda.gov/ScienceResearch/SpecialTopics/RunningClinicalTrials/default.htm

We appreciate the cooperation shown to the FDA Investigator, Ms. Denise Burosh, during the inspection. If you have any questions, please contact Catherine Parker, R.N., at 301-796-5553; FAX 301-847-8748. Your written response and any pertinent documentation should be addressed to:

Catherine Parker, R.N.
Team Lead, Human Subject Protection Branch
Office of Scientific Investigations
Office of Compliance
Center for Drug Evaluation and Research
Food and Drug Administration
Building 51, Room 5247
10903 New Hampshire Avenue
Silver Spring, MD 20993

Sincerely,
{See appended electronic signature page}

Thomas N. Moreno, M.S.
Acting Office Director
Office of Scientific Investigations
Office of Compliance
Center for Drug Evaluation and Research
Food and Drug Administration

Cc: Mr. James P. Mugan
IRB Chairman
Agnesian Healthcare
430 East Division Street
Fond du Lac, WI 54935

[1] Letter from (b)(4), (b)(4), to (b)(4) Site Staff Regarding Deletion of 'Rare but Serious' Risks in Addendum 10 (b)(4) Model Informed Consent (June 18, 2012).
[2] Meeting Minutes of the Agnesian Healthcare Institutional Review Board signed by Chairperson James Mugan (Aug. 21, 2012).
[3] See discussion supra Citation 2, Paragraph 3.

Page Last Updated: 03/29/2013

第8封 给Singing River健康系统伦理委员会的警告信

2013年2月1日

参考号：13-HFD-45-01-01

尊敬的Anderson先生：

2012年7月2日至7月23日，Barbara D. Wright女士代表FDA对贵伦理委员会（IRB）进行了现场检查。这封警告信特告知您现场检查中发现的违规情况。本次现场检查的目的是核实贵伦理委员会受试者保护程序是否符合美国联邦法规（CFR）第21篇第50和第56部分的内容。该法规适用于FDA所监管产品的临床研究。

本次现场检查是FDA的生物研究监查项目的一部分。该项目通过设定的检查方法，对由FDA监管的研究的实施情况进行评估，以确认研究数据在科学上是有效和准确的，并帮助确保这些研究中受试者的权益、安全和福利得到了保护。

在现场检查结束时，Wright女士向伦理委员会主席Angela M. Magee女士出示并讨论了FDA483表，即现场检查发现的问题。伦理委员会2012年8月10日对该FDA483表的书面回复已收悉。

经对现场检查报告、该报告的附件，以及伦理委员会提交的书面回复进行审查，我们认为，贵伦理委员会没有遵循适用的法律要求和监管受试者保护的FDA法规。我们想强调以下几点：

1. IRB未能制定、维护和遵守管理IRB职能和运行的必要的书面程序［21 CFR 56.108（a），21 CFR 56.108（b）和21 CFR56.115（a）（6）］

为满足伦理委员会相关法规的要求，每个伦理委员会都必须制定、维护和遵守书面程序，这些程序描述了法规规定的伦理委员会的职能和运行。伦理委员会未能遵循这项要求，具体而言：

a. 伦理委员会的“方针与规程指南”没有包含所有必需的书面程序。没有关于以下方面的程序：

- 确定哪些项目需要比每年一次更频繁的审查，哪些项目需要从研究者以外的来源进行验证，确认自上次伦理委员会审查以来没有发生材料的改变；
- 确保快速向伦理委员会、适当的机构管理人员、FDA报告关于任何严重或者持续性的不符合法规、要求或伦理委员会决定的情况。

b. 伦理委员会没有遵照“方针与规程指南”中列出的必需的书面程序。例如：

- 标题是“会议前活动”，伦理委员会的“方针与规程指南”中显示：“在安排好的会议前一周，伦理委员会主席要将伦理委员会材料准备好并分发，这些材料包括但是不限于书面的议程、初始审查及跟踪审查申请表的复印件、正被提交审查和批准的任何项目的**所有附件**、上次会议记录的复印件以及任何与将召开的会议有关的其他材料”（增加了强调）。

  我们的现场检查发现，2012年4、5和6月伦理委员会会议前分发的材料包内，都没有包括正被提交审查和批准的任何项目的所有附件。例如，（b）（4），“（b）（4）”的临床研究者提交的研究申请表显示，提交材料包括下列项目“伦理委员会申请表、知情同意文件、试验方案和招募材料。”但提供给伦理委员会委员的材料包没有包括试验方案。然而，这项研究于2012年4月10日被伦理委员会批准。
- 标题是“快速审查”，在伦理委员会的“方针与规程指南”中显示：伦理委员会主席或他（或她）的指定人同意快速审查批准，“主席会告知研究者，写明项目已经获得批准，然后在下次月度会议上将试验方案在整个伦理委员会内传阅”。

我们的现场检查发现，这个流程没有被执行，因为使用快速审查程序批准的项目，所有的伦理委员会委员都没有被征询过研究建议。在现场检查过程中，检查员收到了一个文件夹，该文件夹中的资料涉及已经被快速审查程序批准的研究活动。当FDA检查员询问所有的伦理委员会委员怎样得知被快速审查程序批准的研究活动，她被告知说：伦理委员会已经停止遵照执行这项书面程序。

我们收到了伦理委员会的书面回复，其中包含了下列纠正措施：①修订伦理委员会的流程，确保伦理委员会委员在每次会议开始前都能查看到所有的支持性文件；②修订Singing River Health System（SRHS）伦理委员会政策手册，加入上面列出的缺少的规程；③修订伦理委员会政策手册，要求所有的快速审查都记录在议事日程中，并在下次召集的会议上被伦理委员会审查，伦理委员会审查的快速批准应记录在会议记录中。此外，书面回复显示"所有肿瘤相关的研究，在SRHS伦理委员会开始启动前，通过（b）（4）'s（（b）（4））中心伦理委员会批准，包括对研究人群风险和/或收益的审查"。

伦理委员会的回复是不充分的，因为回复中并没有包含已经修订的程序的复印件。而且，伦理委员会有责任制定、维护和遵守在管理伦理委员会职能和运行方面必需的书面程序。我们还希望强调一下，尽管伦理委员会在特定情况下可以依靠另一个有资质的伦理委员会的审查（详见21 CFR56.114），（b）（4）的伦理委员会进行的审查并不能免除SRHS的伦理委员会在研究审查中遵照书面程序。

请提交一份您的书面程序的复印件，或任何在完善中的草案规程，以及实施任何新规程的时间表。此外，请提供一份简介，说明针对新的规程对伦理委员会员工进行的培训，出席人员名单，或者计划培训的项目时间表。

2. IRB未能满足委员的资格要求［21 CFR 56.107］

伦理委员会不具备必需的专业能力，以对特殊的研究活动进行适当的审查。例如：

伦理委员会的委员名单和会议记录显示，在以下日期里，SRHS的伦理委员会在没有一名医生委员在场的情况下开会、审查，并进行投票：

2010年2月9日、3月9日、5月11日、6月8日、8月10日、9月14日、10月12日、11月9日、12月14日；

2011年1月11日、2月8日、3月4日、5月5日、6月14日、7月12日、8月9日、9月13日、10月11日、11月2日、12月13日；

2012年1月10日、2月14日、3月13日、4月10日、5月7日。

我们要强调的是，在这些会议中，没有一名医生委员出席，使伦理委员会缺少经验和专业知识来审查肿瘤学研究活动。

在现场检查过程中，伦理委员会主席提出，一个新的医生委员、（b）（6）医生已经被招聘进来，并将开始作为投票委员参加2012年8月的伦理委员会会议。我们注意到（b）（6）医生已经被加入到伦理委员会委员名单中，我们认为这种纠正措施是恰当的。

我们注意到伦理委员会的书面回复中声称，伦理委员会具备的专业知识足以审查所有提交的和已经批准的研究，因为科学性审查已经由诸如地区癌症中心（RCC）的医务人员和（b）（4）的伦理委员会等伦理委员会之外的个人或组织实施。我们承认，在特定情况下可以依靠另一个有资质的伦理委员会的审查（详见21 CFR56.114），但是RCC医务人员的审查并不等同于被另一个有资质的伦理委员会审查。此外，伦理委员会的"方针与规程指南"中并没有提到对研究的合作审查，或包含允许SRHS的伦理委员会对某些方面的审查可以依赖（b）（4）的伦理委员会的规程。因此，SRHS伦理委员会对RCC医务人员在科学性审查上的依靠或是对（b）（4）伦理委员会的依靠，都不符合21 CFR56.107的要求。

3. IRB未能在大多数IRB委员出席，其中至少包括一位来自非科学领域委员的召集会议上对拟开展的研究进行审查［21 CFR 56.108（c）］

除了采用快速审查程序以外，伦理委员会仅在召集会议上审查提出的研究，在召集会议上，大多数伦理委员会委员（即法定人数）会到场，并且包括至少一名来自非科学领域的委员。

我们的现场检查发现，伦理委员会在多数委员未到场的会议上审查研究。例如：

a. 2011年8月9日伦理委员会会议记录显示，伦理委员会有12名委员。因此，为了进行审查，至少7名委员需要在场（包括一名非科学领域的委员）。会议记录显示，当FDA监管的临床研究被审查时，有6名委员在场。

b. 2011年10月11日伦理委员会会议记录显示，伦理委员会有13名委员。因此，为了进行审查，至少7名委员需要在场（包括一名非科学领域的委员）。会议记录显示，当FDA监管的临床研究被审查时，有6名委员在场。

我们收到了伦理委员会的书面回复，该回复显示会议记录会反映出大多数伦理委员会委员到场。这样的回复是不充分的，因为其中并没有包括一份简介，说明针对“仅在有多数委员在场的召集会议上对提出的研究进行审查”的要求，对伦理委员会人员进行的任何培训，或者计划培训的项目时间表。仅在有多数委员在场的召集会议上对提出的研究进行审查，这是伦理委员会的责任。

4. IRB未能准备和保存足够的IRB活动记录［21 CFR 56.115（a）］

伦理委员会应当准备和保存伦理委员会活动的足够文件记录，包括但不限于研究者提交的进展报告复印件、伦理委员会会议记录（有足够的细节显示对伦理委员会措施的投票情况）、伦理委员会与研究者之间所有通信的复印件。伦理委员会未能遵循这项要求，尤其是：

a. 在现场检查过程中，FDA检查员发现，像修订的方案、安全性报告等文件在伦理委员会文件中是缺失的。

我们收到了伦理委员会的书面回复，FDA检查之后，肿瘤学研究的电子储存资料被重新组织，以补充保存在RCC办公室中硬拷贝监管活页夹。每项研究的伦理委员会电子文件中都创建了一个单独的文件夹，其中包含了所有监管文件，该系统会维持下去用于将来所有的伦理委员会提交材料。我们认为这种改正措施是恰当的。

b. 有三次（2009年12月14日、2011年6月7日、2012年4月2日）伦理委员会通过远程电话召开会议并批准了FDA监管的临床研究；但是对于远程电话会议没有保存会议记录。

我们收到了伦理委员会的书面回复，显示伦理委员会的政策手册已经进行修订并用来解决如何正确地记录预定的远程电话会议，以全面审查，确保出席人数达到法定人数。这个回复是不充分的，因为“伦理委员会未能准备和保存远程电话会议的会议记录”的这个问题没有解决，而且其中没有包含修订的书面程序的复印件。此外，伦理委员会有责任准备和保存会议记录，并用足够的细节显示对伦理委员会措施的投票情况。请提交一份您的书面程序的复印件，或任何在完善中的草案规程，以及实施任何新规程的时间表。此外，请提供一份简介，说明针对新的规程对伦理委员会员工进行的培训，出席人员签到名单，或者计划培训的项目时间表。

本警告信的目的并非是罗列伦理委员会在审查和批准试验方案时存在的所有缺陷。确保SRHS伦理委员会的实际操作和程序完全符合适用的法律和法规的要求是您的职责。

自收到这封信的15个工作日内，贵伦理委员会应当书面告知本办公室为预防将来发生类似违规情况而采取的措施。如果不能充分、迅速地解释上述违规问题，可能导致我们在不再通知的情况下采取监管措施。如果您认为您已经遵循了FDA的法规要求，请陈述理由，并提供所有支持资料，以供我们参考。

附：英文原文

Singing River Health System IRB

WARNING LETTER

FEB 1，2013

CERTIFIED MAIL
RETURN RECEIPT REQUESTED

Ref: 13-HFD-45-01-01

Mr. Chris Anderson
Chief Executive Officer
Singing River Health System
2809 Denny Avenue
Pascagoula, MS 39581

Dear Mr. Anderson:

This Warning Letter informs you of objectionable conditions observed during the U.S. Food and Drug Administration (FDA) inspection of your Institutional Review Board (IRB) that was conducted between July 2, 2012, and July 23, 2012, by Ms. Barbara D. Wright, representing FDA. The purpose of this inspection was to determine whether the IRB procedures for the protection of human subjects complied with Title 21 of the Code of Federal Regulations (CFR), parts 50 and 56. These regulations apply to clinical investigations of products regulated by FDA.

This inspection is a part of FDA's Bioresearch Monitoring Program, which includes inspections designed to evaluate the conduct of FDA regulated research to help ensure that the data are scientifically valid and accurate, and to help ensure that the rights, safety, and welfare of the human subjects of those studies have been protected.

At the conclusion of the inspection, Ms. Wright presented and discussed Form FDA 483, Inspectional Observations, with Ms. Angela M. Magee, IRB Chairperson. We acknowledge receipt of the IRB's August 10, 2012, written response to the Form FDA 483. From our review of the FDA's establishment inspection report, the documents submitted with that report, and the IRB's written response, we conclude that the IRB did not adhere to the applicable statutory requirements and FDA regulations governing the protection of human subjects. We wish to emphasize the following:

1. The IRB failed to prepare, maintain, and follow required written procedures governing the functions and operations of the IRB [21 CFR 56.108(a), 21 CFR 56.108(b), and 21 CFR 56.115(a)(6)].

In order to fulfill the requirements of the IRB regulations, each IRB must prepare, maintain, and follow written procedures describing IRB functions and operations specified in the regulations. The IRB failed to adhere to this requirement. Specifically:

a. The IRB's "Policy and Procedures Guidebook" does not include all the required written procedures. The IRB does not have procedures for:

- Determining which projects require review more often than annually, and which projects need verification from sources other than the investigator that no material changes have occurred since previous IRB review; and
- Ensuring prompt reporting to the IRB, appropriate institutional officials, and the Food and Drug Administration of any instance of serious or continuing noncompliance with these regulations or the requirements or determinations of the IRB.

b. The IRB does not follow all required written procedures listed in the "Policy and Procedures Guidebook." For example:

- Under the heading, "Pre-Meeting Activities" the IRB's "Policy and Procedures Guidebook" indicates that "one week prior to the scheduled meeting, the Chairperson will develop and distribute the IRB materials. These materials will include, but are not limited to, a written agenda, copies of the initial and continuing review application and all attachments of any projects being presented for review and approval, a copy of the last meeting's minutes and any other material pertinent to the upcoming meeting" (emphasis added).

Our inspection revealed that the packets distributed prior to the April, May, and June 2012 IRB meetings did not include all attachments of any projects being presented for review and approval. For example, the research application submitted by the clinical investigator for (b)(4), "(b)(4)," indicates that the submission included the following items: "IRB application, informed consent document, protocol, and recruitment materials." Packets provided to IRB members did not include the protocol. Nevertheless, this study was approved by the IRB on April 10, 2012.

- Under the heading "Expedited Review," the IRB's "Policy and Procedures Guidebook" indicates that after the Chairperson or his or her designee grants expedited review approval, "the Chairperson will notify the investigator in writing that the project has received approval and then circulate the protocol to the entire IRB Committee at the next monthly meeting." Our inspection revealed that this procedure has not been followed, in that all committee members have not been advised of research proposals that have been approved using the expedited review procedure. During the inspection, our investigator was provided with a binder containing documents that discussed research activities that had been approved by the expedited review procedure. When the FDA investigator asked how all members are informed of research activities that are approved by expedited review, she was informed that the IRB had stopped complying with this written procedure.

We acknowledge the IRB's written response, which includes the following corrective actions: (1) Revising the IRB's process to ensure that IRB members have access to all supporting documents prior to the start of each meeting; (2) revising the Singing River Health System (SRHS) IRB Policy Manual to include the missing procedures listed above; and (3) revising the SRHS IRB Policy Manual to require that all expedited reviews be documented in the agenda and reviewed by the IRB during the next convened meeting, and that the IRB's review of the expedited approvals be documented in the minutes. In addition, the written response indicates that "all cancer related studies are approved through the (b)(4)'s ((b)(4)) central IRB prior to activation at the SRHS IRB, including review of risk and/or benefit to study populations."

The IRB's response is inadequate because it does not include a copy of the revised written procedures. Moreover, it was the IRB's responsibility to prepare, maintain, and follow required written procedures governing the functions and operations of the IRB. We also wish to emphasize that, although an IRB may rely on the review of another qualified IRB under certain circumstances (see 21 CFR 56.114), review by (b)(4)'s IRB does not exempt the SRHS IRB from following its written procedures with respect to review of research.

Please submit a copy of your written procedures, or any draft procedures in development, and a timeline for the implementation of any new procedures. In addition, please provide a description of any training provided to IRB staff on the new procedures and a list of attendees, or a projected timeline of planned training.

2. The IRB failed to fulfill membership requirements [21 CFR 56.107].

The IRB did not possess the professional competence necessary to adequately review the specific research activities. For example:

The IRB's member list and meeting minutes indicate that the SRHS IRB met, reviewed, and voted on oncology research without a physician member present on the following dates:

February 9, 2010	January 11, 2011	January 10, 2012
March 9, 2010	February 8, 2011	February 14, 2012
May 11, 2010	March 4, 2011	March 13, 2012
June 8, 2010	May 5, 2011	April 10, 2012
August 10, 2010	June 14, 2011	May 7, 2012
September 14, 2010	July 12, 2011	
October 12, 2010	August 9, 2011	
November 9, 2010	September 13, 2011	
December 14, 2010	October 11, 2011	
	November 2, 2011	
	December 13, 2011	

We wish to emphasize that without having a physician member present at these meetings, the IRB lacked the experience and expertise to review the oncology research activities.

During the inspection, the IRB Chairperson indicated that a new physician member, Dr. (b)(6), had been recruited and would begin participating as a voting member at the August 2012 IRB meeting. We note that Dr. (b)(6) has been added to the IRB membership list. We find this corrective action to be adequate.

We note that the IRB' s written response asserts that the IRB possessed expertise adequate to review all presented and approved studies because scientific review was conducted by individuals or organizations other than the IRB, such as the medical staff of the Regional Cancer Center (RCC) and (b)(4)'s IRB. We recognize that it is possible to rely on the review of another qualified IRB under certain circumstances (see 21 CFR 56.114). However, review by the medical staff of the RCC does not constitute review by another qualified IRB. Additionally, the IRB' s "Policy and Procedures Guidebook" does not discuss cooperative review of research, or contain procedures that would allow the SRHS IRB to rely on the (b)(4) IRB for certain aspects of the review. Therefore, any reliance of the SRHS IRB on the scientific review conducted by the RCC medical staff or the (b)(4) IRB does not satisfy the requirements of 21 CFR 56.107.

3. The IRB failed to review proposed research at convened meetings at which a majority of the members of the IRB are present, including at least one member whose primary concerns are in nonscientific areas [21 CFR 56.108(c)].

Except when an expedited review procedure is used, the IRB may only review proposed research at convened meetings at which a majority of the IRB members (i.e., a quorum) is present, including at least one member whose primary concerns are in nonscientific areas.

Our inspection revealed that the IRB reviewed research at meetings at which a majority of the IRB members was not present. For example:

a. Minutes of the August 9, 2011, IRB meeting indicate that the IRB had twelve members. Therefore, in order to review research, at least seven members needed to be present (including a nonscientist). The minutes indicate that six members were present when FDA-regulated research was reviewed.

b. Minutes of the October 11, 2011, IRB meeting indicate that the IRB had thirteen members. Therefore, in order to review research, at least seven members needed to be present (including a nonscientist). The minutes indicate that six members were present when FDA-regulated research was reviewed.

We acknowledge the IRB's written response, which indicates that meeting minutes will reflect the presence of a majority of IRB members. The response is inadequate because it does not include a description of any training provided to IRB staff, or a projected timeline of planned training, on compliance with the requirement that proposed research only be reviewed at convened meetings at which a majority of members are present. Moreover, it was the IRB' s responsibility to review proposed research only at convened meetings at which a majority of the IRB members was present.

4. The IRB failed to prepare and maintain adequate documentation of IRB activities [21 CFR 56.115(a)].

An IRB is required to prepare and maintain adequate documentation of IRB activities including, but not limited to, copies of progress reports submitted by investigators, minutes of IRB meetings in sufficient detail to show the vote on IRB actions, and copies of all correspondence between the IRB and the investigators. The IRB failed to adhere to this requirement. Specifically,

a. During the inspection, the FDA inspector noted that documents such as revised protocols and safety reports were missing from the IRB' s files.

We acknowledge the IRB' s written response that subsequent to the FDA inspection, the electronic storage files for the oncology studies were reorganized to complement the hard copy regulatory binders that are maintained in the RCC office. A separate folder containing copies of all regulatory documents was created in the IRB' s electronic file for each study, and this system will be maintained for all future IRB submissions. We find this corrective action to be adequate.

b. On three occasions (December 14, 2009; June 7, 2011; and April 2, 2012), the IRB met by teleconference and approved FDA-regulated research; however, no minutes were kept of these teleconference meetings.

We acknowledge the IRB' s written response indicating that the IRB Policy Manual has been revised to address how to correctly document the scheduled teleconferences for full reviews to ensure the presence of a quorum. The

IRB's response is inadequate because it does not address the IRB' s failure to prepare and maintain minutes of these teleconference meetings, and it does not include a copy of the revised written procedures. Moreover, it was the IRB's responsibility to prepare and maintain minutes of IRB meetings in sufficient detail to show the vote on IRB actions. Please submit a copy of your written procedures, or any draft procedures in development, and a timeline for the implementation of any new procedures. In addition, please provide a description of any training provided to IRB staff on the new procedures and a list of attendees, or a projected timeline of planned training.

This letter is not intended to be an all-inclusive list of deficiencies for the protocols reviewed and approved by the IRB. It is your responsibility to ensure that Singing River Health System IRB's practices and procedures comply fully with all applicable statutes and regulations.

Within fifteen (15) business days of your receipt of this letter, you should notify this office in writing of the actions you have taken to prevent similar violations in the future. Your written response should include any documentation necessary to show that full and adequate correction will be achieved. Please include the projected completion dates for each action to be accomplished. Failure to explain the violations noted above adequately and promptly may result in regulatory action without further notice.

We recommend that you visit the following FDA Web page for information on human subject protections that may assist you in your efforts to bring the IRB into compliance with FDA regulations:
http://www.fda.gov/ScienceResearch/SpecialTopics/RunningClinicalTrials/default.htm1.

We appreciate the cooperation shown to FDA Investigator Wright during the inspection. If you have any questions, please contact Catherine Parker at 301-796-5553; FAX 301-847-8748. Your written response and any pertinent documentation should be addressed to:

Catherine Parker, R.N.
Team Lead, Human Subject Protection Branch
Office of Scientific Investigations
Office of Compliance
Center for Drug Evaluation and Research
Food and Drug Administration
Building 51, Room 5247
10903 New Hampshire Avenue
Silver Spring, MD 20993

Sincerely,

/S/

Thomas Moreno, M.S.
Acting Office Director
Office of Scientific Investigations
Office of Compliance
Center for Drug Evaluation and Research
Food and Drug Administration

Cc: Ms. Angela M. Magee
IRB Chairperson
Singing River Health System
2012 Highway 90, Suite 36
Gautier, MS 39553
Page Last Updated: 02/11/2013

Note: If you need help accessing information in different file formats, see Instructions for Downloading Viewers and Players.

U.S. Food and Drug Administration
10903 New Hampshire Avenue
Silver Spring, MD 20993
Ph. 1-888-INFO-FDA
(1-888-463-6332)

第9封　给Salem医院伦理委员会的警告信

2012年11月29日

参考号：12-HFD-45-11-01

尊敬的Schnabel先生：

2012年6月6日至6月25日，Anita Narula博士和Marijo Kambere博士代表FDA对贵伦理委员会（IRB）进行了现场检查。这封警告信特告知您现场检查中发现的违规情况。本次现场检查的目的是核实贵伦理委员会受试者保护程序是否符合美国联邦法规（CFR）第21篇第50和56部分的要求。该法规适用于FDA所监管产品的临床研究。

本次现场检查是FDA的生物研究监查项目的一部分。该项目通过设定的检查方法，对FDA所监管的相关研究的实施情况进行评估，以确认研究数据在科学上是有效和准确的，并帮助确保这些研究中受试者的权益、安全和福利得到了保护。

在现场检查结束时，Narula和Kambere向Helen A. Hampton女士出示了FDA483表，即现场检查发现的问题，并与您进行了讨论。贵伦理委员会2012年7月11日对该FDA483表的书面回复已收悉。

经对现场检查报告、该报告的附件，以及伦理委员会的书面回复进行审查，我们认为，贵伦理委员会没有遵循适用的法律要求和监管受试者保护的FDA法规。我们想强调以下几点：

1. IRB未能准备和保存足够的IRB活动记录［21 CFR 56.115（a）（1）和（4）］

伦理委员会必须准备和保存伦理委员会活动足够的文件记录，包括但不限于研究建议的复印件、研究者提交的进展报告复印件、伦理委员会与研究者之间所有通信的复印件。贵伦理委员会未能遵循这项要求。

具体而言，伦理委员会未能保存以下方面的复印件：

a. 原始方案；

b. 修订方案；

c. 知情同意文件；

d. 试验方案修正案；

e. 进展报告的提交材料，包括所有的附件；

f. 研究者与伦理委员会之间的通信。

伦理委员会文件的保存是非常重要的，可以确认在审议期间审查了什么材料；也是非常必需的，以确保伦理委员会对研究的审查、对受试者的保护符合21CFR56.111的要求。

2. IRB未能按照21 CFR 56.108（a），（b）的要求，准备和保存足够的IRB书面程序记录［21 CFR56.115（a）（6）］

按照21CFR56.108要求，伦理委员会应当准备、保存与伦理委员会职能和运行有关的书面程序的完整记录。伦理委员会未能遵循这些要求。具体而言，Salem医院伦理委员会的政策和规程中没有包括相关的规程，以充分说明下列职能和操作：

a. 实施初始和跟踪审查或研究；

b. 确保在伦理委员会已经给出批准意见期间，对已经批准的研究中的变更，未经伦理委员会的审查和批准不能启动，除非是需要消除对受试者的明显直接伤害；

c. 确保快速向伦理委员会、适当的机构管理人员、FDA报告，任何严重或者持续性的不符合法规要求或伦理委员会决定的情况，或者任何伦理委员会批准的暂停或终止。

3. IRB未能制定和保存一份IRB委员名单，标识姓名、获得学位、代表资格等足以描述每名委员对IRB审议能带来的主要预期贡献的指标，以及每名委员与机构之间的雇佣或其他关系［21 CFR 56.115（a）（5）］

按照21 CFR 56.115（a）（5）要求，伦理委员会应当保存一份伦理委员会委员的名单。伦理委员会未能遵循这项要求。2008年12月3日至2011年3月21日，伦理委员会委员发生变动，而伦理委员会未对委员名册进行更新。具体而言：

a. 2009年1月21日会议记录显示，（b）（6）作为伦理委员会委员出席。2009年7月22日会议记录宣布（b）（6）退出了伦理委员会。但是，伦理委员会名册中从2008年12月3日到2011年3月21日，都没有把（b）（6）作为伦理委员会委员列出。

b. 2009年10月21日会议记录显示，（b）（6）被批准成为伦理委员会委员。2010年1月20日会议记录把（b）（6）作为伦理委员会委员列出，并显示她在伦理委员会活动中的投票情况。但是，伦理委员会名册中从2008年12月3日到2011年3月21日，都没有把（b）（6）作为伦理委员会委员列出。

当委员情况发生变化，伦理委员会名册没有进行更新。因此，FDA无法确定伦理委员会是否按照21 CFR 56.107的要求正式组成。

4. IRB未能在大多数IRB委员出席，其中至少包括一位来自非科学领域委员的召集会议上对拟开展的研究进行审查［21 CFR 56.108（c）］

除了采用快速审查程序以外，伦理委员会仅在召集会议上审查提出的研究，在召集会议上，大多数伦理委员会委员（即法定人数）会到场，并且包括至少一名来自非科学领域的委员。伦理委员会未能遵循这些要求，具体而言：

a. 2009年3月18日的会议记录显示，8名伦理委员会委员中有6名出席，两名委员在对（b）（4），“（b）（4）”研究的审查和投票中要求回避。因此，这项研究在少于委员会多数委员在场的情况下被批准。

b. 2010年4月21日的会议记录显示，8名伦理委员会委员中有5名出席，1名委员在对（b）（4），“（b）（4）”研究的审查和投票中要求回避。因此，这项研究在少于委员会多数委员在场的情况下被批准。

c. 2010年10月20日的会议记录显示，8名伦理委员会委员中有5名出席，1名委员在对（b）（4），“（b）（4）”试验方案和知情同意文件的修改进行审查和投票中要求回避。因此，这项研究在少于委员会多数人在场的情况下被批准。

5. IRB未能遵守关于快速审查程序的FDA法规［21 CFR 56.110（b）］

FDA法规要求，在快速审查程序中，可以由伦理委员会主席或主席从委员会委员中指定的一个或多个有经验的人员进行审查；伦理委员会可以使用快速审查程序来审查以下两种情况或其中之一：①出现在“适合快速审查的联邦注册研究类别”中，并且被评审人员发现涉及不超过最小风险的部分或所有研究；②在批准授权期间，已批准研究中微小变动。

此外，如联邦注册处告示中规定的，快速审查程序可以用于下列事项的跟踪审查：

a.（ⅰ）当研究将永久性地停止入组新的受试者；（ⅱ）所有的受试者都已经完成了所有研究相关的干预措施；（ⅲ）研究仍在进行，但是只用于对受试者进行长期随访；

b. 当还没有受试者被入组且没有额外的风险被确认；

c. 当仍在进行的研究活动仅限于数据分析。

Salem 医院伦理委员会对不适用于通过快速审查程序批准的研究使用快速跟踪审查程序，未能遵循21 CFR 56.110（b）的要求。具体而言，2009年1月21日的会议记录显示，对研究（b）（4）的跟踪审查通过快速审查实施。然而，来自临床研究者的2008年12月23日的一份备忘录要求对研究（b）（4）进行年度审查，显示这项研究已经开放入组，当前已经入组了4名受试者。因此对研究（b）（4）的跟踪审查不适用于快速审查。

伦理委员会于2012年7月11日对FDA483表的书面回复中承认上述列出的每一条违规行为的有效性。回复中声称，伦理委员会将制定新的书面程序来解决每一项违规。但是，回复中并没有随附提交书面程序的草案，且新的书面程序直到2013年2月28日才可使用。此外，伦理委员会的回复是不充分的，回复中没有任何对过程的描述，说明伦理委员会对新的书面程序，对委员会委员、员工、临床研究者进行培训和教育。没有这些信息，FDA无法准确评估提出的纠正和预防措施的潜在能力，以防止将来这些违规行为或类似违规行为再次发生。

本警告信的目的并非是罗列伦理委员会在审查和批准试验方案时存在的所有缺陷。确保Salem 医院伦理委员会的实际操作和程序完全符合所有适用的法律和法规要求是您的职责。

自收到这封信的15个工作日内，伦理委员会应当书面告知本办公室为预防将来发生类似违规情况而采取的措施。如果不能充分、迅速地解释上述违规问题，可能导致我们在不再通知的情况下采取监管措施。

附：英文原文

Salem Hospital IRB

WARNING LETTER

Nov 29, 2012

VIA UPS

Ref: 12-HFD-45-11-01

Joseph Schnabel, Pharm.D.
Director of Pharmaceutical Care Services
and IRB Chairman
Salem Hospital Campus
890 Oak Street SE, Building B-2-W
Salem, OR 97301

Dear Dr. Schnabel:

This letter informs you of objectionable conditions observed during the U.S. Food and Drug Administration (FDA) inspection conducted at your Institutional Review Board (IRB) between June 6, 2012, and June 25, 2012, by Dr. Anita Narula and Dr. Marijo Kambere, representing FDA. The purpose of this inspection was to determine whether the IRB procedures for the protection of human subjects complied with Title 21 of the Code of Federal Regulations (CFR), Parts 50 and 56. These regulations apply to clinical investigations of products regulated by FDA.

This inspection is a part of FDA's Bioresearch Monitoring Program, which includes inspections designed to evaluate the conduct of FDA-regulated research, to help ensure that the rights, safety, and welfare of the human subjects of those studies have been protected.

At the conclusion of the inspection, Drs. Narula and Kambere presented and discussed with Ms. Helen A. Hampton, the Form FDA 483, Inspectional Observations. We acknowledge receipt of the IRB' s written response dated July 11, 2012, to the Form FDA 483. From our review of the FDA's establishment inspection report, the documents submitted with that report, and the IRB' s written response,we conclude that the IRB did not adhere to the applicable statutory requirements and FDA regulations governing the protection of human subjects. We wish to emphasize the following:

1. The IRB failed to prepare and maintain adequate documentation of IRB activities [21 CFR 56.115(a)(1) and (4)].

An IRB is required to prepare and maintain adequate documentation of IRB activities including, but not limited to, copies of all research proposals, copies of progress reports submitted by investigators, and copies of all correspondence between the IRB and the investigators. The IRB failed to adhere to this requirement.

Specifically, the IRB does not retain copies of the following:

a. Original protocols

b. Revised protocols

c. Informed consent documents
d. Protocol amendments
e. Progress report submissions, including all attachments
f. Correspondence between the investigators and the IRB

The maintenance of IRB documents is important in identifying what materials the IRB has reviewed during its deliberations, and is necessary to ensure that the IRB has met its responsibilities for review of research and protection of human subjects under 21 CFR 56.111.

2. The IRB failed to prepare and maintain adequate documentation of written procedures for the IRB, as required by 21 CFR 56.108(a) and (b) [21 CFR 56.115(a)(6)].

An IRB is required to prepare and maintain adequate documentation of written procedures for a variety of IRB functions and operations, in accordance with 21 CFR 56.108. The IRB failed to adhere to these requirements. Specifically, Salem Hospital IRB policies and procedures do not include written procedures to adequately address the following functions and operations:

a. Conducting initial and continuing review or research;
b. Ensuring that changes in approved research, during the period for which IRB approval has already been given, may not be initiated without IRB review and approval except where necessary to eliminate apparent immediate hazards to the human subjects; and
c. Ensuring prompt reporting to the IRB, appropriate institutional officials, and the FDA of any serious or continuing noncompliance with these regulations or the requirements or determinations of the IRB, or any suspension or termination of IRB approval.

3. The IRB failed to prepare and maintain a list of IRB members identified by name; earned degrees; representative capacity; indications of experience sufficient to describe each member's chief anticipated contributions to IRB deliberations; and any employment or other relationship between each member and the institution [21 CFR 56.115(a)(5)].

An IRB is required to maintain a list of IRB members in accordance with 21 CFR 56.115(a)(5). The IRB failed to adhere to this requirement. The IRB did not update its roster when membership changed between December 3, 2008, and March 21, 2011. Specifically:

a. The IRB meeting minutes dated January 21, 2009, indicate that (b)(6) is present as an IRB member. The IRB meeting minutes dated July 22, 2009, announce (b)(6)'s resignation from the IRB. However, the IRB roster dated December 3, 2008, through March 21, 2011, does not list (b)(6) as a member of the IRB.
b. The IRB meeting minutes dated October 21, 2009, indicate that (b)(6) was approved to become an IRB member. The IRB meeting minutes dated January 20, 2010, list (b)(6) as an IRB member and show her voting on IRB activities. However, the IRB roster dated December 3, 2008, through March 21, 2011, does not list (b)(6) as a member of the IRB.

The IRB membership rosters are not updated as changes in membership occur. Therefore, the FDA may not be able to determine that the IRB is duly constituted, as required by 21 CFR 56.107.

4. The IRB failed to review proposed research at convened meetings at which a majority of the members of the IRB are present, including at least one member whose primary concerns are in nonscientific areas [21 CFR 56.108(c)].

Except when an expedited review procedure is used, the IRB may only review proposed research at convened meetings at which a majority of the IRB members are present, including at least one member whose primary concerns are in nonscientific areas. The IRB failed to adhere to these requirements. Specifically:

a. The IRB minutes dated March 18, 2009, indicate that six of eight IRB members were present. Two IRB members recused themselves during the initial review and vote for Study (b) (4), titled "(b)(4)." Therefore, the study was approved with less than a majority of members being present.
b. The IRB minutes dated April 21, 2010, indicate that five of eight IRB members were present. One IRB member recused himself during the initial review and vote for Study (b)(4), titled "(b)(4)." Therefore, the study was approved with less than a majority of members being present.

c. The IRB minutes dated October 20, 2010, indicate that five of eight IRB members were present. One IRB member recused himself during the review and vote for the protocol and informed consent document changes for Study (b)(4), titled "(b)(4)." Therefore, the changes were approved with less than a majority of members being present.

The maintenance of IRB rosters is an important part of IRB activities in that it provides documentation of current membership. In addition, appropriate roster maintenance helps to ensure that a proper number of members is present at IRB meetings when approving research activities.

5. The IRB failed to follow FDA regulations regarding expedited review procedures [21 CFR 56.110(b)].

FDA regulations require that under an expedited review procedure, the review may be carried out by the IRB chairperson or by one or more experienced reviewers designated by the IRB chairperson from among the members of the IRB; and that the IRB may use the expedited review procedure to review either or both of the following: (1) Some or all of the research appearing on the Federal Register list of categories of research eligible for expedited review and found by the reviewer(s) to involve no more than minimal risk; or (2) minor changes in previously approved research during the period for which approval is authorized.

Furthermore, as stated in the Federal Register notice, an expedited review procedure may be used for continuing review as follows:

a. Where (i) the research is permanently closed to the enrollment of new subjects; (ii) all subjects have completed all research-related interventions; and (iii) the research remains active only for long-term follow-up of subjects; or

b. Where no subjects have been enrolled and no additional risks have been identified; or

c. Where the remaining research activities are limited to data analysis.

The Salem Hospital IRB failed to comply with 21 CFR 56.110(b) when it used expedited continuing review for research that was not eligible for approval through an expedited review procedure. Specifically, the IRB meeting minutes datcd January 21, 2009, indicate that the continuing review for Study (b)(4) was conducted by expedited review. However, a memorandum from the Clinical Investigator, dated December 23, 2008, requesting annual review for the (b)(4) study indicates that this study was open to enrollment and that 4 subjects were currently enrolled. Therefore, the continuing review of Study (b)(4) was not eligible for expedited review.

The IRB' s written response to the Form FDA 483, dated July 11, 2012, acknowledges the validity of each of the violations listed above. The response states that the IRB will develop new written procedures to address each violation. However, the draft procedures were not submitted with this response and will not be available until February 28, 2013. In addition, the IRB's response is inadequate because it does not describe any process that the IRB will use to train and educate IRB members, staff, and clinical investigators with respect to its new written procedures. Without this information, FDA cannot conduct an informed evaluation of the proposed corrective and preventive action's potential ability to prevent the recurrence of these or similar violations in the future.

This letter is not intended to be an all-inclusive list of deficiencies for the protocols reviewed and approved by the IRB. It is your responsibility to ensure that Salem Hospital IRB's practices and procedures comply fully with all applicable statutes and regulations.

Within fifteen (15) business days of your receipt of this letter, you should notify this office in writing of the actions you have taken to prevent similar violations in the future. Failure to explain the violations noted above adequately and promptly may result in regulatory action without further notice.

We recommend that you visit the following FDA webpage for information on human subject protections that may assist you in your efforts to bring the IRB into compliance with FDA regulations:

http://www.fda.gov/ScienceResearch/SpecialTopics/RunningClinicalTrials/default.htm

We appreciate the cooperation shown to FDA Investigators Narula and Kambere during the June 2012 inspection. If you have any questions, please contact Catherine Parker, R.N., at 301-796-5553; FAX 301-847-8748. Your written response and any pertinent documentation should be addressed to:

Catherine Parker, R.N.
Team Lead, Human Subject Protection Branch
Office of Scientific Investigations
Office of Compliance

Center for Drug Evaluation and Research
Food and Drug Administration
Building 51, Room 5247
10903 New Hampshire Avenue
Silver Spring, MD 20993

Sincerely,

/S/

Thomas N. Moreno, M.S.
Acting Office Director
Office of Scientific Investigations
Office of Compliance
Center for Drug Evaluation and Research
Food and Drug Administration

Cc: Ellen A. Hampton
Director of Corporate Integrity,
Safety, and Risk Management
Salem Hospital
Salem, OR 97301

This is a representation of an electronic record that was signed electronically and this page is the manifestation of the electronic signature.

/S/

THOMAS N MORENO
11/29/2012
Close Out Letter
Salem Hospital IRB Close Out Letter 4/25/14
Page Last Updated: 08/15/2014
Note: If you need help accessing information in different file formats, see Instructions for Downloading Viewers and Players.
Accessibility Contact FDA Careers FDA Basics FOIA No FEAR Act Site Map Transparency Website Policies

U.S. Food and Drug Administration
10903 New Hampshire Avenue
Silver Spring, MD 20993
Ph. 1-888-INFO-FDA (1-888-463-6332)

第10封　给Texas应用生物医学服务中心的警告信

2012年9月24日

参考号：CBER- 12- 09

尊敬的Heinrich女士：

这封信特告知您2012年4月25日结束的，FDA对Texas应用生物医学服务中心研究审查委员会（TABS RRC）进行现场检查的结果。FDA 检查员对贵伦理委员会（IRB）进行了现场检查，以确定贵IRB的活动和程序是否符合美国联邦法规21CFR50，56的要求。FDA进行的这次现场检查是FDA的生物研究监查项目的一部分。该项目通过设定的检查方法，对FDA所监管产品相关临床研究的实施情况进行审查，以确保受试者在临床研究过程中不受到不当的危害或风险。

在现场检查结束时，检查员向您出示并讨论了FDA 483表，即现场检查发现的问题。我们审查了现场检查报告、FDA 483表和您2012年5月11日对FDA 483表的书面回复。

我们确定IRB已明显违反了美国联邦政府在21 CFR 56中规定的IRB所应遵从的行为和职责（可在http://www.gpoaccess.gov/cfr/index.html查询）。请尽快对本信所指出的违反项采取适当的纠正措施，并与贵伦理委员会进行讨论，对所指出的违反项提交书面回复。每项违反项对应的CFR条款引用如下：

1. IRB未能确保参与项目初始审查和跟踪审查的委员没有利益冲突［21 CFR 56.107（e）］

TABS RRC程序手册中RRC委员会部分规定，如果存在利益冲突，该RRC委员会委员不得参与项目的初始审查和跟踪审查，除非审查机构需要其提供相关信息。2012年1月26日的会议记录显示，包括身为主席的您在内，两位存在利益冲突的（b）(4）委员会委员参与了由（b）(4）申办的临床研究初始审查和批准活动。您和（b）(6）均投票批准了申办者的方案，而您二位给（b）(4）提供了咨询服务，协助他们撰写方案和知情同意书，并收取了费用。

在您的回复信中，您不同意Texas应用生物医学服务中心伦理委员会委员在审查（b）(4）的临床研究中存在利益冲突。您解释到，其中一位伦理委员会委员协助起草（b）(4）临床研究方案，并由Texas应用生物医学服务中心和/或 J Heinrich咨询公司向（b）(4）提供咨询，不属于利益冲突。您进一步解释到，向（b）(4）提供咨询服务“是独立于任何Texas应用生物医学服务中心研究审查委员会的职能和行为的”。

我们不同意您的解释。问题中涉及的两名委员在参与研究方案和知情同意书的初始审查及批准过程中存在利益冲突，因为他们参与了文件的起草工作。无论是否意识到这一点，同时服务于两家公司可能影响伦理委员会的审议结果。

2. IRB 未能制定、维护并遵守对研究进行初始审查和跟踪审查的书面程序［21 CFR 56.108（a）和56.115（a）(6）］

IRB未建立关于伦理委员会审查方案和知情同意书方法的书面程序，以确保参与临床研究的儿童得到适当的保障措施。2012年1月8日的会议记录显示，伦理委员会批准了涉及（b）(4）岁儿童的（b）(4）研究。

在您的回复函中，您承认Texas应用生物医学服务中心RRC之前未审查涉及儿童受试者的临床研究。您也声明将根据21 CFR50和56的要求起草书面的关于儿童临床研究的SOP（标准操作规程）。请您在对本信的回复函中提交一份新的涉及儿科人群临床研究的SOP。

3. IRB 未能满足委员的资格要求［21 CFR 56.107］

IRB并不具备对具体研究活动开展完整和充分的审查的必要专业能力。例如：

A. 2012年1月8日，伦理委员会审查并批准了一项涉及儿童和成人受试者（b）（4）紊乱的（b）（4）研究。伦理委员会记录显示，伦理委员会缺乏审查该项研究的专业能力，以确保其符合21 CFR 56.111中规定的被批准的标准，包括受试者的风险“与参与者可能获得的预期收益和研究成果中发现知识的重要性相比具合理性”。伦理委员会中没有在（b）（4）紊乱者治疗中具有相关专业能力人员（如医生），也没有任何文件显示伦理委员会如21 CFR 56.107（f）允许的那样邀请了该领域的专家协助审查该项研究。

B. 2012年1月26日，伦理委员会审查并批准了两项涉及（b）（4）受试者的研究。伦理委员会中没有在（b）（4）治疗中具有相关专业能力人员（如医生），也没有任何文件显示伦理委员会如21 CFR 56.107（f）允许的那样邀请了该领域的专家协助审查该项研究。

在您的回复信中，您对此持不同意见。您解释为尽管Texas应用生物医学服务中心伦理委员会未包含一位活跃的定期投票医生委员，但委员会可以获取一个核心医疗团队就任何研究过程中委员会遇到问题所提供的专业知识和意见。您的回复中还指出，在伦理委员会审查和批准两项涉及（b）（4）受试者的研究中，已经咨询了一位在（b）（4）研究领域拥有丰富经验的独立顾问。

我们发现2012年1月26日的会议记录中，未包括任何文件显示伦理委员会在决定批准该项研究时考虑过这位（b）（4）专家的意见。请您在对本信的回复信中提交这份向伦理委员会提供的独立咨询的文件。

4. IRB未能确定儿科研究要遵守50部分D子部分的要求［21 CFR 56.109（h）和56.111（c）］

21 CFR 50（D）中规定，在临床研究中，对于儿童需要额外的保障措施，伦理委员会需要审查关于D子部分适用的涉及儿童受试者的临床研究，并仅批准符合一定风险标准的临床研究，该风险列示在D子部分项下50.51，50.52或50.53。

A. 2012年1月8日的会议记录显示，伦理委员会审查并批准了一项涉及儿童的（b）（4）研究。该会议记录未记录伦理委员会对于相关问题的决定所涉及的风险水平、直接受益的可能性，对受试者的功能障碍或病情可能产生通用的知识，以及了解、预防或减轻影响儿童健康或福利的严重问题的机会。

B. 2012年1月8日的会议记录未显示伦理委员会讨论和（或）决定要制定征求（b）（4）研究中涉及儿童同意的充分条款规定。

在您的回信中，您表示未来所有涉及儿童受试者的项目会加强审查。同时，您在信中引用了FDA关于伦理委员会和临床研究者指南——知情同意文件内容，称FDA并未要求知情同意书留有征求儿童同意的空间。我们不接受您的解释。FDA483表中的问题并不能证明FDA是否要求知情同意书中需要保留征求儿童同意的空间，而是FDA检查员发现伦理委员会在初始审查时未能判断该项研究是否符合21CFR 50（D）的要求。另外，请注意21CFR 50（D）要求伦理委员会能够发现并记录临床研究中的儿童受试者符合D子部分的要求。2012 年 1 月 8 日的会议记录中未记录审查该项涉及儿童受试者项目的额外要求。

5. IRB未能建立和保存足够的IRB活动记录［21CFR56.115］

A. 伦理委员会未保留2011年的会议记录。现场检查过程中，您告诉FDA检查员伦理委员会在2011年开过两次会议。根据您的研究清单，Texas应用生物医学服务中心（b）（4）方案于2011年8月24日被修改且批准，但是未能提供关于伦理委员会审查的会议记录。

在您的回信中，您确认2011年没有会议记录，期间举行过两次会议。您解释由于计算机死机，那段时期内所有会议记录和数据都丢失了。您称您会“重建”这份会议记录，并稍后提供给我们。

这种重写2011年的会议记录的做法不合适且不能被接受。在您对本信的回复中，请提供可行的纠正措施，防止今后再次丢失所需记录。

B. 伦理委员会的会议记录未提供充分的细节证明伦理委员会采取了行动并对这些行动进行投票。2012年1月8日的会议记录未能体现伦理委员会（b）（4）委员中出席会议的人员，投票赞成、反对及弃权的人员。伦理委员会在2012年1月8日的会议上审查并批准了（b）（4）研究，但该会议记录未记录伦理委员会审查并批准了申办者关于该项研究中使用（b）（4）的风险状态的决定。

在您的回复信中，您指出，在对记录每位委员投票总体情况的2012年1月8日会议记录进行誊抄时有疏漏。

您还表示在以后的伦理委员会会议中，会专门指派一名记录员进行记录，确保会议记录信息完整。

在2007年和2000年最近两次FDA的检查中，均发现了伦理委员会会议记录不符合21 CFR 56.115（a）（2）要求的违规情况。鉴于过去未能纠正这种违规情况，请在对本信的回复函中解释伦理委员会具体将采取何种措施确保会议记录符合法规要求。另外，请提供自2012 年4月25日以后所有伦理委员会会议的会议记录复印件。

C. 伦理委员会未根据21 CFR 56.115（a）（5）保留2008 年至 2012 年期间的伦理委员会委员名册。伦理委员会委员名册无法识别委员的代表身份、委员与机构之间的雇佣或其他关系。该违规现象在2000年FDA的检查中重复出现。

在回信中，您提交了一份于2012年5月11日重新修订的委员名册。这份修订的委员名册仍不符合法规要求，因为您是Texas应用生物医学服务中心的总裁和Texas应用生物医学服务中心 RRC的董事长，这份名册中未指出您是一名隶属委员。此外，（b）（6）被列为非隶属委员，但根据56.107（d），机构雇员的直系亲属不得被视作非隶属委员。

本警告信的目的并非是罗列伦理委员会操作中存在的所有缺陷。您和贵伦理委员会应设法纠正本信中提到的违规情况，并全面审查贵伦理委员会的SOP及操作，确保完全符合法规要求，这些是您和伦理委员会的职责。

基于最后三次检查过程中重复出现的缺陷，我们不能确保贵伦理委员会的程序可以为研究过程中的受试者的权益、福利提供适当的保障。因此，根据 21 CFR 56.120（b）（1）和（2），

- FDA 将暂缓批准所有由贵伦理委员会审查的根据21 CFR 56开展的研究；
- 贵伦理委员会批准的根据21 CFR 56开展的研究不得入组新的受试者。

以上限制令立即生效。

在FDA有充分证据显示贵伦理委员会已采取了充分的纠正措施，并以书面形式通知您这些纠正措施满足要求前，这些限制令将持续有效。这些限制令并不免除伦理委员会应继续接受和处理现行研究项目的意外和严重不良反应报告，并进行日常进度报告的职责。

自收到这封信的15个工作日内，您应当书面告知本办公室为促使伦理委员会能够符合FDA要求已采取或计划采取的措施。您应根据上述列出的缺陷项逐条进行回复，并提供必要的文件证明充分并适当的纠正措施已完成，包括列明计划完成纠正措施的日期。如果您认为贵伦理委员会未违反FDA的要求，请陈述理由，并提供所有支持资料，以供我们参考。

在您的回复信中，请提供一份关于伦理委员会与每一个受到影响的申办者和临床研究者书面联系的复印件，告知其FDA目前发布的限制令。同时，请提供一份更新的列表，其中需要涵盖所有正在被贵伦理委员会审查的项目，指出按照21CFR56要求进行的研究，并列出所有受到上述限制令影响的研究清单。

基于21 CFR 56.120，56.121和56.124的授权，如果您不对本警告信内容进行回复，或不能采取适当的纠正措施，FDA可能采取进一步的行政措施。这些措施包括但不限于终止由伦理委员会批准的涉及21 CFR 56的研究，并启动监管程序取消伦理委员会的资格。

根据您的回复，FDA可能会安排一次复查，以确认纠正措施是否充分。

附：英文原文

Texas Applied Biomedical Services

By Facsimile Transmission and Overnight Delivery

CBER- 12-09

Ms. Mildred Joyce Heinrich, President/Chairperson
Texas Applied Biomedical Services
dba Texas Applied Biotechnology Research Review Committee IRB
dba TABS Research Review Committee IRB # 1
12101 Cullen Boulevard, Suite A
Houston, Texas 77048

Warning Letter

September 24, 2012

Dear Ms. Heinrich:

This letter describes the results of a Food and Drug Administration (FDA) inspection of the Texas Applied Biomedical Services Research Review Committee (TABS RRC) that concluded on April 25, 2012. The FDA investigator conducted the inspection of this Institutional Review Board (IRB) to determine if the IRB's activities and procedures for the protection of human subjects comply with FDA regulations published in Title 21, Code of Federal Regulations (CFR), Parts 50 and 56. The FDA conducted this inspection under its Bioresearch Monitoring Program, which includes inspections designed to review IRB operations relating to clinical studies of FDA regulated products and to ensure that human subjects are protected from undue hazard or risk during the course of clinical studies.

At the end of the inspection a Form FDA 483, Inspectional Observations, was issued and discussed with you. We reviewed the inspection report, the Form FDA 483 and your letter dated May 11, 2012, sent in response to the Form FDA 483.

We have determined that the IRB significantly violated applicable federal regulations governing the operation and responsibilities of IRBs as published under 21 CFR Part 56 (available at http://www.gpoaccess.gov/cfr/index.html). This letter requests prompt corrective action to address the violations cited and discusses your IRB's written response to the noted violations.

The applicable provisions of the CFR are cited for each violation.

1. The IRB failed to ensure that no member participated in the initial or continuing review of a project in which the member had a conflicting interest. [21 CFR § 56.107(e)].

The TABS RRC procedures manual, RRC Membership, states that no member of the Committee shall be involved in either the initial or continuing review of an activity in which he or she has a conflicting interest, except to provide information requested by the reviewing body. The meeting minutes dated January 26, 2012, show that two of the (b)(4) committee members, including you as the Chairperson, participated in the initial review and approval of clinical studies sponsored by (b)(4) (hereafter, (b)(4)) in which the members had a conflict of interest. Both you and (b)(6) voted to approve protocols sponsored by (b)(4) even though you had both provided consulting services to (b)(4), assisting with writing protocols and informed consent documents, for which payment was requested.

In your letter, you disagree with the observation that TABS IRB members had a conflict of interest with the review of the (b)(4) clinical studies. You explain that one of the IRB committee members assisted in the initial drafting of the (b)(4) clinical study protocols and that consulting services provided to (b)(4) by Texas Applied Biomedical Services and/or J Heinrich Consulting are not conflicts of interest. You further explain that the consulting services provided to (b)(4) "were maintained separate and apart from any TABS Research Review Committee functions and actions."

We disagree with your explanations. The two members in question had a conflicting interest when they participated in the initial review and approval of the protocols and informed consent documents, which they assisted in drafting. Conflicting loyalties, whether conscious or not, may influence the IRB's deliberations.

2. The IRB failed to prepare, maintain and follow its written procedures for conducting its initial and continuing review of research. [21 CFR §§ 56.108(a) and 56.115(a)(6)].

The IRB does not have a written procedure regarding the IRB's method of reviewing protocols and consent forms to ensure safeguards are in place for children who participate in a clinical study. The meeting minutes dated January 8, 2012, show that the IRB approved an investigational (b)(4) study involving children (b)(4) years old.

In your letter, you acknowledge that TABS RRC had not previously reviewed clinical investigational research studies involving pediatric subjects. You also state that an SOP (standard operating procedure) will be written addressing pediatric clinical studies in accordance with 21 CFR Parts 50 and 56. In your response to this letter please submit a copy of your new SOP addressing clinical studies involving pediatric populations.

3. The IRB failed to fulfill membership requirements. [21 CFR § 56.107].

The IRB did not possess the professional competence necessary to provide complete and adequate review of the specific research activities. For example:

A. On January 8, 2012, the IRB reviewed and approved an investigational (b)(4) study involving pediatric and adult subjects with disorders of the (b)(4). Review of the IRB's records indicates that the IRB lacked the professional competence necessary to review this study and determine whether it met the criteria for approval under 21 CFR 56.111, including whether risks to subjects were "reasonable in relation to anticipated benefits, if any, to subjects, and the importance of the knowledge that may be expected to result." The IRB did not include an individual with professional competence in the treatment of (b)(4) disorders (e.g., a physician), nor is there any documentation to show that the IRB invited individuals with competence in this area to assist in the review of this study, as permitted by 21 CFR 56.107(f).

B. On January 26, 2012, the IRB reviewed and approved two studies involving subjects with (b)(4) The IRB did not include an individual with professional competence (e.g. a physician) in the treatment of (b)(4), nor is there any documentation to indicate that the IRB invited individuals with competence in this area to assist in the review of this study, as permitted by 21 CFR 56.107(f).

In your letter, you disagree with this observation. You explain that TABS IRB does not have a medical doctor as an active, regular voting member of the committee, but the committee has access to a core group of medical advisors that provide expertise and input for any and all clinical research studies the committee encounters. Your letter also states an independent consultant with extensive experience in (b)(4) research was consulted when the IRB reviewed and approved two studies involving subjects with (b)(4).

We note that the meeting minutes dated January 26, 2012, failed to include documentation of any consult with a (b)(4) specialist that was taken into account by the IRB committee in its decision to approve the studies. In your response to this letter please provide documentation of the independent consultation to the IRB.

4. The IRB failed to determine that a pediatric study is in compliance with Part 50 Subpart D. [21 CFR §§ 56.109(h) and 56.111(c)].

Under 21 CFR Part 50 Subpart D, Additional Safeguards for Children in Clinical Investigations, IRBs are required to review clinical investigations involving children as subjects covered by Subpart D and approve only those clinical investigations that satisfy the criteria within certain risk categories identified in sections 50.51, 50.52, or 50.53 under Subpart D.

A. The meeting minutes from January 8, 2012, show that the IRB reviewed and approved an investigational (b)(4) study involving children. The meeting minutes do not document the IRB's determination of the level of risk involved, the potential for direct benefit, the likelihood of yielding generalizable knowledge about the subjects' disorder or condition, and the opportunity to understand, prevent, or alleviate a serious problem affecting the health or welfare of children.

B. The meeting minutes from January 8, 2012, do not document that the IRB discussed and/or determined adequate provisions were made for soliciting the assent of the children involved in the investigational (b)(4) study.

In your letter you state that all future studies involving pediatric subjects will be more closely scrutinized. Also in your letter you reference an FDA Guidance for IRBs and Clinical Investigators - Informed Consent Document Content which provides that FDA does not require the informed consent document to contain a space for assent by children. We do not accept your explanation. The observation on the Form FDA 483 does not speak to whether FDA requires the Informed Consent document to contain a space for assent by children. Instead, the FDA investigator observed that the IRB failed to determine at the time of the initial review that the research study was in compliance with 21 CFR Part 50 Subpart D. Additionally, please note that 21 CFR Part 50, Subpart D requires IRBs to find and then document that the clinical investigations involving children as subjects meets the requirements of Subpart D. The meeting minutes for January 8, 2012, fail to document additional requirements for review of this study involving pediatric subjects.

5. The IRB failed to prepare and maintain adequate documentation of IRB activities. [21 CFR § 56.115].

A. The IRB did not maintain meeting minutes for 2011. During the inspection you told the FDA investigator the IRB met twice in 2011. According to your study list, protocol TABS (b)(4) was modified and approved on August 24, 2011, but no meeting minutes were available for review documenting the IRB's activities.

In your letter, you confirm that there are no meeting minutes for 2011 during which two meetings were held. You explain that due to a computer crash all minutes and data for that time frame were lost. You stated that you would "re-create" the meeting minutes and provide them at a later date.

It is inappropriate and an unacceptable record keeping practice for the IRB to re-create minutes for 2011. In your response to this letter, please provide proposed corrective actions to prevent future occurrence of the loss of required records.

B. The IRB failed to maintain meeting minutes with sufficient detail to show actions taken by the IRB and the vote on these actions. The meeting minutes from January 8, 2012, fail to show which of the (b)(4) IRB members present at the meeting voted for, against or abstained. The IRB reviewed and approved an investigational (b)(4) study during the January 8, 2012, meeting however the meeting minutes do not document that the IRB reviewed and agreed with the sponsor's determination of the risk status of the investigational (b)(4) to be used in that study.

In your letter, you stated there was an oversight in transcription for the January 8, 2012, meeting minutes in recording each member's vote. Your letter also states that you will ensure more complete minutes in future meetings by assigning a clerical person to act as recording secretary for the IRB meeting.

The IRB's failure to maintain meeting minutes in accordance with 21 CFR 56.115(a)(2) is a repeat violation identified in the last two FDA inspections conducted in 2007 and 2000. Given the past failure to correct this deficiency, in your response to this letter please explain what steps the IRB has taken to ensure meeting minutes will be maintained in accordance with the regulations. In addition please submit a copy of the IRB's meeting minutes for all meetings conducted since April 25, 2012.

C. The IRB failed to maintain IRB membership rosters for 2008 through 2012 in accordance with 21 CFR 56.115(a)(5). The IRB membership rosters do not identify members by their representative capacity and any employment or other relationship between each member and the institution. This is a repeat violation identified during the FDA inspection conducted in 2000.

In your letter, you submitted a revised membership roster dated May 11, 2012. The revised roster fails to comply with the regulations because it does not indicate that you are an affiliated member even though you are the president of TABS, Inc. and Chairperson of TABS RRC. In addition, (b)(6) is listed as a non-affiliated member, but immediate family members of an employee of the institution cannot be deemed to be nonaffiliated under 56.107(d).

This letter is not intended to contain an all-inclusive list of deficiencies in the operations of the IRB. It is incumbent upon you and the IRB to correct the violations cited in this letter, and to conduct a thorough review of the IRB's SOPs and practices to ensure full compliance with the regulations.

Based on the repeated deficiencies found during the last three inspections, we have no assurance that the IRB procedures are adequately protecting the rights and welfare of the human subjects of research. For this reason, in accordance with 21 CFR §§ 56.120(b)(1) and (2), and effective immediately,

- FDA will withhold approval of all new studies subject to 21 CFR Part 56 and reviewed by the IRB; and
- No new subjects are to be enrolled in any ongoing studies subject to 21 CFR Part 56 and approved by the IRB.

These restrictions will remain in effect until such time as FDA has evidence of adequate corrective actions and notifies you in writing that the IRB's corrective actions are satisfactory. These restrictions do not relieve the IRB of its responsibility for receiving and reacting to reports of unexpected and serious reactions and routine progress reports from ongoing studies.

You are to notify this office in writing, within fifteen (15) business days of receipt of this letter, of the actions you have taken or plan to take to bring the IRB into compliance with FDA requirements. Your response should address each item listed above, and should include any documentation necessary to show that full and adequate correction has been achieved. Include the projected completion dates for each action to be accomplished. If you do not believe your IRB is in violation of FDA requirements, include your reasoning and any supporting information for our consideration.

Include with your response, a copy of the IRB's written communication to each of the affected sponsors and clinical investigators, notifying them of the current FDA imposed restrictions.

Please also provide an updated list of all studies being reviewed by your IRB, identify those that are subject to 21 CFR Part 56, and list all studies that are affected by the above restrictions.

Your failure to respond to this letter, or implement adequate corrective action, may result in FDA taking further administrative actions, as authorized by 21 CFR 56.120, 56.121, and 56.124. These actions include, but are not limited to, the termination of ongoing studies subject to 21 CFR Part 56 and approved by your IRB, and the initiation of regulatory proceedings for disqualification of your IRB.

On the basis of your response, FDA may schedule a reinspection to confirm the adequacy of your corrective actions.

Please send your written response to:

Lillian Ortega
Division of Inspections and Surveillance (HFM-664)
Office of Compliance and Biologics Quality
Center for Biologics Evaluation and Research
1401 Rockville Pike, Suite 200N
Rockville, MD 20852-1448
Telephone: (301) 827-6335

We request that you send a copy of your response to the FDA District Office listed below.

Sincerely,

/S/

Mary A. Malarkey, Director
Office of Compliance and Biologics Quality
Center for Biologics Evaluation and Research

第11封 给South Bend纪念医院伦理委员会的警告信

2012年9月21日

参考号：12-HFD-45-09-01

尊敬的Gruber先生：

2012年4月11日至4月23日，Myra K. Casey女士代表FDA对贵伦理委员会（IRB）进行了现场检查。这封警告信特告知您现场检查中发现的违规情况。本次现场检查的目的是核实贵伦理委员会受试者保护程序是否符合美国联邦法规（CFR）第21篇第50和第56部分的要求。这些法规均适用于FDA所监管产品的临床研究。

本次现场检查是FDA的生物研究监查项目的一部分。该项目通过设定的检查方法，对FDA所监管的相关研究的实施情况进行评估，以确认研究数据在科学上是有效和准确的，并帮助确保这些研究中受试者的权益、安全和福利得到了保护。

在现场检查结束时，Casey女士向您出示了FDA483表，即现场检查中发现的问题，并与您进行了讨论。您2012年4月23日对该FDA483表的书面回复已收悉。

经对现场检查报告、该报告的附件，以及贵伦理委员会提交的书面回复进行审查，我们认为，贵伦理委员会没有遵循适用的法律要求和监管受试者保护的FDA法规。我们想强调以下几点：

1. IRB未能在初始审查时确定涉及儿童的研究需要依照21 CFR 50（D），临床试验中对儿童的额外保护措施［21 CFR 56.109（h）］

在21 CFR 56.109（h）条款中，当试验中有部分或全部受试者为儿童时，伦理委员会初始审查时应当判断与法规21 CFR 50（D）的符合性（对临床研究中儿童的额外保护），按照21 CFR 50.50的要求，伦理委员会只能批准满足21 CFR 50.51中要求的临床研究（临床研究不涉及高于最小风险），满足21 CFR 50.52中要求的临床研究（临床研究涉及高于最小风险，但能提供给受试者个体直接受益的希望），满足21 CFR 50.53要求的临床研究（临床研究涉及高于最小风险，没有给受试者个体直接受益的希望，但很可能得到有关受试者身体功能紊乱或病情的普遍性认识）。

按照21CFR 50.51、50.52和50.53的要求，伦理委员会必须能发现并记录。我们现场检查发现，在审查和批准涉及儿童受试者的研究中，South Bend纪念医院IRB未能充分发现和记录研究是否符合21 CFR 50.51、50.52或50.53的标准。具体来说，IRB对以下有关儿童的研究进行了审查和批准，但IRB记录未特别说明研究是否按照21 CFR 50.51、50.52或50.53进行批准。

“（b）（4）为预防（b）（4）”

这项试验对于数据分析是开放的。

“（b）（4）”

这是一个开放的试验。

“（b）（4）”

这是一个开放的试验。

我们收到IRB的书面回复，其中包括以下纠正措施：①制定儿科研究检查表；②在IRB会议记录中增加对21 CFR 50（D）的讨论；③在对儿科研究进行跟踪审查时进行Subpart D审查；④将这些措施写进IRB的书面程序。IRB的回复是不充分的，因为它没有包括对以上三个研究是否符合21 CFR 50，（D）的要求进行判断；它不包含书面程序的副本；不包含IRB预计实施这些新措施的时间表。

请IRB提交对这些研究的每一项是否符合Subpart D的判断、一份书面程序的副本或在制定中的任何草案程序，以及对新程序的实施时间表。另外，请提供一份给IRB员工培训新程序的介绍和与会者的名单，或计划培训的项目时间表。

未能对研究中儿童的额外保障措施是否符合进行确定，可能导致这个弱势群体遭受不必要的风险，并导致儿童的父母或监护人对拟进行的研究不能够完全了解。

2. IRB未能制定、维护和遵守管理IRB职能和运行的必要书面程序［21 CFR 56.108（b）和 21 CFR 56.115（a）(6)］

为了满足IRB的法规要求，每个IRB必须制定、维护和遵守管理IRB职能和运行的书面程序。

IRB的“政策和程序手册”未包括所有必需的书面程序。具体而言，IRB没有规程来保证及时将下列情况报告给IRB适当的机构主管人员和FDA。

a. 给受试者或其他人带来风险的非预期问题；

b. 任何严重的或持续不遵守法规、要求或IRB决定的事件；

c. IRB 批准的暂停或终止。

我们注意到，FDA483表不包括缺少报告IRB批准暂停或终止规程的问题，因此，这个问题在您的纠正措施计划中没有得到解决。然而，我们收到IRB的纠正行动计划，承诺立即告知FDA和机构的负责人，修订报告的书面程序：①严重的或持续不遵守FDA规定的问题；②给受试者或其他人带来风险的非预期问题。IRB的回复是不充分的，因为它没有包括一份书面程序。请提交一份书面程序的副本，或完善中的任何草案程序；以及对新程序的实施时间表。另外，请提供一份给IRB员工培训新程序的介绍和与会者的名单，或计划培训的项目时间表。

3. IRB未能准备和保存足够的包括IRB会议记录的IRB活动记录［21 CFR 56.115（a）(2)］

IRB 应准备和保存足够的包括IRB的会议记录的IRB活动记录。该记录应包含充分的信息，显示会议出席情况，IRB采取的行动，对行动投票的赞成、反对和弃权数，要求对研究进行修改或不批准的依据和对争议问题进行讨论及解决的书面总结等。贵IRB未能遵守上述规定。未能遵守的例子，包括但不限于以下：

a. 根据IRB送到临床研究者的两封独立信函，日期均为2009年6月，IRB在2009年6月3日会议中批准了研究（b）(4）知情同意书的两个修订版本（日期为“12/30/2008”和“05/07/2009”），然而没有一个批准记录在2009年6月3日会议记录中。会议记录仅仅是对“对抽血的简化”修正案的批准。

b. 此外，“（b）(4)”研究知情同意书的记录副本“5/7 /2009”版本，加盖批准日期为“8 /5/2009”。如上所述，IRB批准函发出日期为2009年6月3日，提示在2009年6月3日会议上批准了这一文件。此外，对知情同意书的“5/ 7/ 2009”版本审批没有记录在2009年8月5日的IRB会议记录中。该批准记录在与本试验的跟踪审查有关的会议记录中。基于IRB记录的不一致，难以判断此知情同意书是如批准函上所示的在2009年6月3日批准，还是如盖章所示的在2009年8月5日批准。

c. 2009年6月3日会议记录反映了IRB对题为“（b）(4)”的新试验方案的审查。然而，会议记录是提出了一项动议并作出“批准研究延期1年”（作出强调）。基于IRB记录的不一致，难以判断是初始审查还是跟踪审查。

IRB的书面回复表明，这些问题的根源在于未告知委员会通过快速审查程序批准的研究。回复也陈述了自2011年10月以来，所有的快速审查项目在委员会下一次召开的会议中讨论过。回复承诺对书面程序进行修订，以包括这个程序。IRB的回复是不充分的，因为它不包括修改后的书面程序的副本。

请提交一份书面程序的副本，或完善中的任何草案程序；以及对新程序的实施时间表。另外，请提供一份给IRB员工培训新程序的介绍和与会者的名单，或计划培训的项目时间表。

4. IRB未能在大多数IRB委员出席，其中至少包括一位来自非科学领域委员的召集会议上对拟开展的研究进行审查［21CFR 56.108（c）］

除快速审查外，IRB只能在大多数IRB委员出席，其中至少包括一位来自非科学领域委员的召集会议上对拟开展的研究进行审查。IRB不能遵循这些要求。具体来说，2009年2月4日的IRB会议记录表明下列人员出席：（b）（6）（注册护士）、（b）（4）（内科医生）、George Maher（内科医生）、（b）（6）（注册护士）和（b）（6）（药剂师）。所以，关注点为非科学领域委员是缺席的，本次会议中，审查了FDA监管的研究（HUD批准，方案的偏差和不良事件）。

我们已收到IRB的书面回复，从中得知IRB正在招募另外一个非科学领域的委员。IRB承诺修订书面程序来解决这个问题。IRB的回复是不充分的，因为它不包括一份修改后的书面程序的副本。

请提交一份书面程序的副本，或完善中的任何草案程序；以及对新程序的实施时间表。另外，请提供一个给IRB员工培训新程序的介绍和与会者的名单，或计划培训的项目时间表。

5. IRB未能确保没有与项目有利益关系的委员参与IRB初始审查和跟踪审查，除非根据IRB的要求提供信息［21 CFR 56.107（e）］

为了批准研究，IRB必须确保投票人员不能与研究有利益冲突。2008年8月6日的IRB会议记录表明，出席会议的有八名，包括主席George Maher医生，但Maher医生也是研究（b）（4）的临床研究者。IRB的书面程序指出主席除了打破平局外，不参与投票。在这次会议中，IRB投票批准了研究（b）（4），有7票赞成，0票反对，0票弃权。所以，它表明Maher医生参与了审查和批准自己的研究项目。

我们已收到IRB的书面回复，自从2011年10月以来，有利益冲突的IRB所有委员都回避了有关自己的研究项目的讨论和投票表决，IRB承诺修订IRB书面程序，将更详细地解释这个规程。IRB的回复是不充分的，因为它没有提供一份修改后的书面程序的副本。

请提交一份书面程序的副本，或完善中的任何草案程序，以及对新程序的实施时间表。另外，请提供一个给IRB员工培训新程序的介绍和与会者的名单，或计划培训的项目时间表。

6. IRB未能按照不少于一年一次的频次对研究进行跟踪审查［21 CFR 56.109（f）］

为了满足IRB法规的要求，IRB必须按照风险程度每隔适当的时间对研究进行跟踪审查，但不得少于每年一次。

一份签署日期为2010年12月14日的IRB批准文件表明，（b）（4）主要治疗方案被批准，对当前入组的患者进行为期1年的继续治疗，自2010年12月14日开始至2011年12月13日结束。我们的现场检查发生在2012年4月，我们的检查员无法找到任何文件来说明2011年12月13日IRB的批准日期失效后该研究的状态。

IRB的书面回复陈述："这项特别的研究缺失了初始批准的记录，以至于难以确定什么时间该进行跟踪审查。据信，这项研究最初是于2011年6月批准的，这样2012年6月之前应进行跟踪审查"，这一陈述与上述批准函引用的陈述不相符，或与提供给FDA检查员的"开放试验"信息表中的信息不符。根据表中的信息，这项研究最初是在2008年12月3日由IRB批准的。您的书面回复也指出，"2011年10月，IRB开始根据11个月的间隔进行跟踪审查的做法。这将确保不会因会议日期而遗漏跟踪审查。"IRB的回复是不充分的，因为这一纠正措施未能解决有关（b）（4）研究的混乱，并且没有提供修改后的书面程序的副本。

请提交纠正和预防措施（CAPA）的计划，以解决上述问题；同时提交一份书面程序的副本，或制定中的任何草案程序，以及对新程序的实施时间表。另外，请提供一个给IRB员工培训新程序的介绍和与会者的名单，或计划培训的项目时间表。

本警告信的目的并非是罗列贵伦理委员会在审查和批准试验方案时存在的所有缺陷。确保South Bend纪念医院伦理委员会的实际操作和程序完全符合适用法律和法规的要求是您的职责。

自收到这封信的15个工作日内，您应当书面告知本办公室为预防将来发生类似违规情况而采取的措施。您的书面回复应包括必要的文件来表明完全和充分的纠正是可以达到的，另外，对每项措施提供预期完成的日期。如果不能充分、迅速地解释上述违规问题，可能导致我们在不再通知的情况下采取监管措施。

附：英文原文

Memorial Hospital Of South Bend, IRB

WARNING LETTER

SEPT 21, 2012

CERTIFIED MAIL
RETURN RECEIPT REQUESTED

Ref: 12-HFD-45-09-01

Mr. Kreg Gruber,
President Memorial Hospital of South Bend
615 North Michigan Street
South Bend, IN 46601

Dear Mr. Gruber:

This Warning Letter informs you of objectionable conditions observed during the U.S. Food and Drug Administration (FDA) inspection of your Institutional Review Board (IRB) that was conducted between April 11, 2012, and April 23, 2012, by Ms. Myra K. Casey, representing FDA. The purpose of this inspection was to determine whether the IRB procedures for the protection of human subjects complied with Title 21 of the Code of Federal Regulations (CFR), parts 50 and 56. Thcsc regulations apply to clinical investigations of products regulated by FDA.

This inspection is a part of FDA's Bioresearch Monitoring Program, which includes inspections designed to evaluate the conduct of FDA-regulated research to ensure that the data are scientifically valid and accurate, and to help ensure that the rights, safety, and welfare of the human subjects of those studies have been protected.

At the conclusion of the inspection, Ms. Casey presented and discussed with you Form FDA 483, Inspectional Observations. We acknowledge receipt of the IRB's written response dated April 23, 2012, to the Form FDA 483. From our review of the FDA's establishment inspection report, the documents submitted with that report, and the IRB's written response, we conclude that the IRB did not adhere to the applicable statutory requirements and FDA regulations governing the protection of human subjects. We wish to emphasize the following:

1. The IRB failed to determine at the time of initial review that studies involving children are in compliance with 21 CFR Part 50, Subpart D, Additional Safeguards for Children in Clinical Investigations [21 CFR 56.109(h)].

Under 21 CFR 56.109(h), when some or all of the subjects in a study are children, the IRB must determine that the research study is in compliance with 21 CFR part 50, subpart D (Additional Safeguards for Children in Clinical Investigations) at the time of initial review. Under 21 CFR 50.50, an IRB may approve only those clinical investigations that satisfy the criteria described in 50.51 (clinical investigations not involving greater than minimal risk), 50.52 (clinical investigations involving greater than minimal risk but presenting the prospect of direct benefit to individual subjects), or 50.53 (clinical investigations involving greater than minimal risk and no prospect of direct benefit to individual subjects, but likely to yield generalizable knowledge about the subject's disorder or condition).

Under 21 CFR 50.51, 50.52, and 50.53, the IRB must make and document certain findings. Our inspection revealed that in its review and approval of research involving pediatric subjects, Memorial Hospital of South Bend IRB failed to adequately find and document that the research satisfied the criteria of 50.51, 50.52, or 50.53. Specifically, the following pediatric studies were reviewed and approved by the IRB, but the IRB records do not specify whether the study was approved under 50.51, 50.52, or 50.53:

- "(b)(4) for the Prevention of (b)(4)"

This study remains open for data analysis.

- "(b)(4)"

This is an open study.

• “(b)(4)”

This is an open study.

We acknowledge the IRB’s written response, which includes the following corrective actions:(1)Developing a checklist for pediatric studies; (2) including a discussion of 21 CFR 50, Subpart D in the IRB meeting minutes; (3) performing a Subpart D review at the time of continuing review of pediatric research; and (4) incorporating these procedures into the IRB’s written procedures. The IRB’s response is inadequate because it does not contain a 21 CFR 50, Subpart D determination for the three studies listed above; it does not contain copies of the written procedures; and it does not contain a time frame for when the IRB anticipates the implementation of these new procedures.

Please submit the IRB’s Subpart D determinations for each of these studies; a copy of your written procedures, or any draft procedures in development; and a timeline for the implementation of any new procedures. In addition, please provide a description of any training provided to IRB staff on the new procedures and a list of attendees, or a projected timeline of planned training.

Failure to determine that the additional safeguards for children in research are met may expose this vulnerable population to unnecessary risks and result in the child’s parent(s) or guardian(s) not being fully informed about the proposed research.

2. The IRB failed to prepare, maintain, and follow required written procedures governing the functions and operations of the IRB [21 CFR 56.108(b) and 21 CFR 56.115(a)(6)].

In order to fulfill the requirements of the IRB regulations, each IRB must prepare, maintain, and follow written procedures describing IRB functions and operations specified in the regulations. The IRB’s “Policy and Procedures Manual” does not include all the required written procedures. Specifically, the IRB does not have procedures to ensure prompt reporting to the IRB, appropriate institutional officials, and the FDA of:

a. unanticipated problems involving risks to human subjects or others;

b. any instance of serious or continuing noncompliance with these regulations or the requirements or determinations of the IRB; and

c. any suspension or termination of IRB approval.

We note that the Form FDA 483 did not include an observation related to the lack of procedures for the reporting of any suspension or termination of IRB approval, and therefore this issue was not addressed in your corrective action plan. However, we acknowledge the IRB’s corrective action plan that promise prompt notification to FDA and the president of the institution, and revisions to the written procedures, for the reporting of (1) serious or continuing noncompliance with FDA regulations, and (2) unanticipate problems involving risks to human subjects or others. The IRB’s response is inadequate because it does not include a copy of the revised written procedures.

Please submit a copy of your written procedures, or any draft procedures in development, and a timeline for the implementation of any new procedures. In addition, please provide a description of any training provided to IRB staff on the new procedures and a list of attendees, or a projected timeline of planned training.

3. The IRB failed to prepare and maintain adequate documentation of IRB activities, including minutes of IRB meetings [21 CFR 56.115(a)(2)].

An IRB shall prepare and maintain adequate documentation of IRB activities, including minutes of IRB meetings, which shall be in sufficient detail to show attendance at the meetings, actions taken by the IRB, the vote on these actions, including the number of members voting for, against, and abstaining, the basis for requiring changes in or disapproving research, and a written summary of the discussion of controverted issues and their resolution. Your IRB failed to adhere to the above-stated regulations. Examples of this failure include, but are not limited to, the following:

a. According to two separate letters sent by the IRB to the clinical investigator, both dated June 3, 2009, the IRB approved two versions of the revised informed consent documents (dated “12/30/08” and “05/07/09”)for the study “(b)(4)” at the June 3, 2009, meeting. However, neither of these approvals is recorded in the minutes of the June 3, 2009, IRB meeting, which states only that there was approval of an amendment “related to the simplification of blood draws.”

b. Furthermore, the record copy of the “5/7/09” version of the informed consent document for the study “(b)(4)” is stamped with an approval date of "8/5/09." As noted above, the IRB sent an approval letter dated June 3, 2009, indicating approval of this same document at the June 3, 2009, meeting. Moreover, approval of the "5/7/09" version of the informed consent form is not recorded in the minutes of the August 5, 2009, IRB meeting. The approval recorded in the minutes pertains to continuing review of this study. Based on this discrepancy in the IRB's records, it is unclear if this informed consent document was approved on June 3, 2009, as stated in the approval letter, or on August 5, 2009, as stamped on the document.

c. The June 3, 2009, IRB meeting minutes reflect IRB review of a new protocol entitled "(b) (4)." However, the minutes document that a motion was made and seconded "to approve study for an additional year" (emphasis added). Based on this discrepancy in the IRB's records, it is unclear if this the initial review or a continuing review.

The IRB's written response indicates that these problems stemmed from a failure to inform the full board of research approved by the expedited review procedure. The response also states that since October 2011, all expedited review items have been discussed with the full board at the next convened meeting; the response also promised revisions to the written procedures to include this procedure. The IRB's response is inadequate because it does not include a copy of the revised written procedures.

Please submit a copy of your written procedures, or any draft procedures in development, and a timeline for the implementation of any new procedures. Please provide a description of any training provided to IRB staff on the new procedures and a list of attendees, or a projected timeline of planned training.

4. The IRB failed to review proposed research at convened meetings at which a majority of the members of the IRB are present, including at least one member whose primary concerns are in nonscientific areas [21CFR 56.108(c)].

Except when an expedited review procedure is used, the IRB may only review proposed research at convened meetings at which a majority of the IRB members is present, including at least one member whose primary concerns are in nonscientific areas. The IRB failed to adhere to these requirements. Specifically:

Minutes of the February 4, 2009, IRB meeting indicate that the following members were present: (b) (6) (registered nurse); (b)(4) (physician); George Maher (physician); (b)(6) (registered nurse); and (b)(6) (pharmacist). Therefore, a member whose primary concerns are in nonscientific areas was not present at this meeting in which FDA-regulated research (HUD approval, protocol deviations, and adverse events) was reviewed.

We acknowledge the IRB's written response that the IRB is currently recruiting a second nonscientific member, and that the IRB promised that revisions will be made to the written procedures to address this issue. The IRB's response is inadequate because it does not include a copy of the revised written procedures.

Please submit a copy of your written procedures, or any draft procedures in development, and a timeline for the implementation of any new procedures. Please provide a description of any training provided to IRB staff on the new procedures and a list of attendees, or a projected timeline of planned training.

5. The IRB failed to ensure that no member participated in the initial or continuing review of a project in which the member had a conflicting interest, except to provide information requested by the IRB [21 CFR 56.107(e)].

In order to approve research, an IRB must ensure that voting members do not have a conflict of interest in the research. Minutes of the August 6, 2008, IRB meeting indicate that eight members were present, including the Chairman and Dr. George Maher. Dr. Maher was also the clinical investigator fo Study (b)(4). The IRB's written procedures indicate that the Chairman does not vote, except to break tie. At this meeting, the IRB approved Study (b) (4) with a vote of 7 in favor, 0 opposed, and 0 abstentions. Therefore, it appears that Dr. Maher participated in the review and approval of his own research.

We acknowledge the IRB's written response that since October 2011, all members of the IRB with a conflict of interest have excused themselves during discussion and voting on actions related to their research, and that the IRB promised revisions to the IRB's written procedures that will explain this procedure in more detail. The IRB's response is inadequate because it does not include a copy of the revised written procedures.

Please submit a copy of your written procedures, or any draft procedures in development, and a timeline for the implementation of any new procedures. Please provide a description of any training provided to IRB staff on the new procedures and a list of attendees, or a projected timeline of planned training.

6. The IRB failed to conduct continuing review of research at intervals of not less than once per year [21 CFR 56.109(f)].

In order to fulfill the requirements of the IRB regulations, an IRB is required to conduct continuing review of research at intervals appropriate to the degree of risk, but not less than once per year.

An IRB approval letter dated December 14, 2010, indicates that the (b)(4) Master Treatment Protocol was approved for continued treatment of the currently enrolled patient for a one-year period beginning December 14, 2010, and expiring December 13, 2011. Our inspection took place in April 2012, and our investigator could find no documentation to indicate the status of this study after IRB approval expired on December 13, 2011.

The IRB's written response states, "This particular study lacks records of initial approval to determine when continuing review is due. It is believed that the study was initially approved on June 2011 which makes the continuing review due June 2012." This statement does not comport with the statements in the approval letter referenced above, or with the information in the table of "open studies" that was provided to the FDA investigator. According to the information in the table, this study was initially approved by the IRB on December 3, 2008. Your written response also states, "In October 2011, the IRB began the process to review all continuing review on an eleven-month cycle. This will ensure that there are no lapses in continuing review due to meeting dates." The IRB's response is inadequate because this corrective action has failed to address the confusion pertaining to the (b)(4) study, and it does not include a copy of the revised written procedures.

Please submit a corrective and preventive action (CAPA) plan to address the citation above. With your CAPA plan, submit a copy of your written procedures, or any draft procedures in development, and a timeline for the implementation of any new procedures. Please provide a description of any training provided to IRB staff on the new procedures and a list of attendees, or a projected timeline of planned training.

This letter is not intended to be an all-inclusive list of deficiencies for the protocols reviewed and approved by the IRB. It is your responsibility to ensure that Memorial Hospital of South Bend IRB's practices and procedures comply fully with all applicable statutes and regulations.

Within fifteen (15) business days of your receipt of this letter, you should notify this office in writing of the actions you have taken to prevent similar violations in the future. Your written response should include any documentation necessary to show that full and adequate correction will be achieved. Please include the projected completion dates for each action to be accomplished. Failure to explain the violations noted above adequately and promptly may result in regulatory action without further notice.

We recommend that you visit the following FDA Web page for information on human subject protection that may assist you in your efforts to bring the IRB into compliance with FDA regulations:

http://www. fda. aov/SdenceResearch/SoedalToDics/RunninaOinicalTrials/default. htm

We appreciate the cooperation shown to FDA Investigator Casey during the inspection. If you have any questions, please contact Catherine Parker at 301-796-5553; FAX 301-847-8748. Your written response and any pertinent documentation should be addressed to:

Catherine Parker, R.N.
Team Lead, Human Subject Protection Branch
Office of Scientific Investigations
Office of Compliance
Center for Drug Evaluation and Research
Food and Drug Administration
Building 51, Room 5247
10903 New Hampshire Avenue
Silver Spring, MD 20993

Sincerely,

/S/

Thomas Moreno, M.S.
Acting Office Director
Office of Scientific Investigations
Office of Compliance
Center for Drug Evaluation and Research
Food and Drug Administration

Cc: Ms. Alicia Dombkowski
IRB Chairperson
Memorial Hospital of South Bend
615 North Michigan Street
South Bend, IN 46601

第12封　给改善人类功能国际中心伦理委员会的警告信

2012年7月3日

参考号：12-HFD-45-06-01

尊敬的Riordan先生：

2011年7月6日至7月8日，Richard Rutherford先生代表FDA，对贵伦理委员会（IRB）进行了现场检查。这封警告信特告知您现场检查中发现的违规情况。本次检查的目的是核实贵伦理委员会受试者保护程序是否符合联美国邦法规（CFR）第21篇第50和第56部分的要求。这些法规均适用于FDA所监管产品的临床研究。本次现场检查是FDA的生物研究监查项目的一部分。该项目通过设定的检查方法，对FDA监管的相关研究的实施情况进行评估，以确认研究数据在科学上是有效和准确的，并帮助确保这些研究中受试者的权益、安全和福利得到了保护。

在现场检查结束时，Rutherford先生向您出示了FDA483表，即现场检查发现的问题，并与您进行了讨论。您2011年9月29日对该FDA483表的书面回复已收悉。但是您的书面回复超出检查后15个工作日的时间期限。因此，既然我们已经审查了回复，根据2011年8月11日发布的局长执行倡议，我们在本警告信中没有包括对回复的讨论。

此外，2012年1月23日和2月1日期间对三名临床研究者进行了访谈。这些临床研究者曾向贵伦理委员会提交过研究方案。经对现场检查报告、该报告的附件，以及访谈时收集到的文件进行审查，我们认为，贵伦理委员会没有遵循适用的法律要求和监管受试者保护的FDA法规。我们想强调以下几点：

1. IRB未能制定、维护和遵守管理IRB职能和运行的必要书面程序［21 CFR 56.108（a），21 CFR 56.108（b）和21 CFR 56.115（a）（6）］

为了满足IRB监管法规的要求，每个IRB必须制定、维护和遵守管理IRB职能和运行的必要书面程序。我们检查发现IRB没有书面程序，所以未能遵守关于IRB职能和运行的充分书面程序。IRB程序需包括以下：

a. 对研究项目进行初始和跟踪审查，以及将发现的问题和采取的行动报告给研究者和机构的书面程序［21 CFR 56.108（a）（1）］。

b. 确定哪些项目需要至少每年一次进行审查，以及确定哪些项目需要从研究者以外的来源获得验证，自上次伦理审查后没有资料的变更的书面程序［21 CFR 56.108（a）（2）］。

c. 确保将研究活动中的变化及时报告给IRB的书面程序［21 CFR 56.108（a）（3）］。

d. 确保已批准研究中的变更，在被IRB审查和批准期间，未得到IRB审查和批准不能启动，除非是为了消除对受试者造成直接伤害的书面程序［21 CFR 56.108（a）（4）］。

e. 确保及时向IRB、适当的机构人员和FDA报告涉及受试者和其他人员安全的非预期问题的书面程序［21 CFR 56.108（b）（1）］。

f. 确保报告任何严重情况或持续不符合法规要求或IRB决定的任何情况及时向IRB、适当的机构管理人员和FDA的书面程序［21 CFR 56.108（b）（2）］。

g. 确保及时向IRB、适当的机构管理人员和FDA报告暂停或终止IRB批准研究的书面程序［21 CFR 56.108（b）（3）］。

请提交纠正和预防措施（CAPA）计划，以解决上述问题；同时提交一份书面程序，或完善中的任何草案程序，以及对新程序的实施时间表。另外，请提供一个给IRB员工培训新程序的介绍和与会者的名单，或计划培训的项目时间表。

2. IRB 未能准备和保存足够的包括所有审查过的研究方案的副本、批准的知情同意的文件、研究者递交的进展报告在内的IRB活动记录［21 CFR 56.115（a）（1）］

IRB 应准备和保存足够的包括所有审查过的研究报告的副本、批准的知情同意的文件和研究者递交的进展报告等，贵IRB没能遵守这一要求。具体来说：

a. 2007年11月14日，IRB批准了FDA监管试验“（b）（4）”，完整的方案包含127页。然而，IRB的文档只有有限的8页签署日期为2006年5月5日的方案。因此，IRB所保存的文档是不完整的。

b. 一封2008年12月31日来自IRB委员James Jackson博士的信，信中提到批准（b）（4）试验的知情同意书的变更。在IRB的记录中找不到这个试验任何知情同意书的文件副本。

c. 一封2012年12月21日由IRB主席给Hunninghake博士的信，陈述（b）（4）试验被批准继续进行。在IRB的记录中找不到这个试验的任何进展报告。

请提交纠正和预防措施（CAPA）计划，以解决上述问题。CAPA计划中请包含任何预防措施，避免这种违规的再次发生。

3. IRB未能准备和保存足够的包括IRB会议记录的IRB活动记录［21 CFR 56.115（a）（2）］

IRB应准备和保存IRB活动的足够文件，包括IRB会议记录，记录中应有足够的细节来显示出席情况，IRB采取的行动，这些行动的投票情况，投票中赞成、反对和弃权的票数。需要修正或不批准研究的理由，并对有争议问题的讨论和决议的书面总结等。贵IRB未能遵守上述规定。未能遵守的例子包括但不限于以下：

a. 在检查期间，IRB主席表示，每年召开两次会议，并从事业务超过20年。然而现场检查员只能够找到一组日期为1997年6月25日的会议记录。

b. IRB没有关于对（b）（4）试验所采取的措施的会议记录。

请提交纠正和预防措施（CAPA）计划，以解决上述问题。CAPA计划中请包含任何预防措施，避免这种违规的再次发生。

4. IRB未能保存IRB与研究者之间的所有来往信函的副本［21 CFR 56.115（a）（4）］

IRB应准备和保存IRB活动的足够文件，包括所有IRB与研究者之间所有通信的备份。贵IRB未能遵守上述规定。未能遵守的例子包括但不限于以下。

a. 由FDA检查员掌握的，但IRB没有保留以下的通信的有：

i. 一封日期为2007年11月14日由IRB主席James Jackson发给hunninghake博士的信，说明（b）（4）的研究被批准。

ii. 一封日期为2008年12月31日由IRB主席James Jackson发给hunninghake博士的信，说明全体IRB委员批准了（b）（4）试验修改后的知情同意书。

iii. 五封日期为2008年12月31日由IRB主席James Jackson发给IRB委员［（b）（6）博士，（b）（6）先生，（b）（6）先生，（b）（6）博士和（b）（6）］的信，要求他们审查（b）（4）的试验知情同意文件的变更，签名，并传回他们的批准情况。

iv. 一封日期为2009年12月28日由IRB主席James Jackson发给hunninghake博士的信，说明试验被批准继续进行。

b. IRB的记录包括2011年3月23日由现任IRB主席Hinshaw博士发给（b）（4）试验的医学监查员的信，这封信讨论了6个严重不良事件报告和Hinshaw博士对它们归因的关注，但是IRB没有保留原始的严重不良事件报告。

请提交纠正和预防措施（CAPA）计划，以解决上述问题。CAPA计划中请包含任何预防措施，避免这种违规的再次发生。

5. IRB未能制定和保存一份IRB委员的委员名单，标识姓名、获得学位、代表资格等足以描述每个委员对IRB审议能带来的主要预期贡献的指标，以及每个委员与机构之间的雇佣或其他关系［21 CFR 56.115（a）（5）］

IRB应按法规要求制定和保存一份IRB委员的名单。

在现场检查中，贵方提供给FDA的检查员唯一的IRB名册是从一封日期为2007年10月3日的信中拿到的，但名册中并没有包括每个IRB委员获得的学位、代表资格和足以描述每个委员对IRB审议能带来的主要预期贡献的指标。

请提供一份最新的IRB委员的名册，名册中包括IRB委员姓名、获得学位、代表资格和足以描述每个委员对IRB审议能带来的主要预期贡献的指标，以及每个委员和机构之间的雇佣或其他关系。您的回复，请说明贵IRB如何避免这类违规的再次发生。

如上所述，IRB缺乏如何运作的规程，以及未能保存足够的有关IRB开展活动的文件。IRB活动的文档允许FDA检查：①IRB审查了什么材料；②做的初始和跟踪审查；③如果有，进行过什么有争议问题的讨论；④谁审查了试验，以及他们是否有资格审查试验；⑤IRB和研究者之间有什么往来信件。这些信息有助于确保受试者的权利、安全和福利得到保护。

自收到这封信的15个工作日内，您应当书面告知本办公室为预防将来发生类似违规情况而采取的措施。如果不能充分、迅速地解释上述违规问题，可能导致我们在不再通知的情况下采取监管措施。如果您认为您2011年9月29日对FDA483表的书面回复，充分解释了您已采取的措施足以防止类似违规情况的再次发生，请在15个工作日内以书面形式与我们联系。您可参考您2011年9月29日的书面回复，对这封信进行回复。

附：英文原文

Center for the Improvement of Human Functioning International, Inc. IRB

WARNING LETTER

Jul 3, 2012

CERTIFIED MAIL
RETURN RECEIPT REQUESTED

Ref: 12-HFD-45-06-01

Brian Riordan President and CEO
Center for the Improvement of Human Functioning
International, Inc. IRB 822 Greenwich Street, 3C New York,
NY 10014

Dear Mr. Riordan:

This Warning Letter informs you of objectionable conditions observed during the U.S. Food and Drug Administration (FDA) inspection conducted of your Institutional Review Board (IRB) between July 6 and July 8, 2011, by Mr. Richard Rutherford, representing FDA. The purpose of this inspection was to determine whether the IRB procedures for the protection of human subjects complied with Title 21 of the Code of Federal Regulations (CFR), parts 50 and 56. These regulations apply to clinical investigations of products regulated by FDA. This inspection is a part of FDA's Bioresearch Monitoring Program, which includes inspections designed to evaluate the conduct of FDA-regulated research to ensure that the data are scientifically valid and accurate, and to help ensure that the rights, safety, and welfare of the human subjects of those studies have been protected.

At the conclusion of the inspection, Mr. Rutherford presented and discussed with you Form FDA 483, Inspectional Observations. We acknowledge receipt of your September 29, 2011, written response to the Form FDA 483, but note that this response was received past the 15 working days from close of the inspection. Thus, while we have reviewed the response, we have not included a discussion of the response in this letter, as per the Commissioner's Enforcement Initiative announced August 11,2009.

In addition, interviews of three clinical investigators were conducted between January 23 and February 1, 2012. These clinical investigators submitted protocols to your IRB. From our review of the establishment inspection report, the documents submitted with that report, and the documents collected from the clinic investigators interviewed, we conclude that your IRB did not adhere to the applicable statutory requirements and FDA regulations governing the protection of human subjects. We wish to emphasize the following:

1. The IRB failed to prepare, maintain, and follow required written procedures governing the functions and operations of the IRB [21 CFR 56.108(a), 21 CFR 56.108(b), and 21 CFR 56.115(a) (6)].

In order to fulfill the requirements of the IRB regulations, each IRB must prepare, maintain, and follow written procedures describing IRB functions and operations specified in the regulations.

Our inspection revealed that the IRB had no written procedures, and therefore did not follow adequate written procedures for the IRB's functions and operations. IRB procedures need to include the following:

a. Written procedures for conducting its initial and continuing review of research and for reporting its findings and actions to the investigator and the institution [21 CFR 56.108(a)(1)].

b. Written procedures for determining which projects require review more often than annually and which projects need verification from sources other than the investigator that no material changes have occurred since previous IRB review [21 CFR 56.108(a)(2)].

c. Written procedures for ensuring prompt reporting to the IRB of changes in research activities [21 CFR 56.108(a)(3)].

d. Written procedures for ensuring that changes in approved research, during the period for which IRB approval has already been given, may not be initiated without IRB review and approval except where necessary to eliminate apparent immediate hazards to the human subjects [21 CFR 56.108(a) (4)].

e. Written procedures for ensuring prompt reporting to the IRB, appropriate institutional officials, and the FDA of any unanticipated problems involving risks to human subjects or others [21 CFR 56.108(b)(l)].

f. Written procedures for ensuring prompt reporting to the IRB, appropriate institutional officials, and the FDA of any instance of serious or continuing noncompliance with these regulations or the requirements or determinations of the IRB [21 CFR 56.108(b)(2)].

g. Written procedures for ensuring prompt reporting to the IRB, appropriate institutional officials, and the FDA of any suspension or termination of IRB approval [21 CFR 56.108(b)(3)].

Please submit a corrective and preventive action (CAPA) plan to address the citation above. With your CAPA plan, submit a copy of your written procedures, or any draft procedures in development, and a timeline for the implementation of any new procedures.

Please provide a description of any training provided to IRB staff on the new procedures and a list of attendees, or a projected timeline of planned training.

2. The IRB failed to prepare and maintain adequate documentation of IRB activities, including copies of all research proposals reviewed, approved consent documents, and progress reports submitted by investigators [21 CFR 56.115(a)(1)].

An IRB is required to prepare and maintain adequate documentation of IRB activities including, but not limited to, copies of research proposals reviewed, approved consent documents, and progress reports. Your IRB failed to adhere to this requirement.

Specifically:

a. On November 14, 2007, the IRB approved the FDA-regulated study "(b)(4)." The full protocol contained 127 pages. However, the IRB's documentation is limited to eight pages of the protocol dated May 5, 2006. Therefore, the

documentation maintained by the IRB is incomplete.
b. A December 31,2008, letter from Dr. James Jackson, an IRB member, refers to approving a change in the consent form for the (b)(4) study. No copy of any consent form for this study was located among the IRB's records.
c. A December 21, 2010, letter from the IRB Chair to Dr. Hunninghake states that the (b)(4) study is approved to continue. No progress reports for the (b)(4) study were located among the IRB's records.
Please submit a CAPA plan to address the citation above. Please include in your CAPA plan any preventive actions you plan to take to avoid recurrence of this violation.

3. The IRB failed to prepare and maintain adequate documentation of IRB activities, including minutes of IRB meetings [21 CFR 56.115(a)(2)].
An IRB shall prepare and maintain adequate documentation of IRB activities, including minutes of IRB meetings, which shall be in sufficient detail to show attendance at the meetings, actions taken by the IRB, the vote on these actions, including the number of members voting for, against, and abstaining, the basis for requiring changes in or disapproving research, and a written summary of the discussion of controverted issues and their resolution. Your IRB failed to adhere to the above-stated regulations.
Examples of this failure include, but are not limited to, the following:
a. During the inspection, the IRB Chair indicated that the IRB met twice per year and had been in business for over 20 years. However, the field investigator was only able to locate one set of meeting minutes dated June 25, 1997.
b. The IRB had no meeting minutes documenting any action related to the (b)(4) study.
Please submit a CAPA plan to address the citation above. Please include in your CAPA plan any preventive actions you plan to take to avoid recurrence of this violation.

4. The IRB failed to maintain copies of all correspondence between the IRB and investigators [21 CFR 56.115(a)(4)].
An IRB shall prepare and maintain adequate documentation of IRB activities, including copies of all correspondence between the IRB and the investigators. Your IRB failed to adhere to the above-stated regulations. Examples include, but are not limited to, the following:
a. The IRB did not maintain the following items of correspondence that were obtained by the FDA investigator:
1. A letter dated November 14, 2007, from James Jackson, IRB Chair, to Dr. Hunninghake, stating that the (b)(4) study was approved.
2. A letter dated December 31,2008, from James Jackson, IRB Chair, to Dr. Hunninghake, stating that the revised informed consent document for the (b)(4) study had been approved by all IRB members.
3. Five letters dated December 31,2008, from James Jackson, IRB Chair, to IRB members (Dr. (b)(6), Mr. (b)(6), Mr. (b)(6), Dr. (b)(6), and (b)(6)), requesting that they review the changes to the (b)(4) study informed consent document, sign, and send back their approval.
4. A letter dated December 28, 2009, from James Jackson, IRB Chair, to Dr. Hunninghake, stating that the study was approved to continue.
b. The IRB's records include a March 23, 2011, letter from Dr. Hinshaw, the current IRB Chair, to the Medical Monitor for the (b)(4) study. The letter discusses six serious adverse event reports (SAEs) and Dr. Hinshaw's concern over their attributions. However, copies of the original SAEs were not maintained by the IRB.
Please submit a CAPA plan to address the citation above. Please include in your CAPA plan any preventive actions you plan to take to avoid recurrence of this violation.

5. The IRB failed to prepare and maintain a list of IRB members identified by name; earned degrees; representative capacity; indications of experience sufficient to describe each member's chief anticipated contributions to IRB deliberations; and any employment or other relationship between each member and the institution [21 CFR 56.115(a)(5)].
An IRB is required to prepare and maintain a list of IRB members in accordance with the regulations.
During the inspection, the only IRB roster that the FDA Investigator was given was part of a letter dated October 3,

2007, and did not include each IRB member's earned degree, representative capacity, and indications of experience sufficient to describe the member's chief anticipated contributions to the IRB deliberations.

Please submit a current IRB roster that includes names; earned degrees; representative capacities; indications of experience sufficient to describe each member's chief anticipated contributions to IRB deliberations; and any employment or other relationship between each member and the institution. With your response, please address how you will prevent reoccurrence of this violation.

As noted in the citations above, the IRB lacks procedures to define how it operates, and has failed to maintain adequate documentation of its activities. Documentation of an IRB's activities allows FDA to ascertain (1) what material was reviewed by the IRB; (2) that initial and continuing review were performed; (3) what controverted issues were discussed, if any; (4) who reviewed the studies, and whether they were qualified to review the research; and (5) what correspondence took place between the IRB and investigators. Such information helps to ensure that the rights, safety, and welfare of human subjects are protected.

Within fifteen (15) working days of your receipt of this letter, you should notify this office in writing of the actions you have taken to prevent similar violations in the future. Failure to address the violations noted above adequately and promptly may result in regulatory action without further notice. If you believe that your written response to the Form FDA 483 dated September 29, 2011, fully explains the actions you have taken to prevent similar violations in the future, please communicate that to us in writing within fifteen (15) business days. You may reference your written response dated September 29, 2011, in your response to this letter.

We recommend that you visit the following FDA Web page for information on human subject protections. This information may assist you in your efforts to bring the IRB into compliance with FDA regulations:

http.//www.fda.gov/ScienceResearch/SpecialTopics/Running Clinical Trials/default.htm

We appreciate the cooperation shown to FDA Investigator Rutherford during the inspection. If you have any questions, please contact Catherine Parker, R.N., at 301-796-5553; FAX 301-847-8748. Your written response and any pertinent documentation should be addressed to:

Catherine Parker, R.N.
Acting Branch Chief, Human Subject Protection Branch
Office of Scientific Investigations
Office of Compliance
Center for Drug Evaluation and Research
Food and Drug Administration
Building 51, Room 5247
10903 New Hampshire Avenue
Silver Spring, MD 20993

Sincerely,

{See appended electronic signature page}

Leslie K. Ball, M.D.
Acting Office Director
Office of Scientific Investigations
Office of Compliance
Center for Drug Evaluation and Research
Food and Drug Administration

Cc: Charles T. Hinshaw, M.D.
Laboratory Director and IRB Chair
Center for the Improvement of Human Functioning International, Inc. IRB 3100 North
3100 North Hillside Avenue
Wichita, KS 67219

第 13 封　给 Advocate 健康护理中心的警告信

2012年6月1日

参考号：12-HFD-45-05-03

尊敬的Hill博士：

2011年11月7日至11月30日，BradleyJ.Maunder先生代表FDA，对贵伦理委员会（IRB）进行了现场检查。这封警告信特告知您现场检查中发现的违规情况。本次现场检查的目的是核实贵伦理委员会受试者保护程序是否符合美国联邦法规（CFR）第21篇第50和56部分的要求。该法规适用于FDA所监管产品的临床研究。

本次现场检查是FDA的生物研究监查项目的一部分。该项目通过设定的检查方法，对由FDA监管的相关研究的实施情况进行评估，以确认研究数据在科学上是有效和准确的，并帮助确保这些研究中受试者的权益、安全和福利得到了保护。在现场检查结束时，Maunder先生向您出示了FDA483表，即现场检查发现的问题，并与您进行了讨论。

经对现场检查报告、该报告的附件，以及您2011年12月19日、2012年4月26日以及2012年5月8日的书面回复进行审查，我们认为，贵伦理委员会没有遵循适用的法律要求和监管临床研究实施并保护受试者的FDA法规。我们想强调以下几点：

IRB未能确保按照21 CFR 50 的要求并达到所需的程度，获得每个预期受试者或其法律授权代理人的知情同意［21 CFR 56.111（a）（4）］

为了遵从FDA法规，批准一项研究时，伦理委员会必须确定研究满足21 CFR 56.111的所有条款要求。除此之外，伦理委员会必须确定将按照21 CFR 50的要求并达到所需程度，获得每个预期受试者，或其法律授权代理人的知情同意［21 CFR 56.111（a）（4）］。

Advocate健康护理中心伦理委员会在批准研究4257"评估单次推注给予依托咪酯对受试者治疗结果的影响"时未能按照21 CFR 56.111的要求，没有按照21 CFR 50的规定获得知情同意。具体而言，伦理委员会批准了研究4257，未能满足21 CFR 50.24的要求，这项临床试验没有获得潜在的受试者，或其法律认可的代理人的知情同意。

我们注意到，在2011年12月19日针对FDA 483表的书面回复中，您声称，在2011年11月FDA的现场检查之前，伦理委员会没有意识到FDA的法规适用于研究4257。根据2011年11月FDA现场检查期间伦理委员会准备的时间表，伦理委员会对这项研究的审查经过如下：

- 2006年12月11日，作为一项病历回顾研究，伦理委员会批准了研究4257。研究中，急诊室中需要插管的受试者将按照医疗常规进行治疗，将从受试者的医疗记录中收集有关临床治疗结果的数据。伦理委员会2006年12月11日的批件中说明这项研究"以快速审查的方式进行了审查并予以了批准，同时豁免HIPAA和知情同意"。
- 2007年7月11日，研究者提交了研究4257的修正案。修正案提议在插管之前，对受试者进行随机分组，然后给予药物咪达唑仑或依托咪酯。这两种药物均已获批上市。
- 2007年9月7日，伦理委员会批准了研究4257的修正案，并同意该项研究继续豁免知情同意。

当研究者提议研究4257将对受试者进行随机分组后予以咪达唑仑或依托咪酯时，这种药物治疗就不再属于临床医疗的范畴。因此，该项研究应被视为临床试验，但需遵从FDA法规，而伦理委员会应该根据21 CFR 第 56部分的要求审查这项研究，包括确保这项研究将根据21 CFR 第 50 部分的相关要求，获得每个潜在的受试者，或其法律认可的代理人的知情同意。

我们确认收到您在2011年12月19日的书面回复中列出的纠正措施计划，包括：①修改伦理委员会的政策和程序，遵循FDA法规，当发生严重的非预期事件和违规事件时，向FDA、其他政府部门和Advocate健康护理中心领导上报，以及满足FDA有关批准急诊室研究的条件；②根据FDA有关知情同意的法规要求，对伦理委员会委员进行培训；③在IRB的网站上公告培训简报；④在2012年Advocate健康护理中心主题为“Achieving Excellence in Clinical Research”的会议上举办有关急诊室研究的研讨会。此外，我们确认收到您2012年4月26日的信函，其总结了纠正措施的实施情况，提供了修改的伦理委员会的政策和程序，将要或已经开展的培训日期，以及2012年4月伦理委员会的简报复印件。

您在2012年5月8日给FDA的回复中还包括了研究4257的一份方案违背表，以及研究结束后研究者发给该研究受试者的信函复印件。方案违背表中说明研究者给受试者的信函是为了向他们解释该研究。您的回复中说明方案违背表和研究者的信函已归档于伦理委员会的文档中，但还未进入伦理审查流程。您在2012年5月8日的回复中进一步指出，方案违背表和信函已列入2012年5月22日的伦理审查会议的日程中。

然而，您的回复不能被接受，因为从回复中可以看出，伦理委员会并没有审查发给受试者的信函，以确定它是否给受试者提供了有关这项研究的适当信息，以及伦理委员会并没有在信函发给受试者之前或在2011年11月30日伦理委员会办公室收到这封信函时进行伦理审查。此外，我们发现研究者发给受试者的信函中存在不足，其中包括：①没有明确地告诉受试者他/她被纳入了一项研究；②没有告知知情同意书中应该包括的研究的细节以及其他信息，包括有关的研究风险。

此外，伦理委员会有责任按照21 CFR 50的相关要求，在2007年批准研究4257修正案时，确保该研究获得每个潜在的受试者或其法律认可的代理人的知情同意。伦理委员会未能履行这个职责是特别令人担忧的，因为知情同意这一概念对于开展一项伦理研究而言是基本且必要的。

本警告信的目的并非是罗列贵伦理委员会在审查和批准方案中存在的所有缺陷。确保Advocate健康护理中心伦理委员会的实际操作和程序完全符合所有适用的法律和法规是您的职责。

自收到这封信的15个工作日内，您应当书面告知本办公室为预防将来发生类似违规情况而采取的措施。

如果不能充分、迅速地解释上述违规问题，可能导致我们在不再通知的情况下采取监管措施。

附：英文原文

Advocate Health Care

WARNING LETTER

Jun 1, 2012

VIA UPS

Ref: 12-HFD-45-05-03

Joal M. Hill, J.D., M.P.H., Ph.D.
IRB Chairman
Advocate Health Care
205 West Touhy Avenue, Suite 203
Park Ridge, IL 60068-4201

Dear Dr. Hill:

This letter informs you of objectionable conditions observed during the U.S. Food and Drug Administration (FDA) inspection conducted at your Institutional Review Board (IRB) between November 7, 2011, and November 30, 2011, by Mr. Bradley J. Maunder, representing FDA. The purpose of this inspection was to determine whether the IRB procedures for the protection of human subjects complied with Title 21 of the Code of Federal Regulations (CFR), Parts 50 and 56. These regulations apply to clinical investigations of products regulated by FDA.

This inspection is a part of FDA's Bioresearch Monitoring Program, which includes inspections designed to evaluate the conduct of FDA-regulated research, to help ensure that the rights, safety, and welfare of the human subjects of those studies have been protected. We are aware that at the conclusion of the inspection, Mr. Maunder presented and discussed with you Form FDA 483, Inspectional Observations.

From our review of the establishment inspection report, the documents submitted with that report, and your written responses dated December 19, 2011; April 26, 2012; and May 8, 2012, we conclude that the IRB did not adhere to the applicable statutory requirements and FDA regulations governing the protection of human subjects. We wish to emphasize the following:

The IRB failed to ensure that informed consent would be sought from each prospective subject or the subject's legally authorized representative in accordance with and to the extent required by 21 CFR Part 50 [21 CFR 56.111(a)(4)].

In order to approve research subject to FDA's regulations, an IRB must determine that all of the requirements listed under 21 CFR 56.111 are satisfied. Among other things, the IRB must determine that informed consent will be sought from each prospective subject or the subject's legally authorized representative, in accordance with and to the extent required by 21 CFR Part 50. [21 CFR 56.111(a)(4)].

The Advocate Health Care IRB failed to comply with 21 CFR 56.111 when it approved Study 4257, "The Effect of Etomidate on Patient Outcomes after Single Bolus Doses," without requiring that informed consent be sought in accordance with and to the extent required by 21 CFR Part 50. More specifically, the IRB approved Study 4257, a clinical investigation for which informed consent was not sought from prospective subjects or their legally authorized representatives, without satisfying the requirements for approving such an investigation under 21 CFR 50.24.

We note that in your December 19, 2011, written response to the Form FDA 483, you stated that, until FDA's November 2011 inspection, the IRB did not "make a connection" that FDA's regulations applied to Study 4257. According to a timeline prepared by the IRB during the November 2011 inspection, the IRB took the following actions with respect to this study:

- On December 11, 2006, the IRB approved Study 4257 as a chart review study, in which subjects requiring intubation in the emergency room would be treated according to standard of care, and clinical outcome data would be collected from their medical records. The December 11, 2006, IRB approval letter for this chart review study states that the study was "reviewed and approved as expedited, with HIPAA Waiver and Consent Waiver."
- On July 11, 2007, the clinical investigator submitted an amendment to Study 4257. The amendment proposed randomizing study subjects to receive either midazolam or etomidate, which are both approved drugs, prior to intubation.
- On September 7, 2007, the IRB approved the amendment to Study 4257 and allowed the clinical investigation to continue with the waiver of consent left in place.

Once the clinical investigator proposed that Study 4257 would randomize subjects to receive either midazolam or etomidate, the drugs were no longer being used in the course of medical practice. Accordingly, the study became a clinical investigation subject to FDA regulations, and the IRB was required to review the study in accordance with the requirements of 21 CFR Part 56, including determining that informed consent would be sought from each prospective subject or the subject's legally authorized representative, in accordance with and to the extent required by 21 CFR Part 50.

We acknowledge the IRB's corrective action plan as outlined in your December 19, 2011, written response, which includes (1) revising the IRB's Policies and Procedures (P&P) to be consistent with FDA regulations with respect to reporting serious unanticipated problems and noncompliance to FDA, other governmental agencies, and Advocate Health Care institutional officials, and the criteria for the approval of emergency research; (2) educating IRB members with respect to FDA regulatory requirements for informed consent; (3) posting educational newsletters on the IRB's website; and (4) including a workshop on emergency research at Advocate Health Care's 2012 conference on "Achieving Excellence in Clinical Research." In addition, we acknowledge your April 26, 2012, correspondence summarizing the implementation of this corrective action plan, by providing the revisions made to various sections of the IRB's P&P; dates of meetings in which educational sessions have been, or will be, held; and a copy of the April 2012 IRB newsletter.

You also submitted a response to FDA on May 8, 2012, which included a protocol deviation form for Study 4257 and a copy of a letter that the clinical investigator mailed to subjects enrolled in Study 4257 after the study was completed. The protocol deviation form states that the clinical investigator's letter was intended to explain Study 4257 to the subjects. Your response indicated that the protocol deviation form and the clinical investigator's letter were filed with the IRB, but were not routed to the appropriate IRB staff member for processing and review. Your May 8, 2012, response further indicated that the protocol deviation form and the letter would be placed on the agenda for the May 22, 2012, IRB meeting.

However, your response is unacceptable because it indicates that the IRB did not review the letter provided to subjects, to determine whether it provided appropriate information to subjects regarding the study, either before the letter was sent to subjects or upon receipt of the letter in the IRB office on November 30, 2011. In addition, we find the clinical investigator's letter to the subjects to be deficient because, among other things, it did not (1) inform the subject unambiguously that he/she was enrolled in a research study, or (2) include details of the study and other information that should have been contained in the informed consent document, including information about risk to the subject.

Moreover, it was the IRB's responsibility to determine that informed consent would be sought from each prospective subject or the subject's legally authorized representative, in accordance with and to the extent required by 21 CFR Part 50, before approving the 2007 amendment to Study 4257. The IRB's failure to meet this responsibility is particularly concerning because the concept of informed consent is fundamental to the conduct of ethical research.[1]

This letter is not intended to be an all-inclusive list of deficiencies for the protocols reviewed and approved by the IRB. It is your responsibility to ensure that Advocate Health Care IRB's practices and procedures comply fully with all applicable statutes and regulations.

Within fifteen (15) business days of your receipt of this letter, you should notify this office in writing of the actions you have taken to prevent similar violations in the future.

Failure to explain the violations noted above adequately and promptly may result in regulatory action without further notice.

We recommend that you visit the following FDA webpage for information on human subject protections that may assist you in your efforts to bring the IRB into compliance with FDA regulations:

http://www.fda.gov/ScienceResearch/SpecialTopics/RunningClinicalTrials/default.htm

We appreciate the cooperation shown to FDA Investigator Maunder during the November 2011 inspection. If you have any questions, please contact Patrick McNeilly, Ph.D., at 301-796-2941; FAX 301-847-8748. Your written response and any pertinent documentation should be addressed to:

Patrick J. McNeilly, Ph.D.
Acting Branch Chief, Human Subject Protection Branch
Office of Scientific Investigations
Office of Compliance
Center for Drug Evaluation and Research
Food and Drug Administration
Building 51, Room 2266
10903 New Hampshire Avenue
Silver Spring, MD 20993

Sincerely,

/S/

Leslie K. Ball, M.D.
Acting Office Director
Office of Scientific Investigations
Office of Compliance
Center for Drug Evaluation and Research
Food and Drug Administration

Cc: Mr. James H. Skogsbergh
President and Chief Executive Officer
Advocate Health Care Corporation
2025 Windsor Drive
Oak Brook, IL 60523

Ann Errichetti, M.D.
President, Advocate Condell Medical Center
801 South Milwaukee Avenue
Libertyville, IL 60048-3199

1 See, e.g., Protection of Human Subjects; Informed Consent, 44 FR 47713 (Aug. 14, 1979); "The Belmont Report: Ethical Principles and Guidelines for the Protection of Human Subjects of Research" (1979), available at http://ohsr.od.nih.gov/guidelines/belmont.html#gob1.

第14封　给Our Lady of Bellefonte医院的警告信

2012年6月1日

参考号：12-HFD-45-05-02

尊敬的Halter先生：

2012年1月3日至1月6日，Karen Bryerton-Cooper女士代表FDA，对Our Lady of Bellefonte医院伦理委员会进行了现场检查。本次现场检查的目的是核实贵伦理委员会有关受试者保护的程序是否符合美国联邦法规（CFR）第21篇第50和56部分的要求。该法规适用于FDA所监管产品的临床研究。

我们知道在现场检查结束时，我们的检查员向您以及其他工作人员出示了FDA 483表，即现场检查发现的问题，并与您进行了讨论。贵伦理委员会2012年1月20日对该FDA 483表的书面回复已收悉。

经对现场检查报告、该报告的附件进行审查，我们认为，您没有遵循适用的法律要求和监管受试者保护的FDA法规。我们想强调以下几点：

1. IRB未能按照21CFR 56.108（a）（b）的要求，准备并保存足够的IRB书面程序的记录［21CFR56.115（a）（6）］

21 CFR 56.108要求伦理委员会为其各种职能和运行准备并保存足够的书面程序的记录。该伦理委员会未能遵循这些要求。具体而言，Our Lady of Bellefonte医院伦理委员会的政策和程序中没有包括针对以下职能和运行的书面程序：

a. 向研究者和研究机构通报伦理委员会发现的问题和采取的措施；

b. 确定哪些项目的审查频度应多于每年一次，以及确定哪些项目需要从研究者以外的来源获得证实，自上次伦理审查后没有资料的变更；

c. 确保已获得伦理委员会批准的研究，发生变更时必须获得伦理委员会的审查和批准方可实施，除非是为了避免对受试者造成明显的直接伤害；

d. 确保研究活动中出现的变更即刻向伦理委员会报告；

e. 确保当出现严重或持续发生的违背法规以及违背伦理委员会要求或决定的事件时，立刻向伦理委员会、适当的研究机构领导，以及FDA报告；

f. 确保当出现非预期的、可能对受试者造成风险的事件时，立刻向伦理委员会、适当的机构管理人员，以及FDA报告；

g. 确保当暂停或提前终止已获得伦理委员会批准的项目时，立刻向伦理委员会、适当的机构管理人员，以及FDA报告。

伦理委员会在日期为2012年1月20日的针对FDA 483表的书面回复中说明伦理委员会已起草了新的政策和程序，并将对伦理委员会委员进行这方面的培训。然而，与书面回复意见同时提交的政策和程序还没有获得伦理委员会的最终批准。此外，伦理委员会对委员进行流程方面的培训的说明并不充分，因为它没有描述对伦理委员会委员和员工进行这些法规要求培训的过程，并且也没有说明计划完成培训的日期。在上述信息缺失的情况下，FDA无法对提出的预防纠正措施是否能够在将来预防发生类似的违规作出有根据的评估。

2. IRB未能制定和保存一份IRB的委员名单，标识姓名、获得学位、代表资格等足以描述每个委员对IRB审议能带来的主要预期贡献的指标，以及每名委员与研究机构之间的雇佣或其他关系［21CFR56.115（a）（5）］

21 CFR 56，115（a）（5）要求伦理委员会保存一份伦理委员会委员名单。伦理委员会未能遵循这项要求。具体而言：

a. 2009、2010和2011年的委员名册没有标识委员获得的学位、代表资格等足以描述每个委员对伦理委员会审议能带来的主要预期贡献的指标，以及每个委员和研究机构之间的雇佣或其他关系。

b. 2010年1月5日的委员名册中没有包括（b）（6）博士、（b）（6）博士和（b）（6）女士。然而，2010年7月13日的会议记录中显示他们参加了会议并对研究项目进行了表决。

c. 2009年1月21日的委员名册中没有包括（b）（6）博士和（b）（6）女士。然而，2009年10月28日的会议记录中显示他们参加了会议并对研究项目进行了表决。

当委员进行变更时，委员名册没有进行相应的更新。因此，FDA无法判断伦理委员会是否根据21 CFR 56.107的要求而正确地组建。

伦理委员会在签署日期为2012年1月20日的针对FDA 483表的书面回复中说明“已创建了一份包括相关信息的名单，并由临床试验协调员保管”。这个回复是不充分的，因为伦理委员会并没有描述伦理委员会遵循21 CFR 56.115（a）（5）的要求准备和保存一份委员名单的实际流程。因此，FDA无法对提出的预防改正措施是否能够在将来预防发生类似的违规作出有根据的评估。

3. IRB未能准备和保存足够的IRB活动记录［21 CFR 56.115（a）（1），（2）和（4）］

伦理委员会应准备和保存足够的伦理委员会活动记录，包括但不限于：研究者递交的研究进展报告的复印件；充分的伦理委员会会议记录足以显示伦理委员会对伦理审查和表决的过程；伦理委员会和研究者之间的所有往来信函的复印件。贵伦理委员会未能遵循这个要求。具体而言：

a. 伦理委员会没有保留研究者递交的研究进展报告副本。

b. 伦理委员会会议记录没有显示伦理委员会决定的表决结果，包括几票同意，几票反对，几票弃权。

c. 伦理委员会没有保留伦理委员会和研究者之间的通信的复印件。

根据法规要求保存记录，提供了重要的证据说明伦理委员会采用的工作程序是否足以保护伦理委员会审查的临床研究中的受试者。

伦理委员会在签署日期为2012年1月20日的针对FDA 483表的书面回复中，说明伦理委员会已起草了要求研究者递交研究进展报告的新政策和传达伦理委员会决定的政策。此外，伦理委员会的回复中指出对伦理委员会题为“委员资格/会议/总职责”的政策进行了修改。然而，与2012年1月20日的书面回复意见同时提交的新的政策和程序还没有获得伦理委员会的最终批准。此外，伦理委员会有关对委员进行流程方面的培训说明并不充分，因为它没有描述对伦理委员会委员和员工进行这些法规要求培训的过程，并且也没有说明计划完成培训的日期。在上述信息缺失的情况下，FDA无法对提出的预防改正措施是否能够在将来预防发生类似的违规作出有根据的评估。

4. IRB未能在大多数IRB委员出席，其中至少包括一位来自非科学领域的委员的召集会议上对拟开展的研究进行审查［21 CFR 56.108（c）］

除非采用快速审查程序，否则伦理委员会仅在大多数IRB委员出席，其中至少包括一位来自非科学领域的委员召集的会议上对拟开展的研究进行审查。伦理委员会未能遵循这些要求。具体而言：

a. 伦理委员会2010年7月13日的会议记录显示，有五名投票委员参会，而六名投票委员缺席会议。尽管伦理委员会的多数投票委员缺席会议，但伦理委员会仍然审查并批准了研究（**b**）（**4**），所有的严重不良事件，并进行了跟踪审查，批准了研究（**b**）（**4**）。

b. 在召集多数委员参加的会议上，不清楚是否至少有一名投票委员是非科学领域背景。如上述第2点所述，伦理委员会2010年和2011年的委员名册的信息不充分，无法令FDA根据伦理委员会会议记录的信息确定是否有非科学领域背景的委员参加了所有伦理委员会的会议。

伦理委员会在签署日期为2012年1月20日的针对FDA 483表的书面回复中，说明伦理委员会改变了目前的政策，要求必须是多数投票委员参加伦理委员会会议。然而，与该书面回复意见同时提交的新政策和程序还没有获得伦理委员会的最终批准。此外，伦理委员会有关对委员进行流程方面的培训的说明并不充分，因为它没有描述对伦理委员会委员和员工进行这些法规要求培训的过程，并且也没有说明计划完成培训的日期。在上述信息缺失的情况下，FDA无法对提出的预防纠正措施是否能够在将来预防发生类似的违规作出有根据的评估。

5. IRB未能以书面形式通知研究者和机构批准或不予批准被提议的研究的决定，或为确保IRB批准研究而要求的修改意见［21 CFR 56.109（e）］

要求伦理委员会以书面形式告知研究者和机构，批准或不予批准被提议的研究的决定，或为确保IRB批准研究而要求的修改意见。伦理委员会未能遵循这个要求。具体而言，审阅了伦理委员会有关研究（b）（4）的文档，没有发现有记录，研究者被告知伦理委员会批准了研究。

伦理委员会在签署日期为2012年1月20日的针对FDA 483表的书面回复中说明伦理委员会起草了新的政策，并将及时以书面形式告知研究者和研究机构领导其审查决定。然而，与该书面回复意见同时提交的新政策和程序还没有获得伦理委员会的最终批准。此外，伦理委员会对委员进行流程方面的培训的说明并不充分，因为它没有描述对伦理委员会委员和员工进行这些法规要求培训的过程，并且也没有说明计划完成培训的日期。在上述信息缺失的情况下，FDA无法对提出的预防纠正措施是否能够在将来预防发生类似的违规作出有根据的评估。

6. IRB未能遵循关于快速审查程序的FDA法规［21 CFR 56.110（b）］

法规要求快速审查程序中，审查可以由伦理委员会主席或伦理委员会主席在委员中指定的一名或多名有经验的委员完成，伦理委员会可以采取快速审查的方式对以下情况进行审查，具体而言：

（1）联邦注册表上列出的符合快速审查条件的研究，并且审查者发现研究不大于最小风险；或者

（2）对于先前已批准的项目，在批准有效期内进行的较小变更。

此外，根据联邦注册表上所说明的，以下跟踪审查可以采用快速审查的方式：

- （ⅰ）当研究永久地结束而不再纳入新的受试者时；（ⅱ）所有的受试者已完成了研究相关的干预措施；以及（ⅲ）研究活动仅限于长期随访；或者
- 当研究还未纳入新的受试者且未发现有新增加的风险；或者
- 当剩下的研究活动仅限于数据分析。

Lady of Bellefonte医院伦理委员会未能遵循21 CFR 56.110（b）的要求，对不满足快速审查条件的研究的跟踪审查采用了快速审查的程序。

伦理委员会签署日期为2011年7月12日的证书记录了伦理委员会采取了快速审查的流程对研究（b）（4）进行了跟踪审查并予以了批准。证书上记录了对该研究进行快速审查和批准的理由是“采用快速审查是因为多数投票委员不能参加会议。”

我们的现场检查发现，研究（b）（4）的跟踪审查不符合快速审查的条件，因为在快速审查时纳入了一名受试者，而该研究仍可纳入受试者。因此，研究（b）（4）的跟踪审查和批准应采用多数委员参加会议的审查方式。

因为这个发现未被列入FDA 483 表，伦理委员会的书面回复没有涉及这个问题。请提供书面回复，对改正计划予以详细说明，确保伦理委员会的快速审查程序遵循21 CFR 56.110（b）的要求。在这个回复中，提交针对这个问题的新的或修改的标准操作规程（SOP），以及其他将采取的措施，如对委员的培训，说明预防纠正措施能够在将来预防发生类似的违规行为。

本警告信的目的并非是罗列贵伦理委员会在审查和批准试验方案时存在的所有缺陷。确保Our Lady of Bellefonte医院伦理委员会的实际操作和程序完全符合适用的法律与法规要求是您的职责。

自收到这封信的15个工作日内，您应当书面告知本办公室您已采取的促使伦理委员会完全符合FDA法规要求的措施。您的书面回复应解决这封信中提到的所有问题，提供必需的文件证明，将实现完整充分的纠正。请提供纠正措施计划完成的日期。如果不能充分、迅速地解释上述违规问题，可能导致我们在不再通知的情况下采取监管措施。

附：英文原文

Our Lady of Bellefonte Hospital

WARNING LETTER

June 1, 2012

VIA UPS

Ref:12-HFD-45-05-02

Kevin Halter, FACHE
Chief Executive Officer
Our Lady of Bellefonte Hospital
St.Christopher Drive
Ashland, KY41101

Dear Mr. Halter:

Between January 3, 2012, and January 6, 2012, Ms. Karen Bryerton-Cooper, representing the U.S. Food and Drug Administration (FDA), inspected the Institutional Review Board (IRB) at Our Lady of Bellefonte Hospital. The purpose of this inspection was to determine whether the IRB procedures for the protection of human subjects complied with Title 21 of the Code of Federal Regulations (CFR), parts 50 and 56. These regulations apply to clinical investigations of products regulated by FDA. We are aware that at the conclusion of the inspection, our investigator presented and discussed with you and other staff members a Form FDA 483, Inspectional Observations. We acknowledge receipt of the IRB's January 20, 2012, written response to the Form FDA 483.

From our review of the establishment inspection report and the documents submitted with that report, we conclude that the IRB did not adhere to the applicable statutory requirements and FDA regulations governing the protection of human subjects. We wish to emphasize the following:

1. The IRB failed to prepare and maintain adequate documentation of written procedures for the IRB, as required by 21 CFR 56.108(a) and (b) [21 CFR 56.115(a)(6)].

An IRB is required to prepare and maintain adequate documentation of written procedures for a variety of IRB functions and operations, in accordance with 21 CFR 56.108. The IRB failed to adhere to these requirements. Specifically, the Our Lady of Bellefonte Hospital IRB policies and procedures do not include written procedures to address the following functions and operations:

a. Reporting the IRB's findings and actions to the investigator and the institution;

b. Determining which projects require review more often than annually, and which projects need verification from sources other than the investigator that no material changes have occurred since the previous IRB review;

c. Ensuring that changes in approved research, during the period for which IRB approval has already been given, may not be initiated without IRB review and approval except where necessary to eliminate apparent immediate hazards to the human subjects;

d. Ensuring prompt reporting to the IRB of changes in research activity;

e. Ensuring prompt reporting to the IRB, appropriate institutional officials, and the FDA of any instance of serious or continuing noncompliance with these regulations or the requirements or determinations of the IRB;

f. Ensuring prompt reporting to the IRB, appropriate institutional officials, and the FDA of any unanticipated problems involving risks to human subjects or others; and

g. Ensuring prompt reporting to the IRB, appropriate institutional officials, and the FDA of any suspension or termination of IRB approval.

The IRB's written response to the Form FDA 483, dated January 20, 2012, states that the IRB has drafted new policies and procedures, and that it will educate IRB members on these processes. However, the new policies and procedures submitted with this response have not received final approval from the IRB. In addition, the IRB's statement that it will educate IRB members on the processes is inadequate because it does not describe the process that the IRB will use to train and educate IRB members and staff on these regulatory requirements, nor does it provide projected completion dates for the training of the IRB members and staff. Without this information, FDA cannot conduct an informed evaluation of the proposed corrective and preventative action's potential ability to prevent the recurrence of these or similar violations in the future.

2. The IRB failed to prepare and maintain a list of IRB members identified by name; earned degrees; representative capacity; indications of experience sufficient to describe each member's chief anticipated contributions to IRB deliberations; and any employment or other relationship between each member and the institution [21 CFR 56.115(a)(5)].

An IRB is required to maintain a list of IRB members in accordance with 21 CFR 56.115(a)(5). The IRB failed to adhere to this requirement. Specifically:

a. The 2009, 2010, and 2011 membership rosters do not identify members by earned degrees; representative capacity; indications of experience sufficient to describe each member's chief anticipated contributions to IRB deliberations; and any employment or other relationship between each member and the institution.

b. The January 5, 2010, membership roster does not include Dr. (b)(6) Dr. (b)(6), and Ms. (b)(6) as IRB members. However, IRB meeting minutes for the July 13, 2010, meeting indicate that they attended this meeting and voted on research.

c. The January 21, 2009, membership roster does not include Dr. (b)(6) and Ms. (b)(6) as IRB members. However, IRB meeting minutes for the October 28, 2009, meeting indicate that they attended this meeting and voted on research.

The IRB membership rosters are not updated as changes in membership occur. Therefore, the FDA is unable to determine that the IRB is duly constituted, as required by 21 CFR 56.107.

The IRB's written response to the Form FDA 483, dated January 20, 2012, states: "A list containing this information has been created and is now being maintained by the Clinical Trials Coordinator." This response is inadequate because the IRB does not describe the actual process that the IRB will use to ensure that the IRB prepares and maintains a list of IRB members in accordance with the regulations at 21 CFR 56.115(a)(5). As a result, the FDA is unable to undertake an informed evaluation of the proposed corrective and preventative action's potential ability to prevent the recurrence of these or similar violations in the future.

3. The IRB failed to prepare and maintain adequate documentation of IRB activities [21 CFR 56.115(a)(1), (2), and (4)].

An IRB is required to prepare and maintain adequate documentation of IRB activities including, but not limited to, copies of progress reports submitted by investigators; minutes of IRB meetings in sufficient detail to show the vote on IRB actions; and copies of all correspondence between the IRB and the investigators. The IRB failed to adhere to this requirement. Specifically:

a. The IRB does not maintain copies of progress reports submitted by investigators.

b. Minutes of IRB meetings do not show the votes on IRB actions, including the number of members voting for, against, and abstaining.

c. The IRB does not maintain copies of correspondence between the IRB and the investigators.

Maintaining records, as required under the regulations, provides significant evidence of whether the procedures utilized by the IRB are adequately protecting the human subjects of the clinical investigations that the IRB is reviewing.

The IRB's written response to the Form FDA 483, dated January 20, 2012, states that the IRB has drafted new policies requiring progress reports by investigators and the communication of IRB actions. In addition, the IRB's response indicates that it has revised its IRB policy titled "Membership/Meetings/General Functions." However, the new policies and procedures submitted with the January 20, 2012, written response have not received final approval from the IRB. In addition, the IRB's statement that it will educate IRB members on the process is inadequate because it does not describe the process that the IRB will use to train and educate IRB members and staff on these regulatory requirements, nor does it provide projected completion dates for the training of the IRB members and staff. Without this information, FDA cannot conduct an informed evaluation of the proposed corrective and preventative action's potential ability to prevent the recurrence of these or similar violations in the future.

4. The IRB failed to review proposed research at convened meetings at which a majority of the members of the IRB are present, including at least one member whose primary concerns are in nonscientific areas [21 CFR 56.108(c)].

Except when an expedited review procedure is used, the IRB may only review proposed research at convened meetings at which a majority of the IRB members is present, including at least one member whose primary concerns are in nonscientific areas. The IRB failed to adhere to these requirements. Specifically:

a. The IRB meeting minutes for July 13, 2010, indicate that five voting members were present and six voting members were absent at the meeting. Despite the IRB's not having a majority of voting members present, it reviewed and approved a revision to Study (b)(4), all serious adverse events, and conducted continuing review and granted approval for Studies (b)(4).

b. It is unclear if at least one voting member was a nonscientific member at convened IRB meetings. As discussed in Violation 2 above, the IRB membership rosters for 2010 and 2011 are inadequate, and the FDA is unable to determine, based on the IRB meeting minutes, if the required nonscientist was present at all convened IRB meetings.

The IRB's written response to the Form FDA 483, dated January 20, 2012, states that the IRB has changed its existing policy to require that a majority of voting members be present for all meetings. However, the draft policies and procedures submitted with this response have not received final approval from the IRB. In addition, the IRB's statement that it will educate IRB members on the process is inadequate because it does not describe the process that the IRB will use to train and educate IRB members and staff on these regulatory requirements, nor does it provide projected completion dates for the training of the IRB members and staff. Without this information, FDA cannot conduct an informed evaluation of the proposed corrective and preventative action's potential ability to prevent the recurrence of these or similar violations in the future.

5. The IRB failed to notify investigators and the institution in writing of its decision to approve or disapprove proposed research activities, or of modifications required to secure IRB approval of the research activity [21 CFR 56.109(e)].

An IRB is required to notify investigators and the institution in writing of its decision to approve or disapprove proposed research activities. The IRB failed to adhere to this requirement. Specifically, review of the IRB's files for Studies (b)(4) found no documentation that investigators were notified of the IRB approval for those studies.

The IRB's written response to the Form FDA 483, dated January 20, 2012, states that the IRB has drafted a new policy that will notify the investigator and institutional officials of its decisions in a timely manner. However, the new policies and procedures submitted with this response have not received final approval from the IRB. In addition, the IRB's statement that it will educate IRB members on the process is inadequate because it does not describe the process that the IRB will use to train and educate IRB members and staff on these regulatory requirements, nor does it provide projected completion dates for the training of the IRB members and staff. Without this information, FDA cannot conduct an informed evaluation of the proposed corrective and preventative action's potential ability to prevent the recurrence of these or similar violations in the future.

6. The IRB failed to follow FDA regulations regarding expedited review procedures [21 CFR 56.110(b)].

The regulations require that under an expedited review procedure, the review may be carried out by the IRB chairperson or by one or more experienced reviewers designated by the IRB chairperson from among the members of the IRB; and the IRB may use the expedited review procedure to review either or both of the following: (1) Some or all of the research appearing on the Federal Register list of categories of research eligible for expedited review and found by the reviewer(s) to involve no more than minimal risk; or (2) minor changes in previously approved research during the period for which approval is authorized.

Furthermore, as stated in the Federal Register notice, an expedited review procedure may be used for continuing review as follows:

- Where (i) the research is permanently closed to the enrollment of new subjects; (ii) all subjects have completed all research-related interventions; and (iii) the research remains active only for long-term follow-up of subjects; or
- Where no subjects have been enrolled and no additional risks have been identified; or
- Where the remaining research activities are limited to data analysis.

The IRB Lady of Bellefonte Hospital IRB failed to comply with 21 CFR 56.110(b) when it used expedited continuing review for research that was not eligible for approval through an expedited review procedure. Specifically:

The IRB Certification Sheet dated July 12,2011, documents that the IRB used an expedited review procedure for the continuing review and approval of Study (b)(4), titled "(b)(4)." The rationale given on the IRB Certification Sheet for the approval of this study under an expedited review procedure states: "Expedited Review due to majority voting memebers (sic) not available for meeting."

Our inspection revealed that the continuing review of Study (b)(4) was not eligible for expedited review because one subject had been enrolled in the study at the time of the expedited review, and the study was still open for subject accrual. Therefore, Study (b)(4) should have been reviewed and approved at a convened meeting with a majority of the IRB members present.

As this observation was not listed in the Form FDA 483, the IRB's written response did not address this finding. Please provide a written response that details a corrective action plan to ensure that the IRB will use the expedited review procedure in accordance with 21 CFR 56.11 O(b). In this response, submit a copy of any revised or new Standard Operating Procedures (SOPs) developed to address this finding, and any additional actions taken, such as the training of the IRB members, to demonstrate that the proposed corrective action will prevent any future recurrence of this type of violation.

This letter is not intended to be an all-inclusive list of deficiencies for the protocols reviewed and approved by the IRB. It is your responsibility to ensure that Our Lady of Bellefonte Hospital IRB' s practices and procedures comply fully with all applicable statutes and regulations.

Within fifteen (15) business days of your receipt of this letter, you should notify this office in writing of the actions you have taken to bring the IRB into full compliance with FDA regulations. Your written response should address each citation in the letter and include any documentation necessary to show that full and adequate correction will be achieved. Please include the projected completion dates for each action to be accomplished. Failure to explain the violations noted above adequately and promptly may result in regulatory action without further notice.

We recommend that you visit the following FDA webpage for information on human subject protections that may assist you in your efforts to bring the IRB into compliance with FDA regulations:

http://www.fda.gov/ScienceResearch/SpecialTopics/RunningClinicalTrials/default.htm

We appreciate the cooperation shown to Ms. Cooper during the inspection. If you have any questions, please contact Patrick McNeilly, Ph.D., at 301-796-2941; FAX 301-847-8748.

Your written response and any pertinent documentation should be addressed to:

Patrick J. McNeilly, Ph.D.
Acting Branch Chief, Human Subject Protection Branch
Office of Scientific Investigations
Office of Compliance
Center for Drug Evaluation and Research
Food and Drug Administration
Building 51, Room 2266
10903 New Hampshire Avenue
Silver Spring, MD 20993

Sincerely,

/S/

Leslie K. Ball, M.D.
Acting Office Director
Office of Scientific Investigations
Office of Compliance
Center for Drug Evaluation and Research
Food and Drug Administration

Cc: Kevin Howard, D.O.
Chairman, Institutional Review Board
Our Lady of Bellefonte Hospital
St. Christopher Drive
Ashland, KY 41101

第 15 封　给美国生物医学研究所（生物医学伦理委员会）的警告信

2012年3月29日

参考号：CBER-12-0

尊敬的Fox先生：

这封信特告知您FDA对美国生物医学研究所生物医学伦理委员会（IRB）的检查结果。该检查分为两个阶段，分别是2010年9月22日至10月25日和2011年8月8日至8月19日。第一次检查由一名洛杉矶地区FDA检查员执行，重点检查IRB对申报者（b）（4）项目研究挑选的审查过程。鉴于第一次检查中发现的缺陷特点，FDA发起了第二次检查，以对IRB的操作进行更广泛的评估。第二次检查是由同一名地区检查员和一名来自生物制品评价与研究中心（CBER）的检查员执行。FDA检查员进行检查是为了核实IRB保护受试者权益的程序是否符合美国联邦法规第21篇第50和56部分的要求。此次现场检查是FDA的生物研究监查项目的一部分。该项目通过设定的检查方法，审查在使用试验药物的临床研究以及在保护受试者中IRB运行情况。

第一次现场检查重点仅限于以下研究：

- （b）（4）；
- （b）（4）。

第二次现场检查的重点包含：会议记录、委员身份和IRB对研究项目的总体审查情况。

FDA洛杉矶地区检查员在每次检查结束时都向您出示并讨论了FDA483表，即现场检查发现的问题。来自CBER的FDA检查员通过电话参加了第二次检查的末次会议。我们收到并审查了贵IRB日期为2010年11月2日、2011年8月30日、2011年9月1日、2011年9月2日、2011年9月15日以及2012年1月12日对该FDA483表的书面回复。

我们确定IRB明显违反了联邦政府在21 CFR 56中规定的IRB所应遵从的行为和职责（可在http://www.gpoaccess.gov/cfr/index.html查询）。每项违反项所引用的CFR条款已列出。

1. IRB未能满足委员的资格要求［21 CFR 56.107］

A. IRB并不具备必要的专业能力，以充分审查具体研究活动。例如：

i. 2010年1月27日，IRB审查并批准了一项涉及（b）（4）受试者的研究。IRB记录显示，IRB缺乏审查该项研究的专业能力，以确保其符合21 CFR 56.111中规定的被批准的标准，包括受试者的风险"关于参与者的预期收益和获得预期知识的重要性是合理的"。例如，IRB中未包括具备（b）（4）专业能力的委员（如医生），也没有任何文件显示IRB邀请了该领域的专家协助审查该项研究，21 CFR 56.107（f）是允许这种邀请的。

ii. 2010年7月7日，IRB审查并批准了一项受试者使用（b）（4）的研究。IRB既没有在（b）（4）治疗中具有相关专业能力的委员（如医生），也没有任何文件显示IRB邀请了该领域的专家协助审查该项研究，21 CFR 56.107（f）是允许这种邀请的。

iii. 2010年7月14日，IRB审查并批准了一项涉及（b）（4）受试者的研究。IRB中没有在（b）（4）治疗中具有相关专业能力的委员（如医生），也没有任何文件显示IRB邀请了该领域的专家协助审查该项研究，21 CFR 56.107（f）是允许这种邀请的。

B. IRB允许非委员投票。

ⅰ. 2011年4月20日和2011年5月25日的IRB会议记录显示，“（b）（6）”参与了投票。但根据IRB委员名册，在这些会议举行时，（b）（6）并不是IRB的委员。

ⅱ 2010年7月7日和2010年7月14日的IRB会议记录显示，“（b）（6）”参与了投票。但根据IRB委员名册，在这些会议举行时，（b）（6）并不是IRB的委员。

2. IRB未能制定、维护并遵守关于对研究进行初始审查和跟踪审查的足够的书面程序［21 CFR 56.108（a）和56.115（a）（6）］

A. IRB的书面程序是不充分的，因为它没有要求被IRB批准的研究得到多数参会委员的批准。而21 CFR 56.108（c）中规定，如果IRB需要批准一项研究，就需要得到多数参会委员的批准。但是，IRB在标准操作规程（SOP）402“研究的初始审查”（4.1版，2010年1月13日）中规定：

（b）（4）。

根据本SOP，即使没有获得多数参会委员的批准，研究项目仍可以被视为“批准”。例如，如果五个主要的董事会委员出席一个IRB会议，而主席将投票限制为三名委员，那么只需要两个委员批准，研究项目就可被视为通过批准，也就是通过减少出席会议委员数量的方式达到目的。

您在2011年9月1日对2011年8月30日出具的FDA 483表（2011年9月1日的回复函）的回复函中，确认IRB的主席经常不顾出席会议的主要委员的人数，而将投票限制在三个人之间。如下表所示，会议记录显示，至少在11次会议中，一名主要的参会委员未参与投票。

会议日期	有投票或弃权记录的参会者 （候补委员用黑体标注）	无投票或弃权记录的主要参会人员
04/20/2010	（b）（6）	（b）（6）
07/07/2010	（b）（6）	（b）（6）
07/14/2010	（b）（6）	（b）（6）
08/11/2010	（b）（6）	（b）（6） 注：（b）（6）是IRB中唯一的医生委员；（b）（6）是一名制药专业的学生，他的资格与医生没有可比性
08/25/2010	（b）（6）	（b）（6） 注：（b）（6）是IRB中唯一的医生委员；（b）（6）是一名制药专业的学生，他的资格与医生没有可比性
09/01/2010	（b）（6）	（b）（6）
09/08/2010	（b）（6）	（b）（6）
09/15/2010	（b）（6）	（b）（6）
11/03/2010	（b）（6）	（b）（6）
02/23/2011	（b）（6）	（b）（6）

在2011年9月1日的回复函中，您给出的解释是IRB主席：

可以指定投票群体，这样可以确定一个有效的会议的法定人数，如果不是这样，IRB的会议将毫无意义。在每次IRB会议开始前，主席都会提前指定投票或讨论的人数，其目的是保障会议上的投票是一个有约束力的行为。

这种解释是不充分的，因为您的书面程序是允许未获得多数参会委员批准的研究项目得到IRB的批准。

B. BioMed IRB的SOP 402“研究的初始审查”（4.1版，2010年1月13日）中规定，在IRB投票会议前及会议期间应提供相关研究文件。此外，SOP 200“IRB委员”（4.2版，2010年7月29日）第7. H项中也提到了相关规定。

（b）（4）

FDA现场检查中发现几个例子证明了上述材料没有分发给所有IRB的参会委员。例如：

ⅰ. 2011年1月21日的IRB会议“备忘录”显示，2016年1月26日举行会议所需的新研究项目的材料已分发给主要委员（b）(6)，(b）(6）和候补委员（b）(6)。在这次会议上，主要委员（b）(6）和候补委员（b）(6）投票赞成了此项新的研究，但没有文件证明，他们在会议之前或在会议期间已经收到了关于新研究的材料，并有足够的时间审查这些新材料。

ⅱ. 2011年6月22日的IRB会议“备忘录”显示，关于新研究项目的材料提供给了三个主要委员（b）(6)，(b）(6）和候补委员（b）(6)。会议记录显示，一名未收到材料的主要委员（b）(6)，根据“备忘录”进行了投票。而另一位收到材料且出席会议的主要委员（b）(6）却被排除在投票之外。

在您2011年9月1日的回复函中，您解释到，会议材料是发给可能来参加会议的委员，但是他们也可能改变日程，不能参加会议。您声明，您计划将提前向全部委员发送电子版的会议资料，然而您没有提供文件证明这个纠正措施已经实施。

3. IRB的会议记录不足以显示会议的出席情况；IRB采取的行动；对行动的投票情况，包括赞成票数、反对票数和弃权票数；需要修正或不批准研究的理由；对争议问题进行讨论和解决的书面总结［21 CFR 56.115（a）(2)］

A. IRB会议记录信息不充分，不能显示会议出席人员情况，因为在会议记录中经常出现关于会议出席人员矛盾的信息。例如，下面的表格中显示，三个会议记录中的标题为“IRB行动观点”（“行动观点部分”）出现的人员和会议记录中的人员不同。

会议日期	会议记录部分	出席人员
12/09/2009	行动观点	11，22，33，4a，4b，4c，5a，5b，5c，5d
	会议记录	11，33，4a，4c，5c，5d，6e，77，88，99
04/07/2010	行动观点	11，22，33，aa，bb，cc，dd，ee
	会议记录	11，22，33，4a，4c，5d，6e，77，88，99
06/29/2011	行动观点	11，22，33，44，1a，1b，1c，1d
	会议记录	11，22，33，44，1a，1c，AA，AC，DD，1A，1C，1D，(b）(6)

B. 会议记录不能充分显示IRB已经采取的措施和对这些措施进行投票过程中包括的赞成票数、反对票数和弃权票数。

ⅰ. IRB有一项惯例是要求每一名参会委员记录自己的参会情况（或者在某些情况下，由一名会议“观察员”来记录)，然后IRB将这些委员的记录汇总成会议记录。此外，IRB常常会将先前的会议记录合并到后续的会议记录中。因此，会议记录往往超过150页，并且经常无法准确判断IRB采取的某些措施具体是在哪个会议中制定的。例如，2010年4月7日的会议记录显示，在这一天，IRB讨论了关于研究2的修改方案，并有条件地批准了方案修正案。但是与早期的会议记录对比，显示这些讨论和投票早在4个月前，即2009年12月9日就已经进行过了。

ⅱ. 2009年12月9日的会议记录中提到“法定投票数是三张”，但“投票总结”的章节显示只有两张选票。

ⅲ. 2011年1月17日的会议记录显示，至少有三名投票委员在场，但“投票总结”的章节显示只有两张选票。

ⅳ. 2011年1月19日的会议记录显示，至少有三名投票委员在场，但“投票总结”的章节显示只有两张选票。

在您2012年1月12日的回复函中，您提交了一份额外的“节选但仍为正式的会议记录”作为纠正措施以供FDA审查。创建多个版本的会议记录并不是一个可接受的纠正措施。每一份会议记录必须和IRB会议一一对应，而且会议记录必须准确记录每次会议中所采取的措施，包括每次投票的赞成票数、反对票数和弃权票数；需要变更或不批准研究的理由；和一份对争议问题进行讨论和相应解决方案的书面总结。

ⅴ. 会议记录，未能充分显示关于争议问题解决方案的书面总结。例如，2009年10月7日的会议记录显示，IRB在讨论“这家公司修改研究2的方案，急剧增加剂量的行为是否有点过快了”。会议记录还表明会议提出了关于保险支付的争论："会议长时间地讨论了伦理上应支付多少费用"然而，IRB未按要求将这些有争议问题的解决方案进行书面总结，并归类到会议记录中。

本警告信的目的并非是罗列IRB操作中存在的所有缺陷。您和IRB应设法纠正本信中提到的缺陷，并审查IRB的SOP及操作，确保完全符合法规要求，这些是您和IRB的职责。

基于这两次检查过程中发现的缺陷，包括第一次检查中发现的缺陷在第二次检查中被重复发现，我们无法确信IRB的程序足以保护研究中受试者的权益和福利。因此，根据 21 CFR 56.120（b）（1）和（2），

- FDA将不予批准受21 CFR 56管辖并由IRB批准的所有的新研究；
- 任何正在进行的受21 CFR 56管辖并由IRB批准的研究都不得招募新的受试者。

以上的限制令立即生效。

在您收到FDA的书面正式通知告知您已采取了足够的纠正措施之前，这些限制令将持续有效。这些限制令并不免除IRB应从仍在进行的研究项目中接收和应对意外的和严重的不良反应，并进行日常进度报告的职责。

自收到这封信的15个工作日内，您应当书面告知本办公室为促使IRB能够符合FDA法规要求已经或计划采取的具体措施。您应根据上述列出的缺陷项逐条进行回复，并提供必要的文件，证明所有适当的纠正措施已完成，对计划完成的纠正措施列明计划完成日期。

在您的回复函中，请提供一份关于IRB与每一个受到影响的申报者和临床研究者书面联系的副本，告知其FDA目前发布的限制令。

基于21 CFR 56.120和 56.121的授权，如果您不对本信内容进行回复，或不能采取适当的纠正措施，FDA可能采取进一步的监管措施。这些措施包括但不限于终止由IRB批准的涉及21 CFR 56的研究课题，并启动监管程序，取消IRB的资格。

根据您的回复，FDA可能会安排一次复查，确认纠正措施的充分性。

附：英文原文

Biomedical Research Institute of America d/b/a BioMed IRB

Warning Letter
March 29, 2012

CBER-12-0

Fred Fox,J.D.,Chairm an Emeritus, Executive Director
Biomedical Research Institute of America dba BioMed IRB
7676 Hazard Center Drive,Suite 500
San Diego, California92108

Dear Mr.Fox:

This letter describes the results of the Food and Drug Administration (FDA) inspections of the BioMedical Research Institute of America, doing business as BioMed Institutional Review Board (hereafter referred to as "the IRB"), which were conducted from September 22 through October 25, 2010, and from August 8 through August 19, 2011. The first inspection focused on the IRB's review of selected studies for the sponsor (b)(4) and was conducted by a Los Angeles District FDA investigator. Due to the nature of the deficiencies observed in the first inspection, a second inspection was conducted to provide a broader assessment of the IRB's operations. The second inspection was conducted by the same district FDA investigator accompanied by an inspector from the Center for Biologics Evaluation and Research (CBER). The FDA representative(s) conducted the inspections to determine if the IRB's procedures for the protection of human subjects comply with FDA regulations published in the Title 21, Code of Federal Regulations (CFR), Parts 50 and 56. The inspections were part of FDA's Bioresearch Monitoring Program, which includes inspections designed to review IRB operations for clinical studies using investigational products and for the protection of human subjects.

The focus of the first inspection was limited to the following studies: (b)(4) (b)(4)

The focus of the follow-up inspection included meeting minutes, membership, and general review of research by the IRB.

The FDA investigator from the FDA Los Angeles District Office issued and discussed the Forms FDA 483 Inspectional Observations with you at the conclusion of each inspection. The FDA inspector from CBER participated by telephone at the close of the second inspection. We received and reviewed the IRB's responses to the Forms FDA 483, which were dated November 2, 2010, August 30, 2011, September 1, 2011, September 2, 2011, September 15, 2011, and January 12, 2012.

We have determined that the IRB significantly violated applicable federal regulations governing the operation and responsibilities of IRBs as published in Title 21, Code of Federal Regulations (CFR), Part 56 (available at http://www.access.gpo.gov/cgi-bin/cfrassemble.cgi?title=201021). The applicable provisions of the CFR are cited for each violation listed below.

1. The IRB failed to fulfill membership requirements. [21 CFR § 56.107].

A. The IRB did not possess the professional competence necessary to adequately review the specific research activities. For example:

i. On January 27, 2010, the IRB reviewed and approved a study involving subjects with (b) (4). Review of the IRB's records indicates that the IRB lacked the professional competence necessary to review this study and determine whether it met the criteria for approval under 21 CFR 56.111, including whether risks to subjects were "reasonable in relation to anticipated benefits, if any, to subjects, and the importance of the knowledge that may be expected to result." For example, the IRB did not include an individual with professional competence in (b)(4) (e.g., a physician), nor is there any documentation to show that the IRB invited individuals with competence in this area to assist in the review of this study, as permitted by 21 CFR 56.107(f).

ii. On July 7, 2010, the IRB reviewed and approved a study of subjects with (b)(4). The IRB did not include an individual with professional competence in (b)(4) treatment (e.g., a physician), nor is there any documentation to show that the IRB invited individuals with competence in this area to assist in the review of this study, as permitted by 21 CFR 56.107(f).

iii. On July 14, 2010, the IRB reviewed and approved a study involving subjects with (b)(4). The IRB did not include an individual with professional competence in (b)(4) (e.g., a physician) nor is there any documentation to show that the IRB invited individuals with competence in this area to assist in the review of this study, as permitted by 21 CFR 56.107(f).

B. The IRB allowed non-members to vote.

i. IRB meeting minutes from April 20, 2011, and May 25, 2011, show that an attendee identified as "(b)(6)" participated in voting. According to the IRB membership rosters, (b)(6) was not a member of the IRB when these meetings were conducted.

ii. IRB meeting minutes from July 7, 2010, and July 14, 2010, show that an attendee identified as "(b)(6)" participated in voting. According to the IRB membership rosters, (b)(6) was not a member of the IRB when these meetings were conducted.

2. Failure to prepare, maintain, and follow adequate written procedures for conducting th review of research, including initial and continuing review. [21 CFR §§ 56.108(a) and 56.115(a)(6)].

A. The IRB's written procedures are inadequate because they do not require the approval of a majority of those members present at the meeting for research to be approved by the IRB. Under 21 CFR 56.108(c), in order for research to be approved by an IRB, it must receive "the approval of a majority of those members present at the meeting." However, the IRB's Standard Operating Procedure (SOP) 402, Initial Review of Research, (version 4.1 January 13, 2010), provides that:

(b)(4)

Under this SOP, research could be deemed "approved" without the approval of a majority of those members present at the meeting. For example, if five primary Board members are present at an IRB meeting and the Chair limits voting to three members, research could be deemed approved by the IRB with just two approval votes; i.e., by a minority of the members present at the meeting.

Your September 1, 2011 letter responding to the Form 483 issued to you on August 30, 2011 ("September 1, 2011 response letter"), confirms that the IRB Chair "routinely limited voting" to three members regardless of the number of primary Board members who were present at the meeting. As shown in the table below, meeting minutes for at least 11 meetings indicate that the attendees who voted did not include one of the primary members in attendance at the meeting.

Meeting Date	Attendees with recorded vote or abstention("alternate members" in bold)	Primary member in attendance with no recorded vote or abstention
04/20/2010	**(b)(6)**	**(b)(6)**
07/07/2010	**(b)(6)**	**(b)(6)**
07/14/2010	**(b)(6)**	**(b)(6)**
08/11/2010	**(b)(6)**	**(b)(6)**NOTE: (b)(6) is the only physician member of the IRB; (b)(6) is a pharmacy student whose qualifications are not comparable.
08/25/2010	**(b)(6)**	**(b)(6)** NOTE: (b)(6) is the only physician member of the IRB; (b)(6) is a pharmacy student whose qualifications are not comparable.
09/01/2010	**(b)(6)**	**(b)(6)**
11/03/2010	**(b)(6)**	**(b)(6)**
01/26/2011	**(b)(6)**	**(b)(6)**
02/23/2011	**(b)(6)**	**(b)(6)**

In your September 1, 2011 response letter, you explain that the IRB Chair:

…can designate the voting quorum so that there is certainty in an effective quorum for the meeting, and, without that, the IRB meeting would be worthless. The chairman makes that designation in advance of voting or discussion, at the start of any IRB meeting, and the purpose is to safeguard that there will be a binding action voted at the meeting.

This explanation is not adequate because your written procedures would allow research to be approved by the IRB without the approval of a majority of those members present at the meeting.

B. The BioMed IRB's SOP 402, Initial Review of Research (version 4.1 January 13, 2010), states that pertinent study documentation is made available to the IRB voting members prior to and during the meeting. In addition, SOP 200 Membership of the IRB, (version 4.2 July 29, 2010) Item 7.H. states (b)(4)

The FDA inspection noted several instances where the materials described above were not distributed to all IRB members who attended the meeting. Examples include:

i. An IRB meeting "Memorandum" dated January 21, 2011, indicates that the materials for new studies on the agenda for the January 26, 2011, meeting were distributed to primary members (b)(6), and (b)(6) and alternate member (b)(6). At this meeting, primary member (b)(6) and alternate member (b)(6) voted on the new studies but there is no documentation to show that they received the new study materials for review prior to the meeting or had adequate time during the meeting to review the new materials.

ii. An IRB meeting "Memorandum" for a meeting scheduled June 22, 2011, shows that material for new studies were provided to three primary members (b)(6), and (b)(6), and alternate member (b)(6). The meeting minutes show that primary member (b)(6), who did not receive the materials according to the "Memorandum," voted at the meeting. Member (b)(6), a primary member who was present at the meeting and received the materials, was excluded from voting.

In your September 1, 2011, letter, you explain that meeting materials are sent to members who are likely to be available and that their availability may change. You state that your future plans include distributing materials in advance to all members electronically. However, you have not provided documentation to show that this proposed corrective action has been implemented.

3. Minutes of IRB meetings are not sufficient to show attendance at the meetings; actions taken by the IRB; the vote on these actions including the number of members voting for, against, and abstaining; the basis for requiring changes in or disapproving research; and a written summary of the discussion of controverted issues and their resolution. [21 CFR § 56.115(a)(2)].

A. The IRB's meeting minutes are not sufficient to show attendance at meetings because they often contain conflicting information concerning who attended the meeting. For example, as shown in the table below, for three meetings, a summary section of the minutes entitled "IRB Action View" ("Action View section") identified a different group of attendees than the body of the minutes.

Meeting Date	Section of Minutes	Identified Individuals in Attendance
12/09/09	Action View Body	11,22,33,4a,4b,4c,5a,5b,5c,5d 11,33,4a,4c,5c,5d,6e,77,88,99
04/07/10	Action View Body	11,22,33,aa,bb,cc,dd,ee 11,22,33, 4a,4c,5d,6e,77,88,99
06/29/11	Action View Body	11,22,33,44,1a,1b,1c,1d 11,22,33,44,1a,1c,AA,AC,DD,1A,1C,1D, **(b)(6)**

B. Minutes are not sufficient to show actions taken by the IRB and the vote on these actions including the number of members voting for, against, and abstaining.

i. The IRB had a practice of requiring each member present at a meeting to capture his/her own notes on what occurred at the meeting (or in some instances, a meeting "Observer" recorde a member's minutes). The IRB then assembled all of the notes from these multiple individuals into a single document to create minutes for the meeting. Additionally, the IRB often incorporate portions of minutes from previous meetings into the minutes of subsequent meetings. As a result the minutes for any given meeting are often more than 150 pages long, and often do not accurately represent the actions of the IRB at that particular meeting. For example, the meeting minutes for April 7, 2010 indicate that, on that date, the IRB debated proposed protocol amendments to Study 2, and conditionally approved certain protocol amendments. However, comparison with minutes from earlier meetings indicates that the discussion and vote occurred four months earlier, on December 9, 2009.

ii. The meeting minutes for December 9, 2009, state that "a quorum of three members voted," but the "Summary of Votes" section documents only two votes.

iii. The meeting minutes for January 17, 2011, indicate that at least three voting members were present, but the "Summary of Votes" section documents only two votes.

iv. The meeting minutes for January 19, 2011, indicate that at least three voting members were present, but the "Summary of Votes" section documents a total of only two votes.

In your January 12, 2012 letter, as a corrective action you propose generating an additional "truncated yet still an official set of minutes" for FDA's review. Creating multiple versions of meeting minutes is not an acceptable corrective action. One set of minutes should be prepared for each IRB meeting, and the minutes must accurately represent the actions of the IRB at that particular meeting, including the number of members voting for, against, and abstaining from each action; the basis for requiring changes in or disapproving research; and a written summary of the discussion of controverted issues and their resolution.

v. Minutes are not sufficient to show a written summary of the resolution of controverted issues. For example, minutes from a meeting held on October 7, 2009, indicate that the IRB debated whether "it is a little too soon for the company to amend the protocol [for Study 2] to have the dosage so dramatically increased." The minutes also indicate that controversy was raised regarding the insurance payment: "a long conversation addresses the ethical question of price/payment in regards to how much is ethical to ask someone to pay." However, no written summary of the resolution of these controverted issues was included in the meeting minutes as required.

This letter is not intended to contain an all-inclusive list of deficiencies in the operations of the IRB. It is incumbent upon you and the IRB to correct the violations cited in this letter, and to conduct a thorough review of the IRB's SOPs and practices to ensure full compliance with the regulations.

Based on the deficiencies found during these two inspections, including deficiencies observed in the firs inspection that were also found in the second inspection, we have no assurance that the IRB procedure are adequately protecting the rights and welfare of the human subjects of research. For this reason, in accordance with 21 CFR §§ 56.120(b)(1) and (2), and effective immediately,

- FDA will withhold approval of all new studies subject to 21 CFR Part 56 and reviewed by the IRB; and
- No new subjects are to be enrolled in any ongoing studies subject to 21 CFR Part 56 an approved by the IRB.

These restrictions will remain in effect until such time that you have received written notification from this office that adequate corrections have been made. These restrictions do not relieve the IRB of its responsibility for receiving and reacting to reports of unexpected and serious reactions and routine progress reports from ongoing studies.

You are to notify this office in writing, within fifteen (15) business days of receipt of this letter, of the specific actions you have taken or plan to take to bring the IRB into full compliance with FDA regulations. Your response should address each item listed above, and should include any documentation necessary to show that full and adequate correction has been achieved. Include the projected completion dates for each action to be accomplished.

Include with your response, a copy of the IRB's written communication to each of the affected sponsor and clinical investigators, notifying them of the current FDA imposed restrictions.

Your failure to respond to this letter, or to implement adequate corrective action, may result in further administrative actions, as authorized by 21 CFR §§ 56.120 and 56.121. These actions include, but are not limited to, the termination of ongoing studies subject to 21 CFR Part 56 and approved by your IRB, and the initiation of regulatory proceedings for disqualification of your IRB.

On the basis of your response, FDA may schedule a reinspection to confirm the adequacy of your corrective actions.

Please send your written response to:

Christine J. Drabick
Division of Inspections and Surveillance (HFM-664)
Office of Compliance and Biologics Quality Center for Biologics Evaluation and Research
1401 Rockville Pike, Suite 200N
Rockville, Maryland, 20852-1448
Telephone: (301) 827-6336

We request that you send a copy of your response to the FDA District Office listed below.

Sincerely,

/S/

Mary A. Malarkey, Director
Office of Compliance and Biologics Quality
Center for Biologics Evaluation and Research

Cc:Alonza Cruse, District Director, HFR-PA200
Food and Drug Administration
19701 Fairchild
Irvine, CA 92612
Kristina Borror, Ph.D., Director
Division of Compliance Oversight
Office for Human Research Protections
1101 Wooton Parkway, Suite 200
Rockville, MD 20852

第16封　给Northeast-Northwest基督教医院的警告信

2012年3月27日

参考号：CBER-12-02

尊敬的McMullen先生：

这封信特告知您2011年12月2日结束的，FDA对NE-NW基督教医院伦理委员会（IRB）进行现场检查的结果。FDA检查员对伦理委员会进行了现场检查，以核实其保护受试者的程序是否符合发布在美国联邦法规第21篇第50和56部分的FDA法规。FDA实施的这次现场检查属于生物研究监查项目，该项目通过设定的检查方法来检查伦理委员会对试验药物的临床研究和保护受试者的各项操作。

在现场检查结束时，检查员出示了FDA483表，即现场检查发现的问题，并与您和几个伦理委员会委员进行了讨论。我们审查了FDA现场检查报告、FDA483表，以及日期为2011年12月21日对FDA483表的书面回复。

我们认定该伦理委员会严重违反美国联邦法规第21篇第56部分（见http://www.gpoaccess.gov/cfr/index.html）关于伦理委员会运行和责任的适用的联邦规定。每一项违规行为均已标明适用的联邦法规条款。我们写信给您是因为根据21 CFR 56.120（c），上级机构应对该伦理委员会的运行负责。作为上级机构，您的责任应包括确保伦理委员会采取必要的措施，使其完全符合FDA法规。

1. IRB未能制定、维护和遵守关于对研究进行初始审查和跟踪审查的书面程序［21 CFR 56.108（a）和56.115（a）（6）］

伦理委员会没有遵循题为"涉及受试者的临床研究以及伦理委员会政策"书面程序规定的程序和操作。

A. 伦理委员会没有根据其程序的要求保留出席人员的签到表，包括如下会议：11/23/2009，5/19/2010，7/14/2010，3/1/2011，8/25/2011和11/11/2011。

您的回复中提到计划修订伦理委员会的书面程序，终止使用出席签到表，使用由伦理委员会负责人管理的出席工作本替代，并作为所有会议记录附件保存。如果顺利执行，您的纠正措施看来是充分的。考虑到伦理委员会之前没有遵循书面程序，请在对本信的回复中说明贵机构已经采用哪些步骤来确保伦理委员会将遵守修订的规程。

B. 审查2009年到2011年伦理委员会的会议记录发现，伦理委员会始终没有确保至少有一名医师在每次会前审查方案。伦理委员会规程指出，"整个方案应在会前提交给至少一名医师审查"。您的信中包括了修订的议程模板，旨在促使伦理委员会管理者在收到新方案时指定一名初级医师审查员。如果顺利执行，您的纠正措施看来是充分的。

C. 伦理委员会允许委员和其候补人员在同一个召集会议上投票。2011年11月11日会议记录显示，委员（b）（6）和他指定的候补人员（b）（6）同时出席。

在信中您解释这是伦理委员会的记录错误，该期间（b）（6）是一名正式委员。回信的附件中，您提交了修订后的人员名册，其中列出了（b）（6）作为投票委员。这说明在那期间伦理委员会的名册已过期。我们提醒您，伦理委员会的书面程序要求委员名册至少每年更新，并由每一位委员和候补人员的签名与日期。

D. 伦理委员会没有将其在考虑风险程度后认定为合适的拟定研究批准期限记录在2010～2011年的会议

记录中。伦理委员会的书面程序对该项认定做出要求。您12月21日的回复包括了修订后的会议议程模板，模板中有指定区域用于记录批准的期限。如果顺利执行，您的纠正措施看来是充分的。

在2003年的FDA最近一次检查中也指出了伦理委员会未遵循书面程序的违规情况重复出现。在您2011年12月21日的信中，提供了包括伦理委员会书面程序数次修订的纠正计划，预计于2012年1月由伦理委员会批准实行。对这封信的回复中，应提交修订后、已批准的伦理委员会书面程序。

2. IRB未能准备和保存足够的IRB活动记录［21 CFR 56.115（a）］

A. 2009年到2011年，伦理委员会会议记录没有就其所采取的行动投票提供充分细节，包括赞成票数、反对票数和弃权票数。会议记录使用“意见一致”一词来记录投票情况。伦理委员会主席称，（b）（6）委员在单独的投票纸上记录投票情况（赞成、反对或放弃），该投票纸保存在每一个方案中。但是检查期间审查的五份方案中有两份方案的记录中并没有投票纸。

在您的信中，您附上了修订的会议记录/议程模板，以促使伦理委员会管理者在今后的会议记录中能够记录投票人员和讨论的内容。如能顺利执行，您的纠正措施看来是充分的。

伦理委员会未能根据21 CFR 56.115（a）（2）的规定保存会议记录，该违规情况在最近两次2003年和1998年FDA检查中重复出现。

B. 会议记录和签到表中关于出席人员的记录不一致。

ⅰ. 日期为2/3/2010的会议记录列出了包括（b）（6）在内的6位出席委员，但是签到表有5个签名，（b）（6）列为请假。

ⅱ. 日期为11/10/2010的会议记录列出7位出席委员，并且没有请假的委员，但是签到表中有5个签名，（b）（6）和（b）（6）列为请假。

ⅲ. 日期为5/3/2011的会议记录列出6位出席委员，（b）（6）列为请假，但是签到表中有5个签名，（b）（6）和（b）（6）列为请假。

ⅳ. 日期为7/12/2011的会议记录列出（b）（6）作为委员出席，但是签到表中没有他的签名。根据7/12/2011时的委员名册，（b）（6）是（b）（6）的候补。（b）（6）的签名在7/12/2011的签到表上，但是没有作为当天会议记录的出席人员列出。

C. 伦理委员会未能在会议记录中记录一名委员因利益冲突而放弃方案投票。时间为5/3/2011的会议记录没有记录（b）（6）放弃（b）（4）和（b）（4）方案的投票，包括签名和投票情况的方案审查签名表显示，（b）（6）放弃投票。

D. 伦理委员会没有按照21 CFR 56.115（a）（5）规定，保存2010年和2011年伦理委员会委员名册。伦理委员会委员名册不能准确地反映现有的委员会委员。而且，名册无法通过代表职能、雇佣或委员和机构之间其他关系来识别委员。您回复中提供的修订后委员名册缺少2011年的生效日期。此外，没有根据伦理委员会书面程序要求每位委员签名。在本封信的回复中，请提供符合伦理委员会书面程序要求的更新后的委员名册。

伦理委员会未能根据21 CFR 56.115（a）（5）的规定，保存伦理委员会委员名册的违规情况，在2003年和1998年这最近2次的FDA检查中重复出现。

您2011年12月21日的信中提供的纠正计划包括修订的会议记录/议程格式和作为今后伦理委员会记录附件的新的出席记录本。对本封信的回复中，请提交2012年伦理委员会所有会议记录复印件，以证明充分执行了纠正计划。

3. IRB未能在大多数IRB委员出席，其中至少包括一位来自非科学领域的委员的召集会议上，对拟开展的研究进行审查［21 CFR 56.108（c）］

A. 至少在4次大多数伦理委员会委员没有出席的会议上，11/23/2009，5/19/2010，3/1/2011 和 5/3/2011，伦理委员会就新方案进行投票，审查了不良事件报告，并且对研究进行阶段性审查。

名册中伦理委员会委员数量	会议日期	出席的伦理委员会委员数	意见
12	11/23/2009	5	
10	5/19/2010	5	
10	3/1/2011	5	在记录中，（b）（6）作为出席委员列出，但是没有列入那段时期的委员名册中，因此她不能被计票而形成多数
10	5/3/2011	5	在记录中，（b）（6）作为出席委员列出，但是没有列入那段时期的委员名册中，因此她不能被计票而形成多数

B. 伦理委员会在3/1/2011 和 5/3/2011会议上批准了新研究方案，而当时并没有非科学领域的委员参加。在上述表格3.A.项中，（b）（6）出席了3/1/2011和5/3/2011会议，但是实际上在那期间她未包括在委员名册中。因此，（b）（6）不应具有投票权，构成多数派中的一票，或者被认为是伦理委员会非科学领域的委员。我们提醒您，伦理委员会会议记录和委员名册必须准确反映委员会委员。委员名册必须根据变化及时更新。

在您2011年12月21日的信中，提交了新的出席记录本作为此发现项的纠正措施。根据您的回信，将创建出席记录本，以充分解决会议出勤、记录委员进出会议、识别委员作用（如投票或未投票）。如能顺利执行，您的纠正措施看来是充分的。

本警告信的目的并非是罗列贵伦理委员会在运行中存在的所有缺陷。信中我们指出了之前在2003年和1998年检查中，重复出现的违规情况。

在您的回复中，请说明贵机构如何确保贵伦理委员会采取必要的措施使其完全符合FDA法规要求。

自收到这封信的15个工作日内，请书面告知本办公室您为预防将来发生类似违规情况已经或计划采取的措施。回复中请附修订后文件的复印件，如书面程序和近期会议记录。鉴于过去未能按照书面程序执行，也请描述能够确保充分执行修订程序的计划。

如果不能充分地回复本信并采取合适的纠正措施，可能导致我们依照21 CFR 56.120 和 56.121的授权对伦理委员会采取进一步的行政措施，包括根据美国联邦法规第21篇第50和56部分的规定暂缓批准伦理委员会审议的新研究，根据第50和56部分的规定禁止新的受试者入组进行的研究，终止所有伦理委员会已批准的现行研究，并启动取消伦理委员会资格的监管流程。

附：英文原文

Christian Hospital Northeast- Northwest

WARNING LETTER

March 27, 2012

By Facsimile Transmission and Overnight Delivery

CBER- 12- 02

Ronald B. McMullen, President
Christian Hospital Northeast-Northwest
11133 Dunn Road
St. Louis, Missouri 63136

Dear Mr. McMullen:

This letter describes the results of a Food and Drug Administration (FDA) inspection of the Christian Hospital NE-NW Institutional Review Board (IRB) that concluded on December 2, 2011. The FDA investigator conducted the inspection of this Institutional Review Board (IRB) to determine if the IRB's procedures for the protection of human subjects comply with FDA regulations published in Title 21, Code of Federal Regulations (CFR), Parts 50 and 56. The FDA conducted this inspection under its Bioresearch Monitoring Program, which includes inspections designed to review IRB operations for clinical studies of investigational products and for the protection of human subjects.

At the end of the inspection a Form FDA 483, Inspectional Observations, was issued and discussed with you and several IRB staff members. We reviewed the inspection report, the Form FDA 483 and your letter dated December 21, 2011 sent in response to the Form FDA 483.

We have determined that the IRB significantly violated applicable federal regulations governing the operation and responsibilities of the IRBs as published under 21 CFR Part 56 (available at http://www.gpoaccess.gov/cfr/index.html). The applicable provisions of the CFR are cited for each violation. We are addressing this letter to you because, under 21 CFR 56.120(c), the parent institution is presumed to be responsible for the operation of the IRB. As the parent institution, it is within your responsibility to ensure that the IRB takes the actions necessary to bring the IRB into full compliance with FDA regulations.

1. The IRB failed to prepare, maintain and follow its written procedure for conducting its initial and continuing review of research. [21 CFR §§ 56.108(a) and 56.115(a)(6)].

The IRB did not adhere to the procedures and practices established for the IRB in its written procedure entitled "Clinical Research involving Human Subjects and Institutional Review Committee Policy."

A. The IRB failed to maintain attendance sign in sheets as required by the IRB's procedure for the following meetings: 11/23/2009, 5/19/2010, 7/14/2010, 3/1/2011, 8/25/2011 and 11/11/2011.

In your response you proposed to revise the IRB's written procedure to discontinue use of the attendance sign in sheet and replace it with an attendance log managed by the IRB administrator and maintained as an attachment to all meeting minutes. Your corrective actions appear to be adequate if successfully implemented. In your response to this letter please explain what steps the institution has taken to ensure that the revised procedure will be followed given that the IRB did not follow the previous written procedure.

B. A review of the IRB meeting minutes for 2009 through 2011 revealed that the IRB did not consistently have at least one physician member review protocols prior to each meeting. The IRB procedure states, "The entire protocol.... shall be sent for review to at least one (1) physician member reasonably prior to the meeting." In your letter you included a revised agenda template that will prompt the IRB administrator to assign a primary physician reviewer upon receipt of a new protocol. Your corrective actions appear to be adequate if successfully implemented.

C. The IRB allowed a member and his/her alternate to vote at the same convened meeting. The meeting minutes from 11/11/2011 list both the member (b)(6) and his designated alternate (b)(6) as members present.

In your letter you explained this was a clerical error on the IRB's part and that (b)(6) was a regular member during that period. As an attachment to your letter, you submitted a revised membership roster listing (b)(6) as a voting member. This implies that the IRB roster at that time was out of date. We remind you that your IRB written procedures require the membership roster to be updated at least annually, dated, and signed by each member and alternate.

D. The IRB meeting minutes between 2010 and 2011 do not document the period of approval for proposed research determined to be appropriate by the IRB after considering the degree of risk. This determination is required under the IRB's written procedures. In your December 21 response, you included a revised meeting agenda template with a designated area for documenting the period of approval. Your corrective actions appear to be adequate if successfully implemented.

The IRB's failure to follow its written procedures is a repeated violation that was identified during the last FDA inspection in 2003. In your letter dated December 21, 2011, you provided a plan of correction that includes several revisions to the IRB written procedure with an anticipated ratification date by the IRB for January 2012. In your response to this letter include a copy of the current revised and approved IRB written procedure(s).

2. The IRB failed to prepare and maintain adequate documentation of IRB activities. [21 CFR § 56.115(a)].

A. IRB meeting minutes for 2009 through 2011 were not prepared in sufficient detail to show the vote on the actions taken by the IRB, including the number of members voting for, against and abstaining. The meeting minutes used the term "unanimous" to document the vote actions. According to the IRB Chair, (b)(6) the members record their votes (yes, no, or abstain) on a separate voting sheet which is maintained with each protocol. Two of the five protocols reviewed during the inspection did not have voting sheets maintained with the protocol records.

In your letter, you attached a revised meeting minutes/agenda format that will prompt the IRB administrators to record voting numbers and discussion points for future IRB meeting minutes. Your corrective actions appear to be adequate if successfully implemented.

The IRB's failure to maintain meeting minutes in accordance with 21 CFR 56.115(a)(2) is a repeated violation identified in the last two FDA inspections conducted in 2003 and 1998.

B. There are discrepancies between the meeting minutes and the attendance sign-in sheet regarding which members were present.

i. The meeting minutes dated 2/3/2010 list 6 members present including (b)(6), but the attendance sign in sheet has 5 signatures with (b)(6) listed as excused.

ii. The meeting minutes dated 11/10/2010 list 7 members present and no excused members, but the attendance sheet has 5 signatures with (b)(6) and (b)(6) listed as excused.

iii. The meeting minutes dated 5/3/2011 listed 6 members present with (b)(6) listed as excused, the attendance sheet had 5 signatures with (b)(6) and (b)(6) listed as excused.

iv. The meeting minutes dated 7/12/2011 list (b)(6) as a member present but the attendance sheet does not have his signature. According to the membership roster for 7/12/2011, (b)(6) is an alternate member for (b)(6). (b)(6) signature is on the sign in sheet for 7/12/2011 but is not listed as a member present in the meeting minutes for that date.

C. The IRB failed to document in the meeting minutes that a member abstained from voting on a protocol in which the member has a conflict of interest. The meeting minutes dated 5/3/2011 do not document that (b)(6) abstained from voting on protocols (b)(4) and (b)(4). The protocol review signature sheet, which includes members' signatures and their votes, indicates that (b)(6) abstained from voting.

D. The IRB failed to maintain IRB membership rosters for 2010 and 2011 in accordance with 21 CFR 56.115(a)(5). The IRB membership rosters do not accurately reflect current IRB membership. Furthermore, the rosters do not identify members by their representative capacity, and any employment or other relationship between each member and the institution. In your letter, you provided a revised membership roster lacking an effective date in 2011. Additionally, it is not signed by each member as required by the IRB's written procedure. In your response to this letter please provide an updated membership roster that is in compliance with the IRB written procedure.

The IRB's failure to maintain IRB membership rosters in accordance with 21 CFR 56.115(a)(5) is a repeated violation identified in the last two FDA inspections conducted in 2003 and 1998.

In your letter dated December 21, 2011, you provided a plan of correction that included a revised meeting minutes/agenda format and a new attendance log that is a required attachment to the future IRB minutes. In your response to this letter, please submit a copy of the IRB's meeting minutes for all meetings conducted to date in 2012 to demonstrate successful implementation.

3. The IRB failed to review proposed research at convened meetings at which a majority of the members of the IRB were present, including at least one member whose primary concerns are in nonscientific areas. [21 CFR § 56.108(c)].

A. The IRB voted on new protocols, reviewed reports of adverse events, and conducted periodic review of studies on at least four meeting dates, 11/23/2009, 5/19/2010, 3/1/2011 and 5/3/2011, at which a majority of IRB members were not in attendance.

No.of IRB members on roster	Meeting date	No.of IRB members present	Comment
12	11/23/2009	5	
10	5/19/2010	5	
10	3/1/2011	5	**(b)(6)**is listed as a member present in the minutes but was not listed on the membership roster in effect for that time period so she should not have been counted toward a majority
10	5/3/2011	5	**(b)(6)**is listed as a member present in the minutes but was not listed on the membership roster in effect for that time period so she should not have been counted toward a majority

B. The IRB approved new research protocols on 3/1/2011 and 5/3/2011 when there was no member present whose primary concerns are in nonscientific areas. As noted in the table located in Item 3.A., above, (b)(6) is listed as a member present at the meetings held on 3/1/2011 and 5/3/2011 but was not an IRB member according to the membership roster in effect for that time period. As a result, (b)(6) should not have been allowed to vote, count toward a majority, or be considered to be the IRB's nonscientific member. We remind you that the IRB minutes and membership roster must accurately reflect IRB membership. The membership roster must be updated as changes occur.

In your letter dated December 21, 2011, you submitted a new attendance log as the corrective action for this observation. According to your letter, the attendance log was created to sufficiently address meeting attendance, document when individual members log in and out of the meeting as well as to identify individual member roles (i.e. voting or nonvoting). Your corrective actions appear to be adequate, if successfully implemented.

This letter is not intended to contain an all-inclusive list of deficiencies in the operations of the IRB. Throughout this letter we have identified several repeated violations noted during previous FDA inspections conducted in 2003 and 1998. In your response to this letter please explain how the institution will ensure that the IRB takes the actions necessary to bring the IRB into full compliance with FDA regulations.

Please notify this office in writing, within fifteen (15) business days of receipt of this letter, of the actions you have taken or plan to take to bring the IRB into compliance with FDA requirements. Please include a copy of any revised documents, such as written procedures and recent meeting minutes, with your response. Given the past failure to follow written procedures, please also describe your plans to assure compliance with your revised procedures.

Your failure to adequately respond to this letter and take appropriate corrective action may result in further administrative actions against your IRB, as authorized by 21 CFR 56.120 and 56.121. These actions could include FDA withholding approval of new studies reviewed by your IRB that are subject to 21 CFR Parts 50 and 56 of the FDA regulations, prohibiting the admission of new subjects to ongoing studies that are subject to Parts 50 and 56, terminating all ongoing studies approved by your IRB, and initiating regulatory proceedings for disqualification of your IRB.

Please send your written response to:

Lillian Ortega
Division of Inspections and Surveillance (HFM-664)
Office of Compliance and Biologics Quality
Center for Biologics Evaluation and Research
1401 Rockville Pike, Suite 200N
Rockville, MD 20852-1448
Telephone: (301) 827-6335

Sincerely,

/S/

Mary A. Malarkey, Director
Office of Compliance and Biologics Quality
Center for Biologics Evaluation and Research

Cc: John Thorsky, District Director
Food and Drug Administration
11510 West 80th Street
Lenexa, Kansas 66214

Kristina Borror, Ph. D., Director
Division of Compliance Oversight
Office for Human Research Protections
1101 Wootton Parkway, Suite 200
Rockville, Maryland 20852

第17封 给海湾地区医疗中心伦理委员会的警告信

2011年12月20日

参考号：12-HFD-45-12-01

尊敬的Incarnati先生：

2011年6月22日至6月24日，Nancy Bellamy女士代表FDA，对海湾地区医疗中心（以下简称BRMC）伦理委员会（IRB 注册号 00003638）进行了现场检查。本次检查的目的是核实贵伦理委员会对受试者保护的程序是否符合美国联邦法规（CFR）第21篇第50和56部分的要求。这些法规适用于FDA所监管产品的临床研究。我们知道在现场检查结束时，我们的检查员向Alice Gerard女士（主席及首席执行官）和她的员工出示了FDA483表，即现场检查发现的问题，并进行了讨论。经对现场检查报告、该报告的附件，以及BRMC 2011年6月30日针对现场检查发现的问题的书面回复进行审查，我们认为，贵伦理委员会没有遵循适用的法律要求和监管受试者保护的FDA法规。我们想强调如下：

1. IRB未能遵循关于快速审查程序的FDA法规［21 CFR 56.110（b）］

法规要求快速审查可由IRB负责人或由负责人指定的一个或多个有经验的IRB委员来进行。IRB可在以下两种情况或其中之一情况下采用快速审查程序：①联邦注册表上列出的部分或全部研究“受试者保护：可以由IRB通过快速审查程序进行审查的研究类别”[1]，由审查者发现研究大于最小风险；②在先前批准的研究有效期内对批准研究的微小变更。

根据联邦注册通告，快速审查可用于以下情况的跟踪审查：

- （i）研究将永久停止入组新的受试者；（ii）所有的受试者已经完成所有研究相关的干预措施；（iii）研究处于受试者长期随访阶段；或者
- 没有受试者入组，并且没有发现其他风险；或者
- 剩下的研究活动仅限于数据分析。

BRMC的IRB 对不符合快速审查标准的项目采用了快速跟踪审查方式进行了跟踪审查和批准。类似的情况如下，但不仅限于以下所列：

a. 2011年5月 18日，IRB主席采用快速审查程序对研究项目（b）（4）“（b）（4）”进行了跟踪审查和批准。但是，IRB在2011年3月21日被告知，有一个受试者已经在BRMC入组，并且该研究项目仍处于受试者入组阶段。因此研究项目（b）（4）不符合快速跟踪审查的标准。

b. 2010年6月23日，IRB主席采用快速审查程序对研究项目（b）（4）“（b）（4）”进行了跟踪审查和批准。但是，IRB在2010年6月14日被告知，有一个受试者已经在BRMC入组，并且该研究项目仍处于受试者入组阶段。因此研究项目（b）（4）不符合快速跟踪审查的标准。

c. 2010年6月23日，IRB主席采用快速审查程序对研究项目（b）（4）“（b）（4）”进行了跟踪审查和批准。现场检查中发现，在对研究项目（b）（4）进行快速审查时，一些受试者在BRMC已经入组并且试验仍处于受试者入组阶段。因此研究项目（b）（4）不符合快速跟踪审查的标准。

该IRB不恰当地采用快速审查程序进行快速跟踪审查和批准，不符合21 CFR 56.110（b）的要求。（b）（4）试验研究仍处于受试者入组阶段，并且有受试者已经入组，不符合快速跟踪审查的标准。这些试验项目跟踪审查应该通过一个正式召集的、有多数IRB委员参加的会议来审查和批准。

BRMC在 2011年6月30日对FDA483表的书面回复中写到，关于快速审查的相关SOPs已经进行了修订，以纠正这些违规。书面回复中指出，将在下一次IRB会议上针对快速审查的符合标准为IRB工作人员和委员

提供学习资料和培训。书面回复中还进一步提到现场培训将记入会议记录，并且培训材料的复印件也会同会议记录一起保存。我们认为这些回复不够充分，因为修改的SOP并不足以说明如何避免将来发生上述不恰当采用快速审查程序的情况。例如，SOP没有任何管理性审查方式的描述，或是提供工具来确保快速审查程序使用的合理性。因此，BRMC的书面回复不足以纠正违规情况和预防将来再次发生类似的违规。

2. IRB未能按照不少于一年一次的频次对研究进行跟踪审查，并且未能遵守其进行初次审查及跟踪审查的书面程序［21 CFR 56.109（f）和56.108（a）］

IRB应对已经批准的研究基于其风险程度进行一定频率的跟踪审查，审查频率不少于每年一次。此外，IRB应该遵从其关于初始审查和跟踪审查的书面程序。BRMC的IRB书面程序中写到，基于IRB 的政策和规程手册中政策 7.00 的要求，"BRMC的IRB必须对已经批准的试验研究基于其风险程度进行一定频率的跟踪审查，审查频率不少于每年一次"。

BRMC IRB 没有进行每年至少一次的跟踪审查，并且未遵从其书面程序关于进行初始审查和跟踪审查的规定。类似的情况如下，但不仅限于以下所列：

a. 2009年9月11日，BRMC IRB 会议批准了研究项目（b）（4），"（b）（4）" 项目的跟踪审查应于2010年9月11日前完成。然而，该项目的跟踪审查直到2010 年11月12日才进行。因此，IRB并没有在要求的时间内进行跟踪审查，这一做法违背了其书面程序的规定。我们在检查中发现，有一个受试者已经入组并在BRMC进行了随访，同时该试验还在受试者入组阶段。

b. 在2009年9月11日，BRMC IRB 会议批准了研究项目（b）（4），"（b）（4）" 项目的跟踪审查应于2010年9月11日到期。然而，该项目的跟踪审查直到2010 年11月12日才进行。因此，IRB并没有在要求的时间内进行跟踪审查，这一做法违背了其书面程序的规定。我们检查中发现，有一个受试者已经入组并在BRMC进行了随访，同时该试验还在受试者入组阶段。

法规要求IRB进行至少每年一次的跟踪审查，这为IRB提供了机会，得以持续地审查进行中的研究并判断：①其对受试者风险是否最小化；②受试者所承担的风险与预期的可能受益比较是否合理，以及这些风险与预期得到的试验结果的重要性比较是否合理。BRMC的IRB未能进行至少每年一次的审查，导致其未能在研究中保护受试者的权利和福利。

BRMC的IRB 未能按照不少于每年一次的频率进行跟踪审查及未能遵从其关于初始审查和跟踪审查的程序的情况表现为反复发生的违规情况。这些违规在FDA 2010年9月9日给 BRMC的警告信中已经写明。Jay Summer博士，医学事务副总裁，在2010年9月 24日递交的2010年9月9日警告信的书面回复中指出，BRMC已经采取了一些措施支持IRB，以保证其能遵守流程，措施如下：

- BRMC指派另一个人支持IRB，为IRB增加了一个全职工作人员。此外，Summer博士承担对该新增工作人员的直接管理职责，以保证遵循书面程序。
- BRMC对所有的研究项目使用一个简单易懂的跟踪日志，以保证完成这些研究的及时审查。

我们在检查中发现，IRB没能恰当地实施和执行这些纠正预防措施来避免这些违规在将来的再次发生。这导致BRMC的IRB重复地违背法规21 CFR 第 56 部分的要求。这一问题在2011年6月30日的警告信回复中没有纠正。

3. IRB未能准备和保存足够的包括IRB会议记录的IRB活动记录［21 CFR 56.115（a）（2）］

IRB应该准备和保存足够的包括IRB的会议记录在内的IRB活动记录。IRB的会议记录应对会议的出席情况、IRB采取的行动、行动的投票情况，包括赞成票数、反对票数和弃权票数进行足够详细的记录。

BMRC IRB保存了两套2010年11月12日的会议记录，一套会议记录中会议主席是S.S. Ahmad医学博士，另一套会议记录中会议主席是 M. AlQasmi医学博士，这两套会议记录反映了不准确的信息、不准确的投票数，以及不准确的会议出席情况。结论是，BRMC的IRB未能准备和保存足够的IRB活动记录。类似情况如下，但不仅限于以下情况：

a. 2010年11月12日会议主席是S.S. Ahmad医学博士的会议记录说明：

i. IRB的10个投票委员出席了该IRB会议，但会议记录中有5票同意批准研究项目（b）（4）的CRIRB更新内容，0票反对，0票弃权。因此会议记录中记录的投票数没有准确体现参会委员数目。

ⅱ. 2010 年11月12日的会议记录中会议主席是AlQasmi博士，然而AlQasmi博士直到2011年1月才成为IRB委员。因此，记录AlQasmi博士为该次会议的主席表明，IRB活动记录不够准确和充分。

b. 在2010年11月12日Ahmad博士作为会议主席的会议中，记录显示10名IRB投票委员出席了会议，其中Dr.（b）（6）对试验项目（b）（4）弃权，但记录中记载了10名投票委员中9人投了赞成票，2人弃权票。因此，会议记录未能反映准确的出席人数或是准确的票数。

c. 2011年1月的会议记录显示7名IRB投票委员参加了会议，其中 Dr.（b）（6）没有参加对（b）（4）试验的投票。但会议记录亦显示7名委员参加会议并批准了这些试验。因此，会议记录未能反映准确的出席人数或是准确的票数。

该IRB没有充分记录和保存IRB活动的文件记录。2010年11月12日和2011年1月14日的会议记录无法准确地反映委员的会议出席情况或者IRB会议决定的投票情况，包括赞成票数、反对票数和弃权票数。

此外，这些在2010年11月12日会议记录中发现的数据差异令人难以判断该次会议是否自始至终达到了法定人数要求。如果会议中未达到法定人数（例如为避免冲突不能参加，早退，非科学领域委员缺席），IRB则不能采取进一步行动或进行投票，除非法定人数条件重新满足［21 CFR 56.108（c）］。

BRMC在2011年6月30日对FDA警告信的书面回复中写到，IRB主席会在每次会议开始时提醒委员关于投票的规则，并且把这些规则记入会议记录。回复中还提到，会记录一份详细的文件清楚地写明会议中投票数的变化，以此来记录委员的参加和离开情况。我们认为该回复不够充分，因为其没有包括是否对IRB委员进行会议记录要求的培训或是如何对IRB运行进行恰当记录的培训，也未说明如何避免出现内容冲突的会议记录。因此，BRMC的书面回复不能充分纠正偏差和预防此类违规或相似违规情况的再次发生。

FDA对该IRB实施的限制：

本次检查发现了一些新的违规项和一个在2010年9月9日警告信提及的违规项的再次发生。该IRB表现出在过去的连续3次检查过程中一直存在的缺陷，并且没能实施、执行纠正和预防措施防止这些违规行为的再次发生。所以，BRMC的IRB重复出现违反21 CFR 56要求的情况。

考虑到这些违规的严重性及对受试者权益和福利的风险，FDA决定按照法规21 CFR 56.120 和21 CFR 56.110（d）对BRMC的IRB实行两条限制，分别是：

（1）法规21 CFR 56监管范围内的正在进行的试验不允许纳入新的受试者；

（2）FDA将暂停BRMC IRB使用快速审查流程。

这些限制在贵方接到FDA确认充分改正的书面通知之前一直有效。这些限制并没有解除IRB接收和回复在研项目的非预期和严重反应报告，以及常规进展报告的责任。在研的研究将被限制纳入新的受试者，然而，这些限制不影响已经入组的受试者继续留在研究中，只要这些受试者的利益和安全得到了很好的保障。

此外，这些限制不影响在BRMC进行的、那些由Michigan State大学组织和运行的CRIRB审查并批准的研究。

自收到这封信的15个工作日内，您应当书面告知本办公室为使贵伦理委员会完全符合FDA的法规要求您已经采取的措施。您的书面回复应该针对本信中所提到的每一个违规项进行回复，并提供任何必要的文件来证明完全和充分的改正。请注明每一项整改的（计划）完成日期。如果不能充分、迅速地解释上述违规问题，可能导致我们在不再通知的情况下采取监管措施。

您有责任将上述限制通知所有受影响的申办者和临床研究者。在您提供书面回复时，请同时提供一份具有代表性的IRB同受影响的申办者及临床研究者关于当前所受限制进行书面沟通的范例。您还需提供被通知的所有申办者和研究者清单作为通知的证据，其中应包括对方被通知的日期。

请提供一份所有受上述限制影响的当前进行的研究的清单，清单中包括研究的名称（如有IDE或IND号，请写明），受试药物名称，临床研究者姓名，初始审查批准日期和跟踪审查日期。IND和IDE号可从申办者的方案中获知。此外，请提供所有由CRIRB监管的、目前正在BRMC进行的研究项目清单。

如果您未能回复此警告信并采取恰当的纠正措施，可导致FDA在不再通知您的情况下根据21 CFR

56.120，56.121和56.124规定，采取进一步监管行动。这些行动可包括继续上述限制，终止由贵IRB批准的正在进行的受21 CFR 56监管的研究，以及启动取消IRB资格的法律程序。

附：英文原文

Bay Regional Medical Center IRB

WARNING LETTER

December 20, 2011

CERTIFIED MAIL
RETURN RECEIPT REQUESTED

Ref: 12-HFD-45-12-01

Philip Incarnati
President & Chief Executive Officer
McLaren Health Care
G-3245 Beecher Road, Suite 200
Flint, MI 48532

Dear Mr. Incarnati:

Between June 22, 2011, and June 24, 2011, Ms. Nancy Bellamy, representing the U.S. Food and Drug Administration (FDA), inspected the Institutional Review Board (IRB) at Bay Regional Medical Center (BRMC) (IRB Registration Number 00003638). The purpose of this inspection was to determine whether the IRB procedures for the protection of human subjects complied with Title 21 of the Code of Federal Regulations (CFR), parts 50 and 56. These regulations apply to clinical investigations of products regulated by FDA. We are aware that at the conclusion of the inspection, our investigator presented and discussed Form FDA 483, Inspectional Observations, with Ms. Alice Gerard, President and Chief Executive Officer, and her staff. From our review of the establishment inspection report, the documents submitted with that report, and BRMC's June 30, 2011, written response to the inspection findings, we conclude that the IRB did not adhere to the applicable statutory requirements and FDA regulations governing the protection of human subjects. We wish to emphasize the following:

1. The IRB failed to follow FDA regulations regarding expedited review procedures [21 CFR 56.110(b)].

The regulations require that under an expedited review procedure, the review may be carried out by the IRB chairperson or by one or more experienced reviewers designated by the IRB chairperson from among the members of the IRB. An IRB may use the expedited review process to review either or both of the following: (1) Some or all of the research appearing on the Federal Register list, "Protection of Human Subjects: Categories of Research That May Be Reviewed by the Institutional Review Board (IRB) Through an Expedited Review Procedure," [1] and found by the reviewer(s) to involve no more than minimal risk; or (2) minor changes in previously approved research during the period for which approval is authorized.

According to the Federal Register notice, the expedited review procedure may be used for continuing review as follows:

- Where (i) the research is permanently closed to the enrollment of new subjects; (ii) all subjects have completed all research related interventions; and (iii) the research remains active only for long-term follow-up of subjects; or
- Where no subjects have been enrolled and no additional risks have been identified; or
- Where the remaining research activities are limited to data analysis.

The BRMC IRB used expedited continuing review for research that was not eligible for approval through expedited review. Examples of this failure include, but are not limited to, the following:

a. On May 18, 2011, the IRB Chairman used the expedited review procedure for the continuing review and approval of study (b)(4) "(b)(4)." However, on March 21, 2011, the IRB was notified that one subject had been enrolled at BRMC, and the study was still open for subject accrual. Therefore, the (b)(4) study was not eligible for expedited continuing review.

b. On June 23, 2010, the IRB Chairman used the expedited review procedure for the continuing review and approval of study (b)(4) "(b)(4)."However, on June 14, 2010, the IRB was notified that one subject had been enrolled at BRMC, and the study was still open for subject accrual. Therefore, the (b)(4) study was not eligible for expedited continuing review.

c. On June 23, 2010, the IRB Chairman used the expedited review procedure for the continuing review and approval of study (b)(4), "(b)(4)." Our inspection revealed that at the time of the expedited review for study (b)(4), subjects had been enrolled at BRMC and the study was still open for subject accrual. Therefore, the (b)(4) study was not eligible for expedited continuing review.

The IRB inappropriately conducted expedited continuing review and approval of research that did not meet the requirements of 21 CFR 56.110(b). The (b)(4) studies were not eligible for expedited continuing review because the studies were open to subject accrual, and subjects had been enrolled in each study. These studies should have been reviewed and approved at a convened meeting with a majority of the IRB members present.

The BRMC's written response to the Form FDA 483, dated June 30, 2011, notes that written standard operating procedures (SOPs) on expedited review have been modified to address this violation. The written response indicates that the IRB staff and IRB members will be provided with educational material and training on the eligibility criteria for expedited review at the next convened IRB meeting. The written response further notes that the training presentation will be included in the meeting minutes, and a copy of the training material will be kept with the meeting minutes. This response is inadequate because the revised SOP does not address how the inappropriate use of expedited review, as noted above, will be avoided in the future. For example, the revised SOP does not describe any type of administrative review or provide tools to ensure that the use of expedited review is appropriate. As a result, the BRMC's written response is inadequate to correct the violation and prevent the recurrence of these or similar violations in the future.

2. The IRB failed to conduct continuing review of research at intervals of not less than once per year, and failed to follow written procedures for conducting its initial and continuing review of research [21 CFR 56.109(f) and 56.108(a)].

An IRB shall conduct continuing review of previously approved research at intervals appropriate to the degree of risk, but not less than once per year. In addition, an IRB is required to follow written procedures for conducting initial and continuing review of research. The written procedures for BRMC's IRB state, under Policy 7.00 of the IRB's Policy and Procedures Manual, that "BRMC's IRB must conduct continuing review of research at intervals appropriate to the degree of risk, but not less frequently than once per year."

The BRMC IRB failed to conduct continuing review of research at least once per year, and failed to follow their written procedures for conducting initial and continuing review of research. Examples of this failure include, but are not limited to, the following:

a. On September 11, 2009, the BRMC IRB met and approved the study (b)(4), "(b)(4)." Continuing review for this study was due by September 11, 2010. However, continuing review was not conducted until November 12, 2010. As a result, the IRB failed to conduct continuing review within the required interval, and in doing so, failed to follow their written procedures. Our inspection revealed that one subject had been enrolled and followed up at BRMC, and the study was still open for subject accrual.

b. On September 11, 2009, the BRMC IRB met and approved the study (b)(4), "(b)(4)." Continuing review for this study was due by September 11, 2010. However, continuing review was not conducted until November 12, 2010. As a result, the IRB failed to conduct continuing review within the required interval, and in doing so, failed to follow their written procedures. Our inspection revealed that five subjects had been enrolled and followed up at BRMC, and the study was still open for subject accrual.

The regulations require an IRB to conduct continuing review of research at least annually, which provides an IRB with the opportunity to substantively review research in progress and to determine that (1) risks to subjects are minimized, and (2) risks to subjects are reasonable in relation to anticipated benefits to subjects, if any, and the importance of the knowledge that may be expected to result. The BRMC IRB failed to conduct continuing review of research at least annually. As a result, the IRB failed to protect the rights and welfare of human subjects participating in research.

The BRMC IRB's failure to conduct continuing review at intervals of not less than once per year and its failure to follow written procedures for conducting initial and continuing review of research represent repeated occurrences of violations that were cited in the Warning Letter issued to the BRMC IRB on September 9, 2010. On September 24, 2010, Dr. Jay Summer, Vice President of Medical Affairs, submitted the BRMC IRB's written response to the September 9, 2010, Warning Letter. The response stated that BRMC had taken a number of steps to support the IRB and to ensure adherence to the procedures, including the following:

- BRMC assigned a different support person to the IRB and increased the support for a fulltime IRB position staff. In addition, Dr. Summer assumed direct oversight of the new support person, so that the policies would be followed.
- BRMC implemented a simple tracking log for all studies, so that timely review of the studies can be achieved.

Our inspection revealed that the IRB has failed to properly implement and execute corrective and preventive actions in a manner that will prevent the recurrence of these violations in the future. As a result, the BRMC IRB has repeatedly failed to meet the regulatory requirements of 21 CFR Part 56. This issue was not addressed in your June 30, 2011, response to the Form 483.

3. The IRB failed to prepare and maintain adequate documentation of IRB activities, including minutes of IRB meetings [21 CFR 56.115(a)(2)].

An IRB shall prepare and maintain adequate documentation of IRB activities, including minutes of IRB meetings, which shall be in sufficient detail to show attendance at the meetings; actions taken by the IRB; and the vote on these actions, including the number of members voting for, against, and abstaining.

The BRMC IRB maintains two sets of meeting minutes for November 12, 2010. One set of meeting minutes lists S.S. Ahmad, M.D., as Chairman, and the other lists M. Al-Qasmi, M.D., as Chairman. These two sets of minutes reflect inaccurate information, inaccurate numbers of votes, and inaccurate meeting attendance. As a result, the BRMC IRB failed to prepare and maintain adequate documentation of IRB activities. Examples of this failure include, but are not limited to, the following:

a. The November 12, 2010, meeting minutes, which list Dr. Al-Qasmi as Chairman, indicate that:

i. Ten (10) voting IRB members were present at the IRB meeting. However, the meeting minutes document the vote count for CRIRB renewals of studies (b)(4): (b)(4) as having 5 votes for approval, 0 objections, and 0 abstaining. Thus, the vote counts documented in the minutes do not reflect an accurate number of IRB members present at the meeting.

ii. The November 12, 2010, meeting minutes list Dr. Al-Qasmi as the BRMC IRB Chairman. However, Dr. Al-Qasmi was not an IRB member until January 2011. As a result, listing Dr. Al-Qasmi as Chairman for this meeting reflects an inaccurate and inadequate record of IRB activities.

b. The November 12, 2010, meeting minutes, which list Dr. Ahmad as Chairman, indicate that ten (10) voting IRB members were present at the IRB meeting. The minutes document that Dr. (b)(6) and (b)(6) abstained from voting on studies (b)(4); however, the minutes document that 9 of the 10 voting members present at the meeting approved the studies with two abstentions. As a result, the meeting minutes reflect an inaccurate account of meeting attendance or an inaccurate number of votes.

c. The January 14, 2011, meeting minutes indicate that seven (7) voting IRB members were present at the IRB meeting. The minutes document that Dr. (b)(6) did not participate in the voting process on studies (b)(4) and (b)(4); however, the minutes document that 7 of the 7 voting members present at the meeting approved the studies. As a result, the meeting minutes reflect an inaccurate account of meeting attendance or an inaccurate number of votes.

The IRB failed to prepare and maintain adequate documentation of IRB activities. The November 12, 2010, and January 14, 2011, meeting minutes do not accurately reflect the IRB members present at the meeting or the vote on actions taken by the IRB, including the number of members voting for, against, and abstaining.

In addition, the discrepancies found in the November 12, 2010, meeting minutes make it difficult to determine whether a quorum was maintained throughout the convened meeting. If a quorum is lost during a convened meeting (e.g., those with conflicts being excused, early departures, absence of a nonscientist member), the IRB may not take further actions or votes unless the quorum can be restored [21 CFR 56.108(c)].

BRMC's written response to the Form FDA 483, dated June 30, 2011, notes that the IRB Chairman will remind members at the beginning of each convened IRB meeting of the voting rules, and they will be included in the meeting minutes. The written response indicates that a detailed documentation will be recorded to clearly signify the change in vote count during the IRB meeting, thereby tracking when members come and leave. This response is inadequate because it does not include any discussion of training of IRB staff on the requirements of IRB minutes or maintaining appropriate records of IRB operations, nor does it address how the IRB will prevent conflicting meeting minutes. As a result, BRMC's written response is inadequate to correct the violation and to prevent the recurrence of this or similar violations in the future.

FDA Imposed Restrictions on the IRB:

This inspection has identified new violations in addition to the repeated occurrence of a violation cited in & Warning Letter of September 9, 2010. The IRB has demonstrated a continuing pattern of deficiencies in the last three inspections. The IRB has failed to properly implement and execute corrective and preventive actions in a manner that will prevent the recurrence of these violations in the future. As a result, the BRMC IRB has repeatedly failed to meet the regulatory requirements of 21 CFR Part 56.

Given the seriousness of these violations and the risk to the rights and welfare of human research subjects, effective immediately, the FDA is placing the following two restrictions on the Bay Regional Medical Center IRB, according to 21 CFR 56.120 and 21 CFR 56.110(d), respectively:

1. No new subjects will be added to ongoing studies subject to 21 CFR part 56.

2. FDA will suspend the BRMC IRB's use of the expedited review procedure.

These restrictions will remain in effect until such time that you receive written notification from FDA that adequate corrections have been made. These restrictions do not relieve the IRB of its responsibilities to receive and respond to reports of unexpected and serious reactions and routine progress reports from ongoing studies. The restrictions state that no new subjects will be added to ongoing studies; however, this restriction would not affect any subjects already enrolled in ongoing studies, as long as it is in the best interest and safety of individual subjects to remain enrolled.

In addition, these restrictions would not affect those studies being conducted at BRMC but being reviewed and approved by the Community Research Institutional Review Board (CRIRB), which is organized and operated by Michigan State University.

Within fifteen (15) business days of your receipt of this letter, you are to notify this office in writing of the actions you have taken to bring the IRB into full compliance with FDA regulations.Your written response should address each citation in the letter and should include any documentation necessary to show that full and adequate correction will be achieved. Please include the projected completion dates for each action to be accomplished. Failure to adequately and promptly explain the violations noted above may result in regulatory action without further notice.

It is your responsibility to notify all affected sponsors and clinical investigators of the restrictions described above. Include with your response to the FDA a representative sample copy of the IRB's written communication(s) to affected sponsors and clinical investigators, notifying them of the current restrictions. Please also provide a complete list of all sponsors and investigators who were notified as a result of this action, and the date(s) on which they were notified.

Please provide a list of all studies currently being conducted that are affected by the above restrictions, and include the titles of the studies (with IDE or IND numbers, if applicable), the names of the test articles, the names of the clinical investigators, the dates of initial reviews and approvals, and the dates of continuing reviews. IND and IDE numbers can be obtained from the sponsors of the protocols affected by these restrictions. In addition, please provide a complete list of all studies being conducted at BRMC that are continuing under the oversight of CRIRB.

Failure to respond to this letter and to take appropriate corrective action could result in FDA's taking further regulatory actions, as authorized by 21 CFR 56.120, 56.121, and 56.124. These actions could include, but are not limited to, the continuation of the restrictions described above; the termination of ongoing studies subject to 21 CFR part 56 and approved by your IRB; and the initiation of regulatory proceedings for the disqualification of your IRB.

This letter is not intended to be an all-inclusive list of deficiencies for the protocols reviewed and approved by the IRB. It is your responsibility to ensure that the Bay Regional Medical Center IRB's practices and procedures comply fully with all applicable statutes and regulations.

If you have any questions, please contact Patrick J. McNeilly, Ph.D., at 3017962941; FAX 3018478748. Your written response and any pertinent documentation should be addressed to:

Patrick J. McNeilly, Ph.D.
Acting Branch Chief, Human Subject Protection Branch
Division of Safety Compliance
Office of Scientific Investigations
Office of Compliance
Center for Drug Evaluation and Research
Food and Drug Administration
Building 51, Room 2266
10903 New Hampshire Avenue
Silver Spring, MD 20993

Sincerely,

/S/

Leslie K. Ball, M.D.
Acting Director
Office of Scientific Investigations
Office of Compliance
Center for Drug Evaluation and Research
Food and Drug Administration

Cc: Alice Gerard
President & Chief Executive Officer
Bay Regional Medical Center
1900 Columbus Avenue
Bay City, MI 48708

Mohammed Al-Qasmi, M.D.
Chairman, Institutional Review Board
Bay Regional Medical Center
1900 Columbus Avenue
Bay City, MI 48708
Jay L. Summer, M.D.
Vice President of Medical Affairs
Bay Regional Medical Center
1900 Columbus Avenue
Bay City, MI 48708

Ashir Kumar, M.D.
Chairman, Community Research Institutional Review Board
Michigan State University
205 Olds Hall
East Lansing, Michigan 48824

J. Ian Gray, Ph.D.
Vice President for Research & Graduate Studies
Michigan State University
232 Administration Building
East Lansing, Michigan 48824

第 18 封　给 Covenant 健康护理中心的警告信

2011年9月7日

参考号：11-HFD-45-09-01

尊敬的Maidlow先生：

2011年4月4日至4月20日，L'Oreal F. Walke女士代表FDA对Covenant Health Care的伦理委员会（IRB）进行现场检查。本次检查的目的是核实贵伦理委员会（IRB）对受试者保护的程序是否符合美国联邦法规（CFR）第21篇第50和56部分的要求。这些法规均适用于FDA所监管产品的临床研究。我们知道在现场检查结束时，我们的检查员向John M. Kosanovich（M.D.，医学事务部副总裁）出示了FDA 483表，即现场检查发现的问题，并与其进行了讨论。

经对现场检查报告、该报告的附件，以及Kosanovich博士2011年5月10日的书面回复进行审查，我们认为，贵伦理委员会没有遵循适用的法律要求和监管受试者保护的FDA法规。我们想强调以下几点：

1. IRB未能准备和保存足够的包括对争议问题进行讨论和解决的书面总结的IRB活动记录［21 CFR 56.115（a）（2）］，这使得看起来IRB未能确定对受试者风险最小化、受试者的风险与预期收益相比是合理的［21 CFR 56.111（a）（1）和（2）］

如果在IRB审查研究的过程中出现争议问题，他们必须在会议记录中记录讨论过程和决定。

特别是：

IRB于2009年12月16日会上审评项目（b）（4）“（b）（4）”。会议记录显示，一位IRB委员提出问题：“鉴于国家专业协会目前推荐使用（b）（4），是否在该研究中的安慰剂组接受的治疗低于标准治疗？”IRB同时建议修改知情同意书，以及将在完成上述变更后批准该研究。

然而，在关于避免早产儿出生的标准治疗的问题被提出后，没有证据显示IRB与临床研究者就此问题有过通信联系。我们注意到，2009年12月16日，IRB向临床研究者致信（此为IRB书面回复的参考文件）中简要提及此事，但是IRB仅仅要求在知情同意书的“其他治疗”处增加额外信息，并要求知情同意书中声明受试者可以接受安慰剂或研究药物。最终，会议记录未记录2009年12月会议批准该项目之前的任何讨论和决定。IRB在批准此项研究前，发现了潜在风险，却没有记录针对争议问题的讨论和决定。因此，IRB似乎是在未确定风险对于受试者是否为最小化以及相对预期利益来说，风险是否合理的情况下就批准了研究。

2010年2月17日，IRB 批准了修订后的知情同意书文件。修订的知情同意书中增加的内容未解决2009年12月16日会上发现的标准治疗问题。另外，在2010年2月17日的会议记录上，未包括任何关于受试者接受的预防早产儿出生治疗低于标准的讨论。

IRB书面回复显示，IRB审阅并批准了2010年2月15日重新递交的修订的知情同意书及其按照要求做的变更。并且，IRB计划在它的批准函中指明研究者按照要求做了充分地修改，伦理委员会对修改的文件表示满意。

IRB的回复不足以预防将来此类事件或类似违规的再次发生。此回复未针对发现的主要担心的问题提出解决措施。争论的问题是关于弱势群体接受的治疗低于标准治疗。没有关于该问题的讨论和决定的记录。缺乏记录，显示在未决定风险对于受试者是否为最小化以及相对预期收益来说，风险是否合理的情况下，IRB就批准了研究。对此问题的谨慎考量将影响IRB对风险/收益的决定，最终影响到是否批准在弱势群体中开展该研究。

尽管IRB回复中提到修改它的批准函的计划，但Covenant IRB并未提供文件来具体列明这些变更或计划的实施日期。回复中也未解决对有争议问题的讨论和对解决措施进行记录。因此，IRB未能提供充足的纠正和预防措施文件，以使管理部门能够对提出的纠正和预防措施预防将来再次发生类似的违规情况的潜在适当性做出有根据的评估。

2. IRB未能遵循关于快速审查程序的FDA法规［21 CFR 56.110（b）］

法规要求快速审查可由IRB主席或一名或多名指定的资深委员执行，IRB可以使用这种程序来审评满足如下一种或两种条件的申请：①联邦注册表上列出的符合快速审查条件的研究，并且审查者发现研究不大于最小风险；②对于先前已批准的项目，在批准有效期内进行的较小变更。

a. IRB对不满足快速审查条件的研究采用了快速审查。这一点包括但不限于下面列举的情况：

—— 2009年3月24日，IRB主席采用快速审查批准了单例受试者研究IND（b）（4），受试者（b）（6）在2009年3月27日使用了药物（b）（4）。直到2009年4月15日，IRB才通过全体委员会议批准了该项研究。

—— 2009年5月8日，IRB主席采用快速审查批准了单例受试者研究IND（b）（4），受试者（b）（6）似乎在2009年5月11日开始接受了药物（b）（4）治疗（此为签署知情同意书日期，无IRB文件证实给药日期）。（b）（4）作为单例受试者接受了研究新药（b）（4）的治疗，直到2009年6月17日，IRB才通过全体委员会批准了该项研究。

IRB使用快速审查程序来审查批准两项药物（b）（4）的使用（一种试验性的、尚未获得批准的药物）来治疗妊娠妇女近期感染（b）（4）的延伸项目。

对这些研究采用快速审查程序违背了FDA法规，因为它们涉及大于最小风险且并非已批准研究的较小变更。根据FDA规定，最小风险指试验中预期风险的可能性和程度不大于日常生活，或进行常规体格检查，或心理测试的风险。使用研究药物带来的风险是大于日常生活或常规检查带来的风险的。

审阅IRB“关于出于同情/紧急使用试验药物的政策”程序草案时发现，IRB似乎将“紧急使用试验药物”（免除IRB事先审查批准）与“出于同情用药”归成一类，被称为“延长使用”[1]。所有依据“延长使用”程序而获批的项目实际上需要IRB事先审查批准，因为它们不符合快速审查的标准。

b. 2010年7月13日，IRB主席在（b）（4），“（b）（4）”项目的跟踪审查上使用了快速审查程序。在此情况下使用快速审查是不恰当的，因为2010年6月22日研究进展表显示，已经有3位受试者在Covenant入组，且研究仍在开放入组。因此，研究并不符合快速审查中对跟踪审查的规定。

IRB的书面回复指出，他们使用快速审查程序是因为自上次年度更新后无新的信息或出现非预期风险。然而，根据Federal Register通报，“受试者保护：可采用快速审查程序进行审查的研究”[2]指出，针对跟踪审查的快速审查程序只适用于如下情况：

- （ⅰ）当研究永久地结束而不再纳入新的受试者时；（ⅱ）所有的受试者已完成了研究相关的干预措施；（ⅲ）研究活动仅限于长期随访；或者
- 当研究还未纳入新的受试者且未发现有新增加的风险；或者
- 当剩下的研究活动仅限于数据分析。

（b）（4）研究不符合快速审查标准，因为仍在入组受试者且已经入组了3名。

尽管上述3个例子都是研究者要求进行快速审查，但IRB必须确定采用快速审查是否合适。

c. 另外，对（b）（4）的项目采用快速审查也违背了IRB自己的流程，因为涉及妊娠妇女的研究。这个人群是在IRB政策和流程（9：IRB职责：快速审查）中规定的不适用人群，它指出：“涉及弱势群体（妊娠妇女等）或少数族群的研究不能采用快速审查。”IRB的书面回复指出IRB不同意此项发现，坚持认为IRB对这两项研究采用快速审查程序是合适的。这项声明与IRB内部书面程序相矛盾，IRB的书面程序指明，涉及妊娠妇女的研究不适于采用快速审查。

IRB的书面回复是不恰当的，因为它未表现出对快速审查法规的正确理解。特别是，IRB的回复并不承认上述3个例子采用快速审查是不恰当的。因此，Covenant IRB对快速审查法规进行全面了解，对IRB人员进行重新培训是必需的。IRB未能提供足够的足以预防将来再次发生此类或类似违规的纠正和预防措施记录。

3. IRB未能确保提供给受试者作为知情同意书的一部分的信息符合21 CFR 50.25的要求［21 CFR 56.109（b）］

使用（b）（4）治疗的2名受试者签署的知情同意文件（ICD）缺少一些必要的核心内容。

具体而言：

a. 受试者（b）（6）于2009年3月27日/（b）（6）于2009年5月11日签署的题为“同意接受（b）（4）在本人的体内预防（b）（4）”的知情同意书并未说明项目为研究性质，并且缺乏给药治疗的流程描述［21CFR 50.25（a）（1）］。ICD表述为“将与您讨论治疗”，这与法规相比是不充分的。

b. 受试者（b）（6）于2009年3月27日签署的ICD缺少关于如果对研究受试者权利有疑问时该联系谁的描述［21CFR50.25（a）（7）］，Covenant健康护理中心IRB的联系方式为空白。

关于该研究中ICD缺少说明一事，IRB指出，在“知情同意书”第5页第8项“同意声明”中提及了受试者将因参与试验被要求签字以授权使用和公开受保护的健康信息。这个声明本身不足以满足法规所要求的，必须向受试者告知研究属于试验的性质。

未确保知情同意书涵盖所有FDA 要求的要素，可能导致受试者不能获得给予有效知情同意所需的足够的研究信息。

4. IRB未能确保没有与项目有利益关系的委员参与IRB的初始审查或跟踪审查，除非根据IRB的要求提供的信息［21CFR56.107（e）］

为了批准研究，IRB必须确保投票委员与研究无利益冲突。我们检查中发现很多情况下，有利益冲突的IRB委员在自己的研究中投票。这一点包括但不限于下面列举的情况：

a.（b）（4）是IRB委员，又是（b）（4）项目中的研究者，（b）（4）博士在2009年8月19日伦理审查会上对项目（b）（4）的初始审查进行了投票。

Dr.（b）（4）还在2009年10月21日、2010年4月21日、2011年1月19日的会上对（b）（4）项目的SAE报告进行了审查和批准。会议记录显示，所有委员投票通过了SAE报告。

RB书面回复中承认，会议记录未表明（b）（4）博士在投票中弃权。

b. IRB主席DennisBoysen医学博士是研究“（b）（4）”的临床研究者，他在2009年11月16日、2010年2月15日、2010年5月17日、2010年8月16日、2010年11月15日的跟踪审查小组（Continuing Review Subcommittee，CRS）会上，投票批准了（b）（4）研究。在随后的全体会议上，IRB（包括Boysen博士）投票批准如下文件：方案修订、修改的知情同意、年度进展报告、市场手册和修订版研究者手册。

IRB的书面回复承认Boysen博士存在利益冲突，但投了票。

IRB针对这个发现项的纠正措施是，计划在IRB文件上，除了主要研究者还要包括所有合作研究者，通过再次检查，确保有利益冲突的IRB委员都被剔除，不参与审议和投票，这个做法将体现在会议记录中。IRB还声明，将对行政管理人员进行相关培训，我们确认收到了IRB的承诺，在会议记录中加强利益冲突方面的记录。然而，仅培训IRB的管理人员还是不充分。IRB委员也应获得利益冲突培训，包括书面程序的培训，包括存在利益冲突的委员在讨论和投票时应离开房间。最后，我们确认收到了IRB的计划，即在全体会议的会议记录中记录对CRS会议记录批准的投票结果。

IRB的回复是不充分的。IRB未提供纠正和预防措施的有关文件，证明具备足够纠正、预防能力，避免此类或类似违规再次发生。IRB未提供IRB政策和流程变更的记录、实施的时间表以及那些接受政策和流程变更培训的工作人员的培训记录。

此外，我们注意到，IRB快速审查的过程：①一名委员进行初始审查和批准；②在CRS会上审阅和决定；③在全体会上介绍CRS会议记录和决定。IRB可以考虑通过削减，层层审查来简化这个过程。

5. IRB未能遵守对研究进行跟踪审查的书面程序［21 CFR 56.108（a）（1）］

IRB应遵守其关于初始审查和跟踪审查的书面程序。IRB未遵守，特别是：

IRB使用IRB委员组成的跟踪审查小组（CRS）来进行跟踪审查。IRB书面程序显示，“年度更新、更新批件”仅在CRS委员的月度材料中出现。我们并不认为CRS与IRB相同。然而，我们要求IRB以及CRS遵照书面程序来执行研究的跟踪审查。

IRB未遵照其关于CRS跟踪审查的书面程序要求。根据书面程序，CRS包括3~8名IRB委员，每月开会完成跟踪审查。CRS组成包括：一名委员为非科学领域背景（外行），一名委员为科学领域背景（专家），一名委员为药学专业，一名委员不隶属于机构，IRB主席或副主席，以及IRB专员。在下述会议中，CRS没有遵循跟踪审查流程，而IRB投票批准了研究的继续进行。

a. 2010年4月19日会议记录显示，两名委员参加了CRS会议，而IRB的CRS流程要求至少三名委员参会。

b. 2008年7月14日、2008年8月18日、2009年6月15日、2010年4月19日、2010年11月15日会议记录显示，没有非科学领域背景委员参会。而IRB的CRS流程要求1名非科学领域背景委员参会。

c. CRS的任何会议记录中都没有非机构隶属的委员参会的记录。而IRB流程要求1名非机构隶属的委员参会。

我们了解IRB计划在全体会议的会议记录中，记录针对CRS会议记录审查的投票情况。此外，IRB的书面回复显示CRS会议的一般出席情况，平均每次会议有6名委员出席。IRB同意非科学领域委员的出席情况应保持一致。书面回复显示，IRB认为（b）（6）、IRB专员为非科学领域。然而根据2009、2010和2011年度IRB名册显示，（b）（6）女士是科学领域委员。

IRB的回复不足以预防将来此类事件或类似违规的再次发生。此回复未针对发现项中记录的主要担心的问题提出解决措施。此外，回复未解决非机构隶属的委员参加CRS会议的问题。

非预期风险有时是在调查的过程中被发现的，偶然出现的新信息显示，研究中的风险是不合理的。定期审查可以确保这些风险及时地得到IRB的关注，从而给予受试者额外的保护。因此，FDA相信IRB定期审查对于保障研究中受试者权益和福利是必不可少的。

我们希望强调，跟踪审查应遵循和初始审查同样的标准［21 CFR 56.109（f）］。当对那些不适用于快速审查的研究进行跟踪审查时，IRB应获取并审查必要的文件。IRB的流程和操作未考虑到全体会上对于跟踪审查的研究方案应进行讨论，应包括且不限于以下条目：

- 一份研究场所正在使用的当前版本的方案；
- 一份研究场所正在使用的当前版本的知情同意书；
- 研究者手册，如适用；
- 研究进展的状态报告，包括：
  - 受试者数；
  - 退出受试者数；
  - 任何不良事件或非预期问题的描述，包括对受试者或其他人员的风险；
  - 迄今任何发现的汇总；
  - 自上次审查后的修订或变动；
- 任何其他相关信息，尤其是和风险有关的信息。

此方面的更多信息，请参考“IRB/临床研究者和申办者指南：临床研究批准后的IRB跟踪审查”[3]。

本警告信的目的并非是罗列贵伦理委员会在审查和批准研究方案存在的所有缺陷。确保Covenant健康护理中心伦理委员会实际操作和程序完全符合所有适用法律法规的要求是您的职责。

自收到这封信的15个工作日内，您应当书面告知本办公室为预防将来发生类似违规情况已经采取的措施。您的书面回复应对每一个问题逐一答复，并提供所有必要的文件，足以证明已经完成完全和充分的纠正措施。请明确每项措施的计划完成日期。如果不能充分、迅速地解释上述违规问题，可能导致我们在不再通知的情况下采取监管措施。

附：英文原文

Covenant Health Care

WARNING LETTER

Sep 7, 2011

CERTIFIED MAIL
RETURN RECEIPT REQUESTED

Ref: 11-HFD-45-09-01

Mr. Spence Maidlow
President & Chief Executive Officer
Covenant Health Care
1447 North Harrison
Saginaw, MI 48602-5383

Dear Mr. Maidlow:

Between April 4, 2011 and April 20, 2011, Ms. L'Oreal F. Walker, representing the Food and Drug Administration (FDA), inspected the Institutional Review Board (IRB) at Covenant HealthCare. The purpose of this inspection was to determine whether the IRB procedures for the protection of human subjects complied with Title 21 of the Code of Federal Regulations (CFR), parts 50 and 56. These regulations apply to clinical investigations of products regulated by FDA. We are aware that at the conclusion of the inspection, our investigator presented and discussed with John M. Kosanovich, M.D., Vice-President of Medical Affairs, a Form FDA 483, Inspectional Observations.

From our review of the establishment inspection report, the documents submitted with that report, and Dr. Kosanovich's written response dated May 10, 2011, we conclude that the IRB did not adhere to the applicable statutory requirements and FDA regulations governing the protection of human subjects. We wish to emphasize the following:

1. The IRB failed to prepare and maintain adequate documentation of IRB activities including a written summary of the discussion of controverted issues and their resolution [21 CFR 56.115(a)(2)], making it appear that the IRB failed to determine that risks to subjects were minimized and reasonable in relation to anticipated benefits [21 CFR 56.111(a)(1) and(2)].

When a controverted issue arises during the IRB's review of research, they must document the discussion of the issue, and its resolution in the meeting minutes.

Specifically:

The IRB reviewed study # (b)(4) ,"(b)(4)" at the December 16, 2009 IRB meeting. Minutes from this meeting indicate that an IRB member "questioned if the placebo group of the study would be receiving less than the standard of care in this study since the national professional association was recommending the use of (b)(4) currently." The IRB also suggested revisions to the informed consent form, and approved the study pending those changes.

However, after the standard of care for prevention of preterm birth issue was raised, there is no evidence in the correspondence between the IRB and the clinical investigator that the IRB queried the clinical investigator with respect to this issue. We note that a letter dated December 16, 2009 from the IRB to the clinical investigator (that the IRB references in its written response) briefly mentions this issue; however, the IRB merely requests that additional information be added to the "alternative treatments" section of the informed consent form and requests that the informed consent form state that the subject may receive a placebo or the study drug. Finally, the meeting minutes do not document any discussion or its resolution prior to approval at the December 2009 meeting. The IRB identified a potential risk and did not document discussion of the controverted issue, and its resolution, before approving the research. Thus, it appears that the IRB approved research without making a determination that risks to subjects were minimized and reasonable in relation to the anticipated benefit.

On February 17, 2010, the IRB approved the revised informed consent document. The information added to the revised informed consent form did not address the standard of care issue identified at the December 16, 2009 meeting. In addition, the minutes from the February 17, 2010 meeting do not include any discussion with respect to risks associated with subjects receiving less than the standard of care for prevention of preterm birth.

The IRB's written response states that the IRB reviewed and approved the changes requested with the resubmission of the revised informed consent form on February 15, 2010. In addition, the IRB plans to indicate in its approval letters that requested changes have been adequately addressed by the investigator and study documents have been revised to the IRB's satisfaction.

The IRB's response is inadequate to prevent the recurrence of this, or similar violations in the future. The response fails to address the primary concern documented in the observation. There was a controverted issue with respect to members of a vulnerable population receiving less than the standard of care. There was no record of the discussion of this issue or its resolution. The lack of documentation makes it appear that the IRB approved the study without ensuring that risks to subjects are minimized and reasonable in relation to anticipated benefits. Careful consideration of this issue should impact the IRB's risk/benefit determination, and ultimately, approval of this research study in this vulnerable population.

Although the IRB's response describes plans to change its approval letters, Covenant IRB has not provided documentation as to the specifics of those changes or projected implementation dates. Nor does the response address the failure to document discussion and resolution of controverted issues. As a result, the IRB has failed to provide documentation of corrective and preventative actions sufficient to enable the agency to undertake an informed evaluation of the potential adequacy of the proposed corrective and preventative action's ability to prevent the recurrence of these, or similar violations in the future.

2. The IRB failed to follow FDA regulations regarding expedited review procedures [21 CFR 56.110(b)].

The regulations require that under an expedited review procedure, the review may be carried out by the IRB chairperson or by one or more experienced reviewers designated by the IRB chairperson from among the members of the IRB, and the IRB may use the expedited review process to review either or both of the following: (1) some or all of the research appearing on the Federal Register list and found by the reviewer(s) to involve no more than minimal risk, or (2) minor changes in previously approved research during the period for which approval is authorized.

a. The IRB used expedited review for types of research that were not eligible for approval through expedited review. Examples of this failure include, but are not limited to, the following:

- On March 24, 2009, the IRB Chairman granted expedited approval for subject (b)(6) who initiated treatment with (b)(4) on March 27, 2009 under single-patient IND (b)(4). The IRB did not grant full board approval until April 15, 2009.
- On May 8, 2009, the IRB Chairman granted expedited approval for subject (b)(6) who appears to have initiated treatment with (b)(4) on May 11, 2009 (date subject signed the ICD; none of the IRB's documents indicate when treatment was initiated). (b)(4) received treatment under single-patient IND (b)(4). The IRB did not grant full board approval until June 17, 2009.

The IRB used the expedited review procedure to review and approve the use of (b)(4) (an investigational, unapproved drug) in the treatment of pregnant women with recent (b)(4) infection under two expanded access protocols.

The use of expedited review for the approval of these studies violates FDA regulations because they involve more than minimal risk and are not a minor change in previously approved research. According to FDA regulations, minimal risk means that the probability and magnitude of harm or discomfort anticipated in the research are not greater in and of themselves than those ordinarily encountered in daily life or during the performance of routine physical or psychological examinations or tests. The risks associated with receiving an investigational drug are greater than the risks that a person would normally encounter in daily life or when undergoing routine tests.

In reviewing the IRB's draft procedure "Policy for Compassionate/Emergent Use of an Investigational Drug" it appears that the IRB is conflating "emergency use" which is exempt from prospective IRB review and approval, with "compassionate use" now referred to as "Expanded Access."[1] All studies approved under the "Expanded Access" program require prospective IRB review and approval because they are not a type of research eligible for expedited review.

b. On July 13, 2010, the IRB Chairman used the expedited review procedure for the continuing review and approval of study # (b)(4), "(b)(4)." Use of the expedited review procedure was not appropriate in this instance because the June 22, 2010, Research Study Update Form indicated that three subjects had been enrolled at Covenant, and the study was still open for subject accrual; therefore, the study did not meet the requirements for continuing review by an expedited review procedure.

The IRB's written response indicates that they used the expedited review procedure because no new information or unanticipated risks were identified prior to the last annual update. However, according to the Federal Register notice, "Protection of Human Subjects: Categories of Research That May Be Reviewed by the Institutional Review Board (IRB) Through an Expedited Review Procedure,"[2] the expedited review procedure may only be used for continuing review as follows:

- Where (i) the research is permanently closed to the enrollment of new subjects; (ii) all subjects have completed all research-related interventions; and (iii) the research remains active only for long-term follow-up of subjects; or
- Where no subjects have been enrolled and no additional risks have been identified; or
- Where the remaining research activities are limited to data analysis.

The (b)(4) study was not eligible for expedited continuing review because the study was open to subject accrual, and enrolled three subjects.

Even though the clinical investigator requested an expedited review in all three instances discussed above, the IRB must make the determination as to when use of the expedited review procedure is appropriate.

c. In addition, the use of expedited review for the approval of the (b)(4) studies violates the IRB's own procedure because the studies involve pregnant women, a population specifically excluded from expedited review by the IRB's Policy and Procedure #9 "Functions of the IRB: Expedited Review", which states "studies involving vulnerable populations (pregnant women…) or focusing on minority populations may not be expedited." The IRB's written response indicates that the IRB disagrees with this observation and maintains that the IRB used the expedited review procedure appropriately in these two instances. This statement directly contradicts the IRB's own procedure, which states that studies involving pregnant women are not eligible for expedited review.

The IRB's written response is inadequate because it does not represent an accurate understanding of the regulations governing expedited review. Specifically, the IRB's response fails to acknowledge that the use of expedited review was improper in all three instances above. As a result, Covenant IRB conducting a thorough review of the expedited review regulations and the appropriateness of your IRB's expedited review process, and re-training of IRB staff is necessary. The IRB has failed to provide documentation of corrective and preventative actions sufficient to prevent the recurrence of this, or similar violations in the future.

3. The IRB failed to ensure that information given to subjects as part of informed consent is in accordance with 21 CFR Part 50.25 [21 CFR 56.109(b)].

The informed consent documents (ICDs) signed by two subjects who were treated with (b)(4) were lacking some of the required elements of informed consent.

Specifically:

a. The ICD entitled "consent to receive (b)(4) to attempt to prevent (b)(4) in my baby" was signed by subject (b)(6) on March 27, 2009, and subject (b)(6) on May 11, 2009.

The consent forms do not contain statements that the study involves research and lack a description of the procedures to be followed with respect to the investigational drug treatment [21 CFR 50.25(a)(1)]. The statement in the ICD that the "treatment will be discussed with you" does not sufficiently meet the regulatory requirement for a description of procedures.

b. In addition, the ICD signed by subject (b)(6) on March 27, 2009, does not contain an explanation of whom to contact for answers to pertinent questions about research subjects' rights [21 CFR 50.25(a)(7)]. The contact information for Covenant HealthCare IRB was left blank.

In response to the observation that the ICD was lacking a statement that the study involves research, the IRB refers to page 5, item #8 under the "Consent Statement" section of the ICD, which states that the subject will be asked to sign forms authorizing the use and disclosure of protected health information in connection with participation in this research. This statement, on its own, does not sufficiently meet the regulatory requirement of disclosing to the subject that the study involves research.

Failure to ensure that all of the FDA required elements of informed consent are met, may result in human subjects not being provided with enough information about a study so that they can give effective informed consent.

4. The IRB failed to ensure that no member participated in the initial or continuing review of a project in which the member had a conflicting interest, except to provide information requested by the IRB [21 CFR 56.107(e)].

In order to approve research, an IRB must ensure that voting members do not have a conflict of interest in the research. Our inspection revealed that on numerous occasions, IRB members with a conflict of interest voted on their own research. Examples of instances where IRB members voted on their own research include, but are not limited to, the following:

a. (b)(4) is a member of the IRB and a sub-investigator for the (b)(4) study. Dr. (b)(4) voted for the initial approval of the (b)(4) study at the August 19, 2009 IRB meeting.

Dr. (b)(4) also reviewed and approved serious adverse event (SAE) reports for the (b)(4) study at IRB meetings held on October 21, 2009, April 21, 2010, and January 19, 2011. Minutes of these meetings indicate that all members present voted to approve the SAE reports.

The IRB's written response acknowledges that meeting minutes do not indicate that Dr. (b)(4) abstained from voting on the (b)(4) study.

b. IRB Chairman Dennis Boysen, M.D., is the clinical investigator for the study "(b)(4)." Dr. Boysen voted to approve the (b)(4) study at Continuing Review Subcommittee (CRS) meetings held on November 16, 2009, February 15, 2010, May 17, 2010, August 16, 2010, and November 15, 2010. At subsequent full board meetings, the IRB (including Dr. Boysen) voted to approve the following documents: amended protocol, revised ICD, annual progress report, marketing brochure, and revised Investigator Brochure.

The IRB's written response acknowledges that Dr. Boysen had a conflict of interest and voted at these meetings.

The IRB's corrective action for this observation is a plan to include all coinvestigators on IRB documentation, in addition to primary investigators to provide a second check to ensure that IRB members with a conflict of interest are excused from deliberations and vote, and that the minutes will reflect this practice. The IRB also states that IRB administrative support staff will be educated with respect to this issue. We acknowledge the IRB's commitment to improve documentation of conflicts of interest in the minutes; however, it is not sufficient to provide education only to IRB support staff. IRB members also need to be educated with respect to conflict of interest, including education on the IRB's written procedures, which require that members with a conflict of interest leave the room during both discussion and voting. Lastly, we acknowledge the IRB's plan to document vote tallies for approval of CRS meeting minutes in the minutes of full board IRB meetings.

The IRB's response is inadequate because the IRB has failed to provide documentation of corrective and preventative actions sufficient to enable the agency to undertake an informed evaluation of the potential adequacy of the proposed corrective and preventative action's ability to prevent the recurrence of this, or similar violations in the future. The IRB has not provided documentation of the specific changes to the IRB policy and procedure, a timeframe for implementation, and records of the training which staff has received on these planned changes to IRB policy and procedure.

In addition, we note that the IRB's process for expedited review encompasses: (1) an initial review and approval by an IRB member, (2) review and IRB action at a CRS meeting, (3) presentation of the CRS minutes and IRB action at a full board IRB meeting. The IRB may want to simplify this process by eliminating the multiple layers of review.

5. The IRB failed to follow its written procedures for conducting continuing review of research [21 CFR 56.108(a)(1)].

An IRB shall follow its written procedures for conducting its initial and continuing review of research. The IRB has failed to follow their written procedures for continuing review of research. Specifically:

The IRB uses a Continuing Review Subcommittee (CRS) made up of members of the IRB, to accomplish continuing review tasks. The IRB's written procedures state that items such as "annual update/renewal applications" will be presented only in CRS members' monthly materials. We do not consider the CRS to be the same as the IRB. However, we do require that the IRB, and by extension, the CRS, follow written procedures for conducting continuing review of research.

The IRB does not follow its written procedures with respect to CRS continuing review requirements. According to the written procedures, a CRS consisting of three to eight IRB members will meet monthly to accomplish continuing review tasks. The CRS will be comprised of one member whose primary concerns are nonscientific (layperson), one member whose primary concerns are scientific (professional), one pharmacist, one member not affiliated with the institution, the IRB Chairperson or Vice-Chairperson, and the IRB Specialist. The IRB voted to approve the continuation of studies at the following meetings where the CRS did not adhere to the continuing review procedure:

a. Minutes of the April 19, 2010 CRS meeting indicate that two members attended. The IRB's CRS procedure requires a minimum of three members.

b. Minutes of CRS meetings held on July 14, 2008, August 18, 2008, June 15, 2009, April 19, 2010, and November 15, 2010 indicate that a non-scientist did not attend the meetings. The IRB's CRS procedure requires that a nonscientist member be present.

c. There was no documentation of the attendance of an unaffiliated member in any of the CRS minutes. The IRB's CRS procedure requires that an unaffiliated member be present.

We acknowledge the IRB's plan to document vote tallies for review of CRS minutes in the minutes of full board IRB meetings. In addition, the IRB's written response indicates that the general attendance for the CRS meetings averages six members for each meeting and that the IRB agrees that representation of a non-scientific member needs to be consistent. The written response also indicates that the IRB considers (b)(6), IRB Specialist to be a non-scientist. However, according to the 2009, 2010, and 2011 IRB rosters, Ms. (b)(6) is a scientific member.

The IRB's response is inadequate because it does not address the IRB's failure to follow procedures for continuing review. The IRB has failed to provide documentation of corrective and preventative actions to prevent the recurrence of this, or similar violations in the future. In addition, the response does not address the absence of an unaffiliated member from the CRS meetings.

Unanticipated risks are sometimes discovered during the course of an investigation, and new information sometimes comes to light showing that the risks in a study are not justified. Periodic review will assure that these risks are promptly brought to the IRB's attention and will provide extra protection to subjects. Consequently, FDA believes periodic review by an IRB is essential if an IRB is to adequately protect the rights and welfare of the human subjects involved in a clinical investigation.

We wish to emphasize that at continuing review the IRB must apply the same criteria for approval as those for its initial approval of the research [21 CFR 56.109(f)]. In conducting continuing review of research not eligible for expedited review, the IRB should receive and review material necessary for these determinations to be made. It appears that the IRB's procedures and practices fail to allow for discussion among the full IRB on protocols undergoing continuing review. Such items should include, but are not limited to:

- a copy of the current version of the protocol in use at the site
- a copy of the current informed consent document in use at the site
- the Investigator's Brochure, if available
- a status report on the progress of the research to include:
  - the number of subjects accrued
  - the number of subject withdrawals
  - a description of any adverse events or unanticipated problems involving risks to subjects or others

  ○ a summary of any recent literature findings obtained thus far
  ○ amendments or modifications to the research since the last review
- any other relevant information, especially information about risks associated with the research.

For more information on this topic, please refer to the draft guidance, "Guidance for IRBs, Clinical Investigators, and Sponsors: IRB Continuing Review after Clinical Investigation Approval".[3]

This letter is not intended to be an all-inclusive list of deficiencies for the protocols reviewed and approved by the IRB. It is your responsibility to ensure that Covenant Health Care IRB's practices and procedures comply fully with all applicable statutes and regulations.

Within fifteen (15) business days of your receipt of this letter, you should notify this office in writing of the actions you have taken to prevent similar violations in the future. Your written response should address each citation in the letter and include any documentation necessary to show that full and adequate correction will be achieved. Please include the projected completion dates for each action to be accomplished. Failure to adequately and promptly explain the violations noted above may result in regulatory action without further notice.

We recommend that you visit the following FDA web page for information on human subject protections that may assist you in your efforts to bring the IRB into compliance with FDA regulations:
http://www.fda.gov/ScienceResearch/SpecialTopics/RunningClinicalTrials/default.htm

We appreciate the cooperation shown to FDA Investigator Walker during the inspection. If you have any questions, please contact Patrick J. McNeilly, Ph.D., at 301-796-2941; FAX 301-847-8748. Your written response and any pertinent documentation should be addressed to:

Patrick J. McNeilly, Ph.D.
Acting Branch Chief, Human Subject Protection Branch
Office of Scientific Investigations
Office of Compliance
Center for Drug Evaluation and Research
Food and Drug Administration
Bldg 51, Room 2266
10903 New Hampshire Avenue
Silver Spring, MD 20993

Sincerely,

{See appended electronic signature page}

Leslie K. Ball, M.D.
Acting Director
Office of Scientific Investigations
Office of Compliance
Center for Drug Evaluation and Research
Food and Drug Administration

Cc: John M. Kosanovich, M.D.
Vice-President of Medical Affairs
Covenant Health Care
1447 North Harrison
Saginaw, MI 48602-5383

Dennis Boysen, M.D.
IRB Chairman

Covenant HealthCare
1447 North Harrison
Saginaw, MI 48602-5383

This is a representation of an electronic record that was signed electronically and this page is the manifestation of the electronic
signature.

/S/

LESLIE K BALL
09/07/2011
Reference ID: 3011043

1 For information on this topic see:
http://www.fda.gov/For Consumers/By Audience/For Patient Advocates/Accessto Investigational Drugs/ucm176098.htm

2 A link to the Federal Register notice is located at:
http://www.fda.gov/ScienceResearch/SpecialTopics/RunningClinicalTrials/GuidancesInformationSheetsandNotices/ucm118099.htm

3 A link to the draft guidance is located at:
http://www.fda.gov/downloads/RegulatoryInformation/Guidances/UCM197347.pdf

第 19 封　给 Essex 伦理委员会有限公司的警告信

2011年7月26日

参考号：11-HFD-45-07-03

尊敬的Waggoner女士：

2011年3月14日至3月21日，Dawn Wydner女士、Denise Visco博士和Janet Donnelly女士代表FDA，对Essex伦理委员会进行了现场检查。本次现场检查的目的是核实贵伦理委员会受试者保护程序是否符合美国联邦法规（CFR）第21篇第50和56部分的要求。这些法规均适用于FDA所监管产品的临床研究。我们知道在现场检查结束时，我们的检查员向伦理委员会副主席Loretta Szczepanski，R.N.女士和您的员工出示了FDA483表，即现场检查发现的问题，并与其进行了讨论。

如在现场检查中与Glenn Lambert博士（伦理委员会主席）所讨论的，在2011年1月，FDA收到消息举报，有人向数个伦理委员会递交了虚假的研究申请。FDA的调查发现，有一个虚假的申办者向数个伦理委员会递交试验方案（b）(4)[1]，题为"（b）(4)"的试验方案。FDA发现（b）(4）是以前另一个不同的申办者已经完成的真实试验方案。这个虚假申办者还递交了虚假的临床研究者信息。2011年1月27日，FDA在FDA网页上张贴了公告，将这些虚假递交的情况通知各个伦理委员会和其他相关方。2011年2月8日，Lambert 博士通知FDA，称Essex伦理委员会已经审查并批准了这个虚假临床研究者来执行"（b）(4)"试验方案。

经对现场检查报告、该报告的附件，以及Lambert博士2011年4月11日的书面回复进行审查，我们认为，贵伦理委员会没有遵循适用的法律要求和监管受试者保护的FDA法规。我们想强调以下几点：

1. IRB未能确定受试者风险最小化［21 CFR 56.111（a）(1)］

根据21 CFR 56.111（a），伦理委员会批准试验的条件之一是伦理委员会必须确保将受试者的风险控制到最低。Essex伦理委员会在对试验的审查中未能确保将受试者的风险控制到最低。具体而言：

A. 这个虚假申办者递交给Essex伦理委员会的"（b）(4)"的试验方案和研究者手册清楚地指出研究受试制剂是一种（b）(4)。这类药物与增加严重心血管事件风险的关联已经明确。然而，在伦理委员会初始审查试验方案（2010年10月25日）的会议记录中，没有证据显示伦理委员会考虑过这个风险，以确认是否已将对受试者的风险控制到最低。可能关联的心血管风险也没有在伦理委员会批准的知情同意书中体现。

伦理委员会的书面回复显示，伦理委员会事后认为，由虚假申办者提供给伦理委员会的描述风险方面（包括心血管风险）的信息不足。您提出的纠正措施是，对将来递交的申请，伦理委员会将要求申办者和研究者证明递交研究文件的完整性和准确性。这个回复并不充分，因为它没能阐述伦理委员会将采取什么措施来确保对申请研究的相关信息进行全面的审查。

虽说Essex伦理委员会要求递交具体的研究文件供伦理委员会审查，并有赖于申办者和研究者递交的信息，但应由伦理委员会承担起责任，对风险和收益进行彻底、独立、系统、审慎分析。21 CFR 56.107要求伦理委员会运用其经验、专业知识和专业能力来确保申请研究的可接受性。伦理委员会委员需考量递交到伦理委员会的信息，还有伦理委员会委员通过其他资源可获得的信息。

我们注意到，伦理委员会的书面回复中提到，伦理委员会将采取额外的措施来对递交给伦理委员会的研究信息的完整性进行评估，通过参考权威来源如PubMed上已发表的与研究制剂相关的文献来进行审查。您的书面回复中还提到，将给伦理委员会行政管理人员进行如何做此类PubMed文献查阅的培训。虽说伦理委

1 (b) (4) 涉及商业秘密，根据法规内容不予公开。

员会行政管理人员可以协助伦理委员会，但对申请研究的充分性进行评估的整体责任仍有赖于伦理委员会委员的专业知识。

伦理委员会对于申请研究的审查如不能充分将风险控制在最低将导致批准通过不合乎伦理性的研究，并危及受试者的权利和福利。彻底的伦理委员会审查应当确保：受试者得到足够的保护，不将他们暴露在不必要的风险下，并且给他们提供有关研究的充分信息，以便他们给出的知情同意有效。

请提供书面回复，详述Essex伦理委员会打算遵循的确保伦理委员会委员对申请研究进行全面审查的流程，以按照法规要求确保将对受试者的风险控制在最低。请提供更新的或为了解决这一发现新制定的标准操作规程或书面程序。同时我们注意到，您的书面回复中提到了Essex伦理委员会行政管理人员，且我们猜测您指的是支持Essex伦理委员会的工作人员。然而，在现场检查时，FDA检查员审阅了支持伦理委员会的工作人员的职位后发现，没有任何一个Essex伦理委员会工作人员有伦理委员会行政管理人员这个头衔。请解释您所指的伦理委员会行政管理人员是谁，并澄清他们的角色。

B. 我们的现场检查显示，Essex伦理委员会未能恰当运用FDA法规中关于最小风险的定义。21 CFR 56.102（i）将最小风险定义为"在研究中预期的伤害或不适的概率和程度不大于他们自己平时在日常生活中或在常规生理或心理检查时所遇到的。"基于我们审阅过的记录，伦理委员会在审查申请研究运用这一定义和评价风险时未能充分考虑试验药物相关的风险。Essex伦理委员会错误地认定以下两项涉及使用试验药物的研究对受试者的风险不大于最小风险：

（b）（4）［虚假申办者，（b）（4）］；

（b）（4）［（b）（4），试验方案（b）（4）］。

伦理委员会的书面回复表明，伦理委员会承认其错误认定这些研究对受试者的风险不大于最小风险，并且列举了一些纠正措施，包括修改一个标准操作规程，使其包含法规中对最小风险的定义和对伦理委员会委员及行政管理人员进行关于这一更新标准操作规程的培训。伦理委员会同时表明，对于一项研究风险级别的认定，需根据法规中对于最小风险的定义来做出。这一回复是不完整的，因为它没有描述伦理委员会试图建立和遵循的、确保在将来对这一法定定义进行充分理解和运用的标准（即描述伦理委员会如何确定一项研究的风险不大于最小风险的流程）。

伦理委员会未能充分地评估最小风险会导致伦理委员会低估了研究对受试者的风险。虽然如伦理委员会在书面回复中提到的，伦理委员会全体委员均审查了以上所列的两项研究，但任何将来对于最小风险的误用都会导致伦理委员会使用不恰当的审查流程来审查风险大于最小风险的研究，违反伦理委员会相关法规，包括21 CFR 56.110中快速审查的法规。此外，误用最小风险的定义会导致伦理委员会对涉及儿童研究的审查不充分，违反21 CFR 50 D的亚部分中关于对临床试验中儿童的额外保障。

请提供一份书面回复，列举伦理委员会用于确保伦理委员会在将来适当评估研究的最小风险的标准和方法。请提供您回复中提到的更新的标准操作规程的和任何为了解决这一发现而新制定的标准操作规程或书面程序的复印件。

2. IRB未能展示其有能力从制度性承诺、法规、适用法律以及专业的实施和操作标准的角度来确定拟审查研究的可接受性［21 CFR 56.107（a）］

21 CFR 56.107（a）中规定，伦理委员会必须有能力确定申请研究在体制承诺、法规、适用法律、专业执行和实践方面的可接受性。我们的调查显示，贵伦理委员会未能充分地评估据说与由虚假申办者递交试验方案（b）（4）相关的临床研究者的专业资质。我们认可伦理委员会回复中提到的选择合格的研究者是申办者的职责，但伦理委员会未能对临床研究者是合格的研究者这一点进行确证。除了其他事项外，伦理委员会本还应对递交伦理委员会的医疗许可证进行检查，确定其在将开展研究的弗吉尼亚州是有效的。未充分地考虑临床研究者的资质会给受试者带来不必要的风险。

伦理委员会的书面回复指出，Essex伦理委员会已经执行了新的流程，今后，作为审查流程的一部分，将对递交的所有主要研究者的医疗许可文件进行确认，并且会对伦理委员会行政管理人员和委员进行关于更新标准操作规程的培训。这项回复是可以接受的。请提供一份您书面回复中提到的这份更新的标准操作规程的副本。

3. IRB未能在初始审查时确定涉及儿童的研究需要依照21 CFR 50（d）临床试验中对儿童的额外保护措施［21 CFR 56.109（h）］

21 CFR 56.109（h）中规定，当一项研究中有一些或所有的受试者是儿童时，伦理委员会**必须**在初始审查中明确该研究符合21 CFR 50（d）（临床试验中对儿童的额外保护措施）的条款。21 CFR 50.50中规定，伦理委员会仅能批准那些满足50.51（未超过最小风险）、50.52（超过了最小风险，但对受试者个体呈现出直接利益的前景）或50.53（超过了最小风险，对受试者个体不能带来直接利益的前景，但可能归纳出关于受试者疾病的知识）中描述的标准的临床研究。

21 CFR 50.51、50.52和50.53中规定，伦理委员会必须确定并记录这些发现。我们的调查显示，Essex伦理委员会在其对涉及儿童受试者的研究的审查和批准中没有充分确认和记录该研究满足标准50.51、50.52或50.53。尤其是伦理委员会审查和批准了以下这个儿科研究，但伦理委员会的记录中没有具体提到其是否符合50.51、50.52或50.53：

- （b）（4）［（b）（4）试验方案（b）（4）］。

不能明确对研究中儿童的额外保障是否得到满足将会将这类弱势人群置于不必要的风险中，并会导致儿童父母或监护人对该申请研究未能完全知情。

此外，我们注意到，在现场检查中审阅的伦理委员会关于（b）（4）试验方案和另一项儿科研究［儿童便秘研究（b）（4）］的记录中包括大量对21 CFR 50（D）相关法规参考依据不准确的引用。这些记录包括，但不限于以下列举的文件：

- 附在标准操作规程 SX-SOP-10-13的儿科方案清单样本；
- 每项研究用到的儿科方案清单；
- 伦理委员会给申办者关于便秘研究的信函；
- 伦理委员会关于便秘研究的会议记录。

伦理委员会的书面回复称，Essex伦理委员会有一份遵循21 CFR 50（D）的关于评估儿科风险等级的标准操作规程，但是伦理委员会未能记录这个确认过程。该书面回复还称，将向伦理委员会行政管理人员和委员进行培训，强调需要在会议记录中记录风险确认以及根据已知的风险确认而定的其他必要记录。这一回复不充分，因为它没能表述伦理委员会将使用什么流程来确保涉及儿童的研究满足50.51、50.52和50.53的标准。我们的顾虑是，伦理委员会可能还没能理解在审查涉及儿童受试者的研究时必须满足对儿童的额外保障。请提供一份书面回复，详述将用于审查将来涉及儿童受试者的研究时充分评价和记录研究满足50.51、50.52和50.53标准的流程。请提供更新的或为了解决这一发现而新制定的标准操作规程或书面程序的复印件。

最后，伦理委员会的书面回复称，Essex伦理委员会将对所有正在进行的儿科研究进行稽查，以确保已经适当完成并记录了风险确认。请在稽查完成后尽快向FDA提供稽查结果。

4. IRB未能确保IRB批准的知情同意书中包含知情同意的基本要素［21 CFR 56.109（b）］

21 CFR 56.109（b）中规定，伦理委员会必须要求受试者得到的信息作为知情同意的一部分应符合21 CFR 50.25（知情同意的要素）的要求。我们的调查显示，Essex伦理委员会未能确保伦理委员会批准的下列两项研究的知情同意书包括21CFR 50.25（a）（2）要求的关于合理可预见的风险或不适的充分信息。

- （b）（4）［虚假申办者，试验方案（b）（4）］；
- （b）（4）［（b）（4），方案号（b）（4）］。

如上1.中所述，因为伦理委员会似乎未能对（b）（4）研究有增加严重心血管事件风险的可能进行讨论，伦理委员会也未能确保将相关的潜在的心血管风险包含在伦理委员会批准的知情同意书中。

申办者递交给Essex伦理委员会的（b）（4）试验方案将移植排斥反应列为使用（b）（4）的成年受试者中常见的一种不良反应。伦理委员会2010年9月7日的会议记录表明，伦理委员会要求申办者对知情同意书进行重新排版，将移植排斥反应移到知情同意文件的另一个段落中。我们的现场检查显示，伦理委员会未能确保将移植排斥反应包含在伦理委员会批准的知情同意书中，因为这个风险最终完全未被提及。

不能确保满足FDA要求的知情同意的要素会导致不能将足够的信息提供给受试者，以便其给出的知情同意有效。

伦理委员会的书面回复没有具体解决FDA483表上的第三条发现。然而，在对FDA483表1C发现项的回复中，伦理委员会指出，对于（b）（4）研究，伦理委员会确认移植排斥反应的不良事件是被无意删除而未被移动到知情同意文件的新的位置。伦理委员会也表示将修改知情同意表，提示伦理委员会的审查委员和工作人员确保知情同意文件中的风险信息与试验方案、研究者手册或其他相关文件（例如说明书）相一致，也将提示伦理委员会在发现不一致时要求申办者或研究者提供进一步信息。这一回复是可以接受的。请提供修改的知情同意表的副本，且一并提供任何修订或新制定的标准操作规程或书面程序。

本警告信的目的并非是罗列贵伦理委员会在审查和批准试验方案时存在的所有缺陷。确保Essex伦理委员会的实际操作和程序完成符合所有适用的法律和法规的要求是您的职责。

自收到这封信的15个工作日内，您应当书面告知本办公室为预防将来类似违规情况而采取的措施。如果不能充分、迅速地解释上述违规问题，可能导致我们在不再通知的情况下采取监管措施。

附：英文原文

Essex Institutional Review Board, Inc

WARNING LETTER

July 26, 2011

UPS

Ref:11-HFD-45-07-03

Ms.Nancy Waggoner
Chief Executive Officer
Essex Institutional Review Board, Inc.
121Main Street
Lebanon, NJ08833

Dear Ms. Waggoner:

Between March 14, 2011 and March 21, 2011, Ms. Dawn Wydner, Dr. Denise Visco, and Ms. Janet Donnelly, representing the Food and Drug Administration (FDA), inspected Essex Institutional Review Board (IRB), Inc. The purpose of this inspection was to determine whether the IRB procedures for the protection of human subjects complied with Title 21 of the Code of Federal Regulations (CFR), parts 50 and 56. These regulations apply to clinical investigations of products regulated by FDA. We are aware that at the conclusion of the inspection, our investigators presented and discussed with Ms. Loretta Szczepanski, R.N., IRB Vice Chairperson, and your staff, a Form FDA 483, Inspectional Observations.

As discussed during the inspection with Dr. Glenn Lambert, IRB Chairman, in January 2011, FDA received information regarding the submission of fictitious applications for research to several IRBs. FDA's investigation determined that a fictitious sponsor submitted protocol (b)(4) entitled, "(b)(4)" to several IRBs for review. FDA determined that the (b)(4) protocol is an actual protocol that was previously conducted and completed by a different sponsor. The fictitious sponsor also submitted information regarding a fictitious clinical investigator. On January 27,

2011, FDA posted an alert notice on the FDA web page to notify IRBs and other stakeholders of these submissions. On February 8, 2011, Dr. Lambert notified FDA that Essex IRB had reviewed and approved this fictitious clinical investigator to conduct the (b)(4) protocol.

From our review of the establishment inspection report, the documents submitted with that report, and Dr. Lambert's written response dated April 11, 2011, we conclude that the IRB did not adhere to the applicable statutory requirements and FDA regulations governing the protection of human subjects. We wish to emphasize the following:

1. The IRB failed to determine that risks to subjects are minimized [21 CFR 56.111(a)(1)]

Under 21 CFR 56.111(a), one of the criteria for IRB approval of research is that the IRB must determine that risks to subjects are minimized. In its review of proposed research, Essex IRB failed to ensure risks to subjects were minimized. Specifically:

A. The **(b)(4)** protocol and the Investigator's Brochure submitted to Essex IRB by the fictitious sponsor clearly indicate that the test article is a **(b)(4)**. With this drug class, there is a well established association with the potential for increased risk of serious cardiovascular events. However, there is no evidence in the IRB meeting minutes for the initial review of this protocol (October 25, 2010) to indicate that the IRB considered this risk in determining whether risks to subject were minimized. The potential for associated cardiovascular risks was also not included in the IRB-approved informed consent form.

The IRB's written response indicates that the IRB determined, in hindsight, that the information provided to the IRB by the fictitious sponsor was inadequate in describing risk information, including cardiovascular risk. Your proposed corrective action is that for future submissions, the IRB will require sponsors and investigators to attest to the completeness and accuracy of study submissions. This response is inadequate because it fails to address what actions the IRB will take to ensure a comprehensive review of information associated with proposed research.

While Essex IRB requires that specific study documents be submitted for IRB review, and relies on the information submitted by the sponsor and investigator, it is incumbent upon the IRB to conduct a thorough, independent, systematic, non-arbitrary analysis of risks and benefits. The regulations at 21 CFR 56.107 require the IRB to use its experience, expertise, and professional competence to ascertain the acceptability of the proposed research. IRB members should consider the information submitted to the IRB, as well as information accessible to the IRB members through other resources.

We note that the IRB's written response indicates that the IRB will undertake additional measures to assess the completeness of the study information submitted to the IRB by referring to authoritative sources, such as PubMed, for a review of the available published literature related to or concerning the study agent. Your written response also provides that the IRB administrators will be trained on conducting such PubMed reviews. While the IRB administrators may assist the IRB, the overall responsibility for assessment of the adequacy of the proposed research requires the expertise of the IRB members.

An IRB review of proposed research that fails to adequately minimize risk may result in the approval of unethical research and may jeopardize the rights and welfare of human subjects. A thorough IRB review should ensure that human subjects are adequately protected, are not exposed to unnecessary risks, and are provided with enough information about a study so that they can give effective informed consent.

Please provide a written response that details the procedure Essex IRB intends to follow to ensure that the IRB members conduct a comprehensive review of proposed research, in accordance with the regulatory requirements for ensuring that risks to the subjects are minimized. Please submit a copy of any revised or new Standard Operating Procedures (SOPs) or written procedures developed to address this finding. Also, we note that your written response refers to the Essex IRB administrators, and we assume you are referring to the Essex IRB support staff. However, during the inspection, the FDA Investigators reviewed the job descriptions for the IRB support staff and found that none of the Essex IRB staff hold a title of IRB administrator. Please explain who you are referring to as the IRB administrators and clarify their role.

B. Our inspection revealed that Essex IRB failed to appropriately apply the FDA's regulatory definition of minimal risk. The regulations at 21 CFR 56.102(i) define minimal risk as, "*the probability and magnitude of harm or discomfort anticipated in the research are not greater in and of themselves than those ordinarily encountered in daily life or during the performance of routine physical or psychological examinations or tests.*" Based on our review of the available documentation, the IRB's practice of applying this definition and assessing risk in review of proposed research fails to adequately consider the risks associated with an investigational test article. Essex IRB incorrectly determined that the following two studies, which involve the use of investigational test articles, posed no more than minimal risk to subjects:

- **(b)(4)** (fictitious sponsor, **(b)(4)**)
- **(b)(4)** (**(b)(4)**, protocol **(b)(4)**)

The IRB's written response indicates that the IRB agrees that it incorrectly identified these studies as presenting no more than minimal risk to subjects, and outlines proposed corrective actions that include revision of an SOP to include the regulatory definition of minimal risk, and training on the new SOP for IRB members and administrators. The IRB also indicates that all determinations about the degree of risk presented by a study will be made in accordance with the regulatory definition of minimal risk. This response is incomplete because it does not describe the criteria the IRB intends to establish and follow to ensure adequate interpretation and application of this regulatory definition in the future (i.e., the procedure describing how the IRB will determine whether a study involves no more than minimal risk).

The IRB's failure to adequately assess minimal risk may lead the IRB to underestimate risk to subjects. Although, as noted in the IRB's written response the full IRB reviewed both studies listed above, any future misapplication of minimal risk may lead the IRB to review greater than minimal risk studies using an inappropriate review procedure, in violation of the IRB regulations, including the expedited review regulations found at 21 CFR 56.110. In addition, misapplication of the definition of minimal risk may lead the IRB to inadequately review research involving children, in violation of the additional safeguards for children in clinical investigations found at 21 CFR 50, subpart D.

Please provide a written response that outlines the criteria and the method the IRB will use to review proposed research in the future to ensure that the IRB appropriately assesses minimal risk. Please submit a copy of the revised SOP mentioned in your written response and any new SOPs or written procedures developed to address this finding.

2. The IRB failed to demonstrate its ability to ascertain the acceptability of the proposed research in terms of institutional commitments, regulations, applicable law, and standards of professional conduct and practice [21 CFR 56.107(a)].

Under 21 CFR 56.107(a), an IRB must be able to ascertain the acceptability of the proposed research in terms of institutional commitments, regulations, applicable law, and standards of professional conduct and practices. Our inspection revealed that the IRB failed to adequately assess the professional qualifications of the clinical investigator purported to be associated with protocol **(b)(4)** submitted by the fictitious sponsor. While we acknowledge the IRB's written response that it is the sponsor's responsibility to select qualified investigators, the IRB did not corroborate that the clinical investigator was a qualified clinical investigator. The IRB could have checked, among other things, that the medical license submitted to the IRB was valid in the State of Virginia where the research study was purported to be conducted. Failure to adequately consider the qualifications of the clinical investigator may expose subjects to unnecessary risks.

The IRB's written response indicates that, going forward, Essex IRB has implemented new procedures to verify the medical license documents submitted for all principal investigators as part of its review process, and that IRB administrators and IRB members will be trained on the revised SOP. This response is acceptable. Please submit a copy of the revised SOP mentioned in your written response.

3. The IRB failed to determine at the time of initial review that studies involving children are in compliance with 21 CFR Part 50, Subpart D, Additional Safeguards for Children in Clinical Investigations [21 CFR 56.109(h)].

Under 21 CFR 56.109(h), when some or all of the subjects in a study are children, the IRB must determine that the research study is in compliance with 21 CFR part 50, subpart D (Additional Safeguards for Children in Clinical Investigations) at the time of initial review. Under 21 CFR 50.50, an IRB may approve only those clinical investigations that satisfy the criteria described in 50.51 (clinical investigations not involving greater than minimal risk), 50.52 (clinical investigations involving greater than minimal risk but presenting the prospect of direct benefit to individual subjects), or 50.53 (clinical investigations involving greater than minimal risk and no prospect of direct benefit to individual subjects, but likely to yield generalizable knowledge about the subject's disorder or condition). Under 21 CFR 50.51, 50.52, and 50.53, the IRB must make and document certain findings. Our inspection revealed that in its review and approval of research involving pediatric subjects, Essex IRB failed to adequately find and document that the research satisfied the criteria of 50.51, 50.52, or 50.53. Specifically, the following pediatric study was reviewed and approved by the IRB, but the IRB records do not specify whether the study was approved under 50.51, 50.52, or 50.53:

- (b)(4) ((b)(4) protocol (b)(4))

Failure to determine that the additional safeguards for children in research are met may expose this vulnerable population to unnecessary risks, and result in the child's parent(s) or guardian(s) not being fully informed about the proposed research.

In addition, we note that IRB records for this protocol (**(b)(4)**) and a second pediatric study (Pediatric Constipation Study **(b)(4)**) reviewed during the inspection include multiple inaccurate regulatory references with regard to 21 CFR part 50, subpart D. These records include, but are not limited to the following documents:

- The sample pediatric protocol checklist attached to SOP SXSOP1013
- The pediatric protocol checklist used for each study
- The letter to the sponsor from the IRB for the constipation study
- The IRB meeting minutes for the constipation study

The IRB's written response states that Essex IRB has an SOP governing the assessment of the degree of pediatric risk in accordance with 21 CFR part 50, subpart D, but the IRB failed to document that determination. The written response also states that the IRB administrators and IRB members will be retrained on the need to document in the meeting minutes the risk determination, along with other required documentation depending on the identified risk determination. This response is incomplete because it does not describe the actual process the IRB will use to ascertain that the research satisfies the criteria of 50.51, 50.52, or 50.53 for research involving children. We remain concerned that the IRB may not fully understand the additional safeguards for children that must be met in the review of research involving pediatric subjects. Please provide a written response that details the process the IRB will use to adequately evaluate and document that the research satisfies the criteria of 50.51, 50.52, or 50.53 in its review of future research involving pediatric subjects. Please submit a copy of any revised or new SOPs or written procedures developed to address this finding.

Lastly, the IRB's written response says that Essex IRB will also audit all ongoing pediatric studies to assure that the risk determination has been appropriately completed and documented. Please submit the results to FDA as soon as the audit is completed.

4. The IRB failed to ensure that basic elements of informed consent are included in the IRB approved consent form [21 CFR 56.109(b)].

Under 21 CFR 56.109(b), the IRB must require that information given to subjects as part of the informed consent is in accordance with 21 CFR 50.25 (elements of informed consent). Our inspection revealed that Essex IRB failed to ensure that the IRB-approved informed consent forms for the following two studies contained adequate information about reasonably foreseeable risks or discomforts as required by 21 CFR 50.25(a)(2):

- **(b)(4)** (fictitious sponsor, protocol **(b)(4)**)
- **(b)(4)** (**(b)(4)**, protocol number **(b)(4)**)

As described in item #1A above, because it appears that the IRB failed to discuss the potential for increased risk of serious cardiovascular events for the **(b)(4)** study, the IRB failed to ensure that the potential for associated cardiovascular risks was included in the IRB-approved informed consent form.

The protocol provided to Essex IRB by the sponsor for the **(b)(4)** study lists graft rejection as a common adverse reaction in adult patients taking **(b)(4)**. The IRB meeting minutes for September 7, 2010, indicate that the IRB requested that the sponsor reformat the informed consent form to move the risk of graft rejection to a different paragraph in the informed consent document. Our inspection revealed that the IRB failed to ensure that graft rejection was included in the final IRB-approved informed consent form, as this risk was not included at all.

Failure to ensure that all of the FDA required elements of informed consent are met may result in human subjects not being provided with enough information about a study so that they can give effective informed consent.

The IRB's written response does not specifically address Form FDA 483 Observation 3. However, in response to Form FDA 483 Observation 1C, the IRB indicated that for the **(b)(4)** study, the IRB recognizes that the adverse event of graft rejection was inadvertently removed instead of being moved to a new location in the informed consent document. The IRB also indicates that the informed consent checklist will be revised to prompt IRB reviewers and staff to ensure that risk information in the informed consent document is consistent with risk information identified in the protocol, investigator brochure, or other relevant document (e.g. package insert) and will also prompt the IRB to request information from the sponsor or investigator where inconsistencies are identified. This response is acceptable. Please submit a copy of the revised informed consent checklist, and any revised or new SOPs or written procedures developed to accompany the revised form.

This letter is not intended to be an all-inclusive list of deficiencies for the protocols reviewed and approved by the IRB. It is your responsibility to ensure that Essex IRB's practices and procedures comply fully with all applicable statutes and regulations.

Within fifteen (15) business days of your receipt of this letter, you should notify this office in writing of the actions you have taken to prevent similar violations in the future. Your written response should include any documentation necessary to show that full and adequate correction will be achieved. Please include the projected completion dates for each action to be accomplished. Failure to adequately and promptly explain the violations noted above may result in regulatory action without further notice.

We recommend that you visit the following FDA web page for information on human subject protections that may assist you in your efforts to bring the IRB into compliance with FDA regulations:

http://www.fda.gov/ScienceResearch/SpecialTopics/RunningClinicalTrials/default.htm

We appreciate the cooperation shown to FDA Investigators Wydner, Visco and Donnelly during the inspection. If you have any questions, please contact Kevin Prohaska, D.O., M.P.H., at 3017963707; FAX 3018478748. Your written response and any pertinent documentation should be addressed to:

Kevin Prohaska, D.O., M.P.H.
Acting Director, Division of Safety Compliance Office of Scientific Investigations
Office of Compliance
Center for Drug Evaluation and Research Food and Drug Administration
Bldg 51, Room 5356
10903 New Hampshire Avenue Silver Spring, MD 20993

Sincerely,

/S/

Leslie K. Ball, M.D.
Acting Director
Office of Scientific Investigations
Office of Compliance
Center for Drug Evaluation and Research
Food and Drug Administration

Cc: Glenn Lambert, M.D., IRB Chairman
Essex Institutional Review Board, Inc.
121 Main Street
Lebanon, NJ 08833

Loretta Szczepanski, R.N., IRB Vice Chairperson
Essex Institutional Review Board, Inc.
121 Main Street
Lebanon, NJ 08833

Karen Radcliffe, Office Manager and Coordinator
Essex Institutional Review Board, Inc.
121 Main Street
Lebanon, NJ 08833

第20封　给海湾地区医疗中心伦理委员会的警告信

2010年9月9日

参考号：10-HFD-45-09-01

尊敬的Gerard女士：

2010年6月2日至6月4日，Nancy Bellamy 女士代表FDA，对海湾地区医疗中心（以下简称BRMC）的伦理委员会进行了现场检查。本次现场检查的目的是核实贵伦理委员会（IRB）受试者保护程序是否符合美国联邦法规（CFR）第21篇第50和56部分的要求。这些法规适用于FDA所监管产品的临床研究。我们知道，在现场检查结束时，我们的检查员向您出示了FDA 483表，即现场检查发现的问题，并与您进行了讨论。

经对现场检查报告及该报告的附件进行审查，我们认为，贵伦理委员会没有遵循适用的法律要求和监管受试者保护的FDA法规。我们确认，收到了来自医学事务副总裁 Jay Summer 博士对FDA 483表的书面回复，该回复的签署日期为2010年7月20日，超出了现场检查结束后15个工作日回复的期限。因此，尽管我们已经审阅了回复，但根据2009年8月11日公布的局长执行倡议的要求，我们没有就回复内容进行讨论。我们想强调以下几点：

1. IRB未能遵守关于对研究进行初始审查和跟踪审查的书面程序［21 CFR 56.108（a）（1）］

伦理委员会应遵循书面程序和法规对涵盖范围内的研究予以审查和批准。我们的检查发现，伦理委员会未能遵循书面程序的情况如下：

a）伦理委员会政策和程序手册第4页（有关会议部分）规定："每项提交的研究将分配给一名指定的委员进行深入审查，并在伦理委员会会议上陈述。"我们注意到，BRMC伦理委员会实施该程序记录伦理委员会的审查过程的做法，源于2009年3月FDA对BRMC伦理委员会现场检查的结果。我们目前的现场检查发现，BMRC伦理委员会在2009年7月10日、2009年9月11日、2009年11月13日、2010年1月8日和2010年3月12日的伦理委员会会议上并未遵循该程序。现场检查中，伦理委员会秘书确认，伦理委员会没有按照书面程序要求将研究方案分配给一名指定的委员进行深入审查并在会议上陈述。

b）伦理委员会政策和程序手册第7页（有关记录和报告部分）规定："将对伦理委员会跟踪系统进行维护，以完成方案的跟踪审查，包括在知情同意文件上使用标注失效期的印章，以确保遵循联邦法规要求，对方案进行年度审查或按照伦理委员会要求进行更高频度的审查。"我们注意到，伦理委员会政策和程序手册补充了建立和维护跟踪系统这一计划，是2009年3月FDA对BRMC伦理委员会现场检查的结果。我们目前的现场检查发现，BMRC伦理委员会并没有正式的跟踪系统对其职权范围内的方案进行监测，而是依赖于跟踪审查到期时临床研究者的自我报告。而且，我们的现场检查发现，伦理委员会并没有根据如下#2所描述的合适间隔，对方案进行跟踪审查，缺乏发挥功能的跟踪系统，并且完全依赖于临床研究者通知伦理委员会何时进行跟踪审查是不恰当的，并可能导致如以下2.所描述的未进行跟踪审查的事件发生。

2. IRB未能按照不少于一年一次的频次对研究进行跟踪审查［21 CFR 56.109（f）］

2009年5月8日，BRMC伦理委员会开会，对题为"（b）（4）"的方案进行了年度审查并予以了批准。这个方案接下来的年度审查到期日是2010年5月7日。然而，我们的检查员发现，该方案的年度审查直到2010年6月FDA现场检查时仍未进行，该研究并未列在即将于2010年6月4日召开的伦理委员会会议的议程上。

另外，关于试验方案（b）（4），伦理委员会并没有遵循伦理委员会政策和流程手册第六页所述的跟踪审查的流程，“应对研究项目进行至少每年一次的跟踪审查。对于需要进行比每年一次更高频率审查研究项目，应基于受试者的风险而决定审查的频率。”

本警告信的目的并非是罗列贵伦理委员会在审查和批准试验方案时存在的所有缺陷。确保BMRC伦理委员会的操作和规程完全符合所有适用法律法规的要求是您的职责。

自收到这封信的15个工作日内，您应当书面告知本办公室为预防将来发生类似违规情况而采取的措施。您的书面回复应回应这封信中提到的所有问题，提供必需的文件证明将实现的完整充分的纠正。请提供纠正措施计划完成的日期。如果不能充分、迅速地解释上述违规问题，可能导致我们在不再通知的情况下采取监管措施。如果您确信2010年7月20日Summer博士对FDA 483表的书面回复充分地解释了您为避免将来发生类似的违规而已采取的措施，请在15个工作日内以书面的形式与我们沟通。如上所述，我们计划评估您对FDA 483表的书面回复，以及其他作为回复这封警告信的任何书面文件。您在回复这封信的时候可参考2010年7月20日的书面回复。

我们注意到，在现场检查结束时，您告知FDA检查员，在不久的将来，BRMC计划（b）(4）伦理委员会。我们要求您在书面回复中包括对这个计划的描述，包括（b）(4）对BMRC伦理委员会范围内的所有研究承担责任的计划，以及该计划预期的时限。

附：英文原文

Bay Regional Medical Center IRB

WARNING LETTER

September 9, 2010

UPS

Ref: 10-HFD-45-09-01

September 9, 2010
Alice M. Gerard, RN, MSN
President and Chief Executive Officer
Bay Regional Medical Center
1900 Columbus Avenue
Bay City, Michigan 48708

Dear Ms. Gerard:

Between June 2, 2010 and June 4, 2010, Ms. Nancy Bellamy, representing the Food and Drug Administration (FDA), inspected the Institutional Review Board (IRB) at Bay Regional Medical Center (BRMC). The purpose of this inspection was to determine whether the IRB procedures for the protection of human subjects complied with Title 21 of the Code of Federal Regulations (CFR), parts 50 and 56. These regulations apply to clinical investigations of products regulated by FDA. We are aware that at the conclusion of the inspection, our investigator(s) presented and discussed with you, a Form FDA 483, Inspectional Observations.

From our review of the establishment inspection report and the documents submitted with that report, we conclude that the IRB did not adhere to the applicable statutory requirements and FDA regulations governing the protection of human subjects. We acknowledge receipt of the written response from Dr. Jay Summer, Vice President Medical Affairs, dated July 20, 2010 to Form FDA 483 but note that this response was received past the fifteen (15) business days from close of the inspection. Thus, while we have reviewed the response, we have not included a discussion of the response in this letter as per the Commissioner's Enforcement Initiative announced August 11, 2009. We wish to emphasize the following:

1. The IRB failed to follow its written procedures for conducting its initial and continuing review of research [21 CFR 56.108(a)(1)].

The IRB is required to follow written procedures in its review and approval of research covered by the regulations. Our inspection revealed that the IRB failed to follow its written procedures in the following situations:

a) On page 4 of the IRB's Policy and Procedure Manual (under Meetings section) it states "Each study submitted will be assigned to a specific member of the IRB for in-depth review and presentation at the meeting." We note that the BRMC IRB implemented this procedure to document the IRB's review process as a result of the previous FDA inspection of the BRMC IRB conducted in March 2009. Our current inspection revealed that the IRB failed to follow this procedure at IRB meetings held on July 10, 2009, September 11, 2009, November 13, 2009, January 8, 2010 and March 12, 2010. During this inspection, the IRB secretary confirmed that the IRB has not been following its written procedures to assign the review of protocols to a specific member of the IRB for an in-depth review and presentation at IRB meetings.

b) On page 7 of the IRB's Policy and Procedure Manual (under Records and Reports section) it states "An IRB tracking system will be maintained for continuing review of protocols including the use of expiration date stamps on consent documents to ensure that the federal requirement for IRB review of each protocol is done annually or more frequently as required by the IRB." We note that the plan to develop and maintain a tracking system was added to the IRB's Policy and Procedure Manual as a result of the previous FDA inspection of the BRMC IRB conducted in March 2009. Our current inspection revealed that BRMC IRB has no formal tracking system to monitor the status of protocols under its purview and instead relies on clinical investigators to self-report when continuing review is due. Further, our inspection revealed that the IRB failed to conduct continuing review at appropriate intervals as described in item #2 below. The lack of a properly functioning tracking system and the exclusive reliance on clinical investigators to inform the IRB of upcoming continuing review dates is inadequate and has the potential to result in missed continuing review dates as exemplified in item #2 below.

2. The IRB failed to conduct continuing review of research at intervals of not less than once per year [21 CFR 56.109(f)].

On May 8, 2009, BRMC IRB met and approved the annual renewal for Protocol **(b)(4)** entitled "**(b)(4)**." A subsequent continuing review for this protocol was due by May 7, 2010. However, our inspection revealed that continuing review had not been conducted as of the time of the FDA inspection in early June 2010, and that the study was not on the agenda for the upcoming June 4, 2010 IRB meeting.

In addition, with respect to Protocol **(b)(4)**, the IRB did not follow its written procedures for conducting continuing review of research which states on page 6 of the IRB's Policy and Procedure Manual, "Research projects will be reviewed annually. The frequency of reviewing projects, which require review more often than annually, shall be determined individually based on the risk to human subjects involved."

This letter is not intended to be an all-inclusive list of deficiencies for the protocols reviewed and approved by the IRB. It is your responsibility to ensure that BRMC IRB's practices and procedures comply fully with all applicable statutes and regulations.

Within fifteen (15) business days of your receipt of this letter, you should notify this office in writing of the actions you have taken to prevent similar violations in the future. Your written response should include any documentation necessary to show that full and adequate correction will be achieved. Please include the projected completion dates for each action to be accomplished. Failure to adequately and promptly explain the violations noted above may result in regulatory action without further notice. If you believe that Dr. Summer's written response to the Form FDA 483 dated July 20, 2010 fully explains the actions you have taken to prevent similar violations in the future, please communicate that to us in writing within fifteen (15) business days. As noted above, we plan to evaluate your written response to the Form FDA 483 along with any other written material provided as a direct response to this Warning

Letter. You may reference the written response dated July 20, 2010 in your response to this letter.

We note, that during the close of the inspection, you informed the FDA Investigator that Bay Regional Medical Center plans to **(b)(4)** the IRB in the near future. We request you include in your written response to this letter a description of the plan to **(b)(4)** BRMC IRB, including the plan for the responsible **(b)(4)** of all studies under the purview of BRMC IRB and the expected timeline for such actions.

We recommend that you visit the following FDA web page for information on human subject protections that may assist you in your efforts to bring the IRB into compliance with FDA regulations:

http://www.fda.gov/Science Research/Special Topics/Running Clinical Trials/default.html

We appreciate the cooperation shown to FDA Investigator Bellamy during the inspection. If you have any questions, please contact Kevin Prohaska, D.O., M.P.H., at 301-796-3707; FAX 301-847-8748. Your written response and any pertinent documentation should be addressed to:

Kevin Prohaska, D.O., M.P.H.
Human Subjects Protections Team Lead
Division of Scientific Investigations
Office of Compliance
Center for Drug Evaluation and Research
Food and Drug Administration
Bldg 51, Room 5356
10903 New Hampshire Avenue
Silver Spring, MD 20993

Sincerely,

/S/

Leslie K. Ball, M.D.
Director
Division of Scientific Investigations
Office of Compliance
Center for Drug Evaluation and Research
Food and Drug Administration

第21封 给Ephraim McDowell地区医疗中心伦理委员会的警告信

2010年4月26日

参考号：10-HFD-45-04-03

尊敬的Danville女士：

2009年12月21日至2010年1月6日，Karen Bryerton Cooper女士和Craig Rybus先生代表FDA对Ephraim McDowell地区医疗中心的伦理委员会进行了现场检查。此次现场检查的目的是核实伦理委员会受试者保护程序是否符合美国联邦法规第21篇第50和56部分的要求。这些法规适用于FDA所监管产品的临床研究。我们知道在现场检查结束时，我们的检查员向药房主任Joan Haltom博士，研究协调员（b）(6）女士及药房工作人员（b）(6）女士出示并讨论了FDA483表，即现场检查发现的问题。

经对现场检查报告、该报告的附件进行审查，我们认为，贵伦理委员会没有遵循适用的法律要求和监管受试者保护的FDA法规。我们确认收到了2010年2月3日伦理委员会主席Thomas Baeker博士对FDA483表作出的书面回复。但我们是在发出FDA483表后超过15个工作日才收到该书面回复，因此该回复还未予以考虑。我们计划将Baeker博士对FDA483表作出的书面回复以及提交的其他书面资料一起，作为对本警告信的直接回复进行评估。

我们想强调以下几点：

1. IRB未能制定和维护用于IRB的书面程序，未能遵守21 CFR 56.108（a）和（b）要求的书面程序［21 CFR 56.115（a）(6）］

为确保符合伦理委员会相关的法规要求，每个伦理委员会应制定、维护并遵循书面程序，该程序应描述法规具体要求的伦理委员会的职能和运行。我们检查发现，贵伦理委员会未制定和维护实现伦理委员会职能和运行的适当的书面程序，因而也未能遵循此书面程序。贵伦理委员会名为“组织政策”的文件，是伦理委员会工作人员认定为有效的唯一政策性文件，也是已签署的唯一供FDA检查的文件，但该文件未包括下列内容：

a. 对临床研究进行初始伦理审查和跟踪审查的书面程序，及向研究者、研究机构报告审查意见的书面程序［21CFR56.108（a）(1）］。我们承认“组织政策”文件包含了有限的关于审查的规定，如需要超过半数委员投票，规定了法定人数；然而该文件仍然不足以体现法规的要求。

b. 下列工作有关的书面程序：如何确定应对哪些项目进行比年度审查更频繁的审查，以及哪些项目需要从研究者以外的来源获得证实，以确认研究资料自上次伦理审查后未经变更［21 CFR 56.108（a）(2）］。

c. 确保及时向伦理委员会报告研究事项变更的书面程序［21 CFR 56.108（a）(3）］。

d. 书面程序以确保已获得伦理委员会批准的研究发生变更时，未获得伦理委员会审查和批准不能启动，（除非是为了避免对受试者造成明显的直接伤害）［21CFR56.108（a）(4）］。

e. 确保及时向伦理委员会、适当的机构管理人员及FDA报告涉及受试者和其他人员安全的非预期问题的书面程序［21CFR56.108（b）(1）］。

f. 确保及时向伦理委员会、适当的机构管理人员及FDA报告严重或持续地违反法规要求，或伦理委员会决议的书面程序［21CFR56.108（b）(2）］。

g. 确保及时向伦理委员会、适当的机构管理人员及FDA报告暂停或终止伦理委员会批准的书面程序

［21CFR56.108（b）（3）］。

2. IRB未能制定和保存一份IRB的委员名单，标识姓名、获得学位、代表资格等足以描述每位委员对IRB审议能带来的主要预期贡献的指标，以及每位委员和机构之间的雇佣或其他关系［21 CFR 56.115（a）（5）］

作为伦理委员会文档管理的一部分，伦理委员会应根据法规要求保存一份伦理委员会委员名单。

我们现场检查时发现，伦理委员会未能制定和保存一份符合法规要求的伦理委员会委员名单。提供给FDA检查员审查的伦理委员会委员名单（2006~2007年，2007~2008年，2008~2009年）均未注明获得学位、代表资格，不足以描述每位委员对伦理委员会审议能带来的主要预期贡献的指标；或每位委员与机构之间的雇佣或的其他隶属关系。

我们注意到既往于2004年1月对Ephraim McDowell地区医疗中心伦理委员会的检查发现同样的缺陷。

3. IRB未能在大多数IRB委员出席，其中至少包括一名来自非科学领域委员召集的会议上对拟开展的研究进行审查［21 CFR 56.108（c）］

除采用快速审查程序外，伦理委员会是可以只在大多数IRB委员出席（例如，法定人数），其中至少包括一名来自非科学领域的委员的召集会议上对被提议的研究进行审查。

我们检查发现，贵伦理委员会开会审查和批准研究时，缺少大多数委员出席。例如：

a. 2007年4月25日的会议记录显示，有8位伦理委员会委员参加会议审查并批准研究。但同期的伦理委员会委员名单包括17位委员，这意味着至少应有9位委员到会，以达到法定人数的要求。

b. 2009年10月28日的会议记录显示，有8位伦理委员会委员参加会议审查并批准研究。但同期的伦理委员会委员名单包括17位委员，这意味着至少应有9位委员到会，以达到法定人数的要求。

由于上述第二条中提到的关于伦理委员会委员名单的缺陷，导致我们在审查伦理委员会会议记录时无法确认要求出席的非科学领域委员是否到会。

我们注意到既往于2004年1月对Ephraim McDowell地区医疗中心伦理委员会的检查发现同样的缺陷。

4. IRB未能以书面形式通知研究者和机构批准或不予批准被提议的研究的决定，或为保证IRB批准研究而要求的修改意见［21 CFR 56.109（e）］

伦理委员会应将其同意，或不同意，或做必要修正后重审的审查决议以书面形式传达给研究者和研究机构［21 CFR 56.109（e）］。

贵伦理委员会的“组织政策”文件声明，伦理委员会的会议记录将发送给医疗执行委员会。我们检查发现，贵伦理委员会的会议记录未发送给医学执行委员会。没有迹象表明，贵伦理委员会将其发现的问题和措施以书面形式通知研究机构。

本警告信的目的并非是罗列IRB在审查和批准试验方案中存在的所有缺陷。确保Ephraim McDowell地区医疗中心伦理委员会的实际操作和程序完全符合所有适用法律和法规的要求是您的职责。

自收到这封信的15个工作日内，您应当书面告知本办公室为预防将来发生类似违规情况已经采取的措施。您的书面回复应包括所有必要的文件来显示违规行为得到完全和充分的纠正。请包括每一项纠正措施的计划完成日期。如果不能充分、迅速地对上述违规问题进行解释，可能导致我们在不再通知的情况下采取监管措施。

如果您确信Baeker博士于2010年2月3日针对FDA483表的书面回复充分解释了您为预防将来发生类似违规情况已经采取的措施，请您自收到这封信的15个工作日内通知我们。如上所述，我们计划将Baeker博士对FDA483表作出的书面回复以及提交的其他书面资料一起，作为对本警告信的直接回复进行评估。在您回复此信时，请参考您2010年2月3日的书面回复。

附：英文原文

Ephraim McDowell Regional Medical Center IRB

WARNING LETTER

Apr 26, 2010

CERTIFIED MAIL
RETURN RECEIPT REQUESTED

Ref.10-HFD-45-04-03

Ms. Vicki Darnell
President and Chief Executive Officer
Ephraim McDowell Regional Medical Center
217 S. 3rd St.
Danville, KY 40422

Dear Ms. Danville:

Between December 21, 2009 and January6, 2010, Ms. Karen Bryerton Cooper, and Mr. Craig Rybus, representing the Food and Drug Administration(FDA), inspected the Institutional Review Board(IRB) at the Ephraim Mc Dowell Regional Medical Center. The purpose of this inspection was to determine whether the IRB procedures for the protection of human subjects complied with Title 21 of the Code of Federal Regulations(CFR), parts50 and 56.These regulations apply to clinical investigations of products regulated by FDA. We are aware that at the conclusion of the inspection, our investigators presented and discussed with Dr. Joan Haltom, Pharmacy Director, Ms. (b)(6), Study Coordinator, and Ms.(b)(6), Pharmacy Operations Clerk, a Form FDA483, Inspectional Observations.

From our review of the establishment inspection report and the documents submitted with that report, we conclude that the IRB did not adhere to the applicable statutory requirements and FDA regulations governing the protection of human subjects. We acknowledge Dr. Thomas Baeker, IRB Chairman's written response dated February 3, 2010, to the Form FDA483. However, because this written response was received more than fifteen business days after the Form FDA483 was issued, the response has not been considered. We plan to evaluate Dr. Baeker's written response to the Form FDA 483 along with any other written material provided as the direct response to this letter.

We wish to emphasize the following:

1. The IRB failed to prepare and maintain written procedures for the IRB and failed to follow written procedures as required by 21CFR 56.108(a) and (b) [21CFR 56.115(a) (6)].

In order to fulfill the requirements of the IRB regulations, each IRB must prepare, maintain, and follow written procedures describing IRB functions and operations specified in the regulations.

Our inspection revealed that the IRB failed to prepare and maintain, and therefore did not follow, adequate written procedures for the IRB functions and operations. The IRB's Organizational Policy document, the only policy identified by the IRB staff as being in effect, and the only one examined by FDA that is signed, does not include the following:

a. Written procedures for conducting its initial and continuing review of research and for reporting its findings and actions to the investigator and the institution [21CFR 56.108(a)(1)]. We acknowledge some limited references in the Organizational Policy document to certain aspects of review, such as the need for majority vote, and identification of quorum; however, this is not sufficient to address the requirements of this provision.

b. Written procedures for determining which projects require review more often than annually and which projects need verification from sources other than the investigator that no material changes have occurred since previous IRB review [21CFR 56.108(a)(2)].

c. Written procedures for ensuring prompt reporting to the IRB of changes in research activities [21CFR 56.108(a)(3)].

d. Written procedures for ensuring that changes in approved research, during the period for which IRB approval has already been given, may not be initiated without IRB review and approval except where necessary to eliminate apparent immediate hazards to the human subjects [21CFR 56.108(a)(4)].

e. Written procedures for ensuring prompt reporting to the IRB, appropriate institutional officials, and the FDA of any unanticipated problems involving risks to human subjects or others [21CFR 56.108(b)(1)].

f. Written procedures for ensuring prompt reporting to the IRB, appropriate institutional officials, and the FDA of any instance of serious or continuing noncompliance with these regulations or the requirements or determinations of the IRB [21CFR 56.108(b)(2)].

g. Written procedures for ensuring prompt reporting to the IRB, appropriate institutional officials, and the FDA of any suspension or termination of IRB approval [21 CFR 56.108(b)(3)].

2. The IRB failed to prepare and maintain a list of IRB members identified by name; earned degrees; representative capacity; indications of experience sufficient to describe each member's chief anticipated contributions to IRB deliberations; and any employment or other relationship between each member and the institution [21CFR 56.115(a)(5)].

As part of preparing adequate IRB records, the IRB is required to maintain a list of IRB members in accordance with the regulations.

Our inspection revealed that the IRB failed to prepare and maintain an adequate list of IRB member in compliance with the regulations. None of the IRB membership rosters reviewed by the FDA Investigators (years 2006-2007, years 2007-2008, and years 2008-2009) include each IRB member's earned degree, representative capacity, indications of experience sufficient to describe the member's chief anticipated contributions to the IRB deliberations, or any employment or other relationship between the member and the institution.

We note that this finding is a repeat issue from the previous inspection of the Ephraim Mc Dowell Regional Medical Center IRB conducted in January 2004.

3. The IRB failed to review proposed research at convened meetings at which a majority of the members of the IRB are present, including at least one member whose primary concerns are in nonscientific areas [21CFR 56.108(c)].

Except when an expedited review procedure is used, the IRB may only review proposed research at convened meetings at which a majority of the IRB members (i.e., a quorum) is present, including at least one member whose primary concerns are in nonscientific areas.

Our inspection revealed that the IRB reviewed and approved research at meetings at which a majority of the IRB members was not present. For example:

a. Meeting minutes dated April 25, 2007 indicate that eight IRB members were present at the meeting, during which research was reviewed and approved. The IRB membership roster for the noted time period included seventeen members, meaning that at least nine members were required to be present in order to have a quorum.

b. Meeting minutes dated October 28, 2009 indicate that eight IRB members were present at the meeting, during which research was reviewed and approved. The IRB membership roster for the noted time period included seventeen members, meaning that at least nine members were required to be present in order to have a quorum.

The deficiencies found in the IRB membership rosters discussed in item #2 above, made it difficult to determine whether the required nonscientist was present a tall convened IRB meetings when reviewing IRB meeting minutes.

We note that this finding is a repeat issue from the previous inspection of the Ephraim McDowell Regional Medical Center IRB conducted in January 2004.

4. The IRB failed to notify investigators and the institution in writing of its decision to approve or disapprove proposed research activities, or of modifications required to secure IRB approval of the research activity [21 CFR 56.109(e)].

The IRB is required to notify investigators and the institution in writing of its decision to approve or disapprove proposed research, or of modifications required to secure IRB approval.

The IRB Organizational Policy document states that the minutes from the IRB will be forwarded to the Medical Executive Committee. Our inspection revealed that the IRB meeting minutes are not being forwarded to the Medical

Executive Committee. There is no indication that IRB is notifying the institution in writing of its findings and actions. This letter is not intended to be an all-inclusive list of deficiencies for the protocols reviewed and approved by the IRB. It is your responsibility to ensure that the Ephraim McDowell Regional Medical Center IRB's practices and procedures comply fully with all applicable statutes and regulations.

Within fifteen (15) business days of your receipt of this letter, you should notify this office in writing of the actions you have taken to prevent similar violations in the future. Your written response should include any documentation necessary to show that full and adequate correction will be achieved. Please include the projected completion dates for each action to be accomplished. Failure to adequately and promptly explain the violations noted above may result in regulatory action without further notice. If you believe that Dr. Baeker's written response to the Form FDA 483 dated February 3, 2010 fully explains the actions you have taken to prevent similar violations in the future, please communicate that to us in writing within fifteen (15) business days. As noted above, we plan to evaluate your written response to the Form FDA 483 along with any other written material provided as a direct response to this Warning Letter. You may reference the written response dated February 3, 2010 in your response to this letter.

We recommend that you visit the following FDA web page for information on human subject protection that may assist you in your efforts to bring the IRB into compliance with FDA regulations:

http://www.fda.gov/ScienceResearch/SpecialTopics/RunningClinicalTrials/default.htm

We appreciate the cooperation shown to FDA Investigators Bryerton Cooper and Rybus during the inspection. If you have any questions, please contact Kevin Prohaska, D.O., M.P.H., at 301-796-3707; FAX 301-847-8748. Your written response and any pertinent documentation should be addressed to:

Kevin Prohaska, D.O., M.P.H.
Acting Human Subjects Protections Team Lead
Division of Scientific Investigations
Office of Compliance
Center for Drug Evaluation and Research
Food and Drug Administration
Bldg 51, Room 5356
10903 New Hampshire Avenue
Silver Spring, MD 20993

Sincerely yours,

/S/

Leslie K. Ball, M.D.
Director
Office of Scientific Investigations
Office of Compliance
Center for Drug Evaluation and Research
Food and Drug Administration

Cc: Dr. Thomas Baeker
IRB Chairman
Ephraim McDowell Regional Medical Center
217 S.3rd St.
Danville, KY 40422
Dr. Joan Haltom
Pharmacy Director
Ephraim McDowell Regional Medical Center

217 S.3rd St.
Danville, KY 40422

Ms. (b)(6)
Study Coordinator
Ephraim McDowell Regional Medical Center
217 S.3rd St.
Danville, KY 40422

Ms. (b)(6)
Pharmacy Operations Clerk
Ephraim McDowell Regional Medical Center
217 S.3rd St.
Danville, KY 40422

Dr. (b)(6)
Pharmacist
Ephraim McDowell Regional Medical Center
217 S.3rd St.
Danville, KY 40422

第 22 封　给 Brookwood 医疗中心的警告信

2010年4月22日

参考号：10-HFD-45-04-02

尊敬的Gause先生：

2009年11月9日至11月19日，Patricia S.Smith 女士代表FDA，对Brookwood 医疗中心伦理委员会进行了现场检查。本次现场检查的目的是核实伦理委员会保护受试者的程序是否符合美国联邦法规第21篇第50和56部分的要求。这些法规适用于FDA所监管产品的临床研究。我们注意到现场检查结束时，我们检查员向您出示并讨论了FDA483表，即现场检查发现的问题。

经对现场检查报告、该报告的附件进行审查，我们认为，伦理委员会没有遵循适用法律要求和监管受试者保护的FDA法规。我们确认收到了您于2010年1月6日对FDA483表的书面回复。然而，因为我们收到这一书面回复的时间超过FDA483表发布后的15个工作日，所以您的回复不予考虑。我们计划将您对FDA483表的回复，以及任何其他的书面材料一起，作为对警告信的直接回复进行评估。

我们想强调以下几点：

1. IRB未能遵守对研究进行跟踪审查的书面程序［21 CFR 56.108（a）（1）］

我们现场检查中发现伦理委员会未遵守对研究进行跟踪审查书面程序的几个例子。伦理委员会书面程序规定，正在进行的临床研究必须由伦理委员会以至少每年审查一次的频率进行审查，或当IRB发现对受试者的风险程度更高而进行更高频率的审查。这种更新必须在批准的方案上标注的有效期满前实施。否则受试者新增必须停止。如此项研究是卫生和公众服务部发起的，必须通知这个机构。如果在45天内未收到更新报告，将关闭此项研究。我们对伦理委员会记录的审查确定如下：

伦理委员会对试验方案（b）（4）批准存在两项缺陷。

i. 试验方案（b）（4）初始审查批准有效期至2007年5月31日，但是直到2007年7月2日才实施跟踪审查，因此该项目伦理委员会的批准失效超过了1个月。

ii. 随后的跟踪审查有效期至2008年7月1日，然而无文件记录这次审查，直到2009年4月10日递交了终版审查报告，比规定的跟踪审查晚了10个月，伦理委员会跟踪审查批准失效了9个月。

试验方案（b）（4）在2008年7月3日获得增加6个月的再批准。因为有效期到2008年12月31日。这次跟踪审查有效期满到我们现场检查时间相隔10个月时间，FDA 没有见到跟踪审查记录，可见伦理委员会的批准失效10个月。

初始审查试验方案（b）（4）批准的有效期至2009年6月30日，然而直到2009年8月27日才进行再次批准。因此伦理委员会批准失效几乎2个月。

所有3个FDA审查的项目均存在这个严重问题。此外，在2003年2月现场检查时FDA记录下的问题没有得到纠正。

2. IRB未能遵守“确保已批准研究中的变更在被IRB批准期间，未得到IRB审查和批准不能启动，除非是为了消除对受试者造成的直接伤害”的书面程序［21 CFR 56.108（a）（4）］

伦理委员会书面程序规定，实施变更的临床试验方案必须事先获得伦理委员会的批准。我们审查2008年5月22日伦理委员会会议记录，发现伦理委员会记录的下列方案变更没有根据21CFR 56.108（c）要求进行投票表决和获得出席的多数委员批准。

试验方案（b）（4）修正案1包括增加联合用药，如静脉注射阿片类药物、吸入性的类固醇和德美罗；

试验方案（b）（4）修正案2 包括受试者入选标准重大变更，如上调受试者年龄上限从75岁到80岁，并允许招募不同于初始方案规定的受试者类型。

3. IRB未能确定受试者风险最小化［21CFR 56.111（a）（1）］

我们审查伦理委员会2008年4月28日会议记录，FDA注意到，伦理委员会要求提供前2个季度的数据和安全监查委员会审查和统计总结的复印件，因为他们担忧（b）（4）方案发生过流血、栓塞和死亡。尽管有这些担忧，但没有证据表明伦理委员会曾收到了这些文件，这项研究一直允许继续进行，直到试验在2009年4月23日结束。

本警告信的目的并非是罗列对伦理委员会审查和批准试验方案中存在的所有缺陷。确保Brookwood医疗中心伦理委员会的操作和程序符合所有适用法律和法规的要求是您的职责。

自收到这封信的15个工作日内，您应当书面告知本办公室为预防将来发生类似违规情况已经采取的措施。如果不能充分、迅速地解释上述违规问题，可能导致我们在不再通知的情况下采取监管措施。如果您确信在2010年1月6日书面回复中充分解释了您为预防将来发生类似违规行为已经采取的措施，请在15个工作日内以书面形式联系FDA。如上所述，我们计划将您对FDA483表的回复以及任何其他的书面材料一起，作为对警告信的直接回复进行评估。您对本警告信的回复可以参考2010年1月6日的回复。

附：英文原文

Brookwood Medical Center

WARNING LETTER

Apr 22, 2010

CERTIFIED MAIL
RETURN RECEIPT REQUESTED

Ref: 10-HFD-45-04-02

Garry Gause
President and Chief Executive Officer
Brookwood Medical Center
2010 Brookwood Medical Center Drive
Birmingham, AL 35209

Dear Mr. Gause:

Between November 9 and 19, 2009, Ms. Patricia S. Smith, representing the Food and Drug Administration (FDA), inspected the Institutional Review Board (IRB) at Brookwood Medical Center. The purpose of this inspection was to determine whether the IRB procedures for the protection of human subjects complied with Title 21 of the Code of Federal Regulations (CFR), parts 50 and 56. These regulations apply to clinical investigations of products regulated by FDA. We are aware that at the conclusion of the inspection, our investigator presented and discussed with you a Form FDA 483, Inspectional Observations.

From our review of the establishment inspection report and the documents submitted with that report, we conclude that the IRB did not adhere to the applicable statutory requirements and FDA regulations governing the protection of human subjects. We acknowledge your written response, dated January 6, 2010, to the Form FDA 483. However, because this response was received more than 15 business days after the Form FDA 483 was issued, the response has not been considered. We plan to evaluate your response to the Form FDA 483, along with any other written material provided, as a direct response to this Warning Letter.

We wish to emphasize the following:

1. The IRB failed to follow its written procedures for conducting continuing review of research [21CFR 56.108(a)(1)].

Our inspections revealed several instances in which the IRB failed to follow its written procedures for conducting continuing review of research. The IRB's written procedures state: "On-going research studies must be reviewed by the IRB at least annually, or more often if the IRB finds that the degree of risk to subjects warrants more frequent review. This renewal must take place prior to the approval expiration date noted on the approved protocol; otherwise, patient accrual must be suspended and, if the research is HHS-sponsored, the Agency must be notified. If a renewal is not received within 45 days, the study will be closed." Our review of the IRB records determined the following:

- There were two lapses in IRB approval for the (b)(4) protocol.
  - i. The initial approval for the (b)(4) protocol expired on May 31, 2007, but the study was not reapproved until July 2, 2007. Therefore, the study lapsed in IRB approval for more than one month.
  - ii. A subsequent continuing review was due by July 1, 2008; however, there was no documentation of another continuing review. The final report was not submitted until April 10, 2009, more than 10 months after the continuing review was due. It appears that IRB approval lapsed for a period of 9 months.
- Protocol (b)(4) was reapproved for an additional 6 months on July 3, 2008, and was due to expire on December 31, 2008. In our review of the records, FDA did not find any indication that continuing review was done between the expiration date and the time of our inspection 10 months later. Therefore, it appears that there was a lapse in IRB approval for almost 10 months.
- The initial approval for Protocol (b)(4) expired on June 30, 2009; however, the reapproval did not take place until August 27, 2009. As a result, IRB approval lapsed for almost two months.

This significant problem occurred in all three studies that FDA reviewed. Furthermore, this is an uncorrected problem that FDA had noted during our February 2003 inspection.

2. The IRB failed to follow its written procedures for ensuring that changes in approved research, during the period for which IRB approval has already been given, may not be initiated without IRB review and approval except where necessary to eliminate apparent immediate hazards to the human subjects [21 CFR 56.108(a)(4)].

The IRB's written procedures state: "The IRB must approve any protocol changes before they are instituted." Our review of the IRB meeting minutes, dated May 22, 2008, determined that the following protocol changes were noted by the IRB without being voted on and approved by a majority of the members present, as required by 21 CFR 56.108(c):

- Amendment 1 for Protocol (b)(4) included the addition of concomitant medications such as intravenous opioids, inhaled steroids, and Demerol.
- Amendment 2 for Protocol (b)(4) included substantial changes to the inclusion criteria, such as extending the upper age limit from 75 years to 80 years of age and allowing the inclusion of subjects with types of (b)(4) different from those indicated in the initial protocol.

3. The IRB failed to determine that risks to subjects are minimized [21 CFR 56.111(a) (1)].

In our review of the IRB meeting minutes dated April 28, 2008, FDA determined that the IRB requested a copy of the preceding two quarterly Data Safety Monitoring Board reviews along with a statistical summary, because they had concerns about reports of bleeding, embolus formation, and death occurring in the (b)(4) protocol. Despite this concern, there is no evidence that the IRB ever received the requested reports, and the study was permitted to continue until it closed on April 23, 2009.

This letter is not intended to be an all-inclusive list of deficiencies for the protocols reviewed and approved by the IRB. It is your responsibility to ensure that Brookwood Medical Center IRB's practices and procedures comply fully with all applicable statutes and regulations.

Within fifteen (15) working days of your receipt of this letter, you should notify this office in writing of the actions

you have taken to prevent similar violations in the future. Failure to adequately and promptly explain the violations noted above may result in regulatory action without further notice. If you believe that your January 6, 2010, written response to the Form FDA 483 fully explains the actions you have taken to prevent similar violations in the future, please communicate that to us in writing within fifteen (15) working days. As noted above, we plan to evaluate your written response to the Form FDA 483 along with any other written material provided as a direct response to this Warning Letter. You may reference the response dated January 6, 2010, in your response to this letter.

If you have any questions, please contact Kevin Prohaska, D.O., M.P.H., at 301-796-3707; FAX 301-847-8748. Your written response and any pertinent documentation should be addressed to:

Kevin Prohaska, D.O., M.P.H.
Acting Human Subjects Protections Team Lead
Division of Scientific Investigations
Office of Compliance
Center for Drug Evaluation and Research
Food and Drug Administration
Building 51, Room 5356
10903 New Hampshire Avenue
Silver Spring, MD 20993

Sincerely yours,

/S/

Leslie K. Ball, M.D.
Director
Division of Scientific Investigations
Office of Compliance
Center for Drug Evaluation and Research
Food and Drug Administration

Cc: Bradley Dennis, M.D.
Chief Medical Officer and Hospital Administrator
Brookwood Medical Center
2010 Brookwood Medical Center Drive
Birmingham, AL 35209

Armand S. Schachter, M.D.
Chairman
Brookwood Medical Center IRB
2010 Brookwood Medical Center Drive
Birmingham, AL 35209
(b)(4)
Brookwood Medical Center IRB
2010 Brookwood Medical Center Drive
Birmingham, AL 35209

第23封　给Teneo伦理委员会的警告信

2009年11月10日

参考号：CBER-10-01

尊敬的Lamb博士：

2009年3月12日至18日，FDA对Teneo伦理委员会（以下简称伦理委员会，IRB）进行了现场检查，这封信特告知您检查的结果。一名FDA检查员与您会面，并对伦理委员会进行了现场检查，以核实伦理委员会对于受试者保护的程序是否符合发布在美国联邦法规（CFR）第21篇第50和56部分的FDA法规要求。此次现场检查是FDA的生物研究监查项目的一部分，该项目通过设定的检查方法，审查伦理委员会在临床研究中试验产品使用以及受试者保护的实施情况。

在现场检查结束时，FDA检查员向您出示并讨论了FDA 483表，即现场检查发现的问题。此外，FDA还审查了Teneo伦理委员会在（b）（4）[1]中提供的对于FDA问题的回复文件。

我们已经确定，伦理委员会明显违反了颁布在21 CFR 56中的监管伦理委员会运行和职责适用联邦法规（见http://www.fda.gov/ScienceResearch/SpecialTopics/RunningClinicalTrials/default.htm）。

对违规适用的CFR条款引用如下：

Teneo伦理委员会未能准备和保存足够的伦理委员会活动记录［21CFR 56.115（a）（1）、（2）］

在检查Teneo伦理委员会期间，FDA检查员要求提供一套足够的伦理委员会会议记录，您向FDA检查员提供了会议记录，在本封信中指的是“Teneo会议记录（来自Teneo）”。检查期间，Teneo伦理委员会向FDA提供了一些文件的副本，其中一组文件，名为“药物临床试验（IND）申报事宜”，这份文件与“Teneo会议记录（来自Teneo）”是相同的。

第二组文件，名为“医学实践与治疗事宜”，在本封信中指的是“Teneo 会议记录［来自（b）（4）］”，虽然我们把这第二组文件称为“Teneo会议记录［来自（b）（4）］”，以说明会议记录的来源是由我们检查员收集的，但这些会议记录（信头、签名等）记录了Teneo伦理委员会的活动。

FDA审查“Teneo会议记录［来自（b）（4）］”发现，Teneo伦理委员会审查并批准了在“Teneo会议记录（来自Teneo）”中并未包含的（b）（4）研究。“Teneo会议记录（来自Teneo）”仅报告了题为（b）（4）的研究（以下简称为“（b）（4）研究”）。然而，“Teneo会议记录［来自（b）（4）］”记录了Teneo伦理委员会进行了全范围的伦理委员会活动，但在“Teneo会议记录（来自Teneo）”中并未描述：Teneo伦理委员会批准了（b）（4）方案及同意表；进行了跟踪审查；讨论了儿童受试者的登记、治疗及准许；授予紧急批准；评估了不良事件报告；修改了Teneo伦理委员会标准操作规程（SOP），但这些活动都未记录在“Teneo会议记录（来自Teneo）”中。与“Teneo会议记录［来自（b）（4）］”相对照后，可发现“Teneo会议记录（来自Teneo）”是不准确和不完整的，具体如下所示：

1.“Teneo会议记录（来自Teneo）”和“Teneo会议记录［来自（b）（4）］”之间存在差异，具体为以下日期召开的伦理委员会会议：2008年10月23日，2008年9月16日，2008年7月8日，2008年3月4日，2008年2月5日，2007年5月2日，2007年4月3日，2007年3月6日，2007年1月9日，2006年12月5日和2006年10月12日。并且，在“Teneo会议记录（来自Teneo）”中未包括2008年1月8日，2007年7月10日及2007年2月6日的伦理委员会会议内容。

A. 在某些情况下，“Teneo会议记录（来自Teneo）”中没有包括Teneo伦理委员会委员的个人投票记录。

1 （b）（4）涉及商业秘密，根据法规内容不予公开。

例如，2008年10月23日，Teneo伦理委员会投票对（b）（4）程序的知情同意进行修改。个人委员投票被记录在Teneo会议记录表中，但未在“Teneo会议记录（来自Teneo）”中体现。

另外，“Teneo会议记录［来自（b）（4）］”记录了2008年2月5日举行的一次会议，席间进行的休会个人投票显示有一名委员缺席。但“Teneo会议记录（来自Teneo）”中的相同会议却没有显示有委员缺席。

此外，2008年1月8日举行的会议，“Teneo会议记录［来自（b）（4）］”显示有一份关于推迟审议之前的会议记录的记名投票。但“Teneo会议记录（来自Teneo）”却没有记录。

B.“Teneo会议记录（来自Teneo）”省略了向Teneo伦理委员会报告的严重不良事件以及对这些事件的调查。“Teneo会议记录［来自（b）（4）］”显示在2008年9月16日，2008年7月10日，2008年3月4日，2008年2月5日及2008年1月8日举行的会议上讨论了这些不良事件。

C.“Teneo会议记录（来自Teneo）”未包括以下Teneo伦理委员会事项：

i.“Teneo会议记录［来自（b）（4）］”显示Teneo伦理委员会批准了以下事项：到2007年7月10日会议为止的所有有效SOP（标准操作规程）；2008年1月8日的SOP 8；2008年3月4日的SOP 5、7、8和47。“Teneo会议记录（来自Teneo）”但在2008年3月4日的“Teneo会议记录（来自Teneo）”的记录中未包括对SOP 5、7、8和47的批准。

ii.“Teneo会议记录（来自Teneo）”未显示在2008年3月4日会议中增加了一名新的Teneo伦理委员会委员。

D.“Teneo会议记录（来自Teneo）”未显示在2008年9月16日Teneo伦理委员会曾投票修改2008年7月8日召开的会议记录。“Teneo会议记录［来自（b）（4）］”包括了一份修改后的会议记录的副本；然而，“Teneo会议记录（来自Teneo）”未包括这份修正会议记录的任何记录。

2.“Teneo会议记录（来自Teneo）”未包括Teneo伦理委员会在2008年1月8日、2007年7月10日及2007年2月6日召开的会议的任何记录。但这三份会议记录体现在“Teneo会议记录［来自（b）（4）］中”，并显示做了与Teneo伦理委员会运行相关事项的讨论。

例如，“Teneo会议记录［来自（b）（4）］”记录的2008年1月8日会议记录显示，Teneo伦理委员会曾投票推迟对之前伦理委员会会议记录的审查，并讨论了对SOP 8的修改。“Teneo会议记录（来自Teneo）”中无此次会议的记录。

“Teneo会议记录［来自（b）（4）］”在2007年7月10日召开的会议记录显示，伦理委员会讨论了伦理委员会与研究者之间的沟通，研究受试者的补偿以及向受试者提供知情同意书的副本，但“Teneo会议记录（来自Teneo）”中无2007年7月10日会议的记录。

“Teneo会议记录［来自（b）（4）］”在2007年2月6日召开的会议记录显示，Teneo伦理委员会对以下事项进行了讨论：知情同意书的审查、为Teneo伦理委员会委员提供受试者培训课程的可能性、Teneo伦理委员会会员、Teneo伦理委员会网站、Teneo伦理委员会会议记录的形式，以及在下次会议中将进行讨论的新方案。“Teneo会议记录（来自Teneo）”中无此次会议的记录。

3.“Teneo会议记录［来自（b）（4）］”包括的电子信函显示了在2007年8月7日、2007年9月5日以及2007年11月6日会议的议程以及声明“请确认收到此邮件，并确认出席今天的Teneo伦理委员会董事会会议”。“Teneo会议记录（来自Teneo）”中未提到这些日期的会议。

4.“Teneo会议记录（来自Teneo）”未提及Teneo伦理委员会审查并批准了几个（b）（4）研究。

5. Teneo伦理委员会未保存其颁发的批准函的副本。这些批准函通过（b）（4）于2009年8月17日提交至FDA，但并未出现在Teneo记录中。

A. Teneo伦理委员会于2008年11月1日，发布了两封关于研究方案及知情同意书的批准函进入（b）（4），（b）（4）允许儿童受试者入组。这些批准函声明，研究的批准日期为2008年10月23日，跟踪审查的到期日为2009年10月23日。

B. Teneo伦理委员会于2007年11月1日发布给（b）（4）的一封关于（b）（4）研究项目的研究方案和知情同意书的批准函。

6. Teneo伦理委员会未保存“紧急批准”要求的文档或伦理委员会针对这些要求采取的行动。“Teneo会议记录［来自（b）(4)］”显示，在2007年10月25日您与Teneo董事会委员的电子信函中，您曾对（b）(4）的“紧急批准”以及提出的（b）(4）投了赞成票。

7.“Teneo会议记录（来自Teneo）”未能显示在2008年7月8日召开的Teneo伦理委员会会议中，Teneo伦理委员会讨论了儿科知情同意书以及雇佣儿科专家。“Teneo会议记录［来自（b）(4)］”在2008年7月8日的会议记录记录了伦理委员会考虑增加儿科肿瘤学家、儿科心脏病学家或是儿科神经肿瘤学家进入Teneo董事会，因为（b）(4）目前正与一些儿科肿瘤病例合作，预计这类情况未来还会增加。

8. 关于儿童参加（b）(4）研究，部分方案与知情同意书并不一致。在审查及批准过程中，Teneo伦理委员会在没有解决以下不一致的情况下就批准了该研究：

A. 方案中“受试者的治疗标准”部分指定“受试者必须是18岁及以上才适合于此治疗方案。18岁以下的受试者必须征得其法定监护人的同意。”

B. 入选标准没有对18岁以下的受试者进行规定，因为它明确指出“18岁及18岁以上受试者被给予（b）(4)”。

C. 排除标准不包括“小于18岁的受试者（除非有其监护人同意）”。

D. 题为“青少年（12～17）同意接受（b）(4）治疗”及“一般青少年（12～17）同意接受（b）(4)”的知情同意书在12～17岁的受试者中均可获得。

在现场检查过程中，您告诉FDA检查员，伦理委员会未对任何除了（b）(4）研究之外的任何研究进行审查，伦理委员会未收到任何不良事件报告，Teneo伦理委员会审查的任何研究中都不涉及儿童，同时提供给FDA检查员的会议记录都是完整的，请解释。

在现场检查结束时您启动了以下纠正措施：向FDA检查员提供了一份更新后的委员名册，指明哪些是科学领域委员，哪些是非科学领域委员，修正后的SOP #5，将要求每月召开伦理委员会会议改为每年10月召开一次，如需要的话，由执行官安排额外的会议。您也修改了2009年2月11日关于“一项与开放性、单中心、安全性及有效性有关（b）(4）疗效的研究”的批准函。这封批准函最初显示有效期为三年，您修改后的批准函显示批准后的有效期为一年。

此外，我们提醒您的是，有一条法规在Teneo伦理委员会检查期间还没有生效。21 CFR 56.106要求“美国的每个审查临床研究的伦理委员会都按照法案505（i）或520（g）部分的要求受FDA的监管，如打算对FDA监管的产品进行支持应用或市场准入的研究，美国的任何审查临床研究的伦理委员会都必须在卫生和人类服务部（HHS）的网站上进行注册”。每个伦理委员会可通过http://ohrp.cit.nih.gov/file网站进行电子注册，或是寄信至：

Good Clinical Practice Program（HF-34）

Office of Science and Health Coordination

Food and Drug Administration

5600 Fishers Lane

Rockville，MD 20857

本封信的目的并非是罗列所有违规行为。您和伦理委员会有责任对信中指出的违规行为进行改正，并且应彻底审查伦理委员会的SOP以及相关做法，确保完全符合法规要求。

根据21 CFR 56.120（b）(1）和（2）规定，鉴于伦理委员会违背上述FDA法规的情况，以下决定立即生效：

- FDA将暂停批准由此伦理委员会审查的所有新研究，并且
- 根据21 CFR 56要求，任何在研项目都不再入组新的受试者。

这些限制将持续至您收到由本办公室发出的书面通知认定贵伦理委员会作出了适当的纠正为止。这些限制也不减免伦理委员会的责任，即负责接收和反馈在研项目的意外且严重的反应的报告以及日常项目进展并报告。

您应告知本办公室您已经采取特定行动或计划采取的行动，使伦理委员会完全符合FDA法规要求。您的

答复应对上面列出的每一项问题作出回应，并包括所有必需的文档证明已进行全面和恰当的整改，另外，您的回复还要包括每一项纠正措施的预期完成时间。

您的回复中还应包括一份伦理委员会与每一个涉及申办者和临床研究者的书面沟通文件副本，通知他们FDA目前的强制限制措施。请提供一份更新的由Teneo伦理委员会审查的在研项目的列表，根据21 CFR 56的规定，确定并列出哪些研究受到“不批准”及“没有新的受试者入组”的限制。

基于您提供的书面回复，FDA会安排一次复查，以确认您已采取了足够的纠正措施。

附：英文原文

Teneo IRB

Warning Letter

Nov 10, 2009

Craig N. Lamb, Ph.D., President
Teneo Institutional Review Board
2706 South 109th East Avenue
Tulsa, Oklahoma 74129-7634

CBER-10-01

Dear Dr. Lamb:

This letter describes the results of a Food and Drug Administration (FDA) inspection of the Teneo Institutional Review Board (hereafter referred to as “the IRB”) that was conducted from March 12 to 18, 2009. An FDA investigator met with you to conduct an inspection of the IRB to determine if the IRB’s procedures for the protection of human subjects comply with FDA regulations published in Title 21, Code of Federal Regulations (CFR), Parts 50 and 56. The inspection was part of FDA’s Bioresearch Monitoring Program, which includes inspections designed to review IRB operations for clinical studies using investigational products and for the protection of human subjects.

The FDA investigator issued and discussed the Form FDA 483, Inspectional Observations, with you at the end of the inspection. In addition, FDA reviewed Teneo IRB documents provided in response to FDA inquiries during a **(b)(4)**.

We have determined that the IRB significantly violated applicable federal regulations governing the operation and responsibilities of IRBs as published under 21 CFR Part 56 (available at http://www.fda.gov/ScienceResearch/SpecialTopics/RunningClinicalTrials/default.htm).

The applicable provisions of the CFR are cited for the violation.

The Teneo IRB failed to prepare and maintain adequate documentation of IRB activities. [21CFR § 56.115(a)(1) and (2)].

During the Teneo IRB inspection the FDA investigator asked for a complete set of the IRB’s meeting minutes, and you provided the FDA investigator with the minutes we refer to in this letter as the “Teneo Minutes from Teneo.” During the inspection, provided FDA with copies of documents had received from the Teneo IRB. One set of documents, entitled “IND Matters”, is the same as the Teneo Minutes from Teneo.

A second set of documents is entitled “Medical Practice and Treatment Matters” which we refer to in this letter as the “Teneo Minutes from **(b)(4)**. Although we refer to this second set of documents as the Teneo Minutes from **(b)(4)** to reflect the origin of the minutes collected by our investigator, these minutes (letterhead, signatures, etc.) document activities of the Teneo IRB.

FDA's review of the Teneo Minutes from **(b)(4)** show that the Teneo IRB reviewed and approved **(b)(4)** studies that are not included in the Teneo Minutes from Teneo. The Teneo Minutes fromTeneo report activities related only to the study entitled **(b)(4)** (hereafter referred to as the "**(b)(4)** study"). However, the Teneo Minutes from **(b)(4)** document that the Teneo IRB conducted a full range of IRB activities that are not described in the Teneo Minutes from Teneo: the Teneo IRB approved **(b)(4)** protocols and consent forms; conducted continuing review; discussed the enrollment, treatment, and consent of pediatric subjects; granted emergency approvals; evaluated adverse event reports; and revised the Teneo IRB Standard Operating Procedures (SOP) without documenting these activities in the Teneo Minutes from Teneo. Compared to the Teneo Minutes from **(b)(4)**, the Teneo Minutes from Teneo are inaccurate and incomplete, as shown in the following examples.

1. There are discrepancies between the theTeneo Minutes from Teneo and the Teneo Minutes from **(b)(4)** for IRB meetings held on the following dates: October 23, 2008, September 16, 2008, July 8, 2008, March 4, 2008, February 5, 2008, May 2, 2007, April 3, 2007, March 6, 2007, January 9, 2007, December 5, 2006, and October 12, 2006. Also, there are no Teneo Minutes from Teneo for the January 8, 2008, July 10, 2007 or February 6, 2007 IRB meetings.

A. In some cases, the Teneo Minutes from Teneo do not include the individual vote of Teneo IRB members. For example, on October 23, 2008 the Teneo IRB voted to make a change in the informed consent for the **(b)(4)** procedure. The individual member vote was recorded in the Teneo Minutes from , but does not appear in the Teneo Minutes from Teneo.

Also, the Teneo Minutes from **(b)(4)** document an individual vote for adjournment that shows the absence of one member, for a meeting held on February 5, 2008. The Teneo Minutes from Teneo for the same meeting, do not show the absence of a member.

Furthermore, for a meeting conducted on January 8, 2008 the Teneo Minutes from **(b)(4)** show an individual roll call vote for the postponement of review of minutes from the previous meeting. There are no Teneo Minutes from Teneo for this meeting.

B. The Teneo Minutes from Teneo omit serious adverse events reported to the Teneo IRB and investigation of these events. The Teneo Minutes from **(b)(4)** show that adverse events were discussed at meetings held on September 16,2008, July 10, 2008, March 4,2008, February 5,2008 and January 8, 2008.

C. TheTeneo Minutes from Teneo did not include the following Teneo IRB business items:

i. The Teneo Minutes from **(b)(4)** show that the Teneo IRB approved the following: all SOPs that were current as of the July 10, 2007 meeting; SOP 8 on January 8, 2008; and SOPs 5, 7, 8, and 47 on March 4, 2008. The Teneo Minutes from Teneo for March 4, 2008 do not include the approval of SOPs 5, 7,8, and 47.

ii. The Teneo Minutes from Teneo do not show the addition of a new Teneo IRB member at the March 4, 2008 meeting.

D. The Teneo Minutes from Teneo do not show that on September 16, 2008 the Teneo IRB voted to amend the minutes of the meeting held on July 8, 2008. The Teneo Minutes from **(b)(4)** include a copy of the amended minutes; however, the Teneo Minutes from Teneo do not contain any record of such amendment.

2. The Teneo Minutes from Teneo do not include any records for Teneo IRB meetings held on January 8, 2008, July 10, 2007, and February 6, 2007. Minutes for these three meetings exist in the Teneo Minutes from **(b)(4)** and show discussion of items pertinent to Teneo IRB operations.

For example, the Teneo Minutes from **(b)(4)** for the January 8, 2008 meeting show the Teneo IRB voted to postpone review of IRB meeting minutes from the previous meeting and discussed changes to SOP 8. The Teneo Minutes from Teneo have no record of this meeting.

The Teneo Minutes from **(b)(4)** for the meeting held July 10, 2007 show that the IRB discussed communication between the IRB and investigator, compensation for research subjects, and providing subjects with copies of informed consents. The Teneo Minutes **(b)(4)** from Teneo have no record of the July 10, 2007 meeting.

The February 6, 2007 Teneo Minutes from **(b)(4)** show that the Teneo IRB discussed the following: review of informed consent forms, the availability of classes providing Human Subject Training for Teneo IRB members, Teneo IRB membership, the Teneo IRB's website, the format of Teneo IRB's meeting minutes, and new protocols to be discussed at the next meeting. The Teneo Minutes from Teneo have no record of this meeting.

3. The Teneo Minutes from **(b)(4)** include electronic correspondence showing an agenda for meetings on August 7, 2007, September 5, 2007, and November 6, 2007 and the statement "Please acknowledge receipt of this email and

your attendance at the Teneo IRB Board of Directors meeting today". The Teneo Minutes from Teneo do not include any reference to meetings on these dates.

4. The Teneo Minutes from Teneo omit that the Teneo IRB reviewed and approved several **(b)(4)** studies, **(b)(4).**

5. The Teneo IRB did not maintain copies of approval letters that it issued. These approval letters were submitted to FDA on August 17, 2009 by **(b)(4)**. These approvals are not in the Teneo records.

A. Two approval letters were issued to **(b)(4)** by the Teneo IRB on November 1, 2008 for the protocols and informed consents of studies entitled , **(b)(4)** which permits the enrollment of pediatric subjects, and **(b)(4).** The letters state the approval date for both studies is October 23, 2008 and the due date for continuing review is October 23, 2009.

B. The Teneo IRB issued an approval letter to (b)(4) on November 1, 2007 for the protocol and consent form for the study **(b)(4).**

6. The Teneo IRB did not maintain documentation of requests for "emergency approvals" or the IRB action taken on these requests. An electronic communication from you to the members of the Teneo Board of Directors on October 25, 2007 in the Teneo Minutes from **(b)(4)** shows you voted for the "emergency approval" of the "**(b)(4)**" and the proposed "**(b)(4)**".

7. The Teneo Minutes from Teneo for the Teneo IRB meeting held on July 8, 2008 fail to show that the Teneo IRB discussed pediatric consent forms and the hiring of pediatric specialists. The Teneo Minutes from **(b)(4)** for the July 8, 2008 meeting document that the IRB considered the addition of a pediatric oncologist, pediatric cardiologist, or a neuropediatric oncologist to the Teneo Board because **(b)(4)** is currently working with several pediatric cancer cases and expects more in the future."

8. Sections of the protocol and informed consent are inconsistent with regard to the participation of children in the study (b)(4). The Teneo IRB approved the research without resolving the following inconsistencies during the review and approval process:

A. The "Patient Criteria of Treatment" section of the protocol specifies "Patients must be 18 years or older to be eligible for this treatment protocol. Patients under age 18 must have the consent of their legal guardian."

B. The Inclusion Criteria makes no provision for subjects under 18 as it clearly states "Patients 18 and older presenting with **(b)(4)**."

C. The Exclusion Criteria excludes subjects "age less than 18 years (unless consent is given by legal guardian)".

D. Consent Forms entitled "Adolescent (12-17) Agreement to Receive **(b)(4)** "Treatment" and "General Adolescent (12-17) Agreement to Receive **(b)(4)** Treatment" are available for ages 12 to 17.

During the inspection you told the FDA investigator that the IRB did not review any studies other than the **(b)(4)** study, that the IRB received no adverse event reports, that no studies were reviewed by Teneo IRB involving children, and that the minutes provided to the FDA investigator were complete. Please explain.

The following corrective actions were initiated by you at the close of the inspection: an updated membership roster was provided to the FDA investigator that identified members as scientific or non-scientific and SOP #5 was revised to change the requirement for monthly IRB meetings to one meeting in October of each year with additional meetings scheduled by the Chair as needed. You also revised the approval letter dated February 11, 2009 for the study An *Open Label, Single Site,Safety and Efficacy Study of the Effects* of **(b)(4).** The approval letter initially showed an expiration of three years, you revised the letter to show expiration of approval to occur at one year.

In addition, we remind you of a regulation that was not in effect at the time of the Teneo IRB inspection. 21 CFR § 56.106 requires "Each IRB in the United States that reviews clinical investigations regulated by FDA under sections 505(i) or 520(g) of the act and each IRB in the United States that reviews clinical investigations that are intended to support applications for research or marketing permits for FDA-regulated products must register at a site maintained by the Department of Health and Human Services (HHS)." Each IRB may register electronically through http://ohrp.cit.nih.gov/file or in writing at:

Good Clinical Practice Program (HF-34)
Office of Science and Health Coordination
Food and Drug Administration
5600 Fishers Lane
Rockville, MD 20857

This letter is not an all-inclusive list of violations. It is incumbent upon you and the IRB to correct the violations cited in this letter, and to conduct a thorough review of the IRB's SOPs and practices to ensure full compliance with the regulations.

As a result of the IRB's noncompliance with FDA regulations, described above, in accordance with 21 CFR §§ 56.120(b)(1) and (2), and effective immediately,

- **FDA will withhold approval of all new studies reviewed by this IRB; and**
- **No new subjects are to be enrolled in any ongoing studies subject to 21 CFR Part 56.**

These restrictions will remain until such time that you have received written notification from this office that adequate corrections have been made. These restrictions do not relieve the IRB of its responsibility for receiving and reacting to reports of unexpected and serious reactions and routine progress reports from ongoing studies.

You are to notify this office of the specific actions you have taken or plan to take to bring the IRB into full compliance with FDA regulations. Your response should address each item listed above,and should include any documentation necessary to show that full and adequate correction has been achieved. Include the projected completion dates for each action to be accomplished.

Include with your response a copy of the IRB's written communication to each of the affected sponsors and clinical investigators, notifying them of the current FDA imposed restrictions. Please provide an updated list of all studies currently being reviewed by Teneo IRB, identify those that are subject to 21 CFR Part 56, and list all studies that are affected by the "Withhold approval of" and"No new subjects" restrictions.

On the basis of your written response, FDA may schedule a reinspection to confirm the adequacy of your corrective actions.

Christine Drabick
Division of Inspections and Surveillance (HFM-664)
Office of Compliance and Biologics Quality
Center for Biologics Evaluation and Research
1401 Rockville Pike, Suite 200N
Rockville, MD 20852-1448
Telephone: (301) 827-6323

Should you have any questions or comments about the contents of this letter or any aspects of the operations and responsibilities of an Institutional Review Board, you may contact Christine Drabick at (301) 827-6323.

We request that you also send a copy of your response to the FDA District Office listed below.

Sincerely,

/S/

Mary Malarkey, Director
Office of Compliance and Biologics Quality
Center for Biologics Evaluation and Research

Cc: Reynaldo Rodriguez, District Director
Food and Drug Administration
4040 North Central Expressway, Suite 300
Dallas, Texas 75204
Kristina Borror, Ph.D., Chief
Compliance Oversight Branch
Office for Human Research Protections
U.S. Department of Health and Human Services
1101 Wootton Parkway, Suite 200N
Rockville, Maryland 20852

第 24 封　给 MI Hope 股份有限公司（复杂传染病中心）伦理委员会的警告信

2009年10月19日

参考号：10-HFD-45-10-02

尊敬的Martin博士：

2009年5月14日至5月27日，Diane Van Leeuwen女士，Babajide Osunsanmi 先生和Natalie Ayoub 女士代表FDA，对MI Hope 股份有限公司（复杂传染病中心）伦理委员会（IRB）进行了现场检查。本次现场检查的目的是核实伦理委员会受试者保护程序是否符合美国联邦法规第21篇第50和56部分的要求。这些法规适用于FDA所监管产品的临床研究。我们知道，在现场检查结束时，我们的检查员向您出示并讨论了FDA483表，即现场检查发现的问题。

经对现场检查报告、该报告的附件进行审查，我们认为，贵伦理委员会没有遵循适用的法律要求和监管受试者保护的FDA法规。我们想强调以下几点：

1. IRB未能按照法规要求，在合理的时间内以合理的方式将伦理委员会记录提供给FDA授权的代表进行现场检查和复印［21 CFR 56.115（b）］

我们的现场检查发现，伦理委员会的记录保存在W. John Martin博士的私人住所。FDA检查员未能在合理的时间内以合理的方式被允许查阅和复印伦理委员会的记录。现场检查中，拖延了许久之后才提供了非常有限的记录。按要求查阅伦理委员会记录是为了确定伦理委员会保护受试者的程序是否充分，以及是否遵循法规21 CFR 第50和56部分。

2. IRB未能制定和保存一份IRB的委员名单，标识姓名、获得学位、代表资格等足以描述每位委员对IRB审议能带来的主要预期贡献的指标，以及每位委员与机构之间的雇佣或其他关系［21 CFR 56.115（a）（5）］

我们的检查员发现，贵伦理委员会没有遵循法规要求而保存一份伦理委员会委员名单。贵伦理委员会提供的一份题为“参加或愿意参加伦理委员会会议的个人”的名单没有能标识出目前伦理委员会的委员，并且没有显示委员的能力以及与研究机构的雇佣关系。

3. IRB未能在大多数委员出席，且至少包括一位来自非科学领域的委员的召集会议上对拟开展的研究进行审查［21 CFR 56.108（c）］

如2. 所述，贵伦理委员会未能根据法规要求，准备和保存一份委员名单，因此，无法确定目前伦理委员会委员的名字和资质。伦理委员会2006年1月24日的会议记录上显示伦理委员会全体一致批准了主要研究者为W. John Martin医学博士的试验方案（b）（4）。会议记录列出了总计12名参会委员，包括被列为非投票人员的Martin博士，因为所审查的一项研究他是主要研究者。从审阅的文件中，无法确认是否多数委员参加了会议并投票批准了上述研究，以及参会委员中是否有非科学领域的委员。

此外，会议记录中列出的12名参会委员中有3名是委托投票的。为了在会议上批准一项研究，该研究必须获得实际参会人员的多数票批准。允许伦理委员会委员委托投票是不能被接受的做法。

4. IRB未能准备和保存会议记录，用足够的细节显示会议的出席情况；IRB采取的行动；对行动的投票情况，包括赞成票数、反对票数和弃权票数；需要修改或不批准研究的理由；对争议问题讨论和解决的书面总结［21 CFR 56.115（a）（2）］

伦理委员会2006年1月24日的会议记录显示，全体一致批准了一项题为（b）（4）的研究。我们的检查员发现，会议记录没有详细地显示几票赞成、几票反对，以及几票弃权。尽管会议记录显示因为Dr.Martin是主要研究者而未投票，但无法确定哪些委员投票批准了该研究。

此外，伦理委员会的政策和程序要求，与任何提议的项目存在利益冲突的委员，在对该项目讨论和投票前，应离开房间。伦理委员会的会议记录没有详细记录Martin博士是否在讨论和投票决定与他有利益冲突的项目前，离开了房间。

5. IRB未能准备和保存用于IRB的书面程序，未能按照21 CFR 56.108（a）和（b）的要求，遵守书面程序［21 CFR 56.115（a）(6)］

法规要求伦理委员会遵循书面程序批准的研究。我们的检查员发现，伦理委员会的政策和程序没有包括以下法规要求的书面程序：

a. 向研究者和研究机构报告伦理委员会的发现和措施；

b. 决定哪些项目的跟踪审查频次应大于每年一次，哪些项目需要从研究者以外的来源获得证据，确认项目资料自上次伦理委员会审查之后没有发生重大变更；

c. 确保研究的变更立即向伦理委员会报告；

d. 确保伦理委员会批准的项目，在已获得伦理委员会批准期间，所做的变更在获得伦理委员会审查和批准前不得实施，除非是为了消除显而易见的对受试者的即刻伤害；

e. 确保立即向伦理委员会、机构相关管理人员和FDA报告任何使受试者或他人陷于风险的非预期事件；

f. 确保立即向伦理委员会、机构相关管理人员和FDA报告任何严重的或持续发生的违反法规或要求或任何伦理委员会决定的事件；

g. 确保立即向伦理委员会、机构相关管理人员和FDA报告任何暂停和终止伦理委员会批准的项目的情况。

FDA对贵伦理委员会的限制：

基于存在严重的违规以及对受试者的权利和健康的风险，根据21 CFR 56.120（b）(1）和（2)，FDA对MI Hope 股份有限公司（复杂传染病中心）伦理委员会提出以下两项限制：

（1）不得再批准遵从21 CFR 56的新的研究；

（2）进行中的遵从21 CFR 56的研究不得再纳入新的受试者。

这些限制要求将持续有效，直至您收到FDA的通知，确认您采取了充分的纠正措施。这些限制要求并不减免伦理委员会接收和回复来自进行中的研究的非预期的严重反应和常规进展报告的责任。

自收到这封信的15个工作日内，您应当书面告知本办公室您已采取哪些具体措施促使伦理委员会完全符合FDA法规的要求。您的书面回复应提供必需的文件，以证明完整充分的纠正措施，以及提供针对每一个要完成的纠正措施计划完成的日期。

将上述的限制规定通知所有受影响的申办者和研究者是您的责任。在您递交给FDA的回复中，请包括一封贵伦理委员会通知受影响的申办者和研究者的书面沟通函样本，通知他们关于现在所受的限制。请同时提供一份完整的名单，包括所有被告知上述限制要求的申办者和研究者以及日期。

请提供一份所有目前正在进行且受到上述限制规定影响的研究，包括研究名称（IDE或 IND 号，如适用)，受试产品，研究者姓名，初始审查和批准的日期，跟踪审查的日期。IND和IDE号可从那些受到限制规定影响的方案的申办者处获得。

未能回复这封信以及未能采取合适的纠正措施将导致FDA依据21 CFR 56.120，56.121 和56.124的授权采取监管行动。这些行动包括但不仅限于，继续采取上述限制措施，暂停贵伦理委员会批准的、遵从21 CFR 56的进行中的研究，以及启动监管程序取消贵伦理委员会的资质。

本警告信的目的并非是罗列贵伦理委员会在试验方案审查和批准中存在的所有缺陷。确保MI Hope 股份有限公司（复杂传染病中心）伦理委员会的操作和规程完全遵循所有适用的法律和法规是您的职责。

附：英文原文

MI Hope Inc. dba Center for Complex Infectious Diseases IRB

WARNING LETTER

Oct 19，2009

CERTIFIED MAIL
RETURN RECEIPT REQUESTED

Ref.10-HFD-45-10-02

W. John Martin, M.D., Ph.D.
MI Hope Inc. dba Center for Complex Infectious Diseases
1634 Spruce Street
South Pasadena, CA 91030

DearDr.Martin:

Between May 14 and 27, 2009, Ms. Diane Van Leeuwen, Mr. Babajide Osunsanmi, and Ms. Natalie Ayoub, representing the Food and Drug Administration (FDA), inspected the Institutional Review Board (IRB) at MI Hope Inc. dba Center for Complex Infectious Diseases. The purpose of this inspection was to determine whether the IRB procedures for the protection of human subjects complied with Title 21 the Code of Federal Regulations (CFR), parts 50 and 56. These regulations apply to clinical investigations of product regulated by FDA. We are aware that at the conclusion of the inspection, our investigators presented and discussed with you, a Form FDA 483, Inspectional Observations.

From our review of the establishment inspection report and the documents submitted with that report, we conclude that the IRB did not adhere to the applicable statutory requirement and FDA regulations governing the protection of human subjects. We wish to emphasize the following:

1. The IRB failed to make IRB records, required by the regulations, accessible for inspection and copying by authorized representatives of the Food and Drug Administration at reasonable times and in a reasonable manner [21CFR 56.115(b)].

Our inspection revealed that the IRB records are stored at the private residence of Dr. W. John Martin. FDA Investigators were not permitted access to inspect and copy IRB records at reasonable times and in a reasonable manner. Limited records were provided during the inspection, but only after lengthy delays. Access to IRB records is required to determine that IRB procedures for the protection of human subjects are adequate, and that they comply with the regulatory requirements of 21 CFR, part 50 and 56.

2. The IRB failed to prepare and maintain a list of IRB members identified by name; earned degrees; representative capacity; indications of experience sufficient to describe each member's chief anticipated contributions to IRB deliberations; and any employment or other relationship between each member and the institution [21CFR 56.115(a)(5)].

Our inspection revealed that the IRB does not maintain a list of IRB members in compliance with the regulations. The list provided by the IRB entitled, "Individuals who have either participated or indicated their willingness to participate in the IRB meetings, fails to distinguish current IRB members, and fails to identify IRB members by representative capacity or by affiliation with the institution.

3. The IRB failed to review proposed research at convened meetings at which a majority of the members of the IRB are present, including at least one member whose primary concerns are in nonscientific areas [21CFR 56.108(c)].

AS noted in citation #2 above, the IRB did not prepare and maintain a list of IRB members in accordance with the regulations and, as a result, the names and qualifications of the current IRB members cannot be confirmed. The IRB meeting minutes for January 24, 2006, indicate that the IRB unanimously approved the study entitled, (b)(4) with W. John Martin, M.D., Ph.D. as the Principal Investigator. The minutes list a total of twelve individuals in attendance at the meeting, including Dr. Martin, who is listed as nonvoting because of his role as Principal Investigator on the study under review. From the documents reviewed, it cannot be confirmed whether a majority of the IRB members were present at the meeting and voted to approve the noted study, and whether any individual in attendance was a nonscientist member.

In addition, the meeting minutes list three of the twelve individuals as attending the IRB meeting by proxy. In order for research to be approved at a convened meeting, the research must receive the approval of a majority of those members who are actually present at the meeting. Allowing IRB members to attend meetings by proxy is not an acceptable practice.

4. The IRB failed to prepare and maintain minutes of IRB meetings in sufficient detail to show attendance at the meetings; actions taken by the IRB; the vote on these actions including the number of members voting for against, and abstaining; the basis for requiring changes in or disapproving research; and a written summary of the discussion of controverted issues and their resolution [21 CFR 56.115(a)(2)].

The IRB meeting minutes of January 24, 2006, indicate that the study entitled, (b)(4) was approved unanimously by the IRB. Our inspection revealed that the meeting minutes are not sufficiently detailed to indicate the number of members voting for, against, and abstaining. While the meeting minutes indicate Dr. Martin was nonvoting because of his role as Principal Investigator, it is not possible to determine who voted to approve the (b)(4) study.

In addition, the IRB Policies and Procedures require IRB members leave the room before the discussion and voting occur on any proposal in which they have a conflicting interest. The IRB meeting minutes are not sufficiently denied to indicate whether or not Dr. Martin left the room before the discussion and voting occurred on the study in which he had a conflicting interest.

5. The IRB failed to prepare and maintain written procedures for the IRB and failed to follow written procedures as required by 21 CFR 56.108(a) and (b) [21CFR 56.115(a) (6)].

The IRB is required to follow written procedures in order to approve research covered by the regulations. Our inspection revealed that the IRB Policies and Procedures do not include a written procedure to address the following regulatory requirement:

a. Reporting the IRB's findings and actions to the investigator and the institution;

b. Determining which projects require review more often than annually and which projects need verification from sources other than the investigator that no material changes have occurred since previous IRB review;

c. Ensuring prompt reporting to the IRB of changes in research activity;

d. Ensuring that changes in approved research, during the period for which IRB approval has already been given, may not be initiated without IRB review and approval except where necessary to eliminate apparent immediate hazards to human subject;

e. Ensuring prompt reporting to the IRB, appropriate institutional officials, and the FDA of any unanticipated problems involving risks to human subjects or others;

f. Ensuring prompt reporting to the IRB, appropriate institutional officials, and the FDA of any instance of serious or continuing noncompliance with the regulations or the requirements or determinations of the IRB;

g. Ensuring prompt reporting to the IRB, appropriate institutional officials, and the FDA of any suspension or termination of IRB approval.

FDA Imposed Restrictions on the IRB:

Given the seriousness of these violations and the risk to the rights and welfare of human research subjects, the FDA is placing the following two restrictions on MI Hope Inc. dba Center for Complex Infectious Diseases IRB, per 21 CFR 56.120(b)(1) and (2):

1. No new studies subject to the requirements of 21 CFR part 56 will be approved.
2. No new subjects will be added to ongoing studies subject to 21 CFR part 56.

These restrictions will remain in effect until such time that you receive written notification from FDA that adequate corrections have been made. These restrictions do not relieve the IRB of its responsibility for receiving and responding to reports of unexpected and serious reactions and routine progress reports from ongoing studies.

Within fifteen (15) working days of receiving this letter, you are to notify the FDA of the specific actions you have taken or plan to take to bring the IRB into full compliance with FDA regulations. Your response should include any documentation necessary to show that full and adequate correction has been achieved, and should include the projected completion dates for each action to be accomplished.

It is your responsibility to notify all affected sponsors and clinical investigators of the restrictions described above. Include with your response to the FDA a representative sample copy of the IRB's written communication(s) to affected sponsors and clinical investigators, notifying them of the current restrictions. Please also provide a complete list of all sponsors and investigators who were notified as result of this action and the date(s) on which they were notified.

Please provide a list of all studies currently being conducted that are affected by the above restrictions and include the titles of the studies (with IDE or IND numbers, if applicable) , the names of the test articles, the names of the clinical investigators, dates of initial reviews and approvals, and the dates of continuing reviews. IND and IDE numbers can be obtained from the sponsor of the protocols affected by these restrictions.

Failure to respond to this letter and take appropriate corrective action could result in FDA taking regulatory actions, as authorized by 21 CFR 56.120, 56.121, and 56.124. These actions include, but are not limited to, the continuation of the restrictions described above, the termination of ongoing studies subject to 21 CFR part 56 and approved by your IRB, and the initiation of regulatory proceedings for disqualification of your IRB.

This letter is not intended to be an all-inclusive list of deficiencies for the protocols reviewed and approved by the IRB. It is your responsibility to ensure that MI Hope Inc. dba Center for Complex Infectious Diseases IRB's practices and procedures comply fully with all applicable statutes and regulations.

If you have any questions, please contact Kevin Prohaska, D.O., M.P.H., at 301-796-3707; FAX 301-847-8748. Your written response and any pertinent documentation should be addressed to:

Kevin Prohaska D.O., M.P.H.
Acting Human Subjects Protection Team Leader
Division of Scientific Investigations
Office of Compliance
Center for Drug Evaluation and Research
Food and Drug Administration
Building 51, Room 5356
10903 New Hampshire Avenue
SiIver Spring, MD 20993

Sincerely yours,

{See appended electronic signature page}

Leslie K. Ball, M.D.
Director
Division of Scientific Investigations
Office of Compliance
Center for Drug Evaluation and Research

Food and Drug Administration

Cc: Dr. James Julian
IRB Chairman
MI Hope Inc. dba Center for Complex Infectious Diseases IRB
1634 Spruce Street
South Pasadena, CA 91030
Kristina C. Borror, Ph.D.
Director, Division of Compliance Oversight
Department of Health and Human Services
Office for Human Research Protections
The Tower Building
1101 Wootton Parkway, Suite 200
Rockville MD 20852

第 25 封　给 Burzynski 研究所伦理委员会的警告信

2009年10月5日

参考号：10-HFD-45-09-01

尊敬的Hazlewood博士：

2008年12月3日至12月10日，Patrick D. Stone先生代表FDA，对Burzynski 研究所（BRI）的伦理委员会（IRB）进行了检查。本次检查的目的是核实该委员会受试者保护程序是否符合美国联邦法规第21篇第50和第56部分的要求，这些法规适用于FDA所监管产品的临床研究。我们知道在现场检查结束时，我们的检查员向您出示并讨论了FDA483表，即现场检查发现的问题。

经对现场检查报告、该报告的附件，以及2009年4月2日对FDA483表的书面回复进行审查，我们认为，贵IRB没有遵循适用的法律要求和受试者保护的FDA法规。我们想强调以下几点：

1. IRB在未确定是否满足以下标准的情况下批准了临床研究，即受试者风险最小化［21 CFR 56.111（a）（1）］，受试者的风险与预期的利益（如果存在），以及与预期可以获得的重要知识相比是合理的［21 CFR 56.111（a）（2）］

a. 针对试验方案（b）（4）的检查发现如下：

2007年1月10日，（b）（6）医生（IRB委员）向IRB递交了关于该研究的一些意见。该研究的目的是评价（b）（4）对于（b）（4）或（b）（4）受试者的安全性和有效性。（b）（6）医生审阅了研究者手册、临床试验方案和随附的评价后对药物的来源、生产工艺和对受试者潜在的药物影响产生了担忧。他指出，需要更多的信息对风险/受益进行评估。

上述意见被提出一年后，在2008年2月1日IRB会议上该研究被讨论，IRB的文件显示，IRB在2007年1月到2008年2月未收到关于这个研究的任何额外信息。2008年2月1日IRB的会议记录显示，IRB知道临床研究者已经将该试验药物用于受试者。我们的检查发现，在2008年2月1日的会议上，IRB已获得15名注射过（b）（4）的受试者的未注明日期的病例报告。尽管已知（b）（4）医生未遵照21CFR312.66的要求、未经过IRB批准就对受试者用药，IRB却未能按照21CFR56.108（b）（2）的要求向FDA报告（b）（4）医生的违规问题。

2008年2月1日的会议记录中没有记录IRB对（b）（4）研究采取的措施。但是，在一封2008年2月15日给研究者（b）（6）医生的信中，IRB如下写道：

“需要完成额外的动物毒理研究。在人体的（b）（4）研究中，所有的不良反应事件都应尽可能地在最快时间报告给申办者（b）（4）和BRI的IRB。任何可能发生的死亡事件应在24小时内报告给申办者和本办公室。我代表委员会通知您，您可以继续这个研究并希望您在该领域持续的成功”。

当额外的毒理动物研究被要求补充的情况下，不清楚IRB为何允许该研究继续在人体进行。此外，在知道（b）（4）医生在获得IRB批准前就启动了该项试验，即未获得IRB批准就将药物给予受试者的情况下，不清楚IRB为何允许（b）（4）医生继续进行（b）（4）研究。

您在2009年4月2日的书面回复中提到，IRB没有批准（b）（4）研究的受试者入组或其他相关的方案。这与IRB2008年2月15日发给研究者的信函内容不符。

作为2008年8月8日IRB会议结果，IRB发给（b）（4）（研究申办者）一封关于动物毒理研究状态的信函。这封日期为2008年8月18日给（b）（4）的信中提到“此时，我必须提醒您，按照方案，人体临床研究不能继续进行，直到该新药临床试验申请（IND）被FDA批准。”这封给申办者的信与2008年2月15日寄给研究者（b）（6）医生的信中的内容相矛盾，信中IRB同意研究继续进行。

在2008年12月的检查期间，您告诉FDA检查员，您并不知道该IND处于临床试验暂停状态。然而，（b）（4）在2008年9月4日给IRB一封信中提及FDA对该IND给予临床试验暂停。2008年10月24日的IRB会议记录显示“IRB决定起草一封信给（b）（4），说明IRB决定暂停该试验所申请的IRB审批程序，直到IRB收到FDA关于毒理研究结果的表态。届时，IRB将审查毒理研究结果并决定是否继续该项审批。”IRB在一封2008年11月3日的信中表述了这些信息，但这封信只被发给了（b）（6）医生，并没有发给（b）（4）。

在您的书面回复中提到，“IRB被告知申办者正与FDA讨论IND的状态。基于此，IRB认为其与申办者和方案的关系属于待定状态。”如上所述，最后一封IRB发出的关于（b）（4）研究的信函只发给了（b）（6）医生，因此，没有文件证明（b）（4）已经得知IRB暂停该研究的决定。

b. 对试验方案（b）（4）的现场检查发现如下：

作为2005年1月6日IRB会议的会议结果，IRB于2005年2月1日向（b）（6）医生，申办者-研究者发出信函指明，包括知情同意书在内的文件需在最后批准前进行修订，并要求其重新递交方案和知情同意文件供IRB审查。此外，IRB还通知（b）（4）医生必须递交研究者手册。

在2005年3月17日的IRB会议上，IRB决定如果方案和知情同意书文件被适当修订，临床研究将可能被批准。在2005年3月23日给申办–研究者的信中表示，IRB根据修订的内容同意批准方案和知情同意书文件，同时再次要求提供研究者手册。

在2005年4月4日的信中，IRB通知申办–研究者修订的文件已经被批准。本次检查没有在IRB文件中找到研究者手册，因此表明IRB在没有收到研究者手册的情况下批准了研究，这可能影响到IRB判断受试者风险是否最小化和风险是否涉及预期受益的合理性。

在您的书面回复中提到，（b）（4）的临床试验方案一直没有被批准进行患者入组。您的回复与IRB发给申办–研究者的信函沟通内容不一致。在现场检查中，您曾告知FDA检查员该研究被FDA予以临床暂停决定，不清楚IRB何时得知临床暂停状态以及为何在2005年4月4日告知申办–研究者该研究已经被批准。

2. IRB未能制定、维护并遵守关于对研究进行初始审查和跟踪审查的书面程序［21 CFR 56.108（a）和56.115（a）（6）］。具体而言，IRB没有关于进行器械研究审查以判断是否使用了有明显风险的器械，且没有证据表明实际进行过此类审查［21 CFR 812.66］

我们调查发现，IRB在2005年7月21日批准了“（b）（4）”，IRB保存的方案标题为（b）（4）。在与申办者和研究者的沟通信函中，该研究被称作“试验方案（b）（4）”，而在2005年8月10日IRB给申办者的信中，方案被称作（b）（4）。

IRB在按照21 CFR812.2（b）（1）（ⅱ）审查由申办者递交的器械研究时，IRB必须确定申请的研究项目是否使用具有显著风险（SR）的器械［21 CFR 812.66.1］。如果IRB认为812.2（b）（1）（ⅱ）类的研究使用了有显著风险的器械时，IRB应该通知研究者和申办者（如有）［21 CFR 812.66］。

在您的书面回复中提到，IRB阅读了FDA关于显著风险和无显著风险器械研究项目的信息单并确定该研究属于无显著风险（NSR）的器械，可以被批准进行人体试验。在IRB的记录中（2004年9月23日，2005年1月6日，2005年5月26日和2005年7月21日的会议记录或相关IRB沟通信）没有记录显示，IRB曾考虑器械在临床研究中的使用；审阅过器械描述说明和申办者关于为何器械属于无显著风险器械的解释说明；以及如何基于资料审阅做出有显著风险/无显著风险的判断决定。此外，我们注意到IRB的标准操作规程未包含器械研究的审查程序。

3. IRB未能确保按照21 CFR 50的要求并达到所需的程度，获得每一位预期受试者或其法律授权代理人的知情同意［21 CFR 56.111（a）（4）］，以及按照21 CFR 50.27所要求的内容和程度对知情同意进行适当的记录［21 CFR 56.111（a）（5）］

a. 对于（b）（4）研究，我们现场检查发现，在2008年2月1日IRB会议或2008年8月8日和10月24日的后续会议上并没有讨论该研究。在2008年2月15日、8月18日和11月3日的IRB信函沟通中未提及知情同意书，并且在IRB的文件中没有IRB批准的知情同意书文件。由此表明，IRB没有遵照21 CFR 第50部分的要求，在不能确保知情同意被合理取得并记录的情况下，就批准了临床试验。

我们注意到这一发现没有列入FDA483表，因此在您的书面回复中没有关于此项的回复。

b. 对于（b）（4）研究，IRB在2005年7月21日批准的知情同意书文件中未包含21 CFR 50.25要求的所有内容，因此不符合第50部分的要求。以下这些被要求的内容不准确或未包括：

ⅰ）执行操作步骤的和试验性步骤的描述［21CFR 50.25（a）（1）］。知情同意书的“研究步骤”部分没有描述方案中概述的研究步骤。知情同意书中写道“我们会请您每次接受治疗后填写简要的受试者评估表”，但没有描述治疗内容和评估表，也没有写明方案要求的实验室工作和临床、神经学以及功能检测。

ⅱ）对可合理预期的试验研究对受试者或其他人的可能益处的描述［21CFR 50.25（a）（3）］。被批准的知情同意书版本是不准确的，知情同意书中描述道“参加该研究可能对您有直接的好处：减轻（b）（4）”。这个说法与试验方案中的描述不符，方案的描述是“几乎没有公开发表的关于（b）（4）在（b）（4）中有用性的描述…文献搜索没有找到任何科学试验的报告。据我们所知，（b）（4）的使用还没有在（b）（4）受试者中试用”。此外，包含在方案中的知情同意书写到“目前，研究无法保证（b）（4）能帮助我；并且，产生的可能益处该领域作用的确切机制在当下对研究者还不明确”。

ⅲ）关于FDA可能检查这些记录的声明［21CFR 50.25（a）（5）］。知情同意书中没有关于这个内容的声明。

ⅳ）关于试验中患者对于研究和受试者权利有疑问时可以联系并得到解释的联系人信息的说明和万一发生研究相关的患者损害事件时的联系人信息的说明［21CFR 50.25（a）（7）］。知情同意书中没有这些说明。此外，（b）（6）医生被错误地写成研究协调员；（b）（4）医生被写成是临床研究者。

ⅴ）关于受试者有权利随时停止参加该研究并没有任何法律责任和利益损失的描述［21CFR 50.25（a）（8）］。知情同意书中没有关于这个信息的描述。

4. IRB未能确保没有与项目有利益关系的委员参与IRB的初始审查或追踪审查，除非根据IRB的要求提供信息［21 CFR 56.107（e）］

a. 在（b）（4）研究中，您（IRB主席Carlton F. Hazlewood. 博士）在“临床研究者财务利益和分工证明书”中被列为临床研究者；在（b）（4）/IBR的中心注册控制委员会/数据监查委员会中为依职权的顾问。因此，您存在利益冲突。

2008年8月8日的IRB会议记录显示，您参加了这次会议并参与了（b）（4）研究的讨论。本次会议中，IRB对向（b）（4）起草信件问询动物毒理研究状态进行了投票。按照会议记录，所有委员投了赞成票，没有人反对和弃权。2008年10月24日的IRB会议记录显示，您参加了这次会议并参与了（b）（4）研究的审查。这次会议上，IRB对向（b）（4）起草信件通知其申请被暂停进行了投票，对该行动的投票记录为匿名方式。因此，按照这两次的IRB会议记录，您参加了该研究的审查并在您有利益冲突的情况下进行了投票。我们还注意到您签署了所有IRB发给（b）（6）医生和申办者的关于该研究的信函。

我们注意到这一发现没有列入FDA483表，因此在您的书面回复中没有关于此项的回复。

b. 在（b）（4）研究中，（b）（6）在方案中被列为合作研究者。2005年3月17日的IRB会议记录显示10名委员包括（b）（6）参加了这次会议，（b）（6）医生作为一名受邀人员和只作为（b）（4）研究的一名IRB委员参加了这次会议。会议记录显示“（b）（6）医生参加了（b）（4）研究的讨论，并且（b）（6）先生离开了讨论现场。”会议中IRB对于修订方案和知情同意文件要求的信函起草进行了投票。投票记录为“9票同意，0票反对”，没有记录显示（b）（6）离开了会议或弃权。因此，表明（b）（6）在有利益冲突的情况下参加了该研究的审查。

我们注意到这一发现没有列入FDA483表，因此在您的书面回复中没有关于此项的回复。

5. IRB未能对下列批准过的研究进行跟踪审查［21 CFR 56.109（1）］

我们检查发现IRB的文件没有相关记录表明IRB曾进行过以下研究的跟踪审查：

a. IRB2005年3月17日批准的研究“（b）（4）”。

在您2009年4月2日的书面回复中，您写道（b）（4）研究从没被批准进行受试者招募。您的解释与检查期间获得的证据相矛盾。如在本信中前文所述，我们的现场检查发现，IRB在方案和知情同意文件修改后于2005年3月17日批准了（b）（4）研究，并且在2005年4月4日给研究者的信中通知研究者修改后的文件已经被批准。2005年4月4日的信中指出方案（包括知情同意文件）有BRI IRB的批准日期签章。

b. IRB2005年7月21日批准的试验方案（b）（4），即（b）（4）研究。

在您2009年4月2日的书面回复中，您提到试验方案（b）（4）已经被批准进行受试者招募，但由于资金问题没有受试者入组。您的回复没有回应缺乏跟踪审查的问题，回复不够充分。

此外，您的书面回复中提到，IRB没有正式要求报告或审查这两个所提及研究的进展。但确实从研究者和/或申办者处获得了口头的报告。我们认为从研究者和/或申办者处获得的口头报告不能作为可接受的进行跟踪审查的形式，您的回复说到将会纠正这个疏忽，IRB计划在2009年4月要求提供这些报告。

6. IRB未能保存已审查的所有研究提案的复印件、研究提案的科学评估（如果存在，与研究提案一起）、已批准的知情同意样稿、研究者提交的进展报告和受试者受伤害的报告、IRB和研究者之间所有通信的复印件［21 CFR 56.115（a）（1）和56.115（a）（4）］

a. 对于（b）（4）研究，我们的现场检查发现，IRB审阅了研究者手册（IB），但手册没有保留在IRB文件中。您的书面回复中提到研究者手册在FDA检查时存在文件归档错误，现在已经找到并放进了对应的文件中。然而，在您的回复中没有附上这份研究者手册。

b. 对于（b）（4）研究，一封2005年4月4日给申办-研究者的信中提到一份有BRI IRB批准日期签章的方案（包含知情同意文件）复印件。IRB没有保存这份有批准日期印章的方案和知情同意文件。

c. 对于（b）（4）研究的检查发现如下：

ⅰ）在2005年1月6日IRB会议上，IRB要求起草一封信来说明几个问题，问题包括由工程师对设备进行评估。IRB文件中保存了一封2005年5月14日的工程师来信，但IRB要求工程师评估的信没有保存。

ⅱ）IRB文件中方案被定名为（b）（4），因此，好像或者还有其他版本（有不同的标题）IRB没有保存其他版本，或者是IRB混淆了两个研究并错误地归档。

ⅲ）2005年7月21日的IRB会议记录提到了委员会对一个“三折手册”的讨论和不予批准，以及一份2005年7月28日IRB负责人（b）（4）给（b）（4）的关于不接受三折宣传页的备忘录。IRB没有保存该手册/宣传单和拒绝批准宣传单的信函。

您在2009年4月2日的书面回复中提到，（b）（4）单元［试验方案（b）（4）］的描述文件在FDA检查时存在文件归档错误，现在已经找到包括研究者手册在内的完整文件。然而，在您的回复中没有附上任何文件用以支持与该研究相关的文件已经保存在目前的IRB文件中。

7. IRB未能准备和保存IRB会议的会议记录，用足够的细节显示会议的出席情况；IRB采取的行动；对行动的投票情况，包括赞成票数、反对票数和弃权票数；需要修改或不批准研究的理由、对争议问题的讨论和解决的书面总结［21 CFR 56.115（a）（2）］

a. IRB会议采取录音的方式进行记录，并在会后转为硬拷贝格式。因为会议记录没有准确地研究标题或研究编号，很难区分对哪些研究进行了讨论。此外，有记录显示当转录者不清楚某些词时，会用空格或问号代替。由于空格的数量较多，很难判断争议性问题是否被讨论。

b. 研究（b）（4）在2008年2月1日的IRB会议上被进行了讨论。会议记录显示IRB没有采取任何行动，但一封日期为2008年2月1日的批准函发给了临床研究者。

在您的书面回复中，您提到IRB没有批准该研究或其他相关的方案研究以开始人体试验，并且要求研究者完成充分的动物毒理研究。这与IRB2008年2月15日发给（b）（6）医生的信的内容不符，信中IRB提到了人的CIDP研究并指示（b）（6）医生应向申办者和BRI-IRB报告所有的不良事件和死亡情况。该信还进一步指出代表委员会，“您可以继续该研究”。

8. 每个IRB按照要求至少有5位不同背景的委员，以促进对临床研究机构实施的研究进行全面、充分地审查［21 CFR 56.107（a）］

我们的现场检查发现，在有些IRB委员对于个别研究存在利益冲突情况时，其他非IRB委员的人可以代替有冲突的委员参加IRB的行动。在FDA法规中没有关于此做法的规定。例如：

- 2005年3月17日的会议记录显示9名委员参加了这次会议，还有（b）（6）博士，一名非委员只参加了（b）（4）研究的讨论。（b）（6）医生被列为受邀人员。会议记录显示“（b）（6）医生参加（b）（4）的讨论，（b）（6）先生离开了”。（b）（4）的投票记录显示9人赞成，0人反对，因此说明（b）（6）医生参与了关于该研究的决定。

- 2005年5月26日和7月21日的IRB会议记录显示9名委员参加了这些会议，还有（b）（6）博士只参加（b）（4）和（b）（4）研究讨论，（b）（6）医生被列为受邀人员。会议记录显示，“（b）（6）医生作为委员参加（b）（4）的讨论，（b）（6）先生作为该研究的负责人。Hazlewood 医生和（b）（6）医生只参与讨论并不对此研究相关的事情进行投票。”在这些会议中，均对（b）（4）研究进行了讨论，并进行了投票。投票记录显示，8票赞成，0票反对，2票弃权。这表明（b）（6）医生参与了关于该研究的行动决定。

本警告信的目的并非是罗列BRI IRB在方案审查和批准中存在的所有缺陷。确保遵循法律和相关FDA法规的每一项要求是BRI IRB的职责。IRB应纠正这些缺陷，并建立规程，确保所有正在进行和将要进行的研究符合FDA法规要求。

自收到这封信的15个工作日内，您应当书面告知本办公室为预防今后发生类似的违规已经或将要采取的措施。您的书面回复应包括（b）（4）和（b）（4）研究的状态更新。如果不能充分、迅速地解释上述违规问题，可能导致我们在不再通知的情况下采取监管措施。

附：英文原文

Burzynski Research Institute / IRB

WARNING LETTER

OCT 5, 2009

CERTIFIED MAIL
RETURN RECEIPT REQUESTED

Ref: 10-HFD-45-09-01

Carlton F. Hazlewood, Ph.D.
Chairman
Burzynski Research Institute IRB
9432 Katy Freeway #370
Houston, TX 77055-6349

Dear Dr. Hazlewood:

Between December 3 and 10, 2008, Mr. Patrick D. Stone, representing the Food and Drug Administration (FDA), inspected the Burzynski Research Institute (BRI) Institutional Review Board (IRB). The purpose of this inspection was to determine whether the IRB procedures for the protection of human subjects complied with Title 21 of the Code of Federal Regulations (CFR), Parts 50 and 56. These regulations apply to clinical studies of products regulated by FDA. We are aware that at the conclusion of the inspection, our investigator presented and discussed with you, a

Form FDA 483, Inspectional Observations.

From our review of the establishment inspection report, the documents submitted with that report, and your April 2, 2009 written response to Form FDA 483, we conclude that the IRB did not adhere to the applicable statutory requirements and FDA regulations governing the protection of human subjects. We wish to emphasize the following:

1. The IRB approved research without determining that the following criteria were met: that risks to subjects were minimized [21 CFR 56.111(a)(1)] and risks to subjects were reasonable in relation to anticipated benefits, if any, to subjects, and the importance of the knowledge that may be expected to result [21 CFR 56.111(a)(2)].

a. For protocol **(b)(4)** our inspection revealed the following:

On January 10, 2007, **(b)(6)**, Ph.D. (an IRB member) submitted comments to the IRB in regard to this study. The purpose of the study was to evaluate the safety and efficacy of **(b)(4)** in subjects with **(b)(4)** or **(b)(4)** Dr. **(b)(6)** reviewed the investigator's brochure, clinical protocol, and appended evaluation and had concerns related to the source of the drug, the manufacturing process, and the potential effects of the drug on human subjects. He stated more information was needed to make a risk/benefit assessment.

One year elapsed before the IRB discussed this study at a convened meeting on February 1, 2008. There was nothing in the IRB's file to indicate that the IRB received any additional information related to this study between January 2007 and February 2008. Minutes of the February 1, 2008 IRB meeting indicate that the IRB was aware that the clinical investigator had already dosed human subjects with the investigational drug. Our inspection revealed that at the February 1, 2008 meeting, the IRB was in possession of undated case reports on fifteen human subjects who had been injected with **(b)(4)**. Despite knowledge that Dr. **(b)(4)** was dosing human subjects without IRB approval, as required by 21 CFR 312.66, the IRB failed to report Dr. **(b)(4)** noncompliance to the FDA pursuant to 21 CFR 56.108(b)(2).

There is no documentation of an IRB action in regard to the **(b)(4)** study in the minutes of the February 1, 2008 IRB meeting. However, in a letter dated February 15, 2008, the IRB wrote the following to the clinical investigator, **(b)(6)** M.D.

"... additional toxicity studies on animals will need to be completed. In the case of the human **(b)(4)** study, all adverse events are to be reported to the sponsor (**(b)(4)** and to the BRI-IRB as soon as humanly possible. Any deaths that might occur must be reported to the sponsor and our office within 24 hours. On behalf of the Committee, you may go forward with the study and we look forward to your continued success in this area".

It is unclear why the IRB allowed the study to go forward in humans when additional toxicity studies in animals were requested. In addition, it is unclear why the IRB allowed Dr. **(b)(4)** to continue **(b)(4)** the study when it appears that he initiated this research study, i.e., began dosing subjects, prior to obtaining IRB approval.

In your written response of April 2, 2009, you state that the IRB did not approve human enrollment for the **(b)(4)** study or any other related protocol. Your response does not comport with the letter sent by the IRB to the investigator on February 15, 2008.

As a result of an IRB meeting on August 8, 2008, the IRB sent a letter to **(b)(4)** (the study sponsor) regarding the status of the animal toxicity studies. The August 18, 2008 letter to **(b)(4)** stated "At this time, I must remind you that human studies, according to the protocol, cannot proceed until your Investigative [Investigational] New Drug (IND) Application is approved by the FDA." This letter to the sponsor appears to contradict the February 15, 2008 IRB letter sent to Dr. **(b)(6)** in which the IRB permitted the study to go forward.

During the inspection in December 2008, you told the FDA investigator that you were unaware that this IND was on clinical hold. However, **(b)(4)** responded to the IRB in a letter dated September 4, 2008, and referenced the clinical hold placed on the IND by FDA. Minutes of the October 24, 2008 IRB meeting indicate that the IRB decided to "draft a letter to **(b)(4)** stating that their application for this IRB to act as an IRB for their study be placed on hold until such time as we receive information regarding the FDA's position on the Toxicity Studies. At that time we will also review their Toxicity Studies and consider continuing their application." The IRB conveyed this information in a letter dated November 3, 2008; however, the letter was only sent to Dr. **(b)(6)** and not to **(b)(4)**.

In your written response, you state that "the IRB was informed that the sponsors were in discussion with FDA regarding their IND status. Based on this, the IRB considered its relationship to both sponsors and protocols in abeyance." As discussed above, the final piece of correspondence issued by the IRB in regard to the **(b)(4)** study was sent only to Dr. **(b)(6)** therefore, there is no documentation to demonstrate that **(b)(4)** was aware of the IRB's abeyance status of this study.

b. For the protocol **(b)(4)** our inspection revealed the following:

As a result of the January 6, 2005 IRB meeting, the IRB sent a letter on February 1, 2005 to **(b)(6)** M.D., Ph.D., sponsor-investigator, stating that the protocol, including the informed consent document, should be modified before final approval could be granted and asking him to resubmit the protocol and informed consent document to the IRB for review. In addition, the IRB informed Dr. **(b)(4)** that an Investigator's Brochure must be submitted.

At the March 17, 2005 IRB meeting, the IRB decided that if changes were made to the protocol and informed consent document, the clinical investigation could be approved. In a March 23, 2005 letter to the sponsor-investigator, the IRB agreed to approve the protocol and informed consent document contingent upon certain changes and again asked for an Investigator's Brochure.

In an April 4, 2005 letter, the IRB informed the sponsor-investigator that the revised documents had been approved. During the inspection, no Investigator's Brochure was found in the IRB's file. Therefore, it appears that the IRB approved the research without ever receiving one, which could impact an IRB's ability to determine whether risks to subjects were minimized and whether risks were reasonable in relation to anticipated benefits.

In your written response, you state that the clinical protocol for **(b)(4)** was never approved for patient enrollment. Your response does not comport with the correspondence sent by the IRB to the sponsor-investigator. During the inspection, you told the FDA investigator that this study was placed on clinical hold by the FDA. It is unclear when the IRB became aware of the clinical hold status and why the IRB informed the sponsor-investigator on April 4, 2005 that the study had been approved.

2. The IRB failed to prepare, maintain, and follow written procedures for conducting its initial and continuing review of research [21 CFR 56.108(a) and 56.115(a)(6)]. Specifically, the IRB has no written procedures for conducting reviews of device studies to determine whether they involve a significant risk device and had no evidence that it had in fact conducted such reviews [21 CFR 812.66].

Our investigation revealed that the IRB approved the "**(b)(4)** "on July 21, 2005. The protocol in the IRB's file has the following title: **(b)(4)** In correspondence with the sponsor and investigator, the study is referred to as "Protocol **(b)(4)**" and in an August 10, 2005 letter from the IRB to the sponsor, the protocol is referred to as **(b)(4)**

In reviewing a device investigation presented by the sponsor for IRB approval under 21 CFR 812.2(b)(1)(ii), an IRB must determine whether the proposed investigation involves the use of a significant risk (SR) device [21 CFR § 812.66.1]. If an IRB determines that an investigation presented for approval under 812.2(b)(1)(ii) involves an SR device, it shall notify the investigator and, where appropriate, the sponsor [21 CFR 812.66].

In your written response, you state that the IRB reviewed the FDA's Information Sheet for Significant Risk and Nonsignificant Risk Device Studies and made the determination that the study could be approved for human accrual as a nonsignificant risk (NSR) device. There is no documentation in the IRB's records (minutes of the September 23, 2004, January 6, 2005, May 26, 2005, and July 21, 2005 IRB meetings or IRB correspondence) that the IRB considered the use of the device in the clinical investigation, reviewed a description of the device, and the sponsor's explanation as to why the device is NSR, and then made an SR/NSR determination based on this review. In addition, we note that the IRB's Standard Operating Procedures (SOP) do not contain a procedure for the review of investigational device studies.

3. The IRB failed to ensure that informed consent would be sought from each prospective subject or the subject's legally authorized representative in accordance with and to the extent required by 21 CFR Part 50 [21 CFR 56.111(a)(4)] and that informed consent would be appropriately documented in accordance with and to the extent required by 21 CFR 50.27 [21 CFR 56.111(a)(5)].

a. For the **(b)(4)** study, our inspection revealed that there was no discussion about the informed consent document at the February 1, 2008 IRB meeting or at subsequent meetings held on August 8, 2008 and October 24, 2008 in which this study was discussed. There was no mention of the informed consent document in IRB correspondence dated February 15, 2008, August 18, 2008, and November 3, 2008 and there was no IRB-approved informed consent document in the IRB's file. Therefore, it appears that the IRB approved the clinical investigation without ensuring that informed consent would be obtained and documented in accordance with 21 CFR Part 50.

We note that this observation was not listed on Form FDA 483, and therefore, was not addressed in your written response.

b. For the **(b)(4)** Study, the informed consent document approved by the IRB on July 21, 2005 does not contain all of the elements required by 21 CFR 50.25 and therefore is not in compliance with Part 50. The following required elements are inaccurate or missing:

i) A description of the procedures to be followed, and identification of any procedures which are experimental [21 CFR 50.25(a)(1)]. The "Study Procedures" section of the informed consent document does not describe the study procedures outlined in the protocol. The informed consent document states "We will ask you to fill out brief patient assessment form every time you receive therapy"; however, there is no description of the therapy or the assessment forms. In addition, there are no descriptions of the lab work and the clinical, neurological, and functional testing required by the protocol.

ii) A description of any benefits to the subject or to others, which may reasonably be expected from the research [21 CFR 50.25(a)(3)]. The version of the informed consent document approved by the IRB is inaccurate in that it states "There may be direct benefits to you associated with participating in this research study: Relief of **(b)(4)**." This statement is not supported by the protocol which contains the following statements: "Poorly documented reports on the usefulness of **(b)(4)** in **(b)(4)** have been published... a search of the literature does not show any reports of scientific trials. To our knowledge, the use of **(b)(4)** has not been tried on **(b)(4)** patients." In addition, a version of an informed consent document included in the protocol states that "there is no guarantee that **(b)(4)** will help me and that the exact mechanism of action of these fields to produce possible benefits is not known to the investigators at the present time".

iii) A statement that notes the possibility that the Food and Drug Administration may inspect the records [21 CFR 50.25(a)(5)]. There was no such statement in the informed consent document.

iv) An explanation of whom to contact for answers to pertinent questions about the research and research subjects' rights, and whom to contact in the event of a research-related injury to the subject [21 CFR 50.25(a)(7)]. This explanation is missing from the informed consent document. In addition, **(b)(6)**, M.D., is incorrectly identified as the study coordinator; Dr. **(b)(4)** is the clinical investigator.

v) A statement that the subject may discontinue participation at any time without penalty or loss of benefits to which the subject is otherwise entitled [21 CFR 50.25(a)(8)]. There was no such statement in the informed consent document.

4. The IRB failed to ensure that no member participated in the initial or continuing review of a project in which the member had a conflicting interest, except to provide information requested by the IRB [21 CFR 56.107(e)].

a. For the **(b)(4)** study, you (IRB Chairman, Carlton F. Hazlewood, Ph.D.) are listed as a clinical investigator on the "Certification: Financial Interests and Arrangements of Clinical Investigators"; you are also listed as being an ex-officio advisor to the **(b)(4)**/IBR Central Registry Control Committee/Data Monitoring Committee. Therefore, you had a conflict of interest.

Minutes of the August 8, 2008 IRB meeting indicate that you attended this meeting and participated in the discussion of the **(b)(4)** study. At this meeting, the IRB voted to draft a letter to **(b)(4)** to inquire about the status of the animal toxicity studies. According to the minutes, all members were in favor, none were opposed, and none abstained. Minutes of the October 24, 2008 IRB meeting indicate that you attended the meeting and participated in the discussion of the **(b)(4)** study. At this meeting, the IRB voted to draft a letter to **(b)(4)** informing them that their application was on hold. The vote on this action is recorded as unanimous; therefore, according to the minutes of these two IRB meetings, you participated in the review of this study and voted on it even though you had a conflict of interest. We also note that you signed off on all correspondence sent by the IRB to Dr. **(b)(6)** and the sponsor in regard to this study.

We note that this observation was not listed on Form FDA 483, and therefore, was not addressed in your written response.

b. For the **(b)(4)** study, **(b)(6)** is listed on the protocol as a co-investigator. Minutes of the March 17, 2005 IRB meeting indicate that ten IRB members attended the meeting including **(b)(6)** and **(b)(6)**, M.D. was present as an invited guest and as an IRB member for the **(b)(4)** study only. The minutes indicate that "Dr. **(b)(6)** is present for **(b)(4)** discussion and Mr. **(b)(6)** leaves." At this meeting the IRB voted to generate a letter requesting changes to the protocol and informed consent document. The vote is recorded as "nine for and zero against." Nothing in the minutes indicates that **(b)(6)** left the meeting or abstained from voting. Therefore, it appears that **(b)(6)** participated in the review of this study even though he had a conflict of interest.

We note that this observation was not listed on Form FDA 483, and therefore, was not addressed in your written response.

5. The IRB failed to conduct continuing reviews for the following IRB approved studies [21 CFR 56.109(1)]:

Our inspection revealed no documentation in the IRB's files to indicate that the IRB conducted continuing review of the following studies:

a. "**(b)(4)**", approved by the IRB on March 17, 2005.

In your written response of April 2, 2009, you state that the **(b)(4)** study was never approved for patient enrollment. Your explanation is contradicted by evidence obtained during the inspection. As stated earlier in this letter, our inspection revealed that the IRB approved the **(b)(4)** study on March 17, 2005 contingent on changes to the protocol and informed consent document and informed the investigator in an April 4, 2005 letter that the revised documents had been approved. The April 4, 2005 letter states that the protocol (including informed consent documents) has a BRI IRB date stamp of approval.

b. Protocol #**(b)(4)**, also known as the **(b)(4)** Study, approved by the IRB on July 21, 2005.

In your written response of April 2, 2009, you state that protocol **(b)(4)** has been approved for patient enrollment, but no subjects have been enrolled because of funding problems. Your response fails to discuss the lack of continuing review and is inadequate.

In addition, your written response states that the IRB failed to formally request a report or review the progress of these two proposed studies, but did obtain verbal reports from the investigators and/or sponsor. We note that verbal reports from the investigator and/or sponsor are not an acceptable means of conducting continuing review. You state this oversight will be corrected and that the IRB planned to request these reports in April 2009.

6. The IRB failed to maintain copies of all research proposals reviewed, scientific evaluations, if any, that accompany the proposals, approved sample consent documents, progress reports submitted by investigators and reports of injuries to subjects, and correspondence with investigators [21 CFR 56.115(a)(1) and 56.115(a)(4)].

a. For the **(b)(4)** study, our inspection revealed that the Investigator's Brochure. (IB) was reviewed by the IRB, but was not in the IRB's file. In your written response you state that the IB was misfiled at the time of the FDA inspection and that the IB has been located and placed in the file; however, you did not attach the IB to your response.

b. For the **(b)(4)** study, an April 4, 2005 IRB letter to the sponsor-investigator refers to a copy of the protocol (which includes an informed consent document) with a BRI IRB date stamp of approval. The copy of the protocol and informed consent document with the date stamp of approval was not maintained by the IRB.

c. For the **(b)(4)** study our investigation found the following:

i) At the January 6,2005 IRB meeting the IRB requested that a letter be drafted to address several issues, including the evaluation of the device by an engineer. The IRB's file contained a May 14, 2005 letter from an engineer; however, the IRB's letter requesting the engineer's evaluation was not maintained.

ii) The protocol in the IRB's file is entitled **(b)(4)** Therefore, it appears there was either another version of the protocol (with a different title) that was not maintained by the IRB or the IRB has confused these two studies and misfiled documents.

iii) The minutes of the July 21, 2005 IRB meeting, refer to a board discussion and disapproval of a "Tri-Fold Brochure" and a July 28, 2005 memorandum from the IRB administrator, **(b)(4)** to **(b)(4)**, refers to a letter of denial for tri-fold flyer. The IRB did not maintain the brochure/flyer and the IRB letter denying approval of the flyer.

In your written response of April 2, 2009, you state that the description of the **(b)(4)** unit (Protocol #**(b)(4)** was misfiled at the time of the FDA inspection and the complete file, including the Investigator's Brochure, has been found; however, you did not attach any documents to your response to support that all documents pertaining to this study are currently in the IRB's file.

7. The IRB failed to prepare and maintain the minutes of IRB meetings in sufficient detail to show attendance at the meetings; actions taken by the IRB; the vote on these actions including the number of members voting for, against, and abstaining; the basis for requiring changes in or disapproving research; and a written summary of the discussion of controverted issues and their resolution [21 CFR 56.115(a)(2)].

a. It appears that the IRB tape records its meetings, which are then transcribed into a hard copy format. It is difficult to discern what studies are being discussed because the minutes do not reference the exact study titles or study numbers. In addition, it appears that when the transcriptionist does not understand certain words, they are transcribed as either blanks or question marks. Due to the numerous blanks, it is difficult to determine whether controverted issues were discussed.

b. For the **(b)(4)** study that was discussed at the February 1, 2008 IRB meeting, there is no IRB action recorded in the minutes; however, an approval letter, dated February 15, 2008 was sent to the clinical investigator.

In your written response, you state that the IRB did not approve this or any other related protocol to begin human accrual and that investigators were directed to complete adequate animal toxicity studies. This does not comport with the IRB's February 15, 2008 letter to Dr. **(b)(6)** in which the IRB refers to the human CIDP study and instructs Dr. **(b)(6)** to report all adverse events and deaths to the sponsor and BRI-IRB. The letter goes on to state that on behalf of the Committee, "you may go forward with the study".

8. Each IRB is required to have at least five members, with varying backgrounds to promote complete and adequate review of research activities commonly conducted by the institution [21 CFR 56.107(a)].

Our inspection revealed that, in some instances, when an IRB member had a conflict of interest for a particular study, another person, who was not an IRB member, was allowed to take the place of the conflicted member and participate in the IRB's action. There is no provision in FDA regulations for this type of action.

For example:

- Minutes of the March 17, 2005 IRB meeting indicate that nine members were present for this meeting, in addition to **(b)(6)**, M.D. a non-member who was present for the **(b)(4)** study only. Dr. **(b)(6)** is listed as an invited guest. The minutes indicate that "Dr. **(b)(6)** is present for **(b)(4)** discussion and Mr. **(b)(6)** leaves." The vote on the **(b)(4)** study is recorded as nine for and zero against, therefore, it appears that Dr. **(b)(6)** participated in the action on this study.
- Minutes of the May 26, 2005 and July 21, 2005 IRB meetings indicate that nine members were present for these meetings, in addition to, **(b)(6)** M.D. who was present for the **(b)(4)** and **(b)(4)** studies only. Dr. **(b)(6)** is listed as an invited guest. The minutes indicate that "Dr. **(b)(6)** was present as a member for the **(b)(4)** Study. Mr. **(b)(6)** took over as chairman for the study. Dr. Hazlewood and Dr. **(b)(6)** abstain from voting regarding any matter in this study and are only present for discussions." The **(b)(4)** study was discussed at each of these meetings and actions were taken with a vote of eight for, zero against, and two abstained; therefore, it appears that Dr. **(b)(6)** participated in the actions on this study.

This letter is not intended to be an all-inclusive list of deficiencies for the protocols reviewed and approved by BRI IRB. It is the IRB's responsibility to ensure adherence to each requirement of the law and relevant FDA regulations. The IRB should address these deficiencies and establish procedures to ensure that any on-going or future studies will be in compliance with FDA regulations.

Within fifteen (15) working days of your receipt of this letter, you should notify this office in writing of the actions you have taken or will be taking to prevent similar violations in the future. Your response should include an update on the status of the **(b)(4)** and **(b)(4)** studies. Failure to adequately and promptly explain the violations noted above may result in regulatory action without further notice.

If you have any questions, please contact Kevin A. Prohaska, D.O., M.P.H., at 301-796-3707; FAX 301-847-8748.

Your written response and any pertinent documentation should be addressed to:

Kevin A. Prohaska, D.O., M.P.H.
Acting Human Subjects Protections Team Lead
Division of Scientific Investigations
Office of Compliance
Center for Drug Evaluation and Research
Food and Drug Administration
Bldg 51, Room 5356
10903 New Hampshire Avenue
Silver Spring, MD 20993-0002

Sincerely yours,

/S/

Leslie K. Ball, M.D.
Director
Division of Scientific Investigations
Office of Compliance
Center for Drug Evaluation and Research

第26封　给Christus Schumpert健康系统的警告信

2009年7月30日

尊敬的Paine博士：

2008年4月21日至4月25日，Dana Daigle女士代表FDA，对CHRISTUS Schumpert 健康系统的伦理委员会（IRB）进行了现场检查。本次现场检查的目的是核实IRB受试者保护程序是否符合美国联邦法规第21篇第50和56部分的要求，这些法规适用于FDA所监管产品的临床研究。在现场检查结束时，我们的检查员向您出示并讨论了FDA483表，即现场检查发现的问题。

经对现场检查报告、该报告的附件（包括检查收尾时您提供的修订版IRB书面程序）进行审查，我们认为，IRB没有遵循适用的法律要求和受试者保护的FDA法规。我们想强调以下几点：

1. IRB未能要求提供给受试者作为知情同意的一部分的信息符合21 CFR 50.25的要求［21 CFR 56.109（b）］

21 CFR 50.25法规要求在获得知情同意时，每个受试者都应获得知情同意的基本要素［21 CFR 50.25（a）］，如果需要，还应获得额外的知情同意要素［21 CFR 50.25（b）］。

a. 对题为“（b）（4）”的研究项目1125，IRB未审查并批准符合FDA法规要求的知情同意书。我们注意到IRB只审阅批准了三份项目1125相关流程的医院通用知情同意书。它们均不符合21 CFR 50.25的要求。

b. 调查发现，IRB批准的项目1121的知情同意书中未写明如果研究受试者对其权益有疑问时应联系谁，或发生研究相关损害事件时应联系谁，而这是21 CFR 50.25（a）（7）的要求。

2. IRB未能确保参与IRB的初始审查或跟踪审查的委员与项目没有利益冲突关系，除非是根据IRB的要求提供信息［21 CFR 56.107（e）］

我们现场检查发现了5例参与研究的临床研究者在该研究的初始审查或跟踪审查中投票。下表列出了IRB 会议日期和发现的问题的总结：

IRB 会议日期	问题总结
2008年2月6日	（b）（6）医生是项目1055的研究者，IRB会议记录显示他参加了会议。会议通过无记名投票批准了知情同意书变更和该研究的进展报告。没有记录表明他回避了这两个决定的投票过程
2007年2月7日	（b）（6）医生是项目1073和1074的研究者，IRB会议记录显示他参加了会议。会议通过无记名投票批准了这些研究的进展报告。没有记录表明他回避了这两个研究中任一个的投票过程
2005年12月14日	（b）（6）医生是项目1091和1092的研究者，IRB会议记录显示他参加了会议。会议通过无记名投票批准了这两个新的提案。没有记录表明他回避了这两个研究的投票过程
2005年4月6日	（b）（6）医生是项目1055的研究者，IRB会议记录显示他参加了会议。会议通过无记名投票批准了此研究的进展报告。没有记录表明他回避了此研究投票过程
2005年2月2日	（b）（6）医生是项目1073、1074和1075的研究者，IRB 会议记录显示他参加了会议。会议通过无记名投票批准了这些新的提议。没有记录表明他回避了这些研究的投票过程

3. IRB未能遵守关于对研究进行初始审查和跟踪审查的书面程序［21 CFR 56.108（a）（1）］

IRB书面程序要求：议程中的提案的纲要副本应在会前提供给IRB委员。会议记录显示，会前向委员们邮寄了新提案的大纲和知情同意书，但是我们现场检查发现，2007年2月7日和11月1日的会议前，IRB委员并未收到新提案的方案纲要。在检查过程中，IRB 协调员指出，不再常规下发方案纲要。

4. IRB未能按照21 CFR 56.108（a）（b）的要求，准备和保存足够的IRB书面程序的记录［21 CFR 56.115（a）（6）］

具体而言，IRB没有将IRB发现的问题和采取的措施报告给机构的书面程序，而这是21 CFR 56.108（a）（1）所要求的。IRB没有确定哪些项目需要从研究以外的来源获得证实，自上次审查后资料没有变更。这是21 CFR 56.108（a）（2）的要求。

5. IRB 未能在多数委员在场的召集会议上对提交的研究进行审查［21 CFR 56.108（c）］

IRB 2007年11月1日会议记录显示，IRB委员共有10名投票委员和3名依职权（不投票）委员。因此，至少应有6名投票委员出席审评会。我们现场检查发现，2007年11月1日的会议中只有5名投票委员出席。

6. IRB 未能按照与风险程度相对应的，但不少于每年一次的时间间隔对研究进行跟踪审查［21 CFR 56.109（f）］

项目1114的最初被批准是在2007年2月7日。我们现场检查发现，没有IRB记录显示在2008年4月25日前进行过项目1114的跟踪审查。

7. IRB 未能准备和保存足够的、以充分的细节显示IRB采取的行动的会议记录［21 CFR 56.115（a）（2）］

我们现场检查发现，2007年11月1日IRB会议记录中没有关于对项目1051进行跟踪审查的记录，但IRB的项目1051文件中的一份IRB再批准函和进展报告均有IRB主席签字，显示为已经被2007年11月1日IRB会议批准。

本警告信的目的并非是罗列IRB在审查和批准试验方案中存在的所有缺陷。确保CHRISTUS Schumpert健康系统的IRB的操作和程序完全符合法律法规是您的职责。

FDA于2009年2月23日收到IRB对FDA483表的回复，并注意到CHRISTUS Schumpert 健康系统计划于2009年4月18日前正式解散伦理委员会。我们要求您在收到本通知的30个工作日内提供书面文件说明解散活动，以及将现有项目移交给外部IRB的状况。如CHRISTUS Schumpert 健康系统在日后任何时候决定重组IRB，其IRB的流程应符合21 CFR50，56中关于受试者保护的要求。这些法规适用于FDA监管产品的临床研究。

附：英文原文

Christus Schumpert Health System

Untitled Letter

Jul 30, 2009

CERTIFIED MAIL
RETURN RECEIPT REQUESTED

Dr. Charles J. Paine
Chief Executive Officer
CHRISTUS Schumpert Health System
One Saint Mary Place
Shreveport, LA 71101

Dear Dr. Paine:

Between April 21 and 25, 2008, Ms. Dana Daigle, representing the Food and Drug Administration (FDA), inspected the Institutional Review Board (IRB) at the CHRISTUS Schumpert Health System. The purpose of this inspection was to determine whether the IRB procedures for the protection of human subjects complied with Title 21 of the Code of Federal Regulations (CFR), Parts 50 and 56. These regulations apply to clinical studies of products regulated by FDA. We are aware that at the conclusion of the inspection, our investigator presented and discussed with you, a Form FDA 483, Inspectional Observations.

From our review of the establishment inspection report and the documents submitted with that report, including the revised IRB written procedures provided at the close out of the inspection, we conclude that the IRB did not adhere to the applicable statutory requirements and FDA regulations governing the protection of human subjects. We wish to emphasize the following:

1. The IRB failed to require that information given to subjects as part of the informed consent process is in accordance with 21 CFR 50.25 [21 CFR 56.109(b)].

When seeking informed consent, the regulations at 21 CFR 50.25 require that each subject be provided with the basic elements of informed consent [21 CFR 50.25(a)], and when appropriate, one or more of the additional elements of informed consent [21 CFR 50.25(b)].

a. For research Project 1125 entitled, "(b)(4)", our inspection revealed the IRB failed to review and approve an informed consent form that was in compliance with FDA regulatory requirements. We note that the IRB reviewed and approved only three general hospital consent forms for procedures related to Project 1125. None of these consent forms complied with the requirements of 21 CFR Part 50.25.

b. Our inspection revealed the informed consent form approved by the IRB for Project 1121 did not include an explanation of whom the subject should contact for questions about their rights as a research subject, or whom to contact in the event of a research-related injury as required by 21 CFR 50.25(a)(7).

2. The IRB failed to ensure that no member participated in the initial or continuing review of a project in which the member had a conflicting interest, except to provide information requested by the IRB [21 CFR 56.107(e)].

Our inspection revealed five instances in which an IRB member, who was serving as the clinical investigator for a particular research study, voted on the initial or continuing review of that study. The following table lists the dates of the IRB meetings and a brief summary of our findings:

Date of IRB Meeting	Summary of Finding
2/6/2008	Dr. (b) (6) is the clinical investigator for Project 1055. The IRB meeting minutes indicate that he attended the meeting. There was a unanimous vote to approve a consent form change and a unanimous vote to approve the progress report for this study. There is no documentation that Dr. (b) (6) abstained from voting on either action.
2/7/2007	Dr. is the clinical investigator for Projects 1073 and 1074. The IRB meeting minutes indicate that he attended the meeting. There was a unanimous vote to approve the progress reports for these studies. There is no documentation that Dr. (b) (6) abstained from voting on either study.
12/14/2005	Dr. (b) (6) is the clinical investigator for Projects 1091 and 1092. The IRB meeting minutes indicate that he attended the meeting. There was a unanimous vote to approve both of these new proposals. There is no documentation that Dr. (b) (6) abstained from voting on either study.
4/6/2005	Dr. (b) (6) is the clinical investigator for Project 1055. The IRB meeting minutes indicate that he attended the meeting. There was a unanimous vote to approve the progress report for this study. There is no documentation that Dr. (b) (6) abstained from voting on this study.
2/2/2005	Dr. (b) (6) is the clinical investigator for Projects 1073, 1074, and 1075. The IRB meeting minutes indicate that he attended the meeting. There was a unanimous vote to approve these new proposals. There is no documentation that Dr. (b) (6) abstained from voting on any of these studies.

3. The IRB failed to follow its written procedures for conducting its initial and continuing review of research [21 CFR 56.108(a)(1)].

The IRB written procedures require that information, including copies of schemas of all proposals on the agenda, be sent to IRB members prior to the meeting. The meeting minutes indicate members were mailed outlines and consent forms for new proposals prior to the meeting, but our inspection revealed that IRB members were not provided copies of protocol schemas for new proposals for the IRB meetings of February 7, 2007 and November 1, 2007. During the inspection, the IRB Coordinator indicated protocol schemas were no longer routinely distributed.

4. The IRB failed to prepare and maintain adequate documentation of written procedures for the IRB as required by 21 CFR 56.108(a) and (b) [21 CFR 56.115(a)(6)].

Specifically, the IRB does not have written procedures for reporting IRB findings and actions to the institution as required by 21 CFR 56.108(a)(1), and does not have written procedures for determining which projects require verification from sources other than the investigator that no material changes have occurred since previous IRB review as required by 21 CFR 56.108(a)(2).

5. The IRB failed to review proposed research at convened meetings at which a majority of the members of the IRB are present [21 CFR 56.108(c)].

The IRB meeting minutes for November 1, 2007, indicate that the membership of the IRB consisted of ten voting members and three ex-officio (non-voting) members. Accordingly, a minimum of six voting members were required to be present at the meeting to review proposed research. Our inspection revealed that the IRB reviewed and approved research at the November 1, 2007, IRB meeting with only five voting members present.

6. The IRB failed to conduct continuing review of research at intervals appropriate to the degree of risk, but not less than once per year [21 CFR 56.109(f)].

Project 1114 was initially approved by the IRB on February 7, 2007. Our inspection revealed there is no documentation in the IRB files that continuing review of Project 1114 was conducted at any time prior to April 25, 2008.

7. The IRB failed to prepare and maintain adequate minutes of IRB meetings in sufficient detail to show actions taken by the IRB [21 CFR 56.115(a)(2)].

Our inspection revealed the minutes for the November 1, 2007, IRB meeting do not list Project 1051 as being reviewed for continuing review. However, the IRB files for Project 1051 contain an IRB re-approval letter and a progress report signed by the IRB Chair as approved at the November 1, 2007 IRB meeting.

This letter is not intended to be an all-inclusive list of deficiencies for the protocols reviewed and approved by the IRB. It is your responsibility to ensure that CHRISTUS Schumpert Health System IRB's practices and procedures comply fully with all applicable statutes and regulations.

The FDA received the IRB's response dated February 23, 2009 to the FDA Form 483 and noted that CHRISTUS Schumpert Health System planned to formally disband the IRB as of April 18, 2009. We request written documentation within thirty (30) working days of receiving this letter of the status of the plan to disband the IRB and transfer any remaining studies to an external IRB. Should CHRISTUS Schumpert Health System decide to re-establish the IRB at any time in the future, it is expected that IRB procedures comply with the protection of human subjects in accordance with Title 21 of the CFR, Parts 50 and 56. These regulations apply to clinical studies investigations of products regulated by FDA.

If you have any questions, please contact me at 301-796-3707; FAX 301-847-8748. Your response and any pertinent documentation should be sent to me at:

Division of Scientific Investigations
Office of Compliance
Center for Drug Evaluation and Research
Food and Drug Administration
Bldg 51, Room 5356

10903 New Hampshire Avenue
Silver Spring, MD 20993

Sincerely yours,

{See appended electronic signature page}

Kevin Prohaska, D.O., M.P.H.
Acting Human Subjects Protection Team Lead
Division of Scientific Investigations
Office of Compliance
Center for Drug Evaluation and Research

第 27 封　给 Coast 伦理委员会的警告信

2009年4月14日

参考号：09-HFD-46-04-01

尊敬的Dueber先生：

2009年3月26日，美国众议院下属监督委员会与能源商业调查委员会就“监督人体试验的伦理委员会营利性考察”召开了听证会（以下简称听证会）。在听证会上，美国政府问责局（GAO）司法审计和特别调查部门负责人Gregory Kutz先生提供了“秘密调查显示伦理委员会易受非道德操控”的证据[1]。

该证据来自于美国政府问责局于2008年1月至2009年3月进行的一项调查，其一部分目的是考察伦理委员会（IRB）是否对所申请的研究进行了充分的评估。在该项调查中，美国政府问责局杜撰了“一个虚构的医疗器械公司”和“一个具有未经过验证的检测历史且假的质量标准的虚构医疗器械的研究方案”。该方案设计的“使我们提出的研究项目的某些方面仅含有模糊不清的信息”。该“虚构器械是一种针对女性的术后康复设备，该器械符合FDA公开的指导原则中列举的多个具有‘重大风险’案例的特征。”

美国政府问责局通过在线检索选择了3个独立伦理委员会，并向每个伦理委员会均提交了一份虚构的研究方案供其审查。美国政府问责局证实，Coast伦理委员会是唯一一家仅对申报资料进行细微修订就批准的机构。Kutz先生证实，Coast伦理委员会未能核实提交的方案中包含的虚假宣称，即FDA已经允许该器械上市，相关信息可通过搜索FDA在线数据库即可获得。此外，美国政府问责局证实，Coast伦理委员会会议记录显示，委员会委员认为该项研究“可能非常安全”，一致投票通过，即使所提交给IRB的审查材料中的安全信息不足以作出这样的决定。

2009年4月14日，Coast伦理委员会首席执行官Daniel Dueber先生，与FDA 的Leslie Ball博士和Michael Marcarelli博士在电话中讨论了美国政府问责局的书面证词和听证会上公开的其他信息，包括递交给Coast伦理委员会的临床研究方案和其批准的知情同意书[2]。在讨论过程中，FDA确定其严重违反了美国联邦法规（21 CFR）第56部分——伦理委员会、第812部分——器械临床试验豁免（IDE）和第50部分——受试者保护。[3]根据21 CFR 56.111（a）的规定，为使所审查的研究符合上述法律法规，除了其他事项外，IRB必须确定受试者风险最小化，对受试者的风险与受试者的预期获益和预期获得的知识的重要性相比是合理的。FDA并不认为Coast伦理委员符合21 CFR 56.111的规定，有所需的充分信息去批准该项临床研究。下面列举几个严重违反FDA法规21 CFR第50、56和812部分的例子。

1. IRB未能确定受试者风险最小化［21 CFR 56.111（a）（1）］

基于美国政府问责局的书面证词及对所公开信息的审查，Coast伦理委员会没有足够的信息来识别潜在的风险，并没有根据21 CFR 56.111（a）（1）的规定，确认对受试者的风险已降至最低。GAO递交给Coast伦理委员会的资料中，未包括完整的器械信息或临床前研究结果，例如，研究方案中提及ADHESIABLOC®凝胶用于“临床前动物模型”（第3页），但没有提供任何进一步的信息。如果没有一个完整的器械描述信息或临床前研究结果，是无法确认对受试者的风险降至最低。

1　详见http://www.gao.gov/new.items/d09448t.pdf 2009年4月29日披露的信息

2　详见 http://energycommerce.house.gov/index.php?option=com_content&task=view&id=1552

3　详见http://www.gpoaccess.gov/cfr/index.html

2. IRB未能确定对受试者的风险与受试者预期获益（如有）和预期获得知识的重要性相比是合理的［21 CFR 56.111（a）（2）］

如上所述，Coast伦理委员会没有足够的信息来确定受试者的风险；也没有足够的信息来评估预期获益。例如，方案的研究背景信息提到“在Device Med-Systems进行的临床评估中，丙二醇（器械显而易见的组成成分）被证明安全和轻微有效”（第2页），但没有提供这些评估的结果。同样，方案提到ADHESIABLOC®凝胶通过水疗漂浮可防止或减少粘连的形成，与作为起始溶液，在临床前动物模型中有相同效果一样（3页），但未明确什么是“起始溶液”，或者提供临床前试验结果。基于以上有限信息，Coast伦理委员会不可能按照21 CFR 56.111（a）（2）的要求，对受试者面临的风险与预期获益的合理性进行判断。

3. IRB未能确定21 CFR 812的适用性，未能对试验器械研究进行风险确定［21 CFR 812.2（c）（2），812.66，812.20（a）］

Coast伦理委员会没有采取适当的步骤来确定该研究中是否适用21 CFR 812的规定。递交的审查资料显示，该器械曾获得上市前登记［510（k）］。为了该项研究的开展而不需要FDA批准的IDE，Coast伦理委员会需要根据21 CFR 812.2（C）的规定，确定该项器械研究是否可豁免FDA的批准。具体来说，根据所递交的资料，Coast伦理委员会需要确定该临床研究所用的器械的适应症，与已经批准的器械适应症完全一致（即标签载明的适应症，FDA根据21 CFR 第807部分的规定审查过）。Coast伦理委员会未能进行判断。基于美国政府问责局的书面证词和听证会上其他公开的信息，我们可确定，按照21 CFR 812.2（C）的规定，该项器械临床研究不能得到豁免。

根据21 CFR 812的规定，对于不能豁免的临床研究用器械，伦理委员会应按照21 CFR 812.66[1]的规定作出有重大/无重大风险的评估。Coast IRB未能作出上述判断。基于美国政府问责局的书面证词和公开信息，我们确定涉及ADHESIABLOC®凝胶的该项器械临床研究有重大风险[2]，在试验实施前，需要向FDA递交申请，并获得IDE批准，21 CFR 812.20（a）。

4. IRB未能确保其批准的知情同意书中包括知情同意的基本要素［21 CFR 50.25（a）（2），56.109（b）］

根据21 CFR 56.109（b）的规定，IRB应要求知情同意书按21 CFR 50.25的要求提供信息给受试者。根据21 CFR 50.25（a）（2），知情同意书的一个基本要素是将任何合理可预见的风险或不适告知受试者。如上所述，Coast伦理委员会没有足够的信息来判断给受试者带来的合理可预见的风险，也不能从研究方案的背景介绍部分了解该器械的详细介绍或临床前研究资料。伦理委员会批准的知情同意书“该项研究中可能给受试者带来的潜在的风险和不适？”项下申明，“没有ADHESIABLOC®凝胶相关的已知的不良反应或不适，但是可能有罕见的或未知的风险”（第3页）。因为Coast伦理委员会在没有足够信息来确定可预见风险的情况下，批准了该知情同意书，所以没有履行21 CFR 56.109（b）要求的义务，即需将可预计的风险和不适作为知情同意书的一部分告知受试者。

5. IRB未能展示其有能力从法规、适用法律，以及专业的实施和操作标准的角度来确定拟审查研究的可接受性［21 CFR 56.107（a）］

根据21 CFR 56.107（a）的规定，伦理委员会必须能够确定所提交审查研究的可接受性，从法规、适用法律，以及专业的实施和操作标准的角度来，但Coast伦理委员会未能证明具有该能力。如上所述，在受试者风险方面没有充分的信息，没有合格的研究者，未能确定符合21 CFR 812.2（c）（2）规定的豁免条件，未按照21 CFR 50.25（a）（2）的要求将风险作为知情同意书的一部分告知受试者等情况下，Coast伦理委员会批准了该器械的临床研究。综上所述，FDA认为Coast伦理委员会缺乏对适用法规、法律、专业的实施和

1　关于该项判断更多的信息见“Information Sheet Guidance for IRBs, Clinical Investigators, and Sponsors: Significant Risk and Nonsignificant Risk Medical Device Studies,” http://www.fda.gov/oc/ohrt/irbs/devrisk.pdf.

2　重大风险指研究用医疗器械：（1）拟用于植入，且显示对受试者健康、安全或福利有潜在严重风险；（2）拟用于人生命的维持，且显示对受试者健康、安全或福利有潜在严重风险；（3）在诊断、治疗疾病或防止人类健康受害中具有重要作用，且显示对受试者健康、安全或福利有潜在严重风险；（4）其他显示对受试者健康、安全或福利有潜在严重风险的［21 CFR 812.3(m)］。

操作标准的认识。

鉴于上述违规行为的严重性和对研究中受试者的权益和福利带来的风险，2009年4月14日，Coast伦理委员自愿采取如下限制措施：

（1）不批准适用21 CFR 56的新的临床研究。

（2）对于正在进行的、适用21 CFR 56的研究，不再增加新的受试者。

这些限制措施将一直有效，直到您已经采取了足够的纠正措施并收到FDA的书面通知。这些限制措施并不减除Coast伦理委员会有关接收和应对非预期的和严重的不良反应，以及进行中的临床研究的常规进展报告的职责。

自收到这封信后的15个工作日内，您应当书面告知本办公室为使Coast伦理委员会完全符合FDA的法规而采取的措施或计划采取的具体措施。您的回复应包括所有必要的文件，以表明您已采取充分的纠正措施，包括每项整改措施预计完成日期。

将上述限制措施通知所有受影响的申办者和临床研究者是您的职责。请贵方将目前所采取的限制措施通知受影响的申办者和临床研究者的书面样本，一并随整改报告递交。请还提供一份完整的、所需通知的申办者和研究者名单，以及他们被通知的日期。

请提供目前正在进行的受上述限制影响的所有研究项目清单，包括研究标题（IDE或IND申请号，如果可行的话），供试品名称，临床研究者的名字，初始审查和批准的日期，跟踪审查日期。IND和IDE申请号可以通过受上述限制影响的申报者的研究方案获得。

如果不能回复本警告信，并采取适当的纠正措施，FDA会根据21 CFR 56.120、56.124以及56.121的授权，采取进一步的法律措施。这些法律措施包括，但不限于：继续采取上述限制措施，终止贵IRB批准的、适用21 CFR 56规定的正在进行的研究，启动吊销贵方IRB资质的法律程序等。

附：英文原文

Coast Institutional Review Board

WARNING LETTER

April 14, 2009

CERTIFIED MAIL
RETURNED RECEIPT REQUESTED

Ref: 09-HFD-46-04-01

Mr. Daniel Dueber
Chief Executive Officer
Coast IRB, LLC
5475 Mark Dabling Blvd., Suite 351
Colorado Springs, CO 80918

Dear Mr. Dueber:

On March 26, 2009, the U.S. House of Representatives' Subcommittee on Oversight and Investigations of the Committee on Energy and Commerce held a hearing entitled, "Institutional Review Boards that Oversee Experimental Human Testing for Profit" (the Hearing). During the Hearing, Mr. Gregory Kutz, Managing Director, Forensic Audits and Special Investigations Unit of the U.S. Government Accountability Office (GAO), presented the testimony “Undercover Tests Show the Institutional Review Board System is Vulnerable to Unethical Manipulation.”[1] This testimony related to an investigation the GAO conducted between January 2008 and March 2009 to test, in part, whether institutional review boards (IRBs) are adequately evaluating studies submitted for approval. In this test, the GAO created “a bogus medical device company” and “a research protocol for a fictitious medical device with no proven test history and bogus specifications.” The protocol was designed “so that it would contain vague information about certain aspects of our proposed study.” The “fictitious device was a post-surgical healing device for women that matched multiple examples of ‘significant risk’ devices provided in publicly available FDA guidance.”

The GAO selected three independent IRBs from on an online search and submitted a fictitious protocol to each IRB for their review. The GAO testified that Coast IRB, LLC, was the only IRB selected that reviewed and approved the research protocol and did so with only minor edits to the submitted materials. Mr. Kutz testified that Coast IRB failed to verify the false assertion contained in the protocol submission that the Food and Drug Administration (FDA) had already cleared the device for marketing, which could have been accomplished through a search of FDA’s online database. In addition, the GAO testified that Coast IRB meeting minutes showed that the board members thought the protocol was “probably very safe” and voted unanimously to approve it even though the materials submitted to the IRB for review contained insufficient safety information to make such a determination.

In a telephone conversation on April 14, 2009, between Mr. Daniel Dueber, Chief Executive Officer of Coast IRB and Dr. Leslie Ball and Dr. Michael Marcarelli of the FDA, we discussed the GAO’s written testimony and other information made publicly available at the Hearing, including the device clinical study protocol provided to Coast IRB and the informed consent form approved by Coast IRB.[2] During this discussion, FDA identified the following serious violations of Title 21, Code of Federal Regulations (21 CFR) Part 56 – Institutional Review Boards, Part 812 – Investigational Device Exemptions (IDE), and Part 50 – Protection of Human Subjects.[3] Under 21 CFR § 56.111(a), in order to approve research covered by these regulations, the IRB shall determine, among other things, that risks to subjects are minimized and that risks to subjects are reasonable in relation to anticipated benefits, if any, to subjects, and the importance of the knowledge that may be expected to result. FDA does not believe Coast IRB had sufficient information needed in order to make the determinations required for approval of an investigation under 21 CFR § 56.111. Below we have cited applicable provisions of the CFR relevant to this violation. We have also described several other serious violations of FDA regulations at 21 CFR parts 50, 56, and 812.

1. The IRB failed to determine that risks to subjects are minimized. [21 CFR § 56.111(a)(1)].

Based on the GAO’s written testimony and our review of the publicly available information, Coast IRB did not have sufficient information to identify potential risks to subjects and to determine that risks to subjects are minimized, as required under 21 CFR § 56.111(a)(1). The information submitted to Coast IRB by the GAO did not include a complete device description or results from preclinical testing. For example, the protocol provided to Coast IRB mentioned use of the ADHESIABLOC® Gel in “preclinical animal models” (p. 3) without providing any further information. Without a complete device description or results from preclinical testing, a determination that risks to subjects are minimized could not be made.

2. The IRB failed to determine that risks to subjects are reasonable in relation to anticipated benefits, if any, to subjects, and the importance of the knowledge that may be expected to result. [21 CFR § 56.111(a)(2)].

As noted above, Coast IRB did not have sufficient information to identify risks to subjects; nor was sufficient information available to assess anticipated benefits. For example, while the background information in the protocol states, “In clinical evaluations conducted by Device Med-Systems, Propylene Glycol [an apparent component of the device] is found to be safe and marginally effective” (p. 2), the results of these evaluations were not provided. Similarly, the protocol states that the ADHESIABLOC® Gel “has shown to prevent or reduce adhesion formation by hydro floatation and is as effective as the starting solution in preclinical animal models” (p. 3), without identifying the “starting solution” or providing results of this preclinical testing. Based on this limited information, Coast IRB could not determine that the risks to subjects were reasonable in relation to the anticipated benefits, as required under 21 CFR § 56.111(a)(2).

3. The IRB failed to determine the applicability of 21 CFR Part 812 and failed to make a risk determination for the investigational device study. [21 CFR §§ 812.2(c)(2), 812.66, 812.20(a)].

Coast IRB did not take appropriate steps to determine the applicability of 21 CFR Part 812 to the investigation. The information submitted indicated the device had a cleared premarket notification (510(k)). In order for the device investigation to proceed without an FDA-approved IDE, Coast IRB needed to determine that the investigation was exempt under 21 CFR § 812.2(c). Specifically, in light of the information submitted, Coast IRB needed to determine whether the device was being investigated in accordance with the indications for which the device was apparently cleared (i.e., the indications in the labeling that FDA had apparently reviewed under 21 CFR part 807). 21 CFR § 812.2(c)(2). Coast IRB failed to make this determination. Based on the GAO's written testimony and other information made publicly available at the Hearing, we have determined that the investigation would not have been exempt under 21 CFR § 812.2(c).

For device investigations that are not exempt from the submission requirements of 21 CFR Part 812, IRBs are required to make the significant/non-significant risk determination under 21 CFR § 812.66.4 Coast IRB failed to make such a determination. Based on the GAO's written testimony and our review of the publicly available information, we have determined that a study involving the ADHESIABLOC® Gel device would be considered a significant risk device investigation,5 requiring submission to FDA and FDA approval of an IDE before the investigation could be initiated. 21 CFR § 812.20(a).

4. The IRB failed to ensure that basic elements of informed consent are included in the IRB-approved consent form. [21 CFR §§ 50.25(a)(2), 56.109(b)].

Under 21 CFR § 56.109(b), the IRB shall require that information given to subjects as part of informed consent is in accordance with 21 CFR § 50.25. One of the basic elements of informed consent, required under 21 CFR § 50.25(a)(2), is a description of any reasonably foreseeable risks or discomforts to the subject. As discussed above, Coast IRB did not have sufficient information to identify any reasonably foreseeable risks to subjects. Coast IRB did not have a complete device description or results from the preclinical and clinical testing referenced in the background section of the protocol (pp. 2-3). Under the heading "What are the possible risks or discomforts involved with being in the study?" the consent form approved by Coast IRB states, "There are no known side effects or discomforts associated with ADHESIABLOC® Gel, but there may be uncommon or previously unknown risks" (p.3). Because Coast IRB approved this consent form without having sufficient information to identify foreseeable risks to subjects, it did not meet its obligation under 21 CFR § 56.109(b) to require that the information provided to subjects as part of informed consent include a description of any foreseeable risks or discomforts.

5. The IRB failed to demonstrate its ability to ascertain the acceptability of the proposed research in terms of regulations, applicable law, and standards of professional conduct and practice. [21 CFR § 56.107(a)].

Under 21 CFR § 56.107(a), an IRB must be able to ascertain the acceptability of the proposed research in terms of regulations, applicable law, and standards of professional conduct and practices. Coast IRB failed to demonstrate this ability. As discussed above, Coast IRB approved a device investigation without adequate information on the risks posed to subjects, without a qualified clinical investigator, without assuring that the investigation met the exemption criteria under 21 CFR § 812.2(c)(2), and without assuring that the information provided to subjects as part of informed consent is in accordance with 21 CFR § 50.25(a)(2). FDA believes the above findings indicate a lack of understanding of the applicable regulations, law, and standards of professional conduct and practice.

Given the seriousness of these violations and the risk to the rights and welfare of human research subjects, on April 14, 2009 Coast IRB, LLC voluntarily agreed to the following restrictions:

1. No new studies subject to the requirements of 21 CFR Part 56 will be approved; and
2. No new subjects will be added to on-going studies subject to 21 CFR Part 56.

These restrictions will remain in effect until such time that you receive written notification from FDA that adequate corrections have been made. These restrictions do not relieve Coast IRB of its responsibility for receiving and responding to reports of unexpected and serious reactions and routine progress reports from ongoing studies.

Within fifteen (15) working days of receiving this letter, you are to notify the Agency of the specific actions you have taken or plan to take to bring Coast IRB into full compliance with FDA regulations. Your response should include any documentation necessary to show that full and adequate correction has been achieved and include the projected completion dates for each action to be accomplished.

It is your responsibility to notify all affected sponsors and clinical investigators of the restrictions described above. Include with your response to the FDA a representative sample copy of the IRB's written communication(s) to affected sponsors and clinical investigators, notifying them of the current restrictions. Please also provide a complete list of all sponsors and investigators notified as a result of this action and the date on which they were notified.

Please provide a list of all studies currently being conducted that are affected by the above restrictions and include the titles of the studies (with IDE or IND numbers, if applicable), the names of the test articles, the names of the clinical investigators, dates of initial reviews and approvals, and dates of continuing reviews. IND and IDE numbers can be obtained through the sponsor of the protocols affected by these restrictions.

Failure to respond to this letter and take appropriate corrective action could result in FDA taking regulatory actions, as authorized by 21 CFR §§ 56.120, 56.124, and 56.121. These actions include, but are not limited to, continuation of the restrictions described above, the termination of on-going studies subject to 21 CFR Part 56 and approved by your IRB, and the initiation of regulatory proceedings for disqualification of your IRB.

Should you have any questions or comments about the contents of this letter or any aspects of the operations and responsibilities of an Institutional Review Board, you may contact Dr. Leslie Ball at (301) 796-3150.

Please send your written response to:

Leslie K. Ball, M.D.
Director
Division of Scientific Investigations
Office of Compliance
Center for Drug Evaluation and Research
Food and Drug Administration
Bldg 51, Room 5342
10903 New Hampshire Avenue
Silver Spring, MD 20993

Sincerely,

/S/

Deborah M. Autor, Esq.
Director
Office of Compliance
Center for Drug Evaluation and Research

第28封　给Provena St. Joseph's医疗中心伦理委员会的警告信

2009年3月12日

参考号：CBER-09-06

尊敬的Choi博士：

这封信特告知您于2008年11月25日结束的，FDA对Provena St. Joseph's医疗中心伦理委员会（IRB）现场检查的结果。FDA对伦理委员会进行了检查，以核实伦理委员会对于受试者的保护程序是否符合颁布在联邦法规（CFR）第21篇中第50和56部分的FDA法规要求。本次现场检查是FDA的生物研究监查项目的一部分，该项目通过设定的检查方法，来审查涉及试验药物的临床研究并保护受试者。

在现场检查结束时，FDA检查员向您出示并讨论了FDA 483表，即现场检查发现的问题。经对现场检查报告以及该报告的附件进行审查，我们认为，贵伦理委员会违反了在21 CFR 第50和56部分中颁布的监管伦理委员会的运作及责任的适用联邦法规（见http://www.gpoaccess.gov/cfr/index.html）。违反的每一条CFR适用条款在以下列出。基于21 CFR 56.120（a）的要求，我们将这封信发给您，作为现任伦理委员会的主席，确保采取必需的措施使伦理委员会的运作能够完全满足FDA法规的要求是您的职责。我们同时将这封信的副本发送给伦理委员会上级机构的负责人，因为基于21 CFR 56.120（c）的要求，上级机构对伦理委员会的运作也负有责任。

1. IRB未能在大多数IRB委员出席，其中至少包括一名来自非科学领域委员的召集的会议上对拟开展的研究进行审查［21 CFR 56.108（c）］

a. 一份对2005 ~ 2008年的伦理委员会会议记录的审查显示，伦理委员会一直在没有大多数伦理委员会委员出席的情况下审查及批准新研究并进行跟踪审查，包括伦理委员会主席在内的未出现在IRB委员名册上的人参加会议并进行投票。许多会议未包括至少一名非科学领域委员。

会议日期	名册中的伦理委员会委员人数	出席的伦理委员会委员人数	是否有非科学领域委员出席
2008年6月10日，2008年4月28日	6	1	无
2007年12月18日，2007年11月20日	13	6	有
2007年10月16日	13	6	无
2007年9月18日	13	3	无
2007年8月21日	13	5	有
2007年4月17日	13	4	无
2006年11月28日	13	6	有
2006年9月12日，2006年3月28日	14	5	无
2006年7月25日，2006年2月28日	14	4	无
200*年4月26日	14	4	无
2005年8月23日	14	3	无
2005年3月8日	18	6	无
2005年1月11日	18	9	无

b. 2005年1月11日和2005年3月8日的会议记录显示，分别有3名和5名委员通过电子邮件对研究进行投票表决。伦理委员会之前是不允许用电子邮件对讨论事项进行投票表决的，因为这种方法在这些情况下，并不构成召集会议的条件。

2. IRB未能按照与风险程度相对应的，但不少于每年一次的时间间隔对研究进行跟踪审查［21 CFR 56.109（f）］

a. 伦理委员会2006年6月6日对（b）（4）方案的批准函记录显示该项研究批准时间为一年。然而，直到2008年6月10日IRB会议之前也没有任何跟踪审查的文档记录，在2008年6月10日的伦理委员会会议上，讨论了这份方案并批准研究时间到2009年6月10日。这份方案应该在2007年6月6日或之前进行跟踪审查。

b.（b）（4）及（b）（4）方案是在2007年8月21日的伦理委员会会议上批准的。在随后的伦理委员会会议记录中没有关于书面研究进度报告或批准任何一个研究继续的文档记录。而这些研究都在2008年8月21日或之前接受了跟踪审查。

3. IRB未能准备和保存足够的IRB活动记录［21 CFR 56.115（a）］

a. 2005～2008年的会议记录无足够的细节显示伦理委员会进行的活动以及对活动投票表决的情况，包括投票赞成、反对以及弃权的委员人数。56.115（a）（2）。

b. 2005～2008年伦理委员会委员名册未标识获得的学位、代表性能力、经验证明，如委员会资质证明等足以描述每位委员对伦理委员会审议的主要预期贡献，以及能够表明每位委员与机构之间的雇佣或其他任何的关系。56.115（a）（5）。

c. 伦理委员会未能准备或保存于2006年5月23日召开会议的会议记录。2006年7月25日的会议记录声明“……不会再采取进一步的尝试来获得这些会议记录。”56.115（a）（2）。

d. 未对以下列于伦理委员会方针手册上的常见职能建立书面程序。56.115（a）（6）。

ⅰ. 伦理委员会向机构书面汇报关于研究的初始审查中发现的问题和采取的措施。

ⅱ. 确定哪些项目需要从研究者以外的来源获得证实，自上次伦理委员会审查后没有资料的变更。

ⅲ. 根据21 CFR 812.66的要求，重大/非重大风险策略的决定及文档记录。

4. 未能使研究项目中存在利益冲突的委员停止参加对项目的讨论和投票［21 CFR 56.107（e）］

2006年7月25日、2007年10月16日和2007年12月18日的会议记录了同时身为被提议项目的临床研究者的伦理委员会委员，在讨论该提议项目时仍在房间里，并为自己的项目进行了投票表决。

本警告信的目的并非是罗列伦理委员会操作过程中的所有缺陷。

自收到这封信的15个工作日内，您应当书面告知本办公室，为促使伦理委员会符合FDA法规要求您已采取或计划采取的措施。请包括任何修订文档的副本，例如书面程序、名册以及近期的会议记录。同时，对于计划完成的措施，请把计划完成日期也列入其中。

如果您不能充分地回复此封信并采取适当的纠正措施，可能导致我们根据21 CFR 56.120，56.121的要求，对贵伦理委员会作出进一步的行政措施。这些措施包括根据FDA法规21 CFR 50，56，FDA暂停批准由贵伦理委员会审查的新研究项目，禁止新的受试者入组在研项目，终止所有由贵审查委员会批准的在研项目，以及启动取消贵伦理委员会资格的监管行动。

附：英文原文

Provena St. Joseph's Medical Center IRB

Warning Letter

Mar 12, 2009

CBER-09-06

Se H. Choi, Pharm. D., Chair
Institutional Review Board
Provena St. Joseph Medical Center
333 N. Madison Street
Joliet, Illinois 60435

Dear Dr. Choi:

This letter describes the results of a Food and Drug Administration (FDA) inspection of the Provena St. Joseph Medical Center Institutional Review Board (IRB), which concluded on November 25, 2008. The FDA conducted an inspection of the IRB to determine if the IRB's procedures for the protection of human subjects comply with FDA regulations published in Title 21, Code of Federal Regulations (CFR), Parts 50 and 56. The inspection was conducted as part of FDA's Bioresearch Monitoring Program, which includes inspections designed to review research involving investigational products, and for the protection of human subjects.

At the end of the inspection, the FDA investigator issued and discussed with you the Form FDA 483, Inspectional Observations. From our review of the establishment inspection report, and the exhibits submitted with the report, we have determined that the IRB violated applicable regulations governing the operation and responsibilities of IRBs as published under 21 CFR 50 and 56 (available at http://www.gpoaccess.gov/cfr/index.html). The applicable provisions of the CFR are cited for each violation listed below. We are addressing this letter to you under 21 CFR 56.120(a) as the current IRB Chair with responsibility for ensuring that the IRB takes the actions necessary to bring the IRB into full compliance with FDA regulations. Under 21 CFR 56.120(a) we are also sending copies of this letter to the responsible head of the IRB's parent institution because under 21 CFR 56.120(c), the parent institution is presumed to be responsible for the IRB's operations.

1. Failure to review proposed research at convened meetings at which a majority of the IRB membership are present, including at least one nonscientific member. [21 CFR § 56.108(c)].

a. A review of IRB meeting minutes for 2005 through 2008 revealed that the IRB consistently reviewed and approved new studies and conducted continuing review without a majority of the IRB membership present. Individuals not on the IRB membership rosters, including the IRB Chair, attended meetings and voted. Many meetings also failed to include at least one non-scientific member.

Goal	No of IRB members on roster	No of IRB members present	Non-scientific member present
6/10/08, 4/28/08	6	1	No
12/18/07,11/20/07	13	6	Yes
10/16/07	13	6	No
9/18/07	13	3	No
8/21/07	13	5	Yes
4/17/07	13	4	No
11/28/06	13	6	Yes

(Contd.)

Goal	No of IRB members on roster	No of IRB members present	Non-scientific member present
9/12/06,3/28/06	14	5	No
7/25/06,2/28/06	14	4	No
4/26/0	14	4	No
8/23/05	14	3	No
3/8/05	18	6	No
1/11/05	18	9	No

b. The meeting minutes for 1/11/05 and 3/8/05 document that three and five members, respectively, voted on research studies by email. The use of email ballots to vote on issues before the IRB is not permitted because this method, in these instances, does not constitute convened meeting.

2. Failure to conduct continuing review of research at intervals appropriate to the degree of risk, but not less than once per year. [21 CFR § 56.109(f)].

The IRB approval letter dated June 6, 2006 for Protocol **(b)(4)** documents that this study was approved for one year. However, there is no documentation of continuing review until the June 10, 2008 IRB meeting, at which time the protocol was discussed and given approval until June 10, 2009. This protocol should have been subject to continuing review on or before June 6, 2007.

Protocols **(b)(4)** and **(b)(4)** were approved during the August 21, 2007 IRB meeting. There is no documentation of continuing review of written progress reports or approval for continuation of research for either study in subsequent IRB meeting minutes. Both studies should have received continuing review on or before August 21, 2008.

3. Failure to prepare and maintain adequate documentation of IRB activities. [21 CFR § 56.115(a)].

a.Minutes of meetings for the years 2005 through 2008 have not been prepared in sufficient detail to show actions taken by the IRB, and the vote on actions, including the number of members voting for, against and abstaining. 56.115(a)(2).

b.The IRB membership rosters for 2005 through 2008 do not identify members by earned degrees; representative capacity; indications of experience, such as board certifications, licenses, etc., sufficient to describe each members chief anticipated contributions to IRB deliberations; and any employment or other relationship between each member and the institution. 56.115(a)(5).

c.The IRB failed to either prepare or maintain the meeting minutes for the meeting held on May 23,2006. Minutes for July 25, 2006 state "... Further attempts will not be made to receive the minutes." 56.115(a)(2).

There are no written procedures for the following recurring IRB functions listed in the IRB's Policy Manual. 56.115(a)(6).

i. The reporting of the IRB's findings and actions for the initial review of research to the institution in writing.

ii. Determining which projects require verification from sources other than the investigator that no material changes have occurred since previous IRB review.

iii. Significant/non-significant risk device determination and documentation, as required by 21 CFR 812.66.

4. Failure of IRB members to abstain from participating in discussions and voting on projects for which the member has a conflict of interest. [21 CFR 56.107(e)].

Meeting minutes for 7/25/06, 10/16/07 and 12/18/07 document that IRB members who were also the clinical investigator for proposed studies remained in the room during the discussion of the proposed project, and voted on his/her project.

This letter is not intended to contain an all-inclusive list of deficiencies in the operations of the IRB.

Please notify this office in writing, within fifteen (15) business days of receipt of this letter, of the actions you have taken or plan to take to bring the IRB into compliance with FDA requirements. Please include a copy of any revised documents, such as written procedures, roster, and recent meeting minutes with your response. Also, for any plans of action, please include the projected completion dates for actions to be accomplished.

Your failure to adequately respond to this letter and take appropriate corrective action may result in further administrative actions against your IRB, as authorized by 21 CFR 56.120 and 56.121. These actions could include FDA withholding approval of new studies reviewed by your IRB that are subject to Parts 50 and 56 of the FDA regulations, prohibiting the admission of new subjects to ongoing studies that are subject to 21 CFR Parts 50 and 56, terminating all ongoing studies approved by your IRB, and initiating regulatory proceedings for disqualification of your IRB.

Please send your written documentation to:

Robert L. Wesley
Division of Inspections and Surveillance (HFM-664)
Office of Compliance and Biologics Quality
Center for Biologics Evaluation and Research
1401 Rockville Pike, Suite 200N
Rockville, MD 20852-1448
Telephone: (301) 827-6348

We request that you send a copy of your response to the FDA District Office listed below.

Sincerely,

/S/

Mary A. Malarkey Director
Office of Compliance and Biologics Quality
Center for Biologics Evaluation and Research

Cc: Scott MacIntire, District Director
Food and Drug Administration
550 West Jackson Blvd., Suite 1500
Chicago, Illinois 60661

Jeffrey Brickman
Senior VP & Regional CEO
Provena St. Joseph Medical Center
333 N. Madison Street
Joliet, Illinois 60435

Kristina Borror, Ph.D., Director
Division of Compliance Oversight
Office for Human Research Protections 1
101 Wootton Parkway, Suite 200
Rockville, Maryland 20852

第29封　给Brooklyn Kings County健康科学中心的警告信

2009年2月11日

参考号：09-HFD-45-02-02

尊敬的Friedman博士：

2008年9月22日至10月1日，Alia Legaux女士代表FDA，对SUNY Downstate Medical Center/Health Science Center伦理委员会（IRB）进行了现场检查。本次现场检查的目的是核实IRB受试者保护程序是否符合美国联邦法规第21篇第50、56部分。这些法规适用于FDA所监管产品的临床试验。在现场检查结束时，我们的检查员向您出示并讨论了FDA483表，即现场检查发现的问题。

经对FDA现场检查报告、该报告的附件进行审查，我们认为，伦理委员会没有遵循适用的法律要求和监管受试者保护的FDA法规。我们想强调以下几点：

1. IRB未能准备会议记录，以充分的细节显示IRB采取的行动；对行动的投票情况，包括赞成票数、反对票数和弃权票数［21 CFR 56.115（a）（2）］

我们的现场检查发现，伦理委员会E召开会议并实施了重要的伦理委员会活动，但是没有相关的会议记录，这样的情况有7次。下表中列出了会议的时间和支持我们发现问题记录的总结。

日期	记录
2005年12月22日	签到单显示法定人数，伦理委员会信函日期为2005年12月23日，关于研究（b）（4），陈述“您上面提到的沟通内容在2005年12月22日的HSCB/KCHC伦理委员会会议上进行了审查。”
2006年9月12日	签到单显示法定人数及会议的议程
2007年2月8日	签到单显示法定人数
2007年2月28日	签到单显示法定人数，伦理委员会信函日期为2007年3月1日，关于研究（b）（4），陈述“伦理委员会已经收到您关闭上面列出的研究的申请，并在2007年2月28日的HSCB/KCHC伦理委员会会议上进行了审查。”伦理委员会信函日期为2007年3月7日，关于研究（b）（4），陈述“这是为了对日期为2007年1月17日的不良事件进行确认，与上面列出的研究相关的受试者（b）（6）在2007年2月28日的HSCB/KCHC伦理委员会会议上进行了审查。”
2007年7月5日	签到单显示法定人数，会议的议程，伦理委员会信函日期为2007年7月17日，关于研究（b）（4），陈述“您请求批准上面列出的新研究，在2007年7月5日的HSCB/KCHC伦理委员会会议上进行了审查。”
2007年9月18日	签到单显示法定人数，会议的议程，伦理委员会信函日期为2007年9月19日，关于研究（b）（4），陈述“这是为了对日期为2007年7月30日的不良事件进行确认。与上面列出的研究相关的受试者（b）（6）在2007年9月18日的HSCB/KCHC伦理委员会会议上进行了审查。”伦理委员会信函日期为2007年9月26日、关于研究（b）（4），陈述“您请求批准上面列出的新研究，在2007年9月18日的HSCB/KCHC伦理委员会会议上进行了审查。”伦理委员会信函日期为2007年9月27日、关于研究（b）（4），陈述“您请求对上面列出的研究进行跟踪审查，在2007年9月18日的HSCB/KCHC伦理委员会会议上进行了审查。”伦理委员会信函日期为2007年10月11日、关于研究（b）（4），陈述“您请求批准上面列出的新研究，在2007年9月18日的HSCB/KCHC伦理委员会会议上进行了审查。”
2007年11月8日	签到单显示法定人数，伦理委员会信函日期为2007年11月8日，关于研究（b）（4），陈述“您请求重新启动上面列出的研究，在2007年11月8日的HSCB/KCHC伦理委员会会议上进行了审查（委员会E）。”

2. 除了快速审查，IRB未能在大多数IRB委员出席，其中至少包括一位来自非科学领域的委员的召集会议上对拟开展的研究进行审查［21 CFR 56.108（c）］

我们现场检查发现1个实例，伦理委员会在法定人数不足的会议上审查并批准了研究。2007年2月14日伦理委员会A会议记录声明“这次会议上委员会未达到法定人数，因此会议休会”。尽管有这个声明，但是有足够的证据证明伦理委员会的决定就发生在这个会上，表现在下列伦理委员会信函中：2007年3月2日关于研究（b）（4）和研究（b）（4）的信函显示，“您的回复在2007年2月14日的HSCB/KCHC伦理委员会会议上进行了审查”；2007年3月6日关于研究（b）（4）的信函显示，“您请求对上面列出的研究进行跟踪审查，在2007年2月14日的HSCB/KCHC伦理委员会会议上进行了审查”；最后，2007年3月6日和3月8日关于研究（b）（4）的信函显示，“您请求批准上面列出的新研究，在2007年2月14日的HSCB/KCHC伦理委员会会议上进行了审查。”

3. IRB未能遵守关于对研究进行跟踪审查、向研究者和机构报告发现的问题和采取的行动的书面程序［21 CFR 56.108（a）（1）］

我们现场检查发现有几例情况，伦理委员会未能按照自己的书面程序对正在开展的研究进行跟踪审查。

对于方案（b）（4），伦理委员会文件中没有相关记录显示有更新提醒的通知提供给研究者，提醒他们即将到来的跟踪审查日期，而这是书面程序中要求的。伦理委员会书面程序中题为“年度进展报告和跟踪审查”部分写明“更新提醒的通知将由伦理委员会办公室在批准期满前两个月寄给研究者”。

本警告信的目的并非是罗列伦理委员会在审查和批准试验方案中存在的所有缺陷。确保SUNY Down State Medical Center/Health Service Center伦理委员会的实际操作和程序完全符合所有适用法律和法规的要求是您的职责。由于上述讨论的违背FDA法规的行为，伦理委员会或者其上级机构应当自收到这封信的15个工作日内，书面告知本办公室为预防将来发生类似违规情况已经或计划采取的措施。如果不能对上述违规行为进行充分、迅速地解释，可能导致我们在不再通知的情况下采取监管措施。

附：英文原文

Health Science Center Brooklyn Kings County

WARNING LETTER

Feb 11, 2009

CERTIFIED MAIL
RETURN RECEIPT REQUESTED

Ref: 09-HFD-45-02-02

Eli Friedman, M.D.
Chairman, SUNY Downstate Medical Center IRB
Health Science Center
450 Clarkson Ave.
Brooklyn, NY 11203-2056

Dear Dr. Friedman:

Between September 22 and October 1, 2008, Ms. Alia Legaux, representing the Food and Drug Administration (FDA), inspected the Institutional Review Board (IRB) at the SUNY Downstate Medical Center/Health Science Center. The purpose of this inspection was to determine whether the IRB procedures for the protection of human subjects complied with Title 21 of the Code of Federal Regulations (CFR), Parts 50 and 56. These regulations apply to clinical studies of products regulated by FDA. We are aware that at the conclusion of the inspection our investigator presented and discussed with you, a Form FDA 483, Inspectional Observations.

From our review of the establishment inspection report and the documents submitted with that report, we conclude that the IRB did not adhere to the applicable statutory requirements and FDA regulations governing the protection of human subjects. We wish to emphasize the following:

1. The IRB failed to prepare the minutes of IRB meetings in sufficient detail to show actions taken by the IRB, the vote on actions, including the number of members voting for, against and abstaining [21 CFR 56.115(a)(2)].

Our inspection revealed seven instances in which IRB E met and conducted significant IRB activity; however, no meeting minutes could be found. The following table lists the dates of the meetings and a brief summary of the documentation to support our finding.

Date	Documentation
12/22/05	Sign-in sheet demonstrating quorum and IRB letter dated 12/23/05 for study (b)(4), which states "Your communication referenced above was reviewed at the 12/22/2005 meeting of the HSCB/KCHC Institutional Review Board."
9/12/06	Sign-in sheet demonstrating quorum and agenda for the meeting.
2/8/07	Sign-in sheet demonstrating quorum.
2/28/07	Sign-in sheet demonstrating quorum. The IRB letter dated 3/1/07 for study (b)(4) which states "The Board has received your application to close the study listed above. It was reviewed at the 2/28/2007 meeting of the HSCB/KCHC Institutional Review Board." The IRB letter dated 3/7/07 for study (b)(4) which states "This is to confirm that the adverse event dated 1/17/07, Subject (b)(6) related to the study listed above was reviewed at the 2/28/2007 meeting of the HSCB/KCHC Institutional Review Board."
7/5/07	Sign-in sheet demonstrating quorum, agenda for the meeting and IRB letter dated 7/17/07 for study (b)(4) which states "Your request for approval of the new study listed above was reviewed at the 7/5/2007 meeting of the HSCB/KCHC Institutional Review Board."
9/18/07	Sign-in sheet demonstrating quorum. Agenda for the meeting. IRB letter dated 9/19/07 for study (b)(4) which states "This is to confirm that the above adverse event(s) dated July 30, 2007 Subject (b)(6) related to study listed above was reviewed at the 9/18/2007 meeting of the HSCB/KCHC Institutional Review Board." IRB letter dated 9/26/07 for study (b)(4) which states "Your request for approval of the new study listed above was reviewed at the 9/18/2007 meeting of the HSCB/KCHC Institutional Review Board." IRB letter dated 9/27/07 for study (b)(4) which states "Your request for continuing review of the study listed above was reviewed at the 9/18/2007 meeting of the HSCB/KCHC Institutional Review Board." IRB letter dated 10/11/07 for study (b)(4) which states "Your request for approval of the new study listed above was reviewed at the 9/18/2007 meeting of the HSCB/KCHC Institutional Review Board." IRB letter dated 10/11/07 for study (b)(4) which states "Your request for approval of the new study listed above was reviewed at the 9/18/2007 meeting of the HSCB/KCHC Institutional Review Board."
11/8/07	Sign-in sheet demonstrating quorum and IRB letters dated 11/8/07 for study (b)(4) which states "Your request to reopen the study listed above was reviewed at the 11/8/2007 meeting of the HSCB/KCHC Institutional Review Board (Committee E)."

2. For other than expedited reviews, the IRB failed to review proposed research at convened meetings at which a majority of the members of the IRB are present, including at least one member whose primary concerns are in non-scientific areas [21 CFR 56.108(c)].

Our inspection revealed an instance in which the IRB reviewed and approved research at meetings in which a quorum was not present. The meeting minutes for the February 14, 2007 meeting of IRB A state the "committee did not achieve quorum at this meeting so the meeting was adjourned". Despite this statement, there is strong evidence that IRB action occurred on this date as evidenced by the following IRB letters: the March 2, 2007 letters for study (b)(4) and study (b)(4) which states "Your response was reviewed at the 2/14/2007 meeting of the HSCB/KCHC Institutional Review Board."; the March 6, 2007 letter for study (b)(4) which states "Your request for continuing review of the study listed above was reviewed at the 2/14/2007 meeting of the HSCB/KCHC Institutional Review Board.", and finally, the March 6, 2007 letter for study (b)(4) and the March 8, 2007 letter for study (b)(4) which state "Your request for approval of the new study listed above was reviewed at the 2/14/2007 meeting of the HSCB/KCHC Institutional Review Board."

3. The IRB failed to follow its written procedures for conducting its continuing review of research and for reporting its findings and actions to the investigator and the institution [21 CFR 56.108(a)(1)].

Our inspections revealed several instances in which the IRB failed to follow its written procedures for conducting continuing review of ongoing research.

For Protocols (b)(4) there is no documentation in the IRB files that the investigators were ever provided renewal reminder notices alerting them to upcoming continuing review dates as required in the IRB written procedures under the section entitled "Annual Progress Reports and Continuing Review Requirements" which states "Renewal reminder notices will be mailed to investigators by the IRB Office two months prior to expiration of approval".

This letter is not intended to be an all-inclusive list of deficiencies for the protocols reviewed and approved by the IRB. It is your responsibility to ensure that SUNY Down State Medical Center/Health Service Center IRB's practices and procedures fully comply with all applicable statutes and regulations. Because of the departures from FDA regulations discussed above, either the IRB or its parent institution should inform this office, in writing, within fifteen (15) working days of your receipt of this letter, of the actions you have taken or plan to take to prevent similar violations in the future. Failure to adequately and promptly explain the violations noted above may result in regulatory action without further notice.

If you have any questions, please contact Constance Lewin, M.D., M.P.H., at 301-796-3397; FAX 301-847-8748. Your written response and any pertinent documentation should be addressed to:

Constance Lewin, M.D., M.P.H.
Branch Chief, Good Clinical Practice Branch I
Division of Scientific Investigations
Office of Compliance
Center for Drug Evaluation and Research
Food and Drug Administration
Bldg 51, Room 5354
10903 New Hampshire Avenue
Silver Spring, MD 20993

Sincerely yours,

{See appended electronic signature page}

Leslie K. Ball, M.D.
Director
Division of Scientific Investigations
Office of Compliance
Center for Drug Evaluation and Research

第 30 封　给华盛顿医院伦理委员会的警告信

2009年2月5日

参考号：CBER-09-03

尊敬的Weinstein先生：

这封信特告知您2008年10月7日结束的，FDA对华盛顿医院伦理委员会现场检查的结果。FDA检查员检查了贵伦理委员会，以核实其保护受试者的程序是否符合发布在美国联邦法规第21篇50和56部分的FDA法规。FDA实施的这次检查属于生物研究监查项目，该项目通过设定的检查方法来审查伦理委员会的各项操作。

在现场检查结束时，FDA检查员向您出示并讨论了FDA483表，即现场检查发现的问题。经对现场检查报告、该报告提交的附件以及FDA483表的审查，我们认为，贵伦理委员会严重违反了发布在21 CFR 50，56（参见http://www.gpoaccess.gov/cfr/index.html）的、对IRB的运行和职责进行监管的适用法律法规。以下列出的每一项违规都引用了适用的CFR条款。我们根据21 CFR 56.120（a）给您写信，作为现任伦理委员会主席，您有责任确保伦理委员会采取必要措施使伦理委员会完全符合FDA法规。根据21 CFR 56.120（a），我们也会将这封信的复印件寄给伦理委员会上级机构的负责方——华盛顿医院，因为根据21 CFR 56.120（a），上级机构应对伦理委员会的运行负责。

1. IRB未能在大多数IRB委员出席的召集会议上对拟开展的研究进行审查［21 CFR 56.108（c）］

A. 邮寄选票的方式用于以下所有的批准，包括对一项研究的最终批准。这项研究符合21 CFR 50.24紧急研究中知情同意的免除情况，除了对确定的几种涉及不超过最小风险的研究，或对研究中的微小变更可以进行快速审查；必须在大多数伦理委员会委员都出席，其中至少包括一位来自非科学领域的委员的召集会议上对拟开展的研究进行审查。IRB采用邮寄选票对议题进行投票的作法是不能接受的，因为这种方法并不等同于召集会议。

研究	伦理委员会邮件投票批准日期
（b）（4）	2005年4月27日批准额外增加一年（从2005年4月5日到2006年5月3日）
（b）（4）	2005年11月4日批准额外增加一年到2005年12月2日
（b）（4）	2005年11月4日批准额外增加一年到2005年12月2日
（b）（4）	2004年11月30日初始批准
（b）（4）	2005年1月19日批准延长
（b）（4）	2006年10月9日批准到2007年10月8日

B. 根据2006年3月13日和2000年8月9日召集的会议记录，伦理委员会在没有大多数委员出席的情况下，批准了新方案的研究和审查了知情同意书。最新版本为2004年3月8日的现行伦理委员会名册罗列了9人，但是只有4名投票委员出席2006年3月13日会议。没有保留伦理委员会之前的名册，但是2000年8月9日会议记录包括了之后每一次伦理委员会行动，从4个人的记录中看到“批准代理人已收到”。既然在2000年8月9日会议上出现了另外4个人，那么在2000年至少有8人在名册上，因此没有大多数人没有出席此次会议。

2. IRB未能制定、维护和遵守足够的书面程序用以确保受试者权益和福利得到保护［21 CFR 56.102（g），56.108（a）（b），56.109（b），（c），（d）和56.115］

A. 根据伦理委员会书面程序第Ⅵ章——会议的要求，包括一个文件名为“伦理委员会——法律和哲学”，一般会议每年召开或者有需要时由主席召集，但是频率不低于每年。然而，伦理委员会会议记录显示，委员会有时候没有按照这个频率在召集会议上审查研究。正如下表显示，2002 ~ 2008年召开的召集会议没有符合这个要求。

年份	召集会议时间
2002	2002年3月28日，2002年7月2日，2002年11月14日
2003	没有召集会议
2004	没有召集会议
2005	2005年12月16日
2006	2006年3月13日，2006年5月9日，2006年6月23日
2007	2007年3月13日
2008	2008年6月3日

B. 根据书面程序中第Ⅵ章——会议，伦理委员会会根据风险程度定期审查每个研究，但是周期不会超过一年。如下所列，跟踪审查没有在一年内或更短时间内执行。而且，伦理委员会允许批准期限超过一年。伦理委员会经常在效期前几个月或者效期后审查进行中的研究，从之前的效期研究得到额外一年的批准，而不是实际的审查时间。这会导致从委员会审查以后有效期超过12个月和/或者批准作废。这种情况至少在13个研究中的9个发生，在华盛顿医院伦理委员会2008年9月17日的更新报告中有描述。一个医疗器械研究案例见下表。

年	行动	批准期限
2001年5月4日	第一次批准	没有指定
2002年3月28日	批准额外一年	2002年5月4日至2003年5月3日
2003年4月21日	批准额外一年	2003年5月4日至2004年5月3日
2004年6月9日	批准额外一年	2004年5月4日至2005年5月3日
2005年4月27日	批准额外一年	2005年5月4日至2006年5月3日
2006年5月9日	批准额外一年	2006年5月4日至2007年5月3日
2007年3月9日	批准额外一年	2007年5月4日至2008年5月3日
2008年6月30日	批准额外一年	2008年5月4日至2009年5月3日

C. 华盛顿医院伦理委员会的书面程序因为某些原因内容不充分，包括但不仅限于以下：

ⅰ. 以下活动没有书面程序规定：

- 对急救情况下免除知情同意要求的研究进行审查，以确保IRB已发现并记录符合特殊的标准，并确保给受试者的权益和福利提供额外的保护。
- 伦理委员会如何对研究进行跟踪审查。
- 伦理委员会如何决定哪些项目审查频率大于每年一次。
- 伦理委员会如何保证在已批准的期限内，已批准的研究的变更未经伦理委员会审查和批准（除非立即去除对受试者的危害）不会开始进行。
- 伦理委员会如何保证发生任何严重或持续不合规时，及时向适当的机构官员和FDA进行报告。
- 研究审查涉及弱势群体，如孕妇、罪犯、未成年人。

ⅱ. 下列书面程序没有符合21 CFR 56要求：

- 第Ⅴ章——法定人数中定义法定人数为委员会中大多数人或者4（4），取其少数的。21 CFR 56.108（b）要求召集会议上大多数委员出席。
- 第Ⅷ章——快速审查明确所有提交伦理委员会的研究应由全体委员会审查，除非某些研究不超过最少风险，对已批准研究的微小变更，已批准研究的更新。21 CFR 56.110不允许对已批准研究更新采用快速审查，但是在一年或者更短的已授权批准的时间内，快速审查可以用于已批准研究的微小变更。
- 第Ⅹ章——记录，C项规定根据研究完成后保存期限为2年。然而，21 CFR 56.115（b）要求记录应该在研究完成后至少保存3年。
- 伦理委员会程序引用1977年11月11日周五的联邦公报，第Ⅲ部分可作为至少三个程序的参考。这个参考并不合适，因为这是适用于FDA对眼内镜片试验器械豁免要求的最终规定，21 CFR Part 813已经取消了。

ⅲ. 审查知情同意记录的委员会文件并不完全符合21 CFR Part 50要求。比如，程序没有说明知情同意记录必须包括此临床试验涉及研究的声明、对研究目的的解释、受试者参与的预期持续时间并说明哪些程序是试验性的。

3. IRB未能准备和保存足够的IRB活动记录［21 CFR 56.115（a）（2）和50.24］

A. 伦理委员会会议记录没有提供充分的细节表明为采取行动而投票同意、反对和弃权的人数。

B. 2006年5月9日会议记录显示伦理委员会批准（b）（4）研究推进社区咨询，与社区团体公开披露。伦理委员会没有记录充分的细节，以表明伦理委员会根据21 CFR 50.24要求作出特殊决定。社区咨询和公开披露后，伦理委员会在2006年10月9日对（b）（4）项目作出最后决定，但是以邮寄选票方式投票而没有会议记录，就如1.A.所述。

4. 没有达到快速审查的要求［21 CFR 56.1 10（b）（1）］

伦理委员会可能使用快速审查程序审查特定的研究，如果这个研究对受试者不超过最小风险和/或在授权批准阶段内之前对批准的研究微小变更。伦理委员会主席不恰当地对研究的跟踪审查使用了快速审查程序。虽然在2002年11月14日至2005年12月16日没有召集会议，下表显示在此阶段研究按照快速审查程序批准的研究。

研究	日期	行动
（b）（4）	2001年5月4日	伦理委员会批准
（b）（4）	2003年4月21日	批准额外一年
（b）（4）	2004年6月9日	批准额外一年
（b）（4）	2005年4月27日	批准额外一年
（b）（4）	2002年7月2日	伦理委员会批准
（b）（4）	2003年10月14日	批准延长一年
（b）（4）	2004年6月29日	批准额外一年
（b）（4）	2005年1月19日	伦理委员会批准持续进入
（b）（4）	2002年11月14日	伦理委员会批准
（b）（4）	2003年11月26日	持续批准直到研究计划结束（7/1/2005）
（b）（4）	2003年7月8日	伦理委员会批准
（b）（4）	2004年11月1日	批准延长到10/31/2005
（b）（4）	2005年10月26日	批准延长到10/31/2006

5. 对涉及紧急研究中免除知情同意，IRB未能满足对研究审查的要求［21 CFR 56.109（c）和50.24］

根据21 CFR 56.109，伦理委员会必须审查、有权批准、要求修改或拒绝提出的临床研究。根据21 CFR

50.24执行的应急研究，伦理委员会必须评估材料，以决定研究是否满足21 CFR 50.24（a）的标准，发现并记录是否适合进行。具体而言，伦理委员会要审查社区咨询和公众披露计划。必须发现和记录这些应该在研究批准前提供。华盛顿医院伦理委员会2006年10月9日批准（b）（4）研究，没有记录研究满足21 CFR 50.24的标准。此外，尽管临床研究者声称执行了社区咨询和公众披露活动，但是没有记录表明伦理委员会根据21 CFR 50.24要求评估了材料，并且确定了在研究开始之前提供额外的保护。

本警告信并未包含伦理委员会在运行中存在的所有缺陷。

自收到这封信的15个工作日内，您应当书面告知本办公室您为促使伦理委员会符合FDA法规的要求，已经采取或计划采取的措施。回复中请附上已修订文件的复印件，如书面程序和近期会议记录。任何行动计划，请包括每项行动计划预计完成的时间。

如果不能充分地回复本信并采取合适的纠正措施，可能导致我们依照21 CFR 56.120和56.121的授权对伦理委员会采取监管措施。监管措施包括根据21 CFR 50, 56的规定，不予批准伦理委员会审查的新研究项目；根据21 CFR 50, 56的规定，禁止在研项目新受试者入组；终止伦理委员会批准的所有在研项目；启动取消伦理委员会资格的监管程序。

附：英文原文

Washington Hospital IRC

WARNING LETTER

FEB 5, 2009

By Certified Mail - Return Receipt Requested
And Facsimile Transmission

CBER - 09 - 03

Gary B. Weinstein
Executive Vice President and IRC Chair
The Washington Hospital IRC
155 Wilson Avenue
Washington, Pennsylvania 15301-3336

Dear Mr. Weinstein:

This letter describes the results of a Food and Drug Administration (FDA) inspection of The Washington Hospital Institutional Review Committee (IRC) that concluded on October 7, 2008. The FDA investigator conducted an inspection of the IRC to determine whether the IRC's procedures for the protection of human subjects comply with FDA regulations published in Title 21, Code of Federal Regulations (CFR), Parts 50 and 56. FDA conducted this inspection under its Bioresearch Monitoring Program, which includes inspections designed to review IRC operations.

At the end of the inspection, the FDA investigator issued and discussed with you the Form FDA 483, Inspectional Observations. From our review of the establishment inspection report, the exhibits submitted with the report, and the Form FDA 483, we have determined that the IRC significantly violated applicable federal regulations governing the operation and responsibilities of Institutional Review Boards (IRBs) as published under 21 CFR Parts 50 and 56 (available at http://www.gpoaccess.gov/cfr/index.html[1]). The applicable provisions of the CFR are cited for each violation listed below. We are addressing this letter to you under 21 CFR 56.120(a) as the current IRC Chairperson with responsibility for ensuring that the IRC takes the actions necessary to bring the IRC into full compliance with FDA regulations. Under 21 CFR 56.120(a) we are also sending copies of this letter to the responsible head of the IRC's parent institution, The Washington Hospital, because under 21 CFR 56.120(c), the parent institution is presumed to be responsible for the IRC's operations.

1. Failure to review proposed research at convened meetings at which a majority of the members of the IRB are present. [21 CFR § 56.108(c)].

A. Mail ballot voting was used for all of the following approvals including the final approval to a study involving an exception from informed consent requirements for emergency research under 21 CFR 50.24. Except for expedited review of certain kinds of research involving no more than minimal risk, or minor changes in research; review of proposed research must be conducted at a convened meeting at which a majority of the membership of the IRB is present, including one member whose primary concerns are non-scientific. The use of a mail ballot to vote on issues before the IRB is not permitted because this method does not constitute a convened meeting.

Study	Date of IRC Approved by Mail Ballot
(b)(4)	4/27/05 - approved for an additional year (5/4/05 through 5/3/06)
(b)(4)	11/04 - approved for an additional year through 12-2-05
(b)(4)	11/04 - approved for an additional year through 12-2-05
(b)(4)	11/30/04 - initial approval
(b)(4)	1/19/05 - approved extension
(b)(4)	10/9/06 - approved through 10/8/07

B. According to the minutes of meetings convened 3/13/06 and 8/9/00, the IRC approved research on new protocols and reviewed consent forms without the majority of IRC members in attendance. The current IRC roster, last revised 3/8/04, lists nine members, but only four voting members were in attendance at the 3/13/06 meeting. Previous IRC rosters were not retained, but the 8/9/00 meeting minutes include after each IRC action, "proxies for approval were received" from four individuals. Since four other members were present at the 8/9/00 meeting, it can be concluded that there were at least eight members on the roster in 2000 and therefore a majority was not present at this meeting.

2. Failure to prepare, maintain, and follow adequate written procedures designed to assure the protection of the rights and welfare of human subjects. [21 CFR §§ 56.102(g), 56.108(a) and (b), 56.109(b), (c), and (d), and 56.115].

A. According to *ARTICLE VI - MEETINGS* in the IRC's written procedures, contained in a document titled "INSTITUTIONAL REVIEW COMMITTEE BY-LAWS AND PHILOSOPHY," normal meetings will be held annually or as may be required at the call of the Chair, but not less frequently than annually. However, the IRC meeting minutes illustrate that this committee reviews research at convened meetings on a sometimes infrequent basis. As shown in the table below, convened meetings held from 2002 to 2008 did not always meet this requirement.

Year	Date(s) of convened meetings
2002	3/28/02, 7/2/02, 11/14/02
2003	No convened meetings
2004	No convened meetings
2005	12/16/05
2006	3/13/06, 5/9/06, 6/23/06
2007	3/13/07
2008	6/3/08

B. According to *ARTICLE VI - MEETINGS* in the written procedures, the IRB will review each study periodically at intervals appropriate to the degree of risk but not to exceed one year. As shown below, continuing reviews were not always conducted within one year or less. Furthermore, the IRB granted approval periods that exceeded one year. The IRC often reviewed ongoing research several months before the expiration date or after the expiration date, yet the study was given an additional year approval from the previous expiration date, rather than the date it was actually reviewed. This resulted in an expiration date of greater than twelve months from the date of the IRC review and/or a lapse in approval. This practice occurred in at least 9 of 13 studies described in *The Washington Hospital IRC Committee Update* report dated 9/17/08. One medical device study example is shown in the following table.

Year	Action	Approval period
5/4/01	Initial approval	Undesignated
3/28/02	Approved for an additional year	5/4/02 - 5/3/03
4/21/03	Approved for an additional year	5/4/03 - 5/3/04
6/9/04	Approved for an additional year	5/4/04 - 5/3/05
4/27/05	Approved for an additional year	5/4/05 - 5/3/06
5/9/06	Approved for an additional year	5/4/06 - 5/3/07
3/9/07	Approved for an additional year	5/4/07 - 5/3/08
6/30/08	Approved for an additional year	5/4/08 - 5/3/09

C. The Washington Hospital IRC's written procedures are not adequate for a number of reasons, including but not limited to the following:

ⅰ. There are no written procedures for the following activities:

- Review of research involving an exception from informed consent requirements for emergency research to ensure that the IRB has found and documented that specific criteria have been met and to ensure that additional protections of the rights and welfare of the subjects will be provided.
- How the IRC conducts its continuing review of research.
- How the IRC determines which projects require review more often than annually.
- How the IRC ensures that changes in approved research, during the periods for which IRC approval had already been given, are not initiated without IRC review and approval (except where necessary to eliminate apparent immediate hazards to subjects).
- How the IRC ensures prompt reporting to appropriate institutional officials and FDA of any instance of serious or continuing noncompliance.
- Review of research involving vulnerable populations such as pregnant women, prisoners, and minors

ⅱ. The following written procedures do not comply with the requirements of 21 CFR Part 56:

Article Ⅴ- Quorum defines quorum as a majority of the committee members or four (4), whichever is less. 21 CFR 56.108(b) requires that a majority of members be present at convened meetings.

Article Ⅷ - Expedited Review states all studies submitted to the IRC shall be reviewed by the full committee, except for certain studies involving no more than minimal risk, for minor changes in research previously approved by the IRC, and for renewals of studies previously approved by the IRC. 21 CFR 56.110 does not allow for the expedited renewal of previously approved studies, but may be used for minor changes in previously approved research during the period of 1 year or less for which approval is authorized.

- *Article X- Records, Item C* defines a retention period of two years following the date of study completion. However, 21 CFR 56.115(b) requires that records be retained for at least 3 years after completion of the research.
- The IRC procedures cite the Federal Register dated Friday, November 11th, 1977, Part Ⅲ as a reference for at least three of its procedures. This is an inappropriate reference because this is a Food and Drug Administration Final rule for the Investigational Device Exemption Requirements for Intraocular Lenses, 21 CFR Part 813, which has since been rescinded.

ⅲ. The IRC's written procedures for review of informed consent documents do not refer to all provisions required by 21 CFR Part 50. For example, the procedures do not explain that informed consent documents must include a statement that the study involves research, an explanation of the purposes of the research and the expected duration of the subject's participation, and identification of any procedures which are experimental.

3. Failure to prepare and maintain adequate documentation of IRB activities. [21 CFR § 56.115(a)(2) and 50.24].

A. The IRC meeting minutes have not been prepared in sufficient detail to show the number of members voting for, against, and abstaining for the actions taken.

B. The 5/9/06 meeting minutes indicate the IRC approved the (b)(4) study to proceed with community consultation and public disclosure with community groups. The IRC records fail to document in sufficient detail whether the IRC made specific determinations as required by 21 CFR 50.24. Also, the IRC gave the final approval on 10/9/06 for the (b)(4) project after community consultation and public disclosure, but did so by mail ballot so there are no meeting minutes, as referenced in item 1A, above.

4. Failure to fulfill requirements for expedited review. [21 CFR § 56.1 10(b)(1)].

An IRB may review certain research using an expedited review procedure if the research involves no more than minimal risk to subjects and/or there were minor changes in previously approved research during the period for which approval is authorized. The IRC Chair inappropriately used the expedited review process for continuing review of research. Although there were no convened meetings between 11/14/02 and 12/16/05, the following table shows research approved under the expedited review procedure during this period.

Study	Date	Action
(b)(4)	5/4/01	Approved by IRC
(b)(4)	4/21/03	Approved for anadditional year
(b)(4)	6/9/04	Approved for anadditional year
(b)(4)	4/27/05	Approved for anadditional year
(b)(4)	7/2/02	Approved by IRC
(b)(4)	10/14/03	Approved a one year extension
(b)(4)	6/29/04	Approved for an additional year
(b)(4)	1/19/05	Continued access approved by IRC
(b)(4)	11/14/02	Approved by IRC
(b)(4)	11/26/03	Approval will continue until the anticipated end of the study (7/1/05)
(b)(4)	7/8/03	Approved by IRC
(b)(4)	11/1/04	Extension approved through 10/31/05
(b)(4)	10/26/05	Extension approved through 10/31/06

5. Failure to meet the requirements for review of research involving an exception from informed consent for emergency research. [21 CFR § 56.109(c) and 50.24].

Under 21 CFR 56.109, an IRB must review, and has authority to approve, require modifications in, or disapprove a proposed clinical investigation. For emergency research being conducted under 21 CFR 50.24, the IRB must also evaluate materials to determine whether the investigation satisfies the criteria in 21 CFR 50.24(a) and find and document whether it is appropriate to proceed under this section. Specifically, IRBs are expected to review plans for community consultation and public disclosure and must find and document that both of these will be provided prior to the start of the study. The Washington Hospital IRC approved (b)(4) the study on 10/9/06 and failed to document that the study met the criteria set out in 21 CFR 50.24. Additionally, although the clinical investigator states that he conducted the community consultation and public disclosure activities, there is no documentation that the IRC evaluated these materials and determined that these additional protections would be provided prior to start of the study as required by 21 CFR 50.24.

This letter is not intended to contain an all-inclusive list of deficiencies in the operations of the IRB.

Please notify this office in writing, within fifteen (15) business days of receipt of this letter, of the actions you have taken or plan to take to bring the IRB into compliance with FDA requirements. Please include a copy of any revised documents, such as written procedures and recent meeting minutes with your response. Also, for any plans of action, please include the projected completion dates for each action to be accomplished .

Your failure to adequately respond to this letter and take appropriate corrective action may result in further administrative actions against your IRB, as authorized by 21 CFR 56.120 and 56.121. These actions could include FDA withholding approval of new studies reviewed by your IRB that are subject to Parts 50 and 56 of the FDA regulations, prohibiting the admission of new subjects to ongoing studies that are subject to 21 CFR Parts 50 and 56, terminating all ongoing studies approved by your IRB, and initiating regulatory proceedings for disqualification of your IRB.

Please send your written response to:

Janet White
Division of Inspections and Surveillance (HFM-664)
Office of Compliance and Biologics Quality
Center for Biologics Evaluation and Research
1401 Rockville Pike, Suite 200N
Rockville, MD 20852-1488
Telephone: (301) 827-6336

We request that you send a copy of your response to the FDA District Office listed below.

Sincerely,

/S/

Mary A. Malarkey Director
Office of Compliance and Biologics Quality
Center for Biologics Evaluation and Research

Cc: Thomas D. Gardine, District Director
Food and Drug Administration
900 US Customhouse
200 Chestnut Street
Philadelphia, PA 19106

Kristina Borror, Ph.D., Director
Division of Compliance Oversight
Office for Human Research Protections
1101 Wooton Parkway, Suite 200
Rockville, Maryland 20852

Telford W. Thomas, President/CEO
The Washington Hospital
155 Wilson Avenue
Washington, Pennsylvania 15301-3336

第31封　给de San Juan市立医院的警告信

2008年8月15日

参考号：08-HFD-45-0801

尊敬的Medina博士：

2007年11月15日至21日，Lt. Luis O. Rodriguez代表FDA，对de San Juan市立医院伦理委员会（IRB）进行了现场检查。本次现场检查的目的是核实IRB受试者保护的程序是否符合美国联邦法规第21篇50、56部分的要求。这些法规适用于FDA所监管的药物临床研究。我们知道在现场检查结束时，我们的检查员向您出示并讨论了FDA483表，即现场检查发现的问题。

经对FDA现场检查报告（EIR）、该报告的附件以及您2007年12月3日书面回复进行审查，我们认为，IRB没有遵循适用的法律要求和监管受试者保护的FDA法规。我们想强调以下几点：

1. IRB没有准备和保存足够的IRB活动记录，IRB会议记录没有做到用充分的细节显示IRB采取的措施［21 CFR 56.115（a）（2）］

a. 对某试验方案"Ⅰ/Ⅱ期，开放某药物药代动力学和安全性研究"，IRB于2006年8月19日给临床研究者发了一封信，声明IRB重新批准了该试验方案。2006年8月10日的IRB会议的会议记录或其他任何文档中都没有提到该试验方案。因此，由于IRB会议记录及其他文件中都缺乏详细的信息，我们无法确定该研究方案是否按照FDA法规的要求在召集会议上得到重新批准［21 CFR 56.108（c）］。

b. 所有的批准决定都必须在召集会议上或通过快速审查程序作出［详见21 CFR 56.108（c）］。召集会议上的批准决定必须写在IRB会议记录中［21 CFR 56. 115（a）（2）］。

我们现场检查发现，有9处批准日期与IRB会议日期一致，但是IRB的行动没有记录在会议记录中，如下表所示：

试验方案	文件	批准日期	IRB会议日期	批准记录在会议记录中
	西班牙语/英语同意书修正案	2/9/2006	2/9/2006	否
	针对样本储存的西班牙语/英语同意书	2/8/2007	2/8/2007	否
	同意豁免	2/9/2006	2/9/2006	否
	针对样本储存的西班牙语/英语同意书	2/9/2006	2/9/2006	否
	英语/西班牙语信息表	2/9/2006	2/9/2006	否
	#4修正案	8/10/2006	8/10/2006	否
	跟踪审查	2/8/2007	2/8/2007	否
	进展报告	2/8/2007	2/8/2007	否
	同意书中主要研究者变动	9/13/2007	9/13/2007	否

此外，我们现场发现有3处批准日期与IRB会议日期不一致，且没有文件来解释使用了哪种类型的审查程序。San Juan的IRB快速审查程序显示：通过在随后的会议上讨论这些批准，通知所有委员快速审查的批准。因此，任何快速审查批准都应该记录在随后的IRB会议的会议记录中。［详见21 CFR 56. 110（c）和San Juan的IRB书面程序］。

试验方案	文件	批准日期	IRB会议日期	批准记录在会议记录中
	受试者指导	10/3/2005	10/13/2005	否
	跟踪审查	8/19/2006	8/10/2006	否
	跟踪审查	2/16/2007	2/8/2007	否

2. 除了快速审查，IRB并不总是在大多数IRB委员出席，其中至少包括一位来自非科学领域的委员的召集会议上对拟开展的研究进行审查［21 CFR 56. 108（c）］

我们现场检查发现，2006年4月20日会议上IRB审查并批准了一项研究，该会议上没有至少一名来自非科学领域的委员出席。查看2006年4月20日的会议签到表，下列委员出席了会议：Luis A. Medina博士（儿科医生）、[ ] 流行病学家、[ ] 药师、[ ] 注册护士、[ ] 社区代表和 [ ] 法律顾问都缺席了本次会议。

3. IRB未能遵守关于研究审查的FDA法规，这些法规要求IRB应该以书面形式通知研究者和机构批准或不予批准被提议研究的决定，或为保证IRB批准研究而要求进行的修改意见［21 CFR 56. 109（e）］

a. 对于某方案，IRB文件中没有研究者被告知2005年10月3日患者信息表被批准的记录。此外，2006年1月30日，临床研究场所向IRB提交了3份文件，与国家儿童保健和人类发育研究所（NICHD）资助的存储库的样本储存有关：①信息表（西班牙语和英语）；②给父母的存储库同意书（西班牙语和英语）；③给未成年人的存储库同意书（西班牙语和英语）。没有相关的记录显示研究者被告知同意书得到批准。

b. 对于某方案"某药物的药代动力学研究"，IRB文件中没有记录显示研究者被告知：2006年4月20日批准了用于由国家儿童保健和人类发育研究所（NICHD）资助的样本储存的同意书，以及父母情况说明表（英语和西班牙语）。

4. 在批准部分或所有的受试者是儿童的研究时，IRB未能确定所有的研究应符合21 CFR 50（D），临床试验中对儿童的额外保护措施［21 CFR 56. 111（c）］

IRB未能确定研究应遵循21 CFR 50（D），比如 [ ] 研究方案及其他研究方案。D节要求IRB确定临床研究符合这些类别研究之一的要求：[50.51（最低风险）；50.52（风险超过最低风险，但是有希望给受试者带来直接收益）；50.53（超过最低风险的风险而且没有直接收益）]。San Juan的IRB按照与研究者相关的卫生和人类服务部法规45 CFR 46（D）对研究中涉及儿童受试者的额外保护，而没有按照21 CFR 56（D）的要求，作出了的决定。此外，试验方案 [ ] 符合45 CFR 46部分D节的确定在内部是相互矛盾的。

在2007年5月17日IRB为试验方案 [ ]"[ ] 药物安全性、耐受性和药代动力学I期研究"与研究者的通信中，告知研究者IRB批准了2.0版方案、西班牙语和英语知情同意，IRB声称"方案符合45 CFR 46.406，提示'临床研究涉及最低风险，而且对受试者个人没有希望带来直接收益，但是很可能给受试者或他人带来对受试者所患的疾病或状况具有普遍意义的知识'"。IRB写错了这条法规，45 CFR 46.406是关于临床研究涉及超过最低风险的风险而且对受试者个人没有直接收益，但是很可能对受试者所患的疾病或状况产生具有普遍意义的知识。

最低风险指在研究中预期发生伤害或不适感的概率和程度，不能超过日常生活中通常遇到的，或进行常规身体或心理检查测试期间所发生的［21 CFR 56.102（ⅰ）］。2007年9月13日给试验方案 [ ] 与研究者的通信中，IRB批准了主要研究者的变更，IRB声称"方案符合法规45 CFR 46.404，提示临床研究对受试者或他人不涉及比最低风险更高的风险。"但是，作为试验药物的I期研究，试验方案 [ ] 似乎并不符合最低风险的定义。

我们确认收到了您的声明，即您审查了贵伦理委员会的书面程序，修订了部分IRB投票要求，对会议记录实施了内部审查。但是，您的回复并没有充分解决我们现场检查中记录的所有问题。我们要求您实施一项规程，确保对会议记录的准确性进行及时的审查。此外，您必须实施一项规程，确保当使用快速审查程序时所有的委员都能被通知到，做好快速审查的记录。IRB还应当实施一项规程，确保将所有IRB行动的通信内容发布给研究者。最后，IRB必须建立规程，对涉及儿童作为受试者的临床研究进行审查。我们注意到，IRB一直在努力通过应用卫生和人类服务部法规45 CFR 46（D）来做到这一点。对FDA监管的药物临床研究，IRB必须发现和记录临床研究符合FDA法规21 CFR 50（D），对临床研究中儿童的额外保护的要求。IRB应当只批准满足法规标准的临床研究：50.51（临床研究不涉及比最低风险更高的风险）；50.52（临床研究涉及的风险超过最低风险，但是有希望为受试者带来直接收益）；50.53（临床研究涉及超过最低风险的风险而且对受试者个人没有直接收益，但是很可能对受试者所患的疾病或状况产生具有普遍意义的知识）。

本警告信的目的并不是罗列在IRB审查和批准方案时存在的所有缺陷。确保San Juan的IRB的做法和规程完全符合所有适用法律法规的要求是您的职责。

由于上述提到的违背FDA法规的情况，请自收到这封信的15个工作日内，书面告知本办公室为预防将来发生类似违规情况已经或计划采取的措施。如果不能对上述违规行为进行充分、迅速地解释，可能导致我们在不再通知的情况下采取监管措施。

附：英文原文

Hospital Municipal de San Juan

WARNING LETTER

AUG 15, 2008

CERTIFIED MAIL
RETURN RECEIPT REQUESTED

Ref: 08-HFD-45-0801

Luis A. Medina, M.D.
IRB Chairman
Hospital Municipal de San Juan
PMB 498
P.O. Box 70344
San Juan, PR 00936

Dear Dr. Medina:

Between November 15 and 21, 2007, Lt. Luis O. Rodriguez, representing the Food and Drug Administration (FDA), inspected the Institutional Review Board (IRB) at Hospital Municipal de San Juan The purpose of this inspection was to determine whether the IRB procedures for the protection of human subjects complied with Title 21 of the Code of Federal Regulations (CFR), Parts 50 and 56. These regulations apply to clinical studies of products regulated by FDA. We are aware that at the conclusion of the inspection, our investigator presented and discussed with you, a Form FDA 483, Inspectional Observations.

From our review of the establishment inspection report, the documents submitted with that report, and your written response dated December 3, 2007, we conclude that the IRB did not adhere to the applicable statutory requirements and FDA regulations governing the protection of human subjects. We wish to emphasize the following:

1. The IRB has not prepared and maintained adequate documentation of IRB activities. Minutes of IRB meetings have not been prepared in sufficient detail to show actions taken by the IRB [21 CFR 56.115(a)(2)].

a. For protocol [ ] Phase Ⅰ/Ⅱ, Open-Label, Pharmacokinetic and Safety Study of a Novel [ ] the IRB sent a letter to the clinical investigator dated August 19, 2006 stating that the IRB reapproved the protocol. There is no mention of protocol [ ] in the minutes of the August 10, 2006 IRB meeting or in any other documentation. Therefore, due to the lack of adequate detail in the IRB meeting minutes and other documents, we are unable to confirm that the study was re-approved at a convened meeting as required by FDA regulations. [See 21 CFR 56.108(c)].

b. All approval decisions must be made during a convened IRB meeting or through the expedited review process. [See 21 CFR 56.108(c)]. Approval decisions from convened IRB meetings must be in the IRB meeting minutes [21 CFR 56.115(a)(2)].

Our inspection revealed nine instances in which approval dates correspond with IRB meeting dates, but IRB actions are not documented in the minutes as noted in the table below:

Protocol	Document	Date of Approval	IRB Meeting Date	Approval Documented in Minutes?
	Spanish/English Consent Form Amendment	2/9/06	2/9/06	No
	Spanish/English Consent Forms for Specimen Storage	2/8/07	2/8/07	No
	Assent waiver	2/9/06	2/9/06	No
	English/Spanish Consent Forms for Specimen Storage	2/9/06	2/9/06	No
	English/Spanish Information Sheet	2/9/06	2/9/06	No
	Amendment #4	8/10/06	8/10/06	No
	Continuing Review	2/8/07	2/8/07	No
	Progress Report	2/8/07	2/8/07	No
	Change of Principal Investigator in Consent Forms	9/13/07	9/13/07	No

In addition, our inspection revealed three instances in which approval dates do not correspond to IRB meeting dates, and there is no documentation explaining the type of review procedure used. San Juan WB's expedited review procedure states that all members will be informed about expedited review approvals by discussing those approvals at the following meeting; therefore, any expedited review approvals should have been noted in the meeting minutes of the subsequent IRB meeting. [See 21 CFR 56.110(c) and San Juan IRB's Written Procedures].

Protocol	Document	Date of Approval	IRB Meeting Date	Approval Documented in Minutes?
	Patient Instructions	10/3/05	10/13/05	No
	Continuing Review	8/19/06	8/10/06	No
	Continuing Review	2/16/07	2/8/07	No

2. For other than expedited reviews, the IRB does not always review proposed research at convened meetings at which a majority of the members of the IRB are present, including at least one member whose primary concerns are in nonscientific areas [21 CFR 56.108(c)].

Our inspection revealed that the IRB reviewed and approved research at the April 20, 2006, meeting without the presence of at least one member whose primary concerns are in nonscientific areas. According to the Attendance Sheet for the April 20, 2006 meeting, the following members were present: Dr. Luis A. Medina (pediatrician), [ ] (epidemiologist), [ ] (pharmacist) and [ ] (registered nurse), [ ] (community representative) and [ ] (legal advisor) were both excused from this meeting.

3. The IRB failed to follow FDA regulations pertaining to review of research, which require that an IRB shall notify investigators and the institution in writing of its decision to approve or disapprove the proposed research activity, or of modifications required to secure IRB approval of the research activity [21 CFR 56.109(e)].

a. For protocol [ ] there is no documentation in the IRB's files that the investigator was notified of the October 3, 2005 approval of a Patient Information Sheet. In addition, on January 30, 2006, the clinical site submitted three documents to the IRB pertaining to Specimen Storage at Repositories funded by NICFID: 1) Information Sheet (Spanish and English); 2) Repository Consent Form for Parent (Spanish and English); and 3) Repository Consent Form For Youth (Spanish and English). There is no documentation that the investigator was notified of the approval of the consent forms.

b. For protocol [ ] Intensive Pharmacokinectic Studies of [ ] there is no documentation in the IRB's files that the investigator was informed of the April 20, 2006 approvals of Consent Forms for Specimen Storage Funded by the National Institute of Child Health and Human Development (NICHD), and Parent Fact Sheets (English and Spanish).

4. In approving research in which some or all of the subjects are children, the IRB failed to determine that all research is in compliance with 21 CFR Part 50, Subpart D, Additional Safeguards for Children in Clinical Investigations [21 CFR 56.111(c)].

The IRB failed to make determinations that search was in compliance with 21 CFR Part 50, Subpart D, in protocol [ ] among others. Subpart D requires the IRB to make a determination that the clinic investigation meets the requirements of one of these categories of research [50.51 (minimal risk), 50.52 (greater than minimal risk, but presenting the prospect of direct benefit), or 50.53 (greater that minimal risk and no prospect of direct benefit)]. San Juan IRB made determinations under Department of Health and Human Services regulations under Title 45, Part 46, Subpart D - Additional Protections for Children Involved as Subjects in Research in correspondence with investigators without referencing 21 CFR Subpart D. In addition, the determinations of protocol [ ] compliance with Title 45, Part 46, Subpart D are internally inconsistent.

In the IRB's May 17, 2007 correspondence to the investigator for protocol [ ] "A Phase I Study of the Safety, Tolerance and Pharmacokinetics of [ ]" notifying of IRB approval of Version 2.0 of the protocol and the Spanish and English Informed Consents, the IRB states the protocol complies with the regulation 45 CFR §46.406 that implies "research involving minimal risk and no prospect of direct benefit to individual subjects but likely to yield generalizable knowledge about the subject's disorder or condition to subjects or others." The IRB has misstated this regulation, as 45 CFR 46.406 pertains to research involving greater (emphasis added) than minimal risk and no prospect of direct benefit to individual subjects, but likely to yield generalizable knowledge about the subject's disorder or condition.

Minimal risk means that the probability and magnitude of harm or discomfort anticipated in the research are not greater in and of themselves than those ordinarily encountered in daily life or during the performance of routine physical or psychological examinations or tests [21 CFR 56.102(i)]. In September 13, 2007 correspondence to the investigator for protocol [ ] in which the IRB approved a change in principal investigators, the IRB states that "the protocol complies with the regulation 45 CFR §46.404 that implies research not involving greater than minimal risk to subjects or others." However, as a phase I study of investigational drugs, protocol [ ] does not appear to meet the definition of minimal risk.

We acknowledge your statements that you reviewed your written procedures, revised certain IRB voting requirements, and implemented an internal review of the meeting minutes; however, your response does not adequately address all of the observations noted during our inspection. We request that you implement a procedure that will ensure timely review of the meeting minutes for accuracy. In addition, you must implement a procedure to ensure that all IRB members are informed when an expedited review procedure is used and documentation of expedited review. The IRB must also implement a procedure to ensure that correspondence regarding all IRB actions is issued to investigators. Finally, the IRB must develop procedures for review of clinical investigations that involve children as research subjects. We note that the IRB has been attempting to do this using Department of Health and Human Services regulations, 45 CFR Part 46. For clinical investigations of FDA-regulated products, the IRB must find and document that the clinical investigation(s) meet the requirements of FDA regulations, 21 CFR Part 50,

Subpart D - Additional Safeguards for Children in Clinical Investigations. The IRB may approve only those clinical investigations that satisfy the criteria described in 50.51 (clinical investigations not involving greater than minimal risk), 50.52 (clinical investigations involving greater than minimal risk, but presenting the prospect of direct benefit to individual subjects] or 50.53 (clinical investigations involving greater than minimal risk and no prospect of direct benefit to individual subjects, but likely to yield generalizable knowledge about the subjects' disorder or condition).

This letter is not intended to be an all-inclusive list of deficiencies for the protocols reviewed and approved by the IRB. It is your responsibility to assure that San Juan IRB's practices and procedures fully comply with all applicable statutes and regulations. Because of the departures from FDA regulations discussed above, please inform this office, in writing, within fifteen (15) working days of your receipt of this letter, of the actions you have taken or plan to take to prevent similar violations in the future. Failure to adequately and promptly explain the violations noted above may result in regulatory action without further notice.

If you have any questions, please contact Constance Lewin, M.D., M.P.H., at 301-796-3397; FAX 301- 847-8748. Your written response and any pertinent documentation should be addressed to:

Constance Lewin, M.D., M.P.H.
Branch Chief, Good Clinical Practice Branch I
Division of Scientific Investigations Office of Compliance
Center for Drug Evaluation and Research
Food and Drug Administration
Bldg 51, Room 5354
10903 New Hampshire Avenue
Silver Spring, MD 20993

Sincerely yours,

Leslie K. Ball, M.D.
Director
Division of Scientific Investigations
Office of Compliance
Center for Drug Evaluation and Research

第32封 给Coast伦理委员会的警告信

2008年3月11日

参考号：08-HFD-45-11-01

尊敬的McDaniel先生：

2007年7月10日至18日，James Fleckenstein先生代表FDA，对Coast伦理委员会（IRB）进行了现场检查。本次现场检查的目的是核实Coast IRB是否遵循了包含在美国联邦法规第21篇第56和第50部分中的对IRB进行监管并保护临床试验受试者的相关法规。这些法规适用于FDA所监管产品的临床研究。我们知道在这次检查结束时，检查员向您出示并讨论了FDA483表，即现场检查发现的问题。

经对FDA483表、现场检查报告、该报告的附件，以及您2007年8月15日和2007年11月29日的书面回复进行评估，我们认为，Coast IRB未能遵守如下所述的21 CFR 56的某些要求。我们通过审查IRB的书面程序和以下研究，确定了IRB监管的违规行为。

［不公开］试验方案［不公开］：题为1个1期多中心、开放、随机、三臂临床试验，以评估［不公开］在治疗［不公开］。

我们想强调以下几点：

1. IRB未能遵守关于快速审查程序的FDA法规［21 CFR56.110（B）］

该法规要求，根据快速审查程序，审查可由IRB主席或IRB主席从IRB的委员中指定的一个或多个经验丰富的委员进行。IRB可以使用快速审查程序审查以下两者之一或全部情况：①出现在联邦注册名单上的，并由审查员发现涉及不超过最小风险的部分或全部研究；②在批准期内对之前已批准的研究做了微小修改。Coast IRB快速审查的书面程序也反映了这一要求。如下所述，Coast IRB让一个缺乏经验的委员进行了快速审查，且被审查的该项研究未能满足上述条件。

2007年3月19日，贵方任命某先生［不公开］进入IRB董事会，并指示他对上述试验的招募广告进行快速审查。某先生［不公开］缺乏代表IRB进行必要的相关快速审查的经验。此外，2007年3月19日，通过快速审查程序审查的广告也不具备21 CFR56.110（b）中规定的快速审查资格，因为该研究既不是显示在联邦注册名单上，由审查员认定为风险最小的研究，也不是对以前批准的研究的微小改动。最后，该招募广告不适合进行快速审查，因为全体IRB委员曾经开会对此审查过，情况如下。

全体IRB委员曾在2007年3月1日、8日和15日三次召集的会议上讨论了研究招募广告，IRB批准了该广告，但要求修改，并将决定通知了申办者。在申办者重新提交后，IRB分别于2007年3月8日和15日的会议上，对上述研究的招募广告作出不予批准的决定。最初的但要求修改批准和后续的不批准是基于IRB认定该招募广告是强制性的。在两次情况下，IRB或IRB主席均对广告语言提出了董事会可以接受的修改意见。

尽管IRB第一次批准了要求修改的招募广告，但后来又未批准该广告。您于2007年3月19日任命某先生进入IRB董事会，并于同一天指定某先生进行该广告的快速审查。2007年3月19日，某先生经快速审查批准了原始的招募广告，而该广告最初被IRB全体委员批准，但要求修改，后又未予批准。尽管全体董事会在前三次会议中审议这个问题，3月8日和15日的会议记录和电子邮件中记录了未予批准该广告，您声称您不知道董事会对此事的决定。

此外，21 CFR56.110（b）法规要求IRB主席进行快速审查或指定一个有经验的审查员代表IRB进行快速审查。您作为IRB的首席执行官，不具有指定任何人代表IRB进行快速审查的权力。

您在2007年8月15日的书面回复承认，快速审查只能由IRB主席或由主席从IRB委员中指定一名或多名经验丰富的审查员进行审评。该书面回复还指出，某先生快速审查的所有广告/招募资料正在由主席审查，以符合法规要求。您的此次书面回复和2007年11月29日的书面回复都没有解决以下问题，即您在该研究并不符合FDA法规的快速审查资格的情况下对其进行了快速审查，且指定的某先生缺乏快速审查的相关经验。

2. IRB未能遵守关于对研究进行初始审查和跟踪审查、向研究者和机构报告发现的问题和采取的措施的书面程序［121 CFR56.108（a）（1）和56.110（c）］

如前所述，上述研究广告是经快速审查程序批准的。FDA的法规要求采用快速审查程序的IRB需采用方法告知所有委员其已根据规定的程序批准研究提案。Coast IRB的标准操作规程（SOP）手册第4版4.1.1指出，IRB的普通委员应通过Coast IRB议程被告知这些事宜。然而FDA访谈过的IRB委员不能回忆起其被告知该项快速审查，我们无法找到将这个快速审查作为议题的会议议程。如果Coast IRB以公文形式通知了IRB委员该项快速审查，请予以提供。

3. IRB未能保存用充分的细节显示IRB采取的措施的会议记录［21 CFR56.115（a）（2）］

2007年3月1日的会议记录未记录IRB有关批准上述试验广告，但要求修改的事宜。法规要求这些信息需包括在会议记录中。而IRB主席在检查时的口头陈述和由IRB主席修改的广告副本显示，该广告没有被批准。我们接受您的说法，即您修改了有关会议记录需包含21 CFR56.115（a）（2）要求内容的标准操作规程，且雇了一个人专门记录IRB会议记录。

这封信的目的并不是罗列上述由全体IRB和通过快速审查的研究中的所有缺陷。确保Coast IRB的做法和程序完全遵守所有适用的法律和法规是您的职责。

因为Coast IRB未能遵守关于使用快速审查程序的FDA法规，根据21 CFR56.110（d），为了保护受试者权益或福利，FDA将暂停Coast IRB的快速审查，直到得到进一步通知。FDA将在收到该IRB关于解决不当使用快速审查的满意答复和采取纠正措施的细节信息后撤销暂停。

自收到这封信的15个工作日内，请书面告知本办公室您为预防将来发生类似违规情况已经采取或计划采取的措施。如果不能充分、迅速地解释上述违规问题，可能导致我们在不再通知的情况下采取监管措施。

附：英文原文

Coast Institutional Review Board

WARNING LETTER

MAR 11, 2008

CERTIFIED MAIL
RETURN RECEIPT REQUESTED

Ref: 08-HFD-45-1101

Darren McDaniel
Chief Executive Officer
Coast Institutional Review Board
5475 Mark Dabling Blvd, Suite 351
Colorado Springs, CO 80918

Dear Mr. McDaniel:

Between July 10 and 18, 2007, Mr. James Fleckenstein, representing the Food and Drug Administration (FDA), inspected Coast IRB. The purpose of this inspection was to determine whether Coast IRB was incompliance with the regulations governing IRBs and those governing the protection of human subjects participating in clinical trials contained in Title 21 of the Code of Federal Regulations (CFR), Parts 56 and 50.These regulations apply to clinical investigations of products regulated by FDA. We are aware that at the conclusion of this inspection, our investigator presented and discussed with you a Form FDA 483, Inspectional Observations.

From our evaluation of the Form FDA 483, the establishment inspection report, the documents submitted with that report, and your written responses dated August 15 and November 29, 2007, we conclude that the IRB failed to adhere to certain requirements in 21 CFR Part 56 as described below. The regulatory violations were identified from the review of the IRB's written procedures and the review of the following study:

[redacted] Protocol [redacted] entitled "A Phase 1 Multi - Center, Open- Label, Randomized, 3-Arm Clinical Trial to Evaluate [redacted] in the Treatment of [redacted]".

We wish to emphasize the following:

1. The IRB failed to follow FDA regulations regarding expedited review procedures [21 CFR 56.110(b)].

The regulations require that under an expedited review procedure, the review may be carried out by the IRB chairperson or by one or more experienced reviewers designated by the IRB chairperson from among the members of the IRB, and the IRB may use the expedited review process to review either or both of the following:(1) some or all of the research appearing on the Federal Register list and found by the reviewers) to involve no more than minimal risk, or (2) minor changes in previously approved research during the period for which approval is authorized. Coast IRB's written procedures for expedited review also reflect this requirement. As explained below, Coast IRB had an inexperienced member conduct the expedited review and reviewed research under expedited review that did not meet the criteria above.

On March 19, 2007, you appointed Mr. [redacted] to the IRB Board and instructed him to conduct an expedited review of the advertisement for the above referenced study. Mr. [redacted] lacked the requisite relevant experience to conduct expedited review on behalf of the IRB. In addition, the advertisement reviewed under the expedited review procedure on March 19, 2007, did not qualify for expedited review under 21 CFR 56.110(b), as it was neither research appearing on the Federal Register list and found by the reviewer to involve no more than minimal risk nor minor changes to previously approved research. Finally, the advertisement was not appropriate for expedited review because the full IRB had met and reviewed it as discussed below.

The full IRB considered the recruitment advertisement for the study at three previously convened meetings on March 1, 8, and 15, 2007. On March 1, 2007, the IRB approved the advertisement with changes and that decision was communicated to the sponsor. Upon resubmission by the sponsor, the IRB disapproved the recruitment advertisement for the above study on both March 8 and 15, 2007. The initial approval with changes and the subsequent disapprovals were based, on the IRB's determination that the advertisement was coercive in nature. In each case, the IRB or the IRB Chair proposed alternative language which would have been acceptable to the Board.

Despite the advertisement having been first approved with changes and then disapproved by the IRB, you appointed Mr. [redacted] to the IRB Board on March 19, 2007, and then you directed Mr. [redacted] to conduct an expedited review of the advertisement on that same day. On March 19, 2007, Mr. [redacted] via expedited review, approved the advertisement in its original form which had previously been approved with changes and then disapproved as submitted by the full IRB. Despite the full board's consideration of this matter at three previous meetings, documentation of the disapprovals in the minutes of both March 8th and 15th, and e-mails that indicate otherwise, you stated that you were unaware of the Board's decisions on this matter.

Furthermore, the regulations at 21 CFR 56.110(b) require that the IRB chairperson conduct expedited review or designate an experienced reviewer to conduct an expedited review on behalf of the IRB. You in your capacity as the chief executive officer of the IRB, lacked the authority to designate anyone to conduct expedited reviews on behalf of the IRB.

Your written response of August 15, 2007, acknowledges that expedited review may only be conducted by the IRB Chair or by one or more experienced reviewers designated by the Chair from among the IRB members. This written response also states that all advertisement/recruitment materials that underwent expedited review by Mr. [redacted] are being reviewed by the Chair for regulatory compliance. Neither this written response nor your written response of November 29, 2007, addresses the issue that you directed review of the research under expedited review when it did not qualify under FDA regulations for expedited review and that you had Mr. [redacted]conduct an expedited review despite Mr. [redacted]lack of relevant experience.

2. The IRB did not follow written procedures for conducting its initial and continuing review of research and for reporting its findings and actions to the investigator and institution [21 CFR 56.108(a)(1) and 56.110(c)].

As noted, the advertisement for the above referenced study was approved under an expedited review procedure. FDA's regulations require IRBs using an expedited review procedure to adopt a method for keeping all members advised of research proposals which have been approved under the procedure. Coast IRB's Standard Operating Procedure (SOP) Manual, Version 4, Section 4.1.1, stated that a regular members of the IRB were to be informed of such actions via the Coast IRB agenda. However, IRB members interviewed by FDA could not recall being notified about the expedited review and we were not able to locate an agenda with this expedited review listed as an agenda item. If Coast IRB had ocumentation notifying the IRB members about this expedited review, please provide it.

3. The IRB did not maintain minutes of meetings in sufficient detail to indicate the actions taken by the IRB [21 CFR 56.115(a)(2)].

The minutes for the March 1, 2007, meeting do not document the IRB's approval with changes of the advertisement for the above study. Such information is required to be included in the minutes under the regulations. However, verbal statements from the IRB Chair during the inspection and a copy of the advertisement revised by the IRB Chair indicate that the advertisement was not approved as submitted.

We acknowledge your statements that you revised your standard operating procedures regarding minutes to include the meeting minute elements required by 21 CFR 56.115(a)(2), and that you hired an individual to specifically take IRB minutes.

This letter is not intended to be an all-inclusive list of deficiencies for the above referenced study reviewed by the full IRB and through expedited review. It is your responsibility to assure that Coast IRB's practices and procedures fully comply with all applicable statutes and regulations.

Under 21 CFR 56.110(d), FDA, in order to protect the rights or welfare of subjects, is suspending Coast IRB's use of expedited review procedures until further notice because of Coast IRB's failure to follow FDA regulations regarding the use of expedited review procedures. FDA will remove this suspension after receipt of a satisfactory response that addresses the IRB's inappropriate use of expedited review and that provides details concerning the corrective action taken.

Because of the departures from FDA regulations discussed above, please inform this office, in writing, within fifteen (15) working days of your receipt of this letter, of the actions you have taken or plan to take to prevent similar violations in the future. Failure to adequately and promptly explain the violations noted above may result in further regulatory action without further notice.

If you have any questions, please contact Dr. Constance Lewin at (301) 796-3397, FAX (301) 796-8748. Your written response and any pertinent documentation should be addressed to:

Constance Lewin, M.D., M.P.H.
Branch Chief
Good Clinical Practice Branch 1, Bldg. 51, Room. 5354
Division of Scientific Investigations
Office of Compliance
Center for Drug Evaluation and Research
Food and Drug Administration
10903 New Hampshire Avenue

Silver Spring, Maryland 20993-0002

Sincerely yours,
/S/
Leslie K. Ball, M.D.
Director
Division of Scientific Investigations
Office of Compliance
Center for Drug Evaluation and Research
Food and Drug Administration
10903 New Hampshire Avenue
Silver Spring, Maryland 20993-002

Cc:
[ ] M.Ed.
IRB Chair
Coast Institution Review Board
5475 Mark Dabling Blvd., Suite 351
Colorado Springs, CO 80918

第33封　给West Jefferson医疗中心伦理委员会的警告信

2008年2月25日

参考号：08-HFD-45-02-04

尊敬的Abaunza博士：

2007年7月23日至2007年7月26日，Barbara D. Wright女士代表FDA对West Jefferson医疗中心伦理委员会（IRB）进行了现场检查。本次检查的目的是核实伦理委员会保护受试者的程序是否符合联邦法规第21篇第50和56部分的要求。这些法规适用于FDA所监管产品的临床研究。我们知道在现场检查结束时，我们的检查员向您出示了FDA483表，即现场检查发现的问题，并与您进行了讨论。

通过审查现场检查报告、该报告的附件和您2007年8月22日对FDA483表的回复，我们认为，贵IRB未能遵循适用的法律要求和监管保护受试者的FDA法规。我们希望强调以下几点：

1. IRB未能避免有利益冲突的委员不能参与项目的初始审查，除非根据IRB的要求提供信息［21 CFR 56.107（e）］

具体而言，2005年8月9日IRB会议上，［不公开］医生提交了他的题为“一项多中心、随机、双盲静脉使用［不公开］药物与安慰剂比较治疗儿童（6～14岁）急性哮喘有效性的研究”，该医生本人是正式的有投票权的伦理委员会委员。我们发现会议记录中没有声明［不公开］医生回避了此项目的初始审查或投票。会议记录仅提到对该项目进行了动议、附议及批准。

2. IRB未能按照21 CFR 56.115（a）（6），21CFR 56.108（a）（1）和21CFR 812.66的要求，遵守IRB职能和运行的书面程序

根据上述法规，每个IRB在进行项目初始审查和跟踪审查时都应制定、维护并遵循书面程序。“West Jefferson 医疗中心伦理委员会制度和操作规程手册”中缺乏用于判断一项器械研究属于重大风险（SR）还是非重大风险（NSR）的书面程序。具体而言，“Ⅶ章—职责和操作，A节—初始审查程序和B节—IRB批准标准”中未描述IRB作出判断时所参考的标准。

根据21CFR 812.2（b）（1）（ⅱ）条款，对作为NSR的器械研究进行审查时，IRB必须判断到底是SR研究还是NSR研究。IRB在作出SR或NSR决定时，要参考申办者对该器械为什么是非重大风险所做的简要说明。此外，IRB还要参考“重大风险器械”的定义［21 CFR 812.39（m）］、产品和用法描述以及其他IRB要求申办者提供的资料。若经判断的确属NSR研究，IRB将遵照21CFR 56进行操作。若判断是SR研究，按照21CFR 812.66，IRB必须将此判断结果通知研究者，适当情况下也应通知申办者。后一种情况下，申办者需按照21CFR 812.30（a）要求向FDA申请IDE，否则不得开展研究。申办者将IDE批准复印件交给研究者，再由研究者递交给IRB审查证明已得到FDA同意。没有FDA和IRB的批准，不能开展重大风险器械的研究。

3. IRB未能遵守关于对研究进行跟踪审查的书面程序［21 CFR 312.62（b）］

a. IRB制定的书面程序不能准确反映目前跟踪审查行为的状况。现行书面程序提示贵IRB应对项目开展每年至少一次的跟踪审查，以确定研究是否符合标准。但是，我们发现，实际上贵IRB要到每年的11月份才向监管研究者发放书面通知，要求其在12月份内递交书面的研究进展和（或）总结报告。此后，在每年度的第一次伦理委员会会议上完成审查大多数书面研究进展和（或）总结报告。

我们发现，IRB目前采用的跟踪审查方式会导致在通知研究者递交总结报告前有伦理批件的研究已过期。检查员Wright也注意到，贵伦理委员会只给到秋季为止经伦理委员会和医疗执行委员会双方都批准的项目的研究者发出了书面要求。但是，如果项目只是目前已被伦理委员会批准，但还未获得医疗执行委员会的批准，则贵IRB要在下一年度才要求研究者递交书面研究进展和（或）总结报告。因此，在伦理委员会跟踪审查期审查研究前，原研究伦理批件可能已到期。例如，我们发现2005年8月9日伦理委员会会议批准的题为"一项多中心、随机、双盲静脉使用［不公开］药物与安慰剂比较治疗儿童患者（4～14岁）急性哮喘临床有效性的研究"，在伦理委员会批准已期满（失效日2006年8月9日后），2006年11月13日的信中IRB要求研究者递交书面总结报告。

我们也发现，在伦理委员会发通知函的11月至下一年度第一次伦理委员会会议期间审批同意的项目，要到远超首次批准一年后才被再次审查。例如，如果一项研究是在12月1日批准，11月伦理委员会已发出通知函了，那么IRB要在下一年的11月才通知研究者递交研究进展和（或）总结报告。到再下一年的首次伦理委员会会议对研究进行跟踪审查时，IRB首次审查批件此时已过期。因此，贵IRB并未按标准操作规程开展每年至少一次的跟踪审查。

b. IRB跟踪审查书面程序申明，IRB要求研究者至少每年一次向IRB递交书面研究进展报告。我们发现2位研究者未能按您信中要求的12月最后期限内向IRB递交书面报告，贵IRB也未跟踪研究者以确保其符合要求。具体而言：

i. 如上所提及的，IRB于2006年11月13日给"一项多中心、随机、双盲静脉使用［ ］药物与安慰剂比较治疗儿童患者（6～14岁）急性哮喘临床有效性的研究"的研究者寄了一封信，要求研究者在2006年12月22日前递交书面研究进展报告。该研究者，也是伦理委员会投票委员，直到2007年2月6日才递交了书面总结报告。

ii. IRB于2006年11月13日通知"#####"项目的研究者在2006年12月22日前递交书面研究进展报告，FDA检查员Wright发现在FDA现场检查时（2007年7月），研究者未按2006年11月信的要求向IRB递交总结报告。

4. 除了快速审查，IRB未能在大多数委员出席，其中至少包括一名来自非科学领域委员的召集会议上对拟开展的研究进行审查［21 CFR 56.108（c）］

具体而言，我们发现下列会议没有多数委员出席和（或）非科学领域委员没有参会。

a. 2005年1月4日会议，11名委员仅5人出席，因此，没有达到多数人参会的要求。

b. 2005年8月9日会议，非科学领域委员没有出席。此外，我们发现参与投票的［不公开］医生因与他自己的研究项目有利益冲突，他回避了自己项目的审查和投票，因此他不能被计入参会人员数中。所以，他的项目在审查及投票时，伦理委员会出席人员未达多数。

c. 2005年11月3日会议，11名委员仅3人出席，参会人数没有达到多数且没有非科学领域委员参会。

d. 2007年2月7日的会议非科学领域委员没有参会。

5. IRB未能按照不少于一年一次的频次对研究进行跟踪审查［21 CFR 56.109（f）］ 具体而言：

a. 2005年8月9日伦理委员会会议上批准了题为"一项多中心、随机、双盲静脉使用［不公开］药物与安慰剂比较治疗儿童患者（6～14岁）急性哮喘有效性的研究"，到2006年11月伦理委员会才通知研究者递交进展报告，此时批件已过期（失效日期：2006年8月9日）。2007年2月6日研究者递交报告，2007年2月7日IRB才进行了审查。

b. 2005年3月3日的信中，IRB告知研究者题为"研究计划（某研究某阶段）"在跟踪审查中被重新批准。在下一年同一项研究的研究者于2006年2月21日向IRB递交了进展报告。IRB直到2006年9月5日才在跟踪审查中重新批准了该研究。

此外，我们注意到2006年11月7日West Jefferson 医疗中心医疗执行委员会的一封信，通知研究者已通过跟踪审查重新批准了研究，并倒推到IRB跟踪审查并重新批准的日期为2006年3月1日。我们认为，机构倒推伦理委员会批准日期的行为是不合适的。

6. IRB未能在初始审查时确定涉及儿童的研究需要依照21 CFR 50（D），临床研究中对儿童的额外保护措施［21 CFR 56.109（h）］

在2005年8月9日伦理委员会召集的会上批准了“一项多中心、随机、双盲静脉使用［不公开］药物与安慰剂比较治疗儿童患者（6~14岁）急性哮喘临床有效性的研究”，但IRB没有对研究是否遵循21CFR 50（D）进行评判或记录下评判内容。另外，在2007年7月FDA现场检查时，贵伦理委员会秘书强调IRB并不知晓21CFR 50（D）的要求。

7. 跟踪审查时，IRB未能要求充分的信息来确定研究是否满足IRB批准研究的标准［21 CFR 56.111］

IRB的书面程序要求研究者至少每年一次递交书面研究进展报告。在寄给研究者的信中提醒研究者递交书面研究进展报告，IRB仅要求研究者提供当年受试者入组数、入组受试者的结局、已批准项目的任何修订以及其他相关信息。我们发现，由于此信没有详细列明报告所需的细节内容，而由研究者自己决定递交什么，因此可能导致下列信息很有限甚至缺失：AE和/或SAE、方案偏离、现行方案和知情同意书、正在使用的招募材料、研究过程中由研究者或申办者定义的风险/收益变化等。所以，跟踪审查时，IRB要求研究者提供用于批准研究是否达标的材料是不够充分的。

8. IRB未能准备会议记录，用充分的细节显示IRB采取的行动；对行动的投票情况，包括赞成票数、反对票数和弃权票数［21 CFR 56.115（a）（2）］

a. 2005~2006年以及2007年2月的所有伦理委员会会议记录没有充分记录IRB投票细节，包括伦理委员赞成、反对和弃权的票数也没有记录。我们发现所有被IRB批准的研究都被记录为“动议、附议、批准”。

b. IRB会议记录未能详细记录IRB的所有行为，具体而言：

i. 我们发现，2007年2月7日IRB会议审查通过了“一项多中心、随机、双盲静脉使用［不公开］药物与安慰剂比较治疗儿童患者（6~14岁）急性哮喘临床有效性的研究”的总结报告和研究关闭函，IRB将此事以信函形式告知了研究者，但是2007年2月7日的会议记录审查中却没有提及此研究。

ii.［不公开］项目的研究者于2005年2月2日向IRB递交了总结报告，2005年3月3日IRB的信函告知研究者已通过跟踪审查，但2005年3月1日的会议记录中却未提及此研究。

c. 2005年1月4日、2006年1月3日伦理会议记录提到，IRB一次投票批准了正在跟踪审查的所有研究。但是，会议记录中未提及具体每个项目的决议过程，包括伦理委员投赞成、反对和弃权的票数也没有记录。

本警告信的目的并非是罗列贵IRB履行伦理委员会职责过程中的所有缺陷。自收到这封信的15个工作日内，FDA要求您解决这些缺陷，并书面告知本办公室为防止当前或将来的研究中发生类似违规行为，您已经采取或将要采取的措施和程序。请注意，FDA在适当的时间将进行另外的现场检查，以确保已经完成了充分的纠正措施。

附：英文原文

West Jefferson Medical Center IRB

WARNING LETTER

FEB 25, 2008

CERTIFIED MAIL
RETURN RECEIPT REQUESTED

Ref: 08-HFD-45-02-04

Alfred E. Abaunza, M.D.
Chief Medical Officer
West Jefferson Medical Center
Institutional Review Board
1101 Medical Center Boulevard
Marrero, LA 70072

Dear Dr. Abaunza:

Between July 23, 2007 and July 26, 2007, Ms. Barbara D. Wright, representing the Food and Drug Administration (FDA), inspected the Institutional Review Board (IRB) at West Jefferson Medical Center. The purpose of this inspection was to determine whether the IRB procedures for the protection of human subjects complied with Title 21 of the Code of Federal Regulations (CFR), Parts 50 and 56. These regulations apply to clinical studies of products regulated by FDA. We are aware that at the conclusion of the inspection, our investigator presented and discussed with you a Form FDA 483, Inspectional Observations.

From our review of the establishment inspection report, the documents submitted with that report, and your August 22, 2007 letter written in response to the Form FDA 483, Inspectional Observations, we conclude that the IRB did not adhere to the applicable statutory requirements and FDA regulations governing the protection of human subjects. We wish to emphasize the following:

1. The IRB failed to excuse a member from participating in the initial review of a project in which the member had a conflicting interest, except to provide information requested by the IRB [21 CFR 56.107(e)]. Specifically,

At the August 9, 2005 meeting of the IRB, Dr [ ] an official voting member, presented his study entitled "A Multicenter, Randomized, Double Blind Study Comparing the Clinical Effects of Intravenous [ ] with Placebo in Pediatric Patients (Ages 6 to 14 Years) with Acute Asthma." We note that the meeting minutes do not state that Dr. [ ] was excused from participating in the initial review or vote of his study. The minutes only noted that a motion was made, seconded and carried to approve the proposal as presented.

2. The IRB failed to follow written procedures for IRB functions and operations in accordance with 21 CFR Part 56.115(a)(6), 21 CFR 56.108(a)(1), and 21 CFR 812.66.

Pursuant to the above stated regulations, each IRB shall prepare, maintain, and follow written procedures for conducting initial and continuing review of research. The IRB failed to have written procedures in its manual "West Jefferson Medical Center Institutional Review Board Policy and Procedures" to determine if a device investigation is a significant risk (SR) device study or non-significant risk (NSR) device study. Specifically, the "Section Ⅶ - Functions and Operations, subsection A - Initial Review Process and subsection B - Criteria for IRB Approval" does not describe the criteria used by the IRB to .make this determination.

An IRB only has to make a SR or NSR determination for device studies presented as NSR studies to the IRB for review under 21 CFR 812.2(b)(1)(ii). The IRB considers the sponsor's brief explanation (21 CFR 812.2(b) (l)(ii) of why the device is not a significant risk device when making the SR or NSR determination. In addition, in making the SR or NSR determination, the IRB considers the "significant risk device" definition [21 CFR 812.3(m)], the description of the device and how it is used, and any other material that the IRB requests from the sponsor. If the IRB determines the proposed NSR device study to be NSR, the IRB may proceed with its review in accordance with 21 CFR Part 56. However, if the IRB determines that the proposed NSR study is SR, then under 21 CFR 812.66 the IRB must notify the investigator, and where appropriate, the sponsor, about its determination. In this latter case, the sponsor cannot begin the study unless an application for an IDE is provided to FDA as described in 21 CFR 812.30(a). An IRB may verify FDA's approval of a significant risk device study by requesting a copy of the FDA's IDE approval letter from the investigator, who will obtain it from the sponsor. Significant risk device studies cannot proceed without FDA and IRB approval.

3. The IRB failed to follow its written procedure for conducting continuing review of research [21 CFR 56.108(a)(1)].

a. The IRB's written procedures do not accurately reflect the current IRB practices in relation to continuing review. The current written procedures note that your IRB conducts continuing review of studies at least once a year to determine if the investigation still meets IRB approval criteria. In practice, however, we note that, your IRB does not send clinical investigators a written request until November of each year asking them to submit a written progress/summary report to the IRB by a given date in December. Most all written progress/summary reports are then reviewed by the IRB at the first meeting of each calendar year.

We note that the current process used by your IRB for the continuing review of studies allows for studies that had IRB approval to expire before the request is made by the IRB to the investigator to submit a summary report. Investigator Wright also noted that the IRB only sends out the written requests to investigators whose projects have cleared both the IRB and the Medical Executive Committee by the fall. If, however, a project has only recently been approved by the IRB but not the Medical Executive Committee your IRB will not request the investigator to send a written progress/summary report to you until the subsequent calendar year. Thus, a study can reach its expiration prior to the review of the study by the IRB at the continuing review phase. For example, we note that the study entitled "A Multicenter, Randomized, Double-Blind Study Comparing the Clinical Effects of Intravenous [ ] with Placebo in Pediatric Patients (Ages 6 to 14 Years) with Acute Asthma" was approved by the IRB at the August 9, 2005 meeting. In a letter dated November 13, 2006, after the IRB's approval had already expired (i.e. expiration, August 9, 2006), the IRB requested the investigator to submit a written summary report.

Also, we note that any studies that are reviewed and approved by the IRB after the November letter has been sent and before the first IRB meeting of the next calendar year will also not be reviewed until greater than one year after the study was initially approved. For example, if your IRB approves a study on December 1 of a given year after the November letter has been sent, then in November of the next calendar year, you would request that the clinical investigator submit a written progress/summary report by a given date in December. We note that by the time you review the study for continuing review at the first meeting of the subsequent calendar year, the study's original IRB approval would have expired. Thus, your IRB is not conducting continuing review of research at least once a year as described in your written procedure.

b. The IRB written procedures on continuing review state that the IRB requires investigators to submit written progress reports of their investigations to the IRB at least once a year. We note that two investigators failed to submit the written reports to the IRB by the December deadline date stated in your letter and that your IRB did not follow up with the investigators to ensure their compliance with the requirement. Specifically,

i. As noted above, your IRB sent a letter dated November 13, 2006 to the investigator of the study "A Multicenter, Randomized, Double-Blind Study comparing the Clinical Effects of Intravenous [ ] With Placebo in Pediatric Patients (Ages 6 to 14 Years) with Acute Asthma" requesting that the investigator submit a written progress report by December 22, 2006. The investigator, an IRB voting member, did not submit a written summary report to the IRB until February 6, 2007.

ii. The IRB sent, a letter dated November 13, 20, 06 to the investigator of the study "Investigational Plan (Phase [ ] for the [ ] Study)" requesting a written progress report by December 22, 2006. Per the report to the Center, FDA Investigator Wright noted that as of the date of the FDA inspection (i.e. July 2007), the investigator had not submitted a summary report to the IRB as requested in the November 2006 letter.

4. For other than expedited reviews, the IRB failed to review proposed research at convened meetings at which a majority of the members of the IRB are present, including at least one member whose primary concerns are in nonscientific areas [21 CFR 56.108(c)].

Specifically, we note that the meetings below did not have either a majority of members present and/or the presence of a nonscientific member:

a. At the January 4, 2005 meeting only 5 of 11 IRB members were present; thus a majority of the IRB members were not present at the meeting.

b. The nonscientific member was not present at the August 9, 2005 meeting. In addition, we note that Dr. [ ] a voting member was conflicted during the discussion and vote of his study. As Dr. [ ] was conflicted, he was to be excused from participating in the review and approval of his study and thus no longer counted towards the majority of members present. Therefore, during the discussion and vote of his study, the IRB lost a majority of its members present at the meeting.

c. At the November 3, 2005 meeting only 3 of 11 IRB members were present. This meeting did not have a majority of the members present and also did not have a nonscientific member present.

d. At the February 7, 2007 meeting, there was not a nonscientist member in attendance.

5. The IRB failed to conduct continuing review of research at intervals of not less than once per year [21 CFR 56.109(f)]. Specifically,

a. The IRB approved the study entitled "A Multicenter, Randomized, Double Blind Study Comparing the Clinical Effects of Intravenous [ ] with Placebo in Pediatric Patients (Ages 6 to 14 Years) with Acute Asthma" at the August 9, 2005 IRB meeting. The IRB did not request the investigator submit a written progress report until November, 2006 after the study's IRB approval had expired (i.e. expiration, August 9, 2006). The investigator submitted the written progress report to the IRB on February 6, 2007 and the IRB did not review and accept the report until February 7, 2007.

b. In a letter dated March 3, 2005, the IRB informed the investigator that the study entitled an "Investigational plan (Phase [ ] for the [ ] Study)" had been reapproved at continuing review. In the following year the investigator of this same study submitted a written progress report to the IRB on February 21, 2006. The IRB did not re-approve the study for continuing review until September 5, 2006.

In addition, we note that in a letter dated November 7, 2006, the Medical Executive Committee of West Jefferson Medical Center notified the investigator that they had also re approved the study for continuing review and that had retrospectively backdated the IRB's re-approval for continuing review to March 1, 2006. We note that it is inappropriate for an institution to backdate the IRB's approval.

6. The IRB failed to determine at the time of initial review that studies involving children are in compliance with 21 CFR Part 50 Subpart D, "Additional Safeguards for Children in Clinical Investigations" [21 CFR 56.109(h)].

Specifically, the IRB approved the study "A Multicenter, Randomized, Double Blind Study comparing the Clinical Effects of Intravenous [ ] with Placebo in Pediatric Patients (Ages 6 to 14 Years) with Acute Asthma" at the August 9, 2005 convened meeting. The IRB did not make the findings or document that the study was in compliance with 21 CFR 50 Subpart D. In addition, during the FDA inspection of July 2007, your IRB secretary noted that the IRB was not aware of your responsibilities under 21 CFR 50 subpart D.

7. The IRB failed to request sufficient information to determine whether studies meet the criteria for IRB approval of research at continuing review [21 CFR 56.111].

The IRB written procedures note that investigators are to submit a written progress report to the IRB of their investigation at least once a year. In the letter sent to investigators to remind them to submit a written progress report, the IRB only requests information that includes the number of patients enrolled during that year, their outcomes, any changes to the approved research and other pertinent information. We note that because the letter request fails to specify any necessary details concerning these categories of information, the contents of these written progress reports are left to the discretion of the investigator and can include limited to no information about adverse and/or serious adverse events, protocol deviations, current protocol and informed consent document in use, recruitment materials being utilized, changes in risk/benefit identified by the investigator or sponsor during the course of the study, etc. Thus, the IRB failed to request sufficient information to determine whether studies met the criteria for IRB approval under 21 CFR 56.111 at continuing review.

8. The IRB failed to prepare the minutes of IRB meetings in sufficient detail to show actions taken by the IRB, the vote on actions, including the number of members voting for, against and abstaining [21 CFR 56.115(a)(2)]. Specifically,

a. In all the IRB meetings that took place in 2005-2006 and the meeting on February 7,2007, the minutes were not prepared in sufficient detail to show the vote on the IRB actions, including the number of members voting for, against and abstaining on the actions. We note that the statement “motion made, second and carried to approve” was used for all studies that were approved by the IRB.

b. The IRB meeting minutes do not detail all of the actions taken by the IRB. Specifically,

i. In the review of records related to the study “A Multicenter, Randomized, Double-Blind Study Comparing the Clinical Effects of Intravenous [ ] With Placebo in Pediatric Patients (Ages 6 to 14 Years) with Acute Asthma”, we note that the IRB sent a letter to the clinical investigator informing him that the IRB reviewed and accepted his summary report and study closure notification at the February 7, 2007 meeting. However, there was no mention of this study in review of the minutes for the February 7, 2007 meeting.

ii. The investigator for the study “Investigational Plan (Phase [ ] for the [ ] Study)” submitted a summary report to the IRB in a letter dated February 2, 2005. In a letter dated March 3, 2005, the IRB informed the investigator that the study had received continuing approval. There is no mention of this study in the March 1, 2005 IRB meeting minutes.

c. During the January 4, 2005 and January 3, 2006 IRB meetings, the minutes indicate that the IRB held one vote to approve collectively all studies that were undergoing continuing review. However, the minutes for these meetings do not indicate votes for IRB action on the individual studies, including the numbers of members voting for, against, or abstaining.

This letter is not intended to be an all-inclusive list of deficiencies regarding your IRB’s responsibilities. Within fifteen (15) working days of your receipt of this letter, the FDA requests that you address these deficiencies in writing and inform us of corrective actions and procedures that you have or will take to prevent and ensure that similar violations will not occur in any on-going or future studies. Please note that at the appropriate time FDA will conduct additional inspections to ensure that adequate corrective actions have implemented.

We appreciate the cooperation shown Investigator Wright during the inspection. Should you have any questions or concerns regarding this letter or the inspection, please contact me by letter at the address given below.

Sincerely,

{See appended electronic signature page}

Leslie K. Ball, M.D.
Division Director
Division of Scientific Investigations
Office of Compliance
Center for Drug Evaluation and Research
Bldg #51, Room 5342
10903 New Hampshire Ave.
Silver Spring, MD 20993

第二部分

药物 GCP 警告信

——给申办者

FDA

第34封　给Targeted Medical制药有限公司（Physician Therapeutics）的警告信

2017年3月29日

参考号：17-HFD-45-03-02

尊敬的Giffoni先生：

2016年6月14日至7月1日，Diane C. Van Leeuwen女士代表FDA在您的临床研究场所进行了现场检查，对Targeted Medical 制药有限责任公司作为申办者、试验药物为（b）（4）的下列临床研究进行了审查：

- 试验方案（b）（4），“（b）（4）”；
- 试验方案（b）（4），“（b）（4）”。

这封警告信特告知您现场检查中发现的违规情况。

本次检查是FDA的生物研究监查项目的一部分，该项目通过设定的检查方法，以评估研究的实施情况并帮助确保研究中受试者的权益、安全和福利得到保护。

在现场检查结束时，Van Leeuwen女士向您出示了FDA 483表，即现场检查发现的问题，并与您进行了讨论。您2016年7月18日对FDA 483表的书面回复已收悉。

经对FDA现场检查报告、该报告的附件，以及您2016年7月18日对FDA 483表的书面回复进行审查，我们认为，Targeted Medical制药有限责任公司没有遵循适用的法律要求以及监管临床研究实施和受试者保护的FDA法规。我们想强调以下几点：

未能根据21 CFR 312.2（a）的要求对开展新药临床研究提交IND申请［21 CFR 312.20（a），312.20（b）和312.40（a）］

联邦食品药品和化妆品法案（FD&C Act）的相关章节定义药品为："目的是用于诊断、治愈、缓解、治疗或预防疾病的物品"和"除食品外，目的是用于影响人体或其他动物的身体结构或功能的物品"［21 U.S.C. 321（g）］。Targeted Medical制药有限责任公司研究的是（b）（4），因为该产品的目的是为了治疗（b）（4），所以其符合FD&C Act中药品的定义。

为了使新药合法上市，申办者必须依照FD&C Act 505的要求，获得FDA对新药申请或简化新药申请的批准［21 U.S.C 355］。研究新药（IND）申请使申办者获得对这一要求的豁免，得以分发试验药物［21 U.S.C 355（i）］。FDA法规要求，在受试者中开展药物临床研究前，除非该项临床研究符合21 CFR 312.2（b）中IND豁免的情形，否则申办者要递交IND申请。如果满足以下所有豁免标准，该法规对在启动药物临床研究前获得IND的要求提供豁免：

- 该药品在美国已合法上市；
- 所开展的临床研究不打算作为一个完全受控的试验来报告给FDA，用以支持申请新适应症，也不用于支持对该药品标签进行任何其他显著变化；
- 如果是合法上市的处方药，所开展的研究不用于支持药物广告内容的显著变化；
- 所开展的临床研究不涉及给药途径、剂量水平、适用人群或其他显著提高与使用药物相关的风险（或降低风险的可接受性）因素；
- 临床研究的开展符合21 CFR 56中列出的对伦理委员会的要求以及21 CFR 50中列出的对知情同意的要求；
- 临床研究的开展符合21 CFR 312.7中的要求。

Targeted Medical制药有限责任公司对（b）(4）的临床研究至少未能满足第一条标准。用于开展试验方案（b）(4）和（b）(4）的试验药物（b）(4)，是一种新的、未批准的药物，给受试者的用法为每天两次、超过28天。(b）(4）并不是一种在美国已合法上市的药品，因此不免除IND的要求。在临床研究中使用（b）(4）之前，Targeted Medical制药有限责任公司必须向FDA提交IND，并按照21 CFR 312.40的要求使IND生效。FDA的记录显示，Targeted Medical制药有限责任公司未能在使用（b）(4）的方案（b）(4）和（b）(4）的临床研究开展前提交IND。

在2016年7月18日对FDA 483表的书面回复中，您声称“(b）(4）是一个医学用途食品，用于治疗疼痛和感染相关的营养缺乏。我们并没有，也从来没有打算进行新药申请或将（b）(4）作为药品上市”。

孤儿药法案定义医学用途食品为：“在医生的监督下配方为口服或肠内使用，并用于某种疾病或状况的特殊膳食管理的食物，对该疾病或状况的独特的营养需求是通过医学评估，基于公认的科学原理建立的”[21 U.S.C 360ee（b）(3）]。

上面讨论的方案被设计来研究（b）(4)，但是患有（b）(4）的人并没有独特的营养需求。因此，该产品并不是21 U.S.C 360ee（b）(3）所述的医学用途食品。

此外，FD&C Act的相关章节定义药品为：“为了用来诊断、治愈、缓解、治疗或预防疾病的物品”和“除食品外，为了用来影响人体或其他动物的身体结构或功能的物品”[21 U.S.C.321（g）]。我们注意到（b）(4）是试验方案（b）(4）和（b）(4）的研究产品，两个方案都规定临床终点是检查相较于非甾体类抗炎药（NSAID）的“(b）(4)”。

因为Targeted Medical制药有限责任公司在研究（b）(4）对（b）(4）的效用,(b）(4）是为了用来诊断、治愈、缓解、治疗或预防疾病的物品，是为了用来影响人体的结构或任何功能的物品，因此满足FD&C Act中药品的定义。所以，Targeted Medical制药有限责任公司必须提交IND，而且直到IND生效才能开始在受试者中开展（b）(4）的临床研究。

在2016年7月18日的书面回复中，您还提到Targeted Medical制药有限责任公司的一名员工在临床研究开始前与FDA联系，并被建议：“尽管这些是医学用途食品，不需要申请NDA，Targeted Medical制药有限责任公司仍应当申请IND。”您提到针对每一个试验方案都向机关提交了FDA 1571表和FDA 1572表，但是FDA没有收到任何答复。

我们无法对您的书面回复进行知情评价，因为您还没有提供文件以证实FDA收到了（b）(4）的IND申请。当FDA收到IND的时候，FDA给该申请分配了一个IND编号，并将该申请转交给新药办公室内适当的审查部门。审查部门将给Targeted 制药有限责任公司发送信件，提供关于分配的IND编号，收到原始申请的日期，将来提交IND材料的地址，以及FDA联系人（关于该申请的问题应向其提出）的姓名和电话号码的通知。

没有任何FDA记录显示Targeted Medical制药有限责任公司在开展关于（b）(4）的临床研究，方案（b）(4）和（b）(4）的研究前提交了IND申请。我们注意到方案（b）(4）中有129名受试者入组到11个临床研究场所，方案（b）(4）中有122名受试者入组到8个临床研究场所。受试者使用未被批准的产品（b）(4)，每天两次、超过28天治疗（b）(4)。作为申办者，Targeted Medical制药有限责任公司本来应该在启动方案（b）(4）和（b）(4）前、招募受试者进入两个方案前获得IND。

本警告信的目的并非是罗列您在试验药物临床研究中存在的所有缺陷。确保符合法律和相关FDA法规的每一项要求是您的职责。您应当解决这些缺陷，并建立规程，以确保任何正在进行的或将来进行的研究符合FDA法规。

自收到本警告信的15个工作日内，您应当书面告知本办公室您已经采取的预防将来类似违规的措施。未能充分和迅速地对上述违规作出解释，可能导致不再通知的情况下采取监管措施。

[1] 也见于21 CFR 101.9（j）(8）和工业指南关于医疗食品的常见问题，第二版，2016年5月，可从https://www.fda.gov/downloads/Food/GuidanceRegulation/GuidanceDocumentsRegulatoryInformation/UCM50 0094.pdf下载。

附：英文原文

Targeted Medical Pharma, Inc. dba Physician Therapeutics

WARNING LETTER

MAR 29, 2017

CERTIFIED MAIL
RETURN RECEIPT REQUESTED

Ref: 17-HFD-45-03-02

ATTN:
Kim Giffoni, Director
Interim Chief Executive Officer
Targeted Medical Pharma, Inc.
2980 Beverly Glen Circle, Suite 100
Los Angeles, California 90077

Dear Mr. Giffoni:

This Warning Letter informs you of objectionable conditions observed during the U.S. Food and Drug Administration (FDA) inspection conducted at your clinical site between June 14, 2016, and July 1, 2016. Ms. Diane C. Van Leeuwen, representing FDA, conducted an investigation and met with you to review Targeted Medical Pharma, Inc.'s role as the sponsor of the following clinical investigations of the investigational drug (b)(4):

Protocol #(b)(4), "(b)(4)"

Protocol #(b)(4), "(b)(4)"

This inspection is a part of the FDA's Bioresearch Monitoring Program, which includes inspections designed to evaluate the conduct of research and to help ensure that the rights, safety, and welfare of the human subjects of those studies have been protected.

At the conclusion of the inspection, Ms. Van Leeuwen presented and discussed with you Form FDA 483, Inspectional Observations. We acknowledge receipt of your July 18, 2016, written response to the Form FDA 483.

From our review of the FDA Establishment Inspection Report, the documents submitted with that report, and your July 18, 2016, written response to the Form FDA 483, Inspectional Observations, we conclude that Targeted Medical Pharma, Inc., did not adhere to the applicable statutory requirements and FDA regulations governing the conduct of clinical investigations and the protection of human subjects. We wish to emphasize the following:

Failure to submit an IND for the conduct of clinical investigations with an investigational new drug that is subject to 21 CFR 312.2(a) [21 CFR 312.20(a), 312.20(b), and 312.40(a)].

In relevant part, the Federal Food, Drug, and Cosmetic Act (FD&C Act) defines the term drug as "articles intended for use in the diagnosis, cure, mitigation, treatment, or prevention of disease" and "articles (other than food) intended to affect the structure or any function of the body of man or other animals" [21 U.S.C. 321(g)]. Targeted Medical Pharma, Inc., studied the (b)(4). Because the product was intended for the treatment of (b)(4), it meets the definition of a drug under the FD&C Act.

To market a new drug lawfully, a sponsor must obtain FDA approval of either a new drug application or an abbreviated new drug application under Section 505 of the FD&C Act [21 U.S.C. 355]. An Investigational New Drug (IND) application allows a sponsor to obtain an exemption from this requirement in order to distribute an investigational drug [21 U.S.C. 355(i)]. FDA regulations require a sponsor to submit an IND application before conducting a clinical investigation of a drug in human subjects, unless the clinical investigation qualifies for an IND exemption under 21 CFR 312.2(b). That regulation provides an exemption from the requirement to obtain an IND before initiating a clinical investigation of a drug if all of the following exemption criteria are met:

The drug product is lawfully marketed in the United States;

The investigation is not intended to be reported to FDA as a well-controlled study in support of a new indication for use, and there is no intent to use the investigation to support any other significant change in the labeling of the drug;

In the case of a lawfully marketed prescription drug, the investigation is not intended to support a significant change in the advertising for the drug;

The investigation does not involve a route of administration, dosage level, use in a patient population, or other factor that significantly increases the risks (or decreases the acceptability of the risks) associated with the use of the drug product;

The investigation is conducted in compliance with the requirements for institutional review set forth in 21 CFR 56 and with the requirements for informed consent set forth in 21 CFR 50; and

The investigation is conducted in compliance with the requirements of 21 CFR 312.7.

Targeted Medical Pharma, Inc.'s clinical investigations of (b)(4) failed to meet at least the first criterion. The investigational drug (b)(4), used to conduct Protocols (b)(4) and (b)(4), was a new, unapproved drug, administered to human subjects twice daily over 28 days to (b)(4). (b)(4) is not a lawfully marketed drug product in the United States and therefore was not exempt from the IND requirements. Before using (b)(4) in a clinical investigation, Targeted Medical Pharma, Inc., was required to submit an IND to FDA, and to have an IND in effect under 21 CFR 312.40. FDA records indicate that Targeted Medical Pharma, Inc., failed to submit an IND before conducting the clinical investigations with (b)(4) under Protocols (b)(4) and (b)(4).

In your July 18, 2016, written response to the Form FDA 483, you stated, "(b)(4) is a Medical Food used to treat the nutritional deficiencies associated with pain and inflammation. It is not, nor has ever been our intention to apply for a NDA or market (b)(4) as a drug."

The Orphan Drug Act defines medical food as "a food which is formulated to be consumed or administered enterally under the supervision of a physician and which is intended for the specific dietary management of a disease or condition for which distinctive nutritional requirements, based on recognized scientific principles, are established by medical evaluation" [21 U.S.C. 360ee(b)(3)].

The protocols discussed above were designed to investigate the (b)(4). There are, however, no distinctive nutritional requirements for individuals with (b)(4). Thus, this product is not a medical food under 21 U.S.C. 360ee(b)(3).[1]

Furthermore, the FD&C Act defines the term drug (in relevant part) as "articles intended for use in the diagnosis, cure, mitigation, treatment, or prevention of disease" and "articles (other than food) intended to affect the structure or any function of the body of man or other animals" [21 U.S.C. 321(g)]. We note that (b)(4) is the study product for Protocols (b)(4) and (b)(4), and that both protocols specify that the clinical endpoint is to examine the "(b)(4)" compared to a nonsteroidal anti-inflammatory drug (NSAID).

Because Targeted Medical Pharma, Inc., was studying the effects of (b)(4) to (b)(4), (b)(4) is an article intended for use in the diagnosis, cure, mitigation, treatment, or prevention of disease and is intended to affect the structure or any function of the human body, and thus meets the definition of a drug under the FD&C Act. As a result, Targeted Medical Pharma, Inc., was required to submit an IND and not to initiate clinical investigations of (b)(4) in human subjects until the IND was in effect.

In your July 18, 2016, written response, you also indicated that a Targeted Medical Pharma, Inc., employee reached out to the FDA before the initiation of the clinical studies and was advised, "although these were Medical Foods and no NDA would be applied for, Targeted Medical Pharma should still apply for an IND." You stated that a Form FDA 1571 and a Form FDA 1572 were submitted to the Agency for each protocol; however, no response was received by FDA.

We are unable to undertake an informed evaluation of your written response because you have not provided documentation to confirm FDA receipt of an IND submission for (b)(4). When FDA receives an IND, FDA assigns an IND number to the application and forwards the application to the appropriate reviewing division within the Office of New Drugs. The review division would have sent a letter to Targeted Medical Pharma, Inc., providing notification of the IND number assigned, date of receipt of the original application, address where future submissions to the IND should be sent, and the name and telephone number of the FDA contact person to whom questions about the application should be directed.

There are no FDA records to indicate that Targeted Medical Pharma, Inc., submitted an IND application before conducting the investigations under Protocols (b)(4) and (b)(4), a clinical investigation of (b)(4). We note that 129 human subjects were enrolled at 11 clinical sites for Protocol (b)(4), and that 122 human subjects were enrolled at 8 clinical sites for Protocol (b)(4). Subjects were treated with (b)(4), an unapproved product, twice daily over 28 days for the (b)(4). As a sponsor, Targeted Medical Pharma, Inc., should have obtained an IND before initiating Protocols (b)(4) and (b)(4) and before enrolling human subjects into both protocols.

This letter is not intended to be an all-inclusive list of deficiencies with your clinical study of an investigational drug. It is your responsibility to ensure adherence to each requirement of the law and relevant FDA regulations. You should address these deficiencies and establish procedures to ensure that any ongoing or future studies will be in compliance with FDA regulations.

Within fifteen (15) working days of your receipt of this letter, you should notify this office in writing of the actions you have taken to prevent similar violations in the future. Failure to explain the violations noted above adequately and promptly may result in regulatory action without further notice.

If you have any questions, please contact Adam Donat at 301-796-5316; FAX 301-847-8748. Your written response and any pertinent documentation should be addressed to:

Adam Donat, M.S.
Branch Chief
Compliance Enforcement Branch
Division of Enforcement and Postmarketing Safety
Office of Scientific Investigations
Office of Compliance
Center for Drug Evaluation and Research
Food and Drug Administration
Building 51, Room 5352
10903 New Hampshire Avenue
Silver Spring, MD 20993

Sincerely yours,

{See appended electronic signature page}

David C. Burrow, Pharm.D., J.D.
Office Director (Acting)
Office of Scientific Investigations
Office of Compliance
Center for Drug Evaluation and Research
Food and Drug Administration

[1]See also 21 CFR 101.9(j)(8) and the guidance for industry Frequently Asked Questions about Medical Foods; Second Edition, May 2016, available at https://www.fda.gov/downloads/Food/GuidanceRegulation/GuidanceDocumentsRegulatoryInformation/UCM500094.pdf.

This is a representation of an electronic record that was signed electronically and this page is the manifestation of the electronic signature.

/S/

DAVID C BURROW
03/29/2017

第35封　给Oeyama-Moto医疗集团基金会有限责任公司的警告信

2016年3月29日

参考号：16-HFD-45-03-02

尊敬的Liao博士：

2015年8月11日至9月29日，Uttaniti Limchumroon先生、Greg Keshishyan先生和Quynh-Van Tran女士代表FDA，在Oeyama-Moto 医疗集团基金会（Oeyama-Moto）进行了现场检查。这封警告信特告知您现场检查中发现的违规情况。此次现场检查的目的是为了核实（b）(4）作为申办者开展试验药物为（b）(4）临床研究“（b）(4）”的情况。

此次现场检查是FDA的生物研究监查项目的一部分，该项目通过设定的检查方法，对FDA所监管的研究的实施情况进行评估，以确认研究数据在科学上是有效和准确的，并帮助确保这些研究中受试者的权益、安全和福利得到了保护。

在现场检查结束时，Limchumroon 先生和 Keshishyan先生向您出示了FDA483表，即现场检查发现的问题，并与您进行了讨论。您2015年10月12日对该FDA483表的书面回复已收悉。

经对现场检查报告、该报告的附件，以及您2015年10月12日的书面回复进行审查，我们认为，您没有遵守适用的法律要求和监管临床研究实施并保护受试者的FDA法规。我们想强调以下几点：

1. 您违反了临床试验暂停通知，在FDA下令推迟某项申请开展的研究之后，仍然允许一名临床研究者向受试者发放了试验药物［21 CFR312.42（a）］

临床试验暂停是由FDA向申办者颁布的命令，要求推迟一项申请开展的临床研究或者暂停一项正在进行的研究。临床试验暂停的命令可以适用于IND下属的一个或多个研究。当一项申请开展的研究被处以临床试验暂停时，不得将该试验药物发放给受试者。

在2012年12月5日召开的电话会议上，您的IND 申请［IND（b）(4）］，其中包含了此次被现场检查的研究，被处以了全面临床试验暂停，原因是对于受试者有不合理且显著的疾病风险或伤害，并且没有充分的信息来评估申请开展的研究对受试者的风险［21 CFR 312.42（b）(2）(ⅰ）］。作为该电话会议的后续跟进，FDA给您发送了日期为2012年12月20日的全面临床试验暂停函，在信中FDA 反复强调了IND（b）(4）下属的任何研究都不得启动或恢复，并阐明了对该IND处以临床试验暂停的以下原因：

- 对受试者风险评估的信息不充分[21 CFR 312.42（b）(2）(ⅰ）]；
- 对受试者有不合理且显著的疾病风险或伤害［21 CFR 312.42（b）(2）(ⅰ）］；
- 试验计划或者试验方案在设计上有缺陷，不能达到它阐明的目标[21 CFR 312.42（b）(2）(ⅱ）]；
- 研究者手册有误导性、错误的或材料上的不完整［21 CFR 312.42（b）(2）(ⅰ）］。

FDA于2013年8月13日签署了继续临床试验全面暂停函，说明尚无正当理由解除临床试验暂停。基于对您递交资料的跟踪审查，FDA于2014年5月9日签署了一封解除全面临床试验暂停信，允许您可以启动IND（b）(4）下属的临床研究。

您违背了全面临床试验暂停的命令，因为一位临床研究者将试验药物（b）(4）给予了处于临床试验停止期间研究的6位受试者。具体而言，受试者L-3和L-10于2014年5月3日接受了试验药物；受试者L-5，L-6，L-7和L-8于2014年5月7日接受了试验药物。所有这些受试者都在2014年5月9日解除临床试验暂停之前接受了试验药物。

在2015年10月12日对FDA483表的书面回复中，您提及您于2014年3月24日或其前后提交了2期试验方案，并且您一直与血液和肿瘤产品监管项目经理办公室保持紧密的联系，他们"和我们沟通并暗示我们，如果我们没有在30日内接到驳回通知，则我们可在2014年5月初开展研究"。您还提及在FDA1571表上的陈述：您同意在FDA收到该IND后30天后才开展研究，除非您收到FDA的提前通知，说研究可以开始了。您的解释是您因此"在2014年5月的第1周积累了受试者来开始这项临床研究"，并让受试者签署了知情同意文件。但是，您表示为了防止受试者改变参与研究的想法，试验药物没有给其使用。

您的书面回复是不充分的，因为尽管您如此陈述，但是试验记录显示，以上提及的6位受试者在2014年5月9日解除临床试验暂停之前都接受了试验药物。您的书面回复是不充分的，还因为您未能提供一个纠正措施计划，以避免将来发生类似违规。

2. 您未能确保对临床研究进行适当的监查［21 CFR 312.50 和 312.56（a）］

FDA的法规要求申办者对临床研究确保恰当的监查，并确保临床研究者按照IND中的总体研究计划和方案进行临床研究。我们发现贵方并没有确保适当的监查，因为没有与被检查研究相关的任何监查记录。

在您所署日期为2015年10月12日对FDA483表的书面回复中，您表明是通过IRB来监查试验进程，并将其记录在IRB会议记录中。

您的书面回复是不充分的，因为IRB不能承担申办者的职能去确保对临床研究进行适当的监查。另外，请注意，申办者是可以将自己对研究进行监查的责任转交给合同研究组织的，但是任何这样的责任转交都应当以书面方式描述［21 CFR 312.52］。

本警告信的目的并非是罗列您在试验药物临床研究中存在的所有缺陷。确保遵循法律和相关FDA法规的每一项要求是您的职责，您应当解决这些缺陷，并建立规程，以确保任何正在进行或将来进行的研究均符合FDA的法规。

自收到这封信的15个工作日内，您应当书面告知本办公室为预防将来发生类似违规情况而采取的措施。如果不能充分、迅速地解释上述违规问题，可能导致我们在不再通知的情况下采取监管措施。如果您认为您已经遵循了FDA的法规要求，请陈述理由，并提供所有支持资料，以供我们参考。

附：英文原文

Oeyama-Moto Medical Group Foundation, LLC

WARNING LETTER

MAR 29, 2016

CERTIFIED MAIL
RETURN RECEIPT REQUESTED

Ref. 16-HFD-45-03-02

BenedictS. Liao, M.D. Sponsor Representative
Oeyama-Moto Medical Group Foundation
3106 East Garvey Avenue South
West Covina,California 91791-2344

Dear Dr. Liao:

This Warning Letter informs you of objectionable conditions observed during the U.S. Food and Drug Administration (FDA) inspection conducted at Oeyama-Moto Medical Group Foundation (Oeyama-Moto) between August 11 and September 29, 2015, by Mr. Uttaniti Limchumroon, Mr. Greg Keshishyan, and Ms. Quynh-Van Tran, representing FDA. The purpose of this inspection was to review (b)(4) conduct as the sponsor of a clinical investigation ["(b)(4)"] for the investigational drug (b)(4).

This inspection is a part of FDA's Bioresearch Monitoring Program, which includes inspections designed to evaluate the conduct of FDA-regulated research to ensure that the data are scientifically valid and accurate, and to help ensure that the rights, safety, and welfare of the human subjects of those studies have been protected.

At the conclusion of the inspection, Mr. Limchumroon and Mr. Keshishyan presented and discussed with you Form FDA 483, Inspectional Observations. We acknowledge receipt of your October 12, 2015, written response to the Form FDA 483.

From our review of the FDA Establishment Inspection Report, the documents submitted with that report, and your October 12, 2015, written response, we conclude that you did not adhere to the applicable statutory requirements and FDA regulations governing the conduct of clinical investigations and the protection of human subjects. We wish to emphasize the following:

1. You violated a clinical hold by allowing a clinical investigator to give subjects an investigational drug after FDA issued an order to delay a proposed investigation [21 CFR 312.42(a)].

A clinical hold is an order issued by FDA to the sponsor to delay a proposed clinical investigation or to suspend an ongoing investigation. The clinical hold order may apply to one or more of the investigations covered by an IND. When a proposed study is placed on clinical hold, subjects may not be given the investigational drug.

Your IND application (IND (b)(4)), which contained the inspected study, was placed on Full Clinical Hold during a teleconference on December 5, 2012, for unreasonable and significant risk of illness or injury to human subjects, and for insufficient information to assess risks to subjects of the proposed study [21 CFR 312.42(b)(2)(i)]. As a follow-up to this teleconference, FDA sent you a Full Clinical Hold Letter dated December 20, 2012, in which FDA reiterated that no studies under IND (b)(4) could be initiated or resumed, and delineated the following reasons for placing the IND on clinical hold:

Insufficient information to assess risks to human subjects [21 CFR 312.42(b)(2)(i)]

Unreasonable and significant risk of illness or injury to human subjects [21 CFR 312.42(b)(2)(i)]

Plan or protocol is deficient in design to meet its stated objectives [21 CFR 312.42(b)(2)(ii)]

Investigator brochure is misleading, erroneous, or materially incomplete [21 CFR 312.42(b)(2)(i)]

FDA issued a Continue Full Clinical Hold Letter dated August 13, 2013, stating that the removal of the clinical hold was unwarranted. Based on a subsequent review of your submissions, FDA issued a Remove Full Clinical Hold Letter dated May 9, 2014, which permitted you to initiate the clinical investigation under IND (b)(4).

You violated the Full Clinical Hold order when a clinical investigator administered the investigational drug (b)(4) to six subjects participating in an investigation that was currently subject to a clinical hold. Specifically, Subjects L-3 and L-10 received investigational drug on May 3, 2014; and Subjects L-5, L-6, L-7, and L-8 received investigational drug on May 7, 2014. All of these subjects received investigational drug before the clinical hold was removed on May 9, 2014.

In your October 12, 2015, written response to the Form FDA 483, you indicated that you submitted the Phase 2 study protocol on or about March 24, 2014, and that you were in constant contact with the Office of Hematology and Oncology Products Regulatory Project Manager, who "communicated with us and hinted to us that if we did not receive rejection within 30 days, then we can proceed with the Study in early May 2014." You also referred to the statement on the Form FDA 1571 in which you agreed not to begin the study until thirty days after FDA's receipt of the IND unless you received earlier notification by FDA that the study may begin. You explained that you therefore "piled up patients to begin this clinical Study in the first week of May 2014" and had subjects sign informed consent documents. However, you stated that study drug was not administered, in case subjects changed their minds about participating in the study.

Your written response is inadequate because study records show that the six subjects noted above received investigational drug before the clinical hold was removed on May 9, 2014, despite your statement otherwise. Your written response is also inadequate because you have not provided a corrective action plan to prevent the recurrence of similar violations in the future.

2. You failed to ensure proper monitoring of the clinical investigations [21 CFR 312.50 and 312.56(a)].

FDA regulations require that sponsors ensure proper monitoring of clinical investigations and ensure that their clinical investigators conduct the investigations in accordance with the general investigational plan and the protocols contained in the IND application. Our investigation found that you failed to ensure proper monitoring because there are no monitoring records associated with the inspected study.

In your October 12, 2015, written response to the Form FDA 483, you indicated that you monitored the progress of the study through your Institutional Review Board (IRB) and documented this in the IRB meeting minutes.

Your written response is inadequate because an IRB cannot assume the sponsor's responsibility to ensure proper monitoring of clinical investigations. In addition, please note that a sponsor may transfer its obligation to monitor a study to a contract research organization. Any such transfer of obligations shall be described in writing [21 CFR 312.52].

This letter is not intended to be an all-inclusive list of deficiencies with your clinical study of an investigational drug. It is your responsibility to ensure adherence to each requirement of the law and relevant FDA regulations. You should address these deficiencies and establish procedures to ensure that any ongoing or future studies will be in compliance with FDA regulations.

Within fifteen (15) working days of your receipt of this letter, you should notify this office in writing of the actions you have taken to prevent similar violations in the future. Failure to explain the violations noted above adequately and promptly may result in regulatory action without further notice. If you believe that you have complied with FDA regulations, include your reasoning and any supporting information for our consideration.

If you have any questions, please contact Douglas B. Pham, Pharm.D., J.D., at 301-796-1955; FAX 301-847-8748. Your written response and any pertinent documentation should be addressed to:

Douglas B. Pham, Pharm.D., J.D.
Branch Chief (Acting)
Compliance Enforcement Branch
Division of Enforcement and Postmarketing Safety
Office of Scientific Investigations
Office of Compliance
Center for Drug Evaluation and Research
U.S. Food and Drug Administration
Building 51, Room 5348
10903 New Hampshire Avenue
Silver Spring, MD 20993

Sincerely yours,

{See appended electronic signature page}

David C. Burrow, Pharm.D., J.D.
Office Director (Acting)
Office of Scientific Investigations
Office of Compliance
Center for Drug Evaluation and Research
U.S. Food and Drug Administration

第36封　给AB Science的警告信

2015年6月16日

参考号：15-HFD-45-06-01

尊敬的Moussay先生：

2014年9月22日至9月26日，Barbara Wright女士、NiA.Khin医学博士和Michelle Safarik，MSPAS，PA-C，RAC代表FDA进行了现场检查，对AB Science作为申办者开展的试验药物为（b）(4)[1]的以下临床研究进行了现场检查：试验方案（b）(4)，“（b）(4)”；试验方案（b）(4)，“（b）(4)”和试验方案（b）(4)，“（b）(4)”。

这封警告信特告知您现场检查中发现的违规情况。

本次现场检查是FDA的生物研究监查项目的一部分。该项目通过设定的检查方法来评估由FDA监管的相关研究的实施情况，以确认研究数据从科学上是有效和准确的，并帮助确保这些研究中受试者的权益、安全和福利得到了保护。

在现场检查结束时，Wright女士向您出示了FDA483表，即现场检查发现的问题，并与您进行了讨论。您2014年10月10日对该FDA483表的书面回复已收悉。

经对现场检查报告、该报告的附件，以及您2014年10月10日的书面回复进行审查，我们认为，您没有遵循适用的法律要求和监管临床研究实施及受试者保护的FDA法规。我们想强调以下几点：

您未能确保对临床研究进行适当的监查，未能按照IND中的总体研究计划和方案进行临床研究［21 CFR 312.50和312.56（a）］

1. FDA法规要求申办者应确保对临床研究进行适当的监查，并确保临床研究者们依照包含在IND申请中的方案来实施临床研究。

我们的调查发现，您未能确保对试验方案（b）(4)，（b）(4）和（b）(4）实施适当的监查，并且未能确保临床研究者们依照此三个方案实施临床研究。由于您监查不力，临床研究者未按照方案规定的时限报告严重不良事件（SAEs），未进行方案规定的实验室检查，您的监查未能发现并及时纠正。

示例包括但不限于以下内容：

a. 临床研究者未在方案规定的时限内报告SAEs，您的监查未能发现并予以纠正。

试验方案（b）(4）和（b）(4）规定，无论发生的SAE是否被判定与研究药物的使用具有相关性，都需要填写SAE表格，并在发生或者研究者获知24小时内传真给申办者，即使事件看起来不具有治疗相关性仍需要报告。两个方案均定义SAEs为非预期的医学事件，在任何剂量导致死亡、危及生命，需住院治疗或延长住院时间，导致持续的或显著的伤残或影响工作能力，导致先天畸形或出生缺陷，或者其他的重大医学事件，可能影响受试者的健康或者需要干预，以预防以上任何一种情况的发生。试验方案（b）(4）对SAEs的定义中还包括肿瘤的发生。以下的SAEs未能依照方案要求在发生或者研究者获知24小时内报告，监查员未能在监查报告中进行确认。

i. 试验方案（b）(4）受试者03102在2009年5月4日发生了血小板减少，但是试验场所直到2013年4月30日才通过SAE表将血小板减少报告给申办者。

ii. 试验方案（b）(4）受试者03111在2010年6月8日发生了白细胞和中性粒细胞减少，但是试验场所直到

1 (b)(4) 涉及商业秘密，根据法规内容不予公开。

2013年5月2日才通过SAE表将白细胞和中性粒细胞减少报告给申办者。

ⅲ. 试验方案（b）（4）受试者03303因腹痛加重（肠系膜上静脉血栓形成）住院，但是试验场所未使用SAE表报告住院情况。

ⅳ. 试验方案（b）（4）受试者1302住院，并因三级贫血而在（b）（6）接受了输血治疗，一名助理研究者在2010年1月13日的病程记录中记载了受试者住院的情况。试验场所直到2010年8月26日才通过SAE表报告给申办者。

ⅴ. 试验方案（b）（4）受试者1311因膝关节炎合并静脉炎发作进行了手术治疗，研究者在2013年3月15日的病程记录中记载了该受试者的手术，然而，试验场所直到2013年4月10日才通过SAE表将住院情况报告给申办者。

2014年10月10日对FDA483表的书面回复中，您承认这些问题并说明研究者未遵守SAE报告要求。您还指出申办者的监查工作是不充分的，未能发现以上这些研究者的不合规行为。您提出将在2014年第四季度实施纠正措施，包括基于风险的监查培训，重点是SAE和关键不良事件。您提到将在2014年底之前对监查员和试验场所所有参与人员进行安全报告的培训。您的书面回复是不充分的，因为您提到的纠正措施未包含对于培训有效性的评估以及确保监查活动的持续合规性。

b. 有一位临床研究者未能进行方案要求的实验室检查，您的监查未能发现予以纠正。

ⅰ. 试验方案（b）（4）要求对法国的受试者在筛选，基线：1，2，3，4，5，6，7，8，10和12周，后续每4周一次；直到研究结束或末次访视，都需要进行血液学检查。该血液学实验室检查包括红细胞压积和血红蛋白，红细胞计数，白细胞计数和分类，包括中性粒细胞、淋巴细胞、单核细胞、嗜酸性粒细胞、嗜碱性粒细胞，血小板计数，凝血酶原时间，部分凝血活酶时间和国际标准化比值。血液学实验室检查是该研究的安全性评价指标，用于监测（b）（4）相关的不良事件，如中性粒细胞减少，基于发生的严重程度，可能导致药物中断或者停药。不能及时地诊断中性粒细胞减少，受试者将有发生严重感染和脓毒症的风险。因此，遗漏的血液学实验室检查损害了受试者的安全。

以下方案规定的血液学检查未进行，监查员未在检查访视中进行确认。

1）第1周：受试者 033-008-01和033-008-02。

2）第5周：受试者 033-008-05。

3）第6周：受试者 033-008-05。

4）第7周：受试者 033-008-05。

ⅱ. 试验方案（b）（4）要求受试者在筛选，基线：4，8，12，16周，后续每12周一次；直到并包括研究结束或末次访视，都需要进行尿试纸检查，该实验室检查包括红细胞计数、白细胞计数和尿蛋白，如果尿蛋白≥30mg/dL，则需要进行24小时尿蛋白检测。尿试纸检测是该研究的安全性评价指标，用于监测（b）（4）相关的肾功能障碍，研究方案要求基于尿试纸检测尿蛋白≥30mg/dL，并经24小时尿蛋白检测确认＞1.5g的次数，受试者（b）（4）用药将暂停、减量或者停止。因此，未进行方案规定的尿试纸检测，会损害受试者的安全，因为受试者可能会发生（b）（4）相关的肾功能障碍。

受试者033-008-02第36周的尿试纸检测到尿蛋白达到30mg/dL。该受试者未能基于30mg/dL的检测结果完成方案要求的24小时尿蛋白检测，而在监查报告中未记录这个方案违背。您在2014年10月10日对于FDA483表的书面回复中提到，您已经获知了1.b.中提到的问题。您提出2014年10月起将会实施纠正措施，包括建立基于风险的监查策略，质量文件将会更新，AB science的员工和研究者也将会进行相应培训。您指出2014年第四季度起，当地实验室的检测结果将会立即录入到CRF中和发出质疑。

您的书面回复是不充分的，因为所提出的纠正措施未能体现对于您的监查活动有效性的评估，并确保您的监查工作能检查出与安全性评估相关的实验室检查，如血常规和尿常规是否已经按照试验方案要求的时间点实施。您未能确保对这些临床研究进行了适当的监查，因为您未能发现和纠正临床研究者在试验方案规定的时限内未能报告SAEs，未能进行试验方案规定的实验室检查，因此，您未能确认并予以纠正，结果是您未能确保临床研究按照研究计划进行。

2. 由于您未按照您建立的监查计划实施监查，您未能确保INDs中的临床研究得到适当的监查。

a. 您的关于试验方案（b）（4）和（b）（4）的监查指南中要求临床研究检查员（CRA）撰写监查报告，并且在规定的时间内由临床项目经理（CPM）审查批准。然而，有些监查报告未能在监查指南规定的时间内完成和得到批准，有些监查报告根本没有完成。举例包括但不限于以下内容：

i. 遵照试验方案（b）（4）的监查指南，临时的/周期性的监查报告应当在完成监查访视的5个工作日内完成，并由CPM在收到后10个工作日内审查。

1）试验场所31

- 2009年1月22日试验场所启动的访视监查报告应在访视后5个工作日内完成，但是直到2009年3月4日才完成。而CPM的审批直到FDA实施检查时在2014年9月20日才完成。
- 2010年7月8日的监查报告直到2012年11月2日才完成，直到2014年9月FDA检查时CPM才审查。
- 2012年6月19日试验场所关闭访视的监查报告，直到2012年11月2日才完成；并且以下登记在监查日志的访视无监查报告：2009年8月10日，2010年6月7日，2010年11月16日。

2）试验场所33

2009年3月4日的监查报告CPM直到2014年9月FDA检查时才完成审查。

2010年8月30日的监查报告直到2012年11月1日才完成，CPM直到2014年9月FDA检查才完成审查。

2012年5月31日试验场所关闭访视的监查报告直到2012年11月2日才完成，CPM直到FDA检查时才完成审查；并且以下的登记在访视日志上的访视无监查报告：2010年4月2日和2011年6月29~30日。

3）试验场所34

2012年6月28日的试验场所关闭访视监查报告直到2012年10月20日才完成，CPM直到2014年9月FDA核查时才完成审查。

以下登记在监查日志中的访视无监查报告：2009年11月11日和2011年4月29日。

ii. 按照试验方案（b）（4）的监查准则，监查报告应当在完成监查访视的5个工作日内完成，并由CPM在收到后5个工作日内审查。

1）试验场所004

- 以下登记在访视日志上的访视无监查报告：2012年10月19日和2012年11月20日。
- 以下的访视报告未在访视后5个工作日内完成：

访视日期	CRA签署监查报告日期
2013年4月11日	2013年7月1日
2013年5月14日	2013年7月1日
2014年6月11~12日	2014年7月16日
2014年7月29~30日	2014年9月16日

- 以下的监查报告CPM未能在监查指南规定的5个工作日内完成审查：

访视日期	CRA签署监查报告日期	CPM签署监查报告的日期
2012年9月18日	2012年10月4日	2012年11月13日
2012年12月19日	2013年1月13日	2013年8月26日

2）试验场所008

- 以下的访视报告未在访视后5个工作日内完成：

访视日期	CRA签署监查报告日期
2012年11月26日	2013年1月30日
2013年4月9日	2013年9月16日
2013年7月27日	2013年7月16日
2014年7月24-25日	2014年9月16日

- 以下的监查报告CPM未能在监查准则规定的5个工作日内完成审查：

访视日期	CRA签署监查报告日期	CPM签署监查报告的日期
2012年9月21日	2012年10月4日	2013年1月21日
2012年10月2日	2012年10月4日	2013年10月21日
2012年11月21日	2012年11月22日	2013年1月21日
2013年7月27日	2013年9月16日	未签署

2014年10月10日您对FDA483表的书面回复提到，您已经获知以上情况，您声明在2013年1月之前没有电子系统用于跟踪报告完成的时间。您指出自2013年1月起建立了用于跟踪监查电子跟踪系统访视和检查报告审查。您提到CRA会收到自动的邮件提醒，并且CPM和AB science管理团队会每月校对一次。

您的书面回复是不充分的，因为在2013年1月之后，仍然有多次的CRA书写报告的延误以及CPM的审查延误。

b. 研究方案（b）（4）的AB Science 监查指南中要求监查员从试验场所获取实验室结果并提交给数据管理团队。然而，您未能遵照监查指南要求，未收集和递交大量的实验室结果给数据管理团队。例子包括但不限于以下内容：

ⅰ. 受试者033-004-02，第1，5，6，8，10和20周的实验室结果未提交给数据管理团队。

ⅱ. 受试者033-004-03，第2，3，4，5，6，7和10周的实验室结果未提交给数据管理团队。

ⅲ. 受试者033-004-04，基线和第1，2，3，5，6，7，8，10，16，20和24周的实验室结果未提交给数据管理团队。

ⅳ. 受试者033-004-05，第5，20和24周的实验室结果未提交给数据管理团队。

ⅴ. 受试者033-004-06，第1，4，24和36周的实验室结果未提交给数据管理团队。

ⅵ. 受试者033-008-04，基线和第1，2，3，4和8周的实验室结果未提交给数据管理团队。

ⅶ. 受试者033-008-07，基线和第1，5，6，7，8，10，12和16周的实验室结果未提交给数据管理团队。

2014年10月10日您对FDA483表的书面回复显示，您已经获知这个的情况。您提出计划于2014年第四季度实施纠正措施，本实验室的结果将会及时地收集在eCRF表中并发出质疑，并且您还将继续在Ⅲ期试验中使用中心实验室来管理安全性信息。您的书面回复是不充分的，因为您提出的纠正措施未能提供措施有效性的评估并且确保您的监查活动持续合规。

我们已经获知，由于2.b.ⅳ（受试者033-004-05）和2.b.ⅴ（受试者033-004-06）的不合规事项未包含在给您的FDA483表中，因此，书面回复未对此两项进行解释。

本警告信的目的并非是罗列您在试验药物临床研究中存在的所有缺陷。确保遵循法律和相关FDA法规的每一项要求是您的职责，您应当解决所存在的问题，并建立规程，以确保任何正在进行或将来进行的研究均符合FDA法规。

自收到这封信的15个工作日内，您应当书面告知本办公室为预防将来发生类似违规情况而采取的措施。如果不能充分、迅速地解释上述违规问题，可能导致我们在不再通知的情况下采取监管措施。如果您认为您已经遵循了FDA的法规要求，请陈述理由，并提供所有支持资料，以供我们参考。

附：英文原文

AB Science

WARNING LETTER

Jun 16, 2015

CERTIFIED MAIL
RETURN RECEIPT REQUESTED

Ref: 15-HFD-45-06-01

Alain Moussy
Chief Executive Officer
AB Science
3 Avenue George V
Paris, France

Dear Mr. Moussy:

This Warning Letter informs you of objectionable conditions observed during the U.S. Food and Drug Administration (FDA) inspection conducted at AB Science between September 22 and September 26, 2014. Ms. Barbara Wright, Ni A. Khin, M.D., and Michelle Safarik, MSPAS, PA-C, RAC, representing the FDA, reviewed AB Science's conduct as the sponsor of the following clinical investigations for investigational drug **(b)(4)**:

- Protocol **(b)(4)**, "**(b)(4)**";
- Protocol **(b)(4)**, "**(b)(4)**"; and
- Protocol **(b)(4)**, "**(b)(4)**."

This inspection is a part of FDA's Bioresearch Monitoring Program, which includes inspections designed to evaluate the conduct of FDA-regulated research to ensure that the data are scientifically valid and accurate, and to help ensure that the rights, safety, and welfare of the human subjects of those studies have been protected.

At the conclusion of the inspection, Ms. Wright presented and discussed with you Form FDA 483, Inspectional Observations. We acknowledge receipt of your October 10, 2014 written response to the Form FDA 483.

From our review of the FDA Establishment Inspection Report, the documents submitted with that report, and your October 10, 2014 written response, we conclude that you did not adhere to the applicable statutory requirements and FDA regulations governing the conduct of clinical investigations and the protection of human subjects. We wish to emphasize the following:

Failure to ensure proper monitoring of the investigations and failure to ensure that the investigations are conducted in accordance with the general investigational plan and protocols contained in the IND [21 CFR 312.50 and 312.56(a)].

1. FDA regulations require that sponsors ensure proper monitoring of clinical investigations and ensure that their clinical investigators conduct the investigations in accordance with the protocols contained in the Investigational New Drug (IND) application. Our investigation found that you failed to ensure proper monitoring of Protocols **(b)(4)**, **(b)(4)**, and **(b)(4)**, and failed to ensure that clinical investigators conducted investigations in accordance with those three protocols. As a result of your inadequate monitoring, you did not identify, and did not correct in a timely manner, the clinical investigators' failure to report serious adverse events (SAEs) according to protocol-specified timeframes and failure to perform protocol-required laboratory tests. Examples include but are not limited to the following:

a. Your monitoring failed to identify and correct clinical investigators' failure to report SAEs within protocol-specified timeframes.

Protocols **(b)(4)** and **(b)(4)** require that SAEs, whether or not considered related to study drug, be reported on an

SAE form and faxed to the sponsor within 24 hours of occurrence or the investigator's knowledge of the event. Reporting is required even if the event does not appear to be treatment-related. Both protocols define an SAE as any untoward medical occurrence that at any dose results in death, is life-threatening, requires inpatient hospitalization or prolongation of existing hospitalization, results in persistent or significant disability/incapacity; is a congenital anomaly/birth defect, or is another important medical condition that may jeopardize the subject's health or may require intervention to prevent one of the preceding outcomes. Protocol **(b)(4)** also includes emergence of cancer in the definition of an SAE.

The following SAEs were not reported within 24 hours of the occurrence or the investigator's knowledge of the event in accordance with the protocol, and were not identified by the monitor in monitoring visit reports:

i. Subject 03102 in Protocol **(b)(4)** experienced thrombocytopenia on May 4, 2009, but the site did not report the thrombocytopenia to the sponsor on an SAE form until April 30, 2013.

ii. Subject 03111 in Protocol **(b)(4)** experienced leukopenia and neutropenia on June 8, 2010, but the site did not report the leukopenia and neutropenia to the sponsor on an SAE form until May 2, 2013.

iii. Subject 03303 in Protocol **(b)(4)** was hospitalized for worsening abdominal pain (superior mesenteric vein thrombosis) **(b)(6)**, but the site failed to report the hospitalization on an SAE form.

iv.Subject 1302 in Protocol **(b)(4)** was hospitalized and received blood transfusions for grade 3 anemia on **(b)(6)**. A sub-investigator noted the subject's hospitalization in a progress note dated January 13, 2010. However, the site did not report the hospitalization to the sponsor on an SAE form until August 26, 2010.

v. Subject 1311 in Protocol **(b)(4)** had surgery **(b)(6)**, for knee arthritis complicated by an episode of phlebitis. The investigator noted the subject's surgery in a progress note dated March 15, 2013. However, the site did not report the hospitalization to the sponsor on an SAE form until April 10, 2013.

In the October 10, 2014 written response to the Form FDA 483, you acknowledged these observations and stated that investigators did not respect the SAE reporting requirements. You also indicated that sponsor monitoring activities were inadequate to detect non-compliance by investigators as described above. You proposed a corrective action plan for implementation in the fourth quarter of 2014 which included training on risk-based monitoring with a focus on **(b)(4)** SAEs and key adverse events. You noted that you would also train monitors and site staff on safety reporting before the end of 2014. Your written response is inadequate because your proposed corrective actions make no provisions for assessing the effectiveness of and ensuring sustained compliance with your monitoring practices.

b. Your monitoring failed to identify and correct a clinical investigator's failure to perform protocol-required laboratory tests.

i. Protocol **(b)(4)** requires that subjects in France undergo hematologic laboratory tests at Screening; Baseline; Weeks 1, 2, 3, 4, 5, 6, 7, 8, 10, and 12; and then every four weeks thereafter, up to and including the End of Study/Final Visit. The hematologic laboratory tests include hematocrit and hemoglobin; red blood cell count; total and differential white blood cell counts, including neutrophils, lymphocytes, monocytes, eosinophils, and basophils; platelet count; prothrombin time; partial thromboplastin time; and international normalized ratio. These hematologic laboratory tests are safety assessments in the study because they are used to monitor for **(b)(4)**-related adverse events such as neutropenia, for which subjects will have their dose interrupted or discontinued, depending on its severity. Failure to diagnose neutropenia in a timely manner places subjects at increased risk of developing serious infections and sepsis. Therefore, missed hematologic laboratory tests compromise subject safety.

The following protocol-required hematologic laboratory tests were not performed and were not identified by the monitor during monitoring visits:

1) Week 1 for Subjects 033-008-01 and 033-008-02

2) Week 5 for Subject 033-008-05

3) Week 6 for Subject 033-008-05

4) Week 7 for Subject 033-008-05

ii. Protocol **(b)(4)** requires that urine dipstick be performed at Screening; Baseline; Weeks 4, 8, 12, 16, and 24; and then every 12 weeks thereafter, up to and including the End of Study/Final Visit. The urine dipstick test includes measurement of blood, leukocytes, and protein. A 24-hour urine collection to measure protein is performed if protein ≥30 mg/dL is detected on the dipstick. The urine dipstick test is a safety assessment that is used to monitor for **(b)(4)**-related renal disorders, and the study protocol requires that a subject's **(b)(4)** dose be interrupted, reduced, or discontinued based on the number of times a subject experiences protein ≥30 mg/dL on the dipstick and confirmed by 24hour urinary protein >1.5 g/24 hours. Therefore, missed protocol-required urine dipstick tests compromise subject safety, because subjects can develop **(b)(4)**-related renal disorders.

Subject 033-008-02's urine dipstick measured protein to be 30 mg/dL at Week 36. The subject did not complete the protocol-required 24-hour urine collection based on the 30 mg/dL measurement. This protocol deviation was not noted in monitoring reports.

In the October 10, 2014 written response to the Form FDA 483, you acknowledged the observations described in Item1. b. You proposed a corrective action plan which includes instituting a risk-based monitoring strategy starting in October 2014 with new quality documents and training of AB Science personnel and investigators. You indicated that starting in the fourth quarter of 2014, local laboratory values will be captured and queried immediately at the test site in the CFR.

Your written response is inadequate because the proposed corrective actions make no provisions for assessing the effectiveness of your monitoring practices and ensuring that your monitoring practices will detect whether laboratory tests related to safety assessments such as hematology and urinalysis were performed at protocol-specified time points.

You failed to ensure proper monitoring of these clinical investigations because you did not identify and correct clinical investigators' failure to report SAEs and failure to perform protocol-required laboratory tests within timeframes specified in the protocols. As a result, you have failed to ensure that the clinical investigations were conducted in accordance with the investigational plan.

2. You failed to ensure proper monitoring of the investigations contained in your INDs because you did not follow the monitoring guidelines you developed.

a. Your monitoring guidelines for Protocols **(b)(4)** and **(b)(4)** require that monitoring reports be written by the Clinical Research Associate (CRA) and approved by the Clinical Project Manager (CPM) within specific timeframes. However, some monitoring reports were not completed and approved within the timeframes specified in the monitoring guidelines, and in some instances, were not completed at all. Examples include but are not limited to the following:

ⅰ. According to your monitoring guidelines for Protocol **(b)(4)**, interim/periodic monitoring reports should have been prepared within five business days after the corresponding monitoring visit and approved by the CPM within 10 business days after receipt of the report.

1) At Site 31:

• The monitoring report for the January 22, 2009 site initiation visit should have been completed within five business days after the visit, but it was not completed until March 4, 2009. The report had not been approved by the CPM as of September 2014 when FDA conducted its inspection;

• The monitoring report for the July 8, 2010 visit was not completed until November 2, 2012, and the report had not been approved by the CPM as of September 2014 when FDA conducted its inspection;

• The monitoring report for the June 19, 2012 closeout visit was not completed until November 2, 2012; and

• No corresponding monitoring reports were written for the following dates listed on the Site Visit Log: August 10, 2009, June 7, 2010, and November 16, 2010.

2) At Site 33:

• The monitoring report dated March 4, 2009, had not been approved by the CPM as of September 2014 when FDA conducted its inspection;

• The monitoring report for the August 30, 2010 periodic visit was not completed until November 1, 2012, and the report had not been approved by the CPM as of September 2014 when FDA conducted its inspection;

• The monitoring report for the May 31, 2012 closeout visit was not completed until November 2, 2012, and had not been approved by the CPM as of September 2014 when FDA conducted its inspection; and No corresponding monitoring reports were written for the following dates listed on the Site Visit Log: April 2, 2010 and June 29-30, 2011.

3) At Site 34:

• The monitoring report for the June 28, 2012 closeout visit was not completed until October 20, 2012, and the report had not been approved by the CPM as of September 2014 when FDA conducted its inspection; and

• No corresponding monitoring reports were written for the following dates listed on the Site Visit Log: November 11, 2009, and April 29, 2010.

ii. According to your monitoring guidelines for Protocol **(b)(4)**, monitoring reports should have been prepared within five business days after the corresponding monitoring visit and approved by the CPM within five business days after receipt of the report.

1) At Site 004:

• No corresponding monitoring reports were written for the following dates listed on the Site Visit Log: October 19, 2012 and November 20, 2012;

• The following monitoring reports were not completed within five business days of the monitoring visit:

Date of Monitoring Visit	Date CRA Signed Monitoring Report
April 11, 2013	July 1, 2013
May 14, 2013	July 1, 2013
June 11-12, 2014	July 16, 2014
July 29-30, 2014	September 16, 2014

• The following monitoring reports were not approved by the CPM within five business days in accordance with your monitoring guidelines:

Date of Monitoring Visit	Date CRA Signed Monitoring Report	Date CPM Signed Monitoring Report
September 18, 2012	October 4, 2012	December 13, 2012
December 19, 2012	January 13, 2013	August 26, 2013

2) At Site 008:

• The following monitoring reports were not completed within five business days of the monitoring visit:

Date of Monitoring Visit	Date CRA Signed Monitoring Report
November 26, 2012	January 30, 2013
April 9, 2013	July 1, 2013
June 10, 2013	September 16, 2013
July 27, 2013	September 16, 2013
July 24-25, 2014	September 16, 2014

• The following monitoring reports were not approved by the CPM within five business days in accordance with your monitoring guidelines:

Date of Monitoring Visit	Date CRA Signed Monitoring Report	Date CPM Signed Monitoring Report
September 21, 2012	October 4, 2012	January 21, 2013
October 2, 2012	October 4, 2012	October 21, 2013
November 21, 2012	November 22, 2012	January 21, 2013
July 27, 2013	September 16, 2013	Not Signed

In the October 10, 2014 written response to the Form FDA 483, you acknowledged this observation. You stated that prior to January 2013, there was no electronic system to track reporting timelines. You indicated that an electronic tracking system was implemented in January 2013 to track monitoring visits and monitoring report reviews. You noted that CRAs receive automatic e-mail reminders and reconciliation is done once per month by the CPM and AB

Science management team.

Your written response is inadequate because there are still multiple instances of delayed written reports by the CRAs and delayed approval by the CPM after January 2013.

b. AB Science monitoring guidelines for Protocol **(b)(4)** require that monitors retrieve lab results from sites and submit them to the Data Management team. However, you failed to follow your own monitoring guidelines by not collecting and submitting numerous lab results to the Data Management team. Examples include but are not limited to the following:

i. For Subject 033-004-02, no lab results were submitted to the Data Management team for Weeks 1, 5, 6, 8, 10, and 20.

ii. For Subject 033-004-03, no lab results were submitted to the Data Management team for Weeks 2, 3, 4, 5, 6, 7, and 10.

iii. For Subject 033-004-04, no labs were submitted to the Data Management team for Baseline and Weeks 1, 2, 3, 5, 6, 7, 8, 10, 16, 20, and 24.

iv. For Subject 033-004-05, no lab results were submitted to the Data Management team for Weeks 5, 20, and 24.

v. For Subject 033-004-06, no lab results were submitted to the Data Management team for Weeks 1, 4, 24, and 36.

vi. For Subject 033-008-04, no lab results were submitted to the Data Management team for Baseline and Weeks 1, 2, 3, 4, and 8.

vii. For Subject 033-008-07, no lab results were submitted to the Data Management team for Baseline and Weeks 1, 5, 6, 7, 8, 10, 12, and 16.

In the October 10, 2014 written response to the Form FDA 483, you acknowledged this observation. You proposed a corrective action plan for implementation in the fourth quarter of 2014 where local labs will be captured and queried immediately at the site in the eCRF, and you will continue to use the central lab in phase Ⅲ trials in addition to local labs for managing safety information.

Your written response is inadequate because your proposed corrective actions make no provisions for assessing the effectiveness of and ensuring sustained compliance with your monitoring practices.

We acknowledge that the findings noted in Items 2.b.iv (Subject 033-004-05) and 2.b.v (Subject 033-004-06) were not included on the Form FDA 483 that you received, and therefore, the written response does not address these findings.

This letter is not intended to be an all-inclusive list of deficiencies with your clinical study of an investigational drug. It is your responsibility to ensure adherence to each requirement of the law and relevant FDA regulations. You should address these deficiencies and establish procedures to ensure that any ongoing or future studies will be in compliance with FDA regulations.

Within fifteen (15) working days of your receipt of this letter, you should notify this office in writing of the actions you have taken to prevent similar violations in the future. Failure to address the violations noted above adequately and promptly may result in regulatory action without further notice. If you believe that you have complied with FDA regulations, include your reasoning and any supporting information for our consideration.

If you have any questions, please contact Khin M. U, M.D., at 301-796-1156; Fax 301-847-8748. Your written response and any pertinent documentation should be addressed to:

Khin M. U, M.D.
Acting Branch Chief
Compliance Enforcement Branch
Division of Enforcement and Postmarketing Safety
Office of Scientific Investigations
Office of Compliance
Center for Drug Evaluation and Research
Food and Drug Administration
Building 51, Room 5210
10903 New Hampshire Avenue

Silver Spring, MD 20993

Sincerely yours,

{See appended electronic signature page}

Sean Y. Kassim, Ph.D.
Office Director
Office of Scientific Investigations
Office of Compliance
Center for Drug Evaluation and Research
Food and Drug Administration

第37封　给美国CXL有限责任公司的警告信

2015年4月1日
参考号：15-HFD-45-04-01

尊敬的Rubinfeld博士：

2014年8月18日至8月19日，Cynthia Harris女士代表FDA，在美国CXL有限责任公司进行了现场检查，对CXL-USA作为申办者开展的临床试验［试验方案（b）（4）］进行了审查。这封警告信特告知您现场检查中发现的违规情况。

本次现场检查是FDA的生物研究监查项目的一部分。该项目通过设定的检查方法，对研究的实施情况进行评估，并帮助确保这些研究中受试者的权益、安全和福利得到了保护。

在现场检查结束时，Cynthia Harris女士向您出示并讨论了FDA483表，即现场检查发现的问题。您2014年9月19日对该FDA483表的书面回复已收悉。

经对现场检查报告及该报告的附件，以及您2014年9月19日的书面回复进行审查，我们认为，CXL-USA没有遵循适用的法律要求和监管临床试验实施的FDA法规。我们想强调以下几点：

1. 未能根据21 CFR 312.2（a）的要求对开展新药临床研究提交IND申请［21 CFR 312.20（a），（b）和312.40（a），（b）］

在联邦食品药品和化妆品法案（FD&C Act）的相关章节定义了药品是“用于诊断、治愈、缓解、治疗或预防疾病的物品”以及“用于影响人体或其他动物的结构或功能的物品（除食品外）”［21 U.S.C.321（g）］。CXL-USA研究（b）（4）的有效性。因此，由于（b）（4）用于（b）（4）的治疗，所以符合药品的定义。

为了使新药合法上市，申办者必须依照联邦食品药品和化妆品法案［21 U.S.C. 355］第505部分的要求获得新药申请或简化新药申请。新药临床试验申请（IND）使申办者得到对该要求的豁免，从而可以分发试验药物［21 U.S.C 355（i）］。FDA法规要求申办者在人体临床试验开展前递交新药申请，除非属于IND豁免的情形。

如果满足以下所有标准，已上市药品可以豁免该研究IND的要求：

- 该药物已在美国合法上市；
- 所开展的临床研究不打算作为一个完全受控的试验来报告给FDA，用以支持新适应症申请，也不用于支持对该药品说明书内容进行重大的修改；
- 如果是合法上市的处方药，所开展的研究不用于支持药品广告内容的显著改变；
- 所开展的临床研究不涉及给药途径、剂量水平、适用人群，或其他显著提高使用风险（或降低风险接受程度）的因素；
- 所开展的临床研究符合21 CFR 56中规定的伦理审查的要求以及21 CFR 50中规定的要求知情同意的；
- 所开展的临床研究符合21 CFR 312.7中对于试验药物推广的规定。

如果申办者计划开展体外生物利用度或生物等效性研究，属于满足21 CFR 320.31的条款的情形，则无需提交IND的申请。

（b）（4）属于试验药物，（b）（4）目前尚未在美国合法上市，也不符合IND豁免的情形。因此，在（b）（4）用于临床试验前，（b）（4）必须向FDA提交IND申请，并且按照21CFR312.40.要求获得生效的IND证书。

FDA的记录显示（b）（4）在用于临床试验方案（b）（4），一项关于（b）（4）的临床研究，实施前没有

IND递交。我们注意到，有15个不同的参与研究场所入组了（b）（4）药物研究的受试者（自2009年启动）。在FDA的现场检查中，您声明（b）（4）是使用该未获批准的药物的大约（b）（4）个临床研究的申办者。

您在2014年9月19日的书面回复中提到，（b）（4）在2014年9月12日提交了IND申请给FDA，然而，您的回复是不充分的，因为作为申办者，（b）（4）应当在方案启动和受试者入组前获得IND证书。

2. 未能确保对临床研究进行适当的监查［21 CFR 312.50；312.56（a）］

FDA法规要求申办者需确保正确地监查临床研究和确保临床研究者按照包含在IND内的总体研究计划和试验方案实施研究。我们的调查发现，CXL-USA未能正确地对试验方案（b）（4）实施监查。具体而言，在现场检查中，您表示，CXL-USA：（1）未审查研究相关的数据或记录；（2）未对研究场所实施监查任务；（3）依赖于研究场所的"自我监查"。

在您2014年9月19日的书面回复中，您指出，研究场所对于"知情同意书签署、数据收集和其他研究相似的任务"实施自我监查。作为纠正措施，您指出，将制定正式的自我监查方案及正式的申办者监查方案。

您的书面回复是不充分的，因为您未能提交您所提出的监查计划的副本。因此，我们不能判定您的计划是否能充分预防类似违背行为的再次发生。除此之外，请注意申办者仅可以将其监查职责转交给合同研究组织来实施，并且要将转移的职责用书面形式说明［21CFR 312.52］。

本警告信的目的并非是罗列您在试验药物临床研究中存在的所有缺陷。确保遵循法律和相关FDA法规的每一项要求是您的职责。您应当解决这些缺陷，并建立规程，以确保任何正在进行或将来进行的研究均能符合FDA的法规。

自收到这封信的15个工作日内，您应当书面告知本办公室为预防将来发生类似违规情况而采取的措施。如果不能充分、迅速地解释上述违规问题，可能导致我们在不再通知的情况下采取监管措施。如果您认为您已经遵循了FDA的法规要求，请陈述理由，并提供所有支持资料，以供我们参考。

附：英文原文

CXL-USA, LLC

WARNING LETTER

APR 1, 2015

CERTIFIED MAIL
RETURN RECEIPT REQUESTED

Ref: 15-HFD-45-04-01

Roy S. Rubinfeld, M.D.
President, CXL-USA, LLC
11200 Rockville Pike, Suite 150
Rockville, MD 20852

Dear Dr. Rubinfeld:

This Warning Letter informs you of objectionable conditions observed during the U.S. Food and Drug Administration (FDA) inspection at CXL-USA, LLC, conducted August 18 and 19, 2014. Ms. Cynthia Harris, representing the FDA, conducted an investigation and met with you to review CXL-USA's role as the sponsor of a clinical investigation (Protocol **(b)(4).**

This inspection is a part of the FDA's Bioresearch Monitoring Program, which includes inspections designed to evaluate the conduct of research and to help ensure that the rights, safety, and welfare of the human subjects of those studies have been protected.

At the conclusion of the inspection, Ms. Cynthia Harris presented and discussed with you Form FDA 483, Inspectional Observations. We acknowledge receipt of your September 19, 2014, written response to the Form FDA 483.

From our review of the Establishment Inspection Report, the documents submitted with that report, and your September 19, 2014, written response to the Form FDA 483, we conclude that CXL-USA did not adhere to the applicable statutory requirements and FDA regulations governing the conduct of clinical investigations. We wish to emphasize the following:

1. Failure to submit an IND for the conduct of clinical investigations with an investigational new drug that is subject to 21 CFR 312.2(a) [21 CFR 312.20(a), (b) and 312.40(a), (b)].

In relevant part, the Federal Food, Drug, and Cosmetic Act (FD&C Act) defines the term *drug* as "articles intended for use in the diagnosis, cure, mitigation, treatment, or prevention of disease" and "articles (other than food) intended to affect the structure or any function of the body of man or other animals" [21 U.S.C. 321(g)]. CXL-USA studied the efficacy of **(b)(4)**. As a result, because the **(b)(4)** was intended for the treatment of **(b)(4)** meets the definition of a drug under the FD&C Act.

To market a new drug lawfully, a sponsor must obtain approval of a new drug application or abbreviated new drug application under Section 505 of the FD&C Act [21 U.S.C. 355]. An Investigational New Drug (IND) application allows a sponsor to obtain an exemption from this requirement to distribute an investigational drug [21 U.S.C 355(i)]. FDA regulations require a sponsor to submit an IND application before conducting a clinical investigation of a drug in human subjects, unless the clinical investigation qualifies for an IND exemption.

A marketed drug product is exempt from the IND requirements if all of the following exemption criteria are met:

- The drug product is lawfully marketed in the United States;
- The investigation is not intended to be reported to FDA as a well-controlled study in support of a new indication for use and there is no intent to use the investigation to support any other significant change in the labeling of the drug;
- In the case of a lawfully marketed prescription drug, the investigation is not intended to support a significant change in the advertising for the drug;
- The investigation does not involve a route of administration, dosage level, use in a patient population, or other factor that significantly increases the risks (or decreases the acceptability of the risks) associated with the use of the drug product;
- The investigation is conducted in compliance with the requirements for institutional review set forth in 21 CFR 56 and with the requirements for informed consent set forth in 21 CFR 50; and
- The investigation is conducted in compliance with the requirements of 21 CFR 312.7 regarding promotion of investigational drugs.

A person planning to conduct an in vivo bioavailability or bioequivalence study is not required to submit an IND when certain criteria under 21 CFR 320.31 are met.

(b)(4)'s investigational drug, **(b)(4)**, is not a lawfully marketed drug product in the United States, nor is it exempt from the IND requirements. As a result, before using **(b)(4)** in a clinical investigation, **(b)(4)** was required to submit an IND for the drug to FDA, and to have an IND in effect under 21 CFR 312.40.

FDA records indicate that **(b)(4)** did not submit an IND before conducting the investigation under Protocol **(b)(4)**, a clinical investigation of **(b)(4)**. We note that human subjects were enrolled at 15 different sites to participate in clinical investigations (initiated in 2009) with the**(b)(4)**. During FDA's inspection, you stated that **(b)(4)** is the sponsor for approximately **(b)(4)** clinical investigations with this unapproved product.

We acknowledge that in your September 19, 2014, written response, you indicated that **(b)(4)** submitted an IND to the FDA on September 12, 2014. However, your response is inadequate because as a sponsor, **(b)(4)** should have obtained an IND before initiating Protocol **(b)(4)** and enrolling human subjects into Protocol **(b)(4)**.

2. Failure to ensure proper monitoring of the clinical investigations [21 CFR 312.50; 312.56(a)].

FDA regulations require that sponsors ensure proper monitoring of clinical investigations and ensure that their clinical investigators conduct those investigations in accordance with the general investigational plan and protocols contained in the IND. Our investigation found that CXL-USA failed to ensure proper monitoring of Protocol **(b)(4)**. Specifically, during the inspection you indicated that CXL-USA (1) did not review investigation-related data or records, (2) did not perform any site monitoring, and (3) relied on clinical site "self-monitoring."

In your September 19, 2014, written response, you indicated that clinical sites conducted self-monitoring "for informed consent signatures, data collection and other similar study tasks." As a corrective action, you indicated that formal self-monitoring protocols and formal sponsor-monitoring protocols are being developed.

Your written response is inadequate because you did not include a copy of your proposed monitoring plans. As a result, we are unable to determine whether your plans appear sufficient to prevent similar violations in the future. In addition, please note that a sponsor may transfer its obligation to monitor to a contract research organization only, and any such transfer of obligations must be described in writing [21 CFR 312.52].

This letter is not intended to be an all-inclusive list of deficiencies with your clinical study of an investigational drug. It is your responsibility to ensure adherence to each requirement of the law and relevant FDA regulations. You should address these deficiencies and establish procedures to ensure that any ongoing or future studies will be in compliance with FDA regulations.

Within fifteen (15) working days of your receipt of this letter, you should notify this office in writing of the actions you have taken or will take to prevent similar violations in the future. Failure to address the violations noted above adequately and promptly may result in regulatory action without further notice. If you believe you have complied with FDA regulations, include your reasoning and any supporting information for our consideration.

If you have any questions, please contact Chrissy J. Cochran, Ph.D., at 301-796-5633; FAX 301-847-8748. Your written response and any pertinent documentation should be addressed to:

Chrissy J. Cochran, Ph.D.
Branch Chief (Acting)
Compliance Enforcement Branch
Division of Enforcement and Postmarketing Safety
Office of Scientific Investigations
Office of Compliance
Center for Drug Evaluation and Research
Food and Drug Administration
Building 51, Room 5364
10903 New Hampshire Avenue
Silver Spring, MD 20993

Sincerely yours,

{See appended electronic signature page}

Sean Y. Kassim, Ph.D.
Office Director
Office of Scientific Investigations
Office of Compliance
Center for Drug Evaluation and Research
Food and Drug Administration

第38封　给Rogerio Lobo医学博士的警告信

2014年4月18日

参考号：14-HFD-45-04-02

尊敬的Lobo博士：

2013年6月5日至25日，Thomas Hansen先生代表FDA，对您在哥伦比亚大学医学中心（CUMC）的研究场所进行了现场检查，审查了您作为申办者进行的试验药物为（b）（4）、试验方案为（b）（4）的临床研究。这封警告信特告知您现场检查中发现的违规情况。

本次现场检查是FDA的生物研究监查项目的一部分，该项目通过设定的检查方法，对FDA所监管研究的实施情况进行评估，以确认研究数据在科学上是有效和准确的，并帮助确保这些研究中受试者的权益、安全和福利得到了保护。

在现场检查结束时，Hansen先生向您出示了FDA483表，即现场检查发现的问题，并与您进行了讨论。您2013年7月11日对该FDA483表的书面回复已收悉。

经对现场检查报告、该报告的附件，以及您2013年7月11日的书面回复进行审查，我们认为，您没有遵循适用的法律要求和监管临床研究实施及受试者保护的FDA法规。我们想强调以下几点：

未能确保对临床研究进行适当的监查，未能按照IND中的总体研究计划和方案进行临床研究［21 CFR 312.50和312.56（a）］

FDA法规要求申办者确保对临床研究进行适当的监查，并确保临床研究者按照IND中的方案进行临床研究。我们调查发现，您未能确保对方案（b）（4）的研究进行适当的监查，您未能确保临床研究者按照IND中的方案进行临床研究。因为监查不够，研究者未能按照FDA法规的要求获取受试者的知情同意，研究者未能确保伦理委员会对方案的不间断的批准，研究者未能按照方案规定的治疗组给予受试者试验药物剂量的情况，您未能及时发现并予以纠正。

1．作为试验方案（b）（4）的申办者，研究者未能按照21 CFR 321.60和50.20的要求获取受试者的知情同意，您的监查未能发现并予以纠正，具体而言：

a. 入组试验方案（b）（4）的50例受试者中，以下26例受试者研究者未能获取知情同意，您的监查未能发现并予以纠正：C1，C4~C7，C9~C12，C17，C19，C20，C22，C26，C28，C30，C31，C33，C34，C37~C41，C45，A5。

b. 入组试验方案（b）（4）的以下12例受试者，研究者未能在给予试验药物前获取知情同意，您的监查未能发现并予以纠正：C15，C16，C21，C24，C25，C32，C35，C36，C43，C44，C46，C47。

2．研究者未能确保伦理委员会按照21 CFR 56的要求对提出的临床研究进行审查和批准，您的监查未能发现并予以纠正。

具体而言，伦理委员会关于开展试验方案（b）（4）的批准从2011年3月31日到6月3日失效。在失效的这段时间里，研究者入组了6例受试者（受试者C42~C47），并用试验药物对他们进行了治疗。

3．您的监查未能确保临床研究按照研究计划进行。

试验方案（b）（4）包含两个研究治疗组：①“传统”或“标准”的（b）（4）治疗组；②“上楼梯”治疗组。“传统的”治疗组要求受试者在研究期间第一个月经周期的第5~9天接受5天的50mg/d（b）（4）的治疗。如果受试者在第一个月经周期后没有发生阳性反应（即直径至少为17mm的卵泡），方案要求在第二个月经周期将试验药物的剂量增加到100mg。如果受试者在第二个月经周期后没有发生阳性反应，方案要求在第三个月经周期将试验药物的剂量增加到150mg。“上楼梯”治疗组要求受试者接受相同剂量的（b）（4）（即50mg，100mg，150mg）以求引起阳性反应，但是将试验药物的剂量从50mg提高到100mg，或者从100mg提高到150mg要在更短的时限内而且不必等到下一个月经周期。

研究者未能给予4例受试者正确剂量的试验药物，您的监查未能发现并予以纠正，具体而言：

a. 受试者C4在2010年10月10日入组试验方案（b）（4），被分配到“传统/标准”治疗组。受试者给药日志显示，受试者C4在第一周期和第二周期，分别接受了方案要求的50mg和100mg的剂量。但是，给药日志显示在第三周期，受试者依旧接受了5天100mg/d的治疗，而不是按照方案要求的5天150mg/d的治疗。受试者C4的病程记录补遗中说该受试者对50mg的（b）（4）发生反应，不需要进一步的评估，但是这个说法没有得到给药日志的支持。

b. 受试者C6在2010年12月17日入组试验方案（b）（4），被分配到“上楼梯”治疗组。受试者给药日志显示，受试者C6从2011年1月11日到15日接受了50mg/d的（b）（4），从2011年3月31日到4月6日又接受了同样的剂量；然后在2011年4月7日到14日，接受了75mg而不是方案要求的“上楼梯”组给药剂量。受试者C6的病程记录补遗中说该受试者对50mg的（b）（4）发生反应并且成功受孕。但是病程记录补遗与给药日志的内容互相矛盾。

c. 受试者C19在2010年12月13日入组试验方案（b）（4），被分配到“上楼梯”治疗组。受试者给药日志显示，受试者C19从2010年12月13日到17日接受了25mg/d的（b）（4），然后从2011年2月15日到19日接受了同样的剂量，而不是方案要求的“上楼梯”组给药剂量。受试者的病程记录补遗中说该受试者既往对50mg的（b）（4）发生了强烈的反应。

d. 受试者C35在2011年1月21日入组试验方案（b）（4），被分配到“传统/标准”治疗组。根据受试者给药日志，受试者C35在第一周期、第二周期、第三周期，都接受了100mg/d持续5天，而不是在第一周期从方案要求的50mg剂量开始，进展到第二周期100mg、第三周期150mg。病程记录补遗中表明，受试者的第一个治疗周期是50mg，随后按月进行了3个100mg治疗周期。因而，病程记录补遗与给药日志的内容互相矛盾。

我们知道，在发给您的FDA483表上，没有列出以上1~3项内容，所以您的书面回复没有对这些具体问题进行说明。但是在2013年7月11日对FDA483表的书面回复中，您承认您有责任对试验方案（b）（4）的开展进行监查，并且您未能发现临床研究者未按照伦理委员会批准的方案、知情过程、研究过程记录进行。您也承认，一旦发现有不合规，您有责任或者及时确保合规，或者终止该研究者参与该研究。

我们确认在您和哥伦比亚大学医学中心妇产科主任签字的2013年7月11日的书面回复中，您提供了一份纠正措施计划，包含以下内容：

- 应用哥伦比亚大学医学中心临床试验办公室（CTO）的数据监查计划中的模板和表格。
- 完成由哥伦比亚大学医学中心临床试验办公室提供的关于FDA申办者-研究者职责的在线培训；来自哥伦比亚大学的IND / IDE援助项目（IAP）的一对一的培训；由CITI在线受试者研究培训和贵伦理委员会对FDA所监管研究的再次认证。
- 承诺确保今后所有的临床研究都会通过部门质量保证计划受到监查，并且所有参与研究管理的工作人员和研究协调员都会受到适当的培训。
- 与临床试验办公室的IAP合作，提供关于持有IND的职责的培训、教育和指导。
- 采用2011年10月实施的临床试验监查援助计划（CTMAP）的监查计划指南和监查工具。
- 通过对伦理委员会批准的方案、研究计划、法规要求和药物临床试验质量管理规范的理解的表现，确保研究者和研究人员有足够的经验和培训。为了证明对这些要求的理解，研究者和研究人员必须成功完成制度上的培训的要求，例如合作机构培训倡议（CITI）FDA所监管的研究的培训，CITI受试者保护课程，以及2010年10月实施的哥伦比亚大学临床研究合作培训计划。对这些培训要求的完成情况将被记录在培训日志中。

- 通过要求试验药物由研究药房进行发放，要求试验药物供应只能经过培训取得资格的研究者或在FDA157表上授权过的授权研究者才能开具处方。
- 按照哥伦比亚伦理委员会的政策，要求：①必须递交FDA1572表及所有的临床研究方案；②所有最初的IND/IDE申请，在递交到FDA之前，必须经过IAP的审查和批准；③所有终版的FDA申请材料都需要递交一份副本到IAP；④妥善保管一个法规文件检查表文件夹，并且以此来帮助保存相关记录。
- 要求研究者将不良事件都记录在不良事件日志中，以确保对不良事件进行充分、及时地审查和记录。

除了您个人承诺要改变临床研究操作，2013年7月11日的回复中表示哥伦比亚大学医学中心已经实施了以下措施：

- 在伦理委员会批准之前，CUMC的系主任和研究管理高级主任对所有临床研究方案进行批准。
- 实施更加正规化的质量保证（QA）监查计划，包括任命一个QA研究监查员，对研究者发起的临床试验进行跟踪审查和监查。
- 每月定期召开部门教育会议。
- 对于参与临床研究的新人进行入职培训。
- 与哥伦比亚大学CTO和伦理委员会紧密合作，确保符合机构的要求。

以上所述的纠正措施的大部分内容，似乎都是合适的。但是，您计划使用哥伦比亚大学的数据检查计划的模板、指导原则以及对研究者的指示来确保对将来的、您作为申办者的研究进行监查，我们对此感到担忧。具体而言，我们注意到尽管这份文件提供了一个通用的模板来草拟一份数据检查计划，但是它本身并没有提供关于监查时间和频率的指导，要进行的特定监查活动，申办者的检查如何与临床研究者相互配合，以纠正发现的违规情况，并使研究者合规。

鉴于这个缺陷，我们无法确认您将如何确保在您作为申办者的研究中监查能被正确地执行。没有这些细节，我们不能确定是否这个纠正措施足以预防将来类似的违规情况。请注意，作为方案（b）（4）的申办者，您负有最终责任，对研究者、对方案的实施进行监查，以确保临床研究遵循21 CFR 321.50和312.56（a）的规定，按照IND中的研究计划和方案进行。无论您在哪个机构开展临床研究，您都必须确保要遵循适用的FDA法规。

本警告信的目的并非是罗列您在试验药物临床研究中存在的所有缺陷。确保遵循法律和相关FDA法规的每一项要求是您的职责，您应当解决这些缺陷，并建立规程，以确保任何正在进行或将来进行的研究均符合FDA法规。

自收到这封信的15个工作日内，您应当书面告知本办公室为预防将来发生类似违规情况而采取的措施。如果不能充分、迅速地对上述违规情况作出解释，可能导致我们在不再通知的情况下采取监管措施。如果贵方认为已符合FDA法规要求，请陈述理由，并提供所有支持资料，以供我们参考。

附：英文原文

Rogerio Lobo, M.D.

WARNING LETTER

APR 18, 2014

CERTIFIED MAIL
RETURN RECEIPT REQUESTED

Ref:14-HFD-45-04-02

Rogerio A. Lobo, M.D.
Columbia University Medical Center
Department of Obstetricsand Gynecology
622West 168th Street, Room16-65
NewYork, NY 10032

Dear Dr. Lobo:

This Warning Letter informs you of objectionable conditions observed during the U.S. Food and Drug Administration (FDA) inspection conducted at your research office at Columbia University Medical Center (CUMC) between June 5 and June 25, 2013. Mr. Thomas Hansen, representing FDA, reviewed your conduct as the sponsor of a clinical investigation (Protocol (b)(4)) of the investigational drug (b)(4).

This inspection is a part of FDA's Bioresearch Monitoring Program, which includes inspections designed to evaluate the conduct of FDA-regulated research to ensure that the data are scientifically valid and accurate, and to help ensure that the rights, safety, and welfare of the human subjects of those studies have been protected.

At the conclusion of the inspection, Mr. Hansen presented and discussed with you Form FDA 483, Inspectional Observations. We acknowledge receipt of your July 11, 2013, written response to the Form FDA 483.

From our review of the FDA Establishment Inspection Report, the documents submitted with that report, and your July 11, 2013, written response, we conclude that you did not adhere to the applicable statutory requirements and FDA regulations governing the conduct of clinical investigations and the protection of human subjects. We wish to emphasize the following:

Failure to ensure proper monitoring of the investigation and failure to ensure that the investigation is conducted in accordance with the general investigational plan and protocols contained in the IND [21 CFR 312.50 and 312.56(a)].

FDA regulations require that sponsors ensure proper monitoring of clinical investigations and ensure that their clinical investigators conduct the investigations in accordance with the protocols contained in the Investigational New Drug file (IND). Our investigation found that you failed to ensure proper monitoring of Protocol **(b)(4)**, and that you did not ensure that a clinical investigator conducted the investigation in accordance with a protocol contained in the IND. As a result of inadequate monitoring, you did not identify and correct in a timely manner a clinical investigator's failure to obtain informed consent from subjects, in accordance with FDA regulations; a clinical investigator's failure to ensure ongoing Institutional Review Board (IRB) approval of the protocol; and a clinical investigator's failure to administer the dose of investigational drug to subjects, according to their protocol specified treatment arm.

1. As the sponsor for Protocol **(b)(4)**, your monitoring failed to identify and correct a clinical investigator's failure to obtain informed consent from subjects, in accordance with the provisions of 21 CFR 321.60 and 50.20. Specifically:

a. Your monitoring did not identify and correct the clinical investigator's failure to obtain informed consent from the following 26 of 50 subjects who were enrolled into Protocol **(b)(4)**: Subjects C1, C4 through C7, C9 through C12,

C17, C19, C20, C22, C26, C28, C30, C31, C33, C34, C37 through C41, C45, and A5.

b. Your monitoring did not identify and correct the clinical investigator's failure to obtain informed consent before administering investigational drug to the following 12 subjects who were enrolled into Protocol **(b)(4)**: Subjects C15, C16, C21, C24, C25, C32, C35, C36, C43, C44, C46, and C47.

2. Your monitoring did not identify and correct a clinical investigator's failure to ensure that an IRB reviews and approves a proposed clinical investigation, in accordance with 21 CFR part 56.

Specifically, IRB approval to conduct Protocol **(b)(4)** lapsed from March 31 to June 3, 2011. During this lapsed period, the clinical investigator enrolled 6 subjects (Subjects C42 through C47) and treated them with investigational drug.

3. Your monitoring failed to ensure that the investigation was conducted in accordance with the investigational plan. Protocol **(b)(4)** contained two study treatment arms: (1) a "traditional" or "standard" **(b)(4)** treatment arm, and (2) a "stairstep" arm. The "traditional" treatment arm required that the subject receive 50 mg of **(b)(4)** daily for 5 days on Day 5-9 of the first menstrual cycle during the study. If the subject did not develop a positive response (i.e., follicles of at least 17 mm in size) after the first menstrual cycle, the protocol required that the dose be increased to 100 mg on the second menstrual cycle. If the subject did not develop a positive response after the second cycle, the protocol required that the dose be increased to 150 mg on the third cycle. The "stair-step" arm required that the subject receive the same dosing of **(b)(4)** (i.e., 50 mg, 100 mg, and 150 mg) in an attempt to induce a positive response, but within a shorter time frame and without waiting for the next menstrual cycle before increasing the **(b)(4)** dose from 50 mg to 100 mg or from 100 mg to 150 mg.

Your monitoring did not identify and correct a clinical investigator's failure to administer the correct dose of study drug to 4 subjects. Specifically:

a. Subject C4 was enrolled in Protocol **(b)(4)** on October 10, 2010, and was assigned to the "traditional" or "standard" dosing arm. The subject's dosing log shows that Subject C4 received the protocol-required **(b)(4)** doses of 50 mg and 100 mg during Cycles 1 and 2, respectively. However, the dosing log shows that for Cycle 3, the subject again received 100 mg daily for 5 days, rather than 150 mg daily for 5 days, as required by the protocol. The Progress Note Addendum for Subject C4 states that the subject responded to 50 mg of **(b)(4)**, and no further assessment was needed; however, this statement is not supported by the dosing log.

b. Subject C6 was enrolled in Protocol **(b)(4)** on December 17, 2010, and was assigned to the "stair-step" dosing arm. The subject's dosing log shows that Subject C6 received **(b)(4)** 50 mg daily from January 11 to 15, 2011, and the same dose again from March 31 to April 6, 2011; the subject then received 75 mg from April 7 to 14, 2011, rather than the protocol-required stair-step dosing. The Progress Note Addendum for Subject C6 states that the subject responded to 50 mg of **(b)(4)** and became pregnant. Thus, the Progress Note Addendum conflicts with the dosing log.

c. Subject C19 was enrolled in Protocol **(b)(4)** on December 13, 2010, and was assigned to the "stair-step" dosing arm. The subject's dosing log shows that Subject C19 received **(b)(4)** 25 mg daily from December 13 to 17, 2010, and the same dose again from February 15 to 19, 2011, rather that the protocol-required stair-step dosing. The Progress Note Addendum notes that the subject had, in the past, had a strong response to a dose of 50 mg of **(b)(4)**.

d. Subject C35 was enrolled in Protocol **(b)(4)** on January 21, 2011, and was assigned to the "traditional" or "standard" treatment arm. According to the subject's dosing log, Subject C35 received 100 mg daily for 5 days during Cycles 1, 2, and 3, rather than starting with the protocol-required dose of 50 mg in Cycle 1 and progressing to 100 mg in Cycle 2 and 150 mg in Cycle 3. The Progress Note Addendum indicates that the subject's first treatment cycle was for 50 mg, followed monthly by three 100-mg cycles. Thus, the Progress Note Addendum conflicts with the dosing log.

We recognize that the Form FDA 483 issued to you does not include the findings noted in Items 1 through 3 above, and that your written response therefore did not address these specific issues. However, in the July 11, 2013, written response to the Form FDA 483, you acknowledged that you were responsible for monitoring the progress of Protocol **(b)(4)**, and that you failed to discover that the clinical investigator was not complying with the IRB-approved protocol, the consent process, and the documentation of study procedures. You also acknowledged that upon finding noncompliance, you were responsible for either promptly securing compliance or ending the investigator's participation in the study.

We acknowledge that in the July 11, 2013, written response signed by you and the Chair of the Department of Obstetrics and Gynecology at the University of Columbia Medical Center, you provided a corrective action plan that includes the following:

- Use of the Columbia University Clinical Trials Office (CTO) Data Monitoring Plan templates and forms
- Completion of online training about FDA sponsor-investigator responsibilities, given by the Columbia University Clinical Trials Office; one-on-one training from the Columbia University IND/IDE Assistance Program (IAP); and recertification by the CITI online human subjects research training, and by your Institutional Review Board (IRB) for FDA-regulated research
- Commitment to ensure that all future studies will be monitored through the Departmental Quality Assurance Program, and that all staff and research coordinators involved in the management of your studies will be properly trained
- Partnering with the Clinical Trials Office's IAP to provide training, education, and guidance about the responsibilities of holding an IND
- Utilizing the monitoring-plan guidelines and monitoring tools of the Clinical Trials Monitoring Assistance Program (CTMAP), implemented in October of 2011
- Ensuring that investigators and research personnel have adequate experience and training, shown by demonstrating their understanding of the IRB-approved protocol, the investigational plan, regulatory requirements, and Good Clinical Practice (GCP). In order to demonstrate an understanding of these requirements, investigators and research personnel will have to successfully complete institutional training requirements, such as the Collaborative Institutional Training Initiative (CITI) FDA-regulated research training; the CITI Human Subjects Protection course; and the Columbia University Clinical Research Coordinator training program, which was implemented in October 2010. Fulfillment of these training requirements will be documented in a Training Log.
- Ensuring drug accountability by requiring that all investigational drugs be dispensed from the Research Pharmacy, and by requiring that investigational drug supply will be prescribed only by trained qualified investigators and subinvestigators designated on the FDA 1572
- Following the Columbia IRB policy requiring (1) that a Form FDA 1572 be submitted with all protocols; (2) that all initial IND/IDE applications be reviewed and approved by the IAP before they are submitted to FDA; (3) that a final copy of all FDA submissions be submitted to the IAP; and (4) that a Regulatory Binder Checklist be maintained to assist in maintaining these records
- Requiring investigators to record adverse events in an Adverse Events Log to ensure adequate and timely review and recording of adverse events

In addition to your personal commitments to reform research practices, the July 11, 2013, response states that the University of Columbia Medical Center has implemented the following:

- CUMC Department Chair and Senior Director of Research Administration approval of all research protocols before IRB approval
- Implementation of a more formalized Quality Assurance (QA) Monitoring Program, including appointment of a QA Research Monitor to conduct continuing review and monitoring for all investigator initiated trials
- Monthly Departmental educational meetings
- Requiring an orientation program for new personnel involved in clinical research
- Working with the Columbia University CTO and the IRB to ensure compliance with institutional requirements

For the most part, the corrective actions noted above appear to be adequate. However, we are concerned about your plans to use Columbia University's Data-Monitoring Plan Template, Guidance, and Instructions to Investigators to ensure adequate monitoring of future studies for which you are the sponsor. Specifically, we note that while this document provides a general template for drafting a data-monitoring plan, it does not itself provide any guidance on the timing and frequency of monitoring; the specific monitoring activities to be performed; and how the sponsor's monitor will interact with the clinical investigator to correct observed violations and bring the investigator into compliance. In light of this deficiency, we are unable to determine how you will ensure that monitoring is properly carried out in any studies that you may sponsor. Without having these details, we are unable to determine whether this corrective action is sufficient to prevent similar violations in the future. Please note that, as the sponsor of Protocol **(b)(4)**, you were ultimately responsible for monitoring the clinical investigator's conduct of the protocol, to ensure that the investigation was conducted in accordance with the investigational plan and protocols contained in the IND, and in accordance with 21 CFR 312.50 and 312.56(a). You must ensure that you comply with applicable FDA regulations, regardless of the institution where you perform the research.

This letter is not intended to be an all-inclusive list of deficiencies with your clinical study of an investigational drug. It is your responsibility to ensure adherence to each requirement of the law and relevant FDA regulations. You should address these deficiencies and establish procedures to ensure that any ongoing or future studies will be in compliance with FDA regulations.

Within fifteen (15) working days of your receipt of this letter, you should notify this office in writing of the actions you have taken to prevent similar violations in the future. Failure to explain the violations noted above adequately and promptly may result in regulatory action without further notice. If you believe that you have complied with FDA regulations, include your reasoning and any supporting information for our consideration.

If you have any questions, please contact Constance Cullity, M.D., M.P.H., at 301-796-3397; FAX 301-847-8748. Your written response and any pertinent documentation should be addressed to:

Constance Cullity, M.D., M.P.H.
Branch Chief
Good Clinical Practice Reinforcement Branch
Division of Good Clinical Practice Compliance
Office of Scientific Investigations
Office of Compliance
Center for Drug Evaluation and Research
Food and Drug Administration
Building 51, Room 5354
10903 New Hampshire Avenue
Silver Spring, MD 20993

Sincerely yours,

{See appended electronic signature page}

Sean Y. Kassim, Ph.D.
Acting Office Director
Office of Scientific Investigations
Office of Compliance
Center for Drug Evaluation and Research
Food and Drug Administration

第39封　给AMKS TIME RELEASE LAB有限责任公司的警告信

2014年4月10日

参考号：14-HFD-45-04-01

尊敬的Elchagea博士：

2013年6月17日至7月12日，Peter Lenahan先生代表FDA，对AMKS TIME RELEASE LAB有限责任公司（AMKS TRL）进行了检查，审查了AMKS TRL作为申办者进行的试验药物为（b）（4）、试验方案为（b）（4）的临床研究。这封警告信特告知您现场检查中发现的违规情况。

本次现场检查是FDA的生物研究监查项目的一部分，该项目通过设定的检查方法，对FDA所监管的研究的实施情况进行评估，以确认研究数据在科学上是有效和准确的，并帮助确保这些研究中受试者的权益、安全和福利得到了保护。

在现场检查结束时，Lenahan先生向您出示了FDA483表，即现场检查发现的问题，并与您进行了讨论。您于2013年7月30日对该FDA483表的书面回复已收悉。

经对现场检查报告、该报告的附件，以及您2013年7月30日的书面回复进行审查，我们认为，AMKS TRL没有遵循适用的法律要求和监管临床研究实施的FDA法规。我们想强调以下几点：

1. 未能根据21 CFR 312.2（a）的要求对开展新药临床研究提交IND申请［21 CFR 312.20（a）和312.40（a）］

为了使新药合法上市，申办者必须依照联邦食品药品和化妆品法案（FD&Act）第505部分的要求获得新药申请或简化新药申请的批准［21 U.S.C. 355］。试验新药申请（IND）是一种方式，通过它申办者可以获得对这项要求的豁免，以分发试验药物［21 U.S.C. 355（i）］。FDA法规要求申办者在受试者中开展药物临床研究前递交IND申请，除非该项临床研究有资格获得IND豁免。

如果满足以下所有豁免标准，已上市的药品可以豁免IND要求：

- 该药品已在美国合法上市；
- 临床研究的目的不是为了向FDA申请药品新适应症的严格规范的研究，也不是用于支持药品说明书内容的任何重大变更；
- 如是已合法上市的处方药，临床研究的目的不是用于支持对产品广告的重大更改；
- 临床研究不涉及给药途径、剂量水平、在某个受试者群体的使用或其他显著增加用药相关风险（或降低风险接受程度）的因素；
- 临床研究按照符合21 CFR 56提出的伦理审查要求及21 CFR 50提出的知情同意要求进行；
- 临床研究按照符合21 CFR 312.7中关于试验药物推广的要求进行。

如果计划对已批准药品的未批准版本进行生物利用度或生物等效性研究，那么当21 CFR 320.31的某些条款得到满足时，无需提交IND的申请。

AMKS TRL的试验药物（b）（4）不是一个在美国合法上市的药品，也不是正在进行生物利用度或生物等效性研究的已批准药品的未批准版本。因此，在临床研究中使用试验药物（b）（4）之前，AMKS TRL必须向FDA递交该药的IND申请，而且该IND还必须按照21 CFR 312.40的要求生效。

而FDA的记录显示，AMKS TRL在开展（b）（4）临床研究的方案（b）（4）研究之前，没有递交IND申请。

在您2013年7月30日的书面回复中，您声称“我们判断（b）（4）不是药品，我们将（b）（4）用作一种膳食和食品补充剂［原文如此］。”您还说，“我们知道它在21 CFR 182.1中被认为是安全的”而且“为了满足（b）（4）的有效性和安全性［原文如此］，我们做了非临床研究和临床研究来获取足够多的数据递交给FDA。”

在FD&C Act的相关部分，对于“药品”的定义是“用于诊断、治愈、缓解、治疗或者预防疾病的物品”以及“非食品的可以用来影响人体或者动物身体结构或者功能的物品”［21 U.S.C. 321.（g）］。我们注意到，试验方案（b）（4）对于（b）（4）的描述是“研究药物”，而该方案的目的就是为了“在联合感染了丙肝病毒和人免疫缺陷病毒的受试者中，评估（b）（4）抗病毒的效益”。因为AMKS TRL在研究是否（b）（4）在感染免疫缺陷病毒的人群中，可以缓解或者治疗丙肝病毒，它是一种用来诊断、治愈、缓解或预防疾病的物品。（b）（4）符合FD&C Act中对于药品的定义。因此，AMKS TRL必须递交IND申请，并且AMKS TRL启动在受试者中的（b）（4）的任何临床研究之前，IND必须生效。

我们知道在您2013年7月30日的书面回复中，您说“AMKS TRL致力于并正在和FDA合作”，且“不会启动任何进一步研究，除非FDA授权AMKS进行。”如果需要IND申请的临床研究能够正确地开展，AMKS TRL的计划看起来足以预防将来类似的违规情况再次发生。

2. 未能确保对研究进行适当的监查，未能确保临床研究按照IND中的总体研究计划和方案进行［21 CFR 312.50和312.56（a）］

FDA法规要求申办者确保对临床研究进行适当的监查，确保临床研究按照IND中的总体研究计划和方案进行。我们的调查发现，您未能确保对试验方案（b）（4）进行适当的监查，没有确保临床研究者按照方案进行研究。具体而言：

临床研究者未能按照方案（b）（4）的要求，采集研究受试者的数据到方案规定的病例报告表（CRFs）中，AMKS TRL的监查未能发现并予以纠正。我们注意到，在现场检查期间，您说AMKS TRL没有使用任何纸质的CRF或者电子数据采集来记录研究受试者的数据。

在您2013年7月30日的书面回复中，您说AMKS TRL没有对于试验方案（b）（4）的书面监查计划，通过与临床研究者的口头讨论来进行监查。我们确认在那份书面回复中，您指出AMKS TRL已经准备了一个书面的监查计划，并随新的试验方案一同递交给了FDA。

关于缺乏CRFs的问题，我们确认AMKS TRL已经做好准备，并在您2013年7月30日的书面回复中提交了一份CRF的副本。

您的书面回复是不充分的，因为您没有在其中包括一份监查计划的副本，或者提供关于监查计划的任何细节。因此，我们不能确定是否您的监查计划看起来足以预防将来类似的违规情况。另外，您与2013年7月30日的书面回复一起提供的CRF，看起来不像与试验方案（b）（4）有关，因为您提供的CRF上的入选/排除标准和实验室评估项目，与试验方案（b）（4）上的有显著差异。

3. 未能保存显示试验药物接收、转运或其他处置情况的足够记录［21 CFR 312.57（a）］

作为方案（b）（4）的申办者，AMKS TRL必须保存显示试验药物（b）（4）接收、转运或其他处置情况的足够记录。这些记录必须包括，根据情况而定，药物将运送给的临床研究者的姓名，每次运送的日期、数量以及批号或代码标记。AMKS TRL未能保存关于试验药物（b）（4）的充分的记录。具体而言，AMKS TRL未能保存显示试验药物转运或其他处置情况的任何记录。

在您2013年7月30日的书面回复中，您并没有明确说明是否AMKS TRL保存了与试验药物处置有关的书面记录。但是，您坚称“我们过去常常亲自将药品送到医院去，因为医院离我们场所很近。但是现在在新的临床研究中，我们将会按照AMKS TRL已经制定的SOP，保存关于药品运输的准确记录。概要列出临床药物的运送、使用、返还或破损的数量［原文如此］。”您还在书面回复中提到，使用记录都保留在St. Joseph 医院的受试者文件中。

您的回复是不充分的，因为您没有提供回复中提到的关于AMKS TRL标准操作规程（SOP）的文件或细节。因此，我们无法确定是否这个SOP看起来足以预防将来类似的违规情况。

本警告信的目的并非是罗列您在试验药物临床研究中存在的所有缺陷。确保遵循法律和相关FDA法规的每一项要求是您的职责，您应当解决所存在的缺陷，并建立规程，以确保任何正在进行或将来进行的研究均符合FDA法规。

自收到这封信的15个工作日内，您应当书面告知本办公室为预防将来发生类似违规情况而采取的措施。如果不能充分、迅速地解释上述违规问题，可能导致我们在不再通知的情况下采取监管措施。如果贵方认为已符合FDA法规要求，请陈述理由，并提供所有支持资料，以供我们参考。

附：英文原文

AMKS TIME RELEASE LAB, LLC

WARNING LETTER

APR 10, 2014

CERTIFIED MAIL
RETURN RECEIPT REQUESTED

14-HFD-45-04-01

Ismail Elchagea, Ph.D. President
AMKS Time Release Laboratories, LLC
470 Chamberlain Avenue
Paterson,NJ 07522

Dear Dr. Elchagea:

This Warning Letter informs you of objectionable conditions observed during the U.S. Food and Drug Administration (FDA) inspection conducted at AMKS Time Release Laboratories, LLC (AMKS TRL) between June 17 and July 12, 2013. Mr. Peter Lenahan, representing FDA, reviewed AMKS TRL's conduct as the sponsor of a clinical investigation (Protocol **(b)(4)** of the investigational drug **(b)(4)**).

This inspection is a part of FDA's Bioresearch Monitoring Program, which includes inspections designed to evaluate the conduct of FDA regulated research to ensure that the data are scientifically valid and accurate, and to help ensure that the rights, safety, and welfare of the human subjects of those studie have been protected.

At the conclusion of the inspection, Mr. Lenahan presented and discussed with you Form FDA 483, Inspectional Observations. We acknowledge receipt of your July 30, 2013, written response to the Form FDA 483.

From our review of the FDA Establishment Inspection Report, the documents submitted with that report, and your July 30, 2013, written response, we conclude that AMKS TRL did not adhere to the applicable statutory requirements and FDA regulations governing the conduct of clinical investigations. We wish to emphasize the following:

1. Failure to submit an IND application for the conduct of clinical investigations with an investigational new drug that is subject to 21 CFR 312.2(a) [21 CFR 312.20(a) and 312.40(a)].

To market a new drug lawfully, a sponsor must obtain approval of a new drug application or abbreviated new drug application under section 505 of the Federal Food, Drug, and Cosmetic Act (FD&c Act) [21 U.S.C. 355]. An (FD& Act) Investigational New Drug application (IND) is the means through which a sponsor obtains an exemption from this requirement to distribute an investigational drug [21 U.S.C. 355(j)]. FDA regulations require a sponsor to submit an IND application before conducting a clinical investigation of a drug in human subjects, unless the clinical investigation qualifies for an IND exemption.

A marketed drug product is exempt from the IND requirements if all of the following exemption criteria are met:

- The drug product is lawfully marketed in the United States;

- The investigation is not intended to be reported to FDA as a well-controlled study in support of a new indication for use and there is no intent to use the investigation to support any other significant change in the labeling of the drug;
- In the case of a lawfully marketed prescription drug, the investigation is not intended to support significant change in the advertising for the drug;
- The investigation does not involve a route of administration, dosage level, use in a patient population, or other factor that significantly increases the risks (or decreases the acceptability of the risks) associated with the use of the drug product;
- The investigation is conducted in compliance with the requirements for institutional review set forth in 21 CFR part 56 and with the requirements for informed consent set forth in 21 CFR part 50; and
- The investigation is conducted in compliance with the requirements of 21 CFR 312.7 regarding promotion of investigational drugs.

A person planning to conduct a bioavailability or bioequivalence study of an unapproved version of an approved drug product is not required to submit an IND when certain criteria under 21 CFR 320.31 are met.

AMKS TRL's investigational drug **(b)(4)** is not a lawfully marketed drug product in the United States, nor is it an unapproved version of an approved drug product undergoing a bioavailability or bioequivalence study. As a result, before using **(b)(4)** in a clinical investigation, AMKS TRL was required to submit an IND for the drug to FDA, and the IND was required to go into effect under 21 CFR 312.40.

FDA records indicate that AMKS TRL did not submit an IND before conducting the study under Protocol **(b)(4)**, a clinical investigation of **(b)(4)**.

In your July 30, 2013, written response, you state, "Our judgment was that **(b)(4)** was not a drug, we used **(b)(4)** as dietary and food supplement [sic]." You also state, "We know that it is characterized a safe in 21 CFR Section 182.1," and "We did the non-clinical and clinical study to obtain enough data to submit to FDA, in order to satisfy the safety and efficiency [sic] of **(b)(4)**."

In relevant part, the FD&C Act defines the term drug as "articles intended for use in the diagnosis, cure, mitigation, treatment, or prevention of disease" and "articles (other than food) intended to affect the structure or any function of the body of man or other animals" [21 U.S.C. 321(g)]. We note that Protocol **(b)(4)** describes **(b)(4)** as the "study medication," and the protocol's purpose is to "evaluate the antiviral benefit of **(b)(4)** in human subjects coinfected with hepatitis C and human immunodeficiency virus." Because AMKS TRL was studying whether **(b)(4)** mitigates or treats hepatitis C in humans with immunodeficiency virus infection, it is an article intended for use in the diagnosis, cure, mitigation, treatment, or prevention of disease. **(b)(4)** meets the definition of a drug under the FD&C Act; therefore, AMKS TRL was required to submit an IND, which was required to go into effect before AMKS TRL could initiate any clinical investigations of **(b)(4)** in human subjects.

We acknowledge that in your July 30, 2013, written response, you state that AMKS TRL "is committed to and is working with FDA" and "will not initiate any further study unless the FDA authorizes AMKS to proceed." If properly carried out for clinical investigations that require an IND, AMKS TRL's plan appears adequate to prevent the recurrence of similar violations in the future.

2. Failure to ensure proper monitoring of the investigations and failure to ensure that the investigations are conducted in accordance with the general investigational plan and protocols contained in the IND [21 CFR 312.50 and 312.56(a)].

FDA regulations require that sponsors ensure proper monitoring of clinical investigations and ensure that their clinical investigators conduct those investigations in accordance with the general investigational plan and protocols contained in the IND. Our investigation found that you failed to ensure proper monitoring of Protocol **(b)(4)** and did not ensure that a clinical investigator conducted the investigation in accordance with that protocol. Specifically:

AMKS TRL monitoring failed to identify and correct a clinical investigator's failure to collect study subjects' data on protocol specific case report forms (CRFs), as required by Protocol **(b)(4)**. We note that during the inspection, you indicated that AMKS TRL did not use any paper CRFs or electronic data capture to record study subjects' data.

In your July 30, 2013, written response, you indicated that AMKS TRL had no written monitoring plan for Protocol **(b)(4)** and monitored the study's progress through verbal discussions with the clinical investigator. We acknowledge that in that written response, you indicated that AMKS TRL has prepare a written monitoring plan and submitted that plan to FDA, along with a new protocol.

Regarding the lack of CRFs, we acknowledge that AMKS TRL has prepared and provided a copy of a CRF with your July 30, 2013, written response.

Your written response is inadequate because you did not include with it a copy of the monitoring plan o provide any details regarding the monitoring plan. As a result, we are unable to determine whether your written monitoring plan appears sufficient to prevent similar violations in the future. In addition, the CRF you provided with your July 30, 2013, written response does not appear to be related to Protocol **(b)(4)**, because there are significant differences between the inclusion/exclusion criteria and laboratory assessments in the CRF you provided, and those for Protocol **(b)(4)**.

3. Failure to maintain adequate records showing the receipt, shipment, or other disposition of the investigational drug [21 CFR 312.57(a)].

As the sponsor of Protocol **(b)(4)**, AMKS TRL was required to maintain adequate records showing the receipt, shipment, or other disposition of the investigational drug **(b)(4)**. These records were required to include, as appropriate, the name of the clinical investigator to whom the drug was shipped, and the date, quantity, and batch or code mark of each such shipment. AMKS TRL failed to maintain adequate records with respect to the investigational drug **(b)(4)**. Specifically, AMKS TRL did not maintain any records showing the shipment or other disposition of the investigational drug.

In your July 30, 2013, written response, you do not address specifically whether AMKS TRL kept written records of the disposition of investigational drug for Protocol **(b)(4)**. However, you do state, "We used to carry the product to the hospital in person because the hospital is close to our facility. But now in th new study we will keep accurate records for shipment as per AMKS TRL has established an S.O.P. To outline the shipment, quantity used, return or destruction of clinical drug [sic]." You also note in your response that records for use were retained in patient files at St. Joseph Hospital.

Your response is inadequate because you provided no documentation or details regarding the AMKS TR Standard Operating Procedure (SOP) referred to in your response. As a result, we are unable to determine whether this SOP appears sufficient to prevent similar violations in the future.

This letter is not intended to be an all-inclusive list of deficiencies with your clinical study of an investigational drug. It is your responsibility to ensure adherence to each requirement of the law and relevant FDA regulations. You should address these deficiencies and establish procedures to ensure that any ongoing or future studies will be in compliance with FDA regulations.

Within fifteen (15) working days of your receipt of this letter, you should notify this office in writing of the actions you have taken to prevent similar violations in the future. Failure to address the violations noted above adequately and promptly may result in regulatory action without further notice. If you believe you have complied with FDA regulations, include your reasoning and any supporting information for our consideration.

If you have any questions, please contact Constance Cullity, M.D., M.P.H., at 3017963397; FAX 301-847-8748. Your written response and any pertinent documentation should be addressed to:

Constance Cullity, M.D., M.P.H.
Branch Chief
Good Clinical Practice Reinforcement Branch
Division of Good Clinical Practice Compliance
Office of Scientific Investigations
Office of Compliance
Center for Drug Evaluation and Research
Food and Drug Administration
Building 51, Room 5354
10903 New Hampshire Avenue
Silver Spring, MD 20993

Sincerely yours,

{See appended electronic signature page}

Sean Ykassim, Ph.D.
Acting Director
Office of Scientific Investigations
Office of Compliance
Center for Drug Evaluation and Research
Food and Drug Administration

第40封　给Burzynski研究所的警告信

2013年12月3日

参考号：13-HFD-45-11-05

尊敬的Burzynski博士：

2013年1月17日至3月15日，Joel Martinez先生、Hugh McClure先生和Cynthia Kleppinger博士代表FDA，对Burzynski研究所（BRI）进行了现场检查，审查了BRI作为申办者的试验药物为抗瘤酮A10及AS2-1的下列临床研究的进行情况，这封警告信特告知您现场检查中发现的违规情况。

- 试验方案BT-09，“抗瘤酮A10及AS2-1在脑肿瘤受试者中进行的Ⅱ期研究”；
- 试验方案BT-10，“抗瘤酮A10及AS2-1在儿童脑肿瘤受试者中进行的Ⅱ期研究”；
- 试验方案BT-21，“抗瘤酮A10及AS2-1在成人原发性恶性脑肿瘤受试者中进行的Ⅱ期研究”；
- 试验方案BT-22，“抗瘤酮A10及AS2-1在儿童原发性恶性脑肿瘤受试者中进行的Ⅱ期研究”；
- 试验方案AD-02，“抗瘤酮A10及AS2-1在肾上腺癌受试者中进行的Ⅱ期研究”。

本次现场检查是FDA的生物研究监查项目（BIMO）的一部分，BIMO项目通过设定的检查方法，对FDA所监管的相关研究的实施情况进行评估，以确认研究数据在科学上是有效和准确的，并确保这些研究中受试者的权益、安全和福利得到保护。

在现场检查结束时，Martinez先生、McClure先生和Kleppinger博士向您出示了FDA483表，即现场检查发现的问题，并与您进行了讨论。您2013年4月5日对该FDA483表的书面回复已收悉。在2013年4月5日的书面回复中，您说BRI计划在2013年5月15日或之前向FDA提交一份更新，并且之后每月进行报告，直到BRI的纠正措施完成。我们还确认收到了来自您的日期为2013年5月15日、关于对FDA483表回复的进展情况更新。

经对现场检查报告、该报告的附件，以及您2013年4月5日的书面回复进行审查，我们认为BRI没有遵循适用的法律要求和监管临床研究实施及受试者保护的FDA法规。我们想强调以下几点：

1. 未能确保对研究进行适当的监查，未能确保研究根据IND中的总体研究计划和方案来进行［21 CFR 312.50和21 CFR 312.56（a）］

FDA法规要求申办者确保对临床研究进行适当的监查，确保临床研究按照IND中的方案进行。我们的调查发现，BRI未能确保对上述研究进行适当的监查，没有确保临床研究者按照IND中的方案进行研究。因为监查不足，BRI未能及时发现并纠正临床研究者对治疗反应错误分类，未能按照FDA法规要求获取受试者知情同意的情况。具体而言：

a. 试验方案BT-09，BT-10和BT-21定义了每种可能的治疗反应（完全缓解，部分缓解，疾病稳定及疾病进展），并包括了明确的标准，临床研究者必须使用这些标准按照其中一种反应将受试者归类。此次现场检查期间审查了27位受试者的治疗反应分类，其中9位的分类是错误的，而BRI的监查未能发现并予以纠正。具体而言：

ⅰ. 对于完全缓解的分类[1]，试验方案BT-09，BT-10及BT-21要求：①神经影像检查及辅助放射检查（如果有的话）显示所有的对比增强肿瘤完全消失，持续至少4周；②受试者未接受皮质类固醇治疗。

临床研究者将下列受试者错误分类为完全缓解，BRI的监查未能发现并纠正：

1）试验方案BT-10：受试者006389及013660未达到所有对比增强的肿瘤完全消失持续至少4周的标准，但被研究者错误地分类为完全缓解。

a. 受试者006389病例报告表肿瘤测量页以及研究者提供的截至2013年1月7日入组试验方案BT-10受试者

清单均显示该受试者达到完全缓解。但病例报告表肿瘤测量页显示：没有任何一次神经影像检查显示对比增强肿瘤完全消失持续至少4周。因此，该受试者不符合完全缓解的标准。

b. 受试者013660病例报告表肿瘤测量页以及研究者提供的截至2013年1月7日入组试验方案BT-10受试者清单均显示该受试者达到完全缓解。但病例报告表的肿瘤测量页显示：没有任何一次神经影像检查显示对比增强肿瘤完全消失持续至少4周。因此，该受试者不符合完全缓解的标准。

2）试验方案BT-09：受试者007197病例报告表肿瘤测量页显示，根据2001年7月25日、2001年9月11日及2001年11月8日的MRI检查结果，所有对比增强的肿瘤均完全消失至少4周。但病例报告表类固醇报告页及肿瘤血液学流程表显示该受试者于2001年7月25日、2001年9月11日接受MRI检查当天，以及这些MRI检查期间，直至2001年11月8日的MRI检查前一周，都在接受皮质类固醇治疗。因此该受试者不符合完全缓解的标准[2]。

3）试验方案BT-21：受试者009990未停止皮质类固醇治疗，因此被临床研究者错误地分类为完全缓解。

受试者009990病例报告表肿瘤测量页显示，根据正电子发射断层扫描（PET）结果，达到完全缓解。但病例报告表类固醇报告页显示该受试者在接受PET扫描的当天及期间（检查日期为2005年1月4日、2月4日、6月14日及8月16日）均接受了皮质类固醇治疗。因此该受试者不符合完全缓解的标准。

ⅱ. 对于部分缓解的分类，试验方案BT-09要求：①与基线比较，增强肿瘤最大垂直直径乘积的总和减少50%以上并持续至少4周；②没有任何病变大小同时增长，或新病变出现；③受试者皮质类固醇剂量稳定或减少。

临床研究者将下列受试者错误分类为部分缓解，BRI的监查未能发现并纠正：

受试者008765被研究者错误地分类为部分缓解。受试者008765病例报告表肿瘤测量页显示，根据2003年5月1日的放射学检查报告，该受试者被分类为部分缓解。尽管2003年5月1日的放射学检查报告显示肿瘤缩小大于50%，但2002年11月1日（基线MRI）至2003年5月1日放射学检查报告显示，肿瘤缩小大于50%并持续至少4周期间没有进行MRI检查。并且，2003年4月29日的放射学报告（MRI检查日期为2004年4月21日）实际显示肿瘤增大。因此该受试者不符合部分缓解的标准。

ⅲ. 对于疾病稳定的分类[3]，试验方案BT-10要求：①与基线比较，增强肿瘤最大垂直直径乘积的总和变化不足50%（增大或减小）；②这种状态持续至少12周；③皮质类固醇剂量稳定或减少。

临床研究者将下列受试者错误分类为疾病稳定，BRI的监查未能发现并纠正[4]：

1）试验方案BT-10：受试者012184、012206及012252的皮质类固醇剂量未稳定或减少，但被临床研究者错误地分类为疾病稳定。受试者011373没有达到肿瘤大小变化不足50%并持续至少12周，皮质类固醇剂量也未稳定或减少，因此不符合疾病稳定的标准。

a. 受试者012184病例报告表肿瘤测量页显示，根据2009年1月7日、4月20日、6月18日和7月24日的MRI检查，该受试者的肿瘤大小与基线相比变化不足50%，并且这种状态持续了至少12周。但病例报告表类固醇报告页显示，该受试者皮质类固醇剂量未稳定或减少，因此不符合疾病稳定的标准。

b. 受试者012206病例报告表肿瘤测量页显示，根据2009年1月15日和5月6日的MRI检查，该受试者的肿瘤大小与基线相比变化不足50%，并且这种状态持续了至少12周。但病例报告表类固醇报告页显示，该受试者皮质类固醇剂量未稳定或减少，因此不符合疾病稳定的标准。

c. 受试者012252病例报告表肿瘤测量页显示，根据2009年4月20日和8月7日的MRI检查，该受试者的肿瘤大小与基线相比变化不足50%，并且这种状态持续了至少12周。但病例报告表类固醇报告页显示，该受试者皮质类固醇剂量未稳定或减少，因此不符合疾病稳定的标准。

d. 受试者011373病例报告表肿瘤测量页显示，基线MRI检查的日期为2007年4月12日。该受试者于2007年4月13日开始接受试验药物治疗，并于2007年5月18日、7月6日和7月19日再次接受了MRI检查。病例报告表肿瘤测量页记录为2007年5月18日持续至7月19日，该受试者的肿瘤大小与基线相比变化不足50%；然而，自2007年7月19日后没有验证性的MRI或PET检查，因此没有证据表明肿瘤减小持续至少12周。此外，病例报告表类固醇报告页显示，该受试者皮质类固醇剂量未稳定或减少，因此不符合疾病稳定的标准。

BRI未能确保对临床研究进行适当的监查，因为BRI未能发现并纠正研究者对治疗反应的错误分类。因此，BRI未能确保临床研究按照研究计划进行。

BRI 2013年4月5日的书面回复中包括了一个与BRI监查操作相关的概述，也包括对FDA483表所列每个单个部分的专门回复。这封信将按照其在信中的顺序，讨论BRI针对单个部分逐一的回复，以及在违规情况结尾处的总体回复。

BRI 2013年4月5日的书面回复指出，BRI正在保存上述列出的受试者013660、009990、008765、012184、012206、012252及011373相应的完全缓解、部分缓解及疾病稳定（如适用）的原始评估材料。BRI指出，除受试者009990及011373外，临床研究者将根据BRI对肿瘤评估标准提出的修改，对所有受试者维持原始评价，也就是说，不是根据相关受试者被评估时试验方案内的肿瘤评估标准。对于受试者009990，BRI指出，根据BRI对评价标准的修改及中心影像审阅的意见，其建议为代谢完全缓解，研究者维持评价结果为完全缓解。对受试者011373，BRI指出，该受试者连续两次增强MRI的结果丢失，根据相应MRI肿瘤非增强部分定为疾病稳定。

另外，回复指出BRI“对于‘停用皮质类固醇的受试者’的定义为继续使用维持神经稳定性所需的最低剂量的人，维持在他们的舒适和功能的水平”。在回复中，BRI同时引用神经肿瘤工作组的建议：当受试者使用生理替代剂量的皮质类固醇时可以确认为完全及部分缓解。并且，回复指出BRI将修改试验方案BT-09，BT-10及BT-21，“以纠正在方案中规定的对‘停用皮质类固醇’的实际的解释”，并将方案修正案提交伦理委员会（IRB）2013年4月13日的会议进行审查[5]。

BRI的与监查临床研究者治疗反应评估有关的回复不够充分。BRI提出修订方案并未对BRI未能适当地监查临床研究的开展这一情况做出响应。BRI必须确保临床研究者遵循所写的方案，即评价治疗反应时应具体考虑皮质类固醇的使用。另外，BRI关于“停用皮质类固醇的受试者”的定义未包括在上述任何一个方案中。

我们承认使用皮质类固醇来维持生理水平可能是恰当的，尽管方案措辞为完全缓解需要受试者完全停用皮质类固醇。然而，上述所列尽管在使用皮质类固醇、仍分类为完全缓解的所有受试者，他们的皮质类固醇剂量都远远超出所需维持生理水平的剂量。具体而言，这些受试者在使用地卡特隆（地塞米松，一种皮质类固醇）的剂量为4～16mg/d不等，而生理替代的地卡特隆用量为0.25～0.75mg/d。

同时，方案要求受试者“停用皮质类固醇”仅适用于完全缓解的评估。监查为什么没有发现皮质类固醇剂量未稳定或减少的受试者被错误地评估为疾病稳定，BRI的回复未进行说明。另外，如上所述的受试者011373缺乏疾病稳定持续12周，但被错误地评价为疾病稳定，BRI的书面回复也未进行说明。另外，BRI的书面回复不充分，因为回复中未承诺要求临床研究者更正那些包含错误的治疗反应分类的研究记录。请注意对研究记录的所有更正都必须遵循21 CFR 312.62（b），（c），以维持和保留足够及准确的病历。

最后，BRI未能指出其是否计划向FDA提交方案的修正案。所描述的方案修改反映了方案设计上的重大改动。因此，BRI必须将方案的修改提交FDA审查［21 CFR 312.30（b）（1）（ⅱ）和（2）（ⅰ）（a）］。

b. 临床研究者未能按照21 CFR 312.60，50.25（b）（3）及 50.27（b）（1）的要求获得受试者的知情同意，BRI的监查未能发现并纠正。临床研究者使用的用于试验方案BT-10及BT-22的知情同意文件（ICDs）中未包括知情同意所需的所有要素。具体而言，知情同意书中没有包含21 CFR 50.25（b）（3）中要求的，关于参加研究可能导致受试者产生额外费用的描述。研究者已经同意参加临床研究后，费用协议才提供给他们[6]。

临床研究者未能在知情同意中包括所有需要的要素，BRI的监查未能发现并纠正。因此，BRI未能确保对这些临床研究进行适当的监查。此缺陷也导致BRI未能确保临床研究按照研究计划进行。

BRI 2013年4月5日对发现问题的书面回复承认“治疗费用协议仅给予受试者……在签署ICD之后。”并且回复指出“签署ICD和提供治疗费用协议的间隔可能是几小时、几天或几周”。作为纠正措施，BRI提出对知情同意文件的修改措辞，以解决缺少关于参加研究可能产生额外费用的描述的问题。

BRI对于监查临床研究者提供知情同意的相关回复是不充分的。提出的修改措辞不恰当，因为其集中于试验药物是否会收费，仅仅包含了关于产生额外费用可能性的概括描述；将责任加之于受试者，让他自己询问是否有任何增加的费用，而不是提供给受试者可能由于参加研究而产生的具体的额外费用。相反，治疗费用协议确定了受试者由于参加研究而预期将要支付的具体的额外费用。知情同意文件本身必须包括关于受试者可能由于参加研究而导致的额外费用的信息。

BRI 2013年4月5日的书面回复确认了关于BRI一般监查操作的几项纠正措施。回复承认截止2005年，BRI停止使用2004年4月23日的研究监查计划，并且“错误是，我们修订的监查操作未能以修订的监查指南的形式正式确定下来。”此回复包含几个附件，例如，下列新的SOP：

研究监查指南（SOP420）；

GCP监查（SOP421）；

用于材料递交的现场规范性文件的审查及批准（SOP410）；

临床试验资料的管理（SOP430）；

不良事件及严重不良事件的报告及处理（SOP702）。

除了这些新SOP的施行，BRI承诺按照新的SOP审查数据及GCP文件立即重新使用专职监查员。

这些关于BRI一般监查操作的纠正措施，如适当施行，看来会有效预防将来类似的违规情况再次发生。但是，与上述1.a，1.b项相关的纠正措施不充分，应当在您对本警告信的回复中说明。另外，名为“用于材料递交的现场规范性文件的审查及批准”的 BRI的SOP410中的知情同意检查表，仅引用了45 CFR 46中对知情同意的法规要求。作为初始事项，任何BRI提交的IND申请的下属临床研究除了遵循45 CFR 46中的适用法规要求，还要遵循FDA法规中对于知情同意的要求。请修改知情同意检查表（410A）及其他有关SOP，以体现适用的FDA法规要求。并且，我们注意到45 CFR 46.408（c）包括这一条款，据此，伦理委员会可以豁免在儿童作为受试者的临床研究中获得父母许可的要求。在FDA法规21 CFR 50（D)，对临床研究中儿童的额外保护中没有类似条款。因此，在FDA所监管的临床研究中不允许伦理委员会豁免获得父母的许可的要求。请相应地修订知情同意检查表（410A)。

2. 未能从研究者处获取足够的财务信息，供申办者按照21 CFR 54的要求提交足够准确的证明或公开声明［21 CFR 312.53（c）（4）］

FDA法规要求临床试验申办者从研究者处获取足够的财务信息，以供申办者按照FDA法规第54部分的要求提交足够准确的证明或公开声明。BRI未能获得参加试验方案BT-09、BT-10、BT-21及BT-22的122位授权研究者的财务信息，其中参加BT-09的有40位，BT-10的有34位，BT-21的有40位，BT-22的有8位。BRI 2013年4月5日的书面回复指出，BRI认为没必要获得这些授权研究者（都是受试者或受试者的当地的医生）的财务公开声明，因为没有财务关系需要公开。BRI指出：“……我们相信我们有关于临床人员及授权研究者的足够的信息来符合21 CFR 54的要求。BRI进一步指出，作为纠正措施，在递交新药申请时（NDA），BRI将递交FDA3454表，勾选第1格并附上所有当地医生的名单，同时提交一个简要的附件，描述书面回复中展示的情况。

BRI的书面回复不充分，因为BRI在递交NDA申请时作为申请人的职责不同于其作为临床研究申办者的职责。作为申办者，BRI必须遵循21 CFR 312的所有相关要求，包括根据21 CFR 312.53（c）（4）获得财务信息的要求。BRI必须在IND阶段收集这些信息，即使BRI认为没有财务关系需要公开，并且必须获得授权研究者的承诺，在研究期间及研究结束1年内如果有任何情况变化应及时更新这个信息。

本警告信的目的并非是罗列您在试验药物临床研究中存在的所有缺陷。确保遵循法律和相关FDA法规的每一项要求是您的职责，您应当解决这些缺陷，并建立规程，以确保任何正在进行或将来进行的研究均符合FDA法规。

自收到这封信的15个工作日内，您应当书面告知本办公室为预防将来发生类似违规情况而采取的措施。如果不能充分、快速地对上述违规问题作出说明，可能导致我们在不再通知的情况下采取监管措施。如果您认为BRI已符合FDA法规要求，请陈述理由，并提供所有支持资料，以供我们参考。

1. 完全缓解的分类没有反映出在超出作出治疗反应分类的时间点以外，治疗反应是否继续。也就是说，有可能被正确地分类为完全缓解的受试者肿瘤复发。

2. 我们注意到，这与一位先前治疗过的受试者，受试者005297一致。那位受试者的病例报告表肿瘤测量页显示，根据1997年8月11日和10月2日的MRI检查结果，所有对比增强的肿瘤均完全消失至少4周。但病例报告表类固醇报告页及肿瘤血液学流程表显示，该受试者在1997年8月11日MRI检查前，1997年8月11日和10月2日MRI检查期间（包括1997年10月2日），都在接受皮质类固醇治疗。因此受试者005297不符合完全缓解的标准。对于受试者005297，BRI指出已经要求第二次独立放射学审查，以确认正确的治疗反应，并说您将在收到后将这个信息交给FDA。我们注意到截止这封信的日期，FDA仍没有收到这个信息。

3. 我们注意到，是否受试者被按照方案规定的标准正确地分类为疾病稳定这个问题，不同于是否FDA将接受疾病稳定比率作为有效性宣称的基础这个问题。

4. 我们注意到上面引用的例子与先前治疗过的两名试验方案BT-10和试验方案BT-22（该方案关于疾病稳定的分类的标准与试验方案BT-10相同）的受试者一致。试验方案BT-10的受试者005974病例报告表肿瘤测量页显示，根据1999年1月12日和4月6日的MRI检查结果，肿瘤大小与基线相比变化不足50%，且这种状况持续至少12周。但是，病例报告表类固醇报告页显示，该受试者皮质类固醇剂量未稳定或减少，因此不符合疾病稳定的标准。在2013年4月5日的书面回复中，BRI指出根据对肿瘤评估标准提出的修改，正将受试者005974重新分类为疾病进展。试验方案BT-22的受试者004240病例报告表肿瘤测量页显示，其基线MRI检查的日期为1996年2月21日。该受试者于1996年3月6日开始使用试验药物，并于1996年4月10日、5月22日、6月26日和7月31日再次接受了MRI检查。病例报告表肿瘤测量页记录为该受试者的肿瘤大小与基线相比变化不足50%，仅从1996年4月10日持续至5月22日，不足12周。因此该受试者不符合疾病稳定的标准。在2013年4月5日的书面回复中，BRI提出，根据中小者对肿瘤评估标准提出的修改，将保留对该受试者的原始评价。但是，BRI对这位受试者的回复并没有说明由于缺失12周持续期而导致的疾病稳定的错误分类。

5. 我们注意到，试验方案BT-09、BT-10和BT-21都关闭了。BRI的书面回复还提示，BRI已经准备了提交给伦理委员会的试验方案BT-22的修正案草案。试验方案BT-21也关闭了。

6. 我们注意到，根据您2013年4月5日的书面回复，试验方案BT-09使用的知情同意书也没有包含这个信息，受试者在签署了知情同意书以后，费用协议才提供给他们。

附：英文原文

Burzynski Research Institute

WARNING LETTER

Dec 3, 2013

CERTIFIED MAIL
RETURN RECEIPT REQUESTED

Ref:13-HFD-45-11-05

Stanislaw R. Burzynski, M.D., Ph.D.
President
Burzynski Research Institute
9432 Katy Freeway, Suite 200
Houston, TX 77055-6330

Dear Dr. Burzynski:

This Warning Letter informs you of objectionable conditions observed during the U.S. Food and Drug Administration (FDA) inspection conducted at Burzynski Research Institute (BRI) between January 17 and March 15, 2013. Mr. Joel Martinez, Mr. Hugh McClure, and Dr. Cynthia Kleppinger, representing the FDA, reviewed BRI's conduct as the sponsor of the following clinical investigations of the investigational drugs Antineoplastons A10 and AS2-1:

- Protocol BT-09, "Phase Ⅱ Study of Antineoplastons A10 and AS2-1 in Patients with Brain Tumors";
- Protocol BT-10, "Phase Ⅱ Study of Antineoplastons A10 and AS2-1 in Children with Brain Tumors";
- Protocol BT-21, "Phase Ⅱ Study of Antineoplastons A10 and AS2-1 in Adults with Primary Malignant Brain Tumors";
- Protocol BT-22, "Phase Ⅱ Study of Antineoplastons A10 and AS2-1 in Children with Primary Malignant Brain Tumors"; and
- Protocol AD-02, "Phase Ⅱ Study of Antineoplastons A10 and AS2-1 in Patients with Carcinoma of the Adrenal Gland."

This inspection is a part of the FDA's Bioresearch Monitoring Program, which includes inspections designed to evaluate the conduct of FDA-regulated research to ensure that the data are scientifically valid and accurate, and to help ensure that the rights, safety, and welfare of the human subjects of those studies have been protected.

At the conclusion of the inspection, Mr. Martinez, Mr. McClure, and Dr. Kleppinger presented and discussed with you Form FDA 483, Inspectional Observations. We acknowledge receipt of your April 5, 2013 written response to the Form FDA 483.

In your April 5, 2013, written response, you stated that BRI was planning to submit an update to FDA on or before May 15, 2013, and monthly reports thereafter until BRI's corrective actions are completed. We also acknowledge receipt of a progress update from you, dated May 15, 2013, regarding your response to the Form FDA 483.

From our review of the FDA establishment inspection report, the documents submitted with that report, and your April 5, 2013, written response, we conclude that BRI did not adhere to the applicable statutory requirements and FDA regulations governing the conduct of clinical investigations and the protection of human subjects. We wish to emphasize the following:

1. Failure to ensure proper monitoring of the investigations and failure to ensure that the investigations are conducted in accordance with the general investigational plan and protocols contained in the IND [21 CFR 312.50 and 21 CFR 312.56(a)].

FDA regulations require that sponsors ensure proper monitoring of clinical investigations and ensure that their clinical investigators conduct the investigations in accordance with the protocols contained in the Investigational New Drug file (IND). Our investigation found that BRI failed to ensure proper monitoring of the studies referenced above and did not ensure that a clinical investigator conducted the investigations in accordance with the protocols contained in the IND. As a result of inadequate monitoring, BRI did not identify, and correct in a timely manner, a clinical investigator's incorrect classification of therapeutic responses and failure to obtain informed consent from subjects in accordance with FDA regulations. Specifically:

a. Protocols BT-09, BT-10, and BT-21 define each possible therapeutic response (Complete Response, Partial Response, Stable Disease, and Progressive Disease), and include specific criteria the clinical investigator must use to classify a subject as having one of those responses. BRI monitoring failed to identify and correct the clinical investigator's incorrect classification of therapeutic responses for 9 of the 27 subjects whose therapeutic response classifications were reviewed during the inspection. Specifically:

i. For a classification of Complete Response[1], Protocols BT-09, BT-10, and BT-21 required: (1) complete disappearance of all contrast-enhancing tumor on neuroimaging studies and ancillary radiographic studies if appropriate, for a minimum duration of four weeks; and (2) that the subject be off corticosteroids.

BRI monitoring failed to identify and correct the clinical investigator's incorrect classification of the following subjects as having a Complete Response:

1. Protocol BT-10: Subjects 006389 and 013660 did not have complete disappearance of all contrast-enhancing tumors for at least four weeks and, therefore, were incorrectly classified by the clinical investigator as having a

Complete Response.

a. For Subject 006389, both the Tumor Measurements Case Report Form (CRF) and the list that the clinical investigator provided us of subjects enrolled in Protocol BT-10 as of January 7, 2013, identify this subject as having a Complete Response. However, the Tumor Measurements CRF shows that none of the neuroimaging studies showed complete disappearance of contrast-enhancing tumor for at least four weeks. Therefore, the subject did not meet the criteria for Complete Response.

b. For Subject 013660, both the Tumor Measurements CRF and the list that the clinical investigator provided us of subjects enrolled in Protocol BT-10 as of January 7, 2013, identify this subject as having a Complete Response. However, the Tumor Measurements CRF shows that none of the neuroimaging studies showed complete disappearance of contrast-enhancing tumor for at least four weeks. Therefore, the subject did not meet the criteria for Complete Response.

2. Protocol BT-09: For Subject 007197, the Tumor Measurements CRF indicates, based on MRIs taken on July 25, 2001; September 11, 2001; and November 8, 2001, complete disappearance of all contrast-enhancing tumor for a minimum duration of four weeks. However, the Steroids Report CRF and the Oncology-Hematology Flow Sheet show that the subject was on corticosteroids preceding the July 25, 2001 and September 11, 2001 MRIs; during the period between these MRIs; and up to one week prior to the November 8, 2001 MRI. Therefore, the subject did not meet the criteria for Complete Response.[2]

3. Protocol BT-21: Subject 009990 was not off corticosteroids and, therefore, was incorrectly classified by the clinical investigator as having a Complete Response.

For Subject 009990, the Tumor Measurements CRF shows that the subject was classified as having a Complete Response based on Positron Emission Tomography (PET) scan results. However, the Steroids Report CRF shows that the subject was on corticosteroids preceding all of the relevant PET scan dates (January 4, February 4, June 14, and August 16, 2005), as well as during the period between these PET scans. Therefore, the subject did not meet the criteria for Complete Response.

ii. For a classification of Partial Response, Protocol BT-09 required: (1) that subjects have more than 50% reduction in the sum of the products of the greatest perpendicular diameters of contrast-enhancing tumors, compared to the corresponding baseline evaluation, for at least four weeks; (2) that no simultaneous increase in size of any lesion or the appearance of new lesions may occur; and (3) that subjects be on a stable or decreasing dose of corticosteroids.

BRI monitoring failed to identify and correct the clinical investigator's incorrect classification of the following subject as having a Partial Response:

Subject 008765 was incorrectly classified by the clinical investigator as having a partial response. For Subject 008765, the Tumor Measurements CRF shows that the subject was classified as having a Partial Response based on a radiology report dated May 1, 2003. Although the May 1, 2003 radiology report shows a tumor reduction of greater than 50%, there are no MRIs between November 1, 2002 (baseline MRI) and the May 1, 2003 radiology report that show that the tumor reduction of greater than 50% was maintained for at least four weeks during that time period. Further, the April 29, 2003 radiology report (for the April 21, 2003 MRI) actually shows an increase in tumor size. Therefore, the subject did not meet the criteria for Partial Response.

iii. For a classification of Stable Disease[3], Protocol BT-10 required: (1) that subjects have less than 50% change (either greater or smaller) in the sum of the products of the perpendicular diameters of the enhancing tumor compared to the baseline evaluation; (2) that this state be maintained for a minimum of 12 weeks; and (3) that the corticosteroid dose is stable or decreasing.

BRI monitoring failed to identify and correct the clinical investigator's incorrect classification of the following subjects as having Stable Disease[4]:

1. Protocol BT-10: Subjects 012184, 012206 and 012252 were not on stable or decreasing doses of corticosteroids and, therefore, were incorrectly classified by the clinical investigator as having Stable Disease. Subject 011373 did not have a less than 50% change in tumor size maintained for at least 12 weeks and was not on either a stable or decreasing dose of corticosteroids and, therefore, did not meet the criteria for Stable Disease.

a. For Subject 012184, the Tumor Measurements CRF indicates, based on MRIs taken on January 7, April 20, June 18, and July 24, 2009, that the subject had a less than 50% change in tumor size compared to baseline, and that this state was maintained for a minimum of 12 weeks. However, the Steroids Report CRF shows that the subject was not on either a stable or decreasing dose of corticosteroids. Therefore, the subject did not meet the criteria for Stable Disease.

b. For Subject 012206, the Tumor Measurements CRF indicates, based on MRIs taken on January 15 and May 6, 2009, that the subject had a less than 50% change in tumor size compared to baseline, and that this state was maintained for a minimum of 12 weeks. However, the Steroids Report CRF shows that the subject was not on either a stable or decreasing dose of corticosteroids. Therefore, the subject did not meet the criteria for Stable Disease.

c. For Subject 012252, the Tumor Measurements CRF indicates, based on MRIs taken on April 20 and August 7, 2009, that the subject had a less than 50% change in tumor size compared to baseline, and that this state was maintained for a minimum of 12 weeks. However, the Steroids Report CRF shows that the subject was not on either a stable or decreasing dose of corticosteroids. Therefore, the subject did not meet the criteria for Stable Disease.

d. For Subject 011373, the Tumor Measurements CRF shows that a baseline MRI was taken on April 12, 2007. The subject began receiving investigational drug on April 13, 2007, and had additional MRIs taken on May 18, July 6, and July 19, 2007. The Tumor Measurements CRF documents that a change of less than 50% in tumor size, compared to baseline, was maintained from May 18 through July 19, 2007; however, there are no confirmatory MRIs or PET scans after July 19, 2007, and there is therefore no evidence that the reduction was maintained for a minimum of 12 weeks. In addition, the Steroids Report CRF shows that the subject was not on either a stable or decreasing dose of corticosteroids. Therefore, the subject did not meet the criteria for Stable Disease.

BRI failed to ensure proper monitoring of these clinical investigations because BRI did not identify and correct the clinical investigator's incorrect assessments of therapeutic responses. As a result, BRI has failed to ensure that the clinical investigations were conducted in accordance with the investigational plan.

BRI's April 5, 2013 written response included a general section related to BRI's monitoring practices, as well as specific responses to each of the individual sub-parts listed on the Form FDA 483. This letter will discuss the BRI response to the individual sub-parts in the order they appear in the letter, and the general response at the end of this violation.

BRI's April 5, 2013 written response indicated that BRI was retaining the original assessments of Complete Response, Partial Response, and Stable Disease (as applicable) for Subjects 013660, 009990, 008765, 012184, 012206, 012252, and 011373 listed above. BRI indicated that, with the exception of Subjects 009990 and 011373, the clinical investigator will be maintaining the original assessment for all of these subjects based on BRI's proposed changes to the tumor assessment criteria, that is, not based on the tumor assessment criteria as included in the protocol at the time the relevant subjects were evaluated. For Subject 009990, BRI indicated that the clinical investigator was maintaining the assessment as a Complete Response based on BRI's proposed changes to the tumor assessment criteria and based on central radiology review, which suggested a Complete Response metabolically. For Subject 011373, BRI indicated that two consecutive MRIs of the subject using enhancement were unavailable, and that the subject was classified as having Stable Disease based upon the nonenhancement portion of the tumor for the corresponding MRIs.

In addition, the response stated that BRI's "definition of a 'patient off corticosteroids' is one who continues on the lowest dosage necessary for neurologic stability and is maintained at their level of comfort and function." In the response, BRI also cited the Neuro-Oncology Working Group recommendations that complete and partial responses can be determined when a patient is on physiologic replacement doses of corticosteroids. Further, the response stated that BRI will amend Protocols BT-09, BT-10, and BT-21 "to correct the practical interpretation of 'off steroids' as currently specified in the protocols" and will submit the protocol amendments to the Institutional Review Board (IRB) for review and approval at its April 13, 2013 meeting[5].

BRI's response related to monitoring the clinical investigator's therapeutic response assessments is inadequate. BRI's proposal to amend the protocols is not responsive to BRI's failure to monitor the conduct of the clinical investigations properly. BRI was required to ensure that the clinical investigator complied with the protocols as written, which required specific consideration of corticosteroid use when assessing therapeutic response. In addition, BRI's definition of "a patient off corticosteroids" was not included in any of the protocols listed above.

We acknowledge that the use of corticosteroids to maintain physiologic levels may be appropriate, despite protocol wording requiring that subjects be off corticosteroids completely for a Complete Response. However, for all of the subjects listed above as having been classified as a Complete Response despite being on corticosteroids, their corticosteroid doses were well beyond those needed to maintain physiologic levels. Specifically, these subjects were on doses of Decadron (dexamethasone, a corticosteroid) that ranged from 4 mg/day to 16 mg/day, while the physiologic-replacement equivalent of Decadron is in the range of 0.25 mg/day to 0.75 mg/day.

Also, the protocols' requirement that a subject be "off corticosteroids" applies only to the Complete Response assessment. BRI's written response does not address how monitoring failed to detect the incorrect assessments of Stable Disease in cases where subjects were not on stable or decreasing doses of corticosteroids. Further, BRI's written response does not address the incorrect classification of Stable Disease that resulted from lack of a 12-week maintenance period for Subject 011373, as described above. In addition, BRI's written response is inadequate because it does not include a commitment to have the clinical investigator correct the study records that contain these incorrect response classifications. Please note that all corrections to study records must be done in accordance with the requirements of 21 CFR 312.62(b) and (c) to maintain and retain adequate and accurate case histories.

Lastly, BRI has not indicated whether it is planning to submit its proposed protocol amendments to FDA. The described protocol changes reflect a significant change in the design of the protocols. As a result, BRI is required to submit the protocol changes to FDA for review [21 CFR 312.30(b)(1)(ⅱ) and (2)(ⅰ)(a)].

b. BRI monitoring failed to identify and correct the clinical investigator's failure to obtain informed consent from subjects in accordance with the provisions of 21 CFR Parts 312.60, 50.25(b)(3), and 50.27(b)(1). The informed consent documents (ICDs) used by the clinical investigator for Protocols BT-10 and BT-22 did not contain all of the required elements of informed consent. Specifically, the informed consent forms did not contain a statement regarding any additional costs to the subject that may result from participating in the research, as required by 21 CFR 50.25(b)(3). Research subjects were presented with a billing agreement only after they had already consented to participate in clinical research.[6]

BRI's monitoring did not identify and correct the clinical investigator's failure to include all required elements of informed consent. Therefore, BRI failed to ensure proper monitoring of these clinical investigations. As a result of this failure, BRI has also failed to ensure that the clinical investigations were conducted in accordance with the investigational plan.

BRI's April 5, 2013 written response to this observation acknowledged that "a treatment billing agreement is only presented to the patient... after the ICD is signed." In addition, the response stated that "at times, days or weeks may elapse between signing the ICD and presenting the treatment billing agreement." As a corrective action, BRI proposed amended wording to informed consent documents to address the lack of a statement regarding additional costs to the subject that may result from participating in the research.

BRI's response related to monitoring the clinical investigator's provision of informed consent is inadequate. The proposed amended wording is not adequate because it focuses primarily on whether there is a charge for the investigational agent; contains only general statements regarding the possibility of additional costs; and puts the responsibility on the subject to inquire about any expected added costs, rather than providing the subject with specific additional costs that may result from participation in the research. In contrast, the treatment billing agreement identifies the specific additional costs the subject will be expected to pay as a result of participating in research. The informed consent document itself must include the information about the additional costs to the subject that may result from his or her participation in the research.

BRI's April 5, 2013 written response identified several corrective actions related to BRI's general monitoring practices. The response acknowledged that as of 2005, BRI ceased using the Study Monitoring Plan dated 23 April 2004, and that "erroneously our revised monitoring practices were not formally acknowledged in the form of revised monitoring guidelines." The response contained several attachments, including, for example, the following new SOPs:

- Study Monitoring Guidelines (SOP 420)
- GCP Monitoring (SOP 421)
- Review and Approval of Site Regulatory Documents for Submission (SOP 410)
- Clinical Trial Material Management (SOP 430)

- Reporting and Processing Adverse and Serious Adverse Events (SOP 702)

In addition to the implementation of these new SOPs, BRI has committed to immediately reinstituting the use of a dedicated monitor to review data and Good Clinical Practice (GCP) documentation according to the new SOPs.

These corrective actions related to BRI's general monitoring practices, if properly carried out, appear adequate to prevent the recurrence of similar violations in the future. However, the corrective actions related to the specific issues identified in Items 1.a. and 1.b., above, are inadequate and should be addressed in your response to this letter.

In addition, the Informed Consent Checklist for BRI's SOP 410, titled "Review and Approval of Site Regulatory Documents for Submission," only cites the informed consent requirements under 45 CFR part 46. As an initial matter, any clinical investigations conducted under BRI's IND are subject to the informed consent requirements in FDA's regulations, in addition to any applicable regulations in 45 CFR part 46. Please revise the Informed Consent Checklist (410A) and any other SOPs to reflect applicable FDA regulations. Further, we note that 45 CFR 46.408(c) includes a provision whereby an IRB may waive the requirement to obtain parental permission in a clinical investigation that includes children as subjects. There is no analogous provision in FDA's regulations in 21 CFR part 50, subpart D (Additional Safeguards for Children in Clinical Investigations). Therefore, an IRB is not permitted to waive the requirement to obtain parental permission in an FDA-regulated clinical investigation. Please revise the Informed Consent Checklist (410A) accordingly.

2. Failure to obtain from an investigator sufficient financial information to allow the sponsor to submit complete and accurate certification or disclosure statements required under 21 CFR part 54 [21 CFR 312.53(c)(4)].

FDA regulations require that sponsors of clinical investigations obtain sufficient financial information from investigators to allow the sponsor to submit complete and accurate certification or disclosure statements required under part 54 of FDA's regulations. BRI failed to obtain financial information for each of the 122 sub-investigators participating in Protocols BT-09, BT-10, BT-21, and BT-22. There was no financial information for 40 sub-investigators for BT-09; 34 sub-investigators for BT-10; 40 sub-investigators for BT-21; and 8 sub-investigators for BT-22. BRI's April 5, 2013 written response indicated that BRI considered it unnecessary to obtain financial disclosures from these sub-investigators (all of whom were subjects' or patients' local physicians) because there were no financial relationships to disclose. BRI stated, "...we believe that we have sufficient information about both clinic personnel and sub-investigators to be in compliance with 21 CFR part 54." BRI further indicated that as corrective action, when BRI files the New Drug Application (NDA), BRI will submit one Form FDA 3454, will check Box 1, will attach a list of all of the local physicians, and will submit a brief addendum describing the facts set forth in the written response.

BRI's written response is not adequate, because BRI's responsibilities as an applicant at the time of an NDA filing differ from BRI's responsibilities as a sponsor of a clinical investigation. As a sponsor, BRI is required to comply with all of the relevant requirements in 21 CFR part 312, including the requirement to obtain financial information in accordance with 21 CFR 312.53(c)(4). BRI must collect this information at the IND stage even if BRI believes that there are no financial relationships to disclose, and it must obtain the sub-investigators' commitments to update this information promptly if any relevant changes occur during the investigation and for one year following the completion of the investigation.

This letter is not intended to be an all-inclusive list of deficiencies with your clinical study of an investigational drug. It is your responsibility to ensure adherence to each requirement of the law and relevant FDA regulations. You should address these deficiencies and establish procedures to ensure that any ongoing or future studies will be in compliance with FDA regulations.

Within fifteen (15) working days of your receipt of this letter, you should notify this office in writing of the actions you have taken to prevent similar violations in the future. Failure to explain the violations noted above adequately and promptly may result in regulatory action without further notice. If you believe that BRI has complied with FDA regulations, include your reasoning and any supporting information for our consideration.

If you have any questions, please contact Constance Cullity, M.D., M.P.H., at 301-796-3397; FAX 301-847-8748. Your written response and any pertinent documentation should be addressed to:

Constance Cullity, M.D., M.P.H.
Branch Chief
Good Clinical Practice Enforcement Branch
Division of Good Clinical Practice Compliance
Office of Scientific Investigations
Office of Compliance
Center for Drug Evaluation and Research
Food and Drug Administration
Building 51, Room 5354
10903 New Hampshire Avenue
Silver Spring, MD 20993

Sincerely yours,

{See appended electronic signature page}

Thomas N. Moreno, M.S.
Acting Office Director
Office of Scientific Investigations
Office of Compliance
Center for Drug Evaluation and Research
Food and Drug Administration

1. A classification of Complete Response does not reflect whether the response continued beyond the point in time at which the therapeutic response classification was made. That is, it is possible that a subject who is correctly classified as having a Complete Response could have tumor return later.
2. We note that this is consistent with a previously treated subject, Subject 005297. The Tumor Measurements CRF for that subject indicates, based on MRIs taken on August 11, 1997, and October 2, 1997, complete disappearance of all contrast-enhancing tumor for a minimum duration of four weeks. However, the Steroids Report CRF and Oncology-Hematology Flow Sheet show that the subject was on corticosteroids preceding the August 11, 1997 MRI and during the period between August 11, 1997, and the October 2, 1997 MRI (including on October 2, 1997). Therefore, Subject 005297 did not meet the criteria for Complete Response. For Subject 005297, BRI indicated that it had requested a second independent radiology review to confirm the correct response, and stated that you would forward this information to FDA after receipt. We note that as of the date of this letter, FDA has not received this information.
3. We note that the question of whether subjects were appropriately classified as having Stable Disease under protocol-specific criteria is distinct from the question of whether FDA would accept data on Stable Disease rates as the basis of an efficacy claim.
4. We note that the examples cited above are consistent with two previously treated subjects from Protocol BT-10 and Protocol BT-22 (which had the same criteria as Protocol BT-10 regarding classification of Stable Disease). For Subject 005974 in Protocol BT-10, the Tumor Measurements CRF indicates, based on MRIs taken on January 12, 1999, and April 6, 1999, that the subject had less than 50% change in tumor size compared to baseline, and that this state was maintained for a minimum of 12 weeks. However, the Steroids Report CRF shows that the subject was not on either a stable or decreasing dose of corticosteroids. Therefore, the subject did not meet the criteria for Stable Disease. In BRI's April 5, 2013 written response, BRI stated that it was reclassifying Subject 005974 as Progressive Disease, based on the proposed changes to the tumor assessment criteria. For Subject 004240 in Protocol BT-22, the Tumor Measurements CRF shows that the subject had a baseline MRI taken on February 21, 1996. The subject began receiving investigational drug on March 6, 1996, and had additional MRIs taken on April 10, May 22, June 26, and July 31, 1996. The Tumor Measurements CRF documents that a change of less than 50% change in tumor size, compared to baseline, was maintained only from April 10 through May 22, 1996, which is less than 12 weeks. Therefore, the subject did not meet the criteria for Stable Disease. In BRI's April 5, 2013 written response, BRI stated that it was retaining the original assessment for this subject, based on the sponsor's proposed changes to the tumor assessment criteria. However, BRI's response for this subject did not address the incorrect classification of Stable Disease that resulted from lack of a 12-week maintenance period.
5. We note that Protocols BT-09, BT-10, and BT-21 are closed. BRI's written response also indicated that BRI has prepared draft amendments for Protocol BT-22 for submission to the IRB. BT-22 is also closed.
6. We note that, based on your April 5, 2013 written response, the informed consent forms used for Protocol BT-09 also did not contain this information, and subjects were only presented with a billing agreement after they had signed the informed consent forms.

第41封　给辉瑞有限公司的警告信

2010年4月9日

参考号：10-HFD-45-04-01

尊敬的Mackay博士：

2009年5月4日至6月3日，Michelle M. Noe 女士和Cynthia Kleppinger博士代表FDA进行了一次现场检查，与贵公司全球法规事务副总裁John Oidtman会面，并对贵公司作为申办者实施临床研究的情况进行了审查：试验方案（b）（4），标题为“（b）（4）”，试验药物为（b）（4），申办者为辉瑞公司。

本次现场检查是FDA的生物研究监查项目的一部分，该项目通过设定的检查方法，评估研究的实施情况，以确保这些研究中受试者的权益、安全和福利得到了保护。此次现场检查是由于在对实施方案（b）（4）的几个临床研究者的检查中发现了重大违规问题。

在现场检查结束时，Noe女士和Kleppinger博士出示并与John Oidtman讨论了FDA 483表，即现场检查发现的问题。经对FDA现场检查报告、该报告的附件，以及贵公司于2009年7月2日对FDA 483表的书面回复进行审查，我们认为您没有遵循适用的法律要求和监管临床研究实施的FDA法规。我们想强调以下几点：

1. 您未能确保对临床研究进行适当的监查［21 CFR 312.50］

此项违规在2005年4月25日至2005年6月6日间开展的针对Pfizer对临床研究（b）（4）的监查情况的现场检查中已有发现，并已经通过非正式信函与您沟通。

FDA法规要求申办者应确保对临床研究进行适当的监查。我们的调查发现，Pfizer公司没有对上述的研究进行适当的监查，由此导致多个试验场所的受试者普遍用药过量，而未被及时发现并纠正。

a. 研究监查员未能确保临床研究遵照研究计划执行。研究监查员未能及时发现（b）（4）医生的试验场所［试验场所（b）（4）］用药过量情况，也未能及时汇报。

方案规定，在给药第8天之前给药剂量不能超过160mg/d，而且体重45kg及以上的受试者每天试验药物的总剂量不能超过160mg，体重低于45kg的受试者则不能超过80mg。

在贵公司现场检查时发现，（b）（4）医生的试验场所［试验场所（b）（4）］，所有7位儿童受试者持续多天用药错误和过量，其中一例长达22天。以下是现场检查中发现的在（b）（4）医生的试验场所［试验场所（b）（4）］发生的儿童受试者用药过量的实例：

i. 受试者1001文件记录的体重为46.8kg，连续20天过量给予研究药物。在治疗第8天及第9天，受试者被给予180mg/d；在治疗第10天及11天受试者被给予240mg/d；在治疗第12天及13天，受试者被给予320mg/d；在治疗第14天，受试者被给予400mg/d；在治疗第15至27天，受试者被给予180mg/d。

ii. 受试者1003文件记录的体重为65kg，连续21天过量给予研究药物。在治疗第7天，受试者被给予180mg/d；在治疗第8天及第9天，受试者被给予240mg/d；在治疗第10至第26天，受试者被给予400mg/d；在治疗第27天，受试者被给予280mg/d。

iii. 受试者1004连续3天过量给予研究药物。在治疗第9天，受试者被给予320mg/d；在治疗第10和第11天，被给予240mg/d。

iv. 受试者1005连续16天过量给予研究药物。在治疗第8和第9天，受试者被给予180mg/d；在治疗第10天至第14天，被给予240mg/d；在第15天至第20天及第22天至第23天，受试者被给予400mg/d；在治疗第21天，受试者被给予200mg/d。

v. 受试者1006文件记录的体重为低于45kg，连续7天过量给予研究药物。在治疗第16至第22天，此受试者被给予400mg/d的研究药物。

ⅵ. 受试者1007文件记录的体重为39.5kg，连续13天过量给予研究药物。在治疗第16至第28天，此受试者被给予120mg/d的研究药物。

研究监查员对试验场所的访视总共有9天：2006年3月13日和15日，4月25日，5月15～16日，6月6～7日和7月5～6日，然而过量用药的问题直到2006年7月25日由Pfizer的数据管理部门发现，而不是被研究监查员发现。另外，我们调查中发现了一份日期为2006年11月7日的Pfizer内部报告，题为"在辉瑞公司研究（b）（4）中对给药卡的误解导致给药错误的报告"，报告指出，"2006年7月25日，Pfizer临床研究团队才知道可能有给药错误发生"。我们注意到所有三项研究都与有着同样包装的研究（b）（4）有关。

报告表明，Pfizer的研究团队对以上所提的3个临床研究中截至2006年11月7日的所有入组的受试者的给药记录进行了检查，发现有两家试验场所存在给药错误的情况，并采取了多种补救措施，包括在某些等待再次培训的研究场所暂停受试者入组，重新评估这些试验场所遵照试验方案开展研究的能力。值得注意的是，报告指出研究团队"确定给药程序在试验方案、方案附件及给药卡都有清楚地描述，无需对这些文件进行修订。研究团队就正确的给药程序对所有的试验场所和研究监查员进行了重新培训。对所有的试验场所的药物管理的监查增加至100%。对各个试验场所再次强调了必须在试验访视48小时内将所有数据输入至电子病例报告表中的要求"。

b. 我们发现了一份日期为2007年10月3日，题为"受影响受试者的安全信息"的Pfizer内部文件，提及在临床研究（b）（4）两个不同的研究场所另外还有6个儿童受试者有被过量给予研究药物的情况（受试者编号分别为：1170~1001，1170~1002，1170~1003，1136~1001，1136~1002，1136~1003）。这些过量用药发生在2007年的6、7、8月，在Pfizer对所有研究监查员就正确的给药程序再次培训的几个月之后。

ⅶ. 受试者1136~1001经历了30天的过量用药，并出现了中度嗜睡，高催乳素水平，颊面部运动障碍，皮肤瘀点，低碳酸氢，低磷，且有一次心电图Q-TcF区间延长。

ⅷ. 受试者1136~1002经历了22天的过量用药。

ⅸ. 受试者1136~1003经历了17天的过量用药并出现了中度静坐不能，轻微的运动障碍，轻度锥体束外症状。

ⅹ. 受试者1070~1001经历了12天的过量用药并出现了中度静坐不能及严重震颤。

ⅺ. 受试者1070~1002经历了11天的过量用药并出现了中度静坐不能及中度震颤。

ⅻ. 受试者1070~1003经历了7天的过量用药。

2. 您未能确保按照IND中的总体研究计划和试验方案进行研究［21 CFR 312.50］

a. 开展试验方案（b）（4）的多家试验场所的受试者未被给予正确剂量的药物。

ⅰ. 递交给FDA的临床研究总结报告列出了总共有40例受试者发生了与用药错误有关的方案偏离，包括20例受试者超过了方案允许的最大剂量。

ⅱ. 您对用药记录的程序性审核发现，有26例受试者每天给药总剂量超出了方案规定的在其体重范围内允许的各种最大剂量限制。

ⅲ. 基于在贵公司的现场检查发现，在（b）（4）医生的试验场所［试验场所（b）（4）］的所有受试者均发生严重用药错误。所有受试者用药过量持续多天（其中一位受试者最高达到22天）。

ⅳ. 基于在贵公司的现场检查发现，在（b）（4）医生的试验场所［试验场所（b）（4）］，受试者1026经历了两天的过量用药，出现锥体束外症状。

ⅴ. 基于在贵公司的现场检查发现，在（b）（4）医生的试验场所［试验场所（b）（4）］，受试者1005经历了6天的过量用药。

ⅵ. 基于在贵公司的现场检查发现，在（b）（4）医生的试验场所［试验场所（b）（4）］，受试者1010经历了6天的过量用药。

ⅶ. 基于在贵公司的现场检查发现，在（b）（4）医生的试验场所［试验场所（b）（4）］，受试者1001经历了12天的过量用药，出现中度嗜睡及中度躁动；受试者1002经历了14天的过量用药。

b. 试验方案（b）（4）规定，在基线时，研究者应建立一个剂量滴定计划，从20mg的起始剂量（基线访视）逐步增加受试者每天的用药总剂量，经过两周的时间达到目标剂量。试验方案规定，此计划应考虑受试者的既往（b）（4）史、当前（b）（4）状态及体重，且随时根据临床反应及耐受程度进行调整。

ⅰ. 基于在贵公司的现场检查发现，在（b）（4）医生的试验场所［试验场所（b）（4）］，未见对入组的受试者创建剂量滴定计划，同时未按照方案要求给受试者用药。

ⅱ. 基于在贵公司的现场检查发现，在（b）（4）医生的试验场所［试验场所（b）（4）］，未见对入组的受试者创建剂量滴定计划，同时未按照方案要求给受试者用药。

c. 试验方案（b）（4）规定，所有的心电图应由试验场所有资质读取并对结果进行解释的医师来审阅，以确保安全（即儿科心脏病学家或儿科重症监护专家或有解读儿科心电图经验的临床医生）。

ⅰ. 未见充足的文件证明，在所有的试验场所，有儿科心脏病学家或儿科重症护理专家在心电图采集的当天审阅心电图结果。

ⅱ. 在（b）（4）医生的试验场所［试验场所（b）（4）］，有一位经过认证的学生（b）（4）基于其在医学院及住院实习所接受的培训被授权审阅心电图。未见文件显示，其接受了额外培训或/和具备其他资质，足以证明给予其授权是合理的。

d. 试验方案（b）（4）规定，（b）（4）必须由主要研究者或者授权研究者来对受试者实施给药，且其必须是儿童、青少年（b）（4）专家或者具有博士水平的临床（b）（4）专家，并且还必须参加Pfizer公司的人员资质等级评估项目。

ⅰ. 未见文件显示，所有试验场所的主要研究者和/或授权研究者都参加了Pfizer公司的针对（b）（4）的人员资质等级评估项目。此外，在您的书面回复中，您声明Pfizer公司针对（b）（4）人员资质等级评估项目是不存在的，您也没有符合方案要求对（b）（4）开展人员资质等级评估项目的机构。

ⅱ.（b）（4）医生的试验场所［试验场所（b）（4）］，（b）（4）并未由儿童、青少年（b）（4）专家或者具有博士水平的临床（b）（4）专家的主要研究者及/或授权研究者实施给药。另外，对于受试者1008，1010，1011，1012及1013，（b）（4）被用作为诊断仪器，从而代替了（b）（4）。

ⅲ. 在（b）（4）医生的试验场所［试验场所（b）（4）］，受试者1001和1002的（b）（4）并未由儿童、青少年（b）（4）专家或者具有博士水平的临床（b）（4）专家的主要研究者或授权研究者实施给药。

e. 试验方案（b）（4）规定，应该由经过认证或者有资质的儿童或青少年（b）（4）专家来确定本试验的诊断符合要求。

未有充足的文件显示，所有的研究场所都有经过认证或者有资质的儿童或青少年（b）（4）专家来认定诊断符合要求。

f. 试验方案（b）（4）规定，获取知情同意的人应接受足够的有关医学知识培训，能够正确地处理问题，且此人必须是医学博士、哲学博士或者注册护士，不具备上述学位的人员必须获得Pfizer公司的批准。

我们的调查发现，在以下试验场所，知情同意并不是由医学博士、哲学博士或者注册护士获得的，并且/或者无充分文件证明，在对受试者进行知情同意前，因不具备所需学历的人得到了Pfizer的批准。

ⅰ.（b）（4）医生［试验场所（b）（4）］。

ⅱ.（b）（4）医生［试验场所（b）（4）］。

ⅲ.（b）（4）医生［试验场所（b）（4）］。

g. 试验方案（b）（4）规定，知情同意书必须得到Pfizer公司及伦理委员会的同意，且必须符合ICH GCP、当地法律法规的要求。方案规定，用于本试验的知情同意书及其试验期间的任何修改都需在使用前提前获得伦理委员会及Pfizer公司的批准。

在（b）（4）医生的试验场所［试验场所（b）（4）］，受试者 1010签署的知情同意书上有手写增加的信息/语句，说明拒绝支付住院访视的费用。这些手写增加的内容并未经过伦理委员会及Pfizer公司的批准。

3. 您未能确保向每个参与研究的研究者告知申办者发现的或报告给申办者的有关药物的最新观察发现，特别是与不良事件和安全使用相关的发现［21 CFR 312.55（b）］

未见文件显示所有开展试验方案（b）（4）的试验场所都接收到描述发现的用药错误的安全性报告。您的书面回复中也并未提及保持让研究者获得最新观察发现的问题（即用药错误）。

在贵公司2009年7月2日对FDA 483表的回复函中，贵公司承认未按照IND中包含的试验方案进行临床研究。贵公司的回复中声明会实施程序，以确保将来符合FDA法规。我们收到贵公司会采取纠正措施的保证。但是，我们注意到回复中没有包含将被实施的、用以预防这些问题将来再次发生的程序或过程的详细概要。

本警告信的目的并非是罗列您在试验药物临床研究中存在的所有缺陷。确保遵循法律和相关FDA法规的每一项要求是您的职责。您应当解决这些缺陷，并建立规程，以确保任何正在进行或将来的研究均能符合FDA的法规。

自收到这封信的15个工作日内，您应当书面告知本办公室为预防将来发生类似违规情况已经采取的行动（包括纠正措施计划和标准操作规程）。如果不能充分、迅速地解释上述违规问题，可能导致我们在不再通知的情况下采取监管措施。

附：英文原文

Pfizer Inc.

WARNING LETTER

April 9，2010

CERTIFIED MAIL
RETURN RECEIPT REQUESTED

Ref: 10-HFD-45-04-01

Mr. Martin. Mackay, Ph.D.
Senior Vice President
Global Research and Development
Pfizer, Inc.
50 Pequot Avenue
New London, CT 06320

Dear Dr. Mackay:

Between May 4, 2009 and June 3, 2009, Ms. Michelle M. Noe and Dr. Cynthia Kleppinger, representing the Food and Drug Administration (FDA), conducted an investigation and met with John Oidtman, Vice President of Worldwide Regulatory Operations, to review your firm’s practices as the sponsor of the clinical investigation Protocol (b)(4), entitled “(b)(4)” of the investigational drug, (b)(4) performed for Pfizer, Inc.

This inspection is a part of the FDA’s Bioresearch Monitoring Program, which includes inspection designed to evaluate the conduct of research and to ensure that rights, safety, and welfare of the human subjects of those studies have been protected. This inspection was performed due to significant violations found during inspections of several clinical investigators conducting Protocol (b)(4).

We are aware that at the conclusion of the inspection, Ms. Noe and Dr. Kleppinger presented and discussed with John Oidtman Form FDA 483, Inspectional Observations. From our review of the establishment inspection report, the documents submitted with tat report, and your firm’s July 2, 2009 letter written in response to the Form FDA 483, we conclude that you did not adhere to the applicable statutory requirements and FDA regulations governing the conduct of clinical investigations. We wish to emphasize the following:

1. You failed to ensure proper monitoring of the investigation [21 CFR 312.50].

This is a repeat violation of findings communicated to you in an untitled letter generated after an April 25, 2005 to June 6, 2005 inspection of Pfizer's monitoring of clinical investigations for (b)(4)

FDA regulations require that sponsors ensure proper monitoring of clinical investigations. Our investigation found that Pfizer failed to properly ensure monitoring of the study referenced above. As a result of inadequate monitoring, widespread overdosing of study subjects at multiple study sites was neither detected nor corrected in a timely manner.

a. Study monitors failed to ensure that the investigation was conducted in accordance with the investigational plan. Overdosing at Dr.(b)(4) 's site (site (b)(4)) was neither recognized nor reported by study monitors in a timely manner.

The protocol specified that a dose of 160 mg/day was not to be achieved before Day 8 of treatment and that total daily dose of study medication was not to exceed 160 mg for subjects with a body weight 45 kg, or 80 mg for subject with a body weight ＜ 45 kg.

Based on the inspection conducted at your firm, at Dr. (b)(4)'s site (site (b)(4)), dosing errors occurred and overdosing extended over several days for all seven pediatric subjects; in one case for as long as 22 days. The following are some examples of pediatric subject overdosing at Dr. (b)(4)'s site (site (b)(4)) noted during the site inspection:

i. Subject 1001 with a documented weight of 46.8 kg, was overdosed on study medication for 20 consecutive days. On Treatment Days 8 and 9, this subject received 180 mg/day; on Treatment Days 10 and 11, this subject received 240 mg/day; on Treatment Days 12 and 13, this subject received 320 mg/day; on Treatment Day 14, this subject received 400 mg/day; and on Treatment Days 15 through 27, this subject received 180 mg/day.

ii. Subject 1003, with a documented weight of 65 kg, was overdosed on study medication for 21 consecutive days. On Treatment Day 7, this subject received 180 mg/day; on Treatment Days 8 and 9, this subject received 240 mg/day; on Treatment Days 10 through 26, this subject received 400 mg/day; and on Treatment Day 27, this subject received 280 mg/day.

iii. Subject 1004 was overdosed on study medication for 3 consecutive days. On Treatment Day 9, this subject received 320 mg/day; and on Treatment Days 10 and 11, this subject received 240 mg/day.

iv. Subject 1005 was overdosed on study medication for 16 consecutive days. On Treatment Days 8 and 9, this subject received 180 mg/day; on Treatment Days 10 through 14, this subject received 240 mg/day; and on Treatment Days 15 through 20 and Days 22 through 23, this subject received 400 mg/day. On Treatment Day 21 this subject received 200mg/day.

v. Subject 1006, with a documented weight less than 45 kg, was overdosed on study medication for 7 consecutive days. On Treatment Days 16 through 22, this subject received 400 mg/day.

vi. Subject 1007, with a documented weight of 39.5 kg, was overdosed on study medication for 13 consecutive days. On Treatment Days 16 through 28, this subject received 120 mg/day.

Study monitors visited the site on a total of nine days: March 13 and 15, April 25, May 15-16, June 6- 7 and July 5-6, 2006. However, the overdosing was not discovered until July 25, 2006, and not by a study monitor but rather by a Pfizer data management unit. In addition, our investigation found an internal Pfizer report dated November 7, 2006 entitled "Report of Dosing Errors Due to Misunderstanding of Medication Cards in Pfizer Studies **(b)(4)** " that states that "on July 25, 2006, the Pfizer study team became aware of possible dosing errors." We note that all three studies involved the study medication **(b)(4)** with the same packaging.

The report indicated that the Pfizer study team examined the dosing records for all subjects enrolled as of November 7, 2006 in the three referenced studies, identified two sites at which dosing errors occurred, and took various steps to remedy the problem such as suspending enrollment at certain sites pending re-training of the sites, and reassessment of the sites' ability to conduct the studies according to the protocol. It is noteworthy that the report states that the study team "determined that the dosing procedures were clearly described in the protocols, protocol appendix, and medication card, and that no revisions of these documents were required. The study team re-trained all sites and all study monitors on correct dosing procedures. Monitoring of drug accountability was increased to 100% for all sites.

The directive that data be entered into the electronic CRF within 48 hours of study visits was reinforced with all sites."

b. We observe that a Pfizer internal document dated October 3, 2007 and entitled "Safety Information on Affected Subjects" refers to the overdosing of an additional six pediatric subjects in study **(b)(4)** at two different sites (subject #1170-1001, 1170-1002, 1170-1003, 1136-1001, 1136-1002, 1136-1003). These overdoses occurred in June, July and August of 2007, several months after Pfizer retrained study monitors on correct dosing procedures.

vii. Subject 1136-1001 experienced 30 days of overdosing with subsequent moderate somnolence, high prolactin level, buccal facial dyskinesia, skin petechiae, low bicarbonate, low phosphate, and one ECG with prolonged QTcF

viii. Subject 1136-1002 experienced 22 days of overdosing

ix. Subject 1136-1003 experienced 17 days of overdosing with moderate akathisia, mild dyskinesia and mild extrapyramidal symptoms

x. Subject 1070-1001 experienced 12 days of overdosing with moderate akathisia and severe tremor

xi. Subject 1070-1002 experienced 11 days of overdosing with mild akathisia an mild tremor

xii. Subject 1070-1003 experienced 7 days of overdosing

2. You failed to ensure that the investigations were conducted in accordance with the general investigational plan and protocols contained in the IND [21 CFR 312.50].

a. Subjects at multiple sites conducting Protocol (b)(4) were not given the correct doses.

i. The final Clinical Study Report submitted to the FDA lists 40 total subjects reported to have had a protocol deviation related to dosing error, including 20 subjects who exceeded the maximum protocol dose.

ii. Your programmatic review of the dosing records identified 26 subjects whose total daily dose exceeded the maximum allowed by the protocol for their weight range on any occasion.

iii. Based on the inspection conducted at your firm, at Dr. (b)(4)'s site (site **(b)(4)),** there were significant dosing errors for all subjects. The overdosing extended over several days for all subjects (up to 22 days in one subject).

iv. Based on the inspection conducted at your firm, at Dr. (b)(4)'s (site (b)(4)), Subject 1026 experienced two days of overdosing with extrapyramidal symptoms.

v. Based on the inspection conducted at your firm, at Dr. (b)(4)'s (site **(b)(4)),** Subject 1005 experienced six days of overdosing.

vi. Based on the inspection conducted at your firm, at Dr.(b)(4)'s (site **(b)(4)),** Subject 1010 experienced six days of overdosing.

vii. Based on the inspection conducted at your firm, at Dr.(b)(4)'s site (site **(b)(4)),** Subject 1001 experienced 12 days of overdosing with mild somnolence, and mild agitation and Subject 1002 experienced 14 days of overdosing.

b. Protocol (b)(4) specified that, at baseline, the investigator was to develop a titration plan to increase the subject's total daily dose of study medication from a 20 mg starting dose (at the baseline visit) to a target dose achieved over two weeks, in general. The protocol specified that this plan would consider the subject's **(b)(4)** history, current **(b)(4)** status, and weight, and could be modified at any time based on clinical response and toleration.

i. Based on the inspection conducted at your firm, at Dr. (b)(4)'s site (site **(b)(4)),** there was no dosing titration plan developed for enrolled subjects, and subjects were not dosed according to the protocol.

ii. Based on the inspection conducted at your firm, at Dr. (b)(4)' site (site (b)(4)), there was no dosing titration plan developed for enrolled subjects, and subjects were not dosed according to the protocol.

c. Protocol **(b)(4)** specified that all electrocardiograms (ECGs) were to be reviewed for safety at the site by a physician qualified to read and interpret the results (i.e., a pediatric cardiologist or pediatric intensive care specialist or a clinician who was experienced in interpreting pediatric ECGs).

i. There was insufficient documentation to show that all sites had a pediatric cardiologist or pediatric intensive care specialist reading the ECGs on the day performed.

ii. Dr. **(b)(4)** (site **(b)(4)),** a board certified child **(b)(4),** was granted permission, through a Study Issue Form, to read the ECGs based on his training in medical school and residency. There was no documentation to show additional training and/or qualifications to justify this grant of permission.

d. Protocol **(b)(4)** specified that the **(b)(4)** must be administered by the principal investigator or a sub-investigator, who is a child and adolescent **(b)(4)** or Ph.D.-level clinical **(b)(4),** and who has participated in the Pfizer rater qualification program.

i. There was no documentation to show that the principal investigator and/or sub investigators at all sites participated in a Pfizer rater qualification program for the (b)(4). Moreover, in your written response, you stated that a Pfizer rater qualification program does not exist and you have not proposed institution of a rater qualification program for the (b)(4), as required by the protocol.

ii. At Dr. (b)(4)'s site (site(b)(4)), the (b)(4) was not administered by the principal investigator or a subinvestigator, who was a child and adolescent (b)(4) or Ph.D.-level dinical (b)(4). Moreover, for Subjects 1008, 1010, 1011, 1012 and 1013, (b)(4)) was used as the diagnostic instrument in place of the (b)(4).

iii. At Dr. (b)(4)'s site (site (b)(4)), the (b)(4) for Subjects 1001 and 1002 was not administered by the principal investigator or a subinvestigator,who was a child and adolescent (b)(4) or Ph.D. level clinical (b)(4).

e. Protocol (b)(4) specified that diagnostic eligibility for the study was to be determined by a board certified or board eligible child/adolescent (b)(4).

There was insufficient documentation to show that all sites had a board-certified or board-eligible child/adolescent (b)(4) determining diagnostic eligibility.

f. Protocol (b)(4) specified that the person obtaining the informed consent must be sufficiently trained on medical issues so that questions can be adequately addressed and that this person must be an M.D., Ph.D., or R.N., and that persons without one of these degrees must be approved by Pfizer.

Our investigation found that informed consent was not obtained by a M.D., Ph.D., or R.N., and/or there was insufficient documentation to support that persons not otherwise qualified by holding one of the required degrees were approved by Pfizer prior to consenting subjects at the following sites:

i. Dr. (b)(4) (site (b)(4))

ii. Dr. (b)(4) (site (b)(4))

iii. Dr. (b)(4) (site (b)(4))

g. Protocol (b)(4) specified that the informed consent form must be agreed to by Pfizer and the IRB/IEC (Institutional Review Board/Independent Ethics Committee) and must be in compliance with ICH GCP (International Conference on Harmonisation of Technical Requirements for Registration of Pharmaceuticals for Human Use Good Clinical Practice), local regulatory requirements, and legal requirements. The protocol specified that the informed consent form used in this trial, and any changes made during the course of the trial, must be prospectively approved by both the IRB/IEC and Pfizer before use.

At Dr. (b)(4)' site (site (b)(4)), Subject 1010 was consented with a consent form with hand-written information/ language added to the form, which denied payment to subjects for inpatient visits. This additional information/ language was not approved by the IRB/IEC and Pfizer.

3. You failed to keep each participating investigator informed of new observations discovered by or reported to the sponsor on the drug, particularly with respect to adverse effects and safe use [21CFR 312.55(b)].

There is no documentation to show that all sites conducting Protocol (b)(4) received safety reports which describe the dosing errors discovered. Your written response does not address the issue of keeping investigators informed of new observations (i.e., dosing errors).

In your firm's July 2, 2009, letter written in response to the Form FDA 483, inspectional Observations, your firm acknowledged that the clinical investigations were not conducted in accordance with the protocols contained in the IND. Your firm's response stated that procedures will be put into place to ensure compliance with the FDA regulations in the future. We acknowledge your firm's assurance that corrective actions will be implemented to prevent the future occurrence of these observations. be taken. However, we note that the response did not contain a detailed outline of procedures or processes that would be implemented to prevent the future occurrence of these observation.

This letter is not intended to be an all-inclusive list of deficiencies with your clinical study of an investigational drug. It is your responsibility to ensure adherence to each requirement of the law and relevant FDA regulations. You should address these deficiencies and establish procedures to ensure that any on-going or future studies will be in

compliance with FDA regulations.

Within fifteen (15) working days of your receipt of this letter, you should notify this office in writing of the actions you have taken (including corrective action plans and standard operating procedures) to prevent similar violations in the future. Failure to adequately and promptly explain the violations noted above may result in regulatory action without further notice.

If you have any questions, please contact Constance Cullity (formerly Lewin), M.D., M.P.H., at 301-796- 3397; FAX 301-847-8748. Your written response and any pertinent documentation should be addressed to:

Constance Cullity (formerly Lewin), M.D., M.P.H.
Branch Chief, Good Clinical Practice Branch I
Division of Scientific Investigations
Office of Compliance
Center for Drug Evaluation and Research
Food and Drug Administration
10903 New Hampshire Avenue
Bldg 51, Room 5354
Silver Spring, MD 20993

Sincerely yours,

{See appended electronic signature page}

Leslie K. Ball, M.D.
Director Division of Scientific Investigations
Office of Compliance
Center for Drug Evaluation and Research

第三部分

药物 GCP 警告信

——给合同研究组织

第42封　给Semler Research Center Private有限公司的警告信

2016年4月20日

参考号：3917280

尊敬的Bopanna博士：

2015年9月29日至10月9日，检查员Charles Bonapace博士、Arindam Dasgupta博士、Dipesh K. Shah和Daniel J. Roberts代表FDA，对您所开展的以下研究：（b）（4）[1]、（b）（4）和（b）（4）进行了审查。这封警告信特告知您现场检查中发现的违规情况。

本次现场检查是FDA的生物研究监查项目的一部分。该项目通过设定的检查方法，评估由FDA监管研究的实施情况，以确认研究数据在科学上是有效和准确的，并帮助确保受试者的权益、安全和福利得到了保护。

在现场检查结束时，FDA检查员向您出示了FDA483表，即现场检查发现的问题，并与您进行了讨论。您2015年10月29日对该FDA483表的书面回复已收悉。

经对现场检查报告、该报告的附件，以及您2015年10月29日的书面回复和您在2016年1月14日报告的回顾性调查审计结果进行审查，我们认为，您没有遵循适用的法律要求和监管生物等效性研究的FDA法规。我们想强调以下几点：

贵公司未能证明在体内生物利用度或生物等效性研究中，用来测定体液或排泄物中活性药物成分，或治疗组分，或其活性代谢产物浓度的分析方法，有足够的精确度和灵敏度，以及适当的精密度，来测定活性药物成分，或治疗组分，或其活性代谢物在体内达到的实际浓度［21 CFR 320.29（a）］

在对贵公司的现场检查中，FDA发现有证据记录您参与到未合规使用分析方法的行为和过程中，这导致向FDA递交了无效的研究数据。因此，FDA严重关注贵公司向FDA提交所开展的用于支持仿制药申请（ANDAs）或新药申请（NDAs）生物等效性和生物利用度研究数据的有效性和可靠性。

具体而言，在有关（b）（4）研究中，有记录表明，贵公司用已分析的其他受试者样本替换了受试者41～60血浆样本。这种替换样本的行为损害了贵公司所使用的分析方法和研究数据的可靠性和有效性。

举例说明，贵公司服务器上存储的电子表格显示，在（b）（4）研究中如下受试者样本被替换：

（b）（4）	
受试者	替换的受试者
42	16
43	23
44	9
45	28
46	14
47	11
48	8
49	4
50	26

1（b）（4）涉及商业秘密，根据法规内容不予公开。

续表

（b）(4)	
受试者	替换的受试者
51	3
52	25
53	29
54	31
55	32
56	21
57	1
58	20
59	36
60	17

现场检查中，我们要求您绘制各对受试者中记录有被替换样本（b）(4）的药-时曲线，比如上述列举的受试者10和41，用以比较这些受试者的血药浓度曲线。结果表明，记录显示有样本替换的（b）(4）各对受试者几乎都具有完全相同的药-时曲线。现场检查时，您无法解释这些各对受试者之间药物浓度高度相似的现象。您声称，如果受试者样本被替换，样本重现性重分析（incurred sample reanalysis，ISR）将不会得到这样的结果并符合接受标准。然而，FDA不认可您的评估，因为如果是对替换后的样本进行了重分析，ISR结果就应该会符合接受标准。例如，从受试者10中选取2份血浆样本，将其中的一份错误地标为受试者41后进行分析。

现场检查中，我们还要求您将（b）(4）研究人群（n=53）分为三组，计算最大血药浓度（C_{max}）和药-时曲线下面积（$AUC_{0\text{-}inf}$）的几何平均值比值（GMRs）和90%置信区间（CI 90%），用以评估替换血浆样本对生物等效性研究终点判断的影响。根据您提供的分析计算结果表明，替换受试者（41~60）(b）(4）GMRs值与没有记录被替换的受试者（1~40）的（b）(4）GMRs值有显著差异，如下表所示。

(b) (4) 研究 (生物等效性终点)			
受试者	参数	几何均数比值点估计 (%)	90%置信区间
1~20（n=16）	C_{max}	137.69	109.81~172.66
	$AUC_{0\text{-}inf}$	113.62	90.46~142.67
21~40（n=18）	C_{max}	128.95	101.41~163.96
	$AUC_{0\text{-}inf}$	100.51	86.97~116.17
替换的受试者41~60（n=19）	C_{max}	62.18	51.51~75.06
	$AUC_{0\text{-}inf}$	85.93	71.89~102.70
报告给FDA的受试者（n=53）	C_{max}	101.43	87.82~117.15
	$AUC_{0\text{-}inf}$	98.50	89.07~108.92

我们注意到，在检查中您声称研究结果是正确的，(b）(4）GMRs结果的异常趋势是源于该产品所在的生理学条件和化合物分子固有的特性，尤其是在受试者之间存在高变异的药代动力学（PK）结果。然而，FDA不认可您的解释，因为这不能合理解释研究数据的不一致性。特别指出，个体间的PK高变异性不会导致（b）(4）受试者之间几乎完全相同的药-时曲线。另外，PK的高变异性会随机发生在所有受试者之间，而不是在受试者不同分组之间。您也未能解释为什么替换样本受试者的PK数据（C_{max}和$AUC_{0\text{-}inf}$ GMRs）与那些记录中没有替换样本受试者的PK数据之间的不一致。

上述讨论的（b）(4）研究中产生的无效PK数据，已递交给FDA用于支持（b）(4）胶囊的NDA申请。

我们同时也注意到，在您的服务器中有记录表明在（b）(4)，(b）(4）和（b）(4）研究中有替换、可能篡改或稀释受试者样本的情况，而这些数据已递交给FDA用于支持新药申请。在您2015年10月29日的书面回复中，您承认您的服务器中存储了一张电子表格，记录了在贵公司所开展的某些生物等效性研究中，包括（b）（4）、（b）（4）、（b）（4）存在替换和篡改受试者样品的行为。您解释说，您无法确定谁是该文件的创建者或其对研究终点的影响，但是贵公司将会开始随机地检查所有已向FDA申报项目的受试者的药物浓度数据和（或）PK数据。

在您2016年1月14日递交的信中，您递交了一份报告，概述了在一个回顾性调查中可能在调换或替换受试者样本上发现的问题。您声称一个独立的外部顾问公司审计了上述项目涉及的临床、生物分析和PK等各个方面。您也承认存在于您服务器上的电子表格和其对贵公司所产生数据可靠性的影响。该审计报告表明，这些研究的临床部分有较轻的数据转录错误和时间印章的不一致性。该报告也显示，这些研究的生物分析部分存在样本存储问题，手写样本处理系统存在缺陷，以及仪器稳定性的记录不严谨。您的结论是，尽管该审计不能揭示任何有关样本调换或替换的直接证据，但仍然观察到与上述提及的项目中相同的数据趋势问题，但无法从生理学基础上解释该问题。

您的回复是不充分的，因为您未能解释如下问题：①为什么贵公司有记录表明，要通过替换或篡改受试者样本来满足生物等效性标准；②是否在贵公司开展的其他生物利用度或生物等效性研究存在同样的受试者样本替换或篡改问题；③样本替换和篡改对（b）（4），（b）（4），（b）（4）研究的各自影响；④在这些研究中，如何能有多处受试者样本浓度重叠的现象。

本警告信的目的并非是罗列您在生物等效性研究中存在的所有缺陷。确保遵循法律和相关FDA法规的每一项要求是您的职责。您应当解决这些缺陷，并建立规程，以确保任何正在进行或将来的研究均能符合FDA的法规。

我们提醒您，确保贵公司所有取得和递交给FDA的ANDAs或NDAs数据的可靠性是您的职责。上述列举的Semler公司的行为，引起FDA对Semler公司开展的所有生物等效性研究的可靠性和有效性的极大关注。

自收到这封信的30个工作日内，您应当书面告知本办公室对该信中所提及的违规行为或为预防将来发生类似违规行为已采取的或将要采取的纠正措施。

附：英文原文

Semler Research Center Private Limited

CERTIFIED MAIL
RETURN RECEIPT REQUESTED

Ref: 3917280

Krathish Bopanna, Ph.D.
President & Chief Executive Officer
Semler Research Center Private Limited
75 A 15th Cross Road
Bangalore, India 560078

Dear Dr. Bopanna:

This letter informs you of objectionable conditions observed during the U.S. Food and Drug Administration (FDA) inspection conducted at your firm between September 29, 2015 and October 9, 2015. Investigators Charles Bonapace, Pharm.D.; Arindam Dasgupta, Ph.D.; Dipesh K. Shah; and Daniel J. Roberts, representing the FDA, reviewed the conduct of the following studies:

(b)(4)
(b)(4)
(b)(4)

This inspection is part of FDA's Bioresearch Monitoring (BIMO) Program, which includes inspections designed to evaluate the conduct of FDA-regulated research to ensure that the data are scientifically valid and accurate, and to help ensure that the rights, safety, and welfare of the human subjects have been protected.

At the conclusion of the inspection, the FDA investigators presented and discussed with you Form FDA 483, Inspectional Observations. We acknowledge receipt of your October 29, 2015, written response to the Form FDA 483.

From our review of the FDA Establishment Inspection Report, the documents submitted with that report, your October 29, 2015, written response to the Form FDA 483 observations, and your January 14, 2016, letter reporting the results of a retrospective investigative audit, we conclude that you did not adhere to the applicable statutory requirements and FDA regulations governing the conduct of bioequivalence studies. We wish to emphasize the following:

Your firm failed to demonstrate that the analytical method used in an in vivo bioavailability or bioequivalence study to measure the concentration of the active drug ingredient or therapeutic moiety, or its active metabolite(s), in body fluids or excretory products, is accurate and of sufficient sensitivity to measure, with appropriate precision, the actual concentration of the active drug ingredient or therapeutic moiety, or its active metabolite(s), achieved in the body [21CFR 320.29(a)].

During FDA's inspection of your firm, FDA found evidence documenting that you engaged in practices and processes that undermines the analytical methods used at your firm, which resulted in the submission of invalid study data to the FDA. As a result, FDA has significant concerns about the validity and reliability of bioequivalence and bioavailability data generated at your firm that is submitted to the FDA in support of Abbreviated New Drug Applications (ANDAs) or New Drug Applications (NDAs).

Specifically, you documented that for Study (b)(4), your firm replaced plasma samples from Subjects 41-60 with the plasma samples of different subjects that had already been analyzed. This substitution of samples undermines the reliability and validity of the analytical methods used at your firm and the study data produced by your firm.

For example, your server contained a spreadsheet showing that the following subject' samples were substituted in Study (b)(4):

(b) (4)	
Subjects	**Replaced (Substituted)Subjects**
42	16
43	23
44	9
45	28
46	14
47	11
48	8
49	4
50	26
51	3
52	25
53	29
54	31
55	32
56	21
57	1
58	20
59	36
60	17

During the inspection, we requested that you plot the (b) (4) concentration-time profiles for the pairs of subjects that were documented as having their samples substituted (for example, Subjects 10 and 41), as is shown above, to compare the plasma drug profiles for those subjects. The resulting plots from your analysis showed almost identical concentration-time profiles for (b) (4) for each pair of the subjects that you documented as having been substituted. During the inspection, you were unable to explain the similarity in concentration data from these pairs of subjects. You stated that your incurred sample reanalysis (ISR) could not have achieved these results and met the acceptance criteria (that is, the results of a reanalysis of a subset of subject samples are sufficiently consistent with the original results) if the subjects' samples had been substituted. However, FDA does not agree with your assessment, because the acceptance criteria for the ISR would have been met if the same substituted samples were reanalyzed (for example, if two plasma samples from Subject 10, one of which was falsely labeled as Subject 41, were analyzed).

During the inspection, we also requested that you calculate the(b)(4)peak Drug concentration (C_{max}) and area under the plasma concentration-time curve ($AUC_{o\text{-}inf}$) geometric mean ratios (GMRs) with their respective 90% confidence intervals (CI 90%) in three segments of the study population (n=53), to evaluate the impact of substituted plasma samples on the bioequivalence end points. As shown below, the calculations resulting from your analysis indicated that the (b)(4)GMRs data from the substituted subjects (Subjects 41-60) were distinct from the (b)(4)GMRs from subjects that were not documented as having been substituted (Subjects 1-40).

Study (b)(4)(Bioequivalence Endpoints)			
Subjects	**Parameter**	**GMRPoint Estimate(%)**	**90%CI**
1-20(n=16)	C_{max}	137.69	109.81-172.66
	$AUC_{0\text{-}inf}$	113.62	90.46-142.67
21-40 (n=18)	C_{max}	128.95	101.41-163.96
	$AUC_{0\text{-}inf}$	100.51	86.97-116.17
Substituted 41-60 (n=19)	C_{max}	62.18	51.51-75.06
	$AUC_{0\text{-}inf}$	85.93	71.89-102.70
Reported to FDA (n=53)	C_{max}	101.43	87.82-117.15
	$AUC_{0\text{-}inf}$	98.50	89.07-108.92

We note that you indicated during the inspection that the study results were correct, and that the unusual trends with the (b)(4)GMRs were a product of physiological conditions and the intrinsic properties of the molecule, (b)(4) high intrasubject pharmacokinetic (PK) variability in particular. However, FDA does not agree with this explanation because it fails to explain the inconsistencies in the study data adequately. Specifically, high intrasubject PK variability would not produce almost identical (b)(4) concentration-time profiles in study subjects. In addition, PK variability would occur randomly across study subjects, not in distinct subject segments. You also failed to explain why the PK data (the C_{max} and $AUC_{o\text{-}inf}$ GMRs) for subjects with substituted samples are inconsistent with PK data for subjects that were not documented as substituted.

The invalid PK data discussed above for Study(b) (4) were submitted to the FDA insupport of an NDA for(b) (4) capsules.

We also note that your server contained documentation indicating the substitution, and the possible manipulation or dilution, of subject samples for Studies(b) (4) (b) (4) and(b) (4) , which were submitted to FDA in support of drug applications.In your October 29, 2015, written response, you acknowledge that your firm's server contained a spreadsheet that documented the substitution and manipulation of subject samples for certain bioequivalence studies conducted at your firm, including(b) (4) ,(b) (4) , and(b) (4). You explained that you could not determine who created the document or its impact on the study endpoints, but that your firm would begin random reviews of subject concentration data and/or PK data for all studies submitted to FDA.

In your January 14, 2016, letter, you submitted a report that summarizes the findings of a retrospective investigation into the possible switching or substitution of subject samples. You indicated that an independent team of external consultants audited the clinical, bioanalytical, and PK aspects of the studies mentioned above. You also acknowledged the spreadsheet on your server and its implications on the integrity of the data from your firm. The audit report showed that the clinical portions of the studies had minor transcription errors and discrepancies in time stamps. The audit report also showed that the bioanalytical phase of the studies had issues with sample storage, flaws in the handwritten sample-processing system, and poor documentation practices for instrument stabilization. You concluded that, although the audit did not reveal any direct evidence of sample switching or substitution, the audit did observe the same concerning data trends for the studies noted above, but that it was not possible to explain the data trends on a physiological basis.

Your responses are inadequate because you failed to address (1) why your firm had documentation indicating that subject samples were substituted or manipulated in order for studies to meet the bioequivalence criteria; (2) if any other bioequivalence or bioavailability studies conducted at your firm had subject samples substituted or manipulated; (3) what impact the sample substitution and manipulation had on Studies(b) (4), (b) (4) , and(b) (4) ,respectively; and (4) how each of these studies could have multiple instances of overlapping subject sample concentrations.

This letter is not intended to be an all-inclusive list of deficiencies with your bioequivalence studies. It is your responsibility to ensure adherence to each requirement of the law and relevant FDA regulations. You should address these deficiencies and establish procedures to ensure that any ongoing or future studies will comply with FDA regulations.

We remind you that it is your firm's responsibility to ensure the integrity of all data generated at your firm that is submitted to the FDA in ANDAs or NDAs. The manner in which Semler conducted the studies noted above causes FDA to have significant concerns with the reliability and validity of all bioequivalence data generated by Semler.

Within thirty (30) working days of your receipt of this letter, you should notify this office in writing of the actions you have taken or will take to correct the violations noted in this letter and to prevent similar violations in the future.

We appreciate the cooperation shown to FDA investigators Bonapace, Dasgupta, Shah, and Roberts during the inspection. Should you have any questions regarding this letter or the inspection, please call Dr. Chrissy J. Cochran, Division Director, at +1-301-796-5633, Fax +1-301-847-8748, or write to her at this address:

Chrissy J. Cochran, Ph.D.
Division of Enforcement and Postmarketing Safety
Office of Scientific Investigations
Office of Compliance
Center for Drug Evaluation and Research
Food and Drug Administration
Building 51, Room 5364
10903 New Hampshire Avenue
Silver Spring, MD 20993
U.S.A.

Sincerely yours,

{See appended electronic signature page}

David Burrow, Pharm.D., J.D. Acting Director
Office of Scientific Investigations
Office of Compliance
Center for Drug Evaluation and Research
DAVID C BURROW
04/19/2016
Reference ID: 3917280

第43封　给TCA细胞治疗有限责任公司的警告信

2011年8月15日

参考号：CBER－11-03

尊敬的Naparalla先生：

2011年2月22日至2011年3月31日，FDA检查员与您和TCA细胞治疗有限责任公司（TCA）的员工们会面，就TCA作为申办者以及生物制品生产商的临床试验实施情况进行了现场检查。这封警告信特告知您此次FDA现场检查的结果。本次现场检查是FDA的生物研究监查项目的一部分，该项目通过设定的检查方法，审查试验药物临床研究的实施情况。

在现场检查结束时，FDA检查员与您和 TCA的员工们会面，讨论了FDA483表中所列的问题，即现场检查发现的问题。TCA医学总监Gabriel Perez Lasala博士，于2011年4月19日以书信方式对该FDA483表作出了回复（"TCA回复函"）并寄至新奥尔良地区办公室。经对现场检查报告、该报告的附件，其他可获得的相关信息，以及TCA回复信进行审查，我们认为TCA违反了发布在21 CFR 312的监管涉及研究新药的临床研究的正确实施的法规；并违反了21 CFR 1271中监管人类细胞、组织以及基于细胞和组织的产品（HCT/Ps），为防止传染性疾病的引入、传播和蔓延而制定的法规（可通过网站获取http://www.gpoaccess.gov/cfr/index.html）。对以下所列的每一项违规问题，都摘录了适用的CFR条款。

TCA是以下研究新药申请（INDs）的申办者：

IND 11643：自体间充质干细胞体外扩增，混合骨髓衍生单核细胞，以气囊导管或外科手术给药。

适应症：用于治疗心肌梗死。

临床研究者：Gabriel P. Lasala医学博士。

IND 13139：自体骨髓衍生单核细胞和自体骨髓衍生间充质干细胞肌内注射给药。

适应症：用于治疗严重肢体缺血。

临床研究者：Gabriel P. Lasala医学博士。

IND 13562：自体骨髓衍生单核细胞和自体骨髓衍生间充质干细胞扩张导管（导丝）冠状动脉内给药。

适应症：用于治疗严重的冠状动脉缺血。

临床研究者：Gabriel P. Lasala医学博士。

IND 13729：自体骨髓衍生间充质细胞通过腰椎穿刺给药。

适应症：用于治疗肌萎缩性侧索硬化症（ALS）。

临床研究者：Gabriel P. Lasala医学博士。

IND 13981：自体骨髓衍生间充质细胞鞘内注射给药。

适应症：用于治疗脊髓损伤。

临床研究者：Gabriel P. Lasala医学博士。

1. 您未能履行申办者的基本职责以确保各项研究按照研究计划进行，您未能对正在进行中的研究的进展情况进行监查［21 CFR 312.50 和 312.56（a）］

申办者有责任保证对研究实施适当的监查，并保证临床研究按申办者所提交的IND中包含的总体研究计划和试验方案实施。

A. FDA的现场检查显示，自体来源的试验产品被反复使用于未入组TCA的IND研究的患者身上。

自体来源的试验药物被反复使用于未入组IND研究的患者身上，尽管这些患者所接受治疗的适应症与TCA的各项IND研究的适应症相同。更有甚者，至少有5例患者，在相关IND（IND13729和IND13981）已被FDA要求暂停临床试验的情况下，依然接受了自体来源的试验产品治疗。

一些人使用了与IND相同适应症的自体细胞来源药物，但未入组IND研究的患者情况详见下表。

IND	IND中所述适应症	患者身份#	自体注射日期
13139	肢体缺血	(b)(6)	(b)(6)
		(b)(6)	(b)(6)
13981	脊髓损伤	(b)(6)	(b)(6)
13562	冠状动脉缺血	(b)(6)	(b)(6)
		(b)(6)	(b)(6)
		(b)(6)	(b)(6)
		(b)(6)	(b)(6)
11643	心肌梗死	(b)(6)	(b)(6)
		(b)(6)	(b)(6)

TCA回复函试图对这些行为进行辩解，声称这些患者病情危重，极为虚弱，且没有其他的治疗选择，因此Lasala医生出于扩大同情应用的可及性而对这些患者进行了治疗。

B. 尽管TCA的各项IND研究均限于使用自体骨髓衍生细胞，但研究记录显示，未入组TCA的各项IND研究的患者还接受了异体来源细胞治疗。事实上，在FDA的现场检查中，Lasala医生向FDA检查员们承认，他还向不符合临床试验方案入组条件的患者使用了异体来源细胞，他将此行为描述为“出于同情的非法行为”是“完全错误”和“完全非法”的。以下这些患者接受了异体来源细胞而非IND试验方案中要求的自体细胞。

适应症	患者	注射日期
冠状动脉缺血	(b)(6)	(b)(6)
	(b)(6)	(b)(6)
	(b)(6)	(b)(6)
	(b)(6)	(b)(6)
	(b)(6)	(b)(6)
	(b)(6)	(b)(6)
	(b)(6)	(b)(6)
肢体缺血	(b)(6)	(b)(6)
	(b)(6)	(b)(6)
	(b)(6)	(b)(6)
	(b)(6)	(b)(6)
	(b)(6)	(b)(6)
	(b)(6)	(b)(6)
	(b)(6)	(b)(6)
	(b)(6)	(b)(6)
	(b)(6)	(b)(6)

续表

适应症	患者	注射日期
ALS	（b）（6）	（b）（6）
	（b）（6）	（b）（6）
	（b）（6）	（b）（6）
	（b）（6）	（b）（6）
	（b）（6）	（b）（6）
	（b）（6）	（b）（6）
	（b）（6）	（b）（6）
	（b）（6）	（b）（6）
	（b）（6）	（b）（6）
	（b）（6）	（b）（6）
	（b）（6）	（b）（6）
	（b）（6）	（b）（6）
	（b）（6）	（b）（6）
	（b）（6）	（b）（6）
脊髓损伤	（b）（6）	（b）（6）
	（b）（6）	（b）（6）
	（b）（6）	（b）（6）
	（b）（6）	（b）（6）
	（b）（6）	（b）（6）

TCA回复函，试图用上述1.A.段落中所述相同的理由来解释这些行为。

C. 您未能对IND中的所有临床研究的进展情况实施监查。

i. 没有证据表明TCA对以下研究实施了监查：依据IND 13563开展的研究（b）（6），依据IND13729开展的研究（b）（6），以及依据IND13981开展的研究（b）（6）。

在TCA的回复函中，对缺乏监查的解释是，截至2011年1月，原来签订合同的监查员不再执行监查工作，当时正与另一家公司就2011年3月开始执行监查工作进行合同洽谈。TCA回复函中，还进一步解释，在现场检查后，TCA管理层成员Lasala博士发现最后一次监查访视是在2008年8月26日。

ii. 在检查中，我们发现试验中发生了一项严重违背方案的情况，即受试者（b）（6）被注射了不正确的试验药物。研究（b）（6）（IND13981）的方案要求“在签署知情同意书后的10日内安排进行骨髓抽吸”，且正是这些抽吸获得的细胞将被处理后输回受试者体内。受试者（b）（6）在2010年8月4日签署了临床研究知情同意书。而病例报告表访视2——初次骨髓抽吸——显示，这名受试者在（b）（6）接受了（b）（6）药物注射，但这些细胞是在10个月之前，该名受试者在（b）（6）实施骨髓抽吸后收集获得的。

在TCA回复函中，承认了IND13981临床试验方案中未包括注射（b）（6）的条款内容。

iii. 受试者（b）（6）使用了来源于TCA供体库中的异源供体细胞，而非试验方案3.1中要求的自体干细胞。在现场检查中，Lasala博士和Minguell博士告诉FDA检查员，他们不能确认该名受试者所使用细胞的来源。在TCA回复函中，Lasala博士认定供体细胞来源于“（b）（6）”，并且解释了该供体细胞“（b）（6）”原计划供给克罗恩病患者（b）（6），但该受试者的程序被取消了。在TCA的回复函中进一步解释了Lasala博士将供体“（b）（6）”细胞产品注射给了受试者（b）（6），而没有弃置该细胞产品，从而导致了受试者（b）（6）接受了异源细胞。

在TCA的回复函中，试图解释临床研究者是基于该受试者状况的严重性才决定用异源细胞对其进行治疗。

当FDA检查员询问TCA供体库的情况时，Minguell博士开始解释说TCA供体库是指“多余的细胞”，被储存用于校准和测试新批次的胎牛血清。Minguell博士随后又承认，TCA供体库是由同种异体供体骨髓抽吸物组成，并不打算用于特定的接受者。在现场检查期间他还就有意误导了关于供体细胞的情况而向FDA检查员们表示道歉。

2. 您在IND尚未生效的情况下就启动了临床研究［21CFR 312.20 和 312.40］。

2010年11月22日，在与FDA就IND 13139召开的Ⅱ期临床结束会议上，TCA提出了以自体骨髓单核细胞（BM-MNC）联合异源骨髓间充质细胞（BM-MSC）作为试验药物开展Ⅲ期临床研究。开展I期和Ⅱ期临床研究中所用的BM-MNC和BM-MSC均为自体的。FDA在会上建议您如要使用异源骨髓间充质细胞，则需要递交一个新的IND。而根据2010年12月8日签署的会议记录记载，由于您没有安全性或初步的有效性数据，FDA建议您，FDA认为这是一个首次在人体进行的I期临床试验，需要递交一个新的IND，并且在这个IND中需要关注对这种新的异源细胞产品的安全性评估。

尽管FDA的结论是使用异源BM-MSC需要递交一个新的IND，但TCA后来仍然将异源细胞产品使用到了以下患者身上：

患者身份	注射日期	适应症
（b）（6）	（b）（6）	脊髓损伤
（b）（6）	（b）（6）	脊髓性肌肉萎缩
（b）（6）	（b）（6）	脊髓性肌肉萎缩
（b）（6）	（b）（6）	肌营养不良
（b）（6）	（b）（6）	ALS
（b）（6）	（b）（6）	渐进性肌肉萎缩
（b）（6）	（b）（6）	脊髓损伤
（b）（6）	（b）（6）	严重肢体缺血
（b）（6）	（b）（6）	严重肢体缺血
（b）（6）	（b）（6）	脊髓小脑性共济失调
（b）（6）	（b）（6）	脊髓损伤
（b）（6）	（b）（6）	脊髓损伤
（b）（6）	（b）（6）	ALS
（b）（6）	（b）（6）	脊髓损伤
（b）（6）	（b）（6）	创伤性肌肉骨骼损伤

更有甚者，FDA的现场检查还发现，您在2010年11月22日会议之前，就已经启动了使用异源BM-MSC进行的治疗。事实上，在2010年11月22日前，您至少用异源细胞治疗了（b）（4）名受试者，用于多种适应症，包括但不限于严重的冠状动脉缺血、肌肉骨骼异常、肌营养不良、原发性侧索硬化、脊髓小脑性共济失调、脊髓性肌肉萎缩，以及脊髓损伤。

适应症	接受治疗的患者数量
严重的冠状动脉缺血	（b）（6）（b）（4）
ALS	（b）（6）（b）（4）
肢体缺血	（b）（6）（b）（4）
肌肉骨骼异常	（b）（6）（b）（4）
肌营养不良	（b）（6）（b）（4）
原发性侧索硬化	（b）（6）（b）（4）
脊髓小脑性共济失调	（b）（6）（b）（4）
脊髓性肌肉萎缩	（b）（6）（b）（4）
脊髓损伤	（b）（6）（b）（4）
癫痫	（b）（6）（b）（4）

续表

适应症	接受治疗的患者数量
丘脑脓肿	（b）（6）（b）（4）
肾病	（b）（6）（b）（4）
阿尔茨海默病	（b）（6）（b）（4）
渐进性肌肉萎缩	（b）（6）（b）（4）
多发性硬化	（b）（6）（b）（4）
脊髓（卒中）	（b）（6）（b）（4）
神经系统病变	（b）（6）（b）（4）

TCA回复函试图用上述1.A.段落中所述相同的理由来辩解这些行为。

3. 您在未向FDA递交方案修订或新的IND的情况下就启动了临床研究［21 CFR 312.20，312.30和312.40］

您未向FDA递交使用自体BM-MSC治疗新的适应症的试验方案修订或新的IND申请，有关情形列表显示如下。

患者身份	适应症	备注
（b）（6）	肌肉骨骼异常	
（b）（6）	肌肉骨骼异常	
（b）（6）	胃癌	
（b）（6）	肌肉骨骼异常	
（b）（6）	癫痫	该受试者年龄为10岁；在TCA的5个IND中的所有试验方案均要求排除18岁以下的受试者
（b）（6）	视神经萎缩合并脑动静脉畸形	该受试者年龄为24个月；在TCA的5个IND中的所有试验方案均要求排除18岁以下的受试者 此外，眼球内注射试验药物是一种新的给药途径
（b）（6）	神经系统病变	
（b）（6）	创伤性脑损伤	该受试者年龄为14岁；在TCA的5个IND中的所有试验方案均要求排除18岁以下的受试者
（b）（6）	胶质母细胞瘤	

TCA回复函中试图用上述1.A.段落中所述相同的理由来辩解这些行为。

4. 您违反临床试验暂停限制而给予了研究产品［21 CFR 312.42（a）和（e）］

A. IND 13729在2008年7月11日至2010年1月8日，处于临床试验暂停状态。在此期间，以下患者接受了IND 13729中的试验产品，而其适应症与IND申请的相同，也就是ALS。这些患者未入组临床研究，但却在临床试验暂停期间接受了治疗。

患者	骨髓抽吸日期	注射日期
（b）（6）	（b）（6）	（b）（6）
（b）（6）	（b）（6）	（b）（6）
（b）（6）	（b）（6）	（b）（6）

B. IND13981在2009年4月10日至2010年4月14日处于临床试验暂停状态。在此期间，以下患者接受了IND中的13981试验产品，而其适应症与IND申请的相同，也就是脊髓损伤。这些患者未入组临床研究，但却在临床试验暂停期间接受了治疗。

续表

患者	骨髓抽吸日期	注射日期
（b）（6）	（b）（6）	（b）（6）
（b）（6）	（b）（6）	（b）（6）
（b）（6）	（b）（6）	（b）（6）

除了违反FDA关于临床研究实施的法规之外，您还违反了FDA关于确定HCT/P供体资格的法规要求。如上文详述，您重复给患者使用了异源细胞。FDA法规要求您必须在供体筛选以及有关传染性疾病病原体和疾病检测的基础上来决定哪些供体符合这类产品的供体资格。

5. 您未能按照21 CFR 1271.75的要求，根据供体筛选的结果，以及21 CFR 1271.80 和 1271.85的要求，根据供体检测的结果，来确定HCT/P供体是否合格［21 CFR 1271.50（a）］

例如：

供体（b）（6）在（b）（6）接受了初次的骨髓抽吸以收集干细胞。这些细胞后续被输入患者（b）（6）体内用于治疗冠状动脉缺血（CI）。没有证据显示您通过审阅相关医学记录，查找由于有关传染性疾病病原体和疾病引起的感染的风险因素以及临床证据，对供体（b）（6）进行了筛选。也没有记录显示对（b）（6）样本进行了有关传染性疾病病原体的检测以确认其是否被感染。

在TCA回复信中，未能提供任何关于（b）（6）供体或（b）（6）供体细胞接受者就传染性疾病所进行的后续检测或医学随访证据。请您在对本信的回复中，务必提供就传染性疾病所进行的后续检测或医学随访的任何证据。

6. 您未能对供体的标本进行有关传染性疾病病原体检测，以确认其是否被感染，从而充分、适当地降低有关传染性疾病传播的风险［21 CFR 1271.85（a）（5）］

例如：

A. 供体（b）（6）在（b）（6）接受了初次的骨髓抽吸以收集干细胞。这些细胞被处理并被输入（b）（6）个体体内用于治疗脊髓小脑性共济失调。没有证据表明，对供体（b）（6）的标本进行了梅毒螺旋体（梅毒）检测。

B. 供体（b）（6）在（b）（6）接受了初次的骨髓抽吸。这些细胞被输入（b）（6）个体体内用于治疗ALS。没有证据表明对供体（b）（6）的标本进行了梅毒螺旋体（梅毒）检测。

在TCA回复信中，包含的一张表格显示供体（b）（6）和供体（b）（6）梅毒检测结果均为阴性。请您在对这封信的回复中，提供能证明这些检测结果的具体文件。

7. 您未能对供体的标本进行富含白细胞的活细胞检测，从而充分、适当地降低有关细胞相关的传染病，包括人类嗜T淋巴细胞病毒Ⅰ型和Ⅱ型传播的风险（HTLV）［21 CFR 1271.85（b）（1）］

例如：

A. 供体（b）（6）在（b）（6）接受了初次的骨髓抽吸以收集干细胞。这些细胞被处理并被输入患者（b）（6）体内用于治疗肌肉骨骼异常。没有证据表明，对供体（b）（6）的标本进行了HTLV-1和HTLV-2检测。

B. 供体（b）（6）在（b）（6）接受了初次的骨髓抽吸以收集干细胞。这些细胞被处理并被输入患者（b）（6）体内用于治疗肢体缺血（LI）。没有证据表明，对供体（b）（6）的标本进行了HTLV-1和HTLV-2检测。

在TCA回复信中，包含的一张表格显示供体（b）（6）和供体（b）（6）HTLV检测结果均阴性。请您在对这封信的回复中，提供能证明这些检测结果的具体文件。

8. 您未能对供体的标本进行富集白细胞的活力细胞检测，以确认是否避免被巨细胞病毒（CMV）感染，从而充分、适当地降低有传播的风险［21 CFR1271.85（b）（2）］

例如：

A. 供体（b）（6）在（b）（6）接受了初次的骨髓抽吸，以收集干细胞。这些细胞被处理并被输入患者

（b）（6）体内用于治疗肌营养不良（MD）。没有证据表明，对供体（b）（6）的标本进行了CMV检测。

B. 供体（b）（6）在（b）（6）接受了初次的骨髓抽吸，以收集干细胞。这些细胞被处理并被输入患者（b）（6）体内，用于治疗肢体缺血（LI）。没有证据表明，对供体（b）（6）的标本进行了CMV检测。

在TCA的回复函中，包含的一张表格显示供体（b）（6）和供体（b）（6）CMV检测结果为阴性。请您在对这封函的回复中，提供能证明这些检测结果的具体文件。

本警告信的目的并非是罗列所有的缺陷。确保遵循法律和相关FDA法规的每一项要求是您的职责。

我们已经审阅了您2011年4月19日对FDA483表的书面回复，并认为您的回复尚未能充分解释我们的现场检查中发现的、与受试者保护和预防传染性疾病传播相关的多项严重违规。

在收到这封信的15个工作日内，您应当书面告知本部门，作为申办者，您为纠正这些违规行为，以及预防目前和将来的研究中发生类似违规行为，将要采取的具体措施。如果不能对本警告信作出回复或采取恰当的纠正措施，可能导致FDA在不再通知的情况下采取监管措施。

附：英文原文

TCA Cellular Therapy, LLC

Warning Letter

August 15, 2011

By Facsimile Transmission and Overnight Delivery

CBER-11-03

Charles Naparalla, Chief Executive Officer
TCA Cellular Therapy, LLC
101 Judge Tanner Boulevard, Suite 502
Covington, Louisiana 70433

Dear Mr. Naparalla:

This letter describes the results of a Food and Drug Administration (FDA, the Agency) inspection conducted between February 22, 2011, and March 31, 2011. The FDA investigators met with you and the staff of TCA Cellular Therapy, LLC (TCA) to review TCA's conduct as a sponsor and as a biological drug product manufacturer. This inspection was conducted as part of the FDA's Bioresearch Monitoring Program, which includes inspections designed to review the conduct of research involving investigational drugs.

At the end of the inspection, the FDA investigators met with you and TCA staff to discuss the items listed on the Form FDA 483, Inspectional Observations. Dr. Gabriel Perez Lasala, TCA Medical Director, responded to the Form FDA 483 in a letter dated April 19, 2011 ("TCA letter") sent to the New Orleans District Office. Based on our review of the inspection report, the supporting documents submitted with that report, other information available to the Agency, and the TCA letter, we have determined that TCA violated regulations governing the proper conduct of clinical studies involving investigational new drugs, as published in Title 21, Code of Federal Regulations (CFR) Part 312, and violated the regulations governing human cells, tissue, and cellular and tissue based products (HCT/Ps) in 21 CFR Part 1271, which were designed to prevent the introduction, transmission and spread of communicable disease (available at http://www.gpoaccess.gov/cfr/index.html). The applicable provisions of the CFR are cited for each violation listed below.

TCA is the sponsor of the following Investigational New Drug Applications (INDs):

IND 11643: Autologous Mesenchymal Stem Cells Expanded Ex Vivo, Mixed with Bone Marrow-Derived Mononuclear Cells, Administered via Balloon Catheter or Intraoperatively
Indication: Treatment of Myocardial Infarction
Clinical Investigator: Gabriel P. Lasala, M.D.

IND 13139 Autologous Bone Marrow-Derived Mononuclear Cells and Autologous BoneMarrow-Derived Mesenchymal Stem Cells, Administered by Intramuscular Injection
Indication: Treatment of Critical Limb Ischemia
Clinical Investigator: Gabriel P. Lasala, M.D.

IND 13562 Autologous Bone Marrow-Derived Mononuclear Cells and Autologous BoneMarrow-Derived Mesenchymal Stem Cells, Administered Intracoronary by Voyager (Guidant)
Indication: Treatment of Severe Coronary Ischemia
Clinical Investigator: Gabriel P. Lasala, M.D.

IND 13729 Autologous Bone Marrow-Derived Mesenchymal Cells; Administered via LumbarPuncture
Indication: Treatment of Amyotrophic Lateral Sclerosis (ALS)
Clinical Investigator: Gabriel P. Lasala, M.D.

IND 13981 Autologous Bone Marrow-Derived Mesenchymal Cells; Administered Intrathecally
Indication: Treatment of Spinal Cord Injury
Clinical Investigator: Gabriel P. Lasala, M.D.

1. You failed to fulfill the general responsibilities of sponsors to ensure that investigations were conducted according to the investigational plan and you failed to monitor the progress of ongoing investigations. [21 CFR § 312.50 and 312.56(a)].

A sponsor is responsible for ensuring proper monitoring of investigations and ensuring that the investigations are conducted in accordance with the general investigational plan and protocols contained in the sponsor's IND.

A. The FDA inspection revealed that autologous investigational products were repeatedly administered to individuals who were not enrolled in TCA's IND studies.

Autologous investigational products were repeatedly administered to individuals not enrolled in IND studies, even though these individuals were treated for the same indications covered by TCA's INDs. Moreover, in at least five cases, these autologous products were administered while therelevant INDs, (IND 13729 and IND 13981) were on clinical hold as ordered by FDA.

Individuals administered autologous cellular product for the same indications covered by an IND,but not enrolled in the IND studies, are represented in the table below.

IND	IND Indication	Individuals Identification #	Date of Autologous Infusion
13139	Limb Ischemia	(b)(6)	(b)(6)
		(b)(6)	(b)(6)
13981	Spinal Cord Injury	(b)(6)	(b)(6)
13562	Coronary Ischemia	(b)(6)	(b)(6)
		(b)(6)	(b)(6)
		(b)(6)	(b)(6)
		(b)(6)	(b)(6)
11643	Myocardial Infarction	(b)(6)	(b)(6)
		(b)(6)	(b)(6)

The TCA letter attempts to justify these actions by stating that these individuals were terminally ill and severely debilitated with no other options for treatment and, as a result, Dr. Lasala treatedthese patients with intent to expand access for compassionate use.

B. Although TCA's INDs were limited to autologous use of bone marrow-derived cells, study records show that allogeneic cells were administered to patients who were not enrolled as study subjects in any of TCA's INDs. Indeed, during FDA's inspection, Dr. Lasala also admitted to the FDA investigators that he administered allogeneic cells to patients outside of clinical protocols, conduct he described as a "compassionate illegal act," "completely wrong," and "completely illegal." The following individuals received allogeneic cells rather than autologous cells, as required by the IND protocols.

Indication	Individual	Date of Infusion
Coronary Ischemia	(b)(6)	(b)(6)
	(b)(6)	(b)(6)
	(b)(6)	(b)(6)
	(b)(6)	(b)(6)
	(b)(6)	(b)(6)
	(b)(6)	(b)(6)
	(b)(6)	(b)(6)
Limb Ischemia	(b)(6)	(b)(6)
	(b)(6)	(b)(6)
	(b)(6)	(b)(6)
	(b)(6)	(b)(6)
	(b)(6)	(b)(6)
	(b)(6)	(b)(6)
	(b)(6)	(b)(6)
	(b)(6)	(b)(6)
	(b)(6)	(b)(6)
ALS	(b)(6)	(b)(6)
	(b)(6)	(b)(6)
	(b)(6)	(b)(6)
	(b)(6)	(b)(6)
	(b)(6)	(b)(6)
	(b)(6)	(b)(6)
	(b)(6)	(b)(6)
	(b)(6)	(b)(6)
	(b)(6)	(b)(6)
	(b)(6)	(b)(6)
	(b)(6)	(b)(6)
	(b)(6)	(b)(6)
	(b)(6)	(b)(6)
	(b)(6)	(b)(6)
Spinal Injury	(b)(6)	(b)(6)
	(b)(6)	(b)(6)
	(b)(6)	(b)(6)
	(b)(6)	(b)(6)
	(b)(6)	(b)(6)

The TCA letter attempts to justify these actions in the same way as was described in paragraph1.A. above.

C. You failed to monitor the progress of all clinical investigations being conducted under IND.

i. There was no evidence that the following studies were monitored by TCA: Study (b)(6)under IND 13563, Study (b)(6) under IND 13729, and Study (b)(6) under IND 13981.

The TCA letter attempts to justify a lack of monitoring by explaining that the contracted monitor could no longer perform monitoring as of January 2011 and negotiations were ongoing with another company to begin monitoring in March 2011. The TCA letter further explains that after the inspection, Dr. Lasala, TCA Managing Member, discovered that the last monitoring visit was August 26, 2008.

ii. During our inspection, we discovered that a serious protocol violation had occurred regarding the infusion of an incorrect investigational product into subject (b)(6). The protocol for Study (b)(6) (IND 13981) requires that "a Bone Marrow (BM) aspiration be scheduled within 10 days of the signed consent" and that these are the cells that will be processed and reinfused. Subject (b)(6) signed the informed consent for the study on August 4, 2010. The Case Report Forms for Visit 2 - Primary Bone Marrow Aspiration - show that a (b)(6) was infused into this subject on (b)(6) and that these cells were collected from this subject during a bone marrow aspiration performed over ten months earlier, on (b)(6).

The TCA letter acknowledges that the protocol for IND 13981 does not include a provision for the infusion of (b)(6).

iii. Subject (b)(6) was administered allogeneic donor cells from TCA Donor Stock instead of autologous stem cells as required by section 3.1 of the study protocol. During the inspection, Dr.Lasala and Dr. Minguell told the FDA investigators that they could not identify the source of the cells administered to this subject. In the TCA letter, Dr. Lasala identified the donor cell source as"(b)(6)" and explained that donor "(b)(6)" was intended for Crohn's disease patient (b)(6), whose procedure was cancelled. The TCA letter further explains that Dr. Lasala had administered donor "(b)(6)" cellular product to subject (b)(6), rather than discard the cellular product, resulting in subject (b)(6) receiving allogeneic cells.

The TCA letter attempts to justify the Clinical Investigator's decision to treat the subject with allogeneic cells based on the severity of the subject's condition.

When the FDA investigators inquired about TCA Donor Stock, Dr. Minguell originally explained that TCA Donor Stock was a term used to refer to "surplus cells" that were retained for calibrations and testing new lots of fetal bovine serum. Dr. Minguell subsequently admitted that TCA Donor Stock is comprised of allogeneic donor aspirates that are not intended for any specific recipient. He then apologized to the FDA investigators during the inspection for having intentionally misled them inregard to the donor cells.

2. You initiated clinical investigations without an IND in effect. [21 CFR § 312.20 and 312.40].

At the End-of-Phase 2 meeting with FDA for IND 13139 held on November 22, 2010, TCA proposed the use of autologous bone marrow-derived mononuclear cells (BM-MNC) combined with allogeneic bone marrow derived mesenchymal cells (BM-MSC) as the investigational product for a Phase 3 study. The BM-MNC and BM-MSC used to conduct the existing Phase 1 and Phase2 studies were autologous. You were advised by FDA during the meeting that a new IND would be required for the use of allogeneic bone marrow derived mesenchymal cells. As documented in the meeting minutes dated December 8, 2010, you have no safety or preliminary efficacy data, and FDA advised you that the Agency considered this to be a first-in-human Phase 1 study, which would require submission of a new IND, and which should focus on assessment of safety for this new allogeneic product.

Despite FDA's conclusions that a new IND would be required for the use of allogeneic BM-MSC,TCA subsequently administered allogeneic cell products to the following individuals:

Individual	Infusion Date	Indication
(b)(6)	(b)(6)	Spinal cord injury
(b)(6)	(b)(6)	Spinal muscular atrophy
(b)(6)	(b)(6)	Spinal muscular atrophy
(b)(6)	(b)(6)	Muscular dystrophy
(b)(6)	(b)(6)	ALS

(Contd.)

Individual	Infusion Date	Indication
(b)(6)	(b)(6)	Progressed muscular atrophy
(b)(6)	(b)(6)	Spinal cord injury
(b)(6)	(b)(6)	Severe limb ischemia
(b)(6)	(b)(6)	Severe limb ischemia
(b)(6)	(b)(6)	Spinocerebellar ataxia
(b)(6)	(b)(6)	Spinal cord injury
(b)(6)	(b)(6)	Spinal cord injury
(b)(6)	(b)(6)	ALS
(b)(6)	(b)(6)	Spinal cord injury
(b)(6)	(b)(6)	Traumatic musculoskeletal injury

Furthermore, FDA's inspection revealed that you had initiated this treatment with allogeneic BM-MSC even before the November 22, 2010 meeting. In fact, you treated at least -b(4)- individuals with allogeneic cells before November 22, 2010 for a variety of indications, including but not limited to severe coronary is chemia, musculoskeletal disorder, muscular dystrophy, primary lateral sclerosis, spinocerebellar ataxia, spinal muscular atrophy, and spinal injury.

Indication	Number of Individuals Treated
Severe coronary is chemia	(b)(6) (b)(4)
ALS	(b)(6) (b)(4)
Limb is chemia	(b)(6) (b)(4)
Musculoskeletal disorder	(b)(6) (b)(4)
Muscular dystrophy	(b)(6) (b)(4)
Primary lateral sclerosis	(b)(6) (b)(4)
Spinocerebellar ataxia	(b)(6) (b)(4)
Spinal muscular atrophy	(b)(6) (b)(4)
Spinal injury	(b)(6) (b)(4)
Epilepsy	(b)(6) (b)(4)
Thalamic abscess	(b)(6) (b)(4)
Renal Disease	(b)(6) (b)(4)
Alzheimer's	(b)(6) (b)(4)
Progressed muscular atrophy	(b)(6) (b)(4)
Multiple sclerosis	(b)(6) (b)(4)
Spinal (stroke)	(b)(6) (b)(4)
Neuropathy	(b)(6) (b)(4)

The TCA letter attempts to justify these actions in the same way as was described in paragraph1.A. above.

3. You initiated clinical investigations without either submitting a protocol amendment or a new IND to FDA. [21 CFR § 312.20, 312.30 and 312.40].

You failed to either submit a protocol amendment or new IND to FDA for treatment of new indications with autologous BM-MSC, as shown in each of the instances described in the table below.

Identification	Indication	Comments
(b)(6)	Musculoskeletal disorder	
(b)(6)	Musculoskeletal disorder	

(Contd.)

Identification	Indication	Comments
(b)(6)	Stomach cancer	
(b)(6)	Musculoskeletal disorder	
(b)(6)	Epilepsy	This individual was 10 years old; all protocols in TCA's five INDs excluded subjects under the age of 18.
(b)(6)	Optic nerve atrophy, and arteriovenous malformation of the brain	This individual was 24 months old; all protocols in TCA's five INDs excluded subjects under the age of 18. Furthermore, the intraocular injection of the investigational product is a new route of administration.
(b)(6)	Neuropathy	
(b)(6)	Traumatic brain injury	This individual was 14 years old; all protocols in TCA's five INDs excluded subjects under the age of 18.
(b)(6)	Glioblastoma	

The TCA letter attempts to justify these actions in the same way as was described in paragraph1.A. above.

4. You administered an investigational product in violation of a clinical hold. [21 CFR § 312.42(a) and (e)].

A. IND 13729 was on clinical hold from July 11, 2008 through January 8, 2010. During that time period, the following individuals were treated with the investigational product for IND 13729 for the same indication as referenced in the IND, namely, ALS. These individuals were not enrolled in the study and were treated while the study was on hold.

Individual	Date of Aspirate	Date of Infusion
(b)(6)	(b)(6)	(b)(6)
(b)(6)	(b)(6)	(b)(6)
(b)(6)	(b)(6)	(b)(6)

B. IND 13981 was on clinical hold from April 10, 2009 until April 14, 2010. The following individuals were treated with the investigational product for IND 13981 for the same indication as referenced in the IND, namely, treatment of spinal cord injury. These individuals were not enrolled in the study and were treated while the study was on hold.

Individual	Date of Aspirate	Date of Infusion
(b)(6)	(b)(6)	(b)(6)
(b)(6)	(b)(6)	(b)(6)
(b)(6)	(b)(6)	(b)(6)

In addition to these violations of FDA regulations addressing the conduct of clinical studies, you also violated FDA regulations that set forth requirements for determining eligibility of HCT/P donors. You repeatedly administered allogeneic cells to patients, as described in detail above. FDA regulations require you to determine the eligibility of donors of such products based on do nor screening and testing for relevant communicable disease agents and diseases.

5. You failed to determine whether an HCT/P donor is eligible based on the results of donor screening in accordance with 21 CFR § 1271.75 and donor testing in accordance with21 CFR § 1271.80 and 1271.85 [21 CFR § 1271.50(a)].

For example:

Donor (b)(6) underwent a primary bone marrow aspiration to collect stem cells on (b)(6). These cells were subsequently transfused into individual (b)(6) for treatment of Coronary Ischemia(CI). There is no evidence that (b)

(6) was screened, through a review of relevant medical records, for risk factors for, and clinical evidence of, infection due to relevant communicable disease agents and diseases. There are also no records documenting that a specimen from (b)(6) was tested for evidence of infection due to relevant communicable disease agents.

The TCA letter fails to provide any evidence of subsequent testing or medical follow-up in regard to communicable diseases for donor (b)(6) or the recipient of donor (b)(6) cells. Please include any evidence of further testing or medical follow-up in regard to communicable diseases in your response to this letter.

6. You failed to test a specimen from the donor for evidence of infection due to relevantcommunicable diseases agents, to adequately and appropriately reduce the risk of transmission of relevant communicable diseases. [21 CFR § 1271.85(a)(5)].

For example:

A. Donor (b)(6) underwent a primary bone marrow aspiration to collect stem cells on (b)(6). These cells were processed and transfused into individual (b)(6) for treatment of Spinocerebellar Ataxia. There is no evidence that a specimen from (b)(6) was tested for Treponema pallidum (syphilis).

B. Donor (b)(6) underwent a primary bone marrow aspiration on (b)(6). These cells were transfused into individual (b)(6) for the treatment of ALS. There is no evidence that a specimen from (b)(6) was tested for Treponema pallidum (syphilis).

The TCA letter includes a table that shows that donor (b)(6) and donor (b)(6) tested negative for syphilis. Please provide specific documentation of these test results with your response to this letter.

7. You failed to test a specimen from the donor of viable, leukocyte-rich cells to adequately and appropriately reduce the risk of transmission of relevant cell-associated communicablediseases including Human T-lymphotropic virus (HTLV) types Ⅰ and Ⅱ. [21 CFR § 1271.85(b)(1)].

For example:

A. Donor (b)(6) underwent a primary bone marrow aspiration to collect stem cells on (b)(6). These cells were processed and transfused into individual (b)(6) for treatment of amusculoskeletal disorder. There is no evidence that a specimen from (b)(6) was tested for HTLV types Ⅰ and Ⅱ.

B. Donor (b)(6) underwent a primary bone marrow aspiration to collect stem cells on (b)(6). These cells were processed and transfused into individual (b)(6) for treatment of LimbIschemia (LI). There is no evidence that a specimen from (b)(6) was tested for HTLV types Ⅰ and Ⅱ.

The TCA letter includes a table that shows that donor (b)(6) and donor (b)(6) tested negative for HTLV. Please provide specific documentation of these test results with your response to this letter

8. You failed to test a specimen from the donor of viable, leukocyte-rich cells for evidence of infection due to Cytomegalovirus (CMV) to adequately and appropriately reduce the risk of transmission [21 CFR § 1271.85(b)(2)].

For example:

A. Donor (b)(6) underwent a primary bone marrow aspiration to collect stem cells on (b)(6). These cells were processed and transfused into individual (b)(6) for treatment of Muscular Dystrophy (MD). There is no evidence that a specimen from (b)(6) was tested for the presence of CMV.

B. Donor (b)(6) underwent a primary bone marrow aspiration to collect stem cells on (b)(6). These cells were processed and transfused into individual (b)(6) for treatment of LimbIschemia (LI). There is no evidence that a specimen from (b)(6) was tested for CMV.

The TCA letter includes a table that shows that donor (b)(6)and donor (b)(6) tested negative for CMV. Please provide specific documentation of these test results with your response to this letter.

This letter is not intended to be an all-inclusive list of deficiencies. It is your responsibility to ensure adherence to each requirement of the law and relevant FDA regulations.

We have reviewed your April 19, 2011 response to the Form FDA 483 and determined that your response is not adequate to address the serious violations regarding human subject protection and prevention of transmission of communicable diseases that were discovered during our inspection.

Within fifteen (15) business days of receipt of this letter, please provide written documentation of the specific actions you will take to correct these violations and prevent the recurrence of similar violations in current and future studies for which you are the sponsor. Failure to respond to this letter and to take appropriate corrective action could result in FDA taking regulatory action without further notice to you.

Please send your written response to:

Christine Drabick
Division of Inspections and Surveillance (HFM-664)
Office of Compliance and Biologics Quality
Center for Biologics Evaluation and Research
1401 Rockville Pike, Suite 200N
Rockville, Maryland 20852-1488
Telephone: 301-827-6323

We also request that you send a copy of your response to the FDA District Office listed below.

Sincerely,

/S/

Mary A. Malarkey, Director
Office of Compliance and Biologics Quality
Center for Biologics Evaluation and Research

Cc:
District Director
Food and Drug Administration
Building 200, Suite 500
404 BNA Drive
Nashville, Tennessee 37217

第 44 封　给 Cetero 研究公司的警告信

2011年7月26日

参考号：11-HFD-45-07-02

亲爱的Hayes博士：

2010年5月3至7日，检查员Patrick D. Stone先生、Jacqueline A.O’Shaughnessy医生和Carol M. Rivera-Lopez医生；2010年12月6至10日，检查员Albert Peacock、MartinK. Yau、Sam H. Haidar、John Kadavil,和Xikui Chen先生代表FDA，对您位于德克萨斯州休斯顿的生物检测机构进行了现场检查。这封警告信特告知您现场检查中发现的违规情况。FDA检查员发现了严重违反21 CFR 320中关于生物利用度和生物等效性要求的情况。违规行为包括实验室记录中受试者样品提取的日期与时间大量造假，以及明显操纵平衡样品以符合预设的可接受标准。

保证和确认贵公司的检测方法，以及由贵公司采集并作为递交给FDA任何申请材料一部分的生物利用度和生物有效性数据的可靠性是贵公司的职责。贵公司违规行为的普遍性和恶劣性，使得FDA严重怀疑从2005年4月1日至2010年6月15日在Cetero休斯顿机构产生的生物等效性和生物利用度数据，包括在新药申请（NDA）和仿制药申请（ANDA）中递交给FDA作为研究一部分的数据。

如下文所述，FDA的结论基于以下几点：①实验室记录中受试者样品提取的日期与时间大量造假；②明显操纵平衡或“预”批样品，以符合预设的可接受标准；③关于平衡或“预”批记录的缺失，导致您不能进行充分的内部检查，以确定该违规行为的程度和造成的影响。

FDA的现场检查包括对以下研究的不同部分进行审查：

<u>2010年5月检查</u>

- 研究（b）(4)，[（b）(4)]，申办者为（b）(4)。
- 研究（b）(4)，[（b）(4)]，申办者为（b）(4)。
- 研究（b）(4)，[（b）(4)]，申办者为（b）(4)。
- 研究（b）(4)，[（b）(4)]，申办者为（b）(4)。
- 研究（b）(4)，[（b）(4)]，申办者为（b）(4)。

<u>2010年10月检查</u>

- 研究（b）(4)，[（b）(4)]，申办者为（b）(4)。
- 研究（b）(4)，[（b）(4)]，申办者为（b）(4)。
- 研究（b）(4)，[（b）(4)]，申办者为（b）(4)。
- 研究（b）(4)，[（b）(4)]，申办者为（b）(4)。

本次现场检查是FDA的生物研究监查项目的一部分，该项目通过设定的检查方法，对研究的实施情况进行评估，以确认拟向FDA递交的、用以支持FDA批准和监管决定的数据是可靠的，并核实符合21 CFR 320中关于生物利用度和生物等效性的要求。

在日期为2009年4月22日的来信中，您的一位员工（投诉人）对违规和其他不当行为提起正式指控引起了贵公司的注意。该信指出，早在2007年6月，投诉人“在有前任CEO……出席的主管会议上首次提出某些问题。在此会议上，[投诉人]确认了大量的Cetero标准操作规程没有被实验室内的众多化学师遵守。[投诉人]意识到众多化学师在多个项目中伪造和篡改正被使用的样品的数据。”

在收到投诉人2009年4月22日的信之后，贵公司随后启动了关于投诉人主张的内部调查，详见日期为

2009年6月5日题目为“关于2009年4月22日收到的对数据完整性质疑的内部调查”的报告。2009年6月5日，投诉人将对您休斯顿实验室不当行为的质疑报告给FDA达拉斯区域办公室。贵公司在2009年6月10日联系了FDA达拉斯区域办公室，告知FDA有关投诉的内容并提交了贵公司进行内部调查的结果。此外，贵公司寻求独立第三方针对投诉内容进行调查和审查并于2009年7月6日完成。因此，贵公司在题为“关于2009年4月22日收到的对数据完整性质疑的内部调查，2009年7月27日更新”的报告中更新了内部调查的情况。两份内部调查报告及第三方调查报告已收悉。

2010年5月、2010年10月FDA对实验室的现场检查，以及2009年7月的第三方调查，均确认在您的研究场所有关于程序的大量质疑，并且您的内部调查存在缺陷。2010年5月现场检查结束时，贵公司被发放了FDA483表，我们确认贵公司日期为2010年5月24日的回复［以下简称2010年5月24日483表回复函］已收悉。尽管您在回复函中拟定了纠正措施，但是FDA在2010年12月检查中发现在您的研究场所持续的缺陷，并于2010年12月10日发出了另一份FDA 483表［以下简称为2010年12月29日483表回复函］。然而，如下文所述，您的FDA483表回复函并没有充分解决FDA在检查中发现的违规问题。

FDA注意到您的研究场所存在如下违规行为：

贵公司未能证明在体内生物利用度或生物等效性研究中，用来测定体液或排泄物中活性药物成分，或治疗组分，或其活性代谢物浓度的分析方法，有精确度和足够的灵敏度，以及适当的精密度，来测定活性药物成分，或治疗组分，或其活性代谢物在体内达到的实际浓度［21 CFR 320.29(a)］

示例包括，但不限于以下内容：

1. 不当行为的实例

a. 伪造实验室记录

FDA注意到，您内部调查发现与伪造员工时间/日期记录有关的问题。您于2009年7月28日向FDA报告了这些问题。2010年5月和2010年12月的检查中，FDA也发现数个研究的分析程序（AP）原始数据表中关于受试者样品提取时间和日期的不一致或造假。

以下是这类研究的两个举例：

- 研究（b）(4)，分析批5和6测定（b）(4）和分析批4测定（b）(4)。
- 研究（b）(4)，分析批11~16测定（b）(4）和分析批13、14、17和18测定（b）(4)。

在您2010年5月24日对FDA483表回复函中，您同意FDA发现的问题，造假涉及多个申办者多项研究的数据。

您的FDA483表回复函、内部调查以及第三方调查均不足以解决FDA对伪造实验室记录的质疑，详述如下：

（1）您的内部调查范围不够

您的内部调查范围仅限于AP表中日期/时间的造假，而不是整体研究情况和AP表中记录的其他数据；因此，贵公司未能确定是否实验室记录的其他方面也受到损害。因此，这些伪造的真实程度尚未可知。

根据您的内部调查，钥匙卡门禁进入次数的电子记录显示，2005年4月15日至2009年6月30日，大约1900例血液/血浆样品据称是在周末和节假日进行提取，但实验室化学师们的到达时间超过记录的样品提取开始时间1小时。此外，约有875例样品，在记录的样品提取日期实验室化学师并未在研究场所上班。

2010年5月和2010年12月FDA483表的回复函中，贵公司声称化学师们在星期五或节假日前一天提取试验样品，但记录此工作于周末或节假日完成，以获得财务奖励。贵公司还声称，您的调查确认实验室记录的伪造仅限于对提取时间和日期的篡改。

基于您陈述的假设，伪造实验室记录是由于化学师为获取更多的经济补偿，造成不是所有工作都在一天内完成的样子，贵公司起初仅关注周末的提取记录，并且您未考虑是否任何周末的提取记录都是伪造的。继2010年5月现场检查之后，贵公司决定开展进一步调查，并发现员工在周末和工作日伪造考勤卡和实验室记录。

您在2010年5月24日483表回复函中说明如下：

"由于修改AP的原因与财务激励措施相关……没有理由怀疑AP的任何其他部分的有效性。"

然而，既然并没有财务奖励让他们这样做，为什么员工们会伪造工作日记录中的日期和时间？对此您未提出解释。此外，您提出的AP表中周末提取的篡改与财务奖励有关的理论，以及您认为没有理由怀疑AP表的其他部分的有效性的主张，FDA都不同意。贵公司还没有提供任何文件来支持这些主张，或者解释您如何确保您实验室记录的总体可靠性。

（2）您未能提供证据证明在贵公司的质量保证工作将伪造数据的范围限定于样品提取时间和日期

您在2010年5月24日483表回复函中声明，试验前工作（如参照标准品的称量、储备液和同位素标记溶液的制备、大量QC溶液的制备）100%由质量控制/文档管理人员审查。此外，您声明所有试验前工作与20%的受试者分析批已由QA人员进行稽查。您声称，这些例行审查确保试验前工作的完整性，以及确认实验室记录的修改仅限于提取的时间和日期。然而，FDA注意到尽管对研究分析批进行了这些稽查，但是您的QA部门没有发现从2005年4月1日至2009年6月15日超过4年的时间段内对实验室记录的频繁改动，这个时间段内贵公司进行了内部调查。这些问题提示，您的QA部门进行的例行稽查不足以确认或评估您实验室记录的可靠性。

您在2010年5月24日484表回复函中称："我们坚信，因为仅涉及提取步骤中提取日期和时间的不确定，所以每个受影响的研究中报告的浓度数据未受影响。"您在2010年12月29日483表回复函中称："我们进行了非常广泛和深入的调查……因此，我们确信由研究化学师产生的，牵涉到天/日期伪造的数据的完整性并未受到影响或损害。"

FDA不同意您在FDA483表回复函中的上述表述。对伪造实验室记录的内部调查的狭窄的范围，对考勤卡和样品提取的时间和日期不一致缺乏一致的可信的解释，QA规程未能发现伪造的情况，引起对在您的AP表上记录的所有信息，包括用于支持递交给FDA的NDA和ANDA申请的研究结果可靠性的关注。

此外，2009年7月6日来自独立第三方的调查报告指出："疑似有证据显示实验室员工不当行为已发生至少好几年，并一直且持续到至少今年4月份。实验室主管人员疑似已涉入。该不当行为似乎足以对所产生的数据引起质疑。"您的回复并未充分解释第三方调查报告中提出的这些质疑。

实验室记录中任何部分的伪造都会引起对其余部分的可靠性产生怀疑。您未能支持伪造实验室记录仅限于提取的时间和日期这个观点。贵公司对伪造的试验记录的广泛使用，致使FDA对2005年4月1日至2010年6月15日期间您研究场所产生的所有生物分析数据的有效性提出质疑。

b. 操纵样品

FDA已确认贵公司操纵检测的样品符合预设的可接受标准。

根据最初的投诉举报，在将数据纳入正式的研究文件夹之前，平衡或"预"分析批据称通过"固定"分析批来符合可接受标准，而被用于操纵数据。

递交给FDA的最初的投诉举报中列举出这种操作的几个实例。在一个例子中，投诉人提交的照片显示研究（b）（4）第38分析批为2009年1月3日进样，因缺乏内标物而失败（即内标物未按标准的作法，在最初加入至校正标样和质控样品中）。根据照片上明显的记号，在分析批失败后，第38分析批的样品将被放回到冰箱。第二天，第38分析批的样品进样至LC/MS/MS（液相色谱串联质谱）系统，此时内标物出现在校正标样和质控样品中。贵公司的记录没有对这个不一致进行解释，也没有记录内标物是在1月4日重新分析之前才被加入到样品中。

如2009年7月6日第三方调查所述，"疑似标准曲线和质控被其他分析批的替换了。"质控样品为受试者样品中药品浓度的准确性和精密度提供保证。从其他分析批替换质控样品来符合可接受标准是不合适的，这样受试者样品中的药物浓度无法确保。

尽管申诉人提出指控，贵公司的内部调查最初未能发现与第38分析批有关的任何不当行为。直到投诉人提供照片和其他证据，以及第三方稽查发现"指控似乎有道理"，贵公司才在更新的内部调查报告中向FDA承认"有理由假设发生了与第38分析批标准曲线和质控样品有关的不合适的活动。"您未能认识到，关于第

38分析批的不当程序引起了对您内部调查的其他结论的质疑。

2. 平衡样品的使用不当

对活性药物或活性成分浓度的准确测量依赖于正确验证过的分析方法，包括对用于检测的仪器的校准和平衡。使用下列类型的样品用于对LC / MS / MS设备的平衡是不推荐的：

- 尚未被分析的受试者样品；
- 校正标样，质控样品（QCS），以及作为正式运行批一部分的空白样品。

日期为2009年7月6日的第三方调查报告中指出："如果一台仪器需要调试，只能采用专为此目的准备的样品，而且这些样品应当不是用于该分析批的标准品或对照品。绝不能出现这些样品被其他分析批中的标准品和对照品替代的情况"。

根据贵公司提供的信息以及贵公司委托的第三方调查报告，贵公司的LC / MS / MS设备的平衡方法包括使用如校正标样、质控样品、空白样品以及属于当前分析批的一部分的、尚未被分析过的受试者样品。

FDA关注的是，使用尚未被分析过的提取样品来进行系统平衡，可能给化学师们提供了操纵正式研究分析批结果的机会。化学师将有机会在把这些样品作为正式的研究分析批进行分析之前，就确认是否"预"分析批校正标样和质控样品会通过或不通过可接受标准，因而产生了操纵研究分析批的机会，或者通过向样品中添加研究药物或内标物，或者通过用其他先前已经通过的样品来替代该样品。

您2010年5月和2010年10月对FDA483表的回复函，以及您的内部调查和第三方调查，均不足以解决FDA所关注的平衡样品不当使用的问题，详述如下。

（a）2010年5月24日FDA483表回复函中您对此做法提出的解释缺乏可信度

您声称平衡或"预"分析批的目的是为了在开始受试者样品分析之前调试系统和进行必要的故障排除。然而，该观点不能对2010年5月FDA检查期间被评估的，研究（b）（4）第20分析批进行解释。在第20分析批中，"预"分析批在系统95中进行，而实际分析批在系统74中进行。如果"预"分析批的操作确实是为平衡系统，并确保LC/MS/MS系统的最佳性能，那么必须使用同一台平衡过的仪器。

（b）您的对于"预"分析批的内部调查不充分

Cetero的内部调查，包括第三方的调查，并未减少FDA对2005年4月1日至2010年6月15日由贵公司所产生的数据的可靠性的怀疑。缺乏足够的、关于在贵公司使用"预"分析批的文件和SOP，妨碍了您进行充分的调查，以对2010年5月和2010年12月检查期间发放的FDA483表作出反应的能力。

贵公司制定了一份题为"Cetero研究所休斯顿机构研究计划修订版1"、日期为2009年7月28日的研究计划，来针对投诉人"为了获得通过的结果，分析批被多次进样；为了通过，样品不知何故被'固定'了"的指控。

内部调查评估了来自您非正式的电子"预"分析批文件的大约（b）（4）样品，均是2005年4月至2009年6月期间，为大约类似研究（b）（4）进行的。调查确认了三个额外的分析批存在与上面所述的、研究（b）（4）第38分析批类似的不当操作。

在您的内部调查计划中"预分析批决策图表"目的是解决投诉人关于样品被"固定"的指控。根据决策图表，Cetero将评估是否所有样品有内标物或待测药物的响应，是否所有校正标样和质控样品有药物峰，是否空白样品有可接受的响应。您的分析中包含这样的假设："预"分析批的样品与随后在正式的研究分析批中进样的样品是相同的。因为缺乏在贵公司进行的"预"分析批中使用样品的来源文件，FDA不接受这样的假设作为对预分析批作出决定的依据。

您的内部调查中唯一不依赖于样品来源的部分是对所有样品是否有内标物或药物响应的评估。结果，您的内部调查比计划更加局限，因其仅能关注结果，不能被科学地解释的"预"分析批（即最初存在药品或内标物的样品却出现在随后正式分析批的进样中）。调查不能评估是否校准物、质控样品或空白样品可能以及被加入药品或被其他样品替代。此外，您的内部调查不能评估"预"分析批如何被使用，什么被进样以及他们可能会如何影响研究结果。

2010年5月和2010年12月FDA检查结果显示，基本缺乏关于"预"分析批的文件，因此，很明显，贵公司的内部调查不足以彻底解决关于"预"分析批的指控。您的调查未能证明"预"分析批的使用对于被分析的时间段来讲，并未影响试验数据的完整性。文件的缺乏抑制了您充分说明使用样本的实际来源、"预"分析批之间进样不同数量（从4~43）样品，以及是否"预"分析批的结果被用于改变正式分析批结果的能力。

这与2009年7月6日第三方独立调查报告的结论是一致的，其写到"'预'分析批的数据不总是保存在研究文件夹，在准备过程期间对设备或样品可能作出那些调整，但没有任何记录。也没有为什么样品被多次进样的记录。既然样品被重复进样直到获得通过的结果，然后该分析批被正式进样，那么这种过程可以被视为测试到合规。"

在2010年12月29日FDA483表回复函中，您声称化学师对平衡样品的来源是"盲态的"，以限制不当行为的可能性，且描述平衡样品来源和身份的记录没有得到。FDA认为此解释不可信，因为您未提供证据证明化学师对中进样的样品来源不知情。另外，如下文所讨论的，您没有关于这个程序的SOP。

关于"预"分析批文件的缺乏，使贵公司无法进行深入的内部调查并确认您的"预"分析批操作造成的影响。文件的缺乏也使监管部门无法对您实际检测操作进行知情评价。因此，我们无法支持您的内部调查中关于"预"分析批对在您研究场所进行研究的数据的完整性没有影响的结论。

（c）贵公司缺乏针对LC / MS / MS仪器平衡的SOP

在2010年5月24日FDA483表回复函中，您承认实验室过去LC / MS / MS仪器的调试操作就是利用将在当前分析批被分析的样品的一个子集。如上面提到的，投诉人2009年4月22日曾致信Cetero。2009年5月，Cetero管理层发出指令，立即停止使用尚未分析的样品进行LC / MS / MS仪器的调试/平衡，而仅使用之前分析过的样品来达到调试/平衡的目的。但是，贵公司直至2009年12月14日才实施了关于LC / MS / MS仪器调试的书面指导（CET_SOP_04_INS-006，LC / MS / MS仪器的平衡，第1版）。该SOP规定应采用先前进样的校正标样、质控样品以及受试者样品的混合样品平衡LC / MS / MS仪器。FDA注意到SOP第1版并未要求记录平衡样品的识别信息和来源，因此，该SOP不可接受。

日期为2009年7月6日的第三方独立调查报告中提出了下列关于"预"分析批的使用和LC / MS / MS仪器的平衡的建议："对任何分析批进行的使用标准品和对照品的'预备'做法都应该立即停止。如果仪器需要调试，仅应当使用专门制备用于此目的的样品，而且这些样品不应当是用于此分析批的标准品和对照品的一部分。绝不能出现这些样品被其他分析批中的标准品和对照品替代的情况。"从研究开始的每次进样、每个样品制备以及采取的每一个行动均应当被记录。数据应当只被获取到正式的研究文件夹，必须被追溯到文档"。

尽管有这项建议，但是直至2010年6月15日贵公司才实施了一个可接受的SOP，旨在确保休斯顿实验室的LC / MS / MS仪器平衡或"预备"有无偏倚和一致的方法。因此，SOP的制定和实施并不能纠正FDA对于2010年6月15日前您的休斯顿实验室所产生数据的关注。

3. 对Cetero休斯顿实验室数据可靠性的关注

如上所述，FDA严重关注自2005年4月1日至2010年6月15日在德克萨斯休斯顿实验室进行的FDA所监管的研究的数据可靠性，理由如下：

（1）在实验室记录中对受试者样品提取的日期和时间的普遍伪造。

（2）为符合预设的可接受标准，进行平衡或"预"分析样品的明显不当行为。

（3）使您不能进行充分的内部调查，以确定该违规行为的程度和影响的关于"预"分析批的文件缺失。

独立第三方调查提出了与FDA相同的关注，并对数据可靠性的总体影响有如下表述：

"色谱图可能是可接受的，QC可能是通过的，且ISR（生物样本再分析）数据（近期的）可能很好，但由于文件记录的不规范，对分析过程基本要素的完整性仍存怀疑。如果实验室的基础错误百出，那么产生的数据也同样如此。调查发现了显然不可接受的操作。最大的关注是他们可能对产生的数据造成的影响。不可能知道不合理的程度或其最终的影响。"

我们提醒您，确保在ANDA或NDA中提交给FDA的、在贵公司生成的所有数据的真实性是贵公司的职责。鉴于与提取记录有关的伪造和“预”分析批操作的范围和恶劣的性质，我们严重质疑自2005年4月至2010年6月15日第2版CET_SOP_04_INS-006实施期间产生的数据可靠性。

本警告信目的并非罗列贵实验室中存在的所有缺陷。您有责任调查和确定上述发现的违规行为的原因。您必须实施适当的纠正措施预防它们再次发生或其他违规情况的发生。

自收到这封信的15个工作日内，您应当书面回复本办公室，并向FDA提交2005年4月1日至2010年6月15日在Cetero休斯顿实验室进行的、与FDA所监管的研究相关的所有研究的清单，以便监管机关评估对提交的用以支持NDA和ANDA的研究的影响。对每一项研究，我们要求您提供药物名称、研究号码，以及申办者名称。

您还应该包括一份针对这封信提到的纠正违规和预防违规情况再次发生正在采取的步骤说明。请提供支持文件的副本。

附：英文原文

Cetero Research

July 26, 2011

Ref:11-HFD-45-07-02

Roger N. Hayes, Ph.D.
President, Bioanalytical
Cetero Research
10550 Rockley Road, Suite 150
Houston, TX 77099

Dear Dr. Hayes:

This letter is to inform you of objectionable conditions observed during the U.S. Food and Drug Administration (FDA) inspections conducted at your bioanalytical facility, located in Houston, Texas, from May 3-7, 2010, by FDA investigators Mr. Patrick D. Stone, Dr. Jacqueline A. O’Shaughnessy, and Dr. Carol M. Rivera-Lopez; and from December 6-10, 2010, by FDA investigators Drs. Albert Peacock, Martin K. Yau, Sam H. Haidar, John Kadavil, and Xikui Chen. FDA investigators have identified significant violations of the bioavailability and bioequivalence requirements of Title 21, Code of Federal Regulations, Part 320. These violations include the widespread falsification of dates and times in laboratory records for subject sample extractions, and the apparent manipulation of equilibration samples to meet pre- determined acceptance criteria.

It is your firm’s responsibility to ensure and confirm the reliability of your testing methods and the bioequivalence and bioavailability data collected by your firm and presented as part of any applications submitted to the FDA. The pervasiveness and egregious nature of the violative practices by your firm has led FDA to have significant concerns that the bioequivalence and bioavailability data generated at the Cetero Houston facility from April 1, 2005, to June 15, 2010, including data relied on as part of studies submitted in both New Drug Applications (NDA) and Abbreviated New Drug Applications (ANDA) to FDA, are unreliable.

As discussed below, FDA has reached this conclusion based on the following: (1) The widespread falsification of dates and times in laboratory records for subject sample extractions; (2) the apparent manipulation of equilibration or “prep” run samples to meet predetermined acceptance criteria; and (3) the lack of documentation regarding equilibration or “prep” runs that prevented you from conducting an adequate internal investigation to determine the extent and impact of these violations.

The FDA inspections included a review of various portions of the following studies:

May 2010 Inspection

- Study (b)(4) ((b)(4)), sponsored by(b)(4).
- Study (b)(4) ((b)(4)), sponsored by(b)(4).
- Study (b)(4) ((b)(4)), sponsored by(b)(4).
- Study (b)(4) ((b)(4)), sponsored by(b)(4).
- Study (b)(4) ((b)(4)), sponsored by(b)(4).

December 2010 Inspection

- Study (b)(4) ((b)(4)), sponsored by(b)(4).
- Study (b)(4) ((b)(4)), sponsored by(b)(4).
- Study (b)(4) ((b)(4)), sponsored by(b)(4).
- Study (b)(4) ((b)(4)), sponsored by(b)(4).

These inspections are part of FDA's Bioresearch Monitoring (BIMO) Program, which includes inspections to evaluate the conduct of research, to confirm that data intended for submission to FDA are reliable as a basis for FDA approval and regulatory decisions, and to verify compliance with the bioavailability and bioequivalence requirements in 21 CFR Part 320.

In a letter dated April 22, 2009, one of your employees (the complainant) brought formal allegations of regulatory violations and other misconduct to your firm's attention. In this letter, it was noted that as early as June 2007, the complainant "first raised certain issues in a supervisor's meeting in which the former CEO ... attended. During such meeting, [the complainant] identified numerous Cetero Standard Operating Procedures that were not being followed within the lab by many of the chemists. The complainant was aware that many of the chemists were manipulating and falsifying data associated with the samples being used within various projects."

After receipt of the April 22, 2009 letter from the complainant, your firm subsequently initiated an internal investigation regarding the complainant's claims, as detailed in a report titled "Internal Investigation for Data Integrity Concerns Received April 22, 2009," dated June 5, 2009. On June 5, 2009, the complainant notified the FDA Dallas District Office regarding concerns about laboratory misconduct at your Houston facility. Your firm contacted the FDA Dallas District Office on June 10, 2009, to inform FDA of the allegations, as well as to present the outcome of the internal investigation conducted by your firm. Further, your firm sought an independent third party investigation and review of the allegations that was completed July 6, 2009. In addition, your firm updated your internal investigation in a report titled "July 27, 2009 Internal Investigation Update for Data Integrity Concerns Received April 22, 2009." We acknowledge receipt of the two reports of your firm's internal investigation and the report from the third party investigation.

Both the FDA inspections of your facility in May 2010 and December 2010 and the third party investigation in July 2009 identified numerous concerns regarding procedures at your facility, as well as deficiencies with your internal investigation. At the close of the May 2010 inspection, your firm was issued a Form FDA 483, and we acknowledge receipt of your firm's response, dated May 24, 2010 [hereafter referred to as May 24, 2010 483 response letter]. Despite the proposed corrective actions in your letter, FDA found continued deficiencies at your facility during the December 2010 inspection, and another Form FDA 483 was issued on December 10, 2010. We acknowledge the receipt of your December 29, 2010 response to the second Form FDA 483 [hereafter referred to as December 29, 2010 483 response letter]. However, as detailed below, your 483 response letters do not adequately address the violations which FDA discovered during its inspections.

FDA noted the following violations at your facility:

Your firm failed to demonstrate that the analytical method used in an in vivo bioavailability or bioequivalence study to measure the concentration of the active drug ingredient or therapeutic moiety, or its active metabolite(s), in body fluids or excretory products, is accurate and of sufficient sensitivity to measure, with appropriate precision, the actual concentration of the active drug ingredient or therapeutic moiety, or its active metabolite(s), achieved in the body [21 C.F.R. § 320.29(a)].

Examples include, but are not limited to, the following:

1. Instances of misconduct

a. Falsified laboratory records

FDA notes that your internal investigation identified problems related to falsified employee time/date records. You reported these issues to FDA on July 28, 2009. During the course of its inspections in May 2010 and December 2010, FDA also discovered inconsistent and/or falsified Analytical Procedure (AP) raw data sheets for several studies with respect to the times and dates of subject sample extractions.

The following are two examples of such studies:

- Study (b)(4): Analytical Runs 5 and 6 for (b)(4) and analytical Run 4 for (b)(4).
- Study (b)(4): Analytical Runs 11 through 16 for (b)(4) and Runs 13, 14, 17, and 18 for (b)(4)

In your May 24, 2010 483 response letter, you concurred with FDA's observation that the falsifications involve data from multiple studies for multiple sponsors.

As detailed below, your 483 response letters, as well as your internal investigation and the third party investigation, were inadequate to address FDA's concerns regarding the falsified laboratory records.

(1)The scope of your internal investigation was insufficient.

The scope of your internal investigation was limited to only the date/time falsifications on the AP sheets, instead of overall study conduct and other data recorded on the AP sheets; therefore, your firm has failed to determine whether other aspects of the laboratory records might be compromised. The true extent of these falsifications is thus unknown. According to your internal investigation, electronic records of key card building entry times demonstrated approximately 1900 instances of blood/plasma samples allegedly extracted on weekends and holidays between April 15, 2005, and June 30, 2009, where the arrival times of laboratory chemists were greater than one hour after the documented start time of the sample extraction. In addition, there were approximately 875 instances where the laboratory chemists were not present in the facility at the documented sample extraction date.

In your responses to the Forms FDA 483 issued at the close of both the May 2010 and December 2010 inspections, your firm stated that chemists extracted study samples on Fridays or the day before a holiday, and documented the work as completed on the weekend or a holiday to receive financial incentives. Your firm also stated that your investigation determined that falsification of laboratory records was limited to changes to time and date of extractions.

As a result of your stated assumption that laboratory records were falsified due to chemists' incentive to receive increased compensation without the appearance of having done all the work on a single day, your firm focused initially on the weekend extraction records, and you failed to consider whether any weekday extraction records were falsified. Following the May 2010 inspection, your firm decided to investigate further, and you found that employees falsified timecards and laboratory records on both weekends and weekdays.

You stated the following in your May 24, 2010 483 response letter:

"As the reasons for the modifications to the AP were linked to the financial incentive issue ... there was no reason to doubt the validity of any other sections of the AP."

However, you have not provided an explanation regarding why employees would have falsified the dates and times on weekday records, as there was no financial incentive for them to do so. Further, FDA disagrees both with your proposed theory that modifications of the AP sheets were linked to financial incentives for weekend extractions, and with your assertion that there was no reason to doubt the validity of other sections of the AP sheets. Your firm has not provided any documentation to support these claims, or explained how you verified the overall reliability of your laboratory records.

(2) You failed to provide evidence for your assertion that Quality Assurance (QA) activities at your firm limited the scope of the falsification to the time and date of sample extractions.

You stated in your May 24, 2010 483 response that pre-study activities (e.g., weighing of reference standards, preparation of stock and spiking solutions, and preparation of bulk QCs) were reviewed 100% by the Quality Control/Documentation staff. In addition, you stated that all pre-study activities and 20% of the subject runs were audited by Quality Assurance (QA) staff. You claimed that these routine reviews assured the integrity of pre-study events, and by extension, verified that the alterations in laboratory records were limited to time and date of extractions. However, FDA notes that despite these audits of study runs, your QA department did not uncover the frequent alterations in laboratory records that occurred over a four-year period, from April 1, 2005 to June 15, 2009, when your firm conducted an internal investigation. These problems indicate that routine audits conducted by your QA department have been insufficient to verify or assess the reliability of your laboratory records.

You stated the following in your May 24, 2010 483 response letter: "It is our strong belief that the reported concentration data for each of these affected studies was not compromised as only the date and time of extraction was uncertain in the extraction steps involved." You also stated in your December 29, 2010 483 response letter: " we conducted an extremely broad and thorough investigation.... As a result, we are confident that the integrity of the data generated by research chemists implicated in the day/date fraud was not affected or otherwise undermined."

FDA does not agree with the above statements in your 483 response letters. The narrow scope of your internal investigation of the falsification of laboratory records, the lack of a consistent and credible explanation for the time and date discrepancies in timecards and sample extractions, and the failure of your QA procedures to detect the falsification, call into question the validity of all of the information documented on your AP sheets, including study results that were used as the basis for NDAs and ANDAs submitted to FDA.

In addition, the July 6, 2009 report from the independent third party investigation stated that " [t]here appears to be evidence of misconduct among lab staff that has occurred for at least several years and continued until at least April of this year. Laboratory supervisors appear to have been involved. This misconduct appears to be significant enough to cast doubt on the data generated." Your responses have not adequately addressed these concerns raised in the third party investigation report.

The fabrication of any portion of a laboratory record casts doubt upon the reliability of the remaining portions. You failed to support your contention that fabrications of laboratory records were limited to time and date of extractions. The extensive use of falsified laboratory records by your firm has led the FDA to question the validity of all bioanalytical data collected by your facility during the period from April 1, 2005 to June 15, 2010.

b. Manipulation of Samples

FDA has determined that your firm manipulated test samples in order to meet pre- determined acceptance criteria.

According to the original complaint, equilibration or "prep" runs were allegedly used to manipulate data by "fixing" runs to meet acceptance criteria prior to inclusion of data in the official study folder.

The original complaint submitted to FDA described several examples of this practice. In one example, the complainant submitted photographs that showed that Run 38 for Study (b)(4), which was injected on January 3, 2009, failed as a result of lacking the internal standard (i.e., internal standard was not initially added to the calibration standards and quality control samples, as is standard practice). According to the notation evident in the photograph, the Run 38 samples were to be put back in the refrigerator following the failed run. The next day, the Run 38 samples were injected onto the LC/MS/MS (Liquid Chromatography with Tandem Mass Spectrometry) system, and internal standard was now present in the calibration standards and quality control samples. Your firm's records do not explain this discrepancy, nor do they document that internal standard was added to the sample before it was reanalyzed on January 4.

As stated by the third party investigation dated July 6, 2009, " it would appear the standard curve and quality controls were substituted from another run." Quality control samples provide assurance of the accuracy and precision of the drug concentrations in subject samples. Substituting quality control samples from another run to meet acceptance criteria is not appropriate, as the drug concentration of subject samples cannot be ensured.

Your firm's internal investigation initially failed to identify any misconduct related to Run 38, despite the complainant's allegations. It was not until after the complainant provided photographic and other evidence, and the third party audit found that "the allegation appears to have merit," that your firm acknowledged to FDA in the update to the internal investigation that "it is reasonable to assume that inappropriate activities surrounding run 38 standard curve and quality control samples occurred." Your failure to recognize the improper procedures regarding Run 38 calls into question the other conclusions in your internal investigation.

2. Improper use of equilibration samples

Accurate measurement of the concentration of the active drug or active moiety is dependent on a properly validated analytical method, including calibration and equilibration of the instrument used to perform the testing. The use of the following types of samples for equilibration of LC/MS/MS instruments is not recommended:

- Subject samples that have not yet been analyzed, and
- Calibration standards, quality controls (QCs), and blanks that are part of the official run.

The third party investigation report dated July 6, 2009 states: "If an instrument requires conditioning, only samples prepared specifically for this purpose should be used and these samples should not be part of the standards or controls for the run. There must be no manner in which these samples could be substituted for the standards and controls in another run."

Based on the information provided by your firm and the report of the third party investigation contracted by your firm, your firm's method of equilibrating LC/MS/MS instruments consisted of using samples such as calibration standards, quality controls, blanks, and subject samples that were part of the current run and not yet analyzed.

FDA is concerned that the use of extracted samples not yet analyzed for system equilibration can provide opportunities for chemists to manipulate the outcome of the official study run. A chemist would have an opportunity to determine whether the "prep" run calibration standards and quality control samples would pass or fail acceptance criteria prior to analyzing these samples as an official study run, thus creating an opportunity for manipulation of the study run, either by adding study drug or internal standard to the sample, or by substituting the sample with other samples that had previously passed.

Your May 2010 and December 2010 483 response letters, as well as your internal investigation and third party investigation, were inadequate to address FDA's concerns regarding the improper use of equilibration samples, as detailed below.

(a) The explanation you provided for this practice in your May 24, 2010 483 response letter lacks credibility.

You claim that the purpose of an equilibration or "prep" run is to condition the system and perform any necessary troubleshooting prior to starting the subject sample run. However, this contention fails to provide an explanation for Run 20 of Study (b)(4), evaluated during FDA's May 2010 inspection. In Run 20, the "prep" run was performed on system 95, and the actual run was performed on system 74. If the practice of "prep" runs was indeed to equilibrate and to ensure optimal performance of the LC/MS/MS System, then the same equilibrated instrument must be used.

(b) Your internal investigation regarding "prep" runs was inadequate.

Cetero's internal investigation, including the third party investigation, has not reduced FDA's concerns about the reliability of data generated by your firm between April 1, 2005 and June 15, 2010. The lack of sufficient documentation and SOPs regarding the use of "prep" runs at your firm precluded your ability to conduct an adequate investigation to respond to the Forms FDA 483 issued during the May 2010 and December 2010 inspections.

Your firm instituted an investigation plan titled "Cetero Research Houston Facility Investigation Plan Revision 1," dated July 28, 2009, to address the complainant's allegation that runs were injected multiple times in order to obtain a passing result and that samples were somehow "fixed" in order to pass. The internal investigation evaluated approximately (b)(4) samples from your unofficial electronic "prep" run files conducted for approximately studies (b)(4) between the period of April 2005 and June 2009. The investigation identified three additional runs with misconduct similar to Run 38 of Study (b)(4), as described above.

The "Prepping Runs Decision Tree" in your internal investigation plan was intended to address the allegation by the complainant that samples were "fixed." According to the decision tree, Cetero would evaluate whether there was an internal standard or drug response for all samples, whether all calibration standards and quality control samples had drug peaks, and whether blanks had acceptable responses. Your analysis included the assumption that the "prep" run samples were the same as those subsequently injected on the official study run. FDA does not accept this assumption as the basis for making determinations about the prep runs, because you lack documentation of the identity of samples used in the "prep" runs conducted by your firm.

The only part of your internal investigation that does not rely on sample identity is the evaluation of whether there was an internal standard or drug response for all samples. As a result, your internal investigation was more limited than planned, because it was only able to focus on "prep" runs with results that could not be explained scientifically (i.e., samples in which the drug or internal standard was initially absent but appeared in subsequent injections on the official run). The investigation was not able to evaluate whether calibrators, quality control samples, or blanks may have been spiked with drug or substituted with other samples. Further, your internal investigation could not evaluate how the prep runs were used, what was injected, and how they may have impacted the study results.

FDA's May 2010 and December 2010 inspections revealed the fundamental lack of documentation regarding the prep runs, and as such, it became apparent that your firm's internal investigation was insufficient to thoroughly address the allegations regarding "prep" runs. Your investigation failed to demonstrate that the use of "prep" runs did not impact the study data integrity for the period of time analyzed. The lack of documentation inhibited your ability to adequately address the actual identity of the samples used, the varying number (4 to 43) of sample injections between "prep" runs, and whether the "prep" run results were used to alter the results of the official run. This is consistent with the findings from the independent third party investigation report dated July 6, 2009, which noted that " [t]he 'prep' data was not always stored in the study folder and there was no documentation of what changes may have been made during the prepping process to the instrument or samples. Nor was there documentation of why samples were injected multiple times. This process may be seen as testing into compliance since the samples were injected until a passing result was obtained and then the run was formally injected."

In your December 29, 2010 483 response letter, you stated that chemists were "blinded" to the identity of equilibration samples to limit the possibility of misconduct, and that documentation describing the source and identity of equilibration samples was not obtained. FDA does not find this explanation credible, as you provide no evidence to demonstrate that the chemists were blinded to the identity of the samples injected in the "prep" runs. In addition, as discussed below, you had no SOPs regarding this procedure.

The lack of documentation regarding "prep" runs prevents your firm from undertaking a thorough internal investigation and determining the impact of your "prep" run practices. The lack of documentation also prevents the Agency from undertaking an informed evaluation of your actual testing practices. As a result, we are unable to support the conclusion of your internal investigation that the use of "prep" runs had no impact on the data integrity of studies conducted at your facility.

(c) Your firm lacked SOPs for equilibration of LC/MS/MS instruments.

In your May 24, 2010 483 response, you acknowledge that the historical practice of conditioning LC/MS/MS instruments at your facility was to utilize a subset of samples that were to be analyzed on the current run. As noted above, the complainant sent a letter to Cetero on April 22, 2009. In May 2009, Cetero management provided instructions to immediately stop the practice of using samples not yet analyzed to condition/equilibrate the LC/MS/MS instrument, and to use only previously analyzed samples for conditioning/equilibration purposes. However, your firm did not implement written guidance on conditioning LC/MS/MS instruments until December 14, 2009 (CET_SOP_04_INS-006, Equilibration of LC/MS/MS, Version 1). This SOP stated that a pooled sample of previously injected calibration standards, quality controls samples, and subject samples should be used to equilibrate LC/MS/MS instruments. FDA notes that this first version of the SOP did not require documentation of the identification and source of equilibration samples, and therefore, it was not acceptable.

The third party independent investigation report dated July 6, 2009 provided the following recommendation regarding the use of "prep" runs and equilibration of LC/MS/MS instruments: "The practice of "prepping" using standards and controls for any run should be discontinued immediately. If an instrument requires conditioning, only samples prepared specifically for this purpose should be used and these samples should not be part of the standards or controls for the run. There must be no manner in which these samples could be substituted for the standards and controls in another run. Every injection made, every sample prepared and every action taken from the initiation of a study should be documented. Data should only be acquired in the official study folder and it must be traceable to the documentation."

Despite this recommendation, it was not until June 15, 2010 that your firm implemented an acceptable SOP designed to ensure an unbiased and consistent approach to equilibrate or "prep" LC/MS/MS instruments at your Houston facility. Therefore, the development and implementation of your SOP does not remedy FDA's concerns about the data generated at your Houston facility prior to June 15, 2010.

3. Concerns about data reliability at Cetero Houston

As discussed above, FDA has significant concerns that all data relevant to FDA-regulated research conducted at your Houston, Texas, facility from April 1, 2005 to June 15, 2010 are unreliable, based on the following reasons:

(1) The widespread falsification of dates and times in laboratory records for subject sample extractions,

(2) The apparent manipulation of equilibration or "prep" run samples to meet predetermined acceptance criteria, and

(3) The lack of documentation regarding "prep" runs that prevented you from conducting an adequate internal investigation to determine the extent and impact of these violations.

The independent third party investigation shared FDA's concerns, and stated the following with respect to the general impact on data reliability:

"[C]hromatography may have been acceptable, QCs may have passed and ISR [Incurred Sample Reanalysis] data (recent) may be very good, but doubt remains regarding the integrity of the basic elements of the analytical process due to the documentation irregularities. If the foundation of the laboratory is corrupt, then the data generated will be also. The investigation has uncovered practices that are clearly unacceptable. The major concern is the impact they may have had on the data generated. It is not possible to know the extent of the improprieties or their ultimate impact."

We remind you that it is your firm's responsibility to ensure the integrity of all data generated at your firm that is submitted to the FDA in ANDAs or NDAs. Given the scope and the egregious nature of both the fabrications associated with your extraction records and the practice of "prep" runs, we have significant concerns that the data generated between April 2005 and the implementation of CET_SOP_04_INS-006, Version 2, on June 15, 2010, are unreliable.

The violations cited in this letter are not intended to be an all-inclusive statement of violations that exist at your facility. You are responsible for investigating and determining the causes of the violations identified above. You must also implement appropriate corrective actions for preventing their recurrence and the occurrence of other violations.

Within fifteen working days of receipt of this letter, please respond in writing and provide FDA with a list of all studies conducted at Cetero Houston between April 1, 2005 and June 15, 2010 that are relevant to FDA-regulated research, so that the Agency can asscss the impact of studies submitted in support of NDAs and ANDAs. For each study, we request that you provide the drug name, the study number, and the name of the sponsor.

You should also include an explanation of steps being taken to both correct the violations noted in this letter and to prevent the recurrence of violations. Please provide copies of supporting documentation.

If you have any questions or wish to meet with the office of Scientific Investigations, please contact Sam H. Haidar, PH.D.,R.Ph., at 33017963150. Your written response and any pertinent documentation should be addressed to:

Sam H. Haidar, Ph.D., R.Ph.
Chief, Bioequivalence Investigations Branch
Office of Scientific Investigations
Office of Compliance
Center for Drug Evaluation and Research
U.S. Food and Drug Administration
10903 New Hampshire Avenue
Building 51, Room 5210
Silver Spring, MD 20993

Sincerely yours,

{See appended electronic signature page}

Leslie K. Ball, M.D.
Director (Acting)
Office of Scientific Investigations
Office of Compliance
Center for Drug Evaluation and Research
U.S. Food and Drug Administration

第45封　给ICON临床研究有限公司的警告信

2009年11月27日

参考号：10-HFD-45-11-04

尊敬的Hubbard博士：

FDA对ICON临床研究有限公司（以下简称ICON）受（b）（4）委托，作为合同研究组织（CRO）为试验药物（b）（4）的方案编号（b）（4）的临床研究提供的临床研究管理服务进行了现场检查。这封警告信特告知您在此次FDA检查中发现的违规情况。

本次现场检查是FDA的生物研究监查项目的一部分。该项目通过设定的检查方法，评估研究的实施情况，以确保这些研究中受试者的权利、安全和福利得到了保护。该项目的另外一个目的是为了确保提交用于新药申请的数据在科学上是有效和准确的。

第一个临床研究，（b）（4）是由原持有人（b）（4）发起。2005年2月2日，（b）（4）与另一家公司（b）（4）建立了全球伙伴关系，共同进行（b）（4）的研发和上市。根据协议上的条款规定，（b）（4）将由（b）（4）进一步开发，（b）（4）临床试验的所有权利及责任均转移到（b）（4）。值得注意的是，在（b）（4）的转移开发中，ICON与（b）（4）之间所有的临床试验监查协议仍然有效［包括那些在（b）（4）的］。第二个研究，（b）（4）由（b）（4）发起，同样通过合同由ICON为其提供临床试验管理服务。

2007年5月18日，（b）（4）将从（b）（4）和（b）（4）收集的数据提交给FDA，用于支持（b）（4）治疗（b）（4）适应症的审批。在后续对参与这些方案的临床研究者进行的数据有效性检查中，发现了重大的违背FDA法规21 CFR312的情况。

FDA于2008年5月26日至2008年6月12日期间对（b）（4）进行了现场检查。根据（b）（4）与ICON的合同规定，（b）（4）将以下与试验场所监查相关的任务明确地转移给了ICON：

- 根据项目，制定并撰写特定的监查计划；
- 根据监查计划，安排并执行试验场所的现场监查；
- 根据试验及监查计划，安排并进行电话随访；
- 撰写监查访视报告，包括跟进函、电话随访等；
- 通知申办者有关试验场所的任何重要的问题（例如违反GCPP情况、在现场发现的违规的动向）以及提供解决问题的建议计划；
- 每周召开电话会议，审查试验场所监查安排、场所状态以及沟通计划等；
- 提供现场监查、电话随访、监查访视报告以及方案违背进行跟踪。

ICON允诺进行试验现场启动访视、中期盲态/非盲态的监查访视、试验结束访视。对于每一次中期的监查访视，ICON人员允诺："检查病例报告的完整性，对所有数据进行100%原始数据的验证，核实知情同意书的签署，确保正确的AE报告，检查记录的保存、物资供应的充足性以及确保药物保存适当管理"。ICON还允诺"确保试验点依据试验方案及相关法规开展试验，试验人员积极地进行试验研究"，并允诺"将通过给试验场所发送跟进函详细告知发现的不依从情况以及随后将采取的纠正措施。"

在2008年5月26日至2008年6月12日FDA的检查期间，FDA获得了ICON的监查记录，这些记录是ICON在结束临床管理服务时提供给（b）（4）的研究监查记录。

法规允许申办者转移责任至合同研究组织［21 CFR 312.52（a）］，并描述了责任转移后合同研究组织需承担的职责［21 CFR 312.52（b）］。具体来说，当合同研究组织承担申办者的职责时，如未能遵守法规312

部分所规定的责任义务，将受到与申办者同样的监管处罚。根据我们对（b）（4）现场检查报告、该报告的附件、（b）（4）于2008年6月24日对FDA483表作出的书面回复以及2008年9月2日和2008年9月4日对FDA要求的附加信息回复进行的审查，我们的结论是：您没有遵循适用的法律要求和监管临床研究的FDA法规。我们想强调以下几点：

1. 未能确保对临床研究进行适当的监查［21 CFR 312.50和312.56（a）］

FDA法规要求，申办者或者受委托承担申办者责任的合同研究组织需确保对临床研究进行适当的监查。我们调查发现，ICON没有做到确保对上述涉及方案进行适当的监查。监查不足导致了参与上述研究的临床研究人员对病史及药物责任的记录保存存在缺陷。违规行为包括但不限于如下。

a. 病史缺陷

ⅰ. 研究监查员未能发现研究人员在不同场合所记录的不同受试者的给药时间竟完全一致。例如：

a）对于试验场所520的（b）（4）研究，研究监查员未能发现研究协调员在不同场合所记录的2个受试者的给药时间完全一致。根据申办者对试验场所2005年4月27日的审查，以及“门诊患者治疗规范”计划试验场所520被允许从2005年4月27日起开始重新入组受试者。门诊受试者治疗规范计划于2005年4月27日开始执行。门诊受试者治疗规范要求，受试者在试验场所指定的注射中心接受研究药物的首次剂量注射，余下的剂量可以由护士或家庭护理护士在受试者家中注射。根据这些流程，研究监查员应当能够发现在多个场合、作为门诊受试者的受试者，研究协调员记录两个受试者的给药时间一致，研究监查员应要求对这些情况做出解释。具体如下：

ⅰ）记录显示，研究协调员（b）（6）同一天、同一时间给下列受试者使用了研究用药。

（a）2005年7月2日，受试者1266在9:00~10:00及受试者1267在9:00~10:00。

（b）2005年7月3日，受试者1266在9:00~10: 15及受试者1267在9:00~10:15。

（c）2005年7月5日，受试者1266在21:00~22:00及受试者1267在21:00~22:00。

（d）2005年7月6日，受试者1266在21:00~22:00及受试者1267在21:00~22:00。

（e）2005年7月7日，受试者1266在9:00~10:00及受试者1267在9:00~10:15。

ⅱ）记录显示，研究协调员（b）（6）于在2005年7月26日10:00~11:00给受试者2273使用了药物治疗，于10:00~11:00也给受试者2275使用了研究协调员（b）（6）给予的药物治疗。

鉴于试验场所针对门诊受试者进行个体的治疗计划和研究监查，研究监查员应当能够注意到在多次情况下，研究场所的人员记录了不同受试者在同一天完全相同时间接受了试验药物，并应进一步对这一不寻常的现象进行原因的分析调查。而且，基于FDA的现场检查，我们发现，有参加研究的受试者在2005年4月27日仍继续在自己家中自行使用研究药物，而此时该研究场所的研究计划已经执行完毕。此外，即使两个受试者被安排在同一试验场所接受治疗，同一个研究协调员在完全一样的时间内对多个受试者进行研究药物注射也是不可能的。

b）对于试验场所063的（b）（4）研究，研究监查员未能发现，在多个场合“Planilla de estabilidad”被记录了完全相同的时间内给多名受试者使用了研究药物。具体如下：

ⅰ）5月20日，记录了研究护士（b）（6）于8:00~10:00对如下受试者进行药物治疗：

（a）受试者140616［（b）（6）］。

（b）受试者140132［（b）（6）］。

（c）受试者140617［（b）（6）］。

（d）受试者140118［（b）（6）］。

ⅱ）5月20日，记录了同一个研究护士（b）（6）于10:00~11:00对如下受试者开始了安慰剂注射：

（a）受试者140616［（b）（6）］。

（b）受试者140132［（b）（6）］。

（c）受试者140617［（b）（6）］。

（d）受试者140118［（b）（6）］。

研究监查员应当意识到在多个场合、同一个人被记录在完全相同的时间给不同受试者进行药物治疗的情况，并且研究监管实施对这种非正常现象作进一步的原因分析与调查。

ⅱ. 根据ICON监查报告，对于在试验场所551参加试验方案（b）（4）的受试者141050完成了100%原始记录验证。然而，研究监查员没有发现，对这名受试者第8天访视的原始记录和病例报告未能遵循方案要求记录体检、伤情评估或总体临床评估信息。

ⅲ. 临床监查员未能发现试验方案（b）（4）和试验方案（b）（4）两个方案中注射药物送到护理中心的时间没有记录。例如：

a）在试验场所502，根据（b）（4）工作表，受试者1118，至少有4次，配制好的研究药物送到护理中心的时间没有记录。

b）在试验场所508，根据（b）（4）工作表，受试者140005，至少有7次，配制好的研究药物送到护理中心的时间没有记录。

ⅳ. 对于试验场所509的（b）（4）方案，临床监查员未能确保对配制好的研究药物输液剂进行适当储存。试验方案（b）（4）中规定，输液剂应当在常温下（25°C）保存，并且在6小时内使用，在冷藏室（5°C）可以储存达16小时，或是从冷藏库中取出后须在3小时内使用。由于方案并未指出门诊受试者剂量协定，研究监查员为了寻求保证，在2004年10月20日给试验场所509的邮件中要求有记录显示研究药物在受试者家中的保存方法和保存温度是适当的。尽管被ICON的监查员这样要求，但研究中心的人员从来没有提及在受试者家中如何记录储存温度，他们只提出如何记录受试者的体温。研究监查员没有发现试验场所的回复是不完整的，而是将此作为完整回复接受了。之后，试验中心设计并使用的受试者日记上也没有试验可以记录研究药物在受试者的冰箱内储存温度的地方。所以，无法确认这些药物的储存温度是否遵循方案中规定的药物储存条件。2005年5月25日的“（b）（4）门诊患者治疗规范”第三页可证明在受试者家里药物储存温度条件的重要性，它指出研究场所一旦收到研究药物，必须及时确认储存条件。诊所、研究者办公室和/或受试者家储存药物的冰箱温度必须记录下来，并且在计划中需说明储存地点及由谁储存。

ⅴ. 对于试验场所520的（b）（4）方案，临床监查员未能记录该试验场所发生超温读数，且未能就特殊运输的药包的使用给研究场所提供适当的跟进指导。从（b）（4）运输的药品包含了“冷藏装运检验说明”，要求填写包装列表的底部温度记录设备显示的读数，以及如果设备显示屏上显示了一个“警钟”的符号，则意味着该运输温度保持不当，需要将此设备运回（b）（4)。如果没有“警钟”显示，表示运输温度恰当，运输的药品可以使用。2005年4月4日送至试验场所520用于试验方案（b）（4）的编号为1000739的包裹，其底部单子上显示了温度记录超出范围；但是没有任何文档记录显示温度记录设备被返还，或者对超温运输的药品是否可被接受使用有跟进。原始记录显示，这次运输药品已经于2005年4月至6月分发给受试者并已使用。非盲态监查访视报告（2005年5月25日）包含了接受这一批运次药品的时间段内对试验场所520所进行的监查，但监查报告没有记录超温情况，也没有向研究场所提供有关这批药品使用的适当跟进指导。

基于可以取得的那段时间的文件记录，非盲态的临床研究监查员应当发现到订单号1000739中的药包原本不应该分发给受试者。

ⅵ. 对于试验场所146的试验方案（b）（4），所有入组的39名受试者的“Ⅳ稳定性”表格全部缺失，并且研究监查员所采取的纠正措施不足以纠正整个研究中在这方面的缺陷。根据此研究的工作规则，ICON的非盲态监查员应当每10周来访视一次。这个问题在2006年1月27日和2006年9月25日的非盲态监查访视报告中有所记录。此外，监查员要求试验中心人员需填写这些工作表格，并且要求试验中心应制作一份备忘录文件，用于记录之前入组的受试者的Ⅳ温度稳定性情况。然而，这个问题本应该在2006年9月25日非盲态监查前就被解决好。最后在2006年11月16日备忘录文件才被写出来，这时，该试验场所已经完成受试者入组，只是说“已根据Ⅳ标示维持Ⅳ稳定性，标示只包括注射的开始／结束时间及有效期（原文如此），受试者编号”。该说明没有提供足够的细节用于确保药品保存的温度稳定性。

ⅶ. 对于试验中心520的试验方案（b）（4），研究监查员未能发现研究药物发往护理中心的时间与（b）（4）工作表中记录的不一致；而给药时间也与多名受试者“研究药物注射”表格上记录的时间不一致。例如：

a）受试者1187的原始记录指出：

ⅰ）2005年3月1日，研究药物发出时间为19:05，而研究药物的用药时间记录为 18:00~19:00。

ⅱ）2005年3月2日，研究药物发出时间为19:10，而研究药物的用药时间记录为 18:00~19:00。

ⅲ）在2005年3月1日，研究药物发出时间为18:05，而研究药物的用药时间记录为 18:00~19:00。

ⅳ）2005年3月12日，研究药物发出时间为18:45，而研究药物的用药时间记录为 18:00~19:00。

b）受试者1195的原始记录指出：

2005年4月14日，研究药物发出时间为9:00，研究药物的用药时间记录为 8:05~9:05。

c）受试者2671'的原始记录指出：

ⅰ）2005年5月11日，研究药物发出时间为10:00，研究药物的用药时间记录为 9:30~10:30。

ⅱ）2005年5月12日，研究药物发出时间为9:55，研究药物的用药时间记录为 9:30~10:30。

ⅲ）2005年5月13日，研究药物发出时间为9:50，研究药物的用药时间记录为 9:30~10:30。

ⅳ）对于试验方案（b）（4），研究监查员未能发现与观察和研究数据相关的记录不符。例如：

对于试验场所520的试验方案（b）（4），原始记录与研究记录在创口尺寸、创口清创术以及对个受试者注射的标记和符号的信息上存在矛盾。但监查员未能发现这些矛盾的信息。例如：

a）对于受试者1010，根据基线访视的原始记录，创口2被记录作为满足研究纳入资格的创口。而在2005年3月22日，助理研究者的门诊创口治疗的病程记录中，记录了创口尺寸为10mm×4mm，并指出该创口会对清创术非常敏感，但是一份2005年3月23日的创口护理原始文件则记录了该研究创口已于2005年3月22日完成清创，其尺寸大小为25mm×30mm。我们同时注意到，在这份2005年3月23日的“治愈测试临床评估”的原始记录4页中的第二页，助理研究者签的名字缩写和签署的时间为2005年3月5日，这比原始文件注明的访视日期提前了18天。

b）受试者1186，助理研究者于2005年3月7日病程记录中陈述，创口大小为21mm×25mm，而2005年3月7日访视的研究原始文件工作表中记录的创口大小为17mm×15mm，但是在2005年4月18日，这些创口大小数字被线划掉而且更改为21mm×25mm。由于这些原始记录已经注明“已经根据MD完成创口评估及报告至合同研究组织”，不清楚为什么这些创口大小的原始记录与助理研究者病程记录中的大小不一致。与之类似的，2005年3月14日助理研究者的病程记录中记录了创口大小为23mm×29mm。而原始文件创口大小为15mm×10mm，而于2005年4月18日，原始文件报告中的创口大小被划掉更改为23mm×29mm。此外，2005年3月21日助理研究者病程记录中记录创口大小为14mm×23mm，但当天原始文件的2/4页的原始记录为8mm×6mm，在2004年4月18日，原始文件上首次记录的大小被划改为14mm×23mm，但是在2005年4月18日相应的病例报告表页面中关于此创口大小记录为8mm×6mm。另外，2007年3月14日，助理研究者的进展记录“炎症消退，几乎无流液”，而此访视日期的原始文件记录则为流液或浓液处为“无”和红肿处为“无”。

c）对于受试者2274，标注日期为2005年7月26日关于治疗结束访视的原始文件中记录了创口大小为13mm×20mm，创口评估为“未见红肿（原文如此）、疼痛、水肿、发热、胃肠气胀（原文如此）、肝功能损伤及渗水”，但在同一原始文件的另一页则记录为创口大小1mm×0mm，渗水经检查为渗水“改善”，而疼痛或触诊疼痛经诊断为“没有变化”。而相应的治疗结束访视的病例报告表则记录创口大小为80mm×95mm。

b. 药品管理的缺陷

对于试验场所551的试验方案（b）（4），监查员未能发现研究文档中关于药品管理的矛盾信息。拿（b）（4）和药品管理方面的原始工作记录表进行对比，显示在多个场合下，同一支药剂被记录注射给了多个受试者，或/和不止一次地注射给了同一个受试者；或者是试剂瓶的记录的信息不完整。举例包括但不限于如下：

(b) (4) 工作日志 (药物编号) (日期) (受试者编号#)	药物清点表 日志 (药物编号) (日期) (受试者编号#)
21148-8 2006-8-1 #141059	21148-8 2006-7-30 #141052
21148-1 2006-8-1 #141059	21148-1 2006-8-2 #141052
22609-2 2006-8-2 #141059	22609-2 2006-7-27 #141052
10131-8 2006-8-5 #141059	10131-8 2006-8-3 #141059
60126-1 2006-8-3 #141062	60126-1 2006-8-2 #141059
60126-18 2006-8-3 #141062	60126-18 2006-8-8 #141062
60126-7 2006-8-7和2006-8-8 #141062	60126-7 2006-8-4 #141062
23631-15 2006-8-11 #141066	23631-15 2006-8-8 #141066
23631-8 2006-8-11 #141066	23631-8 2006-8-8 #141066
23110-18 2006-8-14 #141067	23110-18 药品未发放
23110-4 2006-8-14 #141067	23110-4 药品未发放

尽管事实是每一单独的小瓶包装是一位受试者一次的用量，但记录显示被使用多次，研究监查员未能发现存在的这些问题。

2. 未能确保按照IND中规定的总体研究计划和方案进行临床研究［21 CFR 312.50］

a. 研究监查员未能确保研究（b）（4）按照研究计划开展。例如：

ⅰ. 在试验场所063，对于研究（b）（4），研究监查员未能确保受试者依据方案接受研究药物。根据临床试验方案（b）（4）评估安排表的脚注1），"所有的筛选／初始剂量评估都将作为基线，且必须在随机化和第一天给药之前完成并进行审查，PK样品收集除外"。基于此说明以及提供给临床研究人员的培训及其他材料，所有受试者应该在随机化当天就开始用药。然而对于在试验场所063的试验方案（b）（4），45个受试者中的9位受试者在随机化超过24小时后还没有被给予试验药物，时间范围为随机化后48小时到11天。例如，受试者140117在2016年5月8日随机，但收到第一次剂量的时间为2006年5月16日。根据2006年9月6日的非盲态监查访视报告，延迟是因为"受试者的个人问题"。这在监查访视后给到非盲态试验场所人员的信函中记录为微小问题，在监查访视后给临床研究者的信中根本没有提及。此外，在监查报告以及发给试验场所063的跟进信中也没有纠正措施记录。

如果事实上9名受试者患有复杂的皮肤和皮肤组织感染，延迟抗菌治疗将会使他们原发感染恶化、感染扩散、败血症和死亡的风险增高。我们已经确认，研究监查员未能充分认识临床研究者随机后一再拖延给药做法。对严重性也未能采取适当的纠正措施，以防这一问题在此试验场所反复出现。

ⅱ. 在试验场所063，对于试验方案（b）(4)，研究监查员未能确保方案设盲计划的正确执行。这个研究是以双盲的方式进行，根据试验方案（6.2 设盲和随机化），"非盲态药剂师将负责以保持研究者和工作人员对药物使用处于盲态的方式为每一位受试者准备方案药物"。

a）在试验场所063，研究护士而不是非盲态的药剂师负责药品溶解和配制，同时负责试验药物注射和看护受试者。因此，监护受试者的护理人员（即研究人员）在研究治疗时未保持盲态，这与试验方案的要求不符。

b）在试验场所063，对于研究（b）(4)，对于治疗组的5个受试者（140103，140107，140114，140111，和140112），研究者可能已被开盲，因为护理日记中包含了注射盲态药品的名称。在试验中心，护理日记是由研究者审查的。根据2006年5月11~12日的非盲态监查访视报告，尽管看起来护士已经使用了修正液来遮盖自己的手写记录，但在某些情况下，这些被遮盖的信息仍然可以解读。与此发现相关，报告中说："医院的记录会被盲态人员看到，我们不确定这些信息是否会被他们看到"。这个报告也清楚地包含了一些ICON监查员给试验场所的建议与ICH GCP指南明显不一致。其中说到："我们告知了研究的主要监查员，她指示我们用黑色标记笔删去这些信息，以防进一步的盲态信息的暴露。这个过程由主要的研究护士完成，并且签了名字和日期"。而"临床试验质量管理规范指南"一般要求，对任何档案的修改或更正都应该签名，注明修改日期，并解释原因，且不可以遮盖原始输入内容。因此试验场所063的人员和ICON监查员至少对入组此场所的5个受试者，均未能采取适当的纠正措施，对原始文件作了修改。

b. 研究监查员未能发现，在试验场所551参加研究（b）(4)的至少14名受试者（141051，140040，140051，140051……）中每天的药物注射顺序#4和#5是相反的。以受试者141051为例，撰写试验方案要求，第四次注射应为安慰剂，输注时间60分钟以上，第五次注射（b）(4)输液时间120分钟以上。然而，试验场所人员将（b）(4)120分钟作为第四次注射，而安慰剂60分钟作为第五次注射。

c. 方案监查员未能发现，两个研究（b）(4)和研究（b）(4)中均有不符合入选标准的受试者。例如：

ⅰ. 对于试验场所520的研究（b）(4)，受试者1011以左足脓肿在2005年3月3日入组。这个受试者不符合满足脓肿诊断入组标准的要求，因为脓肿是在入组前七天发生的。一份2005年5月27日的数据更正表显示，这个受试者在2005年2月21日接受了抗生素复方新诺明治疗。同样地，在原始记录中的一个备注说明此受试者已经接受了复方新诺明抗生素治疗左脚的脓肿。

ⅱ. 对于试验场所551的研究（b）(4)，研究监查员未能发现，有记录表明受试者141061和141074已经接受了妊娠检查，但试验场所在这些受试者入组前没有他们的检测结果及阴性结果的记录，而按照试验方案对可能怀孕的女性是要求做的。

ⅲ. 对于试验场所063的研究（b）(4)，研究监查员未能发现，受试者140107并不符合研究的要求。试验方案要求之前的手术/创伤的局部感染应该发生在手术/创伤的30天内。然而对于受试者140107，之前的手术记录为方案筛选前20个月。此外，从研究场所取得的其他的原始记录显示，对照试验方案规定的其他复杂类型的皮肤和皮肤组织感染的入组标准，该受试者也不符合条件。

d. 对于试验场所551的研究（b）(4)，研究监查员未能发现，非盲态药剂师没有按研究方案的要求及时收到基线肌酐清除率结果，确认合适的药物剂量计算。例如：

ⅰ. 下列基线肌酐清除率结果在2006年8月12日受试者入组和初始剂量之前没有传真给研究药剂师：

a）受试者141060，2006年8月1日随机。

b）受试者141061，2006年8月2日随机。

c）受试者141066，2006年8月7日随机。

d）受试者141067，2006年8月8日随机。

e）受试者141068，2006年8月9日随机。

ii. 下列基线肌酐清除率结果到2006年11月14日，即受试者分别完成治疗的2~3个月之后才传真给方案药剂师：

a）受试者141062。

b）受试者141069。

c）受试者141079。

d）受试者141080。

e）受试者141050。

f）受试者140040。

g）受试者141069。

h）受试者141074。

i）受试者140051。

j）受试者140076。

k）受试者140063。

而2006年8月15日监查报告中却说："给药剂师提供所有受试者的肌酐清除率结果的复印件，已完成。"这个记录是不充分的，因为它不能确保将肌酐清除率结果及时发送给药剂师，以便根据需要适当调整用药剂量。

本警告信的目的并非是罗列您在试验药物临床研究中存在的所有缺陷。确保遵循法律和相关FDA法规的每一项要求是您的职责。您应当解决这些缺陷，并建立规程，以确保任何正在进行或将来进行的研究均能符合FDA的法规。

自收到这封信的15个工作日内，您应当书面告知本办公室为预防将来发生类似违规情况已经或将要采取的措施。如果不能充分、迅速地解释上述违规问题，可能导致我们在不再通知的情况下采取监管措施。

附：英文原文

ICON Clinical Research, Inc.

WARNING LETTER

Nov 27, 2009

CERTIFIED MAIL
RETURN RECEIPT REQUESTED

Ref: #10-HFD-45-11-04

John W. Hubbard,Ph.D.
Global President, CON Clinical Research
c/o CON Clinical Research Limited
212 Church Road
North Wales, PA 19454

Dear Dr. Hubbard:

This Warning Letter is to inform you of regulatory violations found during the U.S. Food and Drug Administration's (FDA) investigation into ICON Clinical Research LTD's (hereafter referred to as ICON) role as the contract monitoring organization (CRO) contracted by (b)(4) (hereafter referred to as (b) (4)) to provide clinical study management services for Study (b)(4) entitled (b)(4) Y and Study (b)(4) entitled (b)(4) of the investigational drug (b)(4). This inspection is a part of the FDA's Bioresearch Monitoring Program, which is designed to evaluate the conduct of research and to ensure that the rights, safety, and welfare of the human subjects of those studies have been protected. Another objective of the program is to ensure that data submitted in support of New Drug Applications are scientifically valid and accurate.

The first study, (b) (4) was initiated by the original holder of (b)(4) (hereafter referred to as (b)(4) On February 2, 2005 (b)(4) entered into a worldwide partnership with (b)(4), a (b)(4) company, to develop and market (b)(4) (referred to as (b)(4) Under the terms of the agreement,(b)(4) was to be developed further by (b)(4) and all rights and responsibilities for (b)(4) clinical trials were transferred to (b)(4). Of note, with the transfer of development to (b)(4), all clinical trial monitoring agreements between (b)(4) and ICON Clinical Research LTD (ICON) remained in effect (including those in place for (b)(4)). The second study, (b)(4) was initiated by (b)(4). As was the case with (b)(4) contracted ICON to provide clinical research management for (b)(4).

On May 18, 2007,(b)(4) submitted the data from (b)(4) and (b)(4) to the FDA to support the approval of (b)(4) for the indication of treatment of (b)(4). Subsequent data validation inspections of clinical investigators participating in these studies revealed significant violations of FDA regulations codified at 21 CFR 312.

Between May 26, 2008 and June 12, 2008 FDA inspected (b)(4). According to contracts between (b)(4) and ICON,(b)(4) specifically transferred the following tasks associated with site monitoring to ICON:

- Develop and write monitoring plan specific to study;
- Schedule and conduct on-site monitoring visits according to monitoring-plan specifications;
- Schedule and conduct telephone follow-up visits according to protocol/monitoring-plan specifications;
- Write monitoring-visit reports, including follow-up letters, telephone contacts, etc.;
- Notify sponsor of any critical site issues (i.e., good clinical practice violations, noncompliance trends noticed at site) and for providing a proposed resolution plan;
- Conduct weekly teleconferences to review site-monitoring schedule, site status, communication plans, etc.; and
- Provide tracking of monitoring visits, telephone follow-up visits, monitoring-visit reports, and protocol violations.

ICON agreed to conduct site-initiation visits, interim blinded and unblinded monitoring visits, and closeout visits. At each interim monitoring visit, ICON personnel agreed to "review CRFs for completion, perform 100% source document verification (SDV) for all data, verify informed consent, ensure proper AE reporting, check record retention and adequacy of supplies and ensure proper drug storage and accountability". ICON also agreed to "ensure that the site is adhering to the protocol and b applicable regulations and that the staff are motivated to conduct the study" and to "send a follow-up letter to the site that detailed any non-conformances [sic] and corrective actions to be taken."

During FDA's inspection of **(b)(4)** between May 26, 2008 and June 12,2008, FDA obtained ICON monitoring records, which were provided to **(b)(4)** at the conclusion of ICON's clinical study management services for these studies.

The regulations permit the transfer of obligations to a CRO by a sponsor [21 CFR 312.52(a)], and describe the responsibilities that the CRO incurs when obligations are transferred [21 CFR 312.52(b)]. Specifically, a CRO that assumes any obligation of a sponsor shall be subject to the same regulatory action as a sponsor for failure to comply with any obligation assumed under part 312. From our review of the **(b)(4)** establishment inspection report and the documents submitted with that report, **(b)(4)** written response to the Form FDA 483,dated June 24, 2008; and **(b)(4)** responses dated September 2, 2008, and September 4, 2008, in response to additional information requests from the FDA, we conclude that you did not adhere to the applicable statutory requirements and FDA regulations governing the conduct of clinical investigations. We wish to emphasize the following:

1. Failure to ensure proper monitoring of the clinical investigations [21CFR 312.50 and 312.56(a)].

FDA regulations require that sponsors, or CROs to whom such responsibilities have been transferred ensure proper monitoring of clinical investigations. Our investigation found that ICON failed to properly ensure monitoring of the studies referenced above. Inadequate monitoring resulted in deficiencies in recordkeeping with respect to case histories and drug accountability by clinical investigators participating in the above-referenced studies. Violations include, but were not limited to, the following:

a. Deficiencies in case histories:

i. Study monitors failed to identify that on multiple occasions, site personnel documented administration of study drug to different subjects at precisely the same time. For example:

a) For Study **(b)(4)** at Site #520,study monitors failed to identify that on multiple occasions, study coordinators documented administration of study drug to two different subjects at the same time. On April 27, 2005, enrollment of subjects at Site # 520 was allowed to resume, based upon the Sponsor's review of the site's April 27, 2005, plan for "Outpatient Treatment Procedures." Implementation of this plan was to begin on April 27, 2005. The Outpatient Treatment Procedures plan called for the first dose of the study drug to be administered in the site's designated infusion center, and for the remaining doses to be administered by a study nurse or a home health nurse in the patient's home. In light of these procedures, study monitors should have identified that on multiple occasions, for subjects being treated as outpatients, study coordinators documented administration of study drug to two different subjects at the same time, and study monitors should have sought an explanation for these observations.

Specifically,

i) Study Coordinator **(b)(6)** was documented as having administered study drug to the following subjects at the same time on the same date:

(a) Subject #1266 at 09:00-10:00 and Subject #1267 at 09:00-10:00 on 7/2/05

(b) Subject #1266 at 09:00-10: 15 and Subject #1267 at 09:00-10: 15 on 7/3/05

(c) Subject #1266 at 21:00-22:00 and Subject #1267 at 21:00-22:00 on 7/5/05

(d) Subject #1266 at 21:00-22:00 and Subject #1267 at 21:00-22:00 on 7/6/05

(e) Subject #1266 at 09:00-10:00 and Subject #1267 at 09:00-10: 15 on 7/7/05

ii) Study Coordinator (b)(6) was documented as having administered study drug to Subject #2273 at 10:00-11:00 and to Subject #2275 at 10:00-11:00 on 7/26/05.

Given the site outpatient treatment plan and study monitoring that was conducted for the identified subjects, study monitors should have noted that on multiple occasions, study site personnel documented administration of study drug to different subjects at precisely the same time, and further investigated the reason for this irregularity. Moreover, based on the FDA investigation conducted at the site, we have determined that subjects enrolled in the study continued to self-administer study medications in their homes beyond the time when the site' April 27, 2005, plan was to have been implemented. In addition, it would not be possible for the same study coordinator to begin study infusions on more than one subject at precisely the same time, even if the two subjects had been treated at the same location.

b) For Study **(b)(4)** at Site #063, study monitors failed to identify that on multiple occasions, the same study nurse, **(b)(6)** was documented in the "Planillade estabilidad" as having administered study drug to different subjects at precisely the same time, as follows:

i) On May 20, the study nurse **(b)(6)** is documented as having administered study drug to the following subjects at 08:00-10:00:

(a) Subject #140616 ((b)(6))

(b) Subject #140132 ((b)(6))

(c) Subject #140617 ((b)(6))

(d) Subject #140118 ((b)(6))

ii) On May 20, the study nurse (b)(6) is documented as starting placebo infusions to the following subjects at 10:00-11:00:

(a) Subject #140616 ((b)(6))

(b) Subject #140132 ((b)(6))

(c) Subject #140617 ((b)(6))

(d) Subject #140118 ((b)(6))

Study monitors should have recognized that on multiple occasions, the same individual was documented as administering study drug to different subjects at precisely the same time, and study monitors should have further investigated the reason for this irregularity.

ii. One hundred percent source documentation verification was completed by study monitors for Subject #141050, enrolled in Study **(b)(4)** at Site #551,according to ICON monitoring reports; however, study monitors failed to identify that no physical examination, wound assessment, or overall clinical assessment was documented in study source documents or on the Case Report Form (CRF) for this subject's Day-8 visit, as required by the protocol.

iii. Study monitors failed to identify that for both Study (b)(4) and Study (b)(4) the times that infusions were "delivered to Nursing Unit" were not recorded. For example:

a)At Site #502, according to the **(b)(4)** worksheet, the times that reconstituted study drug was delivered to the nursing unit were "not recorded" on at least four occasions for Subject #1118.

b)At Site #508 according to the **"(b)(4)** worksheet, the times that reconstituted study drug was delivered to the nursing unit were "not recorded" on at least seven occasions for Subject #140005.

iv. For Study (b)(4) at Site # 509,study monitors failed to ensure that reconstituted study drug infusion solutions were stored appropriately. Protocol (b)(4) stated that reconstituted study drug infusion solutions should "be stored at room temperature (25°C) and used within 6 hours, or stored for up to 16 hours under refrigeration (5°C) and used within 3 hours after removal from the refrigerator." Because the study protocol did not outline outpatient dosing conventions, the study monitor sought assurance, in e-mail correspondence between Site #509 and the study monitor dated October 20, 2004, that there was documentation to show that study medication was being maintained and stored under proper temperature conditions by patients who were to self-administer the study drug in their own homes. Although they were asked by ICON monitors, the personnel at the site never addressed how they would document the temperature storage conditions of the product in subjects' homes; site personnel only addressed how subjects' body temperatures were to be recorded. Study monitors failed to recognize that the site's response was incomplete; rather, they accepted this response as complete. Subject diaries were then created and used by the site that did not include a place to record storage temperatures of study medication that was stored in subjects' refrigerators. Therefore, storage temperatures for these medications could not be confirmed as complying with storage conditions specified by the protocol. The importance of maintaining proper temperature conditions in patients' homes is evidenced by page three of the "(b)(4) Outpatient Study Drug Procedure," dated "25May2005," which stated that the "receiving site storage conditions must be confirmed upon delivery of the study medication. Clinic, investigator office and/or patient refrigerator temperatures must be recorded and the plan must specify where and by whom."

v. For Study (b)(4) at Site #520, study monitors failed to document the out-of-range temperature readings noted at this site, and failed to provide appropriate follow-up instructions to the site regarding the usage of the kits in a particular shipment. Drug shipments from (b)(4) contained "Refrigerated Shipment Inspection Instructions" that included instructions to fill out readings from a temperature-recording device on the bottom of the Packing List, and to return this device to (b)(4) if the device screen displayed a "bell" symbol (potentially signifying that the shipment did not maintain appropriate conditions). If no bell was seen the shipment maintained appropriate temperatures, and the contents could be used. An April 4, 2005, Packing List for Order #1000739, shipped to Site #520 for Study (b)(4) was identified for which temperatures were recorded as being out of range on the bottom of the sheet; however, no documentation was present for the return of the temperature-recording device or for follow-up to the site regarding the acceptability of the use of the kits contained in this shipment. Source documents demonstrated that drug from kits contained in this shipment were dispensed and administered to study subjects between April and June 2005. The Unblinded Monitoring Visit Report (dated May 25, 2005) encompassing monitoring of Site #520 for the time frame when this shipment was received, failed to document the out-of-range temperature readings or the appropriate follow-up instructions to the site regarding the usage of the kits in this shipment.

Based on documentation available at the time, study monitors conducting the Unblinded Monitoring Visit should have recognized that drug kits from Order #1000739 should not have been administered to subjects.

vi. For Study (b)(4) at Site #146, " Ⅳ stability" worksheets were missing for all 39 subjects enrolled, and corrective actions by study monitors were inadequate to correct this deficiency throughout the study. According to the Work Order for this study, unblinded monitoring visits by ICON were to occur every 10 weeks. This issue was documented in the unblinded monitoring visit reports dated 27 January 2006 and 25 September 2006. In addition, the monitor requested that personnel at the site complete these worksheets, and that the site generate a Memo to File that documented the Ⅳ temperature stability conditions for previously enrolled subjects. However, the issue should have been addressed again prior to the 25 September 2006 unblinded monitoring visit. The Memo to File that was finally written on 16 November 2006, after completion of subject enrollment at the site, stated only that "i.v. stability has been maintained according to the IV label, which states start/finish time and the expiry time of the infusion, [sic] patient number." This statement does not provide sufficient detail to ensure that temperature stability conditions for the drug were maintained adequately.

ⅶ. For Study (b)(4) at Site #520,study monitors failed to identify discrepancies in the time of delivery of study drug to the nursing unit, as recorded on (b)(4))" worksheets; and the time of administration of the study drug, as recorded on "Administration of Study Medication" worksheets for multiple subjects. For example:

a) Subject #1187's source documents indicate that:

ⅰ) on 3/1/05, study drug was delivered at 19:05; study drug administration time is documented as 18:00-19:00

ⅱ) on 3/2/05, study drug was delivered at 19: 10; study drug administration time is documented as 18:00-19:00

ⅲ) on 3/11/05, study drug was delivered at 18:05; study drug administration time is documented as 18:00-19:00

ⅳ) on 3/12/05, study drug was delivered at 18:40; study drug administration time is documented as 18:00-19:00.

b) Subject #1195's source documents indicate that:

ⅰ) on 4/14/05, study drug was delivered at 09:00; study drug administration is documented as 08:05-09:05

c) Subject #2671's source documents indicate that:

ⅰ) on 5/11/05, study drug was delivered at 10:00; study drug administration is documented as 09:30-10:30

ⅱ) on 5/12/05, study drug was delivered at 09: 55; study drug administration is documented as 09:30-10:30

ⅲ) on 5/13/05, study drug was delivered at 09:50; study drug administration is documente as 09:30-10:30

ⅷ. For Study (b)(4) study monitors failed to identify discrepancies in study records related to observations and data pertinent to the investigation. For example:

For Study **(b)(4)** at Site #520, source documents and study documents contain conflicting information related to wound dimensions, debridement of wounds, and signs and symptoms of infection for multiple subjects; however, this conflicting information was not identified by the monitors. For example:

a) For Subject #1010, Wound #2 was documented as the qualifying study wound for study enrollment, according to a source document for the baseline visit. In the sub-investigator's "Outpatient Wound Care Progress Note" for 3/22/05, the dimensions of the wound were documented as 10 mm × 4 mm; the progress note also stated that the wound was too sensitive for debridement. However, a wound-care source document dated 3/23/05, documented that the study wound had been debrided on 3/22/05, and that the wound dimensions were 25 mm × 30 mm. We also note that page 2 of 4 of the source document for the "Test of Cure, Clinical Assessment," dated 3/23/05, was initialed and dated "3/5/05" by the sub-investigator; however, this date is 18 days before this source document states that the visit occurred.

b) For Subject #1186, the sub-investigator's progress note for 3/7/05 stated that the wound dimensions were 21mm × 25 mm. Study source document worksheets for the 3/7/05 visit originally documented wound dimensions of 17 mm × 15 mm, but on 4/18/05, those dimensions were lined through and revised to cite the wound dimensions as 21 mm × 25 mm. Because this source document also stated that "wound assessment done per MD + reported to CRC," it is unclear why the originally recorded dimensions were inconsistent with those documented in the sub-investigator's progress note. Similarly, the sub-investigator's progress note for 3/14/2005 stated that the wound dimensions were 23 mm × 29 mm, but the source document for the same day originally documented wound dimensions of 15 mm × 10 mm; then on 4/18/05, the dimensions originally recorded on the source document were lined through an revised to cite the wound dimensions as 23 mm × 29 mm. In addition, the sub-investigator's progress note for 3/21/2005 stated that the wound dimensions were 14 mm × 23 mm; however, page 2 of 4 of the source document for the same day originally documented wound dimensions of 8 mm × 6 mm. On 4/18/04, the dimensions originally appearing on the source document were lined through and revised to cite the wound dimensions as 14 mm × 23 mm. However, the corresponding CRF page for the 4/18/05 visit still documented the wound dimensions as 8 mm × 6 mm. In addition, the sub-investigator's progress note for 3/14/07 documented "much less inflammation and little drainage; however, the source document for the date of this visit documented drainage or discharge as "absent" and erythema as "absent."

c) For Subject # 2274, the source document for the End of Treatment visit, dated 7-26-05, documented wound dimensions of 13 mm × 20 mm and a wound assessment of "absent-reddness [sic], pain, edema, heat, flutuance [sic], funct impair, drainage"; however, on another page of the same source document, wound dimensions were listed as "1 mm × 0 mm," drainage or discharge was checked as "improved," and pain or tenderness to palpation was checked as "unchanged." The corresponding CRF page for the End of Therapy visit documents wound dimensions as "80 mm × 95 mm."

b. Deficiencies in drug accountability:

For Study **(b)(4)** at Site #551, monitors failed to identify that study documents contained conflicting information regarding accountability of the drug. When " **((b)(4))**" and Drug Accountability Form source document worksheets were compared, it appears that on multiple occasions, the same kit vial was recorded as being given to more than one subject; and/or on more than one occasion, to the same subject; or the recorded kit-vial information was incomplete. Examples include, but are not limited to, the following:

(b)(4)Worksheet (Kit-Vial) (Date) (Subject#)	Drug Accountability Form Worksheet (Kit-Vial) (Date) (Subject#)
21148-8 1-Aug-06 #141059	21148-8 30-Jul-06 #141052
21148-1 1-Aug-06 #141059	21148-1 02-Aug-06 #141052
22609-2 2-Aug-06 #141059	22609-2 27-Jul-06 #141052
10131-8 5-Aug-06 #141059	10131-8 03-Aug-06 #141059
60126-1 03-Aug-06 #141062	60126-1 02-Aug-06 #141059
60126-18 03-Aug-06 #141062	60126-18 08-Aug-06 #141062
60126-7 07-Aug-06 and 08-Aug-06 #141062	60126-7 04-Aug-06 #141062
23631-15 11-Aug-06 #141066	23631-15 08-Aug-06 #141066
23631-8 11-Aug-06 #141066	23631-8 08-Aug-06 #141066
23110-18 14-Aug-06 #141067	23110-18 No Record of Being Dispensed
23110-4 14-Aug-06 #141067	23110-4 No Record of Being Dispensed

The study monitors failed to notice these discrepancies, despite the fact that the contents of a single vial,which would constitute a single treatment course for one subject, were documented to have been used multiple times.

2. Failure to ensure that an investigation was conducted in accordance with the general investigational plan and protocols, as specified in the IND [21 CFR 312.50].

a. Study monitors failed to ensure that the investigation was conducted in accordance with the investigational plan for Study **(b) (4)** For example:

i. At Site #063, for Study **(b)(4)** study monitors failed to ensure that subjects received study medication as specified in the protocol. According to footnote 1) of the Schedule of Assessments in Clinical Protocol **(b)(4)** "All screening/ predose assessments will be considered as baseline and must be performed and reviewed before **randomization and dosing on Day 1** [emphasis added], with the exception of the PK sample collections". Based on this statement and on other training and materials made available to clinical investigators, all patients should have begun dosing on the same day as randomization. For Study **(b)(4)** at Site #063, however, nine subjects of fourty-five did not receive study drug for more than 24 hours after randomization, ranging from approximately 48 hours to eleven days post randomization. For example, Subject #140117 was randomized on OS May 2006 and received the first dose of medication on 16 May 2006. According to the Unblinded Monitoring Visit Report dated 06 Sep 2006, the delay was due to "personal problems of the patient." This was noted as a minor issue in the post-monitoring visit letter to unblinded site staff, and was not mentioned at all in the post-monitoring visit letter to the Clinical investigator. In addition, no corrective action was documented in monitoring reports or follow-up letters to Site #063.

The delay in administration of appropriate antibacterial therapy for these nine patients, if in fact they had complicated skin and skin structure infections, would have placed them at increased risk for worsening of primary infection, dissemination of infection, sepsis, and death. We have determined that study monitors failed to fully recognize the significance of the clinical investigator's practice of repeatedly delaying study drug dosing after subject randomization and failed to implement appropriate corrective actions to prevent this issue from recurring at the site.

ii. At Site #063, for Study **(b)(4)** study monitors failed to ensure that planned study blinding procedures were correctly followed. This study was to be conducted in a double-blind fashion. According to the Protocol (Section 6.2 Blinding and Randomization), "The unblinded pharmacist will be responsible for preparing the study medication for each subject in such a way that investigators and staff remain blinded to the medication being administered."

a) At Site #063, study nurses, rather than the unblinded pharmacist, were responsible for completing drug dissolution and reconstitution, as well as administering study drug infusions and caring for the subjects. Therefore, nursing personnel caring for subjects (i.e. study staff) were not blinded to study treatment, as specified by the protocol.

b) At Site #063,for Study **(b)(4)** investigators may have been unblinded to the treatment group for five subjects (#140103, #140107,#140114,#140111,and #140112), because the nursing notes included the name of blinded medication infused. Nursing notes were viewed by clinical investigators at the site. Although it appears that the nurses used correction fluid to cover their handwriting, in some cases the covered handwriting could still be read, according to the ICON Unblinded Monitoring Visit Report, dated 11-12 May 2006. In relation to this finding, this report stated that "the infirmary notes are to be seen by the blinded staff, so we do not know for sure if these notes were seen by them." This report also included instructions that are clearly inconsistent with International Conference on Harmonization Good Clinical Practice (GCP) guidelines, to the site from ICON Monitors, in that it stated, "We called the Lead Study Monitor and she instructed to strike out these inclusions with black marker to prevent further potential of unblinding. This procedure was done by the Lead Study Nurse, who included her initials and date." GCP guidelines generally· state that any change or correction to a document should be dated, initialed, and explained (if necessary), and should not obscure the original entry; therefore, both Site #063 personnel and the ICON monitors assigned to this site failed to make corrections to source documents appropriately for at least five subjects enrolled at the site.

b. Study monitors failed to identify that, for at least fourteen subjects (#141051, #140040, #140051, #141050, #141074, #141080,#141061,#141067,#141066, #141062, #141068, #141059, #141060, and #141079) enrolled in Study (b)(4) at Site # 551, the drug-infusion order was reversed daily for infusions #4 and #5. For example, for Subject #141051 in the (b)(4) arm, the protocol required that the fourth dose be placebo, given over 60 minutes, and that the fifth dose be (b)(4) given over 120 minutes; however, the site personnel administered (b)(4) over 120 minutes as the fourth dose, and placebo was administered over 60 minutes as the fifth dose.

c. Study monitors failed to identify that for both Study (b)(4) and Study (b)(4) subjects who did not meet eligibility criteria were enrolled. For example:

i. For Study **(b)(4)** at Site # 520, Subject #1011 was enrolled on March 3,2005, for treatment of a left-foot abscess. This subject did not meet the inclusion criterion for enrollment of a subject with diagnosis of abscess, because the onset of the abscess was more than seven day before enrollment. A Data Correction Form (DCF) dated May 27, 2005, stated that the subject received antibiotic treatment with Bactrim DS, with the end date "21-FEB-2005"; also, a CI comment in source documents stated that the subject had received the Bactrim for treatment of the left-foot abscess.

ii. For Study (b)(4) at Site #551,study monitors failed to identify that while Subjects # 141061 and # 141074 were documented to have had pregnancy tests done,the site did not have the test results and/or did not document the negative pregnancy test results for these subjects before their enrollment, as was required by the protocol for females of child bearing potential.

iii. For Study **(b)(4)** at Site #063, study monitors failed to identify that Subject #140107 was not eligible for the study. Protocol **(b)(4)** required that infection at a site of previous surgery/trauma occur within 30 days of the surgery/trauma. However, for Subject #140107, the previous surgery was documented as having taken place 20 months prior to the study screening visit. Furthermore, additional source documents obtained from the site demonstrated that this subject also did not qualify for enrollment based on criteria for any of the other types of complicated skin and skin structure infections described in the inclusion criteria.

d. For Study (b)(4) at Site #551, study monitors failed to identify that then blinded site pharmacist did not receive baseline creatinine clearance (CrCl) results in time to ensure appropriate study drug dosing calculations, as required by the protocol. For example,

i. The following CrCls were not faxed to thc study pharmacist until August 12,2006,which was well after subjects' enrollment and start of dosing:

a) Subject #141060, randomized August 1, 2006
b) Subject #141061, randomized August 2, 2006
c) Subject #141066, randomized August 7, 2006
d) Subject #141067, randomized August 8, 2006
e) Subject #141068, randomized August 9, 2006

ii. The following CrCls were not faxed to the study pharmacist until November 14,2006,which was 2-3 months after their respective end of treatment visits:

a) Subject #141062
b) Subject #141069
c) Subject # 141079
d) Subject # 141080
e) Subject # 141050
f) Subject # 140040
g) Subject # 141069
h) Subject #141074
i) Subject #140051
j) Subject #140076
k) Subject #140063

While the monitoring report dated 15 Aug 2006 stated, "Pharmacist to provide copies of CrCl for all patients. Done," this documentation is inadequate, as it does not provide assurance that CrCl values were forwarded to the pharmacist in time to allow appropriate dosing adjustments, if warranted.

This letter is not intended to be an all-inclusive list of deficiencies with your monitoring of clinical studies of an investigational drug. It is your responsibility to ensure adherence to each requirement of the law and relevant FDA regulations. You should address these deficiencies and establish procedures to ensure that any ongoing or future studies will be in compliance with FDA regulations.

Within fifteen (15) working days of your receipt of this letter, you should notify this office in writing of the actions

you have taken or will be taking to prevent similar violations in the future. Failure to adequately and promptly explain the violations noted above may result in regulatory action without further notice.

If you have any questions, please contact Tejashri Purohit-Sheth, M.D., at 301-796-3402; FAX 301-847· 8748. Your written response and any pertinent documentation should be addressed to:

Tejashri Purohit-Sheth,M.D.
Branch Chief
Good Clinical Practice Branch Ⅱ
Division of Scientific investigations
Office of Compliance
Center for Drug Evaluation and Research
Food and Drug Administration
Building 51, Room 5358
10903 New Hampshire Avenue
Silver Spring, MD 20993

Sincerely yours,

{See appended electronic signature page}

Leslie K. Ball M.D
Director
Division of Scientific Investigations
Office of Compliance
Center for Drug Evaluation and Research

第46封　给Johnson & Johnson药物研发有限公司的警告信

2009年8月10日

参考号: 09-HFD-45-07-02

尊敬的Grosser博士：

FDA对强生药物研发有限公司（以下简称J & J PRD）作为申办者的关于试验药物（b）（4）的研究（b）（4）、题目为（b）（4）和研究（b）（4）、题目为（b）（4）的临床研究进行了现场检查，这封警告信特告知您检查中发现的违规的情况。

第一个研究（b）（4），是由IND（b）（4）的原持有者发起的。2005年2月2日，（b）（4）与（b）（4）签署了全球合作伙伴协议，合作来开发和上市（b）（4）。按照协议条款，J & J PRO可以进一步开发（b）（4），关于（b）（4）临床试验的所有权利和责任也转移给您们。第二个研究（b）（4），整体上也是由贵方完成。

本次现场检查是FDA的生物研究监查项目的一部分，该项目通过设定的检查方法，对FDA监管的相关研究的实施情况进行评估，以确保这些研究中受试者的权益、安全和福利得到了保护。这一项目的另一个目标就是要保证为支持新药申请而提交的数据在科学上的有效性和准确性。

通过对现场检查报告、该报告的附件以及您2008年6月24日对FDA483表的书面回复，还有2008年9月2日和2008年9月4日对FDA要求的额外信息所做回复的审查，我们认为，您没有遵循适用的法律要求和监管临床研究实施的FDA法规。我们知道在检查结束时，Wydner女士向您出示并讨论了FDA483表，即现场检查发现的问题，我们想强调以下几点：

1. 没有确保对临床研究进行正确的监查［21 CFR 312.50，312.56（a）］

FDA法规要求申办者要保证对临床研究进行适当的监查。我们的调查发现，J & J PRD没能保证对上述涉及的研究进行充分的监查。尽管J & J PRD与（b）（4）签署了合同，由其对（b）（4）和（b）（4）进行监查访视，（b）（4）没能确保临床研究者被充分地评估，并且也没能确保试验场所遵从（b）（4）的研究；（b）（4）的不充分监查导致了研究者参加的上述研究中在病史和药物清点方面记录保存的缺陷。作为在IND（b）（4）申请下执行（b）（4）和（b）（4）研究的申办者，以及提交给NDA（b）（4）的申办者，您有责任确保这些研究被正确地监查并符合法规要求，以此来保证支持NDA的数据具有良好的质量，并且受试者的权益、福利和安全都得到了充分保护。发现的违规包括，但不限于以下的这些：

a. 病历的缺陷项

i. 研究监查员没有发现，在多个场合，试验场所人员记录的对不同受试者给予试验药物是在完全相同的时间点，例如：

a）对于试验场所520的（b）（4）研究，研究监查员有多个场合都没有发现，研究协调员所记录的两个不同的受试者给药时间是完全相同的。基于对研究场所2005年4月27日“门诊治疗规程”计划的审查，贵方于2005年4月27日同意试验场所520继续开始入组受试者。计划的实施是从2005年4月27日开始的。门诊治疗规程计划要求只有试验药物的第一次剂量注射是在试验场所指定的输液中心，其余剂量的注射将由研究护士或者家庭保健护士在受试者家中进行。按照这些规程，研究监查员应该在多个场合能够发现研究协调员记录的两名不同受试者的给药时间是完全相同的，并且应该对这些发现给予解释。

具体而言：

ⅰ）有记录表明，研究协调员（b）（6）在同一天的同一时间给如下的受试者给予了试验药物。

（a）受试者1266和受试者1267在2005年7月2日9:00~10:00同时给药。

（b）受试者1266和受试者1267在2005年7月3日9:00~10:15同时给药。

（c）受试者1266和受试者1267在2005年7月5日21:00~22:00同时给药。

（d）受试者1266和受试者1267在2005年7月6日21:00~22:00同时给药。

（e）受试者1266在2005年7月7日9:00~10:00给药和受试者1267在2005年7月7日9:00~10:15给药。

ⅱ）有记录表明，研究协调员（b）（6）在2005年7月26日10:00~11:00期间同时给受试者2273和受试者2275使用试验药物。

我们发现，在您提供的2008年6月24日的回复中对这些发现的问题的答复不够充分。您声称原始文件中没有表明输液是在受试者家中进行的，并且试验场所的研究协调员告诉您们这些输液必须在办公室中才能给予。

考虑到中心的门诊治疗计划和对已入组受试者所做的研究监查，研究监查员应该在多种场合下注意到，试验场所人员记录不同受试者给药的时间是在非常准确的同一时间点，并且应该要进一步调查造成这种异常的原因。在您2008年6月24日的信中没有提供任何解释说明为什么没有注意到这些差错，并且在FDA检查发现这些问题之前也没有从中心人员那里寻求合理的解释。

而且，尽管研究协调员声明这些输注必须在办公室完成，根据FDA在试验场所所做检查来看，我们确定入组的受试者除2005年4月27日外都是自己在家里输注试验药物的。并且，即使两位受试者是在同一地点接受治疗，同一个研究协调员也不可能在完全相同的时间点给超过一个以上的受试者开始试验药物的输注。

b）对于试验场所063的（b）（4）研究，研究监查员在多个场合均未发现，同一研究护士（b）（6）被记录在“Planillade estabilidad”中在完全相同的时间点将试验药物用于如下不同的受试者。

ⅰ）5月20日，研究护士（b）（6）被记录在8:00~10:00给下列受试者使用试验药物：

（a）受试者140616（b）（6）;

（b）受试者140132（b）（6）;

（c）受试者140617（b）（6）;

（d）受试者140118（b）（6）。

ⅱ）5月20日，研究护士（b）（6）被记录在10:00~11:00给下列受试者进行安慰剂输注：

（a）受试者140616（b）（6）;

（b）受试者140132（b）（6）;

（c）受试者140617（b）（6）;

（d）受试者140118（b）（6）。

根据您2008年9月2日提交给FDA的每位受试者的“Notas De Enfermeria”的复印件，我们发现护理记录中上述的ⅰ）（a）~（d）和ⅱ）（a）~（d）输液后各相关人员首字母缩写签名与“Planillade estailidad”中每位受试者记录上人员签字完全一致，也与“试验场所人员职责分工表”中记录的研究护士（b）（6）首字母缩写签名一致。您2008年9月2日所提交的文件也因此证明了FDA的发现。项目监查员应该有多个场合会意识到，在完全相同的时间由同一个人给不同的受试者输注了试验药物，并且应该对这种异常进行深入的调查，找出原因。

ⅱ. 试验场所551（b）（4）研究中，入组的受试者141050的原始文件核查是由研究监查员完成的，按照贵方提供的表，上面标注有“受试者原始文件核查100%完成”。但是，研究监查员没有发现在这位受试者的原始文件或病例报告表（CRF）中，没有第8天访视做体格检查、创口评估或者总体临床评价的记录，而这些都是研究方案所要求的。我们注意到，在您2008年6月24日提交给FDA的信中没有提及这一发现。

ⅲ. 项目监查员没有发现在（b）（4）研究和（b）（4）研究中，输液“送到护士站”的时间没有记录。例如：

a）在试验场所502，根据（b）（4）工作表，至少有4次为受试者1118配置的试验药物被送到护士站的时间没有记录。我们注意到在您2008年6月24日提交给FDA的信中没有提及这一发现。

b）在试验场所508，根据（b）（4）工作表，至少有7次为受试者14005配置的试验药物送到护士站的时间没有记录。我们注意到在您2008年6月24日提交给FDA的信中，您确认了发药时间没有记录，而且研究监查员也没有记录这些差错。

ⅳ.（b）（4）试验方案表明，配置处理的试验药物输注溶液应该在25℃室温保存并在6小时内使用，或者在5℃冷藏保存至最多16个小时，并且从冰箱取出后3小时内使用完。因为试验方案没有概述门诊用药的规则，2004年10月20日，在研究监查员与509中心的邮件沟通中，监查员想要保证有文件记录表明由受试者自行在家输注试验药物时这些药物是在正确的温度条件下保存和储藏的。尽管有此要求，但试验场所从未解释他们是如何记录产品在受试者家中的温度保存条件的。试验场所的研究人员只是解释了受试者的体温是如何被记录的。研究监查员没有意识到试验场所的回复是不完整的，并把这样的回复认为是完整的而加以接受。然后就制作了受试者日记并被试验场所使用，但在日记上并没有留出位置用于记录药液在受试者家中冰箱里的存放温度。因此，不能证明这些药液的存放温度是符合试验方案中规定的温度条件的。在受试者家中保证药物合适的温度条件的重要性，已经明显显示在标注日期为2005年5月25日“（b）（4）门诊试验药物处理流程”的第三页上，其中特别强调一旦试验药物发送出去，接受地点的存储条件必须得到确认，诊所、研究者办公室和／或受试者家冰箱的温度必须记录，并且计划中必须说明在哪里由谁来记录。

我们注意到您在2008年6月24日给FDA的信中，辩解说药物在受试者的家中看起来保存稳定，您也确认没有关于受试者家中试验药物的存储条件的记录。

ⅴ. 从（b）（4）运输的药物包含了“冷藏装运检验说明”，要求填写包装列表的底部温度记录设备显示的读数，以及如果设备显示屏上显示了一个“警钟”的符号，则意味着该运输温度保持不当，需要将此设备运回（b）（4）。如果没有“警钟”显示，表示运输温度恰当，运输的药物可以使用。2005年4月4日送至试验场所520用于试验方案（b）（4）的编号为1000739的包裹，其底部单子上显示了温度记录超出范围；但是，没有任何文档记录显示温度记录设备被返还，或者对超温运输的药物是否可被接受使用有跟进。原始记录显示，这一批次的药物已经于2005年4月至6月分发给受试者并已使用。非盲态监查访视报告（2005年5月25日）包含了接受这一批次药物的时间段内对试验场所520进行的监查，但监查报告没有记录超温情况，也没有向研究场所提供有关这批药物使用的适当跟进指导。

在您2008年6月24日的回复函中，声称一项附加的稳定性研究是在这些药物分发给研究受试者之后并且是在2005年5月25日的非盲态监查访视报告之后完成的，稳定性研究表明“温度曲线上最高温度达25℃时容许最多保存2天”。但是，FDA注意到，这项稳定性研究是在参考编号为1000739药物运送到中心后进行的，所以，根据当时的文件记录，项目监查员做非盲态监查时应该意识到来自于此编号的药盒不应该给受试者使用。

ⅵ. 对于试验场所146的试验方案（b）（4），所有入组的39名受试者的“Ⅳ稳定性”表全部缺失，并且研究监查员所采取的纠正措施不足以纠正整个研究中在这方面的缺陷。根据此项研究工作规则，（b）（4）应当每10周来访视一次。FDA注意到，在您2008年6月24日的回复中，这个问题在2006年1月27日和2006年9月29日的非盲态监查访视报告中有所记录。此外，监查员要求试验场所人员需填写这些工作表，并且要求试验场所应制作一份备忘录文件，用于记录之前入组的受试者的Ⅳ温度稳定性情况。然而，这个问题本应该在2006年9月25日非盲态监查前就被解决好。最后在2006年11月16日备忘录文件才被写出来，这时该试验场所已经完成受试者入组，只是说“已根据Ⅳ标示维持Ⅳ稳定性，标示只包括注射的开始／结束时间及有效期，受试者编号”。该说明没有提供足够的细节用于确保药品保存的温度稳定性。

ⅶ. 对于试验场所520的试验方案（b）（4），研究监查员未能发现将试验药物发往护理中心的时间与（b）（4）工作表中记载的不一致；而给药时间也与多名受试者“试验药物注射”表上记录的时间不一致。例如：

a）受试者1187的原始记录指出：

ⅰ）2005年3月1日，试验药物发出时间为19:05，而试验药物的用药时间记录为 18:00~19:00。

ⅱ）2005年3月2日，试验药物发出时间为19:10，而试验药物的用药时间记录为 18:00~19:00。

ⅲ）在2005年3月1日，试验药物发出时间为18:05，而试验药物的用药时间记录为 18:00~19:00。

ⅳ）2005年3月12日，试验药物发出时间为18:45，而试验药物的用药时间记录为 18:00~19:00。

b）受试者1195的原始记录指出:

ⅰ）2005年4月14日，试验药物发出时间为9:00，试验药物的用药时间记录为 8:05~9:05。

c）受试者2671的原始记录指出:

ⅰ）2005年5月11日，试验药物发出时间为10:00，试验药物的用药时间记录为 9:30~10:30。

ⅱ）2005年5月12日，试验药物发出时间为9:55，试验药物的用药时间记录为 9:30~10:30。

ⅲ）2005年5月13日，试验药物发出时间为9:50，试验药物的用药时间记录为9:30~10:30。

我们注意到在您2008年6月24日回复给FDA的信中，声称发生时间上的差异是因为试验场所记录的是预计给药时间，而不是实际给药时间，并且也承认研究监查员没有发现原始文件中的这些差错。

ⅷ. 对于试验方案（b）(4)，研究监查员未能发现与观察和研究数据相关的记录不符。例如：

对于试验场所520的试验方案（b）(4)，原始记录与研究记录在创口尺寸、创口清创术以及对多个受试者注射的标记和符号的信息上存在矛盾。但监查员未能发现这些矛盾的信息。例如：

a）对于受试者1010，根据基线访视的原始记录，创口2被记录作为满足研究纳入资格的创口。而在2005年3月22日，助理研究者的门诊创口治疗的病程记录中，记录了创口尺寸为10mm × 4mm，并指出该创口会对清创术非常敏感，但是一份2005年3月23日的创口护理原始文件则记录了该研究创口已于2005年3月22日完成清创，其尺寸大小为25mm × 30mm。我们同时注意到，在这份2005年3月23日的“治愈测试临床评估”的原始记录4页中的第二页，助理研究者签的名字缩写和签署的时间为2005年3月5日，这比原始文件注明的访视日期提前了18天。

b）受试者1186，助理研究者于2005年3月7日病程记录中陈述，创口大小为21mm × 25mm，而2005年3月7日访视的研究原始文件工作表中记录的创口大小为17mm × 15mm，但是在2005年4月18日，这些创口大小数字被线划掉，而且更改为21mm × 25mm。由于这些原始记录已经注明“已经根据MD以上人员完成创口评估及报告至CRC”，不清楚为什么这些创口大小的原始记录与助理研究者病程记录中的大小不一致。与之类似的，① 2005年3月14日助理研究者的病程记录中记录了创口大小为23mm × 29mm，而原始文件创口大小为15mm × 10mm；而于2005年4月18日，原始文件报告中的创口大小被划掉更改为23mm × 29mm。② 2005年3月21日助理研究者病程记录中记录创口大小为14mm × 23mm，但当天原始文件的2/4页的原始记录为8mm × 6mm。在2004年4月18日，原始文件上首次记录的大小被划改为14mm × 23mm。但是，在2005年4月18日相应的病例报告表页面中关于此创口大小记录为8mm × 6mm。另外，2007年3月14日，助理研究者的进展记录“炎症消退，几乎无流液”，而此访视日期的原始文件记录则为流液或脓液处为“无”和红肿处为“无”。

c）受试者2274，标注日期为2005年7月26日关于治疗结束访视的原始文件中记录了创口大小为13mm × 20mm，创口评估为“未见红肿（原文如此）、疼痛、水肿、发热、胃肠气胀（原文如此）、肝功能损伤及渗水”，但在同一原始文件的另一页则记录为创口大小1mm × 0mm，渗水经检查为渗水“改善”，而疼痛或触诊疼痛经诊断为“没有变化”。而相应的治疗结束访视的病例报告表则记录创口大小为80mm × 95mm。

我们注意到在您2008年6月24日回复给FDA的信中，您们承认研究监查员没有发现原始文件中的这些差错。

b. 药品清点方面的缺陷

对于试验场所551的试验方案（b）(4)，研究文档中关于药品清点方面有相互矛盾的信息。将（b）(4)与药品清点表的原始工作记录表进行对比，显示在多个场合下，同一支药剂被记录注射给了多个受试者，或/和不止一次地注射给了同一个受试者；或者是试剂瓶记录的信息不完整。举例包括但不限于如下：

（b）（4）工作表 （药瓶编号） （使用日期） （受试者编号）	药物清点工作表 （药瓶编号） （使用日期） （受试者编号）
21148-8 2006-8-1 #141059	21148-8 2006-7-30 #141052
21148-1 2006-8-1 #141059	21148-1 2006-8-2 #141052
22609-2 2006-8-2 #141059	22609-2 2006-7-27 #141052
10131-8 2006-8-5 #141059	10131-8 2006-8-3 #141059
60126-1 2006-8-3 #141062	60126-1 2006-8-2 #141059
60126-18 2006-8-3 #141062	60126-18 2006-8-8 #141062
60126-7 2006-8-7和2006-8-8 #141062	60126-7 2006-8-4 #141062
23631-15 2006-8-11 #141066	23631-15 2006-8-8 #141066
23631-8 2006-8-11 #141066	23631-8 2006-8-8 #141066
23110-18 2006-8-14 #141067	23110-18 无分发记录
23110-4 2006-8-14 #141067	23110-4 无分发记录

尽管事实上每一小瓶药剂的剂量就是一位受试者一次的用量，但记录显示被使用多次，研究监查员未能发现存在的这些差异。我们注意到，在您2008年6月24日及随后给FDA的信中都没有提及这些发现。

2. 未能确保研究按照IND中规定的总体研究计划和方案执行［21CFR 312.50］

a. 研究监查员没有保证研究是按照（b）（4）研究的研究计划执行的，例如：

在试验场所063，对于试验方案（b）（4），研究监查员未能确保方案设盲计划的正确执行。这个研究是以双盲的方式进行。根据试验方案（章节6.2 设盲和随机化），“非盲态的药剂师将负责以保持研究者和工作人员对药物使用处于盲态的方式为每一位受试者准备试验药物”。

i. 在试验场所063，研究护士而不是非盲态的药剂师负责药品溶解和配制，同时负责试验药物注射和看护受试者。因此，没有根据，护理人员对受试者的看护对与研究治疗而言是非盲态的。

我们注意到在2008年6月24日给FDA的信中您们没有提及这个发现。

ii. 在试验场所063，对于试验方案（b）（4），对于治疗组的5个受试者（140103，140107，140114，

140111，和140112），研究者可能已被开盲，因为护理日记中包含了注射盲态药物的名称。在试验场所，护理日记是由研究者审查的。根据2006年5月11~12日的（b）（4）非盲态监查访视报告，尽管看起来护士已经使用了修正液来遮盖自己的手写记录，但在某些情况下，这些被遮盖的信息仍然可以辨读。与此发现相关，报告中说“医院的记录会被盲态人员看到，我们不确定这些信息是否会被他们看到”。这个报告也清楚地包含了一些（b）（4）监查员给试验场所的建议，与ICH GCP指南明显不一致。其中说到，“我们告知了研究主要监查员，她指示我们用黑色标记笔删去这些信息，以防将来可能要破盲，而这件事后来由研究护士长去做了，她还留下了姓名首字母及日期”。而GCP指南一般要求，对任何档案的修改或更正都应该签名、注明修改日期并解释原因，且不可以遮盖原始输入内容。因此试验场所063的人员和（b）（4）监查员至少对入组此场所的5个受试者的均未能采取适当的更正措施对原始文件作了修改。

我们注意到在您于2008年6月24日给FDA的信中，您们承认没有遵从GCP指南，未来试验场所经理和研究监查员会被要求要使用特殊的培训模式来强调准确完成原始文件的重要性。

b. 研究监查员未能发现，在试验场所551参加试验方案（b）（4）的至少14名受试者中每天的药物注射顺序#4和#5是相反的。以受试者141051为例，按照试验方案要求，第四次注射应为安慰剂，输液60分钟；第五次注射（b）（4），输液时间120分钟。然而，试验场所人员在将（b）（4）120分钟作为第四次注射，而安慰剂60分钟作为第五次注射。

由您提供的2008年6月24日的信中回复声称试验场所承认第4和第5剂药的每日输液在药物输注顺序和输液持续时间上发生了颠倒，而且还承认研究监查员在试验场所监查访视过程中没有能够发现这一问题。

c. 研究监查员未能发现，研究（b）（4）和研究（b）（4）中均有不符合入组标准的受试者。例如：

i. 对于试验场所520研究（b）（4），受试者1011以足脓肿在2005年3月3日入组。这个受试者不符合入组标准满足脓肿诊断的要求，因为脓肿是在入组前七天发生的。一份2005年5月27日的数据更正表显示，这个受试者在2005年2月21日接受了抗生素复方新诺明治疗。同样，在原始记录中的一个备注说明此受试者已经接受了复方新诺明抗生素治疗左脚的脓肿。因此，在受试者入组前左脚脓肿出现已经超过7天，这名受试者不应该被入组进来。

我们发现在您提供的2008年6月24日回复函中对这一问题的答复是不充分的，您们只是声称这位受试者满足入组标准，但却没有提及感染指数已经出现超过7天的事实，这个事实将会把受试者排除在研究入组之外。

ii. 对于试验场所551研究（b）（4），研究监查员未能发现，有记录表明受试者141061和141074已经接受了妊娠检查，但试验场所在这些受试者入组前没有她们的检测结果及阴性结果的记录，而按照试验方案，对于可能怀孕的女性是要求做的。

我们注意到在您2006年6月24日给FDA的信中，您们确认这些受试者的妊娠检查结果没有被记录，而且研究监查员也没有发现这个问题。

iii. 对于试验场所063的研究（b）（4），研究监查员未能发现受试者140107并不符合研究的要求。试验方案要求之前的手术/创伤的局部感染应该发生在手术/创伤的30天内。然而对于受试者140107，之前的手术记录为方案筛选前20个月。

根据受试者140107相关的原始文件，以及您们于2008年9月2日向FDA提交的对这些文件的解释说明，您们声称这些原始文件不能支持感染是由某一创伤所致的说法。（b）（4）医生还告诉您们，受试者原来手术区会间歇性发炎，并且当受试者入组时，感染的部位正在排脓，已经发炎并疼痛，这次感染是在入组前30天开始的。虽然您在2008年9月2日的提交信中不承认此受试者不适合入组，但在2008年9月2日来信的附加信息也支持，对照研究方案规定的其他复杂类型的皮肤和皮肤组织感染的条件，该受试者也不符合入组标准。

d. 对于试验场所063的研究（b）（4），研究监查员未能发现受试者140107并不符合研究的要求。试验方案要求之前的手术/创伤的局部感染应该发生在手术/创伤的30天内。然而对于受试者140107，之前的手术记录为方案筛选前20个月。此外，从研究场所取得的另外的原始记录显示，对照研究方案规定的其他复杂类型的皮肤和皮肤组织感染的入组标准，该受试者也不符合条件。

d. 对于试验场所551的试验方案（b）（4），研究监查员未能发现非盲态药剂师没有及时收到基线肌酐清除率结果来按研究方案的要求确认合适的药物剂量计算。例如：

i. 下列基线肌酐清除率结果在2006年8月12日受试者入组和初始剂量之前没有传真给研究药剂师：

a）受试者141060，2006年8月1日随机；

b）受试者141061，2006年8月2日随机；

c）受试者141066，2006年8月7日随机；

d）受试者141067，2006年8月8日随机；

e）受试者141068，2006年8月9日随机。

ii. 下列基线肌酐清除率结果到2006年11月14日，即受试者分别完成治疗的2~3个月之后才传真给研究药剂师：

a）受试者141062；

b）受试者141069；

c）受试者141079；

d）受试者141080；

e）受试者141050；

f）受试者140040；

g）受试者141069；

h）受试者141074；

i）受试者140051；

j）受试者140076；

k）受试者140063。

在您2008年6月24日递交给FDA的回复函中，有一份标注日期为2006年8月15日的监查报告中有："药剂师将提供基线肌酐清除率结果的复印件给所有受试者。完成。"这个记录。但是，这个回复是不合适的，因为它不能确保将肌酐清除率结果及时发送给药剂师，以便根据需要及时调整用药剂量。

3. 未能确保研究者遵守研究计划和相关FDA法规［21 CFR 312.56（b）］

按照FDA法规，申办者若发现研究者不遵守已签署的研究者协议（FDA1572表）、总研究计划，或者相关FDA法规的要求，应当立即采取行动确保研究者遵守要求，或者停止给研究者运送药物并且终止研究者继续参加试验。如果研究者被终止试验，申办者应该通知FDA。我们的检查发现，对于研究场所063的（b）（4）研究，您们没有充分适当地执行纠错行动。例如：

根据临床试验方案（b）（4）评估安排表的脚注1），"所有的筛选／初始剂量评估都将作为基线，且必须在随机化和第一天给药之前完成并进行审查，PK样品收集除外"。基于此说明以及提供给临床研究人员的培训及其他材料，所有受试者应该在随机化当天就开始用药。然而对于在试验场所063的试验方案（b）（4），45个受试者中的9位受试者在随机化超过24小时后还没有被给予试验药物，时间范围为随机化后48小时到11天。例如，受试者140117在2016年5月8日随机，但收到第一次剂量的时间为2006年5月16日。根据2006年9月6日的非盲态监查访视报告，延迟是因为"受试者的个人问题"。这在监查访视后给非盲态试验场所人员的信函中记录为微小问题，在监查访视后给临床研究者的信中根本没有提及。此外，在监查报告以及发给试验场所063的跟进信中也没有纠正措施记录。

我们发现由您提供的2008年6月24日回复函中对这些发现的答复是不充分适当的。您们声称在研究方案中没有特别说明研究中开始初始剂量之前的阶段会持续多长时间，也没有说明筛选后多久需要开始进行治疗。但是您们承认"对研究的预期是希望所有的研究治疗将在随机后的1天内开始"。如果事实上这9名受试者有复杂的皮肤和皮肤组织感染，延迟抗菌治疗将会使他们原发感染恶化、感染扩散、败血症和死亡的风险增高。我们已经确认，研究监查员未能充分认识临床研究者随机后一再拖延给药做法的严重性。而且，您们也未能采取适当的纠正措施，以防这一问题在此试验场所反复出现。

4. 未能确保只有经过培训和有经验而取得资格的研究者才能经过选取作为专家来试验药物［21 CFR 312.53（a）］

J & J PRD在551没有挑选出合格的研究者来做试验。特别是，J & J PRD还是选择了Desai博士（试验场所551），尽管研究前的监查访视记录表明“不推荐”此研究者，因其在完成法规文件（包括伦理委员会批件）方面缺乏依从性，在研究启动阶段缺乏积极主动性，而且没有充足的受试者病源人群等。研究监查员还建议不要使用此研究场所，因为此场所拒绝使用西班牙语版的知情同意书，但这一地区的人口构成为大量以西班牙语为母语或者喜欢使用西班牙语的人群。这些问题应该足够提醒您们这样一个事实，此研究者的经验表明她不是一个合格的专家来承当此项研究。

在您2008年6月24日给FDA的回复中，声明当您们质疑（b）（4）代表为什么研究监查员已经建议不选用该研究场所而仍然被选用时，（b）（4）提供了一份2008年6月3日的备忘录，声称CRO的主管否决了研究监查员的建议。但是按照（b）（4）工作流程，应该是J & J PRD而不是（b）（4）负责对参加研究的研究场所进行最后的审批。更有甚者，直到FDA完成此次现场检查之后J & J PRD都没有对此进行调查。根据您的回复，似乎表明您们或者没有积极主动地参加此试验场所的筛选，或者是没有审阅并处理不推荐选用此中心的研究监查报告。

本警告信的目的并不是罗列您在试验药物临床研究中存在的所有缺陷。确保遵循法律和相关FDA法规的每一项要求是您的职责。您应当解决这些缺陷，并建立规程，以确保任何正在进行或将来进行的研究均能符合FDA法规。

自收到这封信的15个工作日内，您应当书面告知本办公室为预防将来发生类似违规情况已经或将要采取的措施。如果不能充分、迅速地解释上述违规问题，可能导致我们在不再通知的情况下采取监管措施。如果您认为您遵循了FDA的法规要求，请陈述您的理由，并提供所有支持资料，以供我们参考。

附：英文原文

Johnson & Johnson Pharmaceutical Research & Development, LLC

WARNING LETTER

Aug 10，2009

CERTIFIED MAIL
RETURN RECEIPT REQUESTED

Ref:09-HFD-45-07-02

Karen Grosser, Ph.D,M.B.A.
Johnson & Johnson Pharmaceutical Research & Development, LLC
920U.S.Highway202
P.O.Box300
Raritan, NJ08869-0602

Dear Dr. Grosser:

This Warning Letter is to inform you of objectionable conditions found during the U.S. Food and Drug

Administration's (FDA) investigation into Johnson & Johnson Pharmaceutical Research & Development's (hereafter referred to as J & J PRD) role as sponsor of Study (b)(4) entitled (b) (4) and Study (b) (4) entitled (b) (4) of the investigational drug, (b) (4).

The first study, **(b)(4)** was initiated by the original holder of IND **(b)(4)** (hereafter referred to as **(b)(4)** On February 2, 2005 **(b)(4)** entered into a worldwide partnership with **(b)(4)**, a **(b)(4)**, to develop and market **(b)(4)** (referred to as **(b)(4)** Under the terms of the agreement, **(b)(4)** was to be developed further by J & J PRD and all rights and responsibilities for **(b) (4)** clinical trials were transferred to you. The second study, **(b)(4)** was conducted in its entirety by you.

This inspection is a part of the FDA's Bioresearch Monitoring Program, which is designed to evaluate the conduct of research and to ensure that the rights, safety, and welfare of the human subjects of those studies have been protected. Another objective of the program is to ensure that data submitted in support of New Drug Applications are scientifically valid and accurate.

From our review of the establishment inspection report and the documents submitted with that report, and your letter written in response to the Form FDA 483, dated June 24, 2008, and your responses dated September 2, 2008 and September 4, 2008 in response to additional information requests from the FDA, we conclude that you did not adhere to the applicable statutory requirements and FDA regulations governing the conduct of clinical investigations. We are aware that at the conclusion of the inspection, Ms. Wydner presented and discussed with you Form FDA 483, Inspectional Observations. We wish to emphasize the following:

1. Failure to ensure proper monitoring of the clinical investigations [21 CFR 312.50; 312.56(a)].

FDA regulations require that sponsors ensure proper monitoring of clinical investigations. Our investigation found that J & J PRD failed to properly ensure monitoring of the studies referenced above. Although J & J PRD contracted with **(b) (4)** (hereafter referred to as **(b) (4)** to conduct monitoring visits for **(b) (4)** and **(b) (4)**, **(b) (4)** did not ensure that the clinical investigators were properly monitored to fully assess and ensure site compliance with Studies **(b) (4)** and **(b) (4)** Inadequate monitoring resulted in deficiencies in recordkeeping with respect to case histories and drug accountability by clinical investigators participating in the above-referenced studies. As sponsor of Studies **(b) (4)** and **(b) (4)** conducted under Investigational New Drug Application **(b) (4)** and submitted in NDA **(b) (4)**, you were responsible for ensuring that these studies were adequately monitored for compliance with regulatory requirements, thereby ensuring that the data supporting the NDA was of good quality, and that the rights, welfare, and safety of study subjects were adequately protected. Violations include, but were not limited to, the following:

a. Deficiencies in case histories:

i. Study monitors failed to identify that on multiple occasions, site personnel documented administration of study drug to different subjects at precisely the same time. For example:

a) For Study **(b) (4)** at Site #520, study monitors failed to identify that on multiple occasions, study coordinators documented administration of study drug to two different subjects at the same time. On April 27, 2005, you allowed enrollment of subjects at Site #520 to resume, based upon your review of the site's April 27, 2005 plan for "Outpatient Treatment Procedures." Implementation of this plan was to begin on April 27, 2005. The Outpatient Treatment Procedures plan called for only the first dose of the study drug to be administered in the site's designated infusion center, and for the remaining doses to be administered by a study nurse or a home health nurse in the patient's home. In light of these procedures, study monitors should have identified that on multiple occasions, study coordinators documented administration of study drug to two different subjects at the same time, and should have sought an explanation for these observations.

Specifically,

i) Study Coordinator **(b)(6)** was documented as having administered study drug to the following subjects at the same time on the same date:

(a) Subject #1266 at 09:00-10:00 and Subject #1267 at 09:00-10:00 on 7/2/05

(b) Subject #1266 at 09:00-10:15 and Subject #1267 at 09:00-10:15 on 7/3/05

(c) Subject #1266 at 21:00-22:00 and Subject #1267 at 21:00-22:00 on 7/5/05

(d) Subject #1266 at 21:00-22:00 and Subject #1267 at 21:00-22:00 on 7/6/05

(e) Subject #1266 at 09:00-10:00 and Subject #1267 at 09:00-10:15 on 7/7/05

ii) Study Coordinator **(b)(6)** was documented as having administered study drug to Subject #2273 at 10:00-11:00 and to Subject #2275 at 10:00-11:00 on 7/26/05.

We find that the response you provided in your June 24, 2008 letter to these observations was inadequate. You stated that source documents did not indicate that infusions were given in subjects' homes, and that the study coordinator at the site told you that these infusions must have been given in the office.

Given the site outpatient treatment plan and the study monitoring that was conducted for the identified subjects, study monitors should have noted that on multiple occasions, study site personnel documented administration of study drug to different subjects at precisely the same time, and should have investigated further the reason for this irregularity. Your June 24, 2008 letter provided no explanation for your failure to notice these discrepancies and to seek an explanation from site staff before FDA's investigation revealed the discrepancies.

Moreover, despite the study coordinator's statement that these infusions must have been given in the office, based on the FDA investigation conducted at the site, we have determined that subjects enrolled in the study continued to self-administer study medications at their homes beyond the time when the site's April 27, 2005 plan was to have been implemented. In addition, it would not be possible for the same study coordinator to begin study infusions on more than one subject at precisely the same time even if the two subjects had been treated at the same location.

b) For Study **(b)(4)** at Site #063, study monitors failed to identify that on multiple occasions, the same study nurse, **(b)(6)** was documented in the "*Planilla de estabilidad*" as having administered study drug to different subjects at precisely the same time as follows:

i) On May 20, the study nurse **(b)(6)** is documented as having administered study drug to the following subjects at 08:00-10:00:

(a) Subject #140616 (b)(6)

(b) Subject #140132 (b)(6)

(c) Subject #140617 (b)(6)

(d) Subject #140118 **(b)(6)**

ii) On May 20, the study nurse **(b)(6)** is documented as having stated placebo infusions to the following subjects at 10:00-11:00:

(a) Subject #140616 **(b)(6)**

(b) Subject #140132 (b)(6)

(c) Subject #140617 (b)(6)

(d) Subject #140118 **(b)(6)**

Based on the copies of the "Notas De Enfermeria" that you provided for each of these subjects in your submission to the FDA dated September 2, 2008, we find that the initials included in the nursing note for each of the doses noted in the bullets i)(a)-(d) and ii)(a)-(d) above are consistent with those recorded on the "Planilla de estabilidad" for each subject, and with the initials (b) (6) for the study nurse recorded on the "Site Personnel Responsibility Log." The documents provided with your September 2, 2008 submission thus confirm the FDA's findings. Study monitors should have recognized that on multiple occasions, the same individual was documented as having administered study drug to different subjects at precisely the same time, and should have investigated further the reason for this irregularity.

ii. Source documentation verification was completed by study monitors for Subject #141050 enrolled in Study **(b)(4)** at Site #551, according to the table you provided that was labeled "Subjects 100% Source Document Verification"; however, study monitors failed to identify that no physical examination, wound assessment, or overall clinical assessment was documented in study source documents or in the Case Report Form (CRF) for this subject's Day 8 visit, as required by the protocol. We note that you did not address this observation in your June 24, 2008 letter to the Agency.

iii. Study monitors failed to identify that for both Study **(b)(4)** and Study **(b)(4)** the times that infusions were "delivered to Nursing Unit" were not recorded. For example:

a) At Site #502, according to the **(b)(4)** worksheet, the times that reconstituted study drug was delivered to the nursing unit were "not recorded" on at least four occasions for Subject #1118. We note that you did not address this observation in your June 24, 2008 letter to the Agency.

b) At Site #508, according to the **(b)(4)** worksheet, the times that reconstituted study drug was delivered to the nursing unit were "not recorded" on at least seven occasions for Subject #140005. We note that in your June 24, 2008 letter to the Agency, you confirmed that delivery times were not documented and that study monitors failed to document these deviations.

ⅳ. Protocol (b)(4) stated that reconstituted study drug infusion solutions should "be stored at room temperature (25°C) and used within 6 hours, or stored for up to 16 hours under refrigeration (5°C) and used within 3 hours after removal from the refrigerator." Because the study protocol did not outline outpatient dosing conventions, in e-mail correspondence between Site #509 and the study monitor dated October 20, 2004, the study monitor sought assurance that there was documentation to show that study medication was being maintained and stored under proper temperature conditions by patients who were to self-administer the study drug in their own homes. Although asked, the site never addressed how they would document the temperature storage conditions of the product in subjects' homes; site personnel only addressed how subject body temperatures were to be recorded. Study monitors failed to recognize that the site's response was incomplete and accepted this response as complete. Subject diaries were then created and used by the site that did not include a place to record storage temperatures of infusions that were stored in subjects' refrigerators. Therefore, storage temperatures for these infusions could not be confirmed to have complied with storage conditions specified by the protocol. The importance of maintaining proper temperature conditions in patients' homes is evidenced by page three of the " (b)(4) Outpatient Study Drug Procedure," dated "25 May 2005," which stated that the "receiving site storage conditions must be confirmed upon delivery of the study medication. Clinic, investigator office and/or patient refrigerator temperatures must be recorded and the plan must specify where and by whom."

We note that in your June 24, 2008 letter to the Agency, while you contended that stability of the drug product was likely maintained in subjects' homes, you also confirmed that there was no documentation of study drug storage conditions in subjects' homes.

ⅴ. Drug shipments from (b)(4) contained "Refrigerated Shipment Inspection Instructions" that included instructions to fill out readings from a temperature-recording device on the bottom of the Packing List and to return this device to (b)(4) if the device screen had a "bell" showing (potentially signifying shipment did not maintain appropriate conditions for some reason). If no bell was seen, the shipment maintained appropriate temperatures and the contents could be used. An April 4, 2005 Packing List for Order #1000739 shipped to Site #520 for Study (b)(4) was identified for which temperatures were recorded as being out of range on the bottom of the sheet; however, no documentation was present for the return of the temperature-recording device or for follow-up to the site regarding the acceptability of use of the kits contained in this shipment. Source documents demonstrated that drug from kits contained in this shipment were dispensed and administered to study subjects between April and June 2005. The Unblinded Monitoring Visit Report (dated May 25, 2005) encompassing monitoring of Site #520 for the time frame when this shipment was received failed to document the out-of-range temperature readings or appropriate follow-up instructions to the site regarding usage of the kits in this shipment.

In your response letter dated June 24, 2008, you stated that an additional stability study, completed after the drugs from this kit were dispensed to study subjects and after the May 25, 2005 Unblinded Monitoring Visit Report, supported "temperature excursions up to maximum 25°C are allowed for up to maximum 2 days." However, FDA notes that this stability study was conducted subsequent to shipment of referenced Order #1000739; therefore, based on documentation available at the time, study monitors conducting the Unblinded Monitoring Visit should have recognized that drug kits from Order #1000739 should not have been administered to subjects.

ⅵ. For Study (b)(4) at Site #146, "Ⅳ stability" worksheets were missing for all 39 subjects enrolled, and corrective actions by study monitors were inadequate to correct this deficiency throughout the study. According to the Work Order for this study, unblinded monitoring visits by (b)(4) were to occur every 10 weeks.

FDA notes that in your response dated June 24, 2008 you state that the issue was recorded in the unblinded monitoring visit reports dated 27 January 2006 and 25 September 2006, along with documentation that the monitor requested completion of these worksheets, and that the site generate a Memo to File that documented the Ⅳ temperature stability conditions for previously enrolled subjects. However, the issue should have been addressed again prior to the 25 September 2006 unblinded monitoring visit. The Memo to File that was finally written on 16 November 2006, after completion of subject enrollment at the site, stated only that "i.v. stability has been maintained according to the IV label, which states start/finish time and the expiry time of the infusion, patient number." This statement does not provide sufficient detail to ensure that temperature stability conditions for the drug were maintained adequately.

ⅶ. For Study (b)(4) at Site #520, study monitors failed to identify discrepancies in the time of delivery of study drug to nursing unit as recorded on (b)(4) worksheets, and the time of administration of the study drug as recorded on "Administration of Study Medication" worksheets for multiple subjects. For example:

a) For Subject #1187, source documents indicate:

ⅰ) on 3/1/05, study drug was delivered at 19:05; study drug administration time is documented as 18:00-19:00

ⅱ) on 3/2/05, study drug was delivered at 19:10; study drug administration time is documented as 18:00-19:00

ⅲ) on 3/11/05, study drug was delivered at 18:05; study drug administration time is documented as 18:00-19:00

ⅳ) on 3/12/05, study drug was delivered at 18:40; study drug administration time is documented as 18:00-19:00.

b) For Subject #1195, source documents indicate:

i) on 4/14/05, study drug was delivered at 09:00; study drug administration is documented as 08:05-09:05

c) For Subject #2671, source documents indicate:

ⅰ) on 5/11/05, study drug was delivered at 10:00; study drug administration is documented as 09:30-10:30

ⅱ) on 5/12/05, study drug was delivered at 09:55; study drug administration is documented as 09:30-10:30

ⅲ) on 5/13/05, study drug was delivered at 09:50; study drug administration is documented as 09:30-10:30

We note that in your June 24, 2008 letter to the Agency, you state that differences in times occurred due to the site recording anticipated times of administration rather than actual times of administration, and you acknowledge that study monitors failed to identify these discrepancies in source documents.

ⅷ. For Study **(b) (4)** and **(b) (4)** study monitors failed to identify discrepancies in study records related to observations and data pertinent to the investigation. For example:

For Study **(b) (4)** at Site #520, source documents and study documents contain conflicting information related to wound dimensions, debridement of wounds, and signs and symptoms of infection for multiple subjects, which were not identified by the monitors. For example:

a) Subject #1010 was enrolled in the study with Wound #2 documented as the qualifying study wound for study enrollment, according to a source document for the baseline visit. In the sub-investigator's "Outpatient Wound Care Progress Note" for 3/22/05, the dimensions of the wound were documented as 10mm × 4mm; also documented was that the wound was too sensitive for debridement. However, a wound care source document dated 3/23/05 documented that the study wound had been debrided on 3/22/05, and that the wound dimensions were 25mm x 30mm. We also note that page 2 of 4 of the source document for the "Test of Cure, Clinical Assessment" dated 3/23/05 was initialed and dated 3/5/05 by the sub-investigator, a date which is 18 days prior to the date that this source document records the visit to have occurred.

b) For Subject #1186, the sub-investigator's progress note for 3/7/05 stated that the wound dimensions were 21mm × 25mm. Study source document worksheets for the 3/7/05 visit originally documented wound dimensions of 17mm × 15mm, but on 4/18/05 dimensions were lined through and revised to 21mm × 25mm. As this source document also stated that "wound assessment done per MD + reported to CRC," it is unclear why originally recorded dimensions were inconsistent with those documented in the sub-investigator's progress note. Similarly: 1) the sub-investigator's progress note for 3/14/2005 stated the wound dimensions were 23mm × 29mm, but the source document for the same day originally documented wound dimensions of 15mm × 10mm; then on 4/18/05, dimensions recorded on the source document were lined through and revised to 23mm × 29mm; and 2) the sub-investigator's progress note for 3/21/2005 stated the wound dimensions were 14mm × 23mm, but page 2 of 4 of the source document for the same day originally documented wound dimensions of 8mm × 6mm. On 4/18/04, the dimensions appearing on the source document were lined through and revised to 14mm × 23mm. On the corresponding CRF page for the 4/18/05 visit, the wound dimensions, however, were still documented as 8mm × 6mm. In addition, the subinvestigator's progress note for the 3/14/07 documents "much less inflammation and little drainage," but the source document for this visit date documents drainage or discharge as absent and erythema as absent.

c) For Subject #2274, the source document for the End of Treatment visit, dated 7-26-05, documented wound dimensions of 13mm × 20mm and a wound assessment of "absent-reddness [sic], pain, edema, heat, flutuance [sic], funct impair, drainage," but on another page of the same source document dimensions were listed as 1mm × 0mm, drainage or discharge was checked as improved, and pain or tenderness to palpation was checked as unchanged. The corresponding CRF page for the End of Therapy visit documents wound dimensions as 80mm × 95mm.

We note that in your June 24, 2008 letter to the Agency, you acknowledge that study monitors failed to identify these discrepancies in source documents.

b. Deficiencies in drug accountability:

For Study **(b) (4)** at Site #551, study documents contained conflicting information regarding accountability of the drug. When **(b) (4)** and Drug Accountability Form source document worksheets were compared, it appears that on multiple occasions, the same kit vial was recorded as having been given to more than one subject, and/or on more than one occasion to the same subject, or the recorded kit vial information was incomplete. Examples include, but are not limited to:

(b)(4)Worksheet (Kit-Vial) (Date) (Subject#)	**Drug Accountability Form Worksheet (Kit-Vial) (Date) (Subject#)**
21148-8 1-Aug-06 #141059	21148-8 30-Jul-06 #141052
21148-1 1-Aug-06 #141059	21148-1 02-Aug-06 #141052
22609-2 2-Aug-06 #141059	22609-2 27-Jul-06 #141052
10131-8 5-Aug-06 #141059	10131-8 03-Aug-06 #141059
60126-1 03-Aug-06 #141062	60126-1 02-Aug-06 #141059
60126-18 03-Aug-06 #141062	60126-18 08-Aug-06 #141062
60126-7 07-Aug-06and08-Aug-06 #141062	60126-7 04-Aug-06 #141062
23631-15 11-Aug-06 #141066	23631-15 08-Aug-06 #141066
23631-8 11-Aug-06 #141066	23631-8 08-Aug-06 #141066
23110-18 14-Aug-06 #141067	23110-18 No Record of Being Dispensed
23110-4 14-Aug-06 #141067	23110-4 No Record of Being Dispensed

The study monitors failed to notice these discrepancies, despite the fact that the contents of a single vial, which would constitute a single treatment course for one subject, were documented to have been used multiple times. We note that you did not specifically address these observations in your June 24, 2008 letter to the Agency, or in any of the subsequent submissions to the Agency.

2. Failure to ensure that an investigation was conducted in accordance with the general investigational plan and protocols as specified in the IND [21 CFR 312.50].

a. Study monitors failed to ensure that the investigation was conducted in accordance with the investigational plan for Study **(b) (4)** For example:

Study monitors failed to ensure that planned study blinding procedures were correctly followed for Study **(b) (4)** at Site #063. This study was to be conducted in a double-blind fashion. According to the Protocol (Section 6.2, Blinding and Randomization), "the unblinded pharmacist will be responsible for preparing the study medication for each subject in such a way that investigators and staff remain blinded to the medication being administered."

i. At Site #063, study nurses, rather than the unblinded pharmacist, were responsible for completing drug dissolution and reconstitution, as well as administering study drug infusions and caring for the subjects. Therefore, nursing personnel caring for subjects (i.e. study staff) were not blinded to study treatment, as specified by the protocol.

We note that you did not address this observation in your June 24, 2008 letter to the Agency.

ii. At Site #063, for Study **(b) (4)** Investigators may have been unblinded to the treatment group for five subjects (#140103, #140107, #140114, #140111, and #140112), since the nursing notes included the name of blinded medication infused. Nursing notes were viewed by clinical investigators at the site. Although it appears that the nurses used correction fluid to cover writing, in some cases the covered writing could still be read, according to the **(b) (4)** Unblinded Monitoring Visit Report, dated 11-12 May 2006. The **(b) (4)** Unblinded Monitoring Visit Report, dated 11-12 May 2006, in relation to this finding, states that "the infirmary notes are to be seen by the blinded staff, so we do not know for sure if these notes were seen by them." This report also includes instructions to the site from **(b) (4)** Monitors that are clearly inconsistent with International Conference on Harmonization Good Clinical Practice (GCP) guidelines, in that it states, " we called the Lead Study Monitor and she instructed to strike out these inclusions with black marker to prevent further potential of unblinding. This procedure was done by the Lead Study Nurse, who included her initials and date." GCP guidelines generally state that any change or correction to a document should be dated, initialed, and explained (if necessary) and should not obscure the original entry; therefore, both Site #063 personnel and **(b) (4)** monitors assigned to this site failed to appropriately make corrections to source documents for at least 5 subjects enrolled at the site.

We note that in your June 24, 2008 letter to the Agency, you acknowledge that GCP guidelines were not followed, and that in the future site managers and study monitors will be reminded through use of specific training modules of the importance of appropriate completion of source documents.

b. Study monitors failed to identify that for at least fourteen subjects (#141051, #140040, #140051, #141050, #141074, #141080, #141061, #141067, #141066, #141062, #141068, #141059, #141060, and #141079) enrolled in Study **(b) (4)** at Site #551, the drug infusion order was reversed for infusions #4 and #5 daily. For example, for Subject #141051 in the **(b) (4)** arm, the protocol required that the 4th dose be placebo given over 60 minutes, and that the 5th dose be **(b) (4)** given over 120 minutes; however, the site administered **(b) (4)** over 120 minutes as the 4th dose and placebo over 60 minutes as the 5th dose.

The response that you provided in your June 24, 2008 letter states that the site acknowledges that the drug infusion order/infusion duration was reversed for daily infusions #4 and #5, and you also acknowledge that the study monitor did not identify this issue during site monitoring visits.

c. Study monitors failed to identify that for both Study **(b)(4)** and Study **(b)(4)** subjects who did not meet eligibility criteria were enrolled. For example:

i. For Study **(b)(4)** at Site #520, Subject #1011 was enrolled on March 3, 2005 for treatment of a left foot abscess. This subject did not meet the inclusion criterion for enrollment of a subject with diagnosis of abscess because the onset of the abscess was greater than 7 days prior to enrollment. A Data Correction Form (DCF) dated 27-May-2005 stated that the subject received antibiotic treatment with Bactrim DS with end date of 21-FEB-2005, and a CI comment in source documents stated that the subject had received the Bactrim for treatment of the left foot abscess.

Therefore, the left foot abscess was present for more than 7 days prior to enrollment, and this subject should not have been enrolled.

We find that the response you provided in your June 24, 2008 letter to this observation was inadequate. You stated only that the subject met inclusion criteria, but you did not address the fact that the index infection had been present for more than 7 days, which would have precluded the subject from study enrollment.

ii. For Study **(b)(4)** at Site #551, study monitors failed to identify that while Subjects #141061 and #141074 were documented to have had pregnancy tests done, the site did not have the test results and/or did not document the negative pregnancy tests results for these subjects prior to enrollment, as was required for females of childbearing potential by the protocol.

We note that in your June 24, 2006 letter to the Agency, you confirmed that pregnancy test results for these subjects were not documented, and that study monitors failed to identify this issue.

iii. For Study **(b)(4)** at Site #063, study monitors failed to identify that Subject #140107 was not eligible for the study. Protocol **(b)(4)** required that infection at a site of prior surgery/trauma occur within 30 days of the surgery/trauma. However, for Subject #140107, the prior surgery was documented as having taken place 20 months prior to the study screening visit.

Based on the source documents for Subject #140107, and translations of those documents that you provided in your submission to the Agency dated September 2, 2008, you stated that the source documents do not support that a specific traumatic event precipitated the infection; and that Dr. **(b)(4)** further told you that this subject's old surgical site was intermittently inflamed, and that when the subject was enrolled, the site of infection was draining pus and was inflamed and painful, and that the infection had begun 30 days prior to enrollment. While you did not concede in your September 2, 2008 submission that this subject did not qualify for enrollment, the additional information included in your September 2, 2008 submission supports that this subject also did not qualify for enrollment based on criteria for any of the other types of complicated skin and skin structure infections described in the inclusion criteria.

d. For Study **(b)(4)** at Site #551, study monitors failed to identify that the unblinded site pharmacist did not receive baseline creatinine clearance (CrCl) results in a time frame adequate to ensure appropriate study drug dosing calculations, as required by the protocol. For example,

i. The following CrCls were not faxed to the study pharmacist until August 12, 2006, which was well after subjects' enrollment and start of dosing:

a) Subject #141060, randomized August 1, 2006
b) Subject #141061, randomized August 2, 2006
c) Subject #141066, randomized August 7, 2006
d) Subject #141067, randomized August 8, 2006
e) Subject #141068, randomized August 9, 2006

ii. The following CrCls were not faxed to the study pharmacist until November 14, 2006, which was 2-3 months after their respective end of treatment visits:

a) Subject #141062
b) Subject #141069
c) Subject #141079
d) Subject #141080
e) Subject #141050
f) Subject #140040
g) Subject #141069
h) Subject #141074
i) Subject #140051
j) Subject #140076
k) Subject #140063

In your June 24, 2008 submission to the Agency, a copy of a monitoring report dated 15 Aug 2006 that stated, "Pharmacist to provide copies of CrCl for all patients. Done" was provided. However, this response is inadequate, as this does not provide assurance that CrCl values were forwarded to the pharmacist in a time frame that would have allowed appropriate dosing adjustments, if warranted.

3. Failure to secure investigator compliance with the investigational plan and applicable FDA regulations [21 CFR 312.56(b)].

Under FDA regulations, a sponsor who discovers that an investigator is not complying with the signed investigator agreement [Form FDA 1572], the general investigational plan, or the requirements of applicable FDA regulations, shall promptly either secure compliance or discontinue shipment of the drug to the investigator and terminate the investigator's participation. If the investigator's participation is terminated, the sponsor shall notify FDA. Our investigation found that you failed to adequately implement corrective actions at Site #063, for Study **(b) (4)** For example:

According to footnote 1) of the Schedule of Assessments in Clinical Protocol **(b) (4)** "all screening/predose assessments will be considered as baseline and must be performed and reviewed before **randomization and dosing on Day 1**, (emphasis added) with the exception of the PK sample collections." Based on this statement and on other training and materials made available to clinical investigators, all patients should have begun dosing on the same day as randomization. For Study **(b) (4)** at Site #063, nine subjects did not receive study drug for more than 24 hours after randomization, ranging from approximately 48 hours to eleven days post randomization. For example, Subject #140117 was randomized on 05 May 2006 and received first dose of medication on 16 May 2006. According to the Unblinded Monitoring Visit Report dated 06 Sep 2006, the delay was due to "personal problems of the patient." This was noted as a minor issue in the post monitoring visit letter to unblinded site staff and was not mentioned at all in the post monitoring visit letter to the Clinical Investigator. In addition, no corrective action was documented in monitoring reports or follow-up letters to Site #063.

We find that the response that you provided in your June 24, 2008 letter to these observations was inadequate. You stated that the protocol did not specify the duration of the predose phase of the study, nor how soon after screening, treatment needed to be started, but you acknowledged that "the expectation for the study was that all study treatments were to begin within 1 calendar day of randomization." The delay in administration of appropriate **(b)(4)** therapy for these nine patients, if they in fact had complicated skin and skin structure infections, would have placed them at increased risk for worsening of primary infection, dissemination of infection, sepsis, and death. We have determined that study monitors failed to fully recognize the significance of the clinical investigator's practice of repetitively delaying study drug dosing post subject randomization. In addition, you failed to implement appropriate corrective actions to prevent this issue from recurring at the site.

4. Failure to ensure that only investigators who were qualified by training and experience were selected as appropriate experts to investigate a drug [21 CFR 312.53(a)].

J&J PRD failed to select a qualified investigator to conduct the study at Site #551. Specifically, J&J PRD selected Dr. Desai (Site #551), despite a pre-study monitoring visit that documented that the investigator "is not recommended" for lack of compliance in completing regulatory documents (including IRB approvals), lack of diligence in study start up procedures and inadequate patient population. This study monitor also recommended that this site not be used because the site declined use of Spanish Informed Consent Forms when demographics of the region indicated a large population with native and preferred language of Spanish. These problems should have alerted you to the fact that this investigator's experience may not have qualified her as an appropriate expert to conduct the study.

In your response to the Agency, dated June 24, 2008, you stated that when you questioned **(b) (4)** representatives regarding why this site was selected despite the study monitor recommendation to not use the site, **(b) (4)** provided a memo dated June 3, 2008 that stated the CRO supervisor overruled the study monitor recommendation. According to the **(b) (4)** Work Order, however, J &J PRD, not **(b) (4)** was responsible for final approval of sites for participation in the study. Furthermore, J&J PRD failed to make this inquiry until after the FDA inspection. Based on your response, it appears that you either failed to actively participate in selection of the site or failed to review and address the study monitoring report that recommended the site not be used.

This letter is not intended to be an all-inclusive list of deficiencies with your clinical studies of an investigational drug. It is your responsibility to ensure adherence to each requirement of the law and relevant FDA regulations. You should address these deficiencies and establish procedures to ensure that any ongoing or future studies will be in compliance with FDA regulations.

Within fifteen (15) working days of your receipt of this letter, you should notify this office in writing of the actions you have taken or will be taking to prevent similar violations in the future. Failure to adequately and promptly explain the violations noted above may result in regulatory action without further notice.

If you have any questions, please contact Tejashri Purohit-Sheth, M.D., at 301-796-3402; FAX 301-847-8748. Your written response and any pertinent documentation should be addressed to:

Tejashri Purohit-Sheth, M.D.
Branch Chief
Good Clinical Practice Branch Ⅱ
Division of Scientific Investigations
Office of Compliance
Center for Drug Evaluation and Research
Food and Drug Administration
Bldg 51, Room 5358
10903 New Hampshire Avenue
Silver Spring, MD 20993

Sincerely yours,

{See appended electronic signature page}

Leslie K. Ball, M.D.
Director
Division of Scientific Investigations
Office of Compliance
Center for Drug Evaluation and Research

第47封　给Travanti Pharma有限公司的警告信

2008年6月30日

参考号：08-HFD-45-0601

尊敬的Cohen先生：

2008年2月19～28日，Sharon Matson女士，代表FDA进行了现场检查，与您会面并审查了您公司作为申办者，为Travanti制药股份有限公司的下列药-械组合产品［ ］所开展临床研究的执行情况。

本次现场检查是FDA的生物研究监查项目的一部分，该项目通过设定的检查方法，评估相关研究的实施情况，以确保这些研究中受试者的权益、安全和福利得到了保护。

我们知道在现场检查结束时，Maston女士向您出示并讨论了FDA483表，即现场检查发现的问题。根据对现场检查报告、该报告的附件和贵公司2008年3月11日对FDA483表的回复进行审查，我们认为，您没有遵循适用的法律要求和监管临床研究的FDA法规。我们想重点强调以下几点：

1. 未能根据21 CFR 312.2（a）的要求对开展新药临床研究提交IND申请［21 CFR 312.20（a）和312.40（a）］

FDA法规21 CFR 312涵括了关于试验新药使用的程序规定和实体要求。21 CFR 312（b）对于临床研究的定义是“任何将药品使用、配给到，或其使用涉及，一个或多个受试者的试验。根据本法这一部分的目的，试验是指除了在医疗活动过程中使用已上市药品以外的任何使用某一药物的行为。”

如果以下的条件能够得到满足，则一种研究新药可以在一项临床研究中使用：申办者为此新药向FDA提交了IND申请，该项IND申请是在FDA的监管之下生效，并且申办者符合21 CFR 50、56和312的所有要求，同时每个参与研究的研究者行为也都应遵从21 CFR 50、56和312以及21 CFR 312.40（a）法规的所有要求。

药-械组合产品［ ］还没有被批准在美国上市。关于药-械组合产品［ ］的临床研究没有从取得21 CFR 312的豁免，必须满足临床研究试验用新药在临床研究中使用的一般要求。参看21 CFR 312.2。上述所列的三项临床研究［ ］显示出不能豁免21 CFR 312.2（a）的要求，也不在21 CFR 312.2（b）的豁免之列，所以必须取得IND批准。因此，Travanti制药股份有限公司是在提交IND申请并在其生效得到批准之前就开始了［ ］的临床研究。

2. 未能在允许某一研究者参加研究之前，取得研究者声明、FDA1572表［21 CFR 31253（c）（1）］

具体而言，Travanti制药股份有限公司在没有获得21CFR312豁免的情况下启动了临床研究，并且允许研究者们在没有取得研究者声明签字之前参加了研究。声明包括以下内容：

a. 研究者姓名和地址；

b. IND中载明将由该研究者执行的临床研究实施方案的名称和编码；

c. 执行临床研究者所在医学院、医院或其他研究设施的名称和地址；

d. 在临床研究中将会使用的任何临床实验室设施的名称和地址；

e. 负责审查和批准研究的IRB的名称和地址；

f. 研究者所做的承诺，她或他：

i. 将会依照相关的、现有的试验方案开展试验，并且只有在通知申办者后，才可以对试验方案进行修改，且必须是为了保护受试者的安全、权利或利益。

ⅱ. 将会遵守关于临床研究者责任的所有要求和法规规定的所有其他相关要求；

ⅲ. 将亲自承担或者监督所述研究的开展；

ⅳ. 将会告知任何潜在受试者即将使用的药品是以研究为目的，并且确保满足获取知情同意（21 CFR 50）及伦理委员会审查和批准（21 CFR 56）的相关要求；

ⅴ. 按照312.64要求，向申办者报告在研究过程中发生的任何不良事件；

ⅵ. 已经阅读并理解研究者手册中的信息，包括潜在的风险和药物的副作用；

ⅶ. 将会确保所有协助试验开展的助手、同事及雇员都了解自己的责任，以此来满足以上的承诺。

g. 研究者承诺，临床研究将21 CFR 56接受IRB的审查，符合本部分要求的以下研究受试者需要伦理审查的要求。符合此部分要求的IRB将会负责启动和持续对临床研究进行审查、审批。研究者需及时向IRB报告在研究活动中的任何变化和所有危及受试者或者其他人的不可预期的问题，未经IRB批准，不得对研究作出任何改变。必须采取措施消除对受试者明显的即时的伤害者除外。

h. 协助研究者开展研究的助理研究者（例如研究助理、住院医生）人员名单。

3. 没有选择已经过培训和有经验的、合格的监查员来监查研究过程［21 CFR 312.53（d）］

FDA 现场检查发现，贵公司没有保留任何文件记录，能够表明上述需要使用试验用新药的临床研究得到充分适当的监查。

4. 没有保留充分、适当的记录来表明试验药物的接收、运送或者其他处置［CFR 312.57（a）］

FDA现场检查披露贵公司没有保留需要试验用新药的上述研究中的药品清点记录。作为申办者，贵公司被要求须保留药品处置记录，并包括，视情况而定，接收药品的研究者姓名，每一运送批次的时间、数量和批号或者编码标记。

5. 未能按照21 CFR 312.57（b）中的要求，保留21 CFR 54中所述的关于研究者的任何财务利益的足够准确的记录

FDA现场检查发现，上述的需要试验用新药的研究中，贵公司并没有保留足够准确的记录来表明21 CFR 54.4（a）（3）（ⅰ），（a）（3）（ⅱ），（a）（3）（ⅲ）和（a）（3）（ⅳ）中规定的，由申办者向有关研究的研究者所支付的任何财务利益。作为申办者，要求贵公司保留的足够准确的记录应包括如下方面：

a. 有关临床试验的申办者与研究者达成的关于开展临床试验的任何财务上的安排，其中对临床试验研究者的补偿值可以受到研究结果的影响［21 CFR 54（a）（3）（ⅰ）］；

b. 来自有关临床研究申办者的任何其他种类的大额报酬，例如对正在进行的研究的奖励，以仪器的形式进行补偿，专家咨询费或谢礼［21 CFR 54（a）（3）（ⅱ）］；

c. 研究者持有的任何与该临床试验产品相关的资本性权益［21 CPR 54（a）（3）（ⅲ）］；

d. 参与有关任何临床试验的任何研究者持有该临床试验申办者的任何重大权益［21 CPR 54（a）（3）（ⅰ）］。

在贵公司2008年3月11日对FDA483表，即现场检查发现问题表的回复中，贵公司承认使用了［ ］的临床研究应该是在IND项下开展，并且也声称，其他的发现确属没有在IND下开展研究的失误。贵公司的回复也宣称，将来会建立相应流程来保证遵从FDA的法规。我们获悉贵公司保证将会采取纠正措施。然而我们注意到在这个回复中并没有包含为避免此类问题继续发生所制定的程序、步骤的详细提纲。

本警告信的目的并非是罗列您在试验药物临床研究中存在的所有缺陷。确保遵循法律和相关FDA法规的每一项要求是您的职责。您应当解决这些缺陷，并建立规程，以确保任何正在进行或将来进行的研究均能符合FDA的法规。

自收到这封信的15个工作日内，您应当书面告知本办公室为预防将来发生类似违规情况已经采取或将要采取的措施。如果不能充分、迅速地解释上述违规问题，可能导致我们在不再通知的情况下采取监管措施。

附：英文原文

Travanti Pharma, Inc

WARNING LETTER

JUN 30, 2008

CERTIFIEDMAIL
RETURN RECEIPT REQUESTED

Ref: 08-HFD-45-0601

Robert Cohen, President & CEO
Travanti Pharma, Inc.
2520 Pilot Knob Rd., Suite 100
Mendota Heights, MN 55120

Dear Mr. Cohen:

Between February 19 and 28, 2008, Ms. Sharon Matson, representing the Food and Drug Administration (FDA), conducted an investigation and met with you to review your firm's practices as the sponsor of the following clinical investigations of the investigational device-drug combination product, [ ] performed for Travanti Pharma, Inc.:

-
-
-

This inspection is a part of the FDA's Bioresearch Monitoring Program, which includes inspections designed to evaluate the conduct of research and to ensure that the rights, safety, and welfare of the human subjects of those studies have been protected.

We are aware that at the conclusion of the inspection, Ms. Matson presented and discussed with you Form FDA 483, Inspectional Observations. From our review of the establishment inspection report, the documents submitted with that report, and your firm's March 11, 2008, letter written in response to the Form FDA 483, we conclude that you did not adhere to the applicable statutory requirements and FDA regulations governing the conduct of clinical investigations. We wish to emphasize the following:

1. Failure to submit an IND for the conduct of clinical investigations with an investigational new drug that is subject to 21 CFR 312.2(a) [21 CFR 312.20(a) and 312.40(a)].

FDA regulations at 21 CFR Part 312 contain procedures and requirements governing the use of investigational new drugs. 21 CFR 312.3(b) defines a clinical investigation as "any experiment in which a drug is administered or dispensed to, or used involving, one or more human subjects. For the purposes of this part, an experiment is any use of a drug except for the use of a marketed drug in the course of medical practice."

An investigational new drug may be used in a clinical investigation if the following conditions are met: the sponsor submits an IND for the drug to FDA, the IND is in effect under FDA regulations, and the sponsor complies with all applicable requirements of 21 CFR Parts 50, 56, and 312; and each participating investigator conducts his investigation in compliance with the requirements of 21 CFR Parts 50, 56, and 312. 21 CFR 312.40(a).

The device-drug combination product of [ ] is not approved for marketing in the U.S.A. Clinical investigations involving the use of the device-drug combination product [ ] that are not exempt from 21 CFR Part 312 must meet the general requirements for use of an investigational new drug in a clinical investigation. See 21 CFR 312.2. The three clinical investigations listed above [ ] appear not to be exempt from 21 CFR 312.2(a) requirements and not within the exemptions of 21 CFR 312.2(b), and therefore required an IND. Thus, Travanti Pharma, Inc., initiated clinical investigations using [ ] prior to submitting, and having in effect, a required IND application.

2. Failure to obtain an investigator statement, Form FDA 1572, before permitting an investigator to participate in an investigation [21 CFR 312.53(c)(1)].

Specifically, Travanti Pharma, Inc., initiated clinical investigations that were not exempt from the requirements of 21 CFR Part 312 and allowed clinical investigators to participate in the investigation prior to obtaining a signed investigator statement containing:

a. The name and address of the investigator;

b. The name and code number, if any, of the protocol(s) in the IND identifying the study(ies) to be conducted by the investigator;

c. The name and address of any medical school, hospital, or other research facility where the clinical investigation(s) will be conducted;

d. The name and address of any clinical laboratory facilities to be used in the study;

e. The name and address of the IRB that is responsible for review and approval of the study(ies); .

f. A commitment by the investigator that he or she:

ⅰ.Will conduct the study(ies) in accordance with the relevant, current protocol(s) and will only make changes in a protocol after notifying the sponsor, except when necessary to protect the safety, the rights, or welfare of subjects;

ⅱ.Will comply with all requirements regarding the obligations of clinical investigators and all other pertinent requirements in this part;

ⅲ.Will personally conduct or supervise the described investigation(s);

ⅳ.Will inform any potential subjects that the drugs are being used for investigational purposes and will ensure that the requirements relating to obtaining informed consent (21 CFR part 50) and institutional review board review and approval (21 CFR part 56) are met;

ⅴ.Will report to the sponsor adverse experiences that occur in the course of the investigation(s) in accordance with 312.64;

ⅵ. Has read and understands the information in the investigator's brochure, including the potential risks and side effects of the drug; and

ⅶ. Will ensure that all associates, colleagues, and employees assisting in the conduct of the study(ies) are informed about their obligations in meeting the above commitments.

g. A commitment by the investigator that. for an investigation subject to an institutional review requirement under part 56, an IRB that complies with the requirements of that part will be responsible for the initial and continuing review and approval of the clinical investigation and that the investigator will promptly report to the IRB all changes in the research activity and all unanticipated problems involving risks to human subjects or others, and will not make any changes in the research without IRB approval, except where necessary to eliminate apparent immediate hazards to the human subjects.

h. A list of the names of the sub-investigators (e.g.• research fellows. residents) who will be assisting the investigator in the conduct of the investigation(s).

3. Failure to select a monitor qualified by training and experience to monitor the progress of the investigation [21 CFR 312.53(d)].

The FDA inspection disclosed that your firm did not maintain any documentation to indicate that the above studies requiring an IND were adequately monitored.

4. Failure to maintain adequate records' showing the receipt, shipment, or other disposition of the investigational drug [CFR 312.57(a)].

The FDA inspection disclosed that your firm did not maintain drug accountability records for the above studies requiring an IND. As a sponsor, your firm is required to maintain drug disposition records to include, as appropriate, the name of the investigator-to whom the drug is shipped, and the date, quantity, and batch or code mark of each such shipment.

5. Failure to maintain complete and accurate records showing any financial interests of investigators under 21 CFR Part 54 as described in 21 CFR 312.57(b).

The FDA inspection disclosed that, for the above studies requiring an IND, your firm did not maintain complete and accurate records showing any financial interest in 21 CFR 54.4(a)(3)(ⅰ), (a)(3)(ⅱ), (a)(3)(ⅲ), and (a)(3)(ⅳ) paid to clinical investigators by the sponsor of the covered studies. As a sponsor, your firm is required to maintain complete and accurate records including the following:

a. Any financial arrangement entered into between the sponsor of the covered study and the clinical investigator involved in the conduct of a covered clinical trial, whereby the value of the compensation to the clinical investigator for conducting the study could be influenced by the outcome of the study [21 CFR 54(a)(3)(ⅰ)];

b. Any significant payments of other sorts from the sponsor of the covered study, such as a grant to fund ongoing research, compensation in the form of equipment, retainer for ongoing consultation, or honoraria [21 CFR 54(a)(3)(ⅱ)];

c. Any proprietary interest in the tested product held by any clinical investigator involved in a study [21 CFR 54(a)(3)(ⅲ)]; and

d. Any significant equity interest in the sponsor of the covered study held by any clinical investigator involved in any clinical study [21 CFR 54(a)(3)(ⅰ)].

In your firm's March 11, 2008, letter written in response to the Form FDA 483, Inspectional Observations, your firm acknowledged that the clinical investigations with the use of [　] Should have been conducted under an IND and stated that the other observations were derivatives of not conducting the study under an IND. Your firm's response stated that procedures will be put into place to ensure compliance with the FDA regulations in the future. We acknowledge your firm's assurance that corrective actions will be taken. However, we note that the response did not contain a detailed outline of procedures or processes that would be implemented to prevent the future occurrence of these observations.

This letter is not intended to be an all-inclusive list of deficiencies with your clinical study of an investigational drug. It is your responsibility to ensure adherence to each requirement of the law and relevant FDA regulations. You should address these deficiencies and establish procedures to ensure that any on-going or future studies will be in compliance with FDA regulations.

Within fifteen (15) working days of your receipt of this letter, you should notify this office in writing of the actions you have taken or will be taking (including corrective action plans and standard operating procedures) to prevent similar violations in the future. Failure to adequately and promptly explain the violations noted above may result in regulatory action without further notice.

If you have any questions, please contact Constance Lewin, M.D., M.P.H., at 301-7963397; FAX 301-847-8747. Your written response and any pertinent documentation should be addressed to:

Constance Lewin, M.D., M.P.H.
Branch Chief, Good Clinical Practice Branch I
Division of Scientific Investigations
Office of Compliance
Center for Drug Evaluation and Research
Food and Drug Administration
Bldg 51, Room 5354
10903 New Hampshire Avenue
Silver Spring, MD 20993

Sincerely yours.

Leslie K. Ball, M.D.
Director
Division of Scientific Investigations
Office of Compliance
Center for Drug Evaluation and Research

第48封　给Replidyne股份有限公司的警告信

2008年1月18日

参考号：08-HFD-45-0117

尊敬的Collins先生：

这封警告信特告知您FDA在对Replidyne公司现场检查中发现的违规情况。Replidyne作为申请人［21 CFR 314.3（b）］提交了上市申请用于支持对［ ］的审批。FDA注意到以下临床研究被提交用于支持［ ］的新药申请（NDA）：

试验方案［ ］：前瞻性，随机，双盲，三臂，多中心的对比临床试验，评估有效性和安全性；［ ］BID7天 vs.［ ］BID10天 vs.［ ］BID10天；治疗［ ］。

试验方案［ ］：前瞻性，随机，双盲，对比研究；［ ］BID10天vs.［ ］BID14天；治疗［ ］受试者。

试验方案［ ］：前瞻性，随机，双盲，对比研究；［ ］BID 5天和vs.［ ］5天；治疗［ ］受试者。

试验方案［ ］：前瞻性，随机，双盲，多中心，对比研究有效性和安全性；［ ］BID7天vs.［ ］BID 7天；治疗［ ］受试者。

本次现场检查是FDA的生物研究监查项目的一部分，该项目评估相关研究的实施情况，以确保这些研究中受试者的权益、安全和福利得到了保护，另一个目的是确保所递交的支持新药申请的研究数据具有科学上的有效性和准确性。

FDA注意到上述关于试验药物［ ］的临床研究系由［ ］公司在递交IND后申办（以下简称［ ］），在2000年至2003年实施。我们进一步发现，研究最初由CRO［ ］或CRO［ ］承担监查任务。之后该产品的所有权由［ ］转移到了［ ］，而Replidyne公司于2004年从［ ］取得了该产品的所有权。2005年2月，美国通用名委员会给该产品赋予一个新的名称［ ］。2005年12月20日，Replidyne公司准备并向FDA递交了［ ］的上市申请（NDA）。

我们注意到，2006年7月19日至8月8日，FDA检查员到访了Replidyne公司，进行了初次的检查；2006年9月11日至2006年10月17日，进行了第二次检查。在每次现场检查结束时，FDA工作人员都向您及您的同事出示并讨论了FDA483表，即现场检查发现的问题。我们审查了Replidyne公司2006年9月11日和2007年2月8日对日期为2006年8月8日和2006年10月17日的FDA483表上所列项目分别进行的书面回复。

根据我们对FDA现场检查报告、该报告的附件和您2006年9月11日及2007年2月8日对FDA483表的书面回复，以及我们对NDA［ ］临床研究者检查的记录所进行的审查，我们认为，Replidyne公司没有遵守相关法律要求和有关申请人向FDA呈交数据及信息的法规。我们想对以上提到的为支持NDA［ ］进行的临床研究中出现偏差强调以下几点：

1. 未能提供隐藏的原始数据给FDA检查［21 CFR 314.3（b）］

Replidyne公司取得了利用或使用最早由［ ］开展的临床研究的权利［21 CFR 314.3（b）］，其后向FDA递交了上市申请。作为取得了利用或使用权利的申请人，Replidyne公司就有责任让在上述临床研究中隐藏原始数据变为可用并提供给FDA检查。我们注意到，您未能提供所有的隐藏原始数据给FDA检查。例如：

a. 在FDA检查期间，当FDA检查员要求提供参加研究人员的培训信息时，Replidyne公司报告称［ ］拒绝向Replidyne提供用于实施和监查临床研究的SOP文件副本，因为已经呈交用于支持NDA［ ］了。

b. 对于试验方案［ ］的临床试验场所36（Dr.［ ］），2001年12月12日的监查访视报告未能提供给FDA审查。

c. FDA曾经要求Replidyne公司提供关于NDA［ ］研究中4位国际研究者接受监查的情况。我们注意到，在日期为2007年9月24日的一封答复信中，您提到您无法找到Dr.［ ］和Dr.［ ］，并且您也没有权限接触这两位研究者的记录。

我们想强调的是，在递交申请之前，应确保所有为支持申请而开展的临床研究的所有潜藏原始数据能够提供给FDA，以备监查，这是Replidyn公司作为申请人的责任。

2. 未能向FDA提供对申请人从任何渠道取得的或接受的国内或国外的、与药物安全和有效性评价相关的其他数据或信息充分适当的描述和分析，包括从临床研究取得的数据［21 CFR 314.50（d）（5）（ⅳ）］

FDA注意到，Replidyne公司作为申请人，被要求在申请中向FDA提交一份从任何渠道取得的或接受的、与该产品安全和有效性评价有关的其他数据或信息的描述和分析资料，包括国内国外，包括在临床研究中生成的［21 CFR 314.50（d）（5）（ⅳ）］，以供FDA作出专业的判断该申请是否可以批准。FDA注意到，Replidyne公司在递交申请时未能提供充分适当的信息。

a. FDA注意到，Replidyne公司提交了来自于几个临床试验场所的数据用以支持NDA［ ］，但是在递交申请前没有对来自这些试验场所的数据的完整性进行充分的确认。例如：

ⅰ. FDA调查了执行试验方案［ ］的Dr.［ ］，结果显示，Dr.［ ］并未亲自与至少2位执行研究的授权研究者见面，也没有查阅他们招募入组的受试者的研究或临床记录。Dr.［ ］告知FDA检查员，他并不知道这两位授权研究者拿到的所有X射线筛选报告在研究结束时都由另一位放射学家进行了再评估，而且他也不知道只有经过这位放射学家再评估的报告才会报告给申办者。Dr.［ ］还声称，他并不审查两位授权研究者招募入组的受试者的入组标准，治疗转归，方案违背，以及不良事件资料进行。FDA调查结论是，该试验场所所产生的数据是不可信的，并对Dr.［ ］寄出警告信。

ⅱ. FDA调查了执行试验方案［ ］的Dr.［ ］，结果显示，大量的受试者没有按照研究计划随机入组。FDA注意到，与随机相关的问题广泛而大量存在，FDA无法确认该试验场所的数据完整性。

ⅲ. FDA调查了执行试验方案［ ］的Dr.［ ］，调查发现他未能按照法规21 CFR 312.62（c）的要求保留研究记录。因而FDA无法确认Replidyne公司向FDA提交的该试验场所的数据完整性。

b. FDA注意到，在对贵公司的两次调查中，FDA检查员无法在几个试验场所找到监查报告（如试验方案［ ］27，Dr.［ ］；试验方案［ ］36，Dr.［ ］；试验方案34，Dr.［ ］和试验方案48，Dr.［ ］；试验方案［ ］36，Dr.［ ］）。我们注意到，您们只在FDA稽查期间或FDA稽查之后对FDA483表作出回复时才获得了拥有这些监查报告的权利。

FDA注意到，在您向FDA提交NDA之前，您并没有拥有全部的监查报告，我们无法检查您是如何能够正确地保证这些从试验场所来源并提交给FDA的数据的完整性，并且还后续提交给FDA一份与该产品安全和有效性评价有关的其他数据或信息的充分适当的描述和分析。

这封信的目的并不是罗列您在向FDA提交的药物上市申请中存在的所有缺陷。确保遵循法律和相关FDA法规的每一项要求是您的职责。您必须解决这些缺陷，并建立规程，以确保任何正在进行或将来进行的研究均能符合FDA法规。

自收到这封信的15个工作日内，您应当书面告知本部门您为预防将来发生类似违规行为已经采取或将要采取的措施。如果不能充分、迅速地解释上述违规问题，可能导致我们在不再通知的情况下采取监管措施。

附：英文原文

Replidyne, Inc.

WARNING LETTER

JAN 18, 2008

CERTIFIED MAIL
RETURN RECEIPT REQUESTED

Ref: 08-HFD-45-0117

Mr. Kenneth Collins
President & CEO
Replidyne, Inc.
1450 Infinite Drive
Louisville, CO 80027

Dear Mr. Collins:

This Warning Letter is to inform you of objectionable conditions found during the U.S. Food and Drug Administration's (FDA) investigations into Replidyne, Inc.'s (hereafter referred to as Replidyne) role as the applicant [21 CFR 314.3(b)] who submitted a marketing application in support of the approval of **[redacted]**. The FDA notes that the following clinical studies were submitted in support of the New Drug Application (NDA) **[redacted]**

Protocol [redacted] "Prospective, randomized, double-blind, three-armed, multi-center comparative trial to evaluate the efficacy and safety of **[redacted]** BID for 7 days vs. **[redacted]** BID for 10 days vs. **[redacted]** BID for 10 days in the treatment of **[redacted]**

Protocol [redacted] "Prospective, randomized, double-blind, study comparing **[redacted]** BID for 10 days with **[redacted]** BID for 14 days in the treatment of patients with **[redacted]**

Protocol [redacted] "Prospective, randomized, double-blind study comparing **[redacted]** BID for 5 days with **[redacted]** for 5 days **[redacted]** in the treatment of patients with **[redacted]**

Protocol [redacted] "Prospective, randomized, double-blind, multi-center, comparative trial to evaluate the efficacy and safety of **[redacted]** BID for 7 days vs. **[redacted]** BID for 7 days in the treatment of **[redacted]**

This investigation is a part of FDA's Bioresearch Monitoring Program which is designed to evaluate the conduct of research and to ensure that the rights; safety, and welfare of the human subjects of those studies have been protected. Another objective of the program is to ensure that data submitted in support of New Drug Applications are scientifically valid and accurate.

The FDA notes that the above mentioned studies of the investigational drug **[redacted]** were sponsored by **[redacted]** (hereafter referred to as **[redacted]** under IND **[redacted]** and the studies were performed between 2000 and 2003. We note further that these studies were originally monitored by **[redacted]** or **[redacted]** agents. The rights for the product were subsequently transferred from **[redacted]** to **[redacted]** and in 2004 Replidyne obtained ownership of the product from **[redacted]** In February 2005, the US Adopted Names Council assigned the new name [redacted] for this product. On December 20, 2005, Replidyne prepared and submitted a marketing application to FDA for **[redacted]** (i.e. NDA **[redacted]**)

We note that FDA investigators visited Replidyne between July 19, 2006 and August 8, 2006 for an initial inspection, and between September 11, 2006 and October 17, 2006 for a second inspection. At the conclusion of each inspection, FDA personnel presented and discussed with you and your staff the Form FDA 483, Inspectional Observations. We have reviewed Replidyne's written responses dated September 11, 2006, and February 8, 2007 to the items listed on the Form FDA 483 dated August 8, 2006 and October 17, 2006, respectively.

From our review of the establishment inspection reports (EIRs), the documents submitted with that report, your written responses dated September 11, 2006 and February 8, 2007 to the inspectional observations, and the EIR. and documents for the clinical investigators that were inspected for NDA **[redacted]** we conclude that Replidyne did not adhere to the applicable statutory requirements and regulations governing an applicant's responsibilities concerning submission of data and information to the FDA. We wish to emphasize the following deficiencies with respect to the above-referenced clinical investigations submitted in support of NDA **[redacted]**

1. Failure to make available the underlying raw data from the investigation for FDA's audit [21 CFR 314.3(b)].

The FDA notes that Replidyne acquired the right of reference or use [21 CFR 314.3(b)] of the clinical investigations originally conducted by **[redacted]** and subsequently submitted a marketing application to the FDA. Thus as the applicant who acquired the right of reference or use, Replidyne was required to make available the underlying raw data from the above clinical investigations for FDA audit. We note that you failed to provide all of the underlying raw data for FDA's audit. For example,

a. During the FDA audit, when FDA investigators asked for information regarding the training of individuals involved in the studies, Replidyne reportedly stated that **[redacted]** refused to provide Replidyne with a copy of the standard operating procedures (SOPs) used for the conduct and monitoring of studies that were submitted in support of NDA **[redacted]**

b. For Protocol **[redacted]** Clinical Site #36 (Dr. **[redacted]** the monitoring visit report for 12 December 2001 was not available for FDA inspection.

c. The FDA had requested information from Replidyne concerning audits that were to take place for 4 international clinical investigators that conducted studies under NDA **[redacted]** We note that in a letter dated September 24, 2007, you noted that you were unable to locate Dr. **[redacted]** and Dr. **[redacted]** and that you also did not have access to the records for these two investigators.

We wish to emphasize that it was the responsibility of Replidyne, as the applicant [21 CFR 314.3(b)], to ensure that prior to submission of the application, all of the underlying raw data from all of the clinical investigations conducted to support the application was to be made available to the FDA for possible auditing.

2. Failure to provide the FDA adequate descriptions and analyses of any other data or information relevant to the evaluation of the safety and effectiveness of the drug product obtained or otherwise received by the applicant from any source, foreign or domestic including information derived from clinical investigations [21 CFR 314.50(d)(5)(iv)].

The FDA notes that as the applicant, Replidyne was required to provide within the application to the FDA, a description and analysis of any other data or information relevant to the evaluation of the safety and effectiveness of the drug product obtained or otherwise received by the applicant from any source, foreign or domestic, including information derived from clinical investigations [21 CFR 314.50(d)(5)(iv)] to permit the FDA to make a knowledgeable judgment about whether or not the application should be approved. The FDA notes that Replidyne failed to provide sufficient information at the time of submission of the application.

a. The FDA notes that Replidyne submitted data from several clinical investigative research sites in support of NDA **[redacted]** but did not adequately verify the integrity of the data at those sites, prior to the submission to the FDA. For example,

i. FDA's investigation of Dr. **[redacted]** for Protocol **[redacted]** revealed that Dr. **[redacted]** did not personally meet with at least two of his sub-investigators who conducted the study, nor did he review the research or clinic records regarding the subjects they enrolled. Dr. **[redacted]** informed FDA investigators that he was not aware that all the screening x-rays obtained by the two sub-investigators were re-interpreted by a second radiologist at the end of the study and that he was not aware that only the results from the second radiologist were reported to the study-sponsor. Dr. **[redacted]** also stated that he did not review the inclusion criteria, treatment outcomes, protocol deviations, or adverse event documentation for the subjects enrolled by these sub-investigators. FDA's inspection concluded that the data generated from the site were unreliable and issued Dr. **[redacted]** a Warning Letter.

ii. FDA's investigation of Dr. **[redacted]** for Protocols **[redacted]** revealed that numerous subjects were not randomized in accordance with the investigational plan. FDA notes that the problems with randomization were so broad and numerous that the FDA was unable to verify the integrity of the data at this site.

iii. FDA's investigation of Dr. **[redacted]** for Protocol **[redacted]** found that he failed to retain research records in accordance with 21 CFR 312.62(c). Thus the FDA was unable to verify the integrity of the data submitted by Replidyne to the FDA from this site.

b. The FDA notes that during the course of both inspections that occurred at your facility, FDA investigators were unable to locate all of the monitoring reports from several clinical investigative sites (e.g. protocol **[redacted]** site #27, Dr. **[redacted]** protocol **[redacted]** site #23, Dr. **[redacted]** site #34, Dr. **[redacted]** and site #48, Dr. **[redacted]** protocol **[redacted]**site #36, Dr. **[redacted]** We note that you only obtained possession of these monitoring reports either during the FDA audits or after the FDA audit and in response to the Form FDA 483 that was issued.

The FDA notes that as you did not have all of the monitoring reports within your possession prior to submission of the NDA to the agency, we cannot assess how you could have properly ensured the integrity of the data that was submitted to the FDA from the clinical investigators sites and have subsequently provided the FDA with an adequate description and analysis of any other data or information relevant to the evaluation of the safety and effectiveness of the drug product.

This letter is not intended to be an all-inclusive list of deficiencies with the submission of a marketing application to the FDA. It is your responsibility to ensure adherence to each requirement of the law and relevant FDA regulations. You must address these deficiencies and establish procedures to ensure that any on-going or future studies will be in compliance with FDA regulations.

Within fifteen (15) working days of your receipt of this letter, you must notify this office in writing of the actions you have taken or will be taking to prevent similar violations in the future. Failure to adequately and promptly explain the violations noted above may result in regulatory action without further notice.

If you have any questions, please contact Dr. Tejashri Purohit-Sheth at (240) 276-8840; FAX (240) 276-8811. Your written response and any pertinent documentation should be addressed to Dr. Leslie Ball at the address below.

Sincerely yours,

/S/

Leslie K. Ball, M.D.
Division Director
Division of Scientific Investigations, HFD-45
Office of Compliance
Center for Drug Evaluation and Research
7520 Standish Place
Rockville, MD 20855

第四部分

药物 GCP 警告信

——给申办-研究者

第49封　给Kang Zhang医学博士的警告信

2017年1月5日

参考号：17-HFD-45-01-01

尊敬的张博士：

2016年7月14日至8月1日，Natalie J. Ayoub女士代表FDA在您的临床试验场所进行了现场检查，对您开展的一项关于试验药物（b）（4）的临床研究［试验方案（b）（4），“（b）（4）”，］进行了审查，该研究您既是申办者，又是临床研究者。这封警告信特告知您现场检查中发现的违规情况。

本次现场检查是FDA的生物研究监查项目的一部分，该项目通过设定的检查方法，对FDA监管的研究的实施情况进行评估，以确认研究数据从科学上是有效和准确的，并帮助确保这些研究中受试者的权益、安全和福利得到了保护。

在现场检查结束时，Natalie J. Ayoub女士向您出示了FDA 483表，即现场检查发现的问题，并与您进行了讨论。您于2016年8月18日对该FDA 483表的书面回复已收悉。

经对现场检查报告、该报告的附件以及您2016年8月18日的书面回复进行审查，我们认为，您没有遵循适用的法律要求和监管临床研究实施的FDA法规。我们想强调以下几点：

1. 您未能确保按照研究计划实施临床研究［21 CFR 312.60］

作为临床研究者，您必须确保临床研究按照研究计划实施。试验方案（b）（4）的研究计划，要求您确保受试者入组前满足方案规定的入选标准。另外，试验方案（b）（4）要求您在规定的时间进行特定的研究程序，如进行眼科评估。您没有遵循这些要求。具体而言：

a. 上述提到的方案研究计划要求，从基线最佳视觉中丧失了超过5个字母的受试者才有入组资格。对于试验方案（b）（4），通过采用早期治疗糖尿病视网膜病研究（ETDRS）的方法，或者在某些情况下，使用斯内伦视力表，评估最佳矫正视力（BCVA）来检测最佳视力。您入组的5名受试者未能满足这项要求。具体而言，尽管下列受试者并没有从基线最佳视觉中丧失了超过5个字母，但是您或者授权研究者允许他们入组：

受试者 C-001，2011年8月15日入组；

受试者 C-006，2012年8月13日入组；

受试者 C-007，2012年8月31日入组；

受试者 C-008，2012年9月18日入组；

受试者 C-009，2012年9月25日入组。

在2016年8月18日对FDA 483表的书面回复中，您表示，根据研究进程，您确定入组从基线最佳视觉中丧失了5个或少于5个字母的受试者是可接受的。您指出，这一入选标准的理由是能更好地评估主要研究目的，即在确诊后早期治疗的受试者是否能够恢复或维持到他们的疾病前的基线视力。您也指出入组这些受试者没有增加风险/收益比率。

b. 研究计划要求，第0天时在4m的距离采用早期治疗糖尿病视网膜病研究的方法（ETDRS法）进行最佳矫正视力（BCVA）评估。可以在两周内两次单独访视过程中完成第0天的研究程序。您必须在第0天评估最佳矫正视力，来确定是否受试者满足入选标准，即要求从基线最佳视觉中丧失了超过5个字母。

对于受试者C-003，您未能在2011年10月6日第0天采用早期治疗糖尿病视网膜病研究的方法进行最佳矫正视力（BCVA）评估。尽管如此，受试者C-003入组本研究并在第0天接受了研究药物。因此，您在该受试者入组研究前未能充分评估其入选资格。

在2016年8月18日对FDA 483表的书面回复中，您表示，您根据要求的研究程序进行了基线记录，并在一张表中标记受试者C-003已经采用早期治疗糖尿病视网膜病研究的方法进行最佳矫正视力（BCVA）评估。特别是，您递交了2011年6月27日的病程记录，表明当天进行了采用早期治疗糖尿病视网膜病研究的方法进行最佳矫正视力（BCVA）评估。我们注意到，该受试者第0天为2011年6月27日病程记录后超过3个多月的2011年10月6日。因此，我们不能确定该例受试者2011年10月6日第0天访视时或2周内是否进行了采用早期治疗糖尿病视网膜病研究的方法进行最佳矫正视力（BCVA）评估。

另外，您表示，您理解应严格地遵循入选和排除标准来评估合格性，对入选和/排除标准的任何修订首先应该获得伦理委员会（IRB）的批准。您还表示，对于所有正在进行和将来的研究，将实施“第二个审阅人筛选程序”，即在知情同意书签订后至少24小时筛选期内审阅每一个新入组的受试者的入选和/排除标准。

由于您未能提供如果正常开展可以预防将来发生类似违规情况的纠正措施计划，我们无法对您对上述1.a.和1.b.项的书面回复进行知情评价。具体而言，您没有提供针对您未能确保只有符合要求的受试者才能入组这一检查发现，而实施的额外措施和程序的计划的充分细节。

我们强调的是，每一项临床研究的合格标准都是设计用来优化收集数据的可理解性和减小对入组受试者的可预见性伤害。入组不满足合格标准的受试者损害了受试者的安全和福利，并引起对在您的研究场所收集的数据的有效性和完整性的关注。FDA特别关注的是，在未能确保受试者符合性的情况下，您将本研究的12名入组受试者中的6名入组这项研究。

c．研究计划规定，在研究完成前退出研究的受试者应该在最后一次注射或访视后的30天（±7天）返回研究场所进行提前终止研究的评估，以监测所有的不良事件（严重的和不严重的）。依据研究计划，在提前终止研究的访视中，您应该进行如下研究程序：眼科检查、采用早期治疗糖尿病视网膜病研究的方法（ETDRS法）进行最佳矫正视力（BCVA）评估、光谱域光学相干层析成像（SD-OCT）和严重不良事件（SAE）监测。受试者C-011于2013年8月13日、入组后1天退出研究，并在第0天服用了研究药物。尽管如此，对于受试者C-011您未进行提前终止研究的访视。

在2016年8月18日对FDA 483表的书面回复中，您承认这名受试者提前终止研究的访视没有完成。您指出该名受试者因个人原因退出研究，并且作为标准治疗患者仍然接受您的治疗。

另外，您指出已经针对提前终止研究评估中不良事件监测的重要性对研究人员进行了再培训。具体而言，您指出研究人员将接受伦理委员会法规、报告时限及其他法规的一对一再培训，您提到的文件应当在30天内递交给FDA。

由于您未能提供如果正常开展可以预防将来发生类似违规情况的纠正措施计划，我们无法对您的书面回复进行知情评价。具体而言，您没有提供针对您未能遵守方案的程序这一检查发现，而实施的额外措施和程序的计划的充分细节。

未能执行方案要求的包括眼科检查和不良事件监测的研究程序，损害了受试者的安全和福利，并引起对在您的研究场所中收集的数据的有效性和完整性的关注。

2. 您未能保持充分的包括日期、数量和受试者的使用情况的药物处置记录［21 CFR 312.62(a)］

作为临床研究者，您必须保持药物处置的充分记录，包括日期、数量和受试者的使用情况。对于试验方案（b）（4），药物处置记录包括研究药物管理日志和未使用研究药物销毁记录。关于这些文件，您未能保持充分的记录。具体而言，您的研究药物管理日志没有记录25个单位未使用的研究药物的处置情况。而且，您未能出示未使用的研究药物，并且没有其他记录显示，这些缺失的、未使用的研究药物的使用或销毁的情况。

在2016年8月18日对FDA 483表的书面回复中，您同意您保持的试验药物的记录是不充分的。您表示药物已经被销毁，但是未使用药物的销毁没有恰当记录。您声明研究药物仅用于这项临床研究。

另外，您表示针对保持准确和充分的试验药物记录的重要性对研究人员进行了再培训。您表示您已经在标准操作规程（SOP）中写明了监查准确和足够的研究药物管理记录的详细计划，并要在递交对FDA 483表的书面回复后的30日内递交给FDA。您还指出，您计划采用研究结束访视来调和药物管理，确保销毁过期的研究药物，确保完成和保存所有的研究记录。

由于您未能提供如果正常开展可以预防将来发生类似违规情况的纠正措施计划，我们无法对您的书面回复进行知情评价。具体而言，您没有提供针对您未能保持充分的药物管理记录这一检查发现，而实施的额外措施和程序的计划的充分细节。

您不能解释25个单位未使用的研究药物的处置情况，这引起了对于您对试验药物的监管和控制是否充足的严重关注。此外，您未能保持全面和准确的药物管理记录引起对您的研究场所收集的数据的有效性和完整性的关注。

本警告信的目的并非是罗列您在试验药物临床研究中存在的所有缺陷。确保遵循法律和相关FDA法规的每一项要求是您的职责，您应当解决这些缺陷，并建立规程，以确保任何正在进行或将来进行的研究均符合FDA的法规。

自收到这封信的15个工作日内，您应当书面告知本办公室您为预防将来发生类似违规情况而采取的措施。如果不能充分、迅速地解释上述违规问题，可能导致我们在不再通知的情况下采取监管措施。如果您认为您已经遵循了FDA的法规要求，请陈述理由，并提供所有支持资料，以供我们参考。

附：英文原文

Kang Zhang, M.D., Ph.D.

WARNING LETTER

Jan 5, 2017

CERTIFIED MAIL
RETURN RECEIPT REQUESTED

Ref: 17-HFD-45-01-01

Kang Zhang, M.D., Ph.D.
9415 Campus Point Drive, Room E214
La Jolla, CA 92093-0946

Dear Dr. Zhang:

This Warning Letter informs you of objectionable conditions observed during the U.S. Food and Drug Administration (FDA) inspection conducted at your clinical site between July 14, 2016, and August 1, 2016. Ms. Natalie J. Ayoub, representing FDA, reviewed your conduct of a clinical investigation (Protocol (b)(4), "(b)(4) ")of the investigational drug (b)(4) for which you were both the sponsor and a clinical investigator.

This inspection is a part of FDA's Bioresearch Monitoring Program, which includes inspections designed to evaluate the conduct of FDA-regulated research to ensure that the data are scientifically valid and accurate, and to help ensure that the rights, safety, and welfare of the human subjects of those studies have been protected.

At the conclusion of the inspection, Ms. Ayoub presented and discussed with you Form FDA 483, Inspectional Observations. We acknowledge receipt of your August 18, 2016, written response to the Form FDA 483.

From our review of the FDA Establishment Inspection Report, the documents submitted with that report, and your written response dated August 18, 2016, we conclude that you did not adhere to the applicable statutory requirements and FDA regulations governing the conduct of clinical investigations. We wish to emphasize the following:

1.You failed to ensure that the investigation was conducted according to the investigational plan [21 CFR 312.60].

As a clinical investigator, you are required to ensure that your clinical studies are conducted in accordance with the investigational plan. The investigational plan for Protocol (b)(4) required you to ensure that subjects met the protocol inclusion criteria before their enrollment. In addition, Protocol (b)(4) required you to perform certain study procedures, such as ophthalmologic evaluations, at specific times. You failed to adhere to these requirements. Specifically:

a.The investigational plan for the above-mentioned protocol required subjects to have lost more than five letters from baseline best vision to be eligible for enrollment. For Protocol (b)(4), best vision was measured by assessing the Best Corrected Visual Acuity (BCVA) using the Early Treatment Diabetic Retinopathy Study (ETDRS) method or, in certain circumstances, the Snellen test. You enrolled five subjects who did not meet this requirement. Specifically, you or a subinvestigator allowed the enrollment of the following subjects even though they did not have a loss of more than five letters from baseline best vision:

Subject C-001, enrolled on August 15, 2011

Subject C-006, enrolled on August 13, 2012

Subject C-007, enrolled on August 31, 2012

Subject C-008, enrolled on September 18, 2012

Subject C-009, enrolled on September 25, 2012

In your August 18, 2016, written response to the Form FDA 483, you indicated that you determined that enrollment of subjects who had lost five or fewer letters from baseline was acceptable for the course of the study. You noted that the rationale for this inclusion criterion was to better assess the primary objective of determining if subjects treated early after diagnosis could return to or maintain their baseline pre-disease visual acuity. You also noted that with inclusion of these subjects, there was no increased risk/benefit ratio.

b.The investigational plan required an assessment of BCVA using the ETDRS method at a distance of 4 meters on Day 0. Day 0 procedures may be carried out over the course of two separate visits within a two-week time period. You were required to assess BCVA on Day 0 to determine whether subjects met the inclusion criterion requiring a loss of more than five letters from baseline best vision.

You failed to perform a BCVA using ETDRS on Day 0 for Subject C-003 on October 6, 2011. However, Subject C-003 was enrolled into the study and received study drug on Day 0. Therefore, you failed to fully evaluate this subject's eligibility before enrolling the subject into this study.

In your August 18, 2016, written response to the Form FDA 483, you indicated that you had baseline records for the required study procedures, and you marked in a table that ETDRS BCVA was performed for Subject C-003. In particular, you submitted a progress note dated June 27, 2011, showing that an ETDRS BCVA was performed on that date. We note that Day 0 for this subject was October 6, 2011, over three months after this June 27, 2011, progress note. We are thus unable to determine whether an ETDRS BCVA was performed on or within 2 weeks of the subject's Day 0 study visit on October 6, 2011.

In addition, you indicated that you understand that stringent adherence to the inclusion and exclusion criteria should be used to assess eligibility, and that any amendment to the inclusion and exclusion criteria should first be approved by the Institutional Review Board (IRB). You also indicated that for all current and future studies, a "Secondary Reviewer Screening Process" will be implemented to review inclusion and exclusion criteria for each newly enrolled subject within at least a 24-hour screening period after informed consent has been obtained.

We are unable to undertake an informed evaluation of your written response to Items 1.a. and 1.b. above because you did not provide a corrective action plan that, if properly carried out, would prevent this type of violation in the future. Specifically, you did not provide sufficient details about your plan for implementing additional measures and procedures, to address the inspection findings concerning your failure to ensure that only eligible subjects were enrolled.

We emphasize that the eligibility criteria for each clinical investigation are designed to optimize interpretability of collected data and to minimize foreseeable harm to enrolled subjects. Enrollment of subjects who do not meet the eligibility criteria jeopardizes subject safety and welfare and raises concerns about the validity and integrity of the data collected at your site. FDA is particularly concerned that you enrolled six of the twelve subjects enrolled into this study without ensuring their subject eligibility.

c. The investigational plan provided that subjects who withdraw from the study before completion should return for an early termination evaluation 30 days (± 7 days) following the last injection or study visit, for monitoring of all adverse events (serious and nonserious). Under the investigational plan, you were to perform the following study procedures at the early termination visit: an ophthalmological exam, ETDRS BCVA, spectral domain optical coherence tomography (SD-OCT), and serious adverse event (SAE) monitoring. Subject C-011 withdrew from the study on August 13, 2013, one day after being enrolled and receiving study drug on Day 0. However, you failed to conduct an early termination visit for Subject C-011.

In your August 18, 2016, written response to the Form FDA 483, you acknowledged that an early termination visit was not completed for this subject. You noted that this subject withdrew for personal reasons and remained under your care as a standard-of-care patient.

In addition, you indicated that study staff has been retrained on the importance of monitoring for adverse events during the early termination assessments. Specifically, you indicated that study staff will receive one-on-one retraining in IRB regulations, reporting timelines, and other regulations, documentation of which you noted should be provided to the FDA in 30 days.

We are unable to undertake an informed evaluation of your written response because you did not provide a corrective action plan that, if properly carried out, would prevent this type of violation in the future. Specifically, you did not provide sufficient details about your plan for implementing additional measures and procedures, to address the inspection findings concerning your failure to follow protocol procedures.

Failure to perform protocol-required study procedures, including ophthalmological evaluations and adverse event monitoring, jeopardizes subject safety and welfare and raises concerns about the validity and integrity of the data collected at your site.

2.You failed to maintain adequate records of the disposition of the drug, including dates, quantity, and use by subjects [21 CFR 312.62(a)].

As a clinical investigator, you are required to maintain adequate records of the disposition of the drug, including dates, quantity, and use by subjects. For Protocol (b)(4), drug disposition records include study drug accountability logs and records documenting the destruction of unused supplies of study drug. You did not maintain adequate records with respect to these documents. Specifically, your study drug accountability logs failed to document the disposition of 25 units of unused supplies of study drug. Further, you were unable to produce the unused supplies of study drug, and there were no other records indicating the use or disposal of these missing unused supplies of study drug.

In your August 18, 2016, written response to the Form FDA 483, you agreed that the investigational drug records were inadequately maintained. You noted that the drug supply had been destroyed, and that the destruction of unused supplies of study drug was not documented adequately. You stated that the study drug was used solely for the purposes of this study.

In addition, you indicated that study staff will be retrained on the importance of maintaining accurate and complete records of the investigational drug. You indicated that you have written a detailed plan for monitoring accurate and complete drug accountability records in a standard operating procedure (SOP), which you intended to provide to FDA within 30 days of the transmittal of your response to the Form FDA 483. You also indicated that you planned to conduct a study closure visit to reconcile drug accountability, ensure destruction of expired supplies of the drug, and ensure completion and retention of all study records.

We are unable to undertake an informed evaluation of your written response because you did not provide a corrective action plan that, if properly carried out, would prevent this type of violation in the future. Specifically, you did not provide sufficient details about your plan for implementing additional measures and procedures, to address the inspection findings concerning your failure to maintain adequate drug accountability records.

Your inability to account for the disposition of 25 units of unused supplies of study drug raises significant concerns regarding the adequacy of your oversight and control of investigational drug. In addition, your failure to maintain adequate and accurate drug accountability records raises concerns about the validity and integrity of the data collected at your site.

This letter is not intended to be an all-inclusive list of deficiencies with your clinical study of an investigational drug. It is your responsibility to ensure adherence to each requirement of the law and relevant FDA regulations. You should address these deficiencies and establish procedures to ensure that any ongoing or future studies will be in compliance with FDA regulations.

Within fifteen (15) working days of your receipt of this letter, you should notify this office in writing of the actions you have taken to prevent similar violations in the future. Failure to address the violations noted above adequately and promptly may result in regulatory action without further notice. If you believe you have complied with FDA regulations, include your reasoning and any supporting information for our consideration.

If you have any questions, please contact Adam Donat, M.S., at 301-796-5316; FAX 301-847-8748. Your written response and any pertinent documentation should be addressed to:

Adam Donat, M.S.
Branch Chief
Compliance Enforcement Branch
Division of Enforcement and Postmarketing Safety
Office of Scientific Investigations
Office of Compliance
Center for Drug Evaluation and Research
Food and Drug Administration
Building 51, Room 5352
10903 New Hampshire Avenue
Silver Spring, MD 20993

Sincerely yours,

{See appended electronic signature page}

David Burrow, Pharm.D., J.D.
Acting Director
Office of Scientific Investigations
Office of Compliance
Center for Drug Evaluation and Research
Food and Drug Administration

This is a representation of an electronic record that was signed electronically and this page is the manifestation of the electronic signature.

/S/

DAVID C BURROW
01/05/2017

第50封 给Lin，Henry医学博士的警告信

2010年3月8日

参考号：10-HFD-45-03-01

尊敬的Lin博士：

2008年9月15日，Teena Aiken女士代表FDA进行了现场检查，与您会面并审查了您作为申办-研究者的实施临床研究［试验方案（b）（4），题为（b）（4），试验药物（b）（4）］的情况。我们接受您的说法：2008年9月15日现场检查之前，（b）（4）医学博士已经担任了上述研究中临床研究者的角色，而您只留作研究申办者。后来，2009年7月1日，Aiken女士与您一起审查了您作为申办者实施上述临床研究的情况。

2008年9月15日和2009年7月1日这两次现场检查，是FDA生物研究监查项目的一部分。该项目通过设定的检查方法，评估研究的实施情况，以确保这些研究中受试者的权益、安全和福利得到了保护。

根据我们对现场检查报告、该报告附件，以及您于2009年7月27日对FDA483表（2009年7月1日现场检查结束时下发）的书面回复进行的审查，我们认为，您没有遵循适用的法律要求和监管临床研究的实施及保护受试者的FDA法规。我们知道在现场检查结束时，Aiken女士向您出示并讨论了FDA483表，即现场检查发现的问题。我们想强调以下与您作为申办者的职责相关的违规情况。

1. 未能确保对临床研究进行适当监查［21 CFR 312.50和312.56（a）］

根据研究记录，试验方案（b）（4）的受试者在2007年2月20日至2008年9月8日被招募。我们的现场检查发现，您没有对该研究的任何方面进行监查。作为试验用新药申请（IND）（b）（4）项下实施的方案（b）（4）的申办者，您有责任确保这项研究得到充分的监查，符合监管要求，从而确保数据的可靠性，以及研究受试者的权益、安全和福利得到了充分的保护（详见21 CFR 312.56，需要申办者监查研究的进展，在监查中发现有违背签署的研究者声明、试验方案、FDA规定时采取具体措施，以及解决发展中的安全性信息）。

在2009年现场检查期间，您告知FDA检查员该研究由（b）（4）数据安全监查委员会（DSMB）进行监查。此外，您告知FDA检查员DSMB每四个月对研究进行监督并发布报告（或者如果有必要的话更快），并且提供了来自临床研究者（b）（4）医生的一封未标明日期的信支持这一说法，而这封信显然是2009年6月29日传真给您的。在2009年7月27日的书面回复中，您重申DSMB对研究进行了监查，并且表明您已经得到了DSMB的审查意见和来自（b）（4）医生为临床研究的监查提供文件的内部稽查报告。您进一步解释，您认为这样符合您监查临床研究的要求。

我们发现您的解释不够充分。您没有随回复一起提供额外的文件，而仅仅依靠2009年现场检查期间收集的日期为2007年2月6日的DSMB研究监查计划和日期为2009年9月9日的DSMB审查意见回顾，来支持这一说法：DSMB提供了充分的监查，来满足您作为申办者确保对研究过程进行适当的监查的义务。那两份文档仅显示DSMB将要监查不良事件，并且截至2009年9月9日，已确定从上次DSMB审查没有新的不良事件被报告。您对FDA检查员的陈述表明，直到受试者招募结束，2008年第一次现场检查期间，您与她一起时，您才明白您有责任对临床研究进行监查。您所提供的信息表明，DSMB的目的是在监查临床研究的某些方面，特别是不良事件和受试者安全方面，发挥不可或缺的作用；我们提醒您，作为申办者，您的责任是监查研究的整个过程，确保研究按照IND及其他FDA规定中包含的总体临床试验计划和试验方案进行。

2. 您未能在允许研究者参加一项研究之前，取得其签署的研究者声明，即FDA1572表［21 CFR 312.53（c）（1）］

具体来说，您所发起的临床试验研究不能作为21 CFR 312要求的例外。但经您同意，在获得（b）（4）博士签署的研究者声明之前，就准许她作为临床研究者参与了研究。

在您2009年7月27日的书面回复中，您说不需要采取进一步的行动，因为您在现场检查期间已提供了一份FDA1572表给FDA检查员。我们发现您的回复是无法接受的。现场检查期间您提供的FDA1572表确定您是主要临床研究者，而不是（b）（4）医生；该表于2009年6月29日、第一批受试者被招募后两年多，由您签署。尽管提供的这个文件已经表明您是这项研究的临床研究者，可您在别处还说您“把研究申办者的角色当作是主要研究者（b）（4）医学博士的研究导师”。但是，由于您没有获得（b）（4）医学博士签署的FDA1572表，所以您在任何时间都不能确认她作为临床研究者，更不用说在她参与试验之前。

3. 您未能给每个参加临床研究的研究者一份含有312.23（a）（5）中描述信息的研究者手册［21 CFR 312.55（a）］

具体来说，21 CFR 312.23（a）（5）要求研究者手册中包含以下信息：

a. 一份关于药物原料药、配方及已知结构式的概述；

b. 一个药物对动物包括对人体已知的药理学和毒理学效应的概述；

c. 药物在动物体内和人体内（如已知）的药代动力学和机体对药物处置的信息；

d. 一个从之前的临床研究获得的、与人体内安全性和有效性相关的信息（有用时，这类研究的已发表的论文的重印件可以附后）。

e. 一份基于前期该药物或相关药物临床之前试验经验所预计可能的风险及副作用的说明，包括对药物试验性应用、需要采取的预防措施或特殊监测的说明。

我们的现场检查发现，在研究开始之前，您未能给每个参加临床试验的研究者提供一份含有21 CFR 312.23（a）（5）中规定信息的研究者手册（招募开始于2007年2月20日）。

在2009年7月27日的书面回复中，您说不需要采取进一步的行动。您在书面回复中附了一份来自（b）（4）医生的传真复印件，证明她在2006年12月6日将研究者手册连同她的伦理委员会（IRB）申请一起提交给IRB。我们发现您的答复不够充分。在您的书面回复和（b）（4）医生传真都没有研究者手册，用以记录研究者手册在研究开始之前就给了（b）（4）医生，或者表明其内容是否满足监管要求。

4. 您未能对从研究者处获得的与试验药物安全性和有效性相关的证据，进行审查和评估［21 CFR 312.56（c）］

我们的现场检查发现，没有证据表明，您对上述提及的研究中试验药物的安全性或有效性进行了审查或评估，或者按照21 CFR 312.32的要求，将关于药物安全性相关信息的这类报告提供给FDA。

5. 您未能向FDA提交临床研究年度报告［21 CFR 312.33和312.56（c）］

作为试验方案的申办者，您需要在IND生效届满1年60天内提交年度报告。您的IND于2006年5月7日生效，但是我们的现场检查没有发现任何向FDA提交年度报告的证据。

6. 您未能保存足够的显示试验药物接收、转运或其他处置的记录［21 CFR 312.57（a）］

作为申办者，您必须保存药物处置记录，包括试验药物送达的研究者的姓名、日期、数量以及每次运送的批次或代码标记。我们的现场检查发现您没有保存这些记录。

在2009年7月27日的书面回复中，您说在FDA现场检查时，您的理解是要向FDA检查员提供一封来自（b）（4）药厂、验证正确的装运的信函。您进一步说，您拿到了显示试验药物收货和发货的记录。但是，您的回复中没有提供文件，来支持您已经获得这些文件的说法。

7. 您未能按照21 CFR 54的要求，保存足够、准确地显示研究者任何利益的记录［21 CFR 312.57（b）］

按照21 CFR 312.57（b），申办者应该保持足够、准确的记录，显示已覆盖的研究中申办者支付给临床研究者们的、21 CFR 54.4（a）（3）（Ⅰ～Ⅳ）中的任何经济利益；申办者也应该保持关于本章第54部分所涉及的所有其他经济利益的完整、准确的记录。我们的现场检查发现，对于上述提及的研究，您没有保持完整、准确的记录，显示这些规定中描述的任何经济利益。

8. 您未能保留记录和报告到药物的运输和发放终止及通知 FDA 后 2 年［21 CFR 312.57（c）］

我们的现场检查发现，对于上述提及的研究，您没有保留任何记录或报告。作为申办者，您需要保留这部分法规要求的记录和报告，直到该药物上市申请获批后2年；或者，如果上市申请没有被批准，直到试验药物终止运输和发放，并且已通知FDA后2年。

在2009年7月27日对FDA483表的书面回复中，您没有提及这个违规问题。

本警告信的目的并非是罗列您在试验药物临床研究中存在的所有缺陷。确保遵循法律和相关FDA法规的每一项要求是您的职责。您应当解决这些缺陷，并建立规程，以确保任何正在进行或将来进行的研究均能符合FDA法规的。

自收到这封信的15个工作日内，您应当书面告知本办公室为预防将来发生类似违规情况已经采取的措施。如果不能充分、迅速地解释上述违规问题，可能导致我们在不再通知的情况下采取监管措施。

附：英文原文

Lin, Henry, M.D.

WARNING LETTER

MAR 8, 2010

CERTIFIED MAIL
RETURN RECEIPT REQUESTED

Ref: 10-HFD-45-03-01

Henry Lin, M.D.
New Mexico Veteran's Administration Health Care System
1501 San Pedro S.E., Mail Code 1115
Albuquerque, New Mexico87108

Dear Dr. Lin:

On September 15, 2008, Ms. Teena Aiken, representing the Food and Drug Administration (FDA), conducted an investigation and met with you to review your conduct as the sponsor-investigator of the clinical investigation (Protocol **(b)(4),** entitled **(b)(4)** of the investigational drug **(b)(4).** We acknowledge your assertion that prior to the September 15, 2008, inspection, **(b)(4)** M.D., had assumed the role of clinical investigator for the above-mentioned study, and that you remained only as the study sponsor. Subsequently, on July 1, 2009, Ms. Aiken met with you to review your conduct as the sponsor of the above clinical investigation.

These two inspections, September 15, 2008 and July 1 2009, are part of the FDA's Bioresearch Monitoring Program, which includes inspections designed to evaluate the conduct of research and to ensure that the rights, safety, and welfare of the human subjects of those studies have been protected.

From our review of the establishment inspection report, the documents submitted with that report, and your July 27, 2009, letter written in response to the Form FDA 483 issued at the conclusion of the July 1, 2009, inspection, we conclude that you did not adhere to the applicable statutory requirements and FDA regulations governing the conduct of clinical investigations and the protection of human subjects. We are aware that at the conclusion of the inspection, Ms. Aiken presented and discussed with you Form FDA 483, Inspectional Observations. We wish to emphasize the following violations related to your responsibilities as sponsor:

1. Failure to ensure proper monitoring of the clinical investigations [21 CFR 312.50 and 312.56(a)].

According to study records, subjects were enrolled in Protocol **(b)(4)** between February 20, 2007 and September 8, 2008. Our inspection found that you did not monitor any aspect of the study. As the sponsor of Protocol **(b)(4)** conducted under Investigational New Drug Application (IND) **(b)(4),** you were responsible for ensuring that this study was adequately monitored for compliance with regulatory requirements, thereby ensuring the data quality, and that the rights, safety, and welfare of study subjects were adequately protected. (See 21 CFR 312.56 (requiring sponsors to monitor the progress of the investigation, and to take specific steps if such monitoring reveals noncompliance with the signed investigator agreement, the investigational plan, or FDA regulations, as well as to address developing safety information.)

During the 2009 inspection, you informed the FDA investigator that the study was monitored by the Data Safety Monitoring Board (DSMB), **(b)(4).** In addition, you informed the FDA Investigator that the DSMB was to oversee the study and issue reports every four months,or sooner if necessary, and supported this statement with an undated letter from the clinical investigator, Dr. **(b)(4),** that was apparently faxed to you on June 29, 2009. In your written response dated July 27, 2009, you reiterated that the DSMB monitored the study, and indicated that you had obtained the DSMB reviews and the internal audit report from Dr. **(b)(4)** to provide documentation for the monitoring of the clinical study. You further explained that you thought this met your requirement for monitoring the clinical study.

We find your explanations to be insufficient. You provided no additional documentation with your response, relying only on the DSMB research monitoring plan dated February 6, 2007, and DSMB Review dated September 9, 2009, collected during the 2009 inspection, to support the assertion that the DSMB provided adequate monitoring to meet your obligations as sponsor to ensure proper monitoring of the progress of the study. Those two documents indicate only that the DSMB was to monitor adverse events, and that as of September 9, 2009, had determined that there had been no new adverse events reported since the last DSMB review. Your statements to the FDA investigator suggest that you were not aware that you were responsible for monitoring the study until you met with her during the first inspection, in 2008, after the last subjects were enrolled. While the information you provided suggests that the DSMB was intended to have an integral role in monitoring some aspects of the clinical trial, specifically, adverse events and subject safety, we remind you that your responsibility as the sponsor was to monitor the overall progress of the investigation and ensure that the investigation is conducted in accordance with the general investigational plan and protocols contained in the IND, as well as other FDA regulations.

2. You failed to obtain a signed investigator statement, Form FDA 1572, before permitting an investigator to participate in an investigation [21 CFR 312.53(c)(1)].

Specifically, you initiated a clinical investigation that was not exempt from the requirements of 21 CFR Part 312, and by your own admission, allowed Dr. **(b)(4)** to participate in the investigation as clinical investigator prior to obtaining a signed investigator statement from her.

In your written response dated July 27, 2009, you stated that no further action is needed because you provided a copy of the Form FDA 1572 to the FDA investigator during the inspection. We find your response unacceptable. The Form FDA 1572 that you provided during the inspection identified **you,** not Dr. **(b)(4),** as the principal clinical investigator, and was signed by you on June 29, 2009, more than two years after the first subjects were enrolled. Despite supplying this documentation that indicates that you were the clinical investigator for this study, elsewhere you stated that you "took on the sponsor role for the study as the research mentor for the principal investigator, **(b)(4)** M.D." You failed, however, to obtain a Form FDA 1572 signed by **(b)(4),** M.D., and identifying her as the clinical investigator at any time, let alone prior to her participation in the investigation.

3. You failed to give each participating investigator an investigator brochure containing the information described in 312.23(a)(5) [21 CFR 312.55(a)].

Specifically, 21 CFR 312.23(a)(5) requires that the investigator brochure contain the following information:

a. A brief description of the drug substance and the formulation, including the structural formula, if known.

b. A summary of the pharmacological and toxicological effects of the drug in animals and, to the extent known, in humans.
c. A summary of the pharmacokinetics and biological disposition of the drug in animals, and if known, in humans.
d. A summary of information relating to safety and effectiveness in humans obtained from prior clinical studies. (Reprints of published articles of such studies may be appended when useful.)
e. A description of possible risks and side effects to be anticipated on the basis of prior experience with the drug under investigation or with related drugs, and of precautions or special monitoring to be done as part of the investigational use of the drug.

Our inspection found that you failed to provide the clinical investigator with an investigator brochure containing the information described in 21 CFR 312.23(a)(5) before the study began. (Enrollment began on February 20, 2007.)

In your written response dated July 27, 2009, you state that no further action is needed. You attached to your written response a copy of a fax from Dr. **(b)(4),** stating that she had submitted the investigator brochure to the Institutional Review Board (IRB) along with her IRB application on 12/6/06. We find your response inadequate. There was no investigator brochure attached to your written response, nor was it attached to the fax from Dr. *(b)(4),* to document that the investigator brochure was given to Dr. **(b)(4)** prior to the start of the study, or to indicate whether its content satisfies the regulatory requirements.

4. You failed to review and evaluate the evidence relating to the safety and effectiveness of the drug as it is obtained from the investigator [21 CFR 312.56(c)].

Our inspection found no evidence that you reviewed or evaluated safety or effectiveness of the drug in the above referenced study, or provided such reports to FDA regarding information relevant to the safety of the drug, as required under 21 CFR 312.32.

5. You failed to submit to the FDA an annual report of the investigation [21 CFR 312.33 &312.56(c)].

As the sponsor of Protocol , you are required to submit an annual report within 60 days of the anniversary date that the IND went into effect. Your IND went into effect on May *7,* 2006; however, our inspection found no evidence that any annual reports were submitted to the FDA.

6. You failed to maintain adequate records showing the receipt, shipment, or other disposition of the investigational drug [21 CFR 312.57(a)].

As a sponsor, you are required to maintain drug disposition records to include, as appropriate, the name of the investigator to whom the drug is shipped, and the date, quantity, and batch or code mark of each such shipment. Our investigation found that you did not maintain these records.

You stated in your written response dated July 27, 2009, that it was your understanding at the time of the FDA inspection that you were to provide a letter from the **(b)(4)** Pharmacy verifying proper shipment to the FDA investigator.

You further stated that you obtained records showing receipt and shipment of the study drug. Your response, however, provided no documentation to corroborate your statements that you had obtained these documents.

7. You failed to maintain complete and accurate records showing any financial interests of investigators subject to 21 CFR Part 54 [21 CFR 312.57(b)].

In accordance with 21 CFR 312.57(b), a sponsor shall maintain complete and accurate records showing any financial interest in 21 CFR 54.4(a)(3)(i-iv) paid to clinical investigators by the sponsor of the covered study and shall also maintain complete and accurate records concerning all other financial interests of investigators subject to part 54 of this chapter. Our inspection found that for the study referenced above you did not maintain complete and accurate records showing any financial interest as described in these regulations.

8. You failed to retain records and reports for two years after shipment and delivery of the drug is discontinued and FDA has been so notified [21 CFR 312.57(c)].

Our inspection found that you did not retain any records or reports for the above referenced study. As the sponsor, you are required to retain the records and reports required by this part for two years after a marketing application is approved for the drug; or, if an application is not approved for the drug, until two years after shipment and delivery of the drug for investigational use is discontinued, and FDA has been so notified.

In your July 27, 2009, letter in response to the Form FDA 483, you did not address this violation.

This letter is not intended to be an all-inclusive list of deficiencies with your clinical study of an investigational drug. It is your responsibility to ensure adherence to each requirement of the law and relevant FDA regulations. You should address these deficiencies and establish procedures to ensure that any ongoing or future studies will be in compliance with FDA regulations.

Within fifteen (15) working days of your receipt of this letter, you should notify this office in writing of the actions you have taken to prevent similar violations in the future. Failure to adequately and promptly explain the violations noted above may result in regulatory action without further notice.

If you have any questions, please contact Constance Lewin, M.D.,at 301-796-3397; FAX 301-847-8748. Your written response and any pertinent documentation should be addressed to:

Constance Cullity (formerly Lewin), M.D., M.P.H.
Branch Chief, Good Clinical Practice Branch I
Division of Scientific Investigations
Office of Compliance
Center for Drug Evaluation and Research
Food and Drug Administration
Building 51, Room 5354
10903 New Hampshire Avenue
Silver Spring, MD 20993

Sincerely yours,

/S/

Leslie K. Ball, M.D.
Director
Division of Scientific Investigations
Office of Compliance
Center for Drug Evaluation and Research

第51封　给Cayman化学公司的警告信

2010年1月19日

参考号：10-HFD-45-01-01

尊敬的Maxey博士：

2009年5月12日至18日，Nancy Bellamy女士代表FDA进行了现场检查，与您会面并对您作为申办者和研究者，对Cayman化学公司/Maxey化妆品有限公司所实施的含前列腺素药物的化合物1、化合物2和化合物3的临床研究进行了审查。

本次现场检查是FDA的生物研究监查项目的一部分。该项目通过设定的检查方法，对研究的实施情况进行评估，以确保这些研究中受试者的权益、安全和福利得到了保护。

根据我们对FDA现场检查报告、该报告附件进行的审查，我们认为您没有遵循适用的法定要求和监管临床研究实施及受试者保护的FDA法规。在现场检查结束时，Bellamy女士向您出示并讨论了FDA483表，即现场检查发现的问题。我们想强调以下几点：

在题为"知情同意"的文件里，贵公司声称"Maxey化妆品（M-化妆品）将使用志愿者来测试一种促使睫毛生长产品……"这段关于眼睫毛生长的声明文字，清楚地表明这个产品试图用于影响人或其他动物身体的结构或功能，并因此导致您的产品将适用于联邦食品药品和化妆品法案（法案）21U.S.C&321（g）（1）中的201（g）（1）下作为药品进行监管。

违背申办者的相关职责［21CFR 312.40，312.8（a）（3）和312.57（a）］

1. 您未能遵循临床研究中使用试验用新药的要求，在IND尚未生效的情况下给予受试者试验用新药化合物1号、2号和3号［21 CFR 312.40］

FDA法规（21CFR 312部分）包含了使用试验用新药的流程和要求。21CFR 312.3（b）定义临床研究为："任何药物给予、发放、使用涉及一个或多个受试者的试验，这部分的目的在于，试验是指任何在医疗实践中使用市售药品以外的药物"。化合物1、2和3在美国没有批准上市，因此，任何使用了上述化合物的临床研究必须符合新药临床研究的基本要求。

在临床研究中使用试验用新药需符合下列条件：①申办者向FDA递交临床研究申请；②这个临床研究申请在FDA法规下是有效的；③申办者符合所有21CFR50、56和312部分适用的规定；④每个参与的研究者按照21CFR50、56和312部分的规定进行研究。

根据21CFR 312.40（b），一个临床研究申请在FDA收到临床研究申请的30天后生效，除非FDA通知申办者这个研究被暂停临床，或FDA提前通知这个临床研究可以开始。您没有递交临床研究申请，但您把新药发放给受试者了。因此，您违背了21CFR 312.40（a）中关于没有有效的临床研究申请但发放化合物1、2、3的试验用新药给受试者。

2. 您未能在对试验药物收取费用前获得FDA预先书面授权［21 CFR 312.8（a）（3）］

FDA法规要求，申办者必须先获得FDA的书面许可，才能收取试验药物费用。您向研究受试者收取了试验用新药，即化合物1、2、3的管理费，而没有事先获得FDA书面许可。

3. 您未能保存足够的显示试验药物接收、转运或其他处置的记录［21 CFR 312.57（a）］

申办者必须保存对试验药物接收、转运或其他处置的足够记录。您没有保留在您的试验中试验药物化合物1、2、3的合适记录。缺少您这边生产的化合物1的分发、受试者药品归还和最终处置的文件。另外，缺少对未发给受试者的化合物2和3处置的文件。

研究者职责的违背［21 CFR 312.60，312.66和312.62（a）］。

4. 您未能按照 21 CFR 50 的要求获得知情同意［ 21 CFR 312.60 ］

除外21CFR50.23和50.24规定的，除非研究者获得了受试者或受试者法定代表人的合法知情同意［21CFR 50.20］，研究者不能把人作为受试者招募进入试验。在获得知情同意的过程中，FDA法规规定以下信息必须提供给每一个受试者［21CFR 50.25］：

a. 研究的试验性，试验的目的，受试者参与的预计持续时间，需要遵循的程序描述，试验性程序的鉴别。

b. 任何对受试者可合理预见的风险或不适的描述。

c. 任何对受试者的收益或可合理期望的描述。

d. 受试者可替代治疗程序或过程，或可能的益处的披露。

e. 能鉴别受试者身份的记录将会一定程度内保密，FDA有可能会检查这些记录。

f. 对于超出最小范围风险的试验，有关于是否有补偿的解释和如果发生伤害，是否有医疗治疗，以及这些治疗包括什么，进一步的信息在哪里可以获得。

g. 需要了解试验相关问题和受试者权利时的联系人，以及试验相关伤害事件的联系人。

h. 参加试验是自愿的，拒绝参加不会受到处罚或损失本来有权得到的利益，受试者可以在任何时候退出试验，而不会受到处罚或损失本来有权得到的利益。

作为研究者，根据21 CFR 50部分获得知情同意是您的职责。除外56.109（c），知情同意需要记录在被伦理委员会批准的书面的知情同意书上，受试者或受试者法定代表人需要当场签名、签日期。一份副本应提供给这个受试者［21 CFR 50.27（a）］。

您没有获得受试者的合法知情同意，然而您给这些受试者发放了试验用新药——化合物1、2、3。您告诉FDA检查员，您获得了这些受试者的知情同意。但是，您提供给FDA检查员作为知情同意的证明文件里没有包含上述必要元素，特别是给予的试验药物。我们承认知情同意书描述了使用药物后"可能的风险"。我们也知道知情同意书写到"这个试验产品的使用结果将不会保密，M-化妆品公司将在合适的地方使用，包括发表、临床研究、对员工或市售产品的说明书上"。这个声明不符合50.25（a）（5）的要求。此知情同意遗漏了50.25（a）其余必要的要求。我们注意到您提供给受试者的知情同意书没有获得伦理委员会的批准。

此外，FDA法规对知情同意［21 CFR 50.20］做了如下规定：无论是口头或书面的知情同意，不能包含任何免责条款，包括受试者或其代表人放弃或可能放弃受试者的法律权益，或免除申办者、试验场所或其代理机构疏忽的责任。您递交给FDA检查员的知情同意书没有符合这条规定，因为其特别包含了如下条款：

我在此解除、放弃以及约定不会控告Maxey化妆品有限公司及其附属机构、负责人、代理人、职员、志愿者和雇员（总称M-化妆品），包括所有使用这个产品后部分或全部责任、索赔、要求损失（原文如此）或对我的伤害或引起的指控；并且我进一步同意，除了这个解除和责任豁免、风险承担和赔偿协议，如果我或任何代表我的人，向以上任何人提出索赔时，我将免除M-化妆品公司承担任何可能由于此类索赔导致的诉讼费用、律师费、损失、责任、损害或费用。

5. 您未能确保 IRB 符合 21 临床研究［ 21 CFR 312.66 ］中列举的要求

FDA法规规定，临床研究只有在符合21CFR第56部分规定的伦理委员会审查和批准后才能启动。临床研究者有责任去确认伦理委员会对临床研究进行了初始审查和跟踪审查［21 CFR 312.66］。您违背了这些要求，因为您没有获得伦理委员会批准，但发放试验用新药——化合物1、2、3给受试者。您向FDA检查员承认，伦理委员会没有批准这个研究。然而，在没有伦理委员会批准下，您启动了研究并且发放了试验用新药——化合物1、2、3给受试者。

6. 您未能保存包括日期、数量和受试者使用情况的关于药物处置情况的足够记录［21 CFR 312.62（a）］

FDA法规规定，研究者需要保存药物处置的足够记录，包括日期、数量和使用者。您没有保存化合物1、2、3药物处置的足够记录，包括日期、数量和使用者。

我们收到您对FDA483表的回复，了解您将会遵从相关法规的声明。但是，您的回复没有明确您将如何确保依从这些法规。

本警告信的目的并非是罗列您在试验药物临床研究中存在的所有缺陷。确保遵循法律和相关FDA法规的每一项要求是您的职责。您应当解决这些缺陷，并建立规程，以确保任何正在进行或将来进行的研究均能符合FDA的法规。

自收到这封信的15个工作日内，您应当书面告知本办公室为预防将来发生类似违规情况已经采取的措施。如果不能充分、迅速地解释上述违规问题，可能导致我们在不再通知的情况下采取监管措施。

附：英文原文

Cayman Chemical Company

WARNING LETTER

JAN 19, 2010

CERTIFIED MAIL
RETURN RECEIPT REQUESTED

Ref: 10-HFD-45-01-01

Kirk M. Maxey, M.D.
President and CEO
Cayman Chemical Company
1180 East Ellsworth Road
Ann Arbor, MI 48108-2419

Dear Dr. Maxey:

Between May 12 and 18,2009, Ms. Nancy Bellamy, representing the Food and Drug Administration (FDA), conducted an investigation and met with you to review your conduct as both sponsor and investigator of clinical investigations of the prostaglandin-containing investigational drugs Compound 1, Compound 2, and Compound 3, performed for Cayman Chemical Company/Maxey Cosmetics, LLC.

This inspection is a part of the FDA's Bioresearch Monitoring Program, which includes inspections designed to evaluate the conduct of research and to ensure that the rights, safety, and welfare of the human subjects of those studies have been protected.

From our review of the establishment inspection report and the documents submitted with that report, we conclude that you did not adhere to the applicable statutory requirements and FDA regulations governing the conduct of clinical investigations and the protection of human subjects. We are aware that at the conclusion of the inspection, Ms. Bellamy presented and discussed with you Form FDA 483, Inspectional Observations. We wish to emphasize the following:

In the document entitled "Informed Consent," your company states, "Maxey Cosmetics (M-Cosmetics) will use volunteers to test an eyelash growth-enhancing product.... " This statement regarding eyelash growth makes clear that this product is intended to affect the structure or function of the body of man or other animals1 and therefore causes your product to be subject to regulation as a drug under Section 201(g)(1) of the Federal Food, Drug, and Cosmetic Act (the Act), 21 U.S.C. § 321(g)(1).

VIOLATIONS RELATED TO SPONSOR RESPONSIBILITIES [21 CFR 312.40, 312.8(a)(3), and 312.57(a)]

1. You failed to comply with the requirements for use of an investigational new drug in a clinical investigation by administering the investigational new drugs Compounds 1,2, and 3 to subjects without an IND in effect [21 CFR 312.40].

FDA regulations (21 CFR part 312) contain procedures and requirements governing the use of investigational new drugs. 21 CFR 312.3(b) defines a clinical investigation as "any experiment in which a drug is administered or dispensed to, or used involving, one or more human subjects. For the purposes of this part, an experiment is any use of a drug except for the use of a marketed drug in the course of medical practice." Compounds 1,2, and 3 are not approved for marketing in the U.S.A; therefore, any clinical investigation involving the use of these compounds must meet the general requirements for the use of an investigational new drug in a clinical investigation.

An investigational new drug may be used in a clinical investigation if the following conditions are met: (1) The sponsor submits an IND for the drug to FDA; (2) the IND is in effect under FDA regulations; (3) the sponsor complies with all applicable requirements of 21 CFR parts 50, 56, and 312; and (4) each participating investigator conducts his investigation in compliance with the requirements of 21 CFR parts 50, 56, and 312. [21 CFR 312.40(a)]

According to 21 CFR 312.40(b), an IND goes into effect thirty days after FDA receives the IND, unless FDA notifies the sponsor that the investigations described in the IND are subject to a clinical hold, or on earlier notification by FDA that the clinical investigations in the IND may begin. You did not submit an IND, yet you administered the new drugs to subjects. Therefore, you violated 21 CFR 312.40(a) by administering the investigational new drugs, Compounds 1, 2, and 3, to subjects without an IND in effect.

2. You failed to obtain prior written authorization from FDA prior to charging for an investigational drug [21 CFR 312.8(a)(3)].

FDA regulations state that a sponsor must obtain prior written authorization from FDA to charge for an investigational drug. You charged the study subjects an administration fee for the investigational new drugs, Compounds 1, 2, and 3 without obtaining prior written authorization from FDA.

3. You failed to maintain adequate records showing the receipt, shipment or other disposition of an investigational drug [21 CFR 312.57(a)].

The sponsor is required to maintain adequate records showing the receipt, shipment, or other disposition of the investigational drug. You did not maintain adequate recordkeeping of the investigational drugs Compounds 1, 2, and 3 used in your studies. There was no documentation of the distribution, return of product from the study subjects, and final disposition of Compound 1 that was manufactured at your firm. Additionally, there was no documentation for disposition of Compounds 2 and 3 that was not distributed to study subjects.

VIOLATIONS RELATED TO INVESTIGATOR RESPONSIBILITIES [21 CFR 312.60, 312.66, and 312.62(a)]

4. You failed to obtain informed consent in accordance with the provisions of 21 CFR part 50, as required by 21 CFR 312.60.

Except as provided in 21 CFR 50.23 and 50.24, no investigator may involve a human being as a subject in research unless the investigator has obtained the legally effective informed consent of the subject or the subject's legally authorized representative [21 CFR 50.20]. In seeking informed consent, the FDA regulations require that the following information must be provided to each subject [21 CFR 50.25]:

a. A statement that the study involves research, an explanation of the purposes of the research and the expected duration of the subject's participation, a description of the procedures to be followed, and identification of any procedures which are experimental.

b. A description of any reasonably foreseeable risks or discomforts to the subject.

c. A description of any benefits to the subject or to others which may reasonably be expected from the research.

d. A disclosure of appropriate alternative procedures or courses of treatment, if any, that might be advantageous to the subject.

e. A statement describing the extent, if any, to which confidentiality of records identifying the subject will be

maintained and that notes the possibility that the Food and Drug Administration may inspect the records.
f. For research involving more than minimal risk, an explanation as to whether any compensation and an explanation as to whether any medical treatments are available if injury occurs and, if so, what they consist of, or where further information may be obtained.
g. An explanation of whom to contact for answers to pertinent questions about the research and research subject's rights, and whom to contact in the event of a research-related injury to the subject.
h. A statement that participation is voluntary, that refusal to participate will involve no penalty or loss of benefits to which the subject is otherwise entitled, and that the subject may discontinue participation at any time without penalty or loss of benefits to which the subject is otherwise entitled.
As an investigator, it is your responsibility to obtain informed consent in accordance with 21 CFR part 50. Except as provided in 56.109(c), informed consent shall be documented by the use of a written consent form approved by the IRB and signed and dated by the subject or the subject's legally authorized representative at the time of consent. A copy shall be given to the person signing the form [21 CFR 50.27(a)].
You failed to obtain legally effective informed consent from subjects to whom you distributed the investigational new drugs, Compounds 1,2, and 3. You told the FDA investigator that you obtained informed consent from subjects to whom you distributed Compounds 1, 2, and 3. However, the documents that you provided as proof of informed consent to the FDA investigator did not contain the required elements described above, specific to the investigational drug product administered. We acknowledge that the informed consent document describes "possible risks" of the using the product. We also acknowledge that the informed consent states that, "The use of the results from the testing of the Product will not be confidential and can be used M-Cosmetics in any way deemed appropriate, including publication, clinical study, instruction of staff and/or marketing materials." This statement is not adequate to meet the requirements of 50.25(a)(5). The informed consent completely omits the remaining required elements of 50.25(a). We note that the informed consent documents you provided to subjects were not approved by an IRB.
Furthermore, FDA regulations governing informed consent [21 CFR 50.20] state that no informed consent, whether oral or written, may include any exculpatory language through which the subject or the representative is made to waive or appear to waive any of the subject's legal rights, or releases or appears to release the investigator, the sponsor, the institution, or its agents from liability for negligence. The informed consent document you submitted to the FDA inspector is not in compliance with this regulation because it specifically includes this statement:
I hereby release, discharge, and covenant not to sue Maxey Cosmetics, LLC, affiliates, directors, agents, officers, volunteers and employees (collectively, "M-Cosmetics"), from all liability, claims, demands losses [sic] or damages on my account caused or alleged to be caused in whole or in part by my use of the Product; and I further agree that if, despite this release and waiver of liability, assumption of risk, and indemnity agreement, I or anyone on my behalf, makes a claim against any, I will indemnify, save and hold harmless M-Cosmetics, from any litigation's expenses, attorney fees, loss, liability, damage or cost which any may incur as a result of such claim.

5. You failed to ensure that an IRB complying with the requirements set forth in 21 clinical study [21 CFR 312.66].

FDA regulations require that clinical investigations not be initiated unless that investigation has been reviewed and approved by an IRB meeting the requirements of 21 CFR Part 56. Clinical investigators are responsible for assuring that an IRB conducts initial and continuing reviews of clinical investigations [21 CFR 312.66]. You violated these requirements by administering the investigational new drugs, Compounds 1,2, and 3, to subjects without obtaining IRB approval. You admitted to the FDA investigator that an IRB had not approved the study. However, you initiated the investigation without IRB approval and proceeded to administer the investigational new drugs, Compounds 1,2, and 3, to subjects.

6. You failed to maintain adequate records of the disposition of the drug, including dates, quantity, and use by subjects [21 CFR 312.62(a)].

FDA regulations state that an investigator is required to maintain adequate records of the disposition of the drug, including dates, quantity, and use by subjects. You did not maintain adequate records of the disposition of the drug, including dates, quantity, and use by subjects, of Compounds 1, 2, and 3.

We acknowledge your response to the FDA Form 483, and note your statement that you will adhere to the required regulations. However, your response does not specify how you will ensure adherence to the regulations.

This letter is not intended to be an all-inclusive list of deficiencies with your clinical study of an investigational drug. It is your responsibility to ensure adherence to each requirement of the law and relevant FDA regulations. You should address these deficiencies and establish procedures to ensure that any on-going or future studies will be in compliance with FDA regulations.

Within fifteen (15) working days of your receipt of this letter, you should notify this office in writing of the actions you have taken to prevent similar violations in the future. Failure to adequately and promptly explain the violations noted above may result in regulatory action without further notice.

If you have any questions, please contact Constance Lewin, M.D., M.P.H., at 301-796-3397; FAX 301-847-8748. Your written response and any pertinent documentation should be addressed to:

Constance Lewin, M.D., M.P.H.
Branch Chief, Good Clinical Practice Branch I
Division of Scientific Investigations
Office of Compliance
Center for Drug Evaluation and Research
Food and Drug Administration
Bldg 51, Room 5354
10903 New Hampshire Avenue
Silver Spring, MD 20993

Sincerely yours,

/S/

Leslie K. Ball, M.D.
Director
Division of Scientific Investigations
Office of Compliance
Center for Drug Evaluation and Research
Food and Drug Administration

1 Products for which hair growth claims are made are drug products subject to FDA regulation. See United States v. Belden, 714 F. Supp. 42, 43-44 (N.D.N.Y. 1987).

第52封　给Brewer, George J. 医学博士的警告信

2009年1月14日

尊敬的Brewer博士：

2008年5月20日至6月9日，Nancy Bellamy女士、Laureen Kononen女士和Virginia Elgin博士代表FDA进行了现场检查，与您会面并对您作为申办-研究者实施的关于［（b）（4）］药物的下列临床研究进行了审查。

- 研究［（b）（4）］：早期治疗的［（b）（4）］临床试验研究［（b）（4）］。
- 研究［（b）（4）］：在［（b）（4）］的（b）（4）］双盲临床试验。
- 研究［（b）（4）］：早期神经性［（b）（4）］中的［（b）（4）］治疗方案Ⅲ期临床试验研究。

本次现场检查是FDA的生物研究监查项目的一部分。该项目通过设定的检查方法，对研究的实施情况进行评估，并确保这些研究中受试者的权益、安全和福利得到了保护。

经对FDA现场检查报告（EIR）、该报告附件进行审查，我们认为，您没有遵循适用的法律要求和监管临床研究实施及受试者保护的FDA法规。我们知道在现场检查结束时，Bellamy女士和Kononen女士向您出示并讨论了FDA483表，即现场检查发现的问题。我们想强调以下几点：

与研究者职责相关的违规［21 CFR 312.60，312.66，312.62（a）和312.62（c）］

1. 您未能按照21 CFR 50的要求，获得参加研究的受试者的知情同意［21 CFR 312.60］

21 CFR 50.20要求，除了50.23和50.24所规定的，除非已取得了受试者或其法定授权代表的具有法律效力的知情同意书，研究者不得将任何人作为受试者纳入临床研究。提供给受试者或其代表的信息应该采用受试者和其代表能够理解的语言。此外，FDA法规要求知情同意应以伦理委员会批准书面同意书的形式记录，并由受试者或其法定授权代表在予以同意时签名并签日期［21 CFR 50.27（a）］。

a. 入组研究［（b）（4）］的受试者［（b）（6）］和[（b）（6）]的文件当中没有签署过姓名和日期的知情同意文件。

b. 在2000年8月31日的访视中入组研究［（b）（4）］的受试者［（b）（6）]，其知情同意文件上没有受试者或其法定授权代表的签字。

c. 在2003年1月14日的访视中入组研究［（b）（4）］的受试者［（b）（4）]，其知情同意文件上没有受试者或其法定授权代表的签字。

d. 关于研究［（b）（4）]，其研究程序在从受试者［（b）（4）］和［（b）（4）］获得知情同意之前就开始实施了。尤其是，对于受试者［（b）（4）]，1988年10月4日进行了脑部MRI检查，而知情同意直到1988年10月8日才由受试者签署。对于受试者［（b）（4）]，1994年10月4日进行了肝活检，而知情同意直到1994年10月5日才由受试者签署。

e. 提供给受试者和其法定授权代表的信息没有用受试者和其代表能够理解的语言。尤其是，提供给非英语母语受试者的知情同意文件用英语书写。实例包括但不限于下列：入组研究［（b）（4）］的受试者［（b）（6）]，入组研究［（b）（4）］的受试者［（b）（6）］。

2. 您未能确保由符合适用法规要求的IRB负责对研究进行跟踪审查和批准［21 CFR 312.66］

在伦理委员会的研究批准已经过期的时限里，您继续开展研究活动。实例包括但不限于下列：

a. 研究［（b）（4）］伦理委员会的批准失效，从1993年3月19日直到1993年4月29日，受试者［（b）（6）］被入组（1993年4月15日）。该研究伦理委员会批准从1995年7月14日到1995年9月28日也失效，在这个

时限内，受试者［（b）（4）］被入组（1995年7月18日）。

b. 研究［（b）（4）］伦理委员会批准失效，从2005年6月30日到2005年9月8日，以及从2006年9月7日到2006年10月5日。在这些时限内，受试者正在接受研究药物治疗或接受评估。

3. 您未能保存对试验药物处置的准确记录［21 CFR 312.62（a）］

就研究［（b）（4）］而论，给数据安全监查委员会（DSMB）和伦理委员会的日期为2004年7月20日的报告显示，［（b）（4）］犯了一个错误，本来只应该含有试验药物的瓶子中包含了安慰剂胶囊。报告显示，这个错误涉及一个受试者、一个星期的时间，在这段时间内该受试者接受了50%～90%的正确的试验药物。一份日期为2004年4月20日的备忘录，描述了2004年2月17日发生的一次发药错误，胶囊被分发给了受试者［（b）（4）］。

4. 您未能按照研究计划进行研究［21 CFR 312.60］

研究［（b）（4）］的研究计划规定，有并行癫痫发作活动的受试者应被排除。受试者［（b）（6）］于1999年5月8日强直-阵挛发作，但是他被违规入组本研究。

与申办者职责相关的违规［21 CFR 312.53（c）（1），312.56（a），312.57（a）和312.57（c）］

5. 您未能在允许研究者参加一项研究之前，取得研究者声明，即FDA1572表［21 CFR 312.53（c）（1）］

尤其是，就研究［（b）（4）］而论，您在取得一份签署过的研究者声明之前，准许一名临床研究者参与药物临床试验，该声明包括以下内容：

a. 研究者的姓名和地址；

b. 研究者实施研究项目在IND内的方案名称和编号（如果存在）；

c. 将进行临床研究的所有医学院、医院或其他研究机构的名称和地址；

d. 研究中用到的所有临床实验室机构的名称和地址；

e. 负责审查和批准研究项目的伦理委员会的名称和地址；

f. 研究者所做的承诺，她或他：

ⅰ. 按照现有相关试验方案执行研究项目，仅在通知申办者后才能对试验方案进行修改，除非为保护研究受试者安全、权益或福利的特殊情况；

ⅱ. 遵循有关临床研究者职责的所有要求以及本部分规定的所有其他相关要求；

ⅲ. 亲自执行或监督该研究的实施；

ⅳ. 告知所有潜在受试者即将使用的药物是以研究为目的，并且确保满足知情同意要求（21 CFR 50部分）和IRB审查和批准的相关要求（21 CFR 56部分）。

ⅴ. 312.64规定向申办者报告研究过程中发生的不良事件；

ⅵ. 已经阅读并理解研究者手册中的信息，包括药物的潜在风险和副作用；

ⅶ. 确保通知所有实施研究项目的人员、同事及员工需履行上述承诺的职责。

6. 您未能对IND下属的所有正在进行的临床研究的进展情况进行监查［21 CFR 312.56（a）］

FDA现场检查发现，您未保留任何记录，以证实在IND项下实施的上述临床研究项目被充分地监控。在2008年8月13日对FDA483表的书面回复中，您声称，您亲自参与到每一名受试者的护理和治疗中，以及在密歇根大学参与到［（b）（4）］研究的每一名受试者的治疗，并且监控他们的进展。您声称，在最近的几年间，DSMB对研究期间的数据进行监控，以确保患者的安全。您声称，确实是这样：您依赖密歇根大学的个人来帮忙确保在Ann Arbor的临床研究项目正确地进行，依赖在［（b）（4）］学术研究机构的一名同事来在他的机构做同样的事。但是，您承认，您未能为监控活动保存足够记录。

7. 您未能保存关于试验药物运输的充足记录［21 CFR 312.57（a）］

对于研究［（b）（4）］来说，在现场检查过程中，您没有任何记录表明，试验药物运输到在［（b）（4）］研究中心的临床研究者。

8. 您未能保存记录到必需的时间段［21 CFR 312.57（c）］

21 CFR 312.62（c）要求，申办者按照21 CFR 312的要求保存记录和报告，直到该药上市申请批准后2年；或者，该药物上市申请如果未被批准，直到临床试验用途的药物装运和交货停止并通知FDA后2年。按照21 CFR 312.53（c）（2）要求，应该获取说明研究者教育程度、培训背景和职业经验、证明其有资格作为专家参与新药临床研究的个人简历或其他资历说明，在［（b）（4）］研究中心实施研究项目［（b）（4）］的临床研究者资料无法找到。在现场检查过程中，您告诉FDA检查员说您确实在研究开始就有临床研究者个人简历的存档，但是找不到它。

本警告信的目的并非是罗列您在试验药物临床试验研究中存在的所有缺陷。确保遵循每一项法律和相关FDA法规的要求是您的职责。您应当解决这些缺陷，建立规程，确保任何正在进行或将来进行的研究都符合FDA法规。

自收到这封信的15个工作日内，您应当书面告知本部门为预防将来发生类似违规情况已经或将要采取的措施。如果不能充分、迅速地解释上述违规行为，可能导致我们在不再通知的情况下采取监管措施。

附：英文原文

Brewer, George J. M.D.

WARNING LETTER

Jan 14, 2009

CERTIFIED MAIL
RETURN RECEIPT REQUESTED

George J. Brewer, M.D.
University of Michigan Medical School
205 Zina Pitcher Rd.
Ann Arbor, MI 48109

Dear Dr. Brewer:

Between May 20 and June 9, 2008, Ms. Nancy Bellamy, Ms. Laureen Kononen, and Dr. Virginia Elgin, representing the Food and Drug Administration (FDA), conducted an investigation and met with you to review your conduct as both sponsor and investigator of the following clinical investigations of the investigational drug [(b)(4)]:

- Study [(b)(4)]: Clinical Trial of [(b)(4)] in the Initial Treatment [(b)(4)]
- Study [(b)(4)]: Double Blind Trial of [(b)(4)] in [(b)(4)]; and
- Study [(b)(4)]: Phase Ⅲ Study of [(b)(4)] Dose Regimen in Initial Neurological [(b)(4)]

This inspection is a part of the FDA's Bioresearch Monitoring Program, which includes inspections designed to evaluate the conduct of research and to ensure that the rights, safety, and welfare of the human subjects of those studies have been protected.

From our review of the establishment inspection report and the documents submitted with that report, we conclude that you did not adhere to the applicable statutory requirements and FDA regulations governing the conduct of clinical investigations and the protection of human subjects. We are aware that at the conclusion of the inspection, Ms. Bellamy and Ms. Kononen presented and discussed with you Form FDA 483, Inspectional Observations. We wish to emphasize the following:

VIOLATIONS RELATED TO INVESTIGATOR RESPONSIBILITIES [21 CFR 312.60, 312.66, 312.62(a), and 312.62(c)]

1. You failed to obtain informed consent of subjects involved in research in accordance with the provisions of 21 CFR Part 50 [21 CFR 312.60].

21 CFR 50.20 requires that except as provided in sections 50.23 and 50.24, no investigator may involve a human being as a subject in research unless the investigator has obtained the legally effective informed consent of the subject or the subject's legally authorized representative. The information that is given to the subject or the representative shall be in language understandable to the subject or the representative. In addition, the FDA regulations require that informed consent be documented by the use of a written consent form approved by the IRB and signed and dated by the subject or the subject's legally authorized representative at the time of consent [21 CFR 50.27(a)].

a. There were no signed and dated informed consent documents on file for subjects [(b)(6)] and [(b)(6)] enrolled in study [(b)(4)].

b. There is no signature of the subject or the subject's legally authorized representative on the informed consent document for subject [(b)(6)] enrolled in study [(b)(4)] at the 8/31/00 visit.

c. There is no signature of the subject or the subject's legally authorized representative on the informed consent document for subject [(b)(4)] enrolled in study [(b)(4)] for the follow-up visit on 1/14/03.

d. Regarding study [(b)(4)], study procedures were conducted prior to obtaining informed consent from subjects [(b)(4)] and [(b)(4)]. Specifically, for subject [(b)(4)], an MRI of the brain was conducted on 10/4/88, but informed consent was not signed by the subject until 10/06/88. For subject [(b)(4)], a liver biopsy was performed on 10/4/94, but informed consent was not signed by the subject until 10/5/94.

e. The information that was given to the subject or the subject's legally authorized representative was not in a language understandable to the subject or the subject's legally authorized representative. Specifically, non-English speaking subjects were given informed consent documents written in English. Examples include, but are not limited to, the following: Subjects [(b)(6)] enrolled in study [(b)(4)] and subjects [(b)(6)] enrolled in study [(b)(4)].

2. You failed to assure that an Institutional Review Board (IRB) complying with applicable regulatory requirements was responsible for the continuing review and approval of a clinical study [21 CFR 312.66].

You continued to perform research activities during timeframes when the IRB's study approval was expired. Examples include, but are not limited to, the following:

a. Study [(b)(4)] lapsed in IRB approval from 3/19/93 until 4/29/93. During this timeframe subject [(b)(6)] was enrolled (4/15/93). The study also lapsed in IRB approval from 7/14/95 until 9/28/95. During this timeframe subject [(b)(4)] was enrolled (7/18/95).

b. Study [(b)(4)] lapsed in IRB approval from 6/30/05 until 9/08/05, and from 9/7/06 until 10/05/06. Subjects were receiving study medications or seen for evaluations during these time periods.

3. You failed to maintain adequate and accurate records for disposition of the investigational drug [21 CFR 312.62(a)].

Regarding study [(b)(4)], a report dated 7/20/04 to the Data Safety Monitoring Board (DSMB) and IRB indicated that the [(b)(4)] made an error by including placebo capsules in a bottle that should have contained only the investigational drug. The report indicated that this involved one subject for a period of one week, during which the subject received between 50% and 90% of the correct investigational drug. A memorandum dated 4/20/04 describes a dispensing error in medication on 2/17/04 when capsules were dispensed for subjects [(b)(4)]

4. You failed to conduct the studies according to the investigational plan [21 CFR 312.60].

The research plan for study [(b)(4)] specified that subjects with concurrent seizure activities should be excluded. Subject [(b)(6)] had tonic-clonic seizures on 5/8/99, but was enrolled in the study in violation of the study.

VIOLATIONS RELATED TO SPONSOR RESPONSIBILITIES [21 CFR 312.53(c)(1), 312.56(a), 312.57(a), and 312.57(c)]

5. You failed to obtain an investigator statement, Form FDA 1572, before permitting an investigator to participate in an investigation [21 CFR 312.53(c)(1)].

Specifically, regarding study [(b)(4)], you allowed a clinical investigator to participate in the investigation prior to obtaining a signed investigator statement containing:

a. The name and address of the investigator;

b. The name and code number, if any, of the study(s) in the IND identifying the study(ies) to be conducted by the investigator;

c. The name and address of any medical school, hospital, or other research facility where the clinical investigation(s) will be conducted;

d. The name and address of any clinical laboratory facilities to be used in the study;

e. The name and address of the IRB that is responsible for review and approval of the study(ies);

f. A commitment by the investigator that he or she:

i. Will conduct the study(ies) in accordance with the relevant, current study(s) and will only make changes in a study after notifying the sponsor, except when necessary to protect the safety, the rights, or welfare of subjects;

ii. Will comply with all requirements regarding the obligations of clinical investigators and all other pertinent requirements in this part;

iii. Will personally conduct or supervise the described investigation(s);

iv. Will inform any potential subjects that the drugs are being used for investigational purposes and will ensure that the requirements relating to obtaining informed consent (21 CFR part 50) and institutional review board review and approval (21 CFR part 56) are met;

v. Will report to the sponsor adverse experiences that occur in the course of the investigation(s) in accordance with 312.64;

vi. Has read and understands the information in the investigator's brochure, including the potential risks and side effects of the drug; and

vii. Will ensure that all associates, colleagues, and employees assisting in the conduct of the study(ies) are informed about their obligations in meeting the above commitments.

6. You failed to monitor the progress of all clinical investigations being conducted under your IND [21 CFR 312.56(a)].

The FDA inspection disclosed that you did not maintain any documentation to indicate that the above studies conducted under an IND were adequately monitored. In your August 13, 2008 response letter to the Form FDA 483, you stated that you were personally involved in the care and treatment of every subject and treatment of every subject who participated in the [(b)(4)] studies at the University of Michigan, and monitored their progress. You stated that during the last several years, a DSMB monitored the data collected during the studies to assure patient safety. You stated that it is true that you relied on individuals at the University of Michigan to help assure that the research was properly conducted in Ann Arbor, and on a colleague at an academic institution in [(b)(4)] to do the same at his site. However, you acknowledged that you failed to document monitoring activities adequately.

7. You failed to maintain adequate records showing the shipment of the investigational drug [21 CFR 312.57(a)].

Regarding study [(b)(4)], during the inspection you did not have any documentation showing the shipment of investigational drugs to the clinical investigator at the [(b)(4)] site.

8. You failed to retain records for the requisite time period 121 CFR 312.57(c)].

21 CFR 312.62(c) requires that a sponsor retain the records and reports required by 21 CFR Part 312 for 2 years after a marketing application is approved for the drug; or, if an application is not approved for the drug, until 2 years after shipment and delivery of the drug for investigational use is discontinued and FDA has been so notified. A curriculum vitae or other statement of qualifications of the investigator showing the education, training, and experience that

qualifies the investigator as an expert in the clinical investigation of the drug for the use under investigation required to be obtain by 21 CFR 312.53(c)(2) could not be located for the clinical investigator conducting study [(b)(4)] at the [(b)(4)] Sites. During the inspection you told the FDA investigators that you did have the clinical investigator's curriculum vitae on file at the start of the study, but could not locate it.

This letter is not intended to be an all-inclusive list of deficiencies with your clinical study of an investigational drug. It is your responsibility to ensure adherence to each requirement of the law and relevant FDA regulations. You should address these deficiencies and establish procedures to ensure that any on-going or future studies will be in compliance with FDA regulations.

Within fifteen (15) working days of your receipt of this letter, you should notify this office in writing of the actions you have taken or will be taking to prevent similar violations in the future. Failure to adequately and promptly explain the violations noted above may result in regulatory action without further notice.

If you have any questions, please contact Constance Lewin, M.D., M.P.H., at 301-796-3397; FAX 301-847-8748. Your written response and any pertinent documentation should be addressed to:

Constance Lewin, M.D., M.P.H.
Branch Chief, Good Clinical Practice Branch I
Division of Scientific Investigations
Office of Compliance
Center for Drug Evaluation and Research
Food and Drug Administration
Bldg 51, Room 5354
10903 New Hampshire Avenue
Silver Spring, MD 20993

Sincerely yours,

{See appended electronic signature page}

Leslie K. Ball, M.D.
Director
Division of Scientific Investigations
Office of Compliance
Center for Drug Evaluation and Research

第53封　给Hsueh, Wila A. 医学博士的警告信

2008年5月30日

参考号：08-HFD-45-0503

尊敬的Hsueh博士：

2007年9月4日至10月9日，Diane C. Van Leeuwen女士 代表FDA进行了现场检查，与您会面并审查了您实施以下临床研究的情况。

试验方案［不公开］药物罗格列酮的“罗格列酮对伴有糖耐量异常的心脏移植患者的心肌纤维化、心肌功能以及动脉粥样硬化的影响”，试验药物［不公开］，试验方案［不公开］糖尿病中的作用和活动［不公开］，［不公开］合并罗格列酮和二甲双胍对比罗格列酮和二甲双胍对2型糖尿病中血糖控制的影响（26周评估安全性和有效性的双盲、平行研究）。

本次现场检查是FDA的生物研究监查项目的一部分。该项目通过设定的检查方法，对研究的实施情况进行评估，并确保这些研究中受试者的权益、安全和福利得到了保护。

经对FDA现场检查报告、该报告的附件，以及您2007年10月22日对FDA 483表的书面回复进行审查，我们认为，您没有遵循适用的法律要求和监管临床研究实施及受试者保护的FDA法规。我们获悉在现场检查结束时，Watson女士向您出示并讨论了FDA483表，即现场检查发现的问题。我们想强调以下几点：

申办者违规

1. 您未能对IND中的所有正在进行的临床研究的进展情况进行监查［21 CFR 312.56（a）］

我们现场检查发现，未对试验方案［不公开］进行监查。如果按照FDA法规要求对研究进行了监查，以下所发现的问题也许就能避免。

2. 在研究开始前，您未能确保FDA 1572表中包括了在研究项目进行过程中协助研究者的助理研究者（例如研究同事、住院医师）的名单［21 CFR 312.53（a）（1）（viii）］

对于试验方案［不公开］，我们检查发现，下列医师在临床研究中承担着重要的角色，但是没有作为助理研究者列在FDA1572表中：［不公开］。尽管医生［不公开］在试验方案［不公开］的FDA1572表上签了名，但作为研究方案［不公开］的申办者-研究者，您有责任确保您已获得一份由协助研究者进行临床研究的助理人员签字确认的研究者申明。

研究者违规

3. 您未能对临床研究进行充分的监管［21 CFR 312.60］

研究者签署研究者声明时，即他（她）同意在他（她）所在的研究场所承担临床研究者的职责。您签署了试验方案［不公开］的FDA1572表，虽然是［不公开］医生签署了试验方案［不公开］的FDA1572表，但您和［不公开］医生都在表中列名为临床研究者。［不公开］医生在受试者入组之前离开了您的部门，您于2005年3月3日告知独立伦理委员会（IRB），您将作为此研究的研究者。因此，我们认为您就是［不公开］试验的研究者。作为研究者的总体职责（21 CFR 312.60），包括确保临床试验按照签署的研究者声明、研究计划和适用的法规执行，在您的监护下保护受试者的权益、安全和福利，确保临床试验中的药品管控。研究者签署FDA1572表时，即他（她）明确同意将亲自进行临床试验或者将对他（她）未能亲自进行的试验部分实施监督。尽管您可以将特定试验任务授权给合格的人来执行，但作为临床研究者，您不能授权您的总体职责。

我们现场检查发现，您对授权了研究任务的人员的监管不够充分，不足以确保临床试验按照签署的研究者声明、研究计划和适用的法规以及从保护受试者的权利、安全和福利的方式来执行。由于您的监管不力，

导致发现问题，讨论如下。

4. 您未能确保符合56部分所列要求的IRB负责对拟进行的临床研究进行初始审查、跟踪审查和批准，您未能确保研究活动的所有更改都及时向IRB报告，而且这些更改得到IRB的批准［21 CFR 312.661］

a. 我们现场检查发现，[不公开] 方案的修改在得到IRB批准前已经执行。检查期间，FDA检查员得知所有和本试验相关的IRB文件复印件未保存在您的研究场所。对IRB关于此研究的文件审查发现，您的研究场所递交了2次试验方案。首次递交由IRB 2004年3月8日接收。IRB 2004年3月8日接收的方案版本中，入组标准规定：受试者应为心脏移植后3个月，并且此类人群中有两组糖尿病患者符合条件：①移植前已存在糖尿病的患者将自动入组；②一次早晨空腹血糖值＞100mmol/dL的患者将进行糖尿病的进一步检查，75g口服糖耐量试验，如果2小时后的血糖值＞200mmol/dL，则他们符合作为糖尿病患者入组试验的条件。

IRB接收第二次递交的时间为2007年2月9日，所有受试者已完成入组（首例受试者知情同意时间为2006年8月3日，末例受试者知情同意时间为2007年1月11日）。虽然看起来这次递交的目的是将［不公开］题目从研究中删除，但该版本的方案却有着不同的入组标准。该版本的方案提出，受试者应为心脏移植后2~6周，且进一步提出，移植前已患糖尿病的患者，如未接受过胰岛素或多于2种口服降糖药治疗，则可入组。空腹血糖＞126或者一次随机血糖＞200的患者，如果OGTT值超过200，则符合标准。IRB于2007年3月7日再次批准了此研究。然而，在FDA检查IRB的过程中，可以确认的是，由于您未按照IRB的流程递交之前已批准研究的修正案，因此IRB不了解对此方案的修订。

由于记录保存的不合理，FDA检查员很难确定试验过程中正在使用哪个版本的方案。对研究记录的审查发现您的试验场所有标识为“版本1”“版本2”“版本3”“版本4”的4个方案复印件。您和［不公开］医生（于2007年3月承担研究者职责）都表示研究过程中使用的是“版本4”。“版本4”中入组标准提示：受试者应为心脏移植术后2周且糖耐量受损，即2次或多次空腹血糖高于或等于100~125mg/dL，以及2次或多次空腹血糖不高于126mg/dL 的frank糖尿病患者。我们现场检查未证实“版本4”方案得到了IRB的审查和批准。

b. 我们调查发现，此研究的IRB批件已于2006年12月14日过期。3名受试者8、9和10于2007年1月通过知情同意进入了研究。2007年2月23日IRB暂停了此研究并向您要求提供信息。直到2007年3月7日IRB才重新批准了此研究。因此，3名受试者是在独立审查委员会批件过期期间入组的。

5. 您未能按照研究计划进行研究［21 CFR 312.60］

独立审查委员会2004年11月17日批准的试验要求［不公开］：

a. 试验方案要求，使用罗格列酮治疗的患者应以4mg/d剂量开始，持续6周后，剂量调整至8mg/d。受试者［不公开］2006年6月17日接受了心脏移植，并于2006年8月3日入组试验，该受试者以2mg/d开始治疗，3个月后即2006年11月剂量调整至6mg/d。受试者［不公开］2006年8月23日接受了心脏移植，2006年9月7日入组。在整个研究期间，受试者的罗格列酮的剂量始终为4mg/d。

b. 试验方案要求，罗格列酮开始治疗后的前6周内需要每周电话联系受试者，以检查过去1周患者体重的变化。没有文件记录该试验方案要求在服用罗格列酮的受试者身上得到了实施。在您的书面回复中，您称因为受试者频繁进行门诊访视，而没有电话联系受试者。这种解释我们不能接受，并认为未电话联系患者这一事实就是违背了试验方案。

c. 试验方案要求，试验药物罗格列酮由［不公开］免费提供给受试者，并且受试者签署的知情同意书中也表明罗格列酮免费。我们调查发现，由［不公开］运输至UCLA药房的用于此研究的罗格列酮并未使用，而受试者都是通过处方被提供了罗格列酮。因此，罗格列酮似乎并未免费提供给受试者。

d. 试验方案［不公开］要求，受试者被随机至试验1.2mg组或1.8mg组，或安慰剂组。受试者381010被随机至试验1.2mg组或安慰剂组。在第6次访视时受试者剂量被错误地调高至1.8mg。

6. 您未能保存充分的包括日期、数量及患者的使用情况的药物处置记录［21 CFR 312.62（a）］

如上第4条所述，试验方案［不公开］中受试者凭处方获得罗格列酮，而并非使用由［不公开］提供的试验药物，且无药物发放记录。在您的回复中，您承认研究者未复印处方，没有数药片，也没有“实时”清点罗格列酮的使用。另外，我们的检查未能确认患者是否按处方拿药。因此，调查未能确认受试者是否按照试验方案要求使用了合适的试验药物及剂量。

7. 您未能按照 21 CFR 50 的要求获得知情同意［21 CFR 50.201］

a. 根据21 CFR50.25（a），在获取知情同意过程中，应向每位受试者提供的信息必须包括应完成的临床试验流程的描述。试验方案［不公开］中，知情同意书中应完成的临床试验流程的描述不准确，受试者被告知参加试验会被随机分配至罗格列酮组或安慰剂组。但我们调查发现，研究中未使用安慰剂。

b. 根据21 CFR 312.60要求，知情同意书中应提及FDA检查此研究记录的可能性。此研究知情同意书中未提及此内容。

c. 21 CFR 50.20要求，提供给受试者或法定代理人的信息必须使用受试者或法定代理人能够理解的语言；知情同意书必须使用IRB批准的版本，并由受试者本人在知情时签名、签日期。FDA法规提供了两种受试者给出知情同意的方式。根据21 CFR 50.27（b）（1）研究者可以使用书面的知情同意文件，其中包括21 CFR 50.25中要求的要素。研究者也可以使用简短的知情同意表，书面记录21 CFR 50.25中要求的要素已经口头通知了受试者。研究者使用简短的知情同意表时，口头讲述时需要一个见证人在场，讲述内容的书面概述需要IRB审批，受试者（或受试者的代表）必须签署此表；见证人也必须签署此表及概述。最后，此表格和概述的副本交给受试者或其代表保存［21 CFR50.27（b）（2）］。试验方案［不公开］的所有受试者均以西班牙语为第一语言，但他们开始签署的知情同意书为英文版本。尽管您在回复函中解释，对受试者的知情讲解使用了西班牙语，但您并未提供遵循了21 CFR50.27（b）（2）的证据。

2007年4月［不公开］医生承担研究者工作后，用西班牙语知情同意书对受试者们进行了重新告知。

8. 您未能保存研究中使用试验药物或对照组的受试者的所有研究观察结果和其他相关数据的足够及准确的病历［21 CFR 312.62（b）］

a. 试验方案中规定，受试者筛选前需要使用一种或多种抗糖尿病药物治疗至少3个月。但［不公开］研究中没有文件记录证明受试者符合这一要求。我们注意到，这些受试者的研究文件中没有病历。您在备忘录中记录，受试者［不公开］既往治疗的医生在墨西哥，因此无法获得受试者的病历。这些备忘录不能充分解决受试者缺少病历的问题。没有病历，受试者是否使用了抗糖尿病药物等信息无法核实，因此无法核实受试者是否符合入组标准。

b. 试验方案［不公开］EKG报告中的日期打印错误，有些报告打印的时间是过去数十年，更多的时间为未来的时间。有些报告打印的时间是正确的，有些报告打印的时间是错误的。

- 受试者［不公开］EKG的日期打印为2038年1月19日，后被划掉修改为2006年12月11日。
- 受试者［不公开］EKG的日期打印为2033年10月18日。
- 受试者［不公开］EKG的日期打印为2033年10月18日，后被划掉修改为2007年1月16日。
- 受试者［不公开］EKG的日期打印为2033年10月18日，后被划掉修改为2006年12月13日。
- 受试者［不公开］EKG的日期打印为2033年10月18日。
- 受试者［不公开］EKG的日期打印为2033年10月18日。
- 受试者［不公开］EKG的日期打印为1970年1月1日。
- 受试者［不公开］EKG的日期打印为1970年1月1日，后被划掉修改为2006年10月20日。

本警告信的目的并非是罗列您在试验药物临床研究中存在的所有缺陷。确保遵循法律和相关FDA法规的每一项要求是您的职责。您应当解决这些缺陷，并建立规程，以确保任何正在进行或将来进行的研究均能符合FDA的法规。

自收到这封信的15个工作日内，您应当书面告知本部门在您书面回复中的纠正措施已经完成。如果不能充分、迅速地解释上述违规问题，可能导致我们在不再通知的情况下采取监管措施。

附：英文原文

Hsueh, Wila A., M.D.

WARNING LETTER

MAY 30, 2008

CERTIFIED MAIL
RETURN RECEIPT REQUESTED

Ref: 08-HFD-45-0503

Willa A. Hsueh, M.D.
David Geffen School of Medicine at UCLA
900 Veteran Avenue, Suite 24-130
Los Angeles, CA 90095

Dear Dr. Hsueh:

Between September 4 and October 9,2007, Ms. Diane C. Van Leeuwen, representing the Food and Drug Administration (FDA), conducted an investigation and met with you, to review your conduct of the following clinical investigations:

Protocol # [ ] "Impact of Rosiglitazone on Cardiac Fibrosis, Function and Atherosclerosis in Cardiac Transplant Patients with Carbohydrate Intolerance", of the investigational drug rosiglitazone; and

Protocol # [ ] Effect and Action in Diabetes [ ] Effect on Glycemic Control of [ ] in Combination with Rosiglitazone plus Metformin versus Rosiglitazone plus Metformin in Type 2 Diabetes (A Twenty-Six Week Double-Blind Parallel Trial to Investigate Safety and Efficacy)", of the investigational drug [ ]

We note that you were the sponsor-investigator for protocol [ ] and [ ] was the sponsor of protocol [ ].

This inspection is a part of the FDA's Bioresearch Monitoring Program, which includes inspections designed to evaluate the conduct of research and to ensure that the rights, safety, and welfare of the human subjects participating in those studies have been protected.

From our review of the establishment inspection report, the documents submitted with that report, and your October 22, 2007 written response to Form FDA 483, we conclude that you did not adhere to the applicable statutory requirements and FDA regulations governing the conduct of clinical investigations and the protection of human subjects. We are aware that at the conclusion of the inspection, Ms. Van Leeuwen presented and discussed with you Form FDA 483, Inspectional Observations. We wish to emphasize the following:

Sponsor Violations

1. You failed to monitor the progress of a clinical investigation being conducted under an IND [21 CFR 312.56(a)].

Our investigation revealed that protocol [ ] was not monitored. It appears that had the study been monitored as required by FDA regulations, the observations discussed below might have been prevented.

2. Before beginning the investigation, you failed to ensure that Form FDA 1572 included the names of the sub-investigators (e.g., research fellows, residents) who will be assisting the investigator in the conduct of the investigation [21 CFR 312.53(c)(1)(ⅷ)].

For protocol [ ] our investigation revealed that the following physicians had a significant role in the conduct of the investigation, but were not listed on Form FDA 1572 as sub-investigators: [ ] Although Dr. [ ] signed Form FDA 1572 for protocol [ ] as the sponsor-investigator of protocol [ ] you were responsible or ensuring that you had obtained a signed investigator statement listing the names of the sub-investigators who would be assisting the investigator in the conduct of the investigation.

Investigator Violations

3. You failed to adequately supervise the investigations [21 CFR 312.60].

When an investigator signs an investigator statement, he or she agrees to take on the responsibilities of a clinical investigator at his or her site. You signed Form FDA 1572 for protocol # [ ] we note that, although Dr [ ] signed Form FDA 1572 for protocol [ ] you and Dr [ ] are listed as the clinical investigators on the form. Dr. [ ] left your division prior to the enrollment of any study subjects, and you informed the IRB on March 3, 2005 that you would be the investigator for the study. Therefore, we consider you to be the investigator for study [ ] Your general responsibilities as an investigator (21 CFR 312.60) include ensuring that the clinical trials are conducted according to the signed investigator statements, the investigational plans, and applicable regulations; protecting the rights, safety, and welfare of subjects under your care; and ensuring control of drugs under investigation. When a clinical investigator signs Form FDA 1572, he or she specifically agrees to personally conduct the clinical trials or to supervise those aspects of the trials that he or she did not personally conduct. While you may delegate certain study tasks to individuals qualified to perform them, as a clinical investigator, you may not delegate your general responsibilities. Our investigation indicates that your supervision of personnel to whom you delegated study tasks was not adequate to ensure that the clinical trials were conducted according to the signed investigator statements, the investigational plans, and applicable regulations, and in a manner that protects the rights, safety, and welfare of human subjects. Your lack of supervision led to the observations discussed below.

4. You failed to assure that an IRB that complies with the requirements set forth in Part 56 was responsible for the initial and continuing review and approval of the proposed clinical study, and you failed to assure that all changes in the research activity were promptly reported to the IRB and that changes to the research received IRB approval [21 CFR 312.661].

a. Our investigation revealed that changes to the # [ ] protocol were implemented without IRB approval. During the inspection, the FDA investigator learned that copies of all IRB documents pertaining to this study were not maintained at your site. A review of the IRB's file for this study revealed two protocol submissions from your site. The first submission was received by the IRB on 3/8/04. In the version of the protocol received by the IRB on 3/8/04, the inclusion criteria stated that subjects would be 3 months post cardiac transplant and that there would be two groups of diabetic patients eligible within this population: l) those who were diabetic before transplantation would be automatically eligible; and 2) subjects who are found to have one fasting morning blood sugar more than 100 mmol/dL would be requested to have further testing for diabetes by doing a 75 gm oral glucose tolerance test, and if their blood sugar is more than 200 mmol/dL after 2 hours, they would be eligible to enter the study as a diabetic.

The second submission was received by the IRB on 2/9/07 after all subjects had been enrolled (initial subjects consented on 8/3/06; last subject consented on 1/11/07). Although it appears that the purpose of this submission was to remove [ ] name from the research, this version of the protocol also has different inclusion criteria. This version of the protocol stated that subjects would be 2-6 weeks post-cardiac transplant. It further stated that patients who were diabetic before transplantation would be eligible if their treatment did not involve insulin or more than 2 oral hypoglycemic agents. Patients who are identified as having fasting blood glucoses of more than 126 or random blood glucose of more than 200 on one occasion would be eligible if their OGTT value exceeded 200. The IRB re-approved the study on 3/7/07; however, during the FDA inspection of the IRB, it was confirmed that the IRB was unaware of modifications to the protocol because you did not follow the IRB's procedures for submitting modifications to previously approved research.

Due to poor recordkeeping, the FDA investigator had difficulty making a determination regarding which version of the protocol was operational during the study. A review of study records revealed 4 copies of the protocol at your site labeled "Version 1", "Version 2", "Version 3", and "Version 4". Both you and Dr. [ ] (who assumed investigator responsibilities in March 2007), stated "Version 4' was the version used during the study. Inclusion criteria in Version 4 stated that patients would be two weeks post cardiac transplant with impaired glucose tolerance, that is a fasting blood glucose of more than or equal to 100-125 mg/dl on 2 or more occasions, as well as frank diabetics with fasting blood glucose of more than 126 mg/dl on 2 occasions or more. Our investigation failed to confirm that "Version 4" of the protocol ever received IRB review and approval.

b. Our investigation revealed that IRB approval for the study expired on 12/14/06. Three subjects (8, 9, and 10) were consented for the study in January 2007. On 2/23/07, the IRB suspended the research study and requested information from you. The IRB did not re-approve the research study until 3/7/07; therefore, these subjects were enrolled during the time-period when IRB approval had expired.

5. You failed to conduct the study according to the investigational plan [21 CFR 312.60].

The version of protocol [ ] approved by the IRB on 11/17/04 required the following:

a. The protocol required that patients placed on rosiglitazone would start at a dose of 4 mg/day and titrate up to 8 mg/day over 6 weeks. Subject 3 underwent cardiac transplant on 6/17/06 and was enrolled in the study on 8/3/06. The subject was started on 2 mg/day and was titrated up to 6 mg/day 3 months later in November 2006. Subject 5 underwent cardiac transplant on 8/23/06 and was enrolled in the study on 9/7/06. The subject was on 4 mg/day of rosiglitazone throughout the study.

b. For the first 6 weeks after initiation of rosiglitazone, the protocol required weekly phone calls to assess variations in the subject's weight during the past week. There was no documentation that this protocol requirement was performed for the subjects on rosiglitazone. In your written response, you state that because of frequent in-person clinic visits by the study subjects, these phone calls were not made. We do not accept your response and consider the fact that these phone call were not made to be a protocol violation.

c. The protocol stated that the study agent rosiglitazone, will be provided to the patient for free by [ ] and subjects signed consent forms that stated rosiglitazone will beprovided at no cost. Our investigation revealed that study drug shipped by [ ] to the UCLA pharmacy for use in this study was not used and that subjects were provided with prescriptions for rosiglitazone. Therefore, it does not appear that rosig1itazone was provided at no cost to study subjects.

d. Protocol [ ] required that subjects be randomized to 1.2 mg or 1.8 mg of [ ] or placebo. Subject was randomized to the 1.2 mg dose of [ ] or placebo. At visit 6, the subject's dose was incorrectly increased to the 1.8 mg dose.

6. You failed to maintain adequate records of the disposition of the drug, including dates, quantity, and use by subjects [21 CFR 312.62(a)].

As stated under item 4 above, for protocol [ ] subjects were provided with prescriptions for rosiglitazone rather than given the study drug provided by [ ] and no drug accountability records were maintained. In your written response, you admitted that the investigators did not xerox the prescriptions and did not count the pills and that there was no "real time" accounting for the use of rosiglitazone. In addition, our investigation failed to reveal that there was any documentation to show that the patients filled their prescriptions. Therefore, our investigation was unable to verify that study subjects received the appropriate study drug in the dosage specified by the protocol.

7. You failed to obtain informed consent in accordance with the provisions of 21 CFR Part 50 [21 CFR 312.60].

a. In seeking informed consent, the information provided to each subject must include a description of the procedures to be followed [21 CFR 50.25(a)(1)]. For protocol [ ] the description of the procedures to be followed that are contained in the consent form are inaccurate in that subjects were told that if they participate in the study, they will either be on the drug rosiglitazone or on a placebo. Our investigation revealed that a placebo was not used in the study.

b. The consent form did not note the possibility that the Food and Drug Administration may inspect the records, as required by 21 CFR 50.25(a)(5).

c. 21 CFR 50.20 requires that the information that is given to the subject or the representative shall be in language understandable to the subject or the representative. Informed consent also must be documented by the use of the written consent form approved by the IRB and signed and dated by the subject at the time of consent [21 CFR 50.27(a)]. FDA regulations provide two mechanisms by which subjects may be provided informed consent.

Investigators may use a written consent document that embodies the elements of informed consent required by 21 CFR 50.25 [21 CFR 50.27(b)(1)]. Alternatively, investigators may use a short form written consent document stating that the elements of informed consent required by § 50.25 have been presented orally. When the short form written consent is used, there shall be a witness to the oral presentation and the IRB shall approve a written summary of what is to be said. The subject (or the subject's representative) must sign the short form. The witness must sign the short form and the summary. Finally, copies of the summary and short form shall be given to the subject or representative [21 CFR 50.27(b)(2)]. For protocol [ ] all enrolled subjects spoke Spanish as their primary language, yet they originally signed English language consent forms. Although you stated in your response letter that the subjects were orally provided informed consent in Spanish, you did not provide information to show that all of the requirements of 21 CFR 50.27(b)(2) were met.

After Dr. [ ] assumed investigator responsibilities in April 2007, the subjects were re-consented with Spanish language consent forms.

8. You failed to maintain adequate and accurate case histories that record all observations and other data pertinent to the investigation on each individual administered the investigational drug or employed as a control in the investigation [21 CFR 312.62(b)].

a. For protocol [ ] there was no documentation that subjects had been treated with one or more oral anti-diabetic drugs for at least 3 months before screening as required by the protocol. We note that there were no medical histories in these subject's research files. For subjects [ ], [ ] , [ ], [ ], and [ ], you created Memos to File stating that medical records were not obtained due to subject's primary care physicians being located in Mexico. These memos do not sufficiently address the issue of the missing medical histories. Without the medical histories, i.e., history of taking an oral anti-diabetic drug, it is not possible to verify if the subjects met inclusion criteria for the study.

b. For protocol [ ] EKG printouts are imprinted with incorrect dates that are off by decades and into the future in most cases. On some printouts the dates are corrected, and on others the dates are not corrected.

- For subject [ ], the EKG is imprinted with the date of Jan. 19, 2038, which has been crossed out and changed to Dec. 11, 2006.
- For subject [ ], the EKG is imprinted with the date of Oct. 18, 2033.
- For subject [ ], the EKG is imprinted with the date of Oct. 18, 2033, which has been crossed out and changed to Jan. 16, 2007.
- For subject [ ], the EKG is imprinted with the date of Oct 18, 2033, which has been crossed out and changed to Dec. 13, 2006.
- For subject [ ], the EKG is imprinted with the date of Oct. 18, 2033.
- For subject [ ], the EKG is imprinted with the date of Jan. 1, 1970.
- For subject [ ], the EKG is imprinted with the date of Jan. 1, 1970, which has been crossed out and changed to Oct. 20, 2006.

This letter is not intended to be an all-inclusive list of deficiencies with your clinical study of an investigational drug. It is your responsibility to ensure adherence to each requirement of the law and relevant FDA regulations. You should address these deficiencies and establish procedures to ensure that any on-going or future studies will be in compliance with FDA regulations.

Within fifteen (15) working days of your receipt of this letter, you should notify this office in writing that the corrective actions outlined in your written response have been implemented. Failure to adequately and promptly explain the violations noted above may result in regulatory action without further notice.

If you have any questions, please contact Constance Lewin, M.D., M.P.H., at (301) 796-3397; FAX (301) 847-8748.

Your written response and any pertinent documentation should be addressed to:

Constance Lewin, M.D., M.P.H.
Branch Chief, Good Clinical Practice Branch I
Division of Scientific Investigations, Bldg. 51, Room 5354
Office of Compliance

Center for Drug Evaluation and Research
Food and Drug Administration
10903 New Hampshire Avenue
Silver Spring, MD 20993

Sincerely yours,

{See appended electronic signature page}

Leslie K. Ball, M.D.
Director
Division of Scientific Investigations
Office of Compliance
Center for Drug Evaluation and Research

第54封　给Mostel, Edward医学博士的警告信

2008年5月16日

参考号：08-HFD-45-0501

尊敬的Mostel博士：

2007年10月17日至10月31日，Albertfiel Salvador先生代表FDA进行了现场检查，与您会面并审查了您实施以下临床研究的情况：在［不公开］进行的以［不公开］为试验药物的在为［不公开］早期介入治疗的患者的随机对照［不公开］与［不公开］试验方案［不公开］。

本次现场检查是FDA的生物研究监查项目的一部分。该项目通过设定的检查方法，评估研究的实施情况，并确保这些研究中受试者的权益、安全和福利得到了保护。

经对FDA现场检查报告、该报告的附件，以及您2007年11月7日对FDA483表的书面回复进行审查，我们认为，您没有遵循适用的法律要求和临床研究实施及受试者保护的FDA法规。我们知道，在现场检查结束时，检查员Salvador向您出示并讨论了FDA483表，即现场检查发现的问题，我们想强调以下几点：

1. 您未能按照21 CFR 50的要求在给药前获得每位受试者的知情同意［21 CFR 50.201］ 具体而言：

a. 受试者［不公开］2004年5月29日签署知情同意书文件，同日临床研究者签署同一份知情同意书文件。然而有记录表明，此受试者于获得知情同意前一天，2004年5月28日入组并于当日下午15：30开始使用试验药物。

b. 受试者［不公开］2004年12月16日签署知情同意书文件，同日临床研究者签署同一份知情同意书文件，然而有记录表明此受试者于获得知情同意前两天，2004年12月14日入组并于当日下午15：30开始使用试验药物。

您的2007年11月7日的回复中声明，这些发现可能是知情同意书文件的记录错误。我们不能接受您的回复，因为实际上无法确认受试者在给予试验药物前已知情同意。

2. 您未能保存足够的试验药物处置记录［21 CFR 312.62（a）］

具体来讲，我们检查发现，2005年10月13日至2005年12月5日，有9位受试者（从［不公开］到［不公开］）的药物的清点记录不全。您回复中声明“医院记录的确证实了受试者每个试验方案接受试验药物”，但您未能为此提供相关的证据。

3. 您未能按照试验方案来进行研究［21 CFR 312.601］ 具体而言：

a. 试验方案15.1部分要求“一旦相关的基本信息给予患者……患者和研究者（或其委任者）应签署伦理委员会或EC批准的知情同意书。”我们检查发现，主要研究者或助理研究者并未在受试者［不公开］2004年10月13日签署的知情同意书上签名和签日期。

b. 试验方案排除了所有之前参加过此研究的受试者。我们检查发现，根据出生日期和社会保障编号，受试者［不公开］和［不公开］是同一个人，且两次入组本研究。此受试者以受试者［不公开］身份于2005年1月4日首次入组研究，再次以受试者［不公开］身份于2005年6月2日入组研究。

您的2007年11月7日的回复承认是您助理研究者的错误。请知悉您作为临床研究者，您有职责监督整个研究在您试验场所的执行。

4. 您未能保存对研究中使用试验药物或对照组的受试者的所有研究观察结果和其他相关数据的足够及准确的病历［21 CFR 312.62（b）］ 具体而言：

a. 根据Cockcroft-Gault公式计算，如果患者血清肌酐清除率＜30mL/min，将被方案排除。我们检查的50名受试者中，原始记录都没有写明计算的血清肌酐清除率的数值。血清肌酐清除率的计算和排除血清肌酐清

除率＜30mL/min的患者，对确保肾功能不全的受试者安全非常关键。您2007年11月7日的回复中声明，这数值有计算但未记录。我们不能接受您的解释。没有记录，我们无法确认受试者是根据计算的血清肌酐清除率被判定合格，入组此研究的。

b. 方案要求患者需要先被判定合格，入组后方能随机。我们检查中发现［不公开］入组记录中有8位受试者没有被记录是否符合所有入组标准。8位受试者如下：［不公开］。

您的2007年11月7日回复中声明，每位受试者，在被考虑纳入研究前，首先要审查所有入组和排除标准。我们不能接受您的解释，因为没有记录，我们无法确认这些受试者是否是合格地入组此研究。

c. 您没有在递交给申办者的12例完成的电子病例报告表上签署姓名和日期。

在您的2007年11月7日回复中，您声明临床研究者可以授权申办者采用代理签名而不用直接签名。您提供了一份2007年1月30日签署的代理委托书副本，而这一天正好是申办者锁定数据库的日期，当时离最后1位受试者入组已超过1年。我们不能接受您的回复，因为您在整个临床研究过程中都没有审阅这些病例报告表。

本警告信的目的并非是罗列您在试验药物临床研究中存在的所有缺陷。确保遵循法律和相关FDA法规的每一项要求是您的职责。您应当解决这些缺陷，并建立规程，以确保任何正在进行或将来进行的研究均能符合FDA的法规。

自收到这封信的15个工作日内，您应当书面告知本办公室为预防将来发生类似违规情况已经采取或将要采取的措施。如果不能充分、迅速地解释上述违规问题，可能导致我们在不再通知的情况下采取监管措施。

附：英文原文

Mostel, Edward, M.D.

WARNING LETTER

MAY 16, 2008

CERTIFIED MAIL
RETURN RECEIPT REQUESTED

Ref.: 08-HFD-45-0501

Edward Mostel, M.D.
Palm Beach Gardens Medical Center
3370 Burns Road
Suite 205
Palm Beach, Florida 33410

Dear Dr. Mostel:

Between October 17 and October 31, 2007, Mr. Albertfiel Salvador, representing the Food and Drug Administration (FDA), conducted an investigation and met with you, to review your conduct of Protocol [ ] A randomized comparison of [ ] versus [ ] in patients undergoing early invasive management for [ ] performed for [ ]
This inspection is a part of FDA's Bioresearch Monitoring Program, which includes inspections designed to evaluate the conduct of research and to ensure that the rights, safety, and welfare of the human subjects of the study have been protected.

From our review of the establishment inspection report, the documents submitted with that report, and your November 7, 2007 letter written in response to the Form FDA 483, we conclude that you did not adhere to the applicable statutory requirements and FDA regulations governing the conduct of clinical investigations and the protection of human subjects. We are aware that at the conclusion of the inspection, Investigator Salvador presented and discussed with you Form FDA 483, Inspectional Observations. We wish to emphasize the following:

1. You failed to obtain informed consent in accordance with 21 CFR Part 50 from each human subject prior to drug administration [21 CFR 50.201]. Specifically,

a. Subject [ ] signed the Informed Consent Document (ICD) on May 29, 2004, and the clinical investigator signed the same ICD on May 29, 2004. However, records document that this same subject was enrolled and administered study drug, starting on May 28, 2004 at 15:30, one day before IC was obtained.

b. Subject [ ] signed the Informed Consent Document on December 16, 2004, and the Clinical Investigator signed the same ICD on December 16, 2004. Records document that this subject was enrolled, and administered study drug starting on December 14, 2004 at 15:30, two days before informed consent was obtained.

Your response letter dated November 7, 2007 states that these findings may have been an error in correctly dating the ICD. Your response is unacceptable, as there is no way to verify whether these subjects in fact gave written informed consent prior to administration of study drug.

2. You failed to maintain adequate drug disposition records [21 CFR 312.62(a)].

Specifically, the investigation found that drug accountability records were missing for nine subjects ([ ] through [ ] between October 13, 2005 and December 5, 2005. You state in your response that "hospital records did confirm the subjects did receive study drug as per the protocol", but you provide no evidence to support your statement.

3. You failed to conduct the study according to the investigational plan [21 CFR 312.60]. Specifically,

a. Protocol Section 15.1 requires that "once the appropriate essential information has been provided to the patient... the patient and the investigator (or designee) shall sign the IRB or EC-approved written informed consent form." The investigation found that the ICD signed by Subject [ ] on October 13, 2004 was not signed or dated by the Principal Investigator or Sub-investigator.

b. The protocol excluded all subjects with prior enrollment in the study. The investigation found that Subject [ ] was the same subject as [ ] and was enrolled twice into this study, as confirmed by matching birthdates and social security numbers. This subject was first enrolled into the study on January 4, 2005 as Subject [ ] and again on June 2, 2005, as Subject [ ]

Your response letter dated November 7, 2007 acknowledges this error by your sub-investigator. Please note as the clinical investigator, you retain responsibility for oversight of the study.

4. You failed to maintain adequate and accurate case histories that record all observations and other data pertinent to the investigation on each individual [21 CFR 312.62(b)]. Specifically,

a. The protocol excluded patients with a calculated serum creatinine clearance <30 mL/min, as determined by the Cockcroft Gault formula. The investigation found that of 50 subjects whose records were audited, source records failed to document the calculated serum creatinine clearance value for all 50 subjects. The calculation of creatinine clearance and exclusion of subjects with creatinine clearance <30 mL/min is crucial to ensure the safety of subjects with renal impairment. Your response letter dated November 7, 2007, states that this value was calculated, but not documented. Your explanation is unacceptable. Without documentation, there is no way to verify that subjects were eligible for enrollment into the study, as determined by calculated serum creatinine clearance.

b. The protocol required that randomization should only occur after patient eligibility is confirmed. The investigation found that the [ ] Enrollment Sheets for eight subjects failed to document if subjects met all inclusion criteria. The eight subjects were as follows: [ ]

Your response letter dated November 7, 2007, states that each subject was considered for the trial by first reviewing all of the inclusion and all the exclusion criteria. Your explanation is unacceptable, as without documentation, there is no way to verify if these subjects were eligible for enrollment into the study.

c. You did not sign and date completed electronic Case Report Forms submitted to the sponsor for 12 subjects.

In your response letter dated November 7, 2007, you state that the clinical investigator could authorize the sponsor to apply a signature by proxy instead direct signature. You provided a copy of a signed proxy dated January 30, 2007, which was the date that the database was locked by the sponsor, and more than 1 year after the last subject was enrolled. Your response is unacceptable, since you did not review these Case Report Forms during the course of the clinical study.

This letter is not intended to be an all-inclusive list of deficiencies with your clinical study of an investigational drug. It is your responsibility to ensure adherence to each requirement of the law and relevant FDA regulations. You must address these deficiencies and establish procedures to ensure that any on-going or future studies will be in compliance with FDA regulations.

Within fifteen (15) working days of your receipt of this letter, you should notify this office in writing of the actions you have taken or will be taking to prevent similar violations in the future. Failure to adequately and promptly explain the violations noted above may result in regulatory action without further notice.

If you have any questions, please contact Tejashri Purohit-Sheth, M.D. at (301) 796-3402 FAX (301) 847-8748. Your written response and any pertinent documentation should be addressed to:

Tejashri Purohit-Sheth, M.D.
Branch Chief (Acting)
Good Clinical Practice Branch 2
Division of Scientific Investigations, Bldg 51, Rm. 5358
Office of Compliance
CDER/FDA
10903 New Hampshire Avenue
Silver Spring, MD 20993

Sincerely yours,

{See appended electronic signature page}

Leslie Ball, M.D.
Director
Division of Scientific Investigations
Bldg 51, Rm. 5342
Office of Compliance
Center for Drug Evaluation and Research

第五部分

药物 GCP 警告信

——给研究者

FDA

第 55 封　给 Sohail M. Khan 医学博士的警告信

2017年10月10日

参考号：17-HFD-45-10-01

尊敬的Khan博士：

2017年7月14日，Cynthia Rakestraw女士代表FDA在您的临床研究场所进行了现场检查，对您开展的下列临床研究进行了审查。

试验方案CQVA149A2336，“一项12周治疗，多中心、随机、双盲、平行组、安慰剂和阳性药物对照的临床研究，评估 QVA149（马来酸茚达特罗/格隆溴铵）对伴有中度至重度气流受限的COPD患者的有效性、安全性和耐受性”。试验药物为马来酸茚达特罗/格隆溴铵（QVA149），申办者为诺华公司。

试验方案（b）(4)，“（b）(4)”，试验药物为（b）(4)，申办者为（b）(4)。

试验方案（b）(4)，“（b）(4)”，试验药物为（b）(4)，申办者为（b）(4)。

这封警告信特告知您现场检查中发现的违规情况。

本次现场检查是FDA的生物研究监查项目的一部分，该项目通过设定的检查方法，评估研究的实施情况，并帮助确保受试者的权益、安全和福利得到保护。

在现场检查结束时，Rakestraw女士向您出示了FDA 483表，即现场检查发现的问题，您于2017年7月25日对FDA 483表的书面回复已收悉。

经对FDA现场检查报告、该报告的附件，以及您2017年7月25日的书面回复进行审查，我们认为，您没有遵循适用的法律要求和监管临床研究实施的FDA法规。我们想强调以下几点：

您未能按照 21 CFR 312 的要求保存需要保存的记录，至试验药物按照被研究的适应症的上市申请获批之日起 2 年；或者，如果未提出申请或者该适应症的申请未获批准，则至研究终止后 2 年［21 CFR 312.62（c）］

作为临床研究者，您必须保存药物的处置记录，包括日期、数量和受试者使用情况，并保存记录研究中使用试验药物或对照组的受试者的所有观察结果和与研究相关的其他数据的足够的、准确的病历。您必须保留这些记录，直至研究药物按照被研究的适应症的上市申请获批之日起2年；或者，如果未提出申请或该适应症的申请未获批准，则至研究终止并通知FDA后2年。

您未能遵守这些要求，具体而言，对于试验方案CQVA149A2336和（b）(4)：

您未能保存包括日期、数量和受试者使用情况的药物处置记录。

您未能保存包括签署了姓名和日期的知情同意书、病例报告表和所有支持数据的全面及准确的病历。

您必须保存在您的研究场所这两项试验方案的研究记录，因为方案CQVA149A233研究的适应症批准后还不到两年，且自申办者终止方案（b）(4)的研究还不到两年。具体而言，对于方案CQVA149A233，对于研究的药物的新药申请（NDA）于2015年10月29日被批准。对于方案（b）(4)，申办者于2015年10月14日告知您，在您的研究场所该研究将终止。

在检查期间，您声称所有与方案CQVA149A2336和方案（b）(4)相关的研究记录已经被工作人员粉碎或销毁，并且您声称，您没有您开展的任何研究的任何纸质或电子记录。

在检查期间，您声称：“我没有任何与方案CQVA149A2336和方案（b）(4)相关的纸质或电子记录，这些记录包括但不限于原始记录、病例报告表、已签署的知情同意书以及试验药物处置记录。我相信这些记录已经被工作人员粉碎或销毁”。

在2017年7月25日提交的书面回复中，您声称，您的理解是这些记录要保存到研究在研究场所终止后两年。您指出，您从研究场所关闭后保存这些记录两年，然后记录被销毁，而且申办者没有通知您“对两年记录保存期的任何延长”。另外，您表示您在将来会遵循研究记录保存指南。您的回复不够充分，因为我们仍然关注到您没有理解您的记录保存要求，而且您没有提供文件表明您保存了要求的记录。具体而言，是否您理解您必须保存在您的研究场所开展的研究记录直到申请批准或研究终止之日起两年。我们还关注的是，您的遵守文件保存指南的计划对于预防将来研究中的类似违规不够详细。

未能按FDA法规的要求保存研究记录严重影响到数据的有效性和完整性。因为您未能保存两项研究的药物管理记录和病历，我们认为在您的研究场所生成的方案CQVA149A2336和方案（b）（4）的数据，在支持临床研究或上市申请上是不可靠的。

本警告信的目的并非是罗列您在试验药物临床研究中存在的所有缺陷。确保遵循法律和相关FDA法规的每一项要求是您的职责。您必须解决这些缺陷，并建立规程，以确保任何正在进行或将来进行的研究均能符合FDA的法规。

自收到这封信的15个工作日内，您应当书面告知本办公室为预防将来发生类似违规情况已经采取的措施。如果不能充分、迅速地解释上述违规问题，可能导致我们在不再通知的情况下采取监管措施。如果您认为已符合FDA法规要求，请陈述理由，并提供所有支持资料，以供我们参考。

附：英文原文

Sohail M. Khan, M.D.

WARNING LETTER

OCT 10, 2017

VIA UNITED PARCEL SERVICE

Ref: 17-HFD-45-10-01

Sohail M. Khan, M.D.
118 Cottonwood Circle
Lynn Haven, Florida 32444

Dear Dr. Khan:

This Warning Letter informs you of objectionable conditions observed during the U.S. Food and Drug Administration (FDA) inspection conducted at your clinical site on July 14, 2017. Ms. Cynthia Rakestraw, representing FDA, reviewed your conduct of the following clinical investigations:

Protocol CQVA149A2336, “A 12-week Treatment, Multi-Center, Randomized, Double-Blind, Parallel-Group, Placebo and Active Controlled Study to Assess the Efficacy, Safety and Tolerability of QVA149 (indacaterol maleate/glycopyrronium bromide) in COPD Patients with Moderate to Severe Airflow Limitation,” of the investigational drug indacaterol maleate/glycopyrronium bromide (QVA149), performed for Novartis

Protocol (b)(4), “(b)(4),” of the investigational drug (b)(4), performed for (b)(4).

Protocol (b)(4), “(b)(4),” of the investigational drug (b)(4), performed for (b)(4).

This inspection is a part of FDA’s Bioresearch Monitoring Program, which includes inspections designed to evaluate the conduct of research and to help ensure that the rights, safety, and welfare of human subjects have been protected. At the conclusion of the inspection, Ms. Rakestraw presented and discussed with you Form FDA 483, Inspectional Observations. We acknowledge receipt of your July 25, 2017, written response to the Form FDA 483.

From our review of the FDA Establishment Inspection Report, the documents submitted with that report, and your written response dated July 25, 2017, we conclude that you did not adhere to the applicable statutory requirements and FDA regulations governing the conduct of clinical investigations. We wish to emphasize the following:

You failed to retain records required to be maintained under 21 CFR Part 312 for a period of two years following the date a marketing application is approved for the drug for the indication for which the drug is being investigated; or, if no application is filed or if the application is not approved for such indication, until two years after the investigation is discontinued [21 CFR 312.62(c)].

As a clinical investigator, you are required to retain records of the disposition of the drug, including dates, quantity, and use by subjects, and to retain adequate and accurate case histories that record all observations and other data pertinent to the investigation on each individual administered the investigational drug or employed as a control in the investigation. You are required to retain these records for a period of two years following the date a marketing application is approved for the drug for the indication for which it is being investigated; or, if no application is to be filed or the application is not approved for such indication, until two years after the investigation is discontinued and FDA is notified.

You failed to adhere to these requirements. Specifically, for Protocols CQVA149A2336 and (b)(4):

You failed to retain records of the disposition of the drug, including dates, quantity, and use by subjects.

You failed to retain adequate and accurate case histories, including signed and dated informed consent forms, case report forms, and all supporting data.

You were required to retain the study records for both protocols because two years had not passed following approval of the indication under study for Protocol CQVA149A2336, and two years had not passed since the sponsor discontinued the study for Protocol (b)(4), at your site. Specifically, for Protocol CQVA149A2336, the New Drug Application (NDA) for the drug under investigation was approved on October 29, 2015. For Protocol (b)(4), the sponsor notified you on October 14, 2015, that the study was being discontinued at your site.

During the inspection, you stated that all study records related to Protocols CQVA149A2336 and (b)(4) had been shredded or destroyed by your staff. You stated that you did not have any paper or electronic records for any study you had conducted.

During the inspection, you stated:

"I do not have any paper or electronic study records related to [Protocols CQVA149A2336 and (b)(4)], including but not limited to source documents, case report forms, signed informed consent forms, and investigational drug disposition records. I believe these records have been shredded or destroyed by my staff."

In your July 25, 2017, written response, you stated that your understanding was that records were to be retained for 2 years following study termination at a site. You indicated that you kept the records 2 years from the date of site closeout, after which the records were destroyed, and that the sponsor did not inform you of "any extension to the two-year record keeping period." In addition, you stated that you will follow the document retention guidelines in the future. Your response is inadequate because we remain concerned that you do not understand your record retention requirements, and because you did not provide any documentation that you retained the required records. Specifically, it is unclear whether you understand that you are required to retain records for studies conducted at your site for 2 years from the date of application approval or study discontinuation. We are also concerned that your plan to follow document retention guidelines is insufficiently detailed to prevent similar violations in future studies.

Failure to retain study records as required by FDA regulations compromises the validity and integrity of data significantly. Because you failed to retain drug accountability records and case histories for both studies, we consider the data generated at your site for Protocols CQVA149A2336 and (b)(4) unreliable in support of a research or marketing application.

This letter is not intended to be an all-inclusive list of deficiencies with your clinical study of an investigational drug. It is your responsibility to ensure adherence to each requirement of the law and relevant FDA regulations. You should address these deficiencies and establish procedures to ensure that any ongoing or future studies will comply with FDA regulations.

Within fifteen (15) working days of your receipt of this letter, you should notify this office in writing of the actions you have taken to prevent similar violations in the future. Failure to address the violations noted above adequately and promptly may result in regulatory action without further notice. If you believe you have complied with FDA regulations, include your reasoning and any supporting information for our consideration.

If you have any questions, please call Adam Donat, M.S., at 301-796-5316. Your written response and any pertinent documentation should be addressed to:

Adam Donat, M.S.
Branch Chief
Compliance Enforcement Branch
Division of Enforcement and Postmarketing Safety
Office of Scientific Investigations
Office of Compliance
Center for Drug Evaluation and Research
Food and Drug Administration
Building 51, Room 5352
10903 New Hampshire Avenue
Silver Spring, MD 20993

Sincerely yours,

{See appended electronic signature page}

David C. Burrow, Pharm.D., J.D.
Acting Director
Office of Scientific Investigations
Office of Compliance
Center for Drug Evaluation and Research
Food and Drug Administration

This is a representation of an electronic record that was signed electronically and this page is the manifestation of the electronic signature.

/S/

DAVID C BURROW
10/10/2017

第56封　给Laveeza（nmi）Bhatti医学博士的警告信

2017年8月4日

参考号：17-HFD-45-07-01

尊敬的Bhatti博士：

2016年10月27日至12月16日，Yvonne T. LaCour女士代表FDA在您的临床研究场所进行了现场检查，对您开展的关于试验药物（b）(4)、由（b）(4）代表（b）(4）的以下临床研究：（b）(4)；（b）(4）进行了审查。

本警告信特告知您现场检查中发现的违规情况。

本次现场检查是FDA的生物研究监查项目的一部分，该项目通过设定的检查方法，对研究的实施情况进行评估，并帮助确保这些研究中受试者的权益、安全和福利得到了保护。

在现场检查结束时，LaCour女士向您出示了FDA 483表，即现场检查发现的问题，并与您进行了讨论。您于2017年1月3日对该FDA 483表的书面回复已收悉。

经对现场检查报告、该报告的附件，以及您2017年1月3日的书面回复进行审查，我们认为您没有遵循适用的法律要求以及监管临床研究实施和受试者保护的FDA法规。我们想强调以下几点：

1. 您未能确保按照研究计划进行研究［21 CFR 312.60］

作为临床研究者，您必须确保临床研究按照研究计划进行。（b）(4）和（b）(4）试验方案的研究计划要求，您在入组前确保受试者满足合格标准（即入组满足入选标准的受试者，而不入组满足排除标准的受试者）。此外，两个试验方案都要求您在规定的时间进行心电图检查（ECGs）。您未能遵守这些要求。具体而言：

a.试验方案（b）(4）的研究计划要求，在筛选或基线心电图（ECG）中存在有任何临床意义问题的受试者将被排除。方案规定QRS间期大于120毫秒和Q-Tc间期大于450毫秒就是这样两项有临床意义的问题。

i. 受试者492在2012年10月1日筛选访视时，QRS间期达到138毫秒，尽管满足排除标准，但是仍于2012年10月22日随机入组并接受研究药物。此外，2012年10月22日的基线访视时，进行的三次心电图（ECGs）结果显示，QRS间期为132毫秒、132毫秒、140毫秒，这证实了该受试者不合格。

在2017年1月3日对FDA 483表的书面回复中，您表示您就这个ECG问题与您研究场所的研究主任、两名其他研究场所的医生以及一名心脏病专家进行了商讨。尽管不正常，但是并不认为具有临床意义，您随后将受试者492入组该研究。您声称该受试者在过去的四年里进展良好，没有任何有临床意义的ECG变化。您还提到，由于这名受试者现在在另一个研究场所入组研究，您与该受试者当前的临床研究者（CI）交谈过，正是这位研究者报告了该受试者进展良好。您解释，您于2016年11月17 日通知了申办者这一事项，而申办者通知当前的临床研究者，该受试者不会被从研究中移出。您承认，尽管ECG问题不具有临床意义，但是它确实使该受试者不合格，并且您应在入组该受试者前得到申办者的许可。

ii. 受试者498尽管符合排除标准，但是仍然随机入组并接受了研究药物。2012年10月30日基线访视进行的三次心电图（ECGs）结果显示，Q-Tc间期为509毫秒、525毫秒和512毫秒。

在2017年1月3日对FDA 483表的书面回复中，您承认受试者498在您审阅心电图（ECGs）前已经接受研究药物的第一次给药。但是您解释说，那天晚些时候审阅完心电图（ECGs）以后，您通知该受试者他不符合合格标准。您声称该受试者将试验药物退回到研究场所，并且他报告已经服用了一剂研究药物。您将受试者送交紧急心脏评估，并且您于2012年10月30日将此事通知了申办者和伦理委员会。

b. 试验方案（b）(4）的研究计划要求您入组（b）(4）确诊［即患有（b）(4）的受试者］后使用任何（b）(4）药剂的提前治疗不超过10天的受试者。方案进一步规定，排除先前有任何（b）(4）或非核苷逆转录酶抑制剂暴露史的受试者。

受试者19先前入组了另一项在您研究场所进行的研究，并接受了（b）（4），因此没有资格进入（b）（4）研究。但是，受试者19在2014年6月19日进行了筛选，并于2014年7月10日（基线/第20周访视）进行随机，而后使用研究药物直到2014年9月8日退出访视。

在2017年1月3日对FDA 483表的书面回复中，您解释，您关注方案中关于受试者使用任何（b）（4）药剂的提前治疗应当不超过10天的语句表述，因此，您忽略了使用（b）（4）就要排除的语句描述；您指出监查员在2014年8月14日发现了这个问题，该受试者的最后一次服用研究药物在2014年9月7日；该受试者于2014年9月8日退出研究，伦理委员会在2014年9月11日收到通知。

为了解决入组不合格受试者的问题，您的书面回复指出您将进行以下作为纠正措施：

对所有研究人员进行方案培训，并强调合格标准。

即便申办者没有提供，也应采用合格标准检查表。

通过原始文件审查和检查是否该信息能够被证实来确定合格性。

采用两个有资质的人员（均在合格标准检查表上首字母签署姓名和日期），其中一个是临床研究者，来证实合格性。

只有在完成合格标准检查表后才将受试者随机。

对研究人员培训修订的关于合格和入组的标准操作规程（2017年2月1日生效）。

如果这些被很好地执行，您的纠正措施似乎足以预防将来类似的违规情况再次发生。

c. 试验方案（b）（4）的研究计划里要求在筛选时、第1天、第2、4、12、24、26、28、36和48周及以后每12周进行心电图检查，一直到从研究中退出，包括退出那天。（b）（4）方案中维持期的研究计划要求，心电图检查在第1天，第1、4、8、24、32、48、64、80和96周，直到从研究中退出。

心电图在（b）（4）和（b）（4）试验方案中都是安全性评价指标，用于监测Q-Tc间期。来自3次或更多次的、间隔不少于5分钟的心电图描记，如果Q-Tc间期平均值＞500 毫秒［对于（b）（4）研究］，如果Q-Tc间期平均值＞500 毫秒或相对于基线有一个大于60毫秒的延长［对于（b）（4）研究］，受试者都将中断使用研究药物。未能及时诊断出延长的Q-Tc间期将导致受试者有发展成尖端扭转型室性心动过速、一个潜在的致命性心律不齐的风险。因此，缺失方案要求的心电图检查将损害受试者的安全。具体而言：

i.（b）（4）研究中的受试者160缺失第4、120和156周的心电图检查。

ii.（b）（4）研究中的受试者491、499、500都缺失第168周的心电图检查。

iii.（b）（4）研究中的受试者492缺失第120周的心电图检查。

在2017年1月3日对试验方案（b）（4）FDA 483表的书面回复中，您指出心电图结果被放在一个单独的文件夹中，您委派一名授权研究者解读心电图。您解释说，只有异常心电图才会提请您注意，并且由于没有按照实验室检查和安全性报告那样放在一个文件夹内供您审阅，这就产生了心电图检查未按要求实施的可能性，或者心电图结果放错位置的可能性。

您声称在发现心电图检查没有进行，或授权研究者没有履行其职责时，受试者被召回到研究场所进行心电图检查。这些心电图结果与之前的心电图结果比较，您注意到没有重大变化。您解释说，所有的受试者都对研究药物进展良好，放错位置的心电图数据已被您的研究协调员录入到受试者医疗记录，并得到了您的签名。

由于您未能提供如果正常开展可以预防将来发生类似违规情况的纠正措施计划，我们无法对您的试验方案（b）（4）的书面回复进行充分的知情评价。具体而言，您没有提供将来研究中您将如何确保执行方案规定的评价的充分细节。

iv.（b）（4）研究中的受试者缺失第64周的心电图检查。

在2017年1月3日对试验方案（b）（4）的FDA 483表的书面回复中，您表明您在日期为2016年4月28日的文件备忘录中将此方案违背报告给伦理委员会。您的研究场所进行了心电图处理的培训，而您于2016年9月

23日建立了纠正措施计划。如果得到正确的实施，您的纠正措施似乎足以预防将来类似违规再次发生。

d. 试验方案（b）（4）的研究计划要求第32周大约服药后2小时并在服药后2小时药代动力学采样前进行心电图检查。如上文讨论的，心电图在该研究中是一项安全性评估指标。

i. 在第32周访视期间，受试者11在13:50接受（b）（4），并在13:52接受（b）（4）。但是，有一份手写的笔记说明"第2次［ECG］（服药后）由于疏忽未做。"

ii. 在第32周访视期间，受试者12在12:40接受（b）（4），并在12:42接受（b）（4）。但是，受试者12在12:20进行了一次心电图检查。

在2017年1月3日对FDA 483表的书面回复中，您表明，您在日期为2016年4月28日的文件备忘录中将这个方案违背报告给伦理委员会。您于2016年9月23日建立了您的纠正措施计划，您的研究场所进行了心电图处理的培训。如果得到正确的实施，您的纠正措施似乎足以预防将来类似违规再次发生。

入组不符合合格标准的受试者，以及未在研究方案要求的时间点进行心电图检查，危害了受试者的安全和福利，也损害了在您的研究场所收集数据的有效性和完整性。

2. 您未能按照 21 CFR 312 的要求保存要求保持的记录，至该研究药物按研究的适应症上市申请获批之日起 2 年；或者，如果未提出上市申请或者该适应症的申请未获批准，则至研究终止后 2 年［21 CFR 312.62(c)］

作为临床研究者，您必须保存记录了对研究中使用试验药物或对照组的受试者的所有观察结果和与研究有关的数据的足够、准确的病历。您必须保存相关记录，至该研究药物按研究的适应症上市申请获批之日起2年；或者，如果未提出上市申请或者该适应症的申请未获批准，则至研究终止并通知FDA后2年。

您未能遵守这些要求。对于（b）（4）研究，您未能保存包括心电图描记和哥伦比亚自杀严重程度评定量表（C-SSRS）的病历。具体而言：

a.以下心电图描记未能保存：

i. 受试者152第60、108、120、132及156周。

ii. 受试者156第72周。

iii. 受试者160第108周。

iv. 受试者491第12、120周。

v. 受试者492第96周。

vi. 受试者499第48周。

vii. 受试者500第28、108、120、132周。

在2017年1月3日对FDA 483表的书面回复中，您表示进行了心电图检查，数据由研究协调员采集到受试者的医疗记录和电子病例报告表（eCRFs）中，但是原始的心电图结果找不到。您解释说心电图由授权研究者审阅，并放置在一个独立的文件夹中，只有异常心电图才会提请您的注意。您声称，您"建立了严格的措施来整改这个程序失误"，但是没有提供细节。您通知了申办者，您没有将缺失心电图描记一事报告给伦理委员会。

b. 受试者152第36周的哥伦比亚自杀严重程度评定量表（C-SSRS）没有保存。

在2017年1月3日对FDA 483表的书面回复中，您承认您之前签署C-SSRS表的流程导致了原始C-SSRS表的缺失。您表示受试者C-SSRS数据已经获取，但是原始的C-SSRS表被放错位置了。您声称，您通知了申办者此项缺失，下一步您将在受试者访视当天签署C-SSRS表，并在签署完立即归档。

我们无法对于您未能保存心电图描记和哥伦比亚自杀严重程度评定量表（C-SSRS）的书面回复做出知情评价，因为您没有提供一个如果适当实施，会预防将来这种类型违规的纠正措施计划。具体而言，就您如何为今后的研究妥善保存足够的、准确的病历，您未能提供充足的细节。

未能按照FDA法规要求保存研究记录，危害了受试者的安全和福利，损害了您研究场所收集数据的有效性和完整性。

本警告信的目的并非是罗列您在试验药物临床研究中存在的所有缺陷。确保遵循法律和相关FDA法规的每一项要求是您的职责。您必须解决这些缺陷，并建立规程，以确保任何正在进行或将来进行的研究均能符合FDA的法规。

自收到这封信的15个工作日内，您应当书面告知本办公室为预防将来发生类似违规情况已经采取的措施。如果不能充分、迅速地解释上述违规问题，可能导致我们在不再通知的情况下采取监管措施。如果您认为已符合FDA法规要求，请陈述理由，并提供所有支持资料，以供我们参考。

附：英文原文

Laveeza (nmi) Bhatti, M.D.

WARNING LETTER

August 4, 2017

CERTIFIED MAIL
RETURN RECEIPT REQUESTED

Ref: 17-HFD-45-07-01

Laveeza Bhatti, M.D., Ph.D.
99 North La Cienga Boulevard
Suite 200
Beverly Hills, California 90211

Dear Dr. Bhatti:

This Warning Letter informs you of objectionable conditions observed during the U.S. Food and Drug Administration (FDA) inspection conducted at your clinical site between October 27 and December 16, 2016. Ms. Yvonne T. LaCour, representing FDA, reviewed your conduct of the following clinical investigations of the investigational drug (b)(4), performed on behalf of (b)(4) by (b)(4):

(b)(4)

(b)(4)

This inspection was conducted as a part of FDA's Bioresearch Monitoring Program, which includes inspections designed to evaluate the conduct of research and to help ensure that the rights, safety, and welfare of the human subjects have been protected.

At the conclusion of the inspection, Ms. LaCour presented and discussed with you Form FDA 483, Inspectional Observations. We acknowledge receipt of your January 3, 2017, written response to the Form FDA 483.

From our review of the FDA Establishment Inspection Report, the documents submitted with that report, and your written response dated January 3, 2017, we conclude that you did not adhere to the applicable statutory requirements and FDA regulations governing the conduct of clinical investigations and the protection of human subjects. We wish to emphasize the following:

1.You failed to ensure that the investigation was conducted according to the investigational plan [21 CFR 312.60].

As a clinical investigator, you are required to ensure that your clinical studies are conducted in accordance with the investigational plan. The investigational plans for the (b)(4) and (b)(4) protocols required you to ensure that subjects met the eligibility criteria before enrollment (that is, to enroll subjects who met inclusion criteria and not to enroll subjects who met exclusion criteria). Further, both protocols also required you to perform electrocardiograms (ECGs) at specific times. You failed to adhere to these requirements. Specifically:

a.The investigational plan for the (b)(4) protocol required that subjects be excluded if there is any clinically significant finding on screening or baseline ECG. The protocol specified that QRS duration >120 milliseconds (msec) and QTc interval >450 msec are two such clinically significant findings.

i. Subject 492 was randomized and received study drug on October 22, 2012, despite meeting the exclusion criteria, with a QRS duration of 138 msec during the screening visit on October 1, 2012. In addition, triplicate ECGs were performed during the baseline visit on October 22, 2012, that demonstrated QRS durations of 132 msec, 132 msec, and 140 msec, thus confirming the subject's ineligibility for the study.

In your January 3, 2017, written response to the Form FDA 483, you indicated that you conferred with your site's Director of Research, two other site clinicians, and a cardiologist about this ECG finding. While abnormal, it was not considered clinically significant, and you subsequently enrolled Subject 492 into the study. You stated that this subject has done well for the past four years, with no significant ECG changes. You also noted that because this subject is now enrolled in the study at a different site, you spoke with the subject's current clinical investigator (CI), who reported that the subject is doing well. You explained that you notified the sponsor of this issue on November 17, 2016, and the sponsor notified the current CI that this subject would not be removed from the study. You acknowledged that while this ECG finding was not clinically significant, it did make the subject ineligible, and you should have received permission from the sponsor before enrolling the subject.

ii. Subject 498 was randomized and received study drug despite meeting the exclusion criteria. Triplicate ECGs were performed during the baseline visit on October 30, 2012, showing QTc intervals of 509 msec, 525 msec, and 512 msec.

In your January 3, 2017, written response to the Form FDA 483, you acknowledged that Subject 498 was given the first dose of study drug before you reviewed the ECGs. You explained, however, that after the ECGs were reviewed later in the day, you notified the subject that he did not meet the eligibility criteria. You stated that the subject brought study drug back to the site, and he reported taking one dose of study drug. You referred the subject for urgent cardiac evaluation, and you notified both the sponsor and the IRB of this issue on October 30, 2012.

b. The investigational plan for the (b)(4) protocol required that you enroll subjects who have taken no more than 10 days of prior therapy with any (b)(4) agent following a diagnosis of (b)(4)(that is, subjects who are (b)(4)). The protocol further specified exclusion of subjects with any previous exposure to an (b)(4) or non-nucleoside reverse transcriptase inhibitor.

Subject 19 was ineligible for the (b)(4) study because she was previously enrolled in another study at your site and received an (b)(4). However, Subject 19 was screened on June 19, 2014, randomized on July 10, 2014 (Baseline/Week 20 Visit), and dosed with study drug until the withdrawal visit on September 8, 2014.

In your January 3, 2017, written response to the Form FDA 483, you explained that you focused on the protocol language stating that subjects should be on no more than 10 days of prior therapy with any (b)(4) agent. Consequently, you overlooked the language stating that use of an (b)(4) was exclusionary. You indicated that the monitor identified this issue on August 14, 2014; the subject's last dose of study drug was on September 7, 2014; the subject was withdrawn from the study on September 8, 2014; and the Institutional Review Board (IRB) was notified on September 11, 2014.

To address the enrollment of ineligible subjects, your written response indicated that you will perform the following as a corrective action:

Train all study staff on the protocol and emphasize eligibility criteria

Use an eligibility criteria checklist even if the sponsor does not provide one

Determine eligibility by source document review and by checking whether that information is verifiable

Confirm eligibility by using two qualified individuals (who will initial and date the eligibility checklist), with one of these individuals being the CI

Randomize subjects only after the eligibility checklist is complete

Train study staff on a revised Standard Operating Procedure (effective date February 1, 2017) for eligibility and enrollment

If they are properly carried out, your corrective actions appear adequate to prevent the recurrence of similar violations in the future.

c. The investigational plan for the (b)(4) protocol required that ECGs be performed at Screening, on Day 1, at Weeks 2, 4, 12, 24, 26, 28, 36, and 48, and every 12 weeks thereafter, up to and including withdrawal from the study. The investigational plan for the Maintenance Period in the (b)(4) protocol required that ECGs be performed on Day 1, at Weeks 1, 4, 8, 24, 32, 48, 64, 80, and 96, and upon withdrawal from the study.

ECGs are safety assessments in both the (b)(4) and (b)(4) protocols because they are used to monitor the QTc interval. Subjects have their study drug discontinued if the average QTc interval >500 msec (for the (b)(4) study), or if the average QTc interval >500 msec or if there is a >60 msec increase from baseline (for the (b)(4) study) from three or more ECG tracings separated by at least five minutes. Failure to diagnose a prolonged QTc interval in a timely manner places subjects at risk of developing torsades de pointes, a potentially fatal arrhythmia. Therefore, missing protocol-required ECGs compromises subject safety. Specifically:

i. Subject 160 in the (b)(4) study missed ECGs at Weeks 4, 120, and 156.

ii. Subjects 491, 499, and 500 in the (b)(4) study all missed an ECG at Week 168.

iii. Subject 492 in the (b)(4) study missed an ECG at Week 120.

In your January 3, 2017, written response to the Form FDA 483 for the (b)(4) protocol, you indicated that ECGs were placed in a separate folder, and that you delegated ECG interpretation to a subinvestigator. You explained that only the abnormal ECGs were brought to your attention, and that this created the potential for ECGs not to be performed as required, or for ECGs to be misplaced because they were not placed in one folder meant for your review, as laboratory and safety reports were.

You stated that subjects were called back to the site to have ECGs performed after it was discovered that either ECGs were not performed or the subinvestigator had not carried out his or her responsibility. These ECGs were compared to previous ECGs, and you noted no significant changes. You explained that all subjects have done well on study drug, and that data from misplaced ECGs were entered by your Study Coordinator into subjects' medical records and were routed for your signature.

We are unable to undertake an informed evaluation of your written response for the (b)(4) protocol because you did not provide a corrective action plan that, if properly carried out, would prevent this type of violation in the future. Specifically, you did not provide sufficient details on how you will ensure the performance of protocol-specific assessments in future studies.

iv. Subject 12 in the (b)(4) study missed an ECG at Week 64.

In your January 3, 2017, written response to the Form FDA 483 for the (b)(4) protocol, you indicated that you reported this protocol violation to the IRB in a memo to file dated April 28, 2016. Your site was trained in ECG processing, and you instituted your corrective action plan on September 23, 2016. If they are properly carried out, your corrective actions appear adequate to prevent the recurrence of similar violations in the future.

d. The investigational plan for the (b)(4) protocol required an ECG approximately two hours post-dose and just before the two-hour post-dose pharmacokinetic sampling at Week 32. As discussed above, an ECG is a safety assessment in this study.

i. During the Week 32 Visit, Subject 11 received (b)(4) at 13:50, and (b)(4) at 13:52. However, there was a handwritten note stating that the "2nd [ECG] (Post Dose) was inadvertently missed."

ii. During the Week 32 Visit, Subject 12 received (b)(4) at 12:40, and (b)(4) at 12:42. However, Subject 12 had an ECG performed at 12:20.

In your January 3, 2017, written response to the Form FDA 483, you indicated that you reported this protocol violation to the IRB in a memorandum to file dated April 28, 2016. You instituted your corrective action plan on September 23, 2016, and your site was trained on ECG processing. If they are properly carried out, your corrective actions appear adequate to prevent the recurrence of similar violations in the future.

Enrollment of subjects who do not meet eligibility criteria, and failure to perform ECGs at protocol-required times, jeopardize subject safety and welfare and compromise the validity and integrity of the data collected at your site.

2.You failed to retain records required to be maintained under 21 CFR Part 312 for a period of two years following the date a marketing application is approved for the drug for the indication for which the drug is being investigated; or, if no application is filed or if the application is not approved for such indication, until two years after the investigation is discontinued [21 CFR 312.62(c)].

As a clinical investigator, you are required to retain records of adequate and accurate case histories that record all observations and other data pertinent to the investigation on each individual administered the investigational drug or employed as a control in the investigation. You are required to retain these records for a period of two years following the date a marketing application is approved for the drug for the indication for which it is being investigated, or if no application is filed or the application is not approved for such indication, until two years after the investigation is discontinued and FDA is notified.

You failed to adhere to these requirements. For the (b)(4) study, you failed to retain case histories that include ECG tracings and the Columbia-Suicide Severity Rating Scale (C-SSRS). Specifically:

a. ECG tracings were not retained for the following:

i. Subject 152 for Weeks 60, 108, 120, 132, and 156
ii. Subject 156 for Week 72
iii. Subject 160 for Week 108
iv. Subject 491 for Weeks 12 and 120
v. Subject 492 for Week 96
vi. Subject 499 for Week 48
vii. Subject 500 for Weeks 28, 108, 120, and 132

In your January 3, 2017, written response to the Form FDA 483, you indicated that ECGs were performed and the data were captured in subjects' medical records and electronic case report forms (eCRFs) by the Study Coordinator, but that the original ECGs could not be located. You explained that ECGs were read by a subinvestigator and were placed in a separate folder, and that only abnormal ECGs were brought to your attention. You stated that you "instituted strict measures to rectify this process failure" but did not provide details. You notified the sponsor that you did not report these missing ECG tracings to the IRB.

b. C-SSRS was not retained for Subject 152 at Week 36.

In your January 3, 2017, written response to the Form FDA 483, you acknowledged that your previous process for signing the C-SSRS led to the loss of the original C-SSRS. You indicated that subjects had the C-SSRS data captured, but the original C-SSRS was misplaced. You stated that you notified the sponsor of this loss, and that going forward, you will sign the C-SSRS on the day of the subject's visit and file it immediately after signing it.

We are unable to undertake an informed evaluation of your written response for your failure to retain ECG tracings and the C-SSRS because you did not provide a corrective action plan that, if properly carried out, would prevent this type of violation in the future. Specifically, you did not provide sufficient details on how you will properly retain records of adequate and accurate case histories for future studies.

Failure to retain study records as required by FDA regulations jeopardizes subject safety and welfare and compromises the validity and integrity of the data collected at your site.

This letter is not intended to be an all-inclusive list of deficiencies with your clinical study of an investigational drug. It is your responsibility to ensure adherence to each requirement of the law and relevant FDA regulations. You should address these deficiencies and establish procedures to ensure that any ongoing or future studies will comply with FDA regulations.

Within fifteen (15) working days of your receipt of this letter, you should notify this office in writing of the actions you have taken to prevent similar violations in the future. Failure to address the violations noted above adequately and promptly may result in regulatory action without further notice. If you believe you have complied with FDA regulations, include your reasoning and any supporting information for our consideration.

If you have any questions, please contact Adam Donat, M.S., at 301-796-5316. Your written response and any pertinent documentation should be addressed to:

Adam Donat, M.S.

Branch Chief
Compliance Enforcement Branch
Division of Enforcement and Postmarketing Safety
Office of Scientific Investigations
Office of Compliance
Center for Drug Evaluation and Research
Food and Drug Administration
Building 51, Room 5352
10903 New Hampshire Avenue
Silver Spring, MD 20993

Sincerely yours,

{See appended electronic signature page}

David C. Burrow, Pharm.D., J.D.
Acting Director
Office of Scientific Investigations
Office of Compliance
Center for Drug Evaluation and Research
Food and Drug Administration

This is a representation of an electronic record that was signed electronically and this page is the manifestation of the electronic signature.

/S/

DAVID C BURROW
08/04/2017

第 57 封　给 Adolfo Kaplan 的警告信

2017年4月20日

参考号：17-HFD-45-04-01

尊敬的Kaplan博士：

2016年11月7日至11月10日，Travis M. Beard先生代表FDA，在您的临床研究场所进行了现场检查，对您所开展的一项临床研究［试验方案（b）（4），试验药物为（b）（4），申办者为（b）（4）］进行了审查。这封警告信特告知您现场检查中发现的违规情况。

本次现场检查是FDA的生物研究监查项目的一部分，该项目通过设定的检查方法，对FDA所监管的相关研究的实施情况进行评估，以确认研究数据在科学上是有效和准确的，并帮助确保这些研究中受试者的权益、安全和福利得到了保护。

在现场检查结束时，Beard先生向您出示了FDA 483表，即现场检查发现的问题，并与您进行了讨论。您2016年11月14日对该FDA 483表的书面回复已收悉。

经对现场检查报告、该报告的附件，以及您2016年11月14日的书面回复进行审查，我们认为，您没有遵守适用的法律要求以及监管临床研究实施和受试者保护的FDA法规。我们想强调以下几点：

您未能确保按照研究计划进行研究［21 CFR 312.60］

作为研究者，您必须确保临床研究按照研究计划进行。试验方案（b）（4）的研究计划要求您确保受试者在入组和治疗随机化前应满足入组标准。试验方案（b）（4）强调不允许偏离入选和排除标准，遵守方案规定的合格标准是非常重要的。此外，试验方案（b）（4）要求您在特定时间执行某些操作，如X射线检查。您未能遵守这些要求，具体而言：

1. 试验方案（b）（4）的研究计划要求受试者必须有以下两种情况之一才符合入组资格：

- 使用支气管扩张剂后，FEV1低于预计正常值的50%，并在前12个月内至少有1次中度或重度（b）（4）加重史；
- 使用支气管扩张剂后，FEV1在预计正常值的50%~ 80%，并在前12个月内至少有2次中度或至少1次重度（b）（4）加重史。

该方案对（b）（4）加重的记录史作了定义，是指（b）（4）症状恶化，需接受全身/口服皮质类固醇和/或抗生素（中度加重）或住院（重度加重）治疗的病历。该方案还规定不接受受试者的口头报告。

在您的研究场所入组的4例受试者中有3例未满足上述标准。具体而言，下列受试者使用支气管扩张剂后，FEV1（第1秒钟用力呼气量）在预计正常值的50% ~ 80%，但在前12个月内没有至少2次中度或至少1次重度加重的记录史，而您允许这些受试者入组研究。

a. 受试者11153使用支气管扩张剂后，FEV1为预计正常值的68%，于2015年6月4日入组。

b. 受试者11154使用支气管扩张剂后，FEV1为预计正常值的62%，于2015年6月15日入组。

c. 受试者11155使用支气管扩张剂后，FEV1为预计正常值的63%，于2015年6月18日入组。（备注：FDA 483表将受试者11155误写为“受试者11555”）

2. 研究计划规定，若受试者在导入期出现肺炎和/或中度或重度（b）（4）加重，将被排除出研究。方案定义，中度（b）（4）加重为（b）（4）症状恶化，需接受全身/口服皮质类固醇和/或抗生素治疗，重度（b）（4）加重为（b）（4）症状恶化，需治疗并住院治疗。

受试者11155在导入期出现中度（b）（4）加重，（b）（4）症状恶化，需要口服皮质类固醇治疗，但该例受试者未被排除出治疗随机化。

3. 研究计划要求，在方案定义的、如上文描述的中度或重度加重时，要尽快行胸部X射线检查，最好在48小时内进行。

下面2例受试者在中度（b）(4）加重后未行胸部 X射线检查：

a. 受试者11152分别在2015年6月31日、2015年9月25日两次出现中度（b）(4）加重，伴有（b）(4）恶化的症状并需抗生素治疗，但任意一次（b）(4）加重，均未行胸部 X射线检查。

b. 受试者11154分别在2016年2月25日、2016年6月14日两次出现中度（b）(4）加重，伴有（b）(4）恶化的症状并需抗生素治疗，但任意一次（b）(4）加重，均未行胸部 X射线检查。

在2016年11月14日对FDA 483表的书面回复中，您说把每日的研究活动委托给了一家独立研究公司。您提到与该独立研究公司定期举行会议，会上您会收到招募和随访的最新信息、签署必要的文件，并对检测进行审核。您也提到在这些定期会面中，该独立研究公司并未将任何上述方案违背告知您引起注意。

我们想强调的是，确保临床研究正确地遵循FDA法规开展，保护受试者权益、安全和福利并保证研究数据有效性和完整性是您作为研究者的基本责任。但是，您的书面回复是不充分的，尽管您在回复中表示“不打算再次参与临床研究”，但是您没有提供细节信息，即如果您改变主意，在将来开展临床研究，您个人将如何计划，以预防类似的违规行为。当考虑到上面提到的违规行为时，您的解释说明您在临床研究中存在系统性失误。

您对临床研究的监督和管理的缺乏，引起对在您的研究场所中开展的上述研究中入组受试者的保护是否充分的严重关注，也引起对您的研究场所生成的数据的完整性的关注。

入组不满足合格标准的受试者和未执行方案要求的包括胸部X射线检查的程序，危害到受试者的安全和福利，并引起对您的研究场所中采集的数据的有效性和完整性的关注。特别值得关注的是，在您的研究场所中，入组到上述研究中的4例受试者中，有3例是没有入组该方案资格的。

本警告信的目的并非是罗列您在试验药物临床研究中存在的所有缺陷。确保遵循法律和相关FDA法规的每一项要求是您的职责。您应当解决这些缺陷，并建立规程，以确保任何正在进行或将来进行的研究均能符合FDA的法规。

自收到这封信的15个工作日内，您应当书面告知本办公室为预防将来发生类似违规情况而采取的措施。如果不能充分、迅速地解释上述违规问题，可能导致我们在不再通知的情况下采取监管措施。如果您认为已符合FDA法规要求，请陈述理由，并提供所有支持资料以供我们参考。

附：英文原文

Adolfo Kaplan

WARNING LETTER

April 20, 2017

CERTIFIED MAIL
RETURN RECEIPT REQUESTED

Ref: 17-HFD-45-04-01

Adolfo E. Kaplan, M.D.
Pulmonary and Sleep Center of the Valley
5300 North McColl Road, Suite 100
McAllen, Texas 78504

Dear Dr. Kaplan:

This Warning Letter informs you of objectionable conditions observed during the U.S. Food and Drug Administration (FDA) inspection conducted at your clinical site between November 7 and November 10, 2016. Mr. Travis M. Beard, representing FDA, reviewed your conduct of a clinical investigation [Protocol (b)(4) of the investigational drug (b)(4), performed for (b)(4)].

This inspection is a part of FDA's Bioresearch Monitoring Program, which includes inspections designed to evaluate the conduct of FDA-regulated research to ensure that the data are scientifically valid and accurate, and to help ensure that the rights, safety, and welfare of the human subjects of those studies have been protected.

At the conclusion of the inspection, Mr. Beard presented and discussed with you Form FDA 483, Inspectional Observations. We acknowledge receipt of your November 14, 2016, written response to the Form FDA 483.

From our review of the FDA Establishment Inspection Report, the documents submitted with that report, and your written response dated November 14, 2016, we conclude that you did not adhere to the applicable statutory requirements and FDA regulations governing the conduct of clinical investigations and the protection of human subjects. We wish to emphasize the following:

You failed to ensure that the investigation was conducted according to the investigational plan [21 CFR 312.60].

As a clinical investigator, you are required to ensure that your clinical studies are conducted in accordance with the investigational plan. The investigational plan for Protocol (b)(4) required you to ensure that subjects met the protocol eligibility criteria before enrollment and treatment randomization. Protocol (b)(4) states that deviations from inclusion and exclusion criteria are not allowed and that adherence to the eligibility criteria as specified in the protocol is essential. In addition, Protocol (b)(4) required you to perform certain procedures, such as chest X-rays, at specific times. You failed to adhere to these requirements. Specifically:

1. The investigational plan for Protocol (b)(4) required that to be eligible for enrollment, subjects must demonstrate either of the following:

- a post-bronchodilator FEV1 less than 50% of predicted normal and a documented history of at least 1 moderate or severe (b)(4) exacerbation in the previous 12 months
- a post-bronchodilator FEV1 between 50% and 80% of predicted normal and a documented history of at least 2 moderate exacerbations or a documented history of at least 1 severe (b)(4) exacerbation in the previous 12 months

The protocol defined a documented history of a (b)(4) exacerbation as a medical record of worsening (b)(4) symptoms that required systemic/oral corticosteroids and/or antibiotics (for a moderate exacerbation) or hospitalization (for a severe exacerbation). The protocol also specified that subjects' verbal reports were not acceptable.

Out of four total subjects enrolled at your site, you enrolled three subjects who did not meet this requirement. Specifically, you allowed the enrollment of the following subjects with a post-bronchodilator FEV1 (forced expiratory volume in 1 second) between 50% and 80% of predicted normal, even though they did not have a documented history of at least 2 moderate (b)(4) exacerbations or at least 1 severe (b)(4) exacerbation in the previous 12 months:

a. Subject 11153, who had a post-bronchodilator FEV1 of 68% of predicted normal, was enrolled on June 4, 2015.

b. Subject 11154, who had a post-bronchodilator FEV1 of 62% of predicted normal, was enrolled on June 15, 2015.

c. Subject 11155, who had a post-bronchodilator FEV1 of 63% of predicted normal, was enrolled on June 18, 2015. (Note that the Form FDA 483 identified Subject 11155 incorrectly as "Subject 11555.")

2. The investigational plan specified that any subject who experienced pneumonia and/or moderate or severe (b)(4) exacerbation during the run-in period would be excluded from the study. The protocol defined moderate (b)(4) exacerbation as worsening symptoms of (b)(4) that require treatment with oral/systemic corticosteroids and/or antibiotics, and severe (b)(4) exacerbation as worsening symptoms of (b)(4) that require treatment and inpatient hospitalization.

Subject 11155 experienced a moderate (b)(4) exacerbation with worsening symptoms of (b)(4) requiring treatment with oral corticosteroids during the run-in period. However, this subject was not excluded from treatment randomization.

3. The investigational plan required a chest X-ray to be performed as soon as possible and preferably within 48 hours of moderate or severe exacerbation, as defined by the protocol and described above.

You failed to perform chest X-rays following moderate (b)(4) exacerbations for the following two subjects:

a. Subject 11152 experienced 2 moderate (b)(4) exacerbations with worsening symptoms of (b)(4) requiring treatment with antibiotics, on July 31, 2015, and on September 25, 2015. However, a chest X-ray was not performed following either (b)(4) exacerbation.

b. Subject 11154 experienced 2 moderate (b)(4) exacerbations with worsening symptoms of (b)(4) requiring treatment with antibiotics, on February 25, 2016, and on June 14, 2016. However, a chest X-ray was not performed following either (b)(4) exacerbation.

In your November 14, 2016, written response to the Form FDA 483, you indicated that you delegated day-to-day research activities to an independent research company. You noted that you held regular meetings with the independent research company, during which you received updates on recruitment and follow-ups, signed required documents, and reviewed tests. You also noted that the independent research company did not bring any of the above-mentioned violations to your attention during these regular encounters.

We wish to emphasize that as the clinical investigator, it was your ultimate responsibility to ensure that clinical studies were conducted properly and in compliance with FDA regulations, both to protect the rights, safety, and welfare of study subjects and to ensure the validity and integrity of study data. However, your response is inadequate because, although you indicate in your response that you "do not plan to get involved in clinical research again," you did not provide details about how you personally plan to prevent similar violations if this decision should change and you conduct clinical research in the future. Your explanation, when taken into consideration with the violations described above, suggests systemic failures in your conduct of this clinical investigation.

Your lack of supervision and oversight of the clinical study raises significant concerns about the adequacy of your protection of the study subjects enrolled at your site in the above-mentioned study, and raises concerns about the integrity of the data generated at your site.

Enrollment of subjects who do not meet eligibility criteria and failure to perform protocol-required procedures, including chest X-rays, jeopardize subject safety and welfare, and raise concerns about the validity and integrity of the data collected at your site. Of particular concern is the fact that three of the four subjects enrolled on the above-mentioned study at your site were ineligible for enrollment into the protocol.

This letter is not intended to be an all-inclusive list of deficiencies with your clinical study of an investigational drug. It is your responsibility to ensure adherence to each requirement of the law and relevant FDA regulations. You should address these deficiencies and establish procedures to ensure that any ongoing or future studies will be in compliance with FDA regulations.

Within fifteen (15) working days of your receipt of this letter, you should notify this office in writing of the actions you have taken to prevent similar violations in the future. Failure to address the violations noted above adequately and promptly may result in regulatory action without further notice. If you believe you have complied with FDA regulations, include your reasoning and any supporting information for our consideration.

If you have any questions, please call Adam Donat, M.S., at 301-796-5316. Your written response and any pertinent documentation should be addressed to:

Adam Donat, M.S.
Branch Chief
Compliance Enforcement Branch
Division of Enforcement and Postmarketing Safety
Office of Scientific Investigations
Office of Compliance
Center for Drug Evaluation and Research
Food and Drug Administration
Building 51, Room 5352
10903 New Hampshire Avenue

Silver Spring, MD 20993

Sincerely yours,

{See appended electronic signature page}

David C. Burrow, Pharm.D., J.D.
Acting Director
Office of Scientific Investigations
Office of Compliance
Center for Drug Evaluation and Research
Food and Drug Administration

This is a representation of an electronic record that was signed electronically and this page is the manifestation of the electronic signature.

/S/

DAVID C BURROW
04/20/2017

第58封　给Merrill D. Benson医学博士的警告信

2017年3月20日

参考号：17-HFD-45-03-01

尊敬的Benson博士：

2016年10月10日至2016年10月11日，Myra K. Casey 女士、Lewis K. Antwi先生和Melanie N. Daniels女士代表FDA在您的临床研究现场进行了现场检查，对您开展的关于试验药物（b）(4）的临床研究［试验方案（b）(4）］进行了审查，该研究您是作为申办-研究者。这封警告信特告知您现场检查中发现的违规情况。

本次检查是FDA的生物研究监查项目的一部分，该项目通过设定的检查方法，对由FDA监管的研究的实施情况进行评估，以确认研究数据在科学上是有效和准确的，并帮助确保这些研究中受试者的权益、安全和福利得到了保护。

在现场检查结束时，Casey女士和Antwi 先生向您出示了FDA 483表，即现场检查发现的问题，并与您进行了讨论。您于2016年11月30日对该FDA 483表的书面回复已收悉。

经对FDA现场检查报告、该报告的附件，以及您2016年11月30日的书面回复进行审查，我们认为您没有遵循适用的法律要求以及监管临床研究实施和受试者保护的FDA法规。我们想强调以下几点：

您未能确保按照研究计划开展研究［21 CFR 312.60］

作为临床研究者，您必须确保按照研究计划开展研究。试验方案（b）(4）的研究计划规定了安全监测的要求，定义了方案特定的停止规则，并要求您在规定的时间执行特定的试验程序，例如血小板计数检测、临床生化指标检测和尿液实验室检测。此外，试验方案（b）(4）的研究计划要求您不能入组符合排除标准的受试者。您未能遵守这些要求。具体而言：

1. 上述方案的研究计划要求，在研究期间，大约每周都需监测血小板；如果由于一些原因，从最后一个可用的血小板值开始已经过去了14天，那么必须暂停给药，直到获得血小板计数结果并由研究者进行了审阅。需要注意的是，在一个单独的随机对照研究中，被给予了试验药物（b）(4）或安慰剂的3名受试者血小板计数暂时性减少，但是不清楚这些减少是否与研究药物有关。因此，经常监测血小板数量和严格遵守方案特定的停止规则，对于保护研究对象的权益、安全和福利非常重要。

a. 对于受试者CM 01, 2016年5月23日至2016年6月12日之间每周一次的血小板检测没有进行。在此期间，超过14天过去了而没有进行血小板检测，但是，研究药物没有暂停。

b. 对于受试者CM 17, 2016年5月24日至2016年6月14日之间每周一次的血小板检测没有进行。在此期间，超过14天过去了而没有进行血小板检测，但是，研究药物没有暂停。

在2016年11月30日对FDA 483表的书面回复中，您认可了发现的问题，即在规定的时间内没有采集血小板检测的血样。您注意到，根据有关（b）(4）治疗的患者发生危及生命的血小板减少的报告，监测受试者的血小板是至关重要的。您指出，研究团队将追踪每个受试者的计划给药日期和所有血小板计数结果，确保每个受试者在每次计划给药之前都有一个被审查过的、可接受的血小板水平。您还注意到，如果这些因素中的任何一个都没有得到满足，受试者将被告知暂停计划的给药，直到临床研究者已收到血小板计数结果并根据方案中的指导原则，确认其是在可接受的范围内为止。

我们无法确定，您书面回复中提供的纠正措施计划如果适当地执行，是否可以预防将来这种类型的违规。具体而言，您没有提供针对您未能遵守方案的程序这一检查发现，而实施的额外措施和程序计划的充分细节。例如，您没有指出，您和您的工作人员是否进行了再培训活动，以预防将来的方案违背。此外，您的书面回复并没有提供关于您个人将如何确保对研究流程的充分监督（例如，方案要求的安全监测和停止规则），以及您和您的研究人员的GCP培训情况的足够细节。没有这些细节，我们无法确定您的纠正措施计划是否足以预防将来类似的违规。

如上所述，经常监测血小板和严格遵守方案特定的停止规则，对于保护参与研究的受试者的权益、安全和福利至关重要。未能遵守方案规定的安全监测和停止规则，特别是与血小板计数结果有关的规则，危害到受试者的安全和福利。

2. 该研究计划要求您将肾功能不全的受试者排除，即排除那些在筛选时24小时尿肌酐清除率（Cockroft-Gault公式）小于35mL/（min·1.73 m^2）的受试者。

尽管受试者CM 04有已知的肾功能不全病史，并在筛选时估测肌酐清除率（Cockroft-Gault公式）为27mL/（min·1.73m^2），但是您仍在2014年12月19日将该受试者入组到试验方案（b）(4）中。

在2016年11月30日对FDA 483表的书面回复中，您承认该受试者的24小时尿肌酐清除率不满足资格要求，并且该受试者的入组是一个方案违背。您还指出，您对这个排除标准做了一次例外，并让该受试者入组，是因为正如您所指出的，您知道该受试者因肾功能不全而被一名肾病专家进行随访，其肾功能不全可能与小动脉肾硬化有关；并且实验室检测表明，受试者的肾功能在受试者进入研究前已经稳定了一年多。

我们无法确定，您书面回复中提供的纠正措施计划如果适当地执行，是否可以预防将来这种类型的违规。具体而言，您没有提供针对您入组了不合格受试者这一检查发现，而实施的额外措施和程序的计划的充分细节。例如，您没有指出您和您的工作人员是否进行了再培训活动，以预防将来的方案违背。此外，您的书面回复并没有提供关于您个人将如何确保对研究流程的充分监督（例如，遵循合格要求），以及您和您的研究人员的方案培训情况的足够细节。没有这些细节，我们无法确定您的纠正措施计划是否足以预防将来类似的违规。

我们强调的是，每一项临床研究的合格标准都是设计用来优化收集数据的可理解性和减小对入组受试者的可预见性伤害。入组不符合合格标准的受试者损害了受试者的安全和福利，并引起对在您的研究场所收集的数据的有效性和完整性的关注。

3. 研究计划要求您在筛选及第1、6、13、26、39、52、78、104和117周进行临床生化指标检查和尿液实验室检测。对于方案（b）(4），临床生化指标包括检测镁、磷和尿酸。您未能按规定的时间间隔进行下列临床实验室检测:

受试者编号	没有执行的实验室检测	检测未进行的研究周数
CM 02	镁和磷	6
	尿酸	52和78
CM 07	尿检	78
CM 10	尿检	6，13和26
CM 11	镁和磷	筛选
	尿酸	13和26
CM 18	镁和磷	1
	尿酸	1和6

我们承认上述项目3.中的关于受试者CM 11的第13周尿酸实验室检测，以及受试者CM 18的第1周尿酸实验室检测的问题未包括在您收到的FDA 483表中，因此，您的书面回复并没有解释这个问题。

在2016年11月30日对FDA 483表的书面回复中，您承认对这些受试者没有进行某些尿液分析和镁、尿酸及磷的实验室检测。您认识到，这些缺陷表明需要培训您的临床研究团队，以确保对所有受试者都按照方案要求进行了检测。作为您纠正措施计划的一部分，您指出，当实验室检测被遗漏时，您的临床研究团队的一名成员将会要求进行该实验室检测，并获得该检测的结果。您还表示，您获得了一个独立的监查员来监查您的临床研究团队对执行实验室检测方案要求的遵循。

我们无法确定，您书面回复中提供的纠正措施计划如果适当地执行，是否可以预防将来这种类型的违规。具体而言，您没有提供针对您未能遵守方案的程序这一检查发现，而实施的额外措施和程序的计划的充分细节。例如，您没有指出您和您的工作人员是否进行了再培训活动，以预防将来的方案违背。此外，您的书面回复并没有提供关于您个人将如何确保对研究流程的充分监督（例如，在规定的时间间隔完成方案要求的检测），以及您和您的研究人员的方案培训情况的足够细节。没有这些细节，我们无法确定您的纠正措施计划是否足以预防将来类似的违规。

未能执行方案要求的程序，包括用于监测受试者安全和耐受性的临床实验室检测，危害了受试者的安全和福利，并会引起对在您的研究场所收集的数据的有效性和完整性的关注。

本警告信的目的并非是罗列您在试验药物临床研究中存在的所有缺陷。确保遵循法律和相关FDA法规的每一项要求是您的职责，您应当解决这些缺陷，并建立规程，以确保任何正在进行或将来进行的研究均符合FDA的法规。

自收到这封信的15个工作日内，您应当书面告知本办公室为预防将来发生类似违规情况而采取的措施。如果不能充分、迅速地解释上述违规问题，可能导致我们在不再通知的情况下采取监管措施。如果您认为已经遵循了FDA的法规要求，请陈述理由，并提供所有支持资料，以供我们参考。

附：英文原文

Merrill D. Benson, M.D.

WARNING LETTER

Mar 20, 2017

CERTIFIED MAIL
RETURN RECEIPT REQUESTED

Ref: 17-HFD-45-03-01

Merrill D. Benson, M.D.
Indiana University
School of Medicine
Department of Pathology
635 Barnhill Drive, MS-128
Indianapolis, Indiana 46202-5126

Dear Dr. Benson:

This Warning Letter informs you of objectionable conditions observed during the Food and Drug Administration (FDA) inspection conducted at your clinical site between October 11, 2016, and November 10, 2016. Ms. Myra K. Casey, Mr. Lewis K. Antwi, and Ms. Melanie N. Daniels, representing FDA, reviewed your conduct of a clinical investigation (Protocol (b)(4)) of the investigational drug (b)(4), which you performed as a sponsor-investigator.

This inspection is a part of FDA's Bioresearch Monitoring Program, which includes inspections designed to evaluate the conduct of FDA-regulated research to ensure that the data are scientifically valid and accurate, and to help ensure that the rights, safety, and welfare of the human subjects in the studies are protected.

At the conclusion of the inspection, Ms. Casey and Mr. Antwi presented and discussed with you Form FDA 483,

Inspectional Observations. We acknowledge receipt of your November 30, 2016, written response to the Form FDA 483. From our review of the FDA Establishment Inspection Report, the documents submitted with that report, and your written response dated November 30, 2016, we conclude that you did not adhere to the applicable statutory requirements and FDA regulations governing the conduct of clinical investigations and the protection of human subjects. We wish to emphasize the following:

You failed to ensure that the investigation was conducted according to the investigational plan [21 CFR 312.60].

As a clinical investigator, you are required to ensure that your clinical studies are conducted in accordance with the investigational plan. The investigational plan for Protocol (b)(4) specifies requirements for safety monitoring, defines protocol-specific stopping rules, and requires you to perform certain study procedures at specific times, such as platelet count measurements, clinical chemistry panel tests, and urinalysis laboratory tests. In addition, the investigational plan for Protocol (b)(4) requires you not to enroll subjects who meet the exclusion criteria. You failed to adhere to these requirements. Specifically:

1. The investigational plan for the above-mentioned protocol requires that platelets be monitored approximately every week for the duration of the study; and if for any reason 14 days has elapsed since the last available platelet value, dosing must be held until a platelet count is obtained and reviewed by the investigator. Of note, in a separate randomized controlled study, three subjects given the study drug (b)(4) or placebo had temporary decreases in their platelet counts; however, it is not known if these decreases were related to the study drug. Therefore, frequent monitoring of platelet counts and strict adherence to protocol-specific stopping rules are important to protect the rights, safety, and welfare of study subjects.

a. For Subject CM 01, weekly platelet measurements were not performed between May 23, 2016, and June 12, 2016. During this time frame, more than 14 days elapsed without platelet testing; however, the study drug was not held.

b. For Subject CM 17, weekly platelet measurements were not performed between May 24, 2016, and June 14, 2016. During this time frame, more than 14 days elapsed without platelet testing; however, the study drug was not held.

In your November 30, 2016, written response to the Form FDA 483, you agreed with the observations that platelets were not drawn during the specified time frames. You noted that in light of the reports concerning life-threatening thrombocytopenia in subjects treated with (b)(4), monitoring of subjects' platelets is of the utmost importance. You indicated that the study team will track scheduled dosing dates and all platelet count results for each subject, ensuring that each subject has a platelet level that has been reviewed and is acceptable on the day before each scheduled dosing. You also noted that if either of these factors is not met, the subject will be informed to hold their scheduled dosing until the clinical investigator has received a platelet count result and confirms that it is acceptable under the guidelines in the protocol.

We are unable to determine if your written response provides a corrective action plan that, if properly carried out, would prevent this type of violation in the future. Specifically, you did not provide sufficient details about your plan for implementing additional measures and procedures to address the inspection findings concerning your failure to follow protocol procedures. For example, you did not indicate whether you and your staff underwent retraining activities to prevent future protocol violations. In addition, your written response does not provide sufficient details about how you personally will ensure adequate oversight of study procedures (for example, protocol-required safety monitoring and stopping rules) and good clinical practice training for you and your study staff. Without these details, we are unable to determine whether your corrective action plan is adequate to prevent similar violations in the future.

As mentioned above, frequent monitoring of platelets and strict adherence to protocol-specific stopping rules are essential to protect the rights, safety, and welfare of subjects participating in the study. Failure to adhere to protocol-required safety monitoring and stopping rules, particularly those related to platelet count results, jeopardizes subject safety and welfare.

2. The investigational plan required you to exclude subjects with renal insufficiency, defined as any subject with an estimated creatinine clearance (Cockroft-Gault formula) for 24-hour urine creatinine clearance <35 mL/min/1.73 m^2 at screening.

You enrolled Subject CM 04 into Protocol (b)(4) on December 19, 2014, even though this subject had a known history of renal insufficiency and an estimated creatinine clearance (Cockroft-Gault formula) of 27 mL/min/1.73 m^2

at screening.

In your November 30, 2016, written response to the Form FDA 483, you acknowledged that this subject's 24-hour urine creatinine clearance did not meet the eligibility requirements, and that enrollment of this subject was a protocol deviation. You also indicated that you made an exception to this exclusion criterion and enrolled this subject because, as you noted, you were aware that the subject was followed by a nephrologist for renal insufficiency, likely related to arteriolar nephrosclerosis; and that laboratory tests indicated that the subject's renal function had been stable for more than one year before the subject entered the study.

We are unable to determine if your written response provides a corrective action plan that, if properly carried out, would prevent this type of violation in the future. Specifically, you did not provide sufficient details about your plan for implementing additional measures and procedures to address the inspection findings regarding the enrollment of ineligible subjects. For example, you did not indicate whether you and your staff underwent retraining activities to prevent future protocol violations. In addition, your written response does not provide sufficient details about how you personally will ensure adequate oversight of study procedures (for example, adherence to eligibility requirements) and protocol training for you and your study staff. Without these details, we are unable to determine whether your corrective action plan is adequate to prevent similar violations in the future.

We emphasize that the eligibility criteria for each clinical investigation are designed both to optimize interpretability of collected data, and to minimize foreseeable harm to enrolled subjects. Enrollment of subjects who do not meet the eligibility criteria jeopardizes subject safety and welfare, and raises concerns about the validity and integrity of the data collected at your site.

3. The investigational plan requires that you perform clinical chemistry panels and urinalysis laboratory tests at Screening and at Weeks 1, 6, 13, 26, 39, 52, 78, 104, and 117. For Protocol (b)(4), clinical chemistry panels include measurement of magnesium, phosphorus, and uric acid. You failed to conduct the following clinical laboratory tests at the specified intervals:

Subject ID	Laboratory tests not performed	Study week(s) when these tests were not performed
CM 02	Magnesium and phosphorus	6
	Uric acid	52 and 78
CM 07	Urinalysis	78
CM 10	Urinalysis	6, 13, and 26
CM 11	Magnesium and phosphorus	Screening
	Uric acid	13 and 26
CM 18	Magnesium and phosphorus	1
	Uric acid	1 and 6

We acknowledge that the findings in Item 3. above for Subject CM 11's Week 13 uric acid laboratory test, and for Subject CM 18's Week 1 uric acid laboratory test, were not included on the Form FDA 483 you received; and that therefore, your written response does not address this finding.

In your November 30, 2016, written response to the Form FDA 483, you acknowledged that certain urinalysis and laboratory tests for magnesium, uric acid, and phosphorus were not performed for these subjects. You noted that these deficiencies demonstrate a need to train your clinical research team, to ensure that all subjects have the required tests performed according to the protocol. As part of your corrective action plan, you indicated that when a laboratory test is missed, a member of your clinical research team will request that laboratory test to be performed and will obtain the result of that laboratory test. You also indicated that you acquired an independent monitor to monitor your clinical research team's adherence to the protocol requirements for laboratory testing.

We are unable to determine if your written response provides a corrective action plan that, if properly carried out, would prevent this type of violation in the future. Specifically, you did not provide sufficient details about your plan for implementing additional measures and procedures to address the inspection findings concerning your failure to follow protocol procedures. For example, you did not indicate whether you and your staff underwent retraining activities to prevent future protocol violations. In addition, your written response does not provide sufficient details about how you personally will ensure adequate oversight of study procedures (for example, completion of protocol-required tests at specified intervals) and protocol training for you and your study staff. Without these details, we are unable to determine whether your corrective action plan is adequate to prevent similar violations in the future.

Failure to perform protocol-required procedures, including clinical laboratory tests used to monitor subject safety and tolerability, jeopardizes subject safety and welfare, and raises concerns about the validity and reliability of the data collected at your site.

This letter is not intended to be an all-inclusive list of deficiencies with your clinical study of an investigational drug. It is your responsibility to ensure adherence to each requirement of the law and relevant FDA regulations. You should address these deficiencies and establish procedures to ensure that any ongoing or future studies will be in compliance with FDA regulations.

Within fifteen (15) working days of your receipt of this letter, you should notify this office in writing of the actions you have taken to prevent similar violations in the future. Failure to address the violations noted above adequately and promptly may result in regulatory action without further notice. If you believe you have complied with FDA regulations, include your reasoning and any supporting information for our consideration.

If you have any questions, please contact Adam Donat, M.S., at 301-796-5316; FAX 301-847-8748. Your written response and any pertinent documentation should be addressed to:

Adam Donat, M.S.
Branch Chief
Compliance Enforcement Branch
Division of Enforcement and Postmarketing Safety
Office of Scientific Investigations
Office of Compliance
Center for Drug Evaluation and Research
Food and Drug Administration
Building 51, Room 5352
10903 New Hampshire Avenue
Silver Spring, MD 20993

Sincerely yours,

{See appended electronic signature page}

David C. Burrow, Pharm.D., J.D.
Acting Director
Office of Scientific Investigations
Office of Compliance
Center for Drug Evaluation and Research
Food and Drug Administration

This is a representation of an electronic record that was signed electronically and this page is the manifestation of the electronic signature.

/S/

DAVID C BURROW
03/20/2017

第59封　给John Gabriel医学博士的警告信

2016年6月28日

参考号：16-HFD-45-06-01

尊敬的Gabriel博士：

2016年2月1日至18日，Travis M. Beard先生代表FDA，在您的临床研究中心，对您实施的临床研究［试验方案（b）（4），关于试验药物（b）（4），申办者为（b）（4）］进行了审查，这封警告信特告知您现场检查中发现的违规情况。

本次现场检查是FDA的生物研究监查项目的一部分。该项目通过设定的检查方法，对FDA所监管的相关研究的实施情况进行评估，以确认研究数据在科学上是有效和准确的，并帮助确保这些研究中的受试者的权益、安全和福利得到了保护。

在现场检查结束时，Beard先生向您出示并讨论了FDA483表，即现场检查发现的问题。我们确认收到您2016年3月4日对FDA483表的书面回复。

经对FDA现场检查报告、该报告的附件，以及您2016年3月4日的书面回复进行审查，我们认为，您没有遵循适用的法律要求和监管临床研究实施及受试者保护的FDA法规。我们想强调以下几方面：

您未能确保研究按照研究计划进行［21 CFR 312.60］

作为临床研究者，您必须确保您的临床研究按照研究计划来实施。研究计划要求您对访视1结束时没有关键实验室检查数据的受试者延迟随机，并且如果受试者的估计肾小球滤过率（eGFR）降到小于30mL/（min·1.73m^2）（基于连续两次血清肌酐测定），（b）（4）剂量将由50mg，一日1次降到25mg，一日2次。您未能遵循这些要求。具体而言：

1. 试验方案要求在访视1（即筛选和随机访视）采集可获取的最近的血清肌酐和eGFR值，并且规定至少这些值中的一个用于在访视1的随机。通过方案规定的肾脏疾病饮食改良（MDRD）方法用血清肌酐值计算eGFR，eGFR值被用于决定受试者的入组资格和初始的试验药物剂量。满足所有入排标准的受试者将在访视1被随机分组，需要再次访视的受试者（例如，到访视1结束时重要的实验室数据还没有获得）将不会被随机，直到已经获得了该信息。

a. 有25名受试者在您收到他们的血清肌酐值之前被随机，且接受了试验药物。具体而言：

受试者	随机并开始试验药物的日期	收到血清肌酐值的日期
110746	2012年1月9日	2012年1月21日
110946	2012年1月23日	2012年1月25日
111043	2012年1月27日	2012年4月19日
111075	2012年1月30日	2012年2月22日
111400	2012年2月17日	2012年4月26日
111448	2012年2月21日	2012年3月15日
111588	2012年2月28日	2012年3月12日
111764	2012年3月7日	2012年3月8日
112138	2012年3月21日	2012年5月4日
112166	2012年3月22日	2012年3月28日
112194	2012年3月23日	2012年4月19日
112542	2012年4月4日	2012年4月5日

续表

受试者	随机并开始试验药物的日期	收到血清肌酐值的日期
110943	2012年1月23日	2012年1月25日
110967	2012年1月24日	2012年4月21日
110991	2012年1月25日	2012年1月27日
111050	2012年1月28日	2012年2月1日
111140	2012年2月2日	2012年4月9日
111206	2012年2月7日	2012年4月24日
111304	2012年2月13日	2012年2月16日
111402	2012年2月17日	2012年5月10日
111521	2012年2月24日	2012年3月15日
111618	2012年2月29日	2012年3月5日
111797	2012年3月8日	2012年3月16日
111853	2012年3月12日	2012年3月21日
112195	2012年3月23日	2012年4月9日

我们承认，受试者112195关于上述第1项发现的问题没有包含在您收到的FDA483表中，因此，您的书面回复没有解决这个问题。

我们注意到，特别是受试者111075于2012年1月30日被随机并接受了试验药物，而2012年2月22日收到的血清肌酐值和eGFR值确定了该受试者不符合入组条件［eGFR ＜30mL/（min·1.73 m^2）］。尽管受试者111075于2012年2月22日退出了研究，但这名受试者原本就不应该入组本研究。

b. 受试者110946和112166开始时就过量服用了试验药物，因为受试者在随机并接受试验药物时您还没有获得血清肌酐值和eGFR值。具体而言：

受试者	随机并开始使用试验药物的日期	初始试验药物剂量	获得血清肌酐值的日期	调低剂量的日期	新的试验药物剂量
110946	2012年1月23日	100mg	2012年1月25日	2012年4月27日	50mg
112166	2012年3月22日	100mg	2012年3月28日	2012年4月25日	50mg

由于一名受试者后来被发现不符合入组本研究的资格，两名受试者接受了不正确的初始试验药物剂量，需要调低剂量。因此，未能在随机时获取血清肌酐值和eGFR值的情况，罔顾了受试者的安全。

在您2016年3月4日对FDA483表的书面回复中，您指出，在研究初期，受试者是从您的临床数据库中被入组，医疗记录是现成的，因此您遵循了研究方案。您指出，在研究后期，受试者被介绍到您的研究中心来使用（b）（4），以促进受试者的招募。就在那时，您提到您不能在访视1确认所需要的血清肌酐值或获取医疗记录，因此您错误地依赖于受试者的口头病史。

而且，您解释说，您联系了受试者并努力去获取有记录的实验室数值。一旦得到这些数值，您指出，如果需要进行调整，受试者将被给予正确剂量的试验药物。您描述受试者的安全如何得到保证：所有的受试者都有肾病专科医生或者主治医生（PCP）进行定期访视。

关于受试者110946和112166过量使用试验药物、需要调低剂量的问题，您指出，您依赖于受试者报告的肾病病史，并且对他们的糖尿病药物作出了如下假设：

- 受试者110946按照她的主治医生（PCP）的医嘱服用2000mg二甲双胍。您解释说，因为那个剂量的二甲双胍只允许用于没有肾功能损害的受试者［即eGFR＞60mL/（min·1.73m^2）］，受试者被分配使用100mg的试验药物，但是后来当您得到她的医疗记录后调低到50mg。
- 受试者112166服用二甲双胍1000mg及格列本脲5mg。您解释说，这种药物和剂量提示没有肾功能损害，因此受试者被分配使用100mg的试验药物，但是后来当您得到她的医疗记录后调低到50mg。

您承认，在没有首先获得所需的实验室结果的情况下，初始的试验药物剂量本来不应该得到确定，在分配试验药物剂量之前，本来应该进行更彻底的筛选过程。您指出，已经对员工进行了分配正确的试验药物剂量、不基于受试者的口头病史就进行随机或者分发试验药物的再次培训。这样一来，您的研究中心将要求受试者在随机和分配试验药物剂量之前，访视1时，把包含当前的血清肌酐值在内的医疗记录带来。我们无法对您的书面回复进行知情评价，因为您并没有提供一份纠正措施计划，来说明如果正确地实施，会在将来预防这种类型的违规。具体而言，您并没有提供关于您将如何确保在将来的其他研究中遵循研究方案规定的要求的足够细节。

2. 试验方案规定，既然（b）（4）主要通过肾脏清除，对肾功能下降的需要进行剂量调整。如果eGFR值下降到小于30mL/（min·1.73m^2），基于两次连续血清肌酐测定，（b）（4）剂量将降至25mg，一日1次。试验方案指出，应该取得最近可用的血清肌酐值和eGFR，作为年度和短期访视的常规护理的一部分，并且如果基于最近得到的血清肌酐值/衍生的eGFR，判断肾功能恶化，研究者将下调盲化试验药物的剂量。如果需要进行剂量调整，受试者需要过来进行计划外的访视（除非是已经计划的访视安排在一个月内），并且剂量调整应通过交互式语音应答系统（IVRS）来进行管理。

尽管受试者112194的两次连续eGFR值小于30mL/（min·1.73m^2），但您未能按照试验方案的要求下调试验药物剂量。2013年3月10日（对应于2013年3月26日的第12个月访视），eGFR值22mL/（min·1.73m^2），受试者112194在使用50mg的试验药物，并且随后在2013年7月18日（对应于2013年9月19日的第18个月访视），eGFR值23mL/（min·1.73m^2）。尽管受试者112194两次连续eGFR值小于30mL/（min·1.73m^2），但您没有按照研究方案的要求，在第18个月访视时将试验药物剂量下调至25mg。研究记录表明，受试者112194在2013年12月3日第21个月访视时还在使用50mg剂量的试验药物。

在您2016年3月4日对FDA483表的书面回复中，您表示受试者112194在研究期间在看肾病专科医生。该肾病专科医生为这名受试者安排了实验室检查，eGFR值如下：

- 2012年3月23日（随机化/访视1）——49mL/（min·1.73m^2）
- 2012年7月23日（第4个月/访视2）——43mL/（min·1.73m^2）
- 2012年11月27日（第8个月/访视3）——39mL/（min·1.73m^2）
- 2013年3月26日（第12个月）——22mL/（min·1.73m^2）

您声称，在2013年9月19日第18个月访视时，该受试者证实肾病专科医生安排了实验室检查，而且这次访视后，您向肾病专科医生索取了实验室检查结果。几周后在收到实验室检查结果时，您注意到eGFR值为23mL/（min·1.73m^2）符合下调试验药物剂量的方案标准。您解释说，您无法联系受试者过来进行试验药物剂量下调，而且受试者在2014年1月15日、剂量下调之前就退出了本研究。

我们无法对您的书面回复进行知情评价，因为您并没有提供一份纠正措施计划，来说明如果正确地实施，会在将来预防这种类型的违规。具体而言，您并没有提供关于您将如何确保在将来的其他研究中遵循研究方案规定的足够细节。

如上所述，您未能按照研究计划实施研究项目。具体而言，您未能对访视1结束时还没有得到血清肌酐值的受试者推迟随机，未能基于eGFR值下降到小于30mL/（min·1.73m^2）（基于两次连续血清肌酐值测定）而下调试验药物的剂量；这种做法危害了受试者的安全和福利，而且使在您的研究中心收集的数据的可释性被削弱。

这封信的目的并非是罗列您在试验药物临床研究过程中存在的所有缺陷。确保遵循法律和相关FDA法规的每一项要求是您的职责。您应当解决这些缺陷，并建立相应规程，以确保任何正在进行或将来进行的研究都符合FDA法规。

自收到这封信的15个工作日内，您应当书面告知本办公室，为预防将来发生类似违规情况已经采取的纠正措施。如果不能充分、迅速地解释上述违规问题，可能导致我们在不再通知的情况下采取监管措施。如果您确信您已符合FDA法规要求，请陈述理由，并提供所有支持资料，以供我们参考。

附：英文原文

John Gabriel, M.D.

WARNING LETTER

JUN 28, 2016

CERTIFIED MAIL
RETURN RECEIPT REQUESTED

Ref: 16-HFD-45-06-01

John D. Gabriel, M.D.
North Hills Medical Research, Inc.
4351 Booth Calloway Road, Suite 101
North Richland Hills, Texas 76180-7319

Dear Dr. Gabriel:

This Warning Letter informs you of objectionable conditions observed during the U.S. Food and Drug Administration (FDA) inspection conducted at your clinical site between February 1 and 18, 2016 Mr. Travis M. Beard, representing FDA, reviewed your conduct of a clinical investigation (Protocol **(b)(4)** for the investigational drug **(b)(4)**, performed for **(b)(4)**.

This inspection is a part of FDA's Bioresearch Monitoring Program, which includes inspections designed to evaluate the conduct of FDA-regulated research to ensure that the data are scientifically valid and accurate, and to help ensure that the rights, safety, and welfare of the human subjects of those studies have been protected.

At the conclusion of the inspection, Mr. Beard presented and discussed with you Form FDA 483, Inspectional Observations We acknowledge receipt of your March 4, 2016 written response to the Form FDA 483.

From our review of the FDA Establishment Inspection Report, the documents submitted with that report, and your March 4, 2016 written response, we conclude that you did not adhere to the applicable statutory requirements and FDA regulations governing the conduct of clinical investigations and the protection of human subjects We wish to emphasize the following:

You failed to ensure that the investigation was conducted according to the investigational plan [21 CFR 312.60].

As a clinical investigator, you are required to ensure that your clinical studies are conducted in accordance with the investigational plan The investigational plan requires that you delay randomization for subjects who do not have key laboratory data by the end of Visit 1, and that if the subject's estimated glomerular filtration rate (eGFR) drops to <30 mL/min/1.73 m^2 (based on two consecutive serum creatinine determinations) the **(b)(4)** dose will be reduced from 50 mg once daily to 25 mg once daily You failed to adhere to these requirements Specifically:

1. The protocol requires collection of the most recent available serum creatinine and eGFR values at Visit 1 (i.e., the screening and randomization visit), and states that at least one of these values is required for randomization at Visit 1 Serum creatinine is used to calculate eGFR via the protocol-specified Modification of Diet in Renal Disease (MDRD) method, and the eGFR value is used to determine a subject's eligibility [1] and initial study drug dose. [2] Subjects who satisfy all inclusion and exclusion criteria will be randomized at Visit 1; subjects who require a repeat visit (for example, key laboratory data are not available by the end of Visit 1) will not be randomized until that information is available.

a. Twenty-five subjects were randomized and received study drug prior to your receipt of their serum creatinine values Specifically:

Subject	Date of Randomization and Start of Study Drug	Date Serum Creatinine Received
110746	January 9, 2012	January 21, 2012
110946	January 23, 2012	January 25, 2012
111043	January 27, 2012	April 19, 2012
111075	January 30, 2012	February 22, 2012
111400	February 17, 2012	April 26, 2012
111448	February 21, 2012	March 15, 2012
111588	February 28, 2012	March 12, 2012
111764	March 7, 2012	March 8, 2012
112138	March 21, 2012	May 4, 2012
112166	March 22, 2012	March 28, 2012
112194	March 23, 2012	April 19, 2012
112542	April 4, 2012	April 5, 2012
110943	January 23, 2012	January 25, 2012
110967	January 24, 2012	April 21, 2012
110991	January 25, 2012	January 27, 2012
111050	January 28, 2012	February 1, 2012
111140	February 2, 2012	April 9, 2012
111206	February 7, 2012	April 24, 2012
111304	February 13, 2012	February 16, 2012
111402	February 17, 2012	May 10, 2012
111521	February 24, 2012	March 15, 2012
111618	February 29, 2012	March 5, 2012
111797	March 8, 2012	March 16, 2012
111853	March 12, 2012	March 21, 2012
112195	March 23, 2012	April 9, 2012

We acknowledge that the finding in Item 1 above for Subject 112195 was not included on the Form FDA 483 you received and therefore, your written response does not address this finding.

We note it is particularly concerning that Subject 111075 was randomized and received study drug on January 30, 2012, when the serum creatinine and eGFR values, received on February 22, 2012, determined the subject to be ineligible (eGFR <30 mL/min/1.73 m^2). While Subject 111075 was discontinued from the study on February 22, 2012, this subject should never have been enrolled in the study.

b. Subjects 110946 and 112166 were initially overdosed with study drug because you did not have required serum creatinine and eGFR values at the time the subjects were randomized and received study drug Specifically:

Subject	Date of Randomization and Start of Study Drug	Initial Study Drug Dose	Date Serum Creatinine Received	Date of Down Titration	New Study Drug Dose
110946	January 23, 2012	100 mg	January 25, 2012	April 27, 2012	50 mg
112166	March 22, 2012	100 mg	March 28, 2012	April 25, 2012	50 mg

The failure to have serum creatinine and eGFR values at the time of randomization compromises subject safety as one subject was later found to be ineligible for the study and two other subjects received incorrect initial doses of study drug and required down titration.

In your March 4, 2016 written response to the Form FDA 483, you indicate that during the early part of the study, subjects were enrolled from your own clinic database and medical records were readily available so you followed the protocol You state that in the later part of study, subjects were referred to your site using **(b)(4)** to help facilitate subject recruitment At that point, you state you could not confirm the required serum creatinine value or obtain medical records at Visit 1, so you erroneously relied on subject verbal history

Further, you explain that you contacted subjects and made efforts to obtain documented laboratory values. Once these values were obtained, you indicate that subjects were placed on the correct dose of study drug if adjustment was necessary You describe how subject safety was ensured as all enrolled subjects had regular visits with their nephrologist or primary care physician (PCP).

With regard to Subjects 110946 and 112166 being overdosed with study drug and requiring down titration, you indicate that you relied on subject-reported kidney history and made the following assumptions about their diabetes medications:

- Subject 110946 was taking metformin 2000 mg as prescribed by her PCP You explain that because that dose of metformin is only permissible in subjects with no renal impairment (i.e., eGFR >60 mL/min/1.73m^2), the subject was assigned 100 mg of study drug, but was later down titrated to 50 mg when you received her medical records.
- Subject 112166 was taking metformin 1000 mg with glyburide 5 mg You explain that these medications and doses are indicative of no renal impairment, so the subject was assigned 100 mg of study drug, but was later down titrated to 50 mg when you received the medical records.

You acknowledge that the initial study drug dose should not have been determined without first obtaining the required laboratory results, and that a more thorough screening process should have been done prior to assigning study drug dose You state that staff has been retrained on assigning correct study drug dose and to not randomize or dispense study drug based on subjects' verbal history Such that, your site will require subjects to have medical records in-hand at Visit 1, including current serum creatinine values, before randomization and assignment of study drug dose.

We are unable to undertake an informed evaluation of your written response because you did not provide a corrective action plan that, if properly carried out, would prevent this type of violation in the future Specifically, you did not provide sufficient details on how you will ensure adherence to protocol-specific requirements for other future studies.

2. The protocol states that since **(b)(4)** is cleared primarily through the kidneys, a dose adjustment is required for reduced renal function If the eGFR drops to <30 mL/min/1.73m^2, based on two consecutive serum creatinine determinations, the **(b)(4)** dose will reduced to 25 mg once daily The protocol specifies that the most recent available serum creatinine and eGFR values should be obtained as part of usual care at Annual and Brief Visits, [3] and that study investigators will down-titrate the dose of blinded study medication if renal function deteriorates based on the most recently available serum creatinine/derived eGFR If a dose adjustment is needed, the subject will be brought in for an unscheduled visit (unless a scheduled visit is planned within one month), and the dose adjustment managed through the Interactive Voice Response System (IVRS).

Despite two consecutive eGFR values $<$ 30mL/min/1.73m^2 for Subject 112194, you failed to down titrate study drug as required by the protocol Subject 112194 was taking 50 mg of study drug with an eGFR of 22 mL/min/1.73 m^2 on March 10, 2013 (corresponding to the Month 12 Visit that occurred on March 26, 2013) and subsequently, had an eGFR of 23 mL/min/1.73 m^2 on July 18, 2013 (corresponding to the Month 18 Visit that occurred on September 19, 2013) Despite this subject having two consecutive eGFR values $<$30 mL/min/1.73m^2, you did not down titrate Subject 112194 to 25 mg of study drug at the Month 18 Visit as required by the protocol Study records indicate that Subject 112194 was still taking 50 mg of study drug at the Month 21 Visit that occurred on December 3, 2013

In your March 4, 2016, written response to the Form FDA 483, you indicate that Subject 112194 was seeing his nephrologist during the study The nephrologist ordered labs for this subject with the following eGFR values:

- March 23, 2012 (randomization/Visit 1) – 49 mL/min/1.73 m^2

- July 23, 2012 (Month 4/Visit 2) – 43 mL/min/1.73 m^2
- November 27, 2012 (Month 8/Visit 3) – 39 mL/min/1.73 m^2
- March 26, 2013 (Month 12) – 22 mL/min/1.73 m^2

You state that at the Month 18 Visit on September 19, 2013, the subject confirmed that his nephrologist ordered labs and after the visit, you requested the laboratory results from the nephrologist Upon receiving the laboratory results several weeks later, you noted that the eGFR was 23 mL/min/1.73 m^2, which met the protocol criteria for down titration of study drug You explain that you were not able to contact the subject to come in for down titration of study drug, and that the subject withdrew from the study on January 15, 2014, prior to being down titrated

We are unable to undertake an informed evaluation of your written response because you did not provide a corrective action plan that, if properly carried out, would prevent this type of violation in the future Specifically, you did not provide sufficient details on how you will ensure adherence to protocol-specific requirements for other future studies

As discussed above, you failed to conduct the investigation in accordance with the investigational plan Specifically, your failure to delay randomization for subjects who did not have serum creatinine by the end of Visit 1 and your failure to reduce the dose of study drug based on a drop in eGFR to less than 30 mL/min/1.73m^2 (based on two consecutive serum creatinine determinations), jeopardized subject safety and welfare, and compromised the interpretability of the data collected at your site

This letter is not intended to be an all-inclusive list of deficiencies with your clinical study of an investigational drug It is your responsibility to ensure adherence to each requirement of the law and relevant FDA regulations You should address these deficiencies and establish procedures to ensure that any ongoing or future studies will be in compliance with FDA regulations

Within fifteen (15) working days of your receipt of this letter, you should notify this office in writing of the actions you have taken to prevent similar violations in the future Failure to explain the violations noted above adequately and promptly may result in regulatory action without further notice If you believe you have complied with FDA regulations, include your reasoning and any supporting information for our consideration

If you have any questions, please contact Douglas B. Pham, Pharm.D., J.D., at 301-796-1955; FAX 301-847-8748 Your written response and any pertinent documentation should be addressed to:

Douglas B. Pham, Pharm.D., J.D.
Branch Chief (Acting)
Compliance Enforcement Branch
Division of Enforcement and Postmarketing Safety
Office of Scientific Investigations
Office of Compliance
Center for Drug Evaluation and Research
U.S. Food and Drug Administration
Building 51, Room 5348
10903 New Hampshire Avenue
Silver Spring, MD 20993

Sincerely yours,

{See appended electronic signature page}

David C. Burrow, Pharm.D., J.D.
Office Director (Acting)
Office of Scientific Investigations
Office of Compliance
Center for Drug Evaluation and Research

U.S. Food and Drug Administration

This is a representation of an electronic record that was signed electronically and this page is the manifestation of the electronic signature.

/S/

DAVID C BURROW
06/28/2016

1 Subjects with an eGFR <30 mL/min/1.72 m^2 must be excluded from enrollment in the study

2 Initial dose of **(b)(4)** or placebo (taken once daily in morning) is as follows: If eGFR $\geqslant 50$ mL/min/1.73 m^2, determined via the MDRD method, starting dose is 100 mg If eGFR is 30 to <50 mL/min/1.73 m^2, starting dose is 50 mg Subjects with eGFR $<$ 30 mL/min/1.73 m^2 at screening are excluded.

3 Annual Visits occur at Months 12, 24, 36, 48, 60, and 72 Brief Visits occur at Months 18, 30, 42, 54, and 66 Study drug is dispensed via IVRS at Annual and Brief Visits Phone contacts occur at Month 15 and every 6 months thereafter.

第60封　给Jose Giron的警告信

2016年5月19日

参考号：16-HFD-45-05-01

尊敬的Giron博士：

2015年9月1日至10月8日，Brunilda Torres女士代表FDA，在您的临床研究中心，对您实施的下列临床研究进行了审查，这封警告信特告知您现场检查中发现违规情况。

- 试验方案（b）（4），“（b）（4）”，关于试验药物（b）（4），申办者为（b）（4）；
- 试验方案（b）（4），“（b）（4）”，关于试验药物（b）（4），申办者为（b）（4）。

本次现场检查是FDA的生物研究监查项目的一部分。该项目通过设定的检查方法，对FDA所监管的相关研究的实施情况进行评估，以确认研究数据在科学上是有效和准确的，并帮助确保这些研究中的受试者的权益、安全和福利得到了保护。

在现场检查结束时，Torres女士向您出示并与您讨论了FDA483表，即现场检查发现的问题。我们已经收到您2015年10月27日对FDA483表的书面回复，以及您同一日期、提供附加注释的第二封信函。

经对FDA现场检查报告、该报告的附件，以及您2015年10月27日的书面回复、2015年10月27日的附加注释进行审查，我们认为，您没有遵循适用的法律要求和监管临床研究实施的FDA法规。我们想强调以下几点：

您未能确保按照研究计划进行研究［21 CFR 312.60］

作为临床研究者，您必须确保您的临床研究按照研究计划来进行。试验方案（b）（4）的研究计划要求您采集入组受试者的粪便和血液样本用于中心实验室进行评估。此外，试验方案（b）（4）的研究计划要求受试者接受正确剂量的试验药物。您未能遵循这些要求，具体而言：

1. 试验方案（b）（4）要求，最好是输液前，但至少在输液（访视1）72小时内，采集粪便样本用于厌氧菌培养和其他辅助微生物学评估（包括微生物鉴定、产毒菌株分型和抗菌药物敏感性试验），并送往中心实验室。值得注意的是，试验方案（b）（4）规定这个粪便样本是必需的要求。

14名受试者中有13名（即受试者106409，106489，106514，106555，106593，106595，106601，106655，106660，106712，106742，106743和 106801），您未按照要求，将访视1的粪便样本送往中心实验室进行厌氧菌培养评价。

由于您未能遵循试验方案，引起我们对在您的研究中心获取的数据的可靠性的关注。

在检查期间，您表示您想当然地认为，既然所有参与的受试者都有来自本地实验室关于（b）（4）的阳性粪便检查，所以访视1的粪便样本没有采集。但是，与Torres女士一起对试验方案进行回顾后，您同意基线粪便样本是方案必要条件。在2015年10月27日的书面回复中，您表示您知道至少部分粪便样本已经采集，您并没有预料到那些样本竟然没有运送。作为一项预防措施，您表示您正在您的研究中心实施一套体系来确保样本的获取、贮存和运送。此外，您表示您将每周与场所人员召开会议，对任何潜在的研究问题进行回顾，并且“对于将来的任何研究，我们都将竭尽全力遵循规定的程序，并作为一项保证措施，确保这些程序确实被遵循了”。

我们无法对您的书面回复进行全面评估，因为您没有提供一份纠正措施的计划，来说明如果正确地实施，会在将来防止这种类型的违背。具体而言，您并没有提供关于您用来解决检查中发现的、您未能遵循方案规定程序的问题所实施的额外的措施和程序的充足细节。例如，您没有表明是否您和您的员工进行了再培训活动，以防止将来的方案违背。此外，您的书面回复没有提供足够的细节，关于您本人如何确保对研究过程、研究协调员的行动、对您和您的工作人员的培训方案进行充分的监督。没有这些细节，我们无法确定是否您的纠正措施计划足以防止将来发生类似的违规情况。

2. 研究方案（b）（4）要求，下列血液样本要进行采集并送往指定的中心实验室：

- 对（b）（4）的（b）（4）水平的评估，在第1天（访视1）、第4周（访视4）、第12周（访视6），以及任何非计划访视时进行；
- （b）（4）（b）（4）和（b）（4）（b）（4）的药物代谢动力学（PK）评估，在第1天（访视1）（输液前和输液后）、第1周（访视2）、第2周（访视3）、第4周（访视4）、第8周（访视5）、第12周（访视6）进行。
- 抗药抗体（ADA）（包括中和抗体）水平的检测，在第1天（访视1）、第2周（访视3）、第4周（访视4）、第8周（访视5）、第12周（访视6）进行。

您未能遵循这些要求。具体而言，您未能评估内源性（b）（4）和（b）（4）抗体；（b）（4）的药代动力学，或者两者都没有进行；以及下列受试者和研究访视的ADA水平：

a. 受试者106408，您未能向中心实验室提供血液样本进行（b）（4）抗体检测（访视4）；（b）（4）药代动力学评估（访视1输液前和输液后，访视2、3、4、6）和（b）（4）药代动力学评估（访视1输液前和输液后，访视2、3、4、5、6）；ADA水平［访视1（仅（b）（4））、3、4、5和6（两者都有）］。受试者106408于2012年2月21日进行了随机。

b. 受试者106409，您未能向中心实验室提供血液样本进行（b）（4）和（b）（4）抗体检测（访视4）；（b）（4）药代动力学评估（访视1输液前，访视4、5）和（b）（4）药代动力学评估（访视1输液前和输液后，访视3、4、5）；ADA水平［访视3（仅（b）（4））、4和5（两者都有）］。受试者106409于2012年2月27日进行了随机。

c. 受试者106489，您未能向中心实验室提供血液样本进行（b）（4）和（b）（4）抗体检测（访视4）；（b）（4）药代动力学评估（访视1输液后，访视4、6）和（b）（4）药代动力学评估（访视1输液前，访视4、6）；ADA水平（访视1、3、4、6）。受试者106489于2012年3月7日进行了随机。

d. 受试者106514，您未能向中心实验室提供血液样本进行（b）（4）和（b）（4）抗体检测（访视1、4）；（b）（4）药代动力学评估（访视3、4）和（b）（4）药代动力学评估（访视1输液前和输液后，访视2、3、4、5）；ADA水平（访视1、4、5）。受试者106514于2012年3月16日进行了随机。

e. 受试者106555，您未能向中心实验室提供血液样本进行（b）（4）和（b）（4）抗体检测（访视1）；（b）（4）药代动力学评估（访视1输液后、访视3）和（b）（4）药代动力学评估（访视1输液前，访视2、3、5）；ADA水平（访视1、5）。受试者106555于2012年5月19日进行了随机。

f. 受试者106593，您未能向中心实验室提供血液样本进行（b）（4）抗体检测（访视1）和（b）（4）抗体检测（访视1、4）；（b）（4）药代动力学评估（访视1输液前和输液后，访视2、3、4）；ADA水平（访视1、4）。受试者106593于2012年5月23日进行了随机。

g. 受试者106595，您未能向中心实验室提供血液样本进行（b）（4）和（b）（4）抗体检测（访视1、4）；（b）（4）药代动力学评估（访视3、4）和（b）（4）药代动力学评估（访视1输液前和输液后，访视2、3、4、5）；ADA水平（访视1、4、5）。受试者106595于2012年5月30日进行了随机。

h. 受试者106601，您未能向中心实验室提供血液样本进行（b）（4）和（b）（4）抗体检测（访视1、4）；（b）（4）药代动力学评估（访视3、4）和（b）（4）药代动力学评估（访视1输液前和输液后，访视2、3、4、5）；ADA水平［访视1（仅（b）（4））、访视4和5（两者都有）］。受试者106601于2012年6月16日进行了随机。

i. 受试者106655，您未能向中心实验室提供血液样本进行（b）（4）抗体检测（访视4）和（b）（4）抗体检测（访视1、4、6）；（b）（4）药代动力学评估（访视2、3、5）和（b）（4）药代动力学评估（访视1输液前和输液后，访视4、5、6）；ADA水平［访视1（两者都有）、访视4、5和6（仅（b）（4））］。受试者

106655于2012年7月8日进行了随机。

j. 受试者106660，您未能向中心实验室提供血液样本进行（b）（4）抗体检测（访视1、4）和（b）（4）抗体检测（访视1、6）；（b）（4）药代动力学评估（访视4、5）和（b）（4）药代动力学评估（访视1输液前和输液后，访视2、3、4、5、6）；ADA水平［访视1（两者都有）、访视4（仅（b）（4））、访视5和6（两者都有）］。受试者106660于2012年7月22日进行了随机。

k. 受试者106712，您未能向中心实验室提供血液样本进行（b）（4）抗体检测（访视1）；（b）（4）药代动力学评估（访视4）和（b）（4）药代动力学评估（访视1输液前和输液后，访视2、3、4）；ADA水平（访视1、4）。受试者106712于2012年9月4日进行了随机。

l. 受试者106742，您未能向中心实验室提供血液样本进行（b）（4）抗体检测（访视1、4）；（b）（4）药代动力学评估（访视1输液前）和（b）（4）药代动力学评估（访视1输液前和输液后，访视2、3、4）；ADA水平［访视1（仅（b）（4））、访视4（两者都有）］。受试者106742于2012年8月21日进行了随机。

m. 受试者106743，您未能向中心实验室提供血液样本进行（b）（4）抗体检测（访视1）和（b）（4）抗体检测（访视1、4）；（b）（4）药代动力学评估（访视3）和（b）（4）药代动力学评估（访视1输液前和输液后，访视2、3、4、5）；ADA水平［访视1、4、5（仅（b）（4））］。受试者106743于2012年8月27日进行了随机。

n. 受试者106801，您未能向中心实验室提供血液样本进行（b）（4）抗体检测（访视4）；（b）（4）药代动力学评估（访视3、5）和（b）（4）药代动力学评估（访视1输液前和输液后，访视2、4、5）；ADA水平［访视1、4、5（仅（b）（4））］。受试者106801于2012年10月2日进行了随机。

在2015年10月27日对FDA483表的书面回复中，您承认样本缺失了，但是您指出，您在每次访视时都看到受试者，观察到血液样本的采集。您提到，您在研究过程很晚的时候才知道样本的缺失。作为一项预防性措施，您指出，正在您的研究中心实施一套体系来确保样本的获取、贮存和运送。此外，您表示，您将每周与场所人员召开会议，对任何潜在的研究问题进行回顾，并且“对于将来的任何研究，我们都将竭尽全力遵循规定的程序，并作为一项保证措施，确保这些程序确实被遵循了”。

我们无法对您的书面回复进行全面评估，因为您并没有提供一份纠正措施的计划，来说明如果正确地实施，会在将来防止这种类型的违背。具体而言，您并没有提供关于您用来解决检查中发现的、您未能遵循方案规定程序的问题所实施的额外的措施和程序的足够细节。

例如，您没有表明是否您和您的员工进行了再培训活动（例如样本的采集、处理和运送），以防止将来的方案违背。此外，您的书面回复没有提供足够的细节，关于您本人如何确保对研究过程、研究协调员的行动、对您和您的工作人员的培训方案进行充分的监督。结果就是，我们无法确定是否您的纠正措施计划足以防止将来发生类似的违规情况。

3. 试验方案（b）（4）要求，受试者早晨服用（b）（4）400mg（2片），晚上服用（b）（4）400mg（2片），每天服用（b）（4）的总量为800mg。您未能遵循这些方案要求。具体而言，自2013年2月28日（首次用药）开始，受试者557早晨、晚上各给药（b）（4）600mg（3片），每天服用（b）（4）的总量为1200mg。研究记录显示，这起过量用药事件发生在2013年2月28日，2013年3月31日得到解决。

您未能确保受试者得到正确剂量的试验药物的行为，引起我们对来自您研究中心数据可靠性的高度关注。

在2015年10月27日的书面回复中，您指出这起方案违背得到纠正，且报告给申办者，并且“就我所知，没有对受试者造成危害”。

您的回复是不充分的，因为您没有提供预防将来发生类似违背情况的任何纠正措施。

未能遵循研究方案的要求危害了受试者的安全和福利，引起我们对您研究中心数据可靠性的关注。

本警告信的目的并非是罗列您在试验药物临床研究过程中存在的所有缺陷。确保遵循法律和相关FDA法规的每一项要求是您的职责。您应当解决这些缺陷并建立相应规程来确保任何正在进行或将要进行的研究都将符合FDA的法规。

自收到这封信的15个工作日内，您应当书面告知本办公室为预防将来发生类似违规情况而采取的纠正措施。如果不能充分、迅速地解释上述违规问题，可能导致我们在不再通知的情况下采取监管措施。如果您认为已符合了FDA法规要求，请陈述理由，并提供所有相关支持信息，以供我们参考。

附：英文原文

Jose Giron, M.D.

WARNING LETTER

MAY 19, 2016

CERTIFIED MAIL
RETURN RECEIPT REQUESTED

Ref: 16-HFD-45-05-01

Jose Giron, M.D.
4401 S. Orange Avenue, Suite 118
Orlando, Florida 32806

Dear Dr. Giron:

This Warning Letter informs you of objectionable conditions observed during the U.S. Food and Drug Administration (FDA) inspection conducted at your clinical site between September 1, 2015, and October 8, 2015. Ms. Brunilda Torres, representing FDA, reviewed your conduct of the following clinical investigations:

- Protocol **(b)(4)**, "**(b)(4)**," of investigational drug **(b)(4)**, performed for **(b)(4)**
- Protocol **(b)(4)**, "**(b)(4)**," of investigational drug **(b)(4)**, performed for **(b)(4)**

This inspection is a part of FDA's Bioresearch Monitoring Program, which includes inspections designed to evaluate the conduct of FDA-regulated research to ensure that the data are scientifically valid and accurate, and to help ensure that the rights, safety, and welfare of the human subjects of those studies have been protected.

At the conclusion of the inspection, Ms. Torres presented and discussed with you Form FDA 483, Inspectional Observations. We acknowledge receipt of your October 27, 2015, written response to the Form FDA 483, and of your second letter of the same date providing additional comments.

From our review of the FDA Establishment Inspection Report, the documents submitted with that report, your written response dated October 27, 2015, and your additional comments dated October 27, 2015, we conclude that you did not adhere to the applicable statutory requirements and FDA regulations governing the conduct of clinical investigations. We wish to emphasize the following:

You failed to ensure that the investigation was conducted according to the investigational plan [21 CFR 312.60].

As a clinical investigator, you are required to ensure that your clinical studies are conducted in accordance with the investigational plan. The investigational plan for Protocol **(b)(4)** requires that you collect stool and blood samples from enrolled subjects for central laboratory assessment. In addition, the investigational plan for Protocol **(b)(4)** requires that subjects receive the correct dose of investigational drug. You failed to adhere to these requirements. Specifically:

1. Protocol **(b)(4)** required that, optimally before infusion but at least within 72 hours of infusion (Visit 1), a stool sample for anaerobic culture and other ancillary microbiological assessments (including microbial identification, toxigenic strain typing, and antibacterial susceptibility testing) be collected and sent to a central laboratory. Notably,

Protocol **(b)(4)** specified that this stool sample was an absolute requirement.

For 13 out of 14 enrolled subjects (i.e., Subjects 106409, 106489, 106514, 106555, 106593, 106595, 106601, 106655, 106660, 106712, 106742, 106743, and 106801), you failed to send Visit 1 stool samples to the central laboratory for anaerobic culture assessment, as required.

Your failure to follow the protocol raises concerns about the reliability of the data collected at your site.

During the inspection, you indicated you were under the assumption that the Visit 1 stool sample was not required, since all participating subjects had a positive stool test for **(b)(4)** from a local laboratory. However, after reviewing the protocol with Ms. Torres, you agreed that the baseline stool sample was a protocol requirement. In your October 27, 2015, written response, you indicated you knew that at least some stool samples were collected, and that you did not suspect those samples would not be shipped. As a preventive action, you indicated you were implementing a system at your site to verify sample acquisition, storage, and shipment. In addition, you indicated you will have weekly meetings with site staff to go over any potential study issues, and "for any protocols in the future, we will be diligent to follow the procedures as outlined and, as a check, verify that indeed, such procedures are followed."

We are unable to undertake an informed evaluation of your written response because you did not provide a corrective action plan that, if properly carried out, would prevent this type of violation in the future. Specifically, you did not provide sufficient details about your plan for implementing additional measures and procedures to address the inspection findings about your failure to follow protocol procedures. For example, you did not indicate whether you and your staff underwent retraining activities to prevent future protocol violations. In addition, your written response does not provide sufficient details about how you personally will ensure adequate oversight of study procedures, the activities of study coordinators, and protocol training for you and your study staff. Without these details, we are unable to determine whether your corrective action plan is adequate to prevent similar violations in the future.

2. Protocol **(b)(4)** required that the following blood samples be collected and sent to designated central laboratories:

- An assessment of **(b)(4)** levels to **(b)(4)**, performed at Day 1 (Visit 1), Week 4 (Visit 4), Week 12 (Visit 6), and at any unscheduled visits
- A pharmacokinetic (PK) assessment of **(b)(4)** (**(b)(4)**) and **(b)(4)** (**(b)(4)**), performed at Day 1 (Visit 1) (pre- and post-infusion), Week 1 (Visit 2), Week 2 (Visit 3), Week 4 (Visit 4), Week 8 (Visit 5), and Week 12 (Visit 6)
- A test for anti-drug antibody (ADA) (including neutralizing antibody) levels performed at Day 1 (Visit 1), Week 2 (Visit 3), Week 4 (Visit 4), Week 8 (Visit 5), and Week 12 (Visit 6)

You failed to adhere to these requirements. Specifically, you failed to assess endogenous **(b)(4)** and **(b)(4)**antibodies; PKs for **(b)(4)**, or both; and ADA levels for the following subjects and study visits:

a. For Subject 106408, you failed to provide the central laboratory blood samples for **(b)(4)** antibody testing (Visit 4); for PK assessments of **(b)(4)** (Visit 1 pre- and post-infusion, 2, 3, 4, and 6) and of **(b)(4)**(Visit 1 pre- and post-infusion, 2, 3, 4, 5, and 6); and for ADA levels [Visit 1 ((**b)(4)** only), 3, 4, 5, and 6 (both)]. Subject 106408 was randomized on February 21, 2012.

b. For Subject 106409, you failed to provide the central laboratory blood samples for **(b)(4)** and **(b)(4)**antibodies testing (Visit 4); for PK assessments of **(b)(4)** (Visit 1 pre-infusion, 4, and 5) and of **(b)(4)** (Visit 1 pre- and post-infusion, 3, 4, and 5); and for ADA levels [Visit 3 ((**b)(4)** only), 4, and 5 (both)]. Subject 106409 was randomized on February 27, 2012.

c. For Subject 106489, you failed to provide the central laboratory blood samples for **(b)(4)** and **(b)(4)**antibodies testing (Visit 4); for PK assessments of **(b)(4)** (Visit 1 post-infusion, 4, and 6) and of **(b)(4)** (Visit 1 pre-infusion, 4, and 6); and for ADA levels (Visit 1, 3, 4, and 6). Subject 106489 was randomized on March 7, 2012.

d. For Subject 106514, you failed to provide the central laboratory blood samples for **(b)(4)** and **(b)(4)**antibodies testing (Visit 1 and 4); for PK assessments of **(b)(4)** (Visit 3 and 4) and **(b)(4)** (Visit 1 pre- and post-infusion, 2, 3, 4, and 5); and for ADA levels (Visit 1, 4, and 5). Subject 106514 was randomized on May 16, 2012.

e. For Subject 106555, you failed to provide the central laboratory blood samples for **(b)(4)** and **(b)(4)**antibodies testing (Visit 1); for PK assessments of **(b)(4)** (Visit 1 post-infusion and 3) and **(b)(4)** (Visit 1 pre-infusion, 2, 3, and 5); and for ADA levels (Visit 1 and 5). Subject 106555 was randomized on May 19, 2012.

f. For Subject 106593, you failed to provide the central laboratory blood samples for **(b)(4)** antibody testing (Visit 1) and **(b)(4)** antibody testing (Visit 1 and 4); for PK assessments of **(b)(4)** (Visit 1 pre- and post-infusion, 2, 3, and 4);

and for ADA levels (Visit 1 and 4). Subject 106593 was randomized on May 23, 2102.

g. For Subject 106595, you failed to provide the central laboratory blood samples for **(b)(4)** and **(b)(4)**antibodies testing (Visit 1 and 4); for PK assessment of **(b)(4)** (Visit 3 and 4) and **(b)(4)** (Visit 1 pre- and post-infusion, 2, 3, 4, and 5); and for ADA levels (Visit 1, 4, and 5). Subject 106595 was randomized on May 30, 2102.

h. For Subject 106601, you failed to provide the central laboratory blood samples for **(b)(4)** and **(b)(4)**antibodies testing (Visit 1 and 4); for PK assessments of **(b)(4)** (Visit 3 and 4) and **(b)(4)** (Visit 1 pre- and post-infusion, 2, 3, 4, and 5); and for ADA levels [Visit 1 (**(b)(4)** only), 4, and 5 (both)]. Subject 106601 was randomized on June 16, 2012.

i.For Subject 106655, you failed to provide the central laboratory blood samples for **(b)(4)** antibody testing (Visit 4) and **(b)(4)** antibody testing (Visit 1, 4, and 6); for PK assessments of **(b)(4)** (Visit 2, 3, and 5) and **(b)(4)** (Visit 1 pre- and post-infusion 4, 5, and 6); and for ADA levels [Visit 1 (both) and Visit 4, 5, and 6 (**(b)(4)** only)]. Subject 106655 was randomized on July 8, 2012.

j. For Subject 106660, you failed to provide the central laboratory blood samples for **(b)(4)** antibody testing (Visit 1 and 4) and **(b)(4)** antibody testing (Visit 1 and 6); for PK assessments of **(b)(4)** (Visit 4 and 5) and **(b)(4)** (Visit 1 pre- and post-infusion, 2, 3, 4, 5, and 6); and for ADA levels [Visit 1 (both), 4 (**(b)(4)**only), 5, and 6 (both)]. Subject 106660 was randomized on July 22, 2012.

k. For Subject 106712, you failed to provide the central laboratory blood samples for **(b)(4)** antibody testing (Visit 1); for PK assessments of **(b)(4)** (Visit 4) and **(b)(4)** (Visit 1 pre- and post-infusion, 2, 3, and 4); and for ADA levels (Visit 1 and 4). Subject 106712 was randomized on September 4, 2012.

l. For Subject 106742, you failed to provide the central laboratory blood samples for **(b)(4)** antibody testing (Visit 1 and 4); for PK assessments of **(b)(4)** (Visit 1 pre-infusion) and **(b)(4)** (Visit 1 pre- and post-infusion, 2, 3, and 4); and for ADA levels [Visit 1 (**(b)(4)** only) and 4 (both)]. Subject 106742 was randomized on August 21, 2012.

m. For Subject 106743, you failed to provide the central laboratory blood samples for **(b)(4)** antibody testing (Visit 1) and **(b)(4)** antibody testing (Visit 1 and 4); for PK assessments of **(b)(4)** (Visit 3) and **(b)(4)**(Visit 1 pre- and post-infusion, 2, 3, 4, and 5); and for ADA levels [Visit 1, 4, and 5 (**(b)(4)** only)]. Subject 106743 was randomized on August 27, 2012.

n. For Subject 106801, you failed to provide the central laboratory blood samples for **(b)(4)** antibody testing (Visit 4); for PK assessments of **(b)(4)** (Visit 3 and 5) and **(b)(4)** (Visit 1 pre- and post-infusion, 2, 4, and 5); and for ADA levels [Visit 1, 4, and 5 (**(b)(4)** only)]. Subject 106801 was randomized on October 2, 2012.

In your October 27, 2015, written response to the Form FDA 483, you acknowledged the missing blood samples, but you also indicated that you saw subjects at every visit, and that you observed the collection of blood samples. You noted that you learned of the missing samples much later in the course of the study. As a preventive action, you indicated that you were implementing a system at your site to verify sample acquisition, storage, and shipment. In addition, you indicated you will have weekly meetings with site staff to go over any potential study issues, and "for any protocols in the future, we will be diligent to follow the procedures as outlined and, as a check, verify that indeed, such procedures are followed."

We are unable to undertake an informed evaluation of your written response because you did not provide a corrective action plan that, if properly carried out, would prevent this type of violation in the future. Specifically, you did not provide sufficient details about your plan for implementing additional measures and procedures to address the inspection findings about your failure to follow protocol procedures.

For example, you did not indicate whether you and your staff underwent retraining activities (such as sample collection, handling, and shipment) to prevent future protocol violations. In addition, your written response does not provide sufficient details on how you personally will ensure adequate oversight of study procedures, the activities of study coordinators, and protocol training for you and your study staff. As a result, we are unable to determine whether your corrective action plan is adequate to prevent similar violations in the future.

3. Protocol **(b)(4)** requires that subjects take **(b)(4)** 400 mg (2 tablets) in the morning and 400 mg (2 tablets) in the evening, for a total of 800 mg of **(b)(4)** per day. You failed to adhere to these protocol requirements. Specifically, starting on February 28, 2013 (first dose), Subject 557 was dosed with 600 mg of **(b)(4)** (3 tablets) in the morning and the evening, for a total of 1200 mg of **(b)(4)** per day. Study records indicate that this overdose event occurred on February 28, 2013, and was resolved on March 31, 2013.

Your failure to ensure that subjects received the correct doses of investigational drug raises significant concerns about the reliability of the data from your site.

In your October 27, 2015, written response, you indicated that this violation was corrected and reported to the sponsor, and "to the best of my knowledge, no harm has come to" the subject.

Your response is inadequate because you did not provide any corrective actions to prevent similar violations in the future.

Failure to follow the protocol requirements jeopardizes subject safety and welfare, and raises concerns about the reliability of the data collected at your site.

This letter is not intended to be an all-inclusive list of deficiencies with your clinical study of an investigational drug. It is your responsibility to ensure adherence to each requirement of the law and relevant FDA regulations. You should address these deficiencies and establish procedures to ensure that any ongoing or future studies will comply with FDA regulations.

Within fifteen (15) working days of your receipt of this letter, you should notify this office in writing of the actions you have taken to prevent similar violations in the future. Failure to address the violations noted above adequately and promptly may result in regulatory action without further notice. If you believe you have complied with FDA regulations, include your reasoning and any supporting information for our consideration.

If you have any questions, please contact Douglas B. Pham, Pharm.D., J.D., at 301-796-1955; FAX 301-847-8748. Your written response and any pertinent documentation should be addressed to:

Douglas Pham, Pharm.D., J.D.
Branch Chief (Acting)
Compliance Enforcement Branch
Division of Enforcement and Postmarketing Safety
Office of Scientific Investigations
Office of Compliance
Center for Drug Evaluation and Research
U.S. Food and Drug Administration
Building 51, Room 5348
10903 New Hampshire Avenue
Silver Spring, MD 20993

Sincerely yours,

{See appended electronic signature page}

David C. Burrow, Pharm.D., J.D.
Acting Office Director
Office of Scientific Investigations
Office of Compliance
U.S. Food and Drug Administration

This is a representation of an electronic record that was signed electronically and this page is the manifestation of the electronic signature.

/S/

DAVID C BURROW
05/19/2016

第61封　给Benedict S. Liao医学博士的警告信

2016年3月29日

参考号：16-HFD-45-03-03

尊敬的Liao博士：

2015年8月11日和9月29日，Uttaniti Limchumroon先生、Greg K. Keshishyan先生与Quynh-Van Tran女士代表FDA，在贵临床研究场所，对您所开展的试验药物（b）（4）[1]临床研究“（b）（4）”，申办者为（b）（4）进行了审查。这封警告信特告知您现场检查中发现的违规情况。

本次现场检查是FDA的生物研究监查项目的一部分。该项目通过设定的检查方法，对FDA监管的相关研究的实施情况进行评估，以确保研究数据在科学上是有效和准确的，并确保这些研究中受试者的权益、安全和福利得到了保护。

在现场检查结束时，Limchumroon先生与Keshishyan先生向您出示了FDA483表，即现场检查发现的问题，并与您进行了讨论。您2015年10月6日对FDA483表的书面回复已收悉。

经对现场检查报告、该报告的附件，以及您2015年10月6日的书面回复进行审查，我们认为，您没有遵循适用的法律要求和监管临床研究实施及受试者保护的FDA法规。我们想特强调以下几点：

1. 您未能确保按照研究计划进行研究［21 CFR 312.60］

作为临床试验研究者，您必须确保临床研究按照研究计划［21 CFR 312.60］进行。该研究计划要求受试者有1～15个可测量的肿瘤（即大小介于0.2～10 cm），以便符合研究与实验室检查的条件，每四周进行1次实验室检查包括促甲状腺激素（TSH）和甲胎蛋白（AFP）检测，以及每3个月做一次计算机断层扫描（CT）与/或正电子发射断层扫描（PET）。您未能遵循这些试验方案要求，具体而言：

a. 您未能遵守试验方案中受试者入组标准。受试者L-36入组时，在基线上没有可测量的肿瘤。尽管没有满足试验方案要求，但该受试者仍于2014年7月22日接受了试验药物。

b. 您没有在要求的时间间隔内（即每4周）对标注时间段的下述受试者的TSH和AFP进行实验室检查。

i. 2014年5月3日至2014年11月15日，您未对受试者L-10进行任何所要求的TSH与AFP实验室检查。

ii. 2014年5月3日至2014年12月17日，您未对受试者L-20进行任何所要求的TSH与AFP实验室检查。

iii. 2014年5月7日至2014年12月3日，您未对受试者L-21进行任何所要求的TSH与AFP实验室检查。

iv. 2014年5月6日至2015年1月28日，您未对受试者L-35进行任何所要求的TSH与AFP实验室检查。

v. 2014年5月29日至2015年12月12日，您未对受试者H-67进行任何所要求的TSH与AFP实验室检查。

我们承认在上述第1条a项（受试者L-36）的调查结果与第1条b项（受试者L-10，L-20，L-21，L-35以及H-67）AFP调查结果未包含在出具给您的FDA 483表中，因此，您的书面回复中未触及这些调查结果。

c. 2014年7月8日至2015年2月17日，您未能在规定的时间间隔内（即每3个月）对受试者L-36进行CT和/或PET扫描。

您2015年10月6日对FDA 483表的书面回复中，指出因试验药物（b）（4）是非毒性的，故认为并无严格遵守试验方案的必要。此外，您称一些受试者不遵守试验方案说明进行实验室检查和CT扫描。您还表明，对于未患甲状腺癌的受试者，没有必要进行TSH评估；且对于全部受试者，均采用了适当的癌症标志物予以替代［如对前列腺癌受试者检测前列腺特异性抗原（PSA）］。您还称，部分受试者每4个月做CT扫描而非每

---

1 (b) (4) 涉及商业秘密，根据法规内容不予公开。

3个月，且部分受试者在后续测试中除了接受骨盆和直肠超声检查外，还接受了阴道镜检查，而非（方案中写明的）CT扫描、PET扫描或者两者均进行。

您的书面回复并不充分，因为即便假定试验药物及研究受试者声称的应答是安全的，您也必须遵守方案要求的评估。尽管您以癌症特异性血液标志物来随访受试者，但方案要求所有受试者均需进行下述的实验室检查：全血细胞计数、Chemistry-7、Chemistry-24、肝肾功能、癌胚抗原、癌抗原125、癌抗原153、癌抗原199、TSH、AFP和“其他肿瘤标志物”。此外，您没有提供预防将来类似违规事项再次发生的纠正措施计划。

您未能实施方案要求的实验室检查和扫描，损害了受试者的安全与福利，影响了在贵试验场所收集数据的有效性与完整性。

2. 您未能保存对试验中使用试验药物或对照组的受试者的所有研究观察结果和其他相关数据的足够及准确的病历［21 CFR 312.62（b）］

作为临床研究者，您必须准备和保存对研究中使用试验药物的受试者或对照受试者的所有研究观察结果和其他相关数据足够和准确的病历。病历中包括证明受试者符合方案所规定的入排标准的记录。您未能保存包括这些记录的足够和准确的病历。具体而言：

a. 您未能保存好证明受试者L-10、L-21、L-26与 L-36在研究入组前接受传统放疗和/或化疗两种疗法失败，从而满足试验方案入组标准的研究记录。

在您2015年10月6日对FDA 483表的书面回复中，您指出以下几点：

- 受试者L-10 与 L-26接受了6个疗程的卡铂/紫杉醇。
- 受试者L-21自2012年8月至2013年2月，每3～4周在其他医院接受盐酸阿霉素、博莱霉素、硫酸长春碱以及达卡巴嗪（ABVD）的治疗，且您已获取这些记录。
- 受试者L-36接受了6个疗程的丝裂霉素/紫杉醇®。

您没能提交上述受试者先前接受化疗的记录，故我们无法对该答复进行合理的评价。未能保存对上述入组标准的研究记录，极大地影响了在贵试验现场所收集数据的有效性与完整性；缺少这些研究记录，我们无法确认这些受试者是否符合研究入组标准。此外，您未能提供预防类似违规事项再次发生的纠正措施计划。

b. 您没能保存表明受试者L-3，L-10，L-20，L-21，L-35和H-67符合方案所规定的下述实验室入组标准的研究记录。

- 入组标准：血小板计数高于100 000/mL，血红蛋白高于9.0 g/dL且无“明显的肝和/或肾功能异常”。
- 排除标准：血红蛋白低于9.0 g/dL，白细胞计数低于4000/μL，血小板计数低于100 000/mL，国际标准化比值大于1.5。

在您2015年10月6日对FDA 483表的书面回复中，您指出以下几点：

- 受试者L-3的实验室检查是在附属设施中进行的。您试图收集实验室报告，但或许文件放错了地方（而丢失）。
- 受试者L-10, L-20以及H-67的实验室检查是在贵诊所和/或附属设施中进行的。您试图收集实验室报告，但或许错放了文件位置（而丢失）。
- 您或许放错了受试者L-21的实验室报告，故试图找到它们并放入该受试者的记录档案中。
- 您有受试者L-35的部分实验室报告，并试图补上遗漏的部分。

您没能提交任何维护贵试验现场的实验室报告，故我们无法对您的回复进行合理的评价。此外，您未能提供预防类似违规事项再次发生的纠正措施计划。

您未能保存充足和准确的病史，损害了受试者的安全与福利，影响了在贵试验场所所采集数据的有效性与完整性。

3. 您未能保存足够的包括日期、数量以及受试者使用情况的药物处置记录［21 CFR 312.62（a）］

作为临床试验研究者，必须保存足够的包括日期、数量以及受试者的使用情况的药物处置记录。您未能遵守这一要求。具体来说，对于在贵研究中心入组该研究并接受小剂量与/或大剂量（b）（4）的所有受试者，您没有保存任何药物处置记录。

在您2015年10月6日对FDA 483表的书面回复中，您表明在“一般病史与体格检查概要表”中提供了治疗计划，给予每位受试者试验药物的剂量和数量以及研究的访视频次。您还提供了发放给受试者的药片数与瓶数的总量及剩余在库房中余量的计算方法，以及表明受试者计划治疗的组别及特定时间段内预计的药片数量的记录。

您未能提交表明实际给予每位受试者的及退回的药片数量的证明文件、相应的日期和剂量规格。因此，我们无法对该回复进行合理的评价。此外，您未能提供预防将来类似违规事项再次发生的纠正措施计划。

您未能保存充足和准确的药物责任记录，影响了贵试验场所数据的有效性和完整性。

本警告信的目的并非是罗列您在试验药物临床研究中存在的所有缺陷。确保遵循法律和FDA相关法规的每一项要求是您的职责，您应当解决这些缺陷，并建立规程，以确保任何正在进行或将来进行的研究均符合FDA法规。

自收到这封信的15个工作日内，您应当书面告知本办公室为预防将来发生类似违规情况而采取的措施。如果不能充分、迅速地解释上述违规问题，可能导致我们在不再通知的情况下采取监管措施。如果您认为您已经遵守了FDA法规的要求，请陈述理由，并提供所有支持资料，供我们参考。

附：英文原文

Benedict S. Liao, M.D.

WARNING LETTER

MAR 29, 2016

CERTIFIED MAIL
RETURN RECEIPT REQUESTED

Ref: 16-HFD-45-03-03

Benedict S. Liao, M.D.
3106 East Garvey Avenue South
West Covina, California 91791-2344

Dear Dr. Liao:

This Warning Letter informs you of objectionable conditions observed during the U.S. Food and Drug Administration (FDA) inspection conducted at your clinical site between August 11 and September 29, 2015. Mr. Uttaniti Limchumroon, Mr. Greg K. Keshishyan, and Ms. Quynh-Van Tran, representing FDA, reviewed your conduct of a clinical investigation (“**(b)(4)**”) for the investigational drug **(b)(4)**, performed for **(b)(4)**.

This inspection is a part of FDA’s Bioresearch Monitoring Program, which includes inspections designed to evaluate the conduct of FDA-regulated research to ensure that the data are scientifically valid and accurate, and to help ensure that the rights, safety, and welfare of the human subjects of those studies have been protected.

At the conclusion of the inspection, Mr. Limchumroon and Mr. Keshishyan presented and discussed with you Form FDA 483, Inspectional Observations. We acknowledge receipt of your October 6, 2015 written response to the Form FDA 483.

From our review of the FDA Establishment Inspection Report, the documents submitted with that report, and your

October 6, 2015, written response, we conclude that you did not adhere to the applicable statutory requirements and FDA regulations governing the conduct of clinical investigations and the protection of human subjects. We wish to emphasize the following:

1. You failed to ensure that the investigation was conducted according to the investigational plan [21 CFR 312.60].

As a clinical investigator, you are required to ensure that your clinical studies are conducted in accordance with the investigational plan. The investigational plan requires that subjects have between 1 and 15 measurable tumor(s) (i.e., between 0.2-10 cm in size) in order to be eligible for the study, and that laboratory tests, including thyroid stimulating hormone (TSH) and alpha-fetoprotein (AFP), be conducted every four weeks, and computed tomography (CT) and/or positron emission tomography (PET) scans be conducted every three months. You failed to adhere to these protocol requirements. Specifically:

a. You failed to follow the protocol for subject eligibility when you enrolled Subject L-36, who did not have a measurable tumor at baseline. Subject L-36 received investigational drug on July 22, 2014, even though the subject did not meet this protocol requirement.

b. You failed to conduct TSH and AFP laboratory tests at required time intervals (i.e., every 4 weeks) for the following subjects during the noted time periods:

i. Between May 3, 2014, and November 15, 2014, you failed to conduct any required TSH and AFP laboratory tests for Subject L-10.

ii. Between May 3, 2014, and December 17, 2014, you failed to conduct any required TSH and AFP laboratory tests for Subject L-20.

iii. Between May 7, 2014, and December 3, 2014, you failed to conduct any required TSH and AFP laboratory tests for Subject L-21.

iv. Between May 6, 2014, and January 28, 2015, you failed to conduct any required TSH and AFP laboratory tests for Subject L-35.

v. Between May 29, 2014, and December 12, 2014, you failed to conduct any required TSH and AFP laboratory tests for Subject H-67.

We acknowledge that the finding noted in Item 1.a. above (Subject L-36) and the AFP findings in Item 1.b. above (Subjects L-10, L-20, L-21, L-35, and H-67) were not included on the Form FDA 483 you received, and that therefore, your written response does not address these findings.

c. Between July 8, 2014, and February 17, 2015, you failed to conduct a CT and/or PET scan at any of the required time intervals (i.e., every 3 months) for Subject L-36.

In your October 6, 2015, written response to the Form FDA 483, you indicated that because **(b)(4)** is nontoxic, you did not see the need to follow the protocol strictly. In addition, you stated that some subjects were noncompliant with the protocol instructions to have laboratory tests and CT scans performed. You also indicated that for subjects who did not have thyroid carcinoma, TSH assessment was unnecessary; and that for all subjects, appropriate cancer markers were used instead [e.g., prostate-specific antigen (PSA) for subjects with prostate cancer]. You also stated that some subjects had CT scans every 4 months instead of every 3 months, and some subjects were followed by vaginal colposcopy in addition to pelvic and rectal ultrasound examinations, rather than by CT scan, PET scan, or both.

Your written response is inadequate because you must adhere to protocol-required assessments despite the presumed safety of the investigational drug, and study subjects' purported responses to it. Although you followed subjects with cancer-specific blood markers, the protocol requires all subjects to undergo the following laboratory tests: complete blood count,chemistry-7, chemistry-24, liver and renal function, carcinoembryonic antigen, cancer antigen 125, cancer antigen 153, cancer antigen 199, TSH, AFP, "and other tumor markers." Further, you have not provided a corrective action plan to prevent the recurrence of similar violations in the future.

Your failure to perform protocol-required laboratory tests and scans jeopardizes subject safety and welfare, and compromises the validity and integrity of the data collected at your site.

2. You failed to maintain adequate and accurate case histories that record all observations and other data pertinent to the investigation on each individual administered the investigational drug or employed as a control in the investigation [21 CFR 312.62(b)].

As a clinical investigator, you are required to prepare and maintain adequate and accurate case histories that record all observations and other data pertinent to the investigation on each individual administered the investigational drug or employed as a control in the investigation. Case histories include records demonstrating that subjects met protocol-specified inclusion and exclusion criteria. You failed to maintain adequate and accurate case histories that included these records. Specifically:

a. You failed to maintain study records demonstrating that Subjects L-10, L-21, L-26, and L-36 met the protocol-specified inclusion criterion of failure to be helped by two separate regimens of conventional radiation therapy and/or chemotherapy before study enrollment.

In your October 6, 2015, written response to the Form FDA 483, you indicated the following:

- Subjects L-10 and L-26 received 6 courses of carboplatin/Taxol®.
- Subject L-21 received the doxorubicin hydrochloride/Adriamycin®, bleomycin, vinblastine sulfate, and dacarbazine (ABVD) regimen every 3 to 4 weeks from August 2012 through February 2013 at other hospitals, and you obtained those records.
- Subject L-36 received 6 courses of mitomycin/Taxol®.

We are unable to perform an informed evaluation of your response because you did not submit documentation of these subjects' prior courses of chemotherapy. Failure to maintain study records for the above-mentioned inclusion criterion compromises significantly the validity and integrity of data collected at your site; without these study records, we cannot confirm these subjects' eligibility for enrollment in the study. In addition, you have not provided a corrective action plan to prevent the recurrence of similar violations in the future.

b. You failed to maintain study records demonstrating that Subjects L-3, L-10, L-20, L-21, L-35, and H-67 met the following protocol-specified laboratory eligibility criteria:

- Inclusion criteria of platelet count greater than 100,000/mL, hemoglobin greater than 9.0 g/dL, and no "significant abnormal hepatic and/or renal function."
- Exclusion criteria of hemoglobin less than 9.0 g/dL and white blood cell count less than 4.0 k/μL, platelet count less than 100,000/μL, and international normalized ratio greater than 1.5.

In your October 6, 2015 written response to the Form FDA 483, you indicated the following:

- Laboratory tests for Subject L-3 were performed at affiliated facilities. You tried to collect the laboratory reports but may have misplaced them.
- Laboratory tests for Subjects L-10, L-20, and H-67 were performed by your clinic and/or affiliated facilities. You tried to collect the laboratory reports but may have misplaced them.
- You may have misplaced some of the laboratory reports for Subject L-21, so you tried to recover them and place them in the subject's record.
- You had some of the laboratory reports for Subject L-35 and tried to obtain the missing ones.

We are unable to perform an informed evaluation of your response because you did not submit any laboratory reports maintained at your site. In addition, you have not provided a corrective action plan to prevent the recurrence of similar violations in the future.

Your failure to maintain adequate and accurate case histories jeopardizes subject safety and welfare, and compromises the validity and integrity of data captured at your site.

3. You failed to maintain adequate records of the disposition of the drug, including dates, quantity, and use by subjects [21 CFR 312.62(a)].

As a clinical investigator, you are required to maintain adequate records of the disposition of the drug, including dates, quantity, and use by subjects. You failed to comply with this requirement. Specifically, for all subjects at your site who enrolled in the study and received low-dose and/or high-dose **(b)(4)**, you failed to maintain any drug disposition records.

In your October 6, 2015, written response to the Form FDA 483, you indicated that you have General History and Physical Examination Summary Forms that provide treatment planning, the study-drug dose and quantity to be given to each subject, and study-visit frequency. You also provided calculations of the overall number of tablets and bottles given to subjects and remaining in the warehouse, and you provided records stating subjects' planned treatment groups and projected number of tablets over certain time periods.

We are unable to perform an informed evaluation of your response because you did not submit documentation showing how many tablets were actually given to and returned by each subject, with corresponding dates and dosage strengths. In addition, you have not provided a corrective action plan to prevent the recurrence of similar violations in the future.

Your failure to maintain adequate and accurate drug accountability records compromises the validity and integrity of the data at your site.

This letter is not intended to be an all-inclusive list of deficiencies with your clinical study of an investigational drug. It is your responsibility to ensure adherence to each requirement of the law and relevant FDA regulations. You should address these deficiencies and establish procedures to ensure that any ongoing or future studies will be in compliance with FDA regulations.

Within fifteen (15) working days of your receipt of this letter, you should notify this office in writing of the actions you have taken to prevent similar violations in the future. Failure to explain the violations noted above adequately and promptly may result in regulatory action without further notice. If you believe that you have complied with FDA regulations, include your reasoning and any supporting information for our consideration.

If you have any questions, please contact Douglas B. Pham, Pharm.D., J.D., at 301-796-1955; FAX 301-847-8748. Your written response and any pertinent documentation should be addressed to:

Douglas B. Pham, Pharm.D., J.D.
Branch Chief (Acting)
Compliance Enforcement Branch
Division of Enforcement and Postmarketing Safety
Office of Scientific Investigations
Office of Compliance
Center for Drug Evaluation and Research
U.S. Food and Drug Administration
Building 51, Room 5348
10903 New Hampshire Avenue
Silver Spring, MD 20993

Sincerely yours,

{See appended electronic signature page}

David C. Burrow, Pharm.D., J.D.
Office Director (Acting)
Office of Scientific Investigations
Office of Compliance
Center for Drug Evaluation and Research
U.S. Food and Drug Administration

This is a representation of an electronic record that was signed electronically and this page is the manifestation of the electronic signature.

/S/

DAVID C BURROW
03/29/2016

第62封　给Cheta Nand医学博士的警告信

2016年3月10日

参考号：16-HFD-45-03-01

尊敬的Nand博士：

2015年10月6日至10月30日，Tracy K. Li 女士与Sherri N. Rohlf女士代表FDA，在您的临床研究机构，对您所开展的以下临床研究：试验方案（b）(4)，试验药物的（b）(4)“（b）(4)”，（b）(4）试验，进行了审查。这封警告信特告知您现场检查中发现的违规情况。

本次现场检查是FDA的生物研究监查项目一部分。该项目通过设定的检查方法，对由FDA监管的相关研究的实施情况进行评估，以确认研究数据在科学上是有效和准确的，并帮助确保这些研究中受试者的权益、安全和福利得到了保护。

在现场检查结束时，Li女士与Rohlf女士向您出示了FDA483表，即现场检查发现的问题，并与您进行了讨论。您2015年11月19日和2015年12月18日对该FDA483表的书面回复已收悉。

经对现场检查报告、该报告的附件，以及您2015年11月19日与2015年12月18日的书面回复进行审查，我们认为，您没有遵循适用的法律要求和监管临床研究实施的FDA法规。我们想强调以下几点：

您未能确保按照研究计划研究进行［21 CFR 312.60］

作为临床研究者，必须确保临床研究按照研究计划进行。试验方案（b）(4）的研究计划要求您确保研究受试者在入组前满足试验方案的入组排除标准。您未能遵循该要求，具体而言：

1. 试验方案（b）(4）规定，受试者将接受阿托伐他汀、辛伐他汀或瑞舒伐他汀的治疗，且阿托伐他汀的剂量不得低于20mg，辛伐他汀的剂量不得低于20mg，瑞舒伐他汀的剂量不得低于40mg。方案中还规定所有受试者在筛选前，稳定维持剂量至少达6周。

您未能遵守研究计划，如您于2014年7月31日、2014年9月3日和2014年9月15日分别随机入组了受试者1004，1023与1037，尽管这几位受试者所接受的瑞舒伐他汀剂量低于40mg。在筛选检查前至少六周内，受试者1004，1023，1037每日服用20mg维持剂量的瑞舒伐他汀。

在2015年10月6日对FDA 483表的书面回复中，您承认受试者1004，1023与1037瑞舒伐他汀的所服剂量为20mg，且被错误地随机入组研究。您表示，作为纠正和预防措施计划中的一部分，在您的带领下，研究人员将完成有关NIH和GCP的继续教育培训。您同样提到，将对该研究记录进行两步核校程序，以监控其完整性、质量与准确性。

我们无法对您的书面回复进行合理的评价，因为您没能提供如果正确执行可防止此类违规再次发生的纠正措施计划。具体来说，您既没有提供任何防止未来同类违规事项再次发生的纠正措施计划的细节或说明，又没有提供实施追加措施和程序解决现场检查中发现的未能保证入组受试者合格的计划细节。

2. 试验方案（b）(4）规定，筛查时肌酸激酶（CK）值＞正常值上限（ULN）3倍的受试者不得入组该临床研究。然而，方案同时允许＞3倍ULN值（的受试者）在筛选期间可以进行再次检测。若重测结果＜3倍ULN值，受试者是符合入组条件的。

试验方案（b）(4）也规定，如果在筛选检查后的任何研究访视中，发现受试者有原因不明的CK值＞5倍ULN的情况，那么该受试者必须重新检测CK，最好在研究者获知结果的48小时内。若复测结果确认了升高的CK值，未伴随有肌肉痛、肌肉压痛和/或肌无力，或新发的肾功能不全，如果申办者的医学监护获得批准，受试者可以继续接受试验药物。

a. 您未能遵循研究计划。2014年8月22日随机入组的受试者1014，2014年8月4日筛查时的CK值为1074 U/L，即>3倍ULN（198U/L）。2014年8月6日，您草签了实验室报告，并在其中注明“↑CK不明显——或许是临床诊断上的实验室值，而非通过观察患者得出”。无论您的临床评价如何，该方案要求您或是重新检测CK值（您未做过），或是按照排除标准，不让该受试者入组。

b. 您未能遵守研究计划。受试者1041没有进行最好在48小时内的CK重新检测，尽管在随机化访视时其有原因不明的（即没有暂时与之关联的近期外伤、肌内注射、剧烈运动或繁重的体力活动）高于ULN 5倍的CK值（2014年8月22日检测值为992U/L）。

c. 您未能遵守研究计划。受试者1014没有进行最好在48小时内的CK重新检测，尽管第11次访视/365天时其有原因不明>5倍ULN的CK值（2015年9月10日，3168U/L）。我们确认，您于2015年9月18日手写注明，您曾致电受试者预定复测日期，但因受试者工作无法安排复测计划。

在您2015年11月19日对FDA 483表的书面回复中表明，您认为受试者1014升高的CK值无临床意义，因为受试者非常活跃，定期做举重训练，未表现出任何临床症状。您批注，您的研究协调员曾收到一位研究监查员的口头确认，说根据您对受试者1014升高的CK值无临床意义的判断，该受试者符合随机入组研究的条件。

此外，您表示作为纠正和预防措施计划的一部分，在您的带领下，您的研究人员将完成NIH与GCP的继续教育培训。您注明研究记录将经过两步核校程序，以监督其完整性、质量与准确性。您还表明与研究监查员的口头对话将以邮件的方式跟进，以便口头对话以文件形式存档。

我们无法对您的书面回复进行合理的评价，因为您没能提供一份正确实施可防止未来此类违规再次发生的预防纠正措施计划。具体来说，您既没能提供任何防止未来同类违规事项再次发生的纠正措施计划细节或说明，也没有提供实施追加措施和程序解决现场检查中发现的未能保证入组受试者合格的计划细节。

3. 试验方案（b）（4）规定，受试者在随机入组7日内（±3日）的第二次筛查访视时，空腹甘油三酯（TG）值必须≤400mg/dL。

a. 您未能遵守研究方案。受试者1005于2014年7月31日随机入组，尽管该受试者于2014年7月24日的第二次筛选访视时，TG值为456mg/dL，超出了合格受试者空腹TG值标准。

b. 您未能遵守研究方案。受试者1006于2014年8月4日随即入组，尽管该受试者于2014年7月28日的第二次筛选访视时，TG值为701mg/dL，超出了合格受试者空腹TG值标准。

2015年11月19日在对FDA 483表的书面回复中，您承认，TG值超出入组标准的受试者1005与1006随机进入研究。您注明，贵方的研究协调员曾收到一位研究监查员允许受试者1005和1006继续参与研究的口头确认。您表示，那位研究协调员已经就遵守入/排标准及可接受的报告期限，接受了再培训。您还称，作为纠正和预防措施计划中的一部分，在您的带领下，研究人员将完成NIH和GCP的继续教育培训。您注明研究记录将经过两步核校程序，以监督其完整性、质量与准确性。您还表明，与研究监查员的口头对话，将进一步以邮件的方式进行跟进，以便口头对话以文件形式存档。

我们无法对您的书面回复进行合理的评价，因为您没能提供一份正确实施可防止未来此类违规再次发生的纠正措施计划。具体来说，您既没能提供任何防止未来同类违规事项再次发生的纠正措施计划细节或说明，也没有提供实施追加措施和程序解决检查中发现的未能保证入组合格受试者的计划的细节。

4. 试验方案（b）（4）规定，乙肝表面抗原（HBsAg）、乙肝核心抗体（HBcAb）检测阳性的受试者，或者丙型肝炎抗体显示，目前或先前受到感染的受试者不得入组本临床研究。然而，方案允许HBsAg检测阴性而乙型肝炎表面抗原抗体呈阳性的HBcAb阳性受试者入组。

您未能遵守研究计划。受试者1014于2014年8月12日随机入组，尽管该受试者在筛查时HBcAb检测呈阳性，HBsAg检测呈阴性，乙型肝炎表面抗原抗体呈阴性。

2015年11月19日在对FDA 483表的书面回复中，您承认，基于受试者1007 HBcAb检测呈阳性，让该受试者入组研究是错误的。回复指出，您在获知该受试者不符标准后，研究协调员将这次方案违背报告了IRB，并试图联系该受试者回收所有研究药物。您表明，研究场所的所有员工均就密切监测实验室结果和遵守所有入排标准的重要性接受了再培训。您称，作为纠正和预防措施计划中的一部分，在您的带领下，研究人员将完成有关NIH与GCP的继续教育培训。您注明研究记录将经过两步核校程序以监测其完整性、质量与准确性。您还表明与研究监查员的口头对话将以邮件的方式跟进，以便以文件方式将口头对话存档。

我们无法对您的书面回复进行合理的评价，因为您没能提供一份正确实施可防止未来此类违规再次发生的纠正措施计划。具体来说，您既没能提供任何防止未来此类违规事项再次发生的纠正措施计划细节或说明，也没有提供实施追加措施和程序解决检查中发现的有关不合格受试者入组的计划的细节。

5. 试验方案（b）（4）规定，在两次筛选访视中，已知有（b）（4）等同状况的服用最高批准剂量的受试者空腹低密度脂蛋白胆固醇（LDL-C）值≥70mg/dL（1.81mmol/L），且第二次筛选访视（在随机后7日内，±3日）的检测值不得低于或高于其起始空腹LDL-C值的20%。

您未能遵守研究计划。受试者1026于2014年9月19日随即入组，尽管该受试者在2014年9月12日的第二次筛查访视时的LDL-C值为125mg/dL，高于其起始LDL-C值的20%（2014年9月5日检测值为97mg/dL）。

2015年11月19日在对FDA 483表的书面回复中，您承认受试者1026 LDL水平升高。回复指出您对试验结果进行了审查并标注研究协调员对有关LDL值的合格入组标准进行审查。您进一步指出，研究协调员没有对实验室报告进行审查，导致未进行第二次标准资格审查的受试者随机入组。

您声明，研究场所的所有员工均就密切监测实验结果和遵守入排标准的重要性，以及符合方案报告时限的审查进行了再次培训。您对所有研究受试者的实验室检测值进行了审计，以再次检查LDL值与方案的符合性。此外，您表示，作为纠正预防措施计划中的一部分，在您的带领下，研究人员将完成关于NIH与GCP的继续教育培训。您注明研究记录将经过两步核校程序以监测其完整性、质量与准确性。

我们想强调，作为临床试验研究者，您有确保这些研究正确实施、遵守FDA保护研究受试者权益、安全和福利的法规要求，以及确保研究数据的完整性的最终责任。我们无法对您的书面回复进行合理的评价，因为您既没能提供预防将来此类违规再次发生的纠正措施计划，又没能提供拟实施的附加措施与程序，以解决检查中发现的不合格受试者入组的详细信息。

6. 试验方案（b）（4）指明，已知有（b）（4）等同状况，或存在多个（即三个或三个以上）在列的危险因素的受试者，处于发生（b）（4）的高或非常高风险的状态。该方案所定义的患有已知的（b）（4）等同状况如有既往冠心病史，其他临床动脉粥样硬化疾病，（b）（4）或慢性肾病。

您未能遵守研究计划。受试者1029于2014年9月12日随即入组，没有已知的（b）（4）等同状况［方案中描述的如既往冠心病史，其他临床动脉粥样硬化疾病，（b）（4）或慢性肾病］且仅存在两个在列的危险因素。根据方案中的定义，该受试者没有发生CV事件的高或者非常高的风险，不应入组。

2015年11月19日在对FDA 483表的书面回复中，您指出受试者1029仅存在两个引发心血管疾病的危险因素。答复还指出，您的研究协调员收到了一位研究监查员的口头确认，允许受试者1029继续参与研究。答复中表示，作为纠正和预防措施计划中的一部分，在您的带领下，研究人员将完成关于NIH与GCP的继续教育培训。您注明研究记录将经过两步核校程序以监查其完整性、质量与准确性。

我们无法对您的书面回复进行合理的评价，因为您没能提供一份如果正确实施可防止未来此类违规发生的纠正措施计划。具体来说，您既没有提供任何防止未来同类违规事项再次发生的纠正措施计划细节或说明，又没能提供拟实施的附加措施与程序，以解决检查中发现的不合格受试者入组的详细信息。

每个临床研究入组标准的制定，都是为了最优化所收集数据的可解释性，以及对入组受试者的可预见性伤害最小化。入组不符合标准的受试者，将损害受试者的安全与福利，并引发（我们）对您研究场所所收集数据的有效性与完整性的关注。FDA尤其关注的是您研究场所随机入组方案（b）（4）的23位受试者中有9位并未确定是否满足入组标准。

本警告信的目的并非是罗列您在试验药物临床研究中存在的所有缺陷。确保遵循法律和相关FDA法规的每一项要求是您的职责，您应当解决这些缺陷，并建立规程，以确保任何正在进行或将来进行的研究均符合

FDA的法规。

自收到这封信的15个工作日内，您应当书面告知本办公室为预防将来发生类似违规情况而采取的措施。如果不能充分、迅速地解释上述违规问题，可能导致我们在不再通知的情况下采取监管措施。如果您认为您已经遵循了FDA的法规要求，请陈述理由，并提供所有支持资料，以供我们参考。

附：英文原文

Cheta Nand, M.D.

WARNING LETTER

Mar 10, 2016

CERTIFIED MAIL
RETURN RECEIPT REQUESTED

Ref.: 16-HFD-45-03-01

Cheta Nand, M.D.
2630 N. Columbia Center Boulevard
Richland, Washington 99352-4853

Dear Dr. Nand:

This Warning Letter informs you of objectionable conditions observed during the U.S. Food and Drug Administration (FDA) inspection conducted at your clinical site between October 6 and October 30, 2015. Ms. Tracy K. Li and Ms. Sherri N. Rohlf, representing FDA, reviewed your conduct of the following clinical investigations:

- Protocol **(b)(4)**, "**(b)(4)**," of the investigational drug **(b)(4)**, performed for **(b)(4)**.
- Protocol **(b)(4)**, "**(b)(4)**," of the investigational drug **(b)(4)**, performed for **(b)(4)**.

This inspection is a part of FDA's Bioresearch Monitoring Program, which includes inspections designed to evaluate the conduct of FDA-regulated research to ensure that the data are scientifically valid and accurate, and to help ensure that the rights, safety, and welfare of the human subjects of those studies have been protected.

At the conclusion of the inspection, Ms. Li and Ms. Rohlf presented and discussed with you Form FDA 483, Inspectional Observations. We acknowledge receipt of your November 19, 2015, written response to the Form FDA 483, and your written response dated December 18, 2015.

From our review of the FDA Establishment Inspection Report, the documents submitted with that report, and your written responses dated November 19, 2015, and December 18, 2015, we conclude that you did not adhere to the applicable statutory requirements and FDA regulations governing the conduct of clinical investigations. We wish to emphasize the following:

You failed to ensure that the investigation was conducted according to the investigational plan [21 CFR 312.60].

As a clinical investigator, you are required to ensure that your clinical studies are conducted in accordance with the investigational plan. The investigational plan for Protocol **(b)(4)** required you to ensure that study subjects met the protocol inclusion and exclusion criteria before their enrollment. You failed to adhere to this requirement. Specifically:

1. Protocol **(b)(4)** specified that subjects were to be treated with atorvastatin, simvastatin, or rosuvastatin, and that no dose should be lower than atorvastatin 20 mg, rosuvastatin 20 mg or simvastatin 40 mg. It also stated that all subjects must be on a stable dose at least 6 weeks before screening.

For example, you failed to follow the investigational plan when you randomized subjects 1004, 1023, and 1037 on July 31, 2014; September 3, 2014; and September 15, 2014, respectively, despite these subjects' receiving a dose of simvastatin lower than 40 mg. For at least six weeks before screening, Subjects 1004, 1023, and 1037 were on stable doses of simvastatin 20 mg once daily.

In your November 19, 2015, written response to the Form FDA 483, you agreed that Subjects 1004, 1023, and 1037 were on 20 mg of simvastatin and were randomized into the study in error. You indicated that as part of your corrective and preventive action plan, your study staff will complete continuing education training regarding NIH and GCP practices, which you will lead. You also noted that study records will undergo a two-step verification process to monitor for completion, quality, and accuracy.

We are unable to undertake an informed evaluation of your written response because you did not provide a corrective action plan that, if properly carried out, would prevent this type of violation in the future. Specifically, you did not provide any details or descriptions of a corrective action plan to prevent similar violations in the future, nor did you provide sufficient details about your plan to implement additional measures and procedures to address the inspection findings regarding your failure to ensure the eligibility of enrolled subjects.

2. Protocol **(b)(4)** specified that subjects with creatinine kinase (CK) values > 3.0 times the upper limit of normal (ULN) at screening cannot be enrolled into this clinical investigation. However, the protocol also permitted a measurement of > 3.0 times ULN to be repeated once during screening. If the repeat measurement was < 3.0 times ULN, the subject was eligible for enrollment.

Protocol **(b)(4)** also specified that if at any study visit after screening, a subject experiences unexplained CK values > 5 times ULN, that subject must return for a repeat CK, preferably within 48 hours of when results are made available to the investigator. If the repeat testing confirms the elevated CK value, without associated muscle pain, muscle tenderness, and/or muscle weakness, or new-onset renal dysfunction, the subject may continue to receive investigational drug if the sponsor's medical monitor provides approval.

a. You failed to follow the investigational plan when Subject 1014 was randomized on August 22, 2014, with a CK of 1074 U/L, which is > 3 times ULN (198 U/L), at screening on August 4, 2014. You initialed the laboratory report on August 6, 2014, and noted that "↑CK is not visible – clinically on lab values it might be, but not by looking at the patient." Regardless of your clinical evaluation, the protocol required either that you repeat the CK test, which you did not do, or that you not enroll the subject, as required by this exclusion criterion.

b. You failed to follow the investigational plan when Subject 1014 did not undergo a repeat CK test, preferably within 48 hours, despite having an unexplained (i.e., not associated temporally with recent trauma, intramuscular injections, heavy exercise, or physically strenuous activity) elevated CK value > 5 times ULN at the randomization visit (992 U/L on August 22, 2014).

c. You failed to follow the investigational plan when Subject 1014 did not undergo a repeat CK test, preferably within 48 hours, despite having an unexplained elevated CK value > 5 times ULN at Visit 11/Day 365 (3168 U/L on September 10, 2015). We acknowledge your handwritten note on September 18, 2015, which appears to state that the subject was called to schedule a repeat test, but the subject was unable to schedule a repeat test due to the subject's work schedule.

In your November 19, 2015, written response to the Form FDA 483, you indicated that you determined Subject 1014's elevated CK values not to be clinically significant because the subject was highly active, does regular weight training, and did not present with any clinical symptoms. You noted that your study coordinator had received verbal confirmation from a study monitor that Subject 1014 was eligible to be randomized on the study, based on your determination that the elevated CK value was not clinically significant.

In addition, you indicated that as part of your corrective and preventive action plan, your study staff will complete continuing education training regarding NIH and GCP practices, which you will lead. You noted that study records will undergo a two-step verification process to monitor for completion, quality, and accuracy. You also noted that verbal conversations with the study monitor will be followed up with e-mail correspondence to document the verbal conversations.

We are unable to undertake an informed evaluation of your written response because you did not provide a corrective action plan that, if properly carried out, would prevent this type of violation in the future. Specifically, you did not provide any details or descriptions of a corrective action plan to prevent similar violations in the future, nor did you provide sufficient details about your plan to implement additional measures and procedures to address the inspection findings regarding your failure to ensure the eligibility of enrolled subjects.

3. Protocol **(b)(4)** specified that subjects must have a fasting triglyceride (TG) value of ≤ 400 mg/dL at the second screening visit within 7 days (± 3 days) of randomization.

a. You failed to follow the investigational plan when Subject 1005 was randomized on July 31, 2014, despite having a TG value of 456 mg/dL at the second screening visit on July 24, 2014, which exceeded the fasting TG value for subject eligibility.

b. You failed to follow the investigational plan when Subject 1006 was randomized on August 4, 2014, despite having a TG value of 701 mg/dL at the second screening visit on July 28, 2014, which exceeded the fasting TG value for subject eligibility.

In your November 19, 2015, written response to the Form FDA 483, you agreed that Subjects 1005 and 1006 were randomized into the study with exclusionary TG levels. You noted that your study coordinator had received verbal confirmation from a study monitor to allow Subjects 1005 and 1006 to continue on the study. You indicated that study coordinators have been re-educated on following inclusion/exclusion criteria and acceptable reporting timelines. You also stated that as part of your corrective and preventive action plan, your study staff will complete continuing education training regarding NIH and GCP practices, which you will lead. You noted that study records will undergo a two-step verification process to monitor for completion, quality, and accuracy. You also noted that verbal conversations with the study monitor will be followed up with e-mail correspondence to document the verbal conversations.

We are unable to undertake an informed evaluation of your written response because you did not provide a corrective action plan that, if properly carried out, would prevent this type of violation in the future. Specifically, you did not provide any details or descriptions of a corrective action plan to prevent similar violations in the future, nor did you provide sufficient details about your plan to implement additional measures and procedures to address the inspection findings regarding your failure to ensure the eligibility of enrolled subjects.

4. Protocol **(b)(4)** specified that subjects cannot be enrolled into this clinical investigation with tests positive for hepatitis B surface antigen (HBsAg), HB core antibody (HBcAb), or hepatitis C antibody indicative of present or prior infection. However, the protocol permitted the enrollment of subjects who test positive for HBcAb if the subject tests negative for HBsAg and positive for antibody to HB surface antigen.

You failed to follow the investigational plan when Subject 1007 was randomized on August 12, 2014, despite testing positive for HBcAb, negative for HBsAg, and negative for antibody to HB surface antigen at screening.

In your November 19, 2015, written response to the Form FDA 483, you agreed that Subject 1007 was enrolled into the study in error, based on the subject's having tested positive for HBcAb. You indicated that, upon learning that the subject was ineligible, the study coordinator reported the protocol deviation to the IRB and attempted to get the subject to return all study medication. You noted that all site staff were re-educated on the importance of closely monitoring laboratory values and following all inclusion/exclusion criteria. You stated that, as part of your corrective and preventive action plan, your study staff will complete continuing education training regarding NIH and GCP practices, which you will lead. You noted that study records will undergo a two-step verification process to monitor for completion, quality, and accuracy. You also noted that verbal conversations with the study monitor will be followed up with e-mail correspondence to document the verbal conversations.

We are unable to undertake an informed evaluation of your written response because you did not provide a corrective action plan that, if properly carried out, would prevent this type of violation in the future. Specifically, you did not provide any details or descriptions of a corrective action plan to prevent similar violations in the future, nor did you provide sufficient details about your plan to implement additional measures and procedures to address the inspection findings regarding the enrollment of ineligible subjects.

5. Protocol **(b)(4)** specified that subjects with known **(b)(4)** equivalents at the highest approved dose of statins have a fasting low-density lipoprotein cholesterol (LDL-C) value of ≥70 mg/dL (1.81 mmol/L) at both screening visits, and that the value at the second screening visit (within 7 days of randomization, ± 3 days) must not be lower or higher than 20% of the initial fasting LDL-C value.

You failed to follow the investigational plan when Subject 1026 was randomized on September 19, 2014, despite having an LDL-C value of 125 mg/dL at the second screening visit on September 12, 2014, which is higher than 20% of the initial LDL-C value (97 mg/dL on September 5, 2014).

In your November 19, 2015, written response to the Form FDA 483, you agreed that Subject 1026 had elevated LDL levels. You noted that you reviewed the results and made a notation for the study coordinator to review the eligibility criteria pertaining to LDL values. You further noted that your study coordinator failed to review the lab reports and consequently randomized the subject without a second review of the eligibility criteria.

You stated that all site staff were re-educated on the importance of closely monitoring laboratory values and following all inclusion/exclusion criteria, along with review of reporting timelines per protocol. Your site audited the lab values for all the study subjects to re-check LDL values for compliance with the protocol. In addition, you indicated that as part of your corrective and preventive action plan, your study staff will complete continuing education training regarding NIH and GCP practices, which you will lead. You noted that study records will undergo a two-step verification process to monitor for completion, quality, and accuracy.

We wish to emphasize that as the clinical investigator, it was your ultimate responsibility to ensure that these studies were conducted properly and in compliance with FDA regulations to protect the rights, safety, and welfare of study subjects and to ensure the integrity of study data. We are unable to undertake an informed evaluation of your written response because you did not provide any details or descriptions of a corrective action plan to prevent similar violations in the future, nor did you provide sufficient details about your plan to implement additional measures and procedures to address the inspection findings regarding the enrollment of ineligible subjects.

6. Protocol **(b)(4)** specified that subjects must be at a high or very high risk of incurring a **(b)(4)**, as defined either by known **(b)(4)** equivalents, or by the presence of multiple (that is, three or more) listed risk factors. The protocol defined having known **(b)(4)** equivalents as having a history of coronary heart disease, other clinical atherosclerotic diseases, **(b)(4)**, or chronic kidney disease.

You failed to follow the investigational plan when Subject 1029 was randomized on September 12, 2014, without known **(b)(4)** equivalents (described in the protocol as a known history of coronary heart disease, other clinical atherosclerotic diseases, **(b)(4)**, or chronic kidney disease) and with the presence of only two of the listed risk factors. By definition of the protocol, this subject did not have a high or very high risk of incurring a CV event and should not have been enrolled.

In your November 19, 2015, written response to the Form FDA 483, you indicated that Subject 1029 had only two CV risk factors. You also noted that your study coordinator had received verbal confirmation from a study monitor to allow Subject 1029 to continue in the study. You indicated that as part of your corrective and preventive action plan, your study staff will complete continuing education training regarding NIH and GCP practices, which you will lead. You noted that study records will undergo a two-step verification process to monitor for completion, quality, and accuracy.

We are unable to undertake an informed evaluation of your written response because you did not provide a corrective action plan that, if properly carried out, would prevent this type of violation in the future. Specifically, you did not provide any details or descriptions of a corrective action plan to prevent similar violations in the future, nor did you provide sufficient details about your plan to implement additional measures and procedures to address the inspection findings regarding the enrollment of ineligible subjects.

The eligibility criteria for each clinical investigation are designed to optimize the interpretability of the collected data and to minimize foreseeable harm to enrolled subjects. Enrollment of subjects who do not meet the eligibility criteria jeopardizes subject safety and welfare, and raises concerns about the validity and integrity of the data collected at your site. Particularly concerning to FDA is that you enrolled 9 of the 23 subjects randomized into Protocol **(b)(4)** at your site without having ensured their eligibility to be enrolled as subjects.

This letter is not intended to be an all-inclusive list of deficiencies with your clinical study of an investigational drug. It is your responsibility to ensure adherence to each requirement of the law and relevant FDA regulations. You should address these deficiencies and establish procedures to ensure that any ongoing or future studies will be in compliance with FDA regulations.

Within fifteen (15) working days of your receipt of this letter, you should notify this office in writing of the actions

you have taken to prevent similar violations in the future. Failure to address the violations noted above adequately and promptly may result in regulatory action without further notice. If you believe you have complied with FDA regulations, include your reasoning and any supporting information for our consideration.

If you have any questions, please contact Douglas Pham at 301-796-1955; FAX 301-847-8748. Your written response and any pertinent documentation should be addressed to:

Douglas B. Pham, Pharm.D., J.D.
Branch Chief (Acting)
Compliance Enforcement Branch
Division of Enforcement and Postmarketing Safety
Office of Scientific Investigations
Office of Compliance
Center for Drug Evaluation and Research
U.S. Food and Drug Administration
Building 51, Room 5348
10903 New Hampshire Avenue
Silver Spring, MD 20993

Sincerely yours,

{See appended electronic signature page}

David Burrow, Pharm.D., J.D.
Acting Director
Office of Scientific Investigations
Office of Compliance
Center for Drug Evaluation and Research
U.S. Food and Drug Administration

This is a representation of an electronic record that was signed electronically and this page is the manifestation of the electronic signature.

/S/

DAVID C BURROW
03/10/2016

第63封　给Alexander Neumeister的警告信

2016年2月19日

参考号：16-HFD-45-02-01

尊敬的Neumeister博士：

2015年7月16日至8月5日，Iram R. Hassan医生代表FDA对您所开展的以下临床研究进行了审查：

- 试验药物（b）（4）的试验方案（b）（4），“（b）（4）”，申办者（b）（4）；
- 试验方案（b）（4），“（b）（4）”。

这封警告信特告知您现场检查中发现的违规情况。

本次现场检查是FDA的生物研究监查项目的一部分。该项目通过设定的检查方法，对FDA所监管的相关研究的实施情况进行评估，以确认研究数据在科学上是有效和准确的，并确保这些研究中受试者的权益、安全和福利得到了保护。

在现场检查结束时，Iram R. Hassan医生向您出示了FDA483表，即现场检查发现的问题，并与您进行了讨论。您的律师Georges G. Lederman先生代贵方于2015年8月19日对该FDA483表的书面回复已收悉。

经对现场检查报告、该报告的附件、2015年7月22日Lederman先生对Hassan医生于2015年7月16日同您会谈要旨的信函，以及2015年8月29日书面回复进行审查，我们认为，您没有遵循适用的法律要求和监管临床研究实施的FDA法规。我们想强调以下几点：

1. 您未能保存研究中使用试验药物或对照组的受试者的所有观察结果和其他相关数据的足够及准确的病历［21 CFR 312.62（b）］

作为临床试验研究者，您必须准备和保存研究中使用试验药物或对照组的受试者的所有观察结果和其他相关数据的足够及准确的病历。病历包括病例报告表以及支持数据，其中支持数据包括，如签名并注明日期的同意书、医疗记录等；医疗记录又包括，如医生写的病程记录、个人检查记录图表、护理记录等。对于方案（b）（4），病历包括所要求程序的研究记录，例如病史、精神状况评估、体检和神经系统检查结果及自杀风险评估。您未能保存足够和准确的病历，在曾实施特定要求研究程序中记录了您的助理研究者的名字，但事实上，这是您或其他研究人员做的。下列此类失误的案例，包括但不限于：

a. 病史、体格检查和神经系统检查的工作表中，您亲自手签了助理研究者的名字，以表示这些研究程序是您的助理研究者实施的。然而事实上，真正实施这些研究程序的是您或者其他研究人员，而非您的助理研究者。示例如下：

i. 两位受试者病史筛查（受试者1和2）。

ii. 所有14位入组受试者的体检筛查（受试者1、2、3、4、6、7、8、10、11、12、13、14、15和16）。

iii. 所有14位入组受试者的神经系统检查的筛查（受试者1、2、3、4、6、7、8、10、11、12、13、14、15和16）。

iv. 11位受试者第8天的简单体检（受试者1、2、3、4、6、8、10、11、12、13和14）。

v. 8位受试者的随访简单体检（受试者1、2、3、6、7、8、10和12）。

b. 在下列研究记录中，您的助理研究者作为实施各项研究的程序人员签字。然而，事实上您或其他研究人员，而非您的助理研究者，实施了如下研究程序：

i. 所有14位入组受试者的精神状况评估筛查（受试者1、2、3、4、6、7、8、10、11、12、13、14、15和16）。

ⅱ. 一位受试者的自杀风险评估筛查（受试者15）。

在2015年8月19日对FDA 483表的书面回复中，Lederman先生承认是您执行的这些程序，并签了您的助理研究者的名字，而不是您自己的名字。Lederman先生表示，方案中并未规定获取病史及执行体检和神经系统检查的责任可以委派给谁，也未规定执业的精神病医师必须对精神状况的评估形成文件。此外，Lederman称，在您的研究人员收集资料而完善这些研究记录后，您与您的助理研究者就受试者的资格进行了仔细的审查与讨论。

Lederman先生进一步表示，上述工作表为申办者并未提供的病例报告表。他指出，这些研究记录“仅仅被认为是正在进行中的工作，从未被认为是最终文件。

您的回复并不符合要求，尽管试验方案并未规定这些研究活动的职责可以委派给谁，但许多研究记录中的信息都不准确，这些都被错误地归咎于您执行研究程序的助理研究者。

在您书面回复的总结中，Lederman先生表示，您不同意检查中所发现缺陷的认定依据，这些缺陷的责任应归咎于您的员工而不是您。我们想强调，当您为上述临床研究签署研究者声明（FDA 1572表）时，您就已经同意承担作为您研究场所的一位临床试验研究者的责任。您对这些事项的解释，与上述违规事项联系在一起，提示在该临床研究中您的行为出现系统性失职。作为临床试验研究者，您有承担确保研究的正确执行、遵守FDA的法规要求，既要保护研究受试者权益、安全和福利，又要确保研究数据的完整性的最终责任。

您没能保存足够和准确的病历，包括上述执行特定研究程序人员指派中的不符合项，从而引发了我们对您研究场所所采集数据有效性与完整性的关注。

2. 您未能确保研究按照研究计划进行［21 CFR 312.60］

作为临床试验研究者，您需确保临床研究按照研究计划进行。方案（b）（4）的研究计划要求研究受试者在入组前符合方案的入排标准。方案（b）（4）的研究计划要求在服药约24小时后实施研究（b）（4）。您未能遵循方案要求，具体表现为：

a. 对于方案（b）（4），您未能确保研究受试者在入组前符合方案的入排除标准。方案（b）（4）规定（b）（4），经DSM-IV临床定式检查评估、研究版本、患者版本（SCID-RV/P）证实，必须是原发性精神疾患的受试者才符合入组本研究的条件。然而，13位受试者在筛选访视阶段没能完成SCID中（b）（4）模块评估。因此，14位受试者中有13位无法以SCID-RV/P来诊断（b）（4）是否为原发精神疾病。

具体如下：

ⅰ. 2014年10月16日，受试者1在筛选阶段没完成SCID中（b）（4）模块评估。在记录中有“请见（b）（4）”的注释。该受试者于2014年11月13日随机入组。

ⅱ. 2014年10月20日，受试者2接受了筛选阶段的SCID检查。然而，该受试者只完成了（b）（4）模块“创伤性事件清单简介”中的一部分检查。该受试者于2015年2月2日随机入组。

ⅲ. 2014年11月13日，受试者3在筛选阶段没完成SCID中（b）（4）模块评估。在记录中有“请见（b）（4）”的注释。该受试者于2014年11月17日随机入组。

ⅳ. 2014年12月1日，受试者6在筛选阶段没完成SCID中（b）（4）模块评估。在记录中有“请见（b）（4）”的注释。该受试者于2014年12月10日随机入组。

ⅴ. 2014年12月11日，受试者7在筛选阶段没完成SCID中（b）（4）模块评估。该受试者于2014年12月15日随机入组。

ⅵ. 2014年12月12日，受试者8在筛选阶段没完成SCID中（b）（4）模块评估。在记录中有“请见（b）（4）”的注释。该受试者于2015年1月7日随机入组。

ⅶ. 2014年1月16日，受试者10在筛选阶段没完成SCID中（b）（4）模块评估。在记录中有“请见（b）（4）”的注释。该受试者于2015年1月20日随机入组。

ⅷ. 2015年1月20日，受试者11在筛选阶段没完成SCID中（b）（4）模块评估。在记录中有“请见（b）

（4）”的注释。该受试者于2015年1月22日随机入组。

ⅸ. 2015年1月26日，受试者12在筛选阶段没完成SCID中（b）（4）模块评估。在记录中有“请见（b）（4）”的注释。该受试者于2015年2月2日随机入组。

x. 受试者13在筛选阶段没完成SCID中（b）（4）模块评估（具体日期不详）。在记录中有“请见（b）（4）”的注释。该受试者于2015年2月4日随机入组。

xi. 2015年2月12日，受试者14在筛选阶段没完成SCID中（b）（4）模块评估。在记录中有“请见（b）（4）”的注释。该受试者于2015年2月17日随机入组。

xii. 2015年2月17日，受试者15在筛选阶段没完成SCID中（b）（4）模块评估。在记录中有“请见（b）（4）”的注释。该受试者于2015年2月19日随机入组。

xiii. 2015年2月25日，受试者16在筛选阶段没完成SCID中（b）（4）模块的检查。在记录中有“请见（b）（4）”的注释。该受试者于2015年3月4日随机入组。

如上所述，13位受试者中11位的SCID（b）（4）模块记录中都有“请见（b）（4）”的标注。我们注意到，方案要求在筛选阶段SCID和（b）（4）检查要同时实施，且方案不允许以其中一项检查替代另外一项。您未提供任何说明，以解释没能对13位受试者中的2位进行SCID（b）（4）模块评估的情况。

我们还注意到，您是用SCID患者版本（SCID-I/P）来管理全部入组受试者，而非方案所规定的研究版本（SCID-RV/P）。

2015年8月19日的书面回复中，Lederman先生承认没能完成对上述受试者的SCID（b）（4）模块检查。Lederman先生表示，您的研究人员采用源于（b）（4）评估的有关信息确认（b）（4）的诊断，而不是采用源于SCID的信息。Lederman先生同时声称，您从以前的研究了解所有入组受试者，他们均完成了SCID评估。Lederman先生指出，在进行研究的时候，您并不知道这些受试者的SCID评估没能妥善完成，且贵方研究人员或申办者的监查员均没有让您注意到此违规事项。

我们希望强调，作为临床试验研究者，您有确保研究正常进行，遵守FDA保护研究受试者的权利、安全和福利的法规要求，以及确保研究数据完整性的法规要求的最终责任。您的回复并不充分，因为您没有说明纠正措施计划的落实情况，以预防未来类似违规情况再次发生。您对这些事项的解释，当与上述违规事项相联系时，提示您在本次临床研究中的行为存在系统性失职。

您对临床研究在监督管理上的不足，引发了我们对上述研究中您研究场所在对入组受试者的保护能力上的严重关注，也引发了对您研究场所收集数据的有效性和完整性的关注。

b. 试验方案（b）（4）规定，在此研究开始前30天内或5个半衰期之内（以时间较长的为准），或在参与此研究期间，参与任何其他涉及试验药物的临床试验的受试者，不得入组此临床研究。

受试者13之前曾入组试验方案（b）（4），并于2015年1月20日完成最后一次研究访视。然而，该受试者于2015年2月4日被随机入组试验方案（b）（4），距其之前最后一次研究访视只有15天，且距服用之前的试验药物只有16天。

2015年8月19日的书面回复中，Lederman先生承认，受试者13参与另一项临床研究的30天之内入组了此临床研究。他表示，该受试者在两项临床研究中均没有任何不良事件报告，且在整个研究过程中始终受到严密的监测。

您的回复并不充分，因为您没能说明纠正措施计划的落实情况，以预防未来类似违规情况的再次发生。您对临床研究在监督管理上的不足，引发了我们对上述研究中您研究场所在对入组受试者保护能力上的严重关注，也引发了对您研究场所收集数据的有效性和完整性的关注。

每个临床研究入组标准的制定，都是为了最优化所收集数据的可释性，以及为了对入组受试者可预见性的危害减少到最小。入组不符合标准的受试者，将损害受试者的安全与福利，并引发我们对您研究场所所收集数据的有效性与完整性的关注。我们尤其关注的是您研究场所入组方案（b）（4）的14位受试者中的13位并未确定是否满足入组标准。

c. 方案（b）（4）要求，在服药后24小时的第二次访视时，要求对受试者进行（b）（4）评估，以评价受试者的情绪与健康状况，同时监测他们是否有不良事件。我们注意到，在服药后24小时的（b）（4）评估还要求一次用疗效变量来估量（b）（4）症状的整体严重性。

您没能对至少下列三位受试者进行服药后24小时（b）（4）评估：

i. 受试者9于2015年2月3日服用研究药物，但在服药后24小时的第二次访视时，没能进行（b）（4）评估。

ii. 受试者11于2015年2月10日服用研究药物，但在服药后24小时的第二次访视时，没能进行（b）（4）评估。

iii. 受试者14于2015年3月3日服用研究药物，但在服药后24小时的第二次访视时，没能进行（b）（4）评估。

2015年8月19日的书面回复中，Lederman先生表示，根据方案要求，应在短时间内服用两次（b）（4）（服药后4小时与服药后24小时），"要求员工与受试者以自己的评估进行时间安排。"

您的回复并不充分，因为您没能说明纠正措施计划的落实情况，以预防未来类似违规情况再次发生。您对临床研究在监督管理上的不足，引发了我们对上述研究中您研究场所在对入组受试者的保护能力上的严重关注，也引发了对您研究场所数据有效性和完整性的关注。

如上详述，您没能按照研究计划进行研究。具体来说，您未能遵守试验方案要求来实施研究程序，且您入组受试者没能符合入组标准，损害了受试者的安全与福利，引发了我们对您研究场所所收集数据有效性与完整性的关注。

本警告信并非是罗列您在试验药物临床研究中存在的所有缺陷。确保遵循法律和相关FDA法规的每一项要求是您的职责，您应当解决这些缺陷，并建立规程，以确保任何正在进行或将来进行的研究均符合FDA法规。

自收到这封信的15个工作日内，您应当书面告知本办公室为预防将来发生类似违规情况而采取的措施。如果不能充分、迅速地解释上述违规问题，可能导致我们在不再通知的情况下采取监管措施。如果您认为您已经遵循了FDA法规要求，请陈述理由，并提供所有支持资料，以供我们参考。

附：英文原文

Alexander Neumeister

WARNING LETTER

FEB 19，2016

CERTIFIED MAIL
RETURN RECEIPT REQUESTED

Ref: 16-HFD-45-02-01

Alexander Neumeister, M.D.
c/o Georges G. Lederman, Attorney at Law
52 Duane Street
7th Floor
New York, NY 10007

Dear Dr. Neumeister:

This Warning Letter informs you of objectionable conditions observed during the U.S. Food and Drug Administration (FDA) inspection conducted from July 16 to August 5, 2015. Dr. Iram R. Hassan, representing FDA, reviewed your conduct of the following clinical investigations:

- Protocol **(b)(4)**, "**(b)(4)**," of the investigational drug **(b)(4)**, performed for **(b)(4)**.
- Protocol **(b)(4)**, "**(b)(4)**

This inspection is a part of FDA's Bioresearch Monitoring Program, which includes inspections designed to evaluate the conduct of FDA-regulated research to ensure that the data are scientifically valid and accurate, and to help ensure that the rights, safety, and welfare of the human subjects of those studies have been protected.

At the conclusion of the inspection, Dr. Iram R. Hassan presented and discussed with you Form FDA 483, Inspectional Observations. We acknowledge receipt of the August 19, 2015, written response to the Form FDA 483 submitted on your behalf by your attorney, Mr. Georges G. Lederman.

From our review of the FDA Establishment Inspection Report; the documents submitted with that report; the July 22, 2015, letter from Mr. Lederman, memorializing the substance of Dr. Hassan's interview with you on July 16, 2015; and the written response dated August 29, 2015, we conclude that you did not adhere to the applicable statutory requirements and FDA regulations governing the conduct of clinical investigations. We wish to emphasize the following:

1. You failed to maintain adequate and accurate case histories that record all observations and other data pertinent to the investigation on each individual administered the investigational drug or employed as a control in the investigation [21 CFR 312.62(b)].

As a clinical investigator, you are required to prepare and maintain adequate and accurate case histories that record all observations and other data pertinent to the investigation on each individual administered the investigational drug or employed as a control in the investigation. Case histories include the case report forms and supporting data including, for example, signed and dated consent forms and medical records, including, for example, progress notes of the physician, the individual's hospital chart(s), and the nurse's notes. For Protocol**(b)(4)**, case histories include study records of required procedures such as medical history, psychiatric evaluations, physical and neurological examinations, and suicide risk assessments. You failed to maintain adequate and accurate case histories when your subinvestigator's name was recorded as having conducted certain required study procedures that, in fact, you or another study employee conducted. Examples of this failure include, but are not limited to, the following:

a. On worksheets for medical history, physical examinations, and neurological examinations, you personally hand-printed the name of your subinvestigator to indicate that these study procedures were conducted by your subinvestigator. However, in fact, you or another study employee actually conducted these study procedures, not your subinvestigator. Examples include the following:

i. Screening medical history for 2 subjects (Subjects 1 and 2)

ii. Screening physical examinations for all 14 enrolled subjects (Subjects 1, 2, 3, 4, 6, 7, 8, 10, 11, 12, 13, 14, 15, and 16)

iii. Screening neurological examinations for all 14 enrolled subjects (Subjects 1, 2, 3, 4, 6, 7, 8, 10, 11, 12, 13, 14, 15, and 16)

iv. Day 8 brief physical examinations for 11 subjects (Subjects 1, 2, 3, 4, 6, 8, 10, 11, 12, 13, and 14)

v. Follow-up Visit brief physical examinations for 8 subjects (Subjects 1, 2, 3, 6, 7, 8, 10, and 12)

b. On the following study records, your subinvestigator signed as having performed the respective study procedures. However, in fact, you or another study employee, not your subinvestigator, performed these study procedures:

i. Screening psychiatric evaluations for all 14 enrolled subjects (Subjects 1, 2, 3, 4, 6, 7, 8, 10, 11, 12, 13, 14, 15, and 16)

ii. Screening suicide risk assessment for 1 subject (Subject 15)

In the August 19, 2015, written response to the Form FDA 483, Mr. Lederman agreed that you had performed these procedures and had your subinvestigator's name added instead of your own. Mr. Lederman noted that the protocol did not specify to whom the responsibility of obtaining medical history and performing physical and neurological examinations could be delegated, nor did it specify that a licensed psychiatrist must document the psychiatric evaluations. In addition, Mr. Lederman stated that after your study staff collected the information to complete these study records, you and your subinvestigator carefully reviewed and discussed the eligibility of the subjects.

Mr. Lederman indicated further that the above-mentioned worksheets were case report forms that the sponsor did not provide. He noted that these study records were “merely considered a work in progress” and were never considered final documents.

This response is inadequate because, although the protocol did not specify to whom the responsibility of these study activities could be delegated, inaccurate information was recorded in numerous study records, which falsely attributed the conduct of study procedures to your subinvestigator.

In the conclusion of the written response, Mr. Lederman indicated that while you do not agree with the basis for the assertion of the deficiencies observed during the inspection, the responsibility for these deficiencies rests with your employer and not with you. We wish to emphasize that when you signed the Statement of the Investigator (Form FDA 1572) for the above-referenced clinical investigation, you agreed to take on the responsibilities of a clinical investigator at your site. Your explanation of these matters, when taken in conjunction with the violations described above, suggests systemic failures in your conduct of this clinical investigation. As a clinical investigator, it was ultimately your responsibility to ensure that these studies were conducted properly and in compliance with FDA regulations, both to protect the rights, safety, and welfare of study subjects and to ensure the integrity of study data.

Your failure to maintain adequate and accurate case histories, including the aforementioned discrepancies in the designation of the person who performed certain study procedures, raises concerns about the validity and integrity of the data captured at your site.

2. You failed to ensure that the investigation was conducted according to the investigational plan [21 CFR 312.60].

As a clinical investigator, you are required to ensure that your clinical studies are conducted in accordance with the investigational plan. The investigational plan for Protocol **(b)(4)** required you to ensure that study subjects met the protocol inclusion and exclusion criteria before their enrollment. The investigational plan for Protocol **(b)(4)** required that you perform the **(b)(4)** approximately 24 hours after dosing. You failed to adhere to these requirements. Specifically:

a. For Protocol **(b)(4)**, you failed to ensure that study subjects met the protocol inclusion and exclusion criteria before their enrollment. Protocol **(b)(4)** specified that **(b)(4)**, confirmed by the Structured Clinical Interview for DSM-IV, Research Version, Patient Edition (SCID-RV/P), must be the primary psychiatric disorder present for the subject to be eligible for enrollment into the study. However, **(b)(4)** modules of the SCID were not completed at the screening visit for 13 subjects. Therefore, you failed to confirm a **(b)(4)** diagnosis as the primary psychiatric disorder using the SCID-RV/P for 13 of the 14 enrolled subjects.

Specifically:

i. For Subject 1, the **(b)(4)** module of the SCID was not completed at screening on October 16, 2014. A notation, “See **(b)(4)**,” was recorded in its place. Subject 1 was randomized on November 13, 2014.

ii. For Subject 2, the SCID was administered at screening on October 20, 2014. However, only a portion of the Brief Description of the Traumatic Events List of the **(b)(4)** module was completed. Subject 2 was randomized on November 17, 2014.

iii. For Subject 3, the **(b)(4)** module of the SCID was not completed at screening on November 13, 2014. A notation, “See **(b)(4)**,” was recorded in its place. Subject 3 was randomized on November 17, 2014.

iv. For Subject 6, the **(b)(4)** module of the SCID was not completed at screening on December 1, 2014. A notation, “See **(b)(4)**,” was recorded in its place. Subject 6 was randomized on December 10, 2014.

v. For Subject 7, the **(b)(4)** module of the SCID was not completed at screening on December 11, 2014. Subject 7 was randomized on December 15, 2014.

vi. For Subject 8, the **(b)(4)** module of the SCID was not completed at screening on December 12, 2014. A notation, “See **(b)(4)**,” was recorded in its place. Subject 8 was randomized on January 7, 2015.

vii. For Subject 10, the **(b)(4)** module of the SCID was not completed at screening on January 16, 2015. A notation, “See **(b)(4)**,” was recorded in its place. Subject 10 was randomized on January 20, 2015.

viii. For Subject 11, the **(b)(4)** module of the SCID was not completed at screening on January 20, 2015. A notation, “See **(b)(4)**,” was recorded in its place. Subject 11 was randomized on January 22, 2015.

ix. For Subject 12, the **(b)(4)** module of the SCID was not completed at screening on January 26, 2015. A notation,

"See **(b)(4)**," was recorded in its place. Subject 12 was randomized on February 2, 2015.

x. For Subject 13, the **(b)(4)** module of the SCID was not completed at screening (date not indicated). A notation, "See **(b)(4)**," was recorded in its place. Subject 13 was randomized on February 4, 2015.

xi. For Subject 14, the **(b)(4)** module of the SCID was not completed at screening on February 12, 2015. A notation, "See **(b)(4)**," was recorded in its place. Subject 14 was randomized on February 17, 2015.

xii. For Subject 15, the **(b)(4)** module of the SCID was not completed at screening on February 17, 2015. A notation, "See **(b)(4)**," was recorded in its place. Subject 15 was randomized on February 19, 2015.

xiii. For Subject 16, the **(b)(4)** module of the SCID was not completed at screening on February 25, 2015. A notation, "See **(b)(4)**," was recorded in its place. Subject 16 was randomized on March 4, 2015.

As described above, for 11 of the 13 subjects, a notation, "See **(b)(4)**," was recorded under the **(b)(4)** module of the SCID. We note that the protocol required the administration of both the SCID and the **(b)(4)** at screening, and that the protocol did not allow for the substitution of one assessment for the other. There was no explanation provided for the failure to perform the **(b)(4)** module of the SCID for 2 of the 13 subjects.

We also note that you used the Patient Version (SCID-I/P) of the SCID to administer the SCID for all enrolled subjects, rather than the Research Version (SCID-RV/P), as the protocol specified.

In the August 19, 2015, written response, Mr. Lederman agreed that the **(b)(4)** module of the SCID was not completed for these subjects. Mr. Lederman indicated that your study staff used the relevant information derived from the **(b)(4)** assessment to confirm diagnosis of **(b)(4)**, rather than using the information from the SCID. Mr. Lederman also stated that you knew all of the enrolled subjects from previous studies, for which SCID interviews were completed. In addition, Mr. Lederman noted that you were unaware at the time of the study that the SCID assessments for these subjects were not completed properly, and that this violation was not brought to your attention by either your study staff or sponsor monitors.

We wish to emphasize that as the clinical investigator, it was your ultimate responsibility to ensure that these studies were conducted properly and in compliance with FDA regulations, both to protect the rights, safety, and welfare of study subjects and to ensure the integrity of study data. Your response is inadequate because you did not indicate that you have put a corrective action plan in place to prevent similar violations in the future. Your explanation of these matters, when taken in conjunction with the violations described above, suggests systemic failures in your conduct of this clinical investigation.

Your lack of supervision and oversight of the clinical studies raises significant concerns about the adequacy of your protection of study subjects enrolled at your site in the studies mentioned above, and also raises concerns about the integrity of the data generated at your site.

b. Protocol **(b)(4)** specified that subjects who participated in any other clinical study involving an investigational drug within 30 days or 5 half-lives (whichever is longer) before the current study begins and/or during study participation cannot be enrolled into this clinical investigation.

Subject 13 was previously enrolled in Protocol **(b)(4)** and completed the last study visit on January 20, 2015. However, this subject was randomized into Protocol **(b)(4)** on February 4, 2015, which is only 15 days after the last study visit for the previous study, and only 16 days from drug administration in the previous study.

In the August 19, 2015, written response, Mr. Lederman agreed that Subject 13 was enrolled in this clinical investigation within 30 days of participating in another clinical study. He noted that this subject did not report any adverse events in either of the clinical studies, and that he was closely monitored throughout the course of the study.

Your response is inadequate because you did not indicate that you have put a corrective action plan in place to prevent similar violations in the future. Your lack of supervision and oversight of the clinical studies raises significant concerns about the adequacy of your protection of study subjects enrolled at your site in the studies mentioned above, and also raises concerns about the integrity of the data generated at your site.

The eligibility criteria for each clinical investigation are designed to optimize the interpretability of the collected data and to minimize foreseeable harm to enrolled subjects. Enrollment of subjects who do not meet the eligibility criteria jeopardizes subject safety and welfare, and raises concerns about the validity and integrity of the data collected at your site. Particularly concerning to us is that you enrolled 13 of the 14 subjects into Protocol **(b)(4)**at your site without having ensured their subject eligibility.

c. Protocol **(b)(4)** required that the **(b)(4)** assessment be performed 24 hours post-dose at Visit 2 to assess the mood and well-being of the subjects, as well as to monitor them for adverse events. We note that the 24 hours post-dose **(b)(4)** assessment was also required as a secondary efficacy variable to measure the overall severity of **(b)(4)** symptoms. You failed to perform the **(b)(4)** assessment at 24 hours post-dose for at least the following three subjects:

i. Subject 9 was administered study drug on February 3, 2015; however, the **(b)(4)** assessment was not conducted 24 hours post-dose at Visit 2.

ii. Subject 11 was administered study drug on February 10, 2015; however, the **(b)(4)** assessment was not conducted 24 hours post-dose at Visit 2.

iii. Subject 14 was administered study drug on March 3, 2015; however, the **(b)(4)** assessment was not conducted 24 hours post-dose at Visit 2.

In the August 19, 2015, written response, Mr. Lederman indicated that, given the protocol requirement for the **(b)(4)** to be administered twice within a short period of time (at 4 hours post-dose and at 24 hours post-dose), "the staff and subjects were instructed to rate these timeframes [*sic*] in their assessments."

Your response is inadequate because you did not indicate that you have put a corrective action plan in place to prevent similar violations in the future. Your lack of supervision and oversight of the clinical studies raises significant concerns about the adequacy of your protection of study subjects enrolled at your site in the studies mentioned above, and also raises concerns about the integrity of the data generated at your site.

As detailed above, you failed to conduct the investigation in accordance with the investigational plan. Specifically, your failure to adhere to protocol requirements for performing study procedures and your enrollment of subjects who did not meet eligibility criteria jeopardize subject safety and welfare, and raise concerns about the validity and integrity of the data collected at your site.

This letter is not intended to be an all-inclusive list of deficiencies with your clinical study of an investigational drug. It is your responsibility to ensure adherence to each requirement of the law and relevant FDA regulations. You should address these deficiencies and establish procedures to ensure that any ongoing or future studies will be in compliance with FDA regulations.

Within fifteen (15) working days of your receipt of this letter, you should notify this office in writing of the actions you have taken or will take to prevent similar violations in the future. Failure to address the violations noted above adequately and promptly may result in regulatory action without further notice. If you believe you have complied with FDA regulations, include your reasoning and any supporting information for our consideration.

If you have any questions, please contact Douglas Pham at 301-796-1955; FAX 301-847-8748. Your written response and any pertinent documentation should be addressed to:

Douglas B. Pham, Pharm.D., J.D.
Acting Branch Chief
Compliance Enforcement Branch
Division of Enforcement and Postmarketing Safety
Office of Scientific Investigations
Office of Compliance
Center for Drug Evaluation and Research
U.S. Food and Drug Administration
Building 51, Room 5348
10903 New Hampshire Avenue
Silver Spring, Maryland 20993

Sincerely yours,

{See appended electronic signature page}

David Burrow, Pharm.D., J.D.

Acting Director
Office of Scientific Investigations
Office of Compliance
Center for Drug Evaluation and Research
U.S. Food and Drug Administration

This is a representation of an electronic record that was signed electronically and this page is the manifestation of the electronic signature.

/S/

DAVID C BURROW
02/19/2016

第 64 封　给 Gregory J. Tracey 医学博士的警告信

2015年12月16日

参考号：16-HFD-45-10-01

尊敬的Tracey博士：

2015年3月25日至4月15日，Jonee J. Mearns女士和Byungja E. Marciante女士代表FDA，在贵临床研究现场，对您所开展的以下临床研究：试验方案（b）(4)[1]，"（b）(4)"和试验方案（b）(4)，"（b）(4)"，进行了现场审查。这封警告信特告知您现场检查中发现的违规情况。

本次现场检查是FDA的生物研究监查项目的一部分。该项目通过设定的检查方法，对FDA所监管的相关研究的实施情况进行评估，以确保研究数据在科学上是有效和准确的，并帮助确保这些研究中受试者的权益、安全和福利得到了保护。

在现场检查结束时，Mearns女士和Marciante女士向您出示了FDA483表，即现场检查发现的问题，并与您进行了讨论。您2015年4月29日对该FDA483表的书面回复已收悉。

经对现场检查报告、该报告的附件，以及您2015年4月29日的书面回复进行审查，我们认为，您没有遵循适用的法律要求和监管临床研究实施的FDA法规。我们想强调以下几点：

您未能确保研究按照研究计划进行［21 CFR 312.60］

作为临床研究者，您必须确保临床研究按照研究计划进行。（b）(4)的研究计划要求您需确认受试者符合所有规定的入组标准，尤其是在筛选或入组时应排除血清妊娠试验阳性的受试者，但您未能遵循这些要求。

试验方案（b）(4)规定在筛选或入组时血清妊娠试验阳性的受试者不能入组，并要求您或者您指定的人在筛选或入组时核实受试者是否符合所有规定的入组标准。受试者1214入组时是一名22岁的育龄女性，在筛选和入组时血清妊娠试验均为阳性，入组时您未能遵循上述要求，具体而言：

筛查检验报告：2014年12月4日，受试者1214的筛查检验报告清楚地显示，受试者人绒毛膜促性腺激素（hCG）水平为70.8mIU/mL，该数值显著高于提示怀孕的参考hCG水平。您于2014年12月4日签署了该检验报告，表明您已经审查过报告上的内容。

复筛检验报告：2014年12月19日，受试者1214的复筛检验报告清楚地显示，受试者hCG水平为34833.0mIU/mL，该数值仍然显著高于提示怀孕的参考hCG水平。您于2014年12月22日签署了该检验报告，表明您已经审查过报告上的内容。

筛查合格表：尽管几次检查的血清hCG水平升高，2015年1月2日，您仍然签署了受试者1214的筛查合格表，认为受试者1214有资格参加研究。该筛查合格表上显示，受试者无论在筛查或入组时"血清妊娠试验是否阳性（也就是血清hCG水平高于参考水平）"项标记为"No"。但是，受试者1214有资格参加研究的决定违背了试验方案的规定，因为您签署的实验室报告表明，受试者1214在筛查或入组时血清妊娠试验均为阳性。

入组检验报告：2015年1月4日，受试者1214的入组检验报告清楚地显示，受试者血清hCG为135828.0mIU/mL。这个数值再次仍然显著高于提示怀孕的参考hCG水平。您于2015年1月5日签署了实验室报告，表明您已经审查过报告上的内容。

---

1 (b) (4) 涉及商业秘密，根据法规内容不予公开。

研究第1天入组/排除小结：2015年1月5日您签署了意见，声明您已经审阅了该研究的受试者入组/排除标准和原始文件；您承认，为确认受试者接受研究药物资格已经审查了相关记录，并且您已经确认受试者符合接受研究药物的要求。但是，如上所述，受试者1214有资格接受研究药物的决定违背了试验方案，因为您签署的记录表明受试者1214在筛选、复筛以及入组时血清妊娠试验均为阳性。

结果是，2015年1月5日（研究第1天），该受试者接受两个口服（b）（4）剂量的研究药物（b）（4）；2015年1月6日至8日（研究第2至4天），该受试者每天接受1粒（b）（4）胶囊。

该受试者没有再回诊所，于2015年1月9日停止了此项研究。2015年1月22日，该受试者完成了提前退出的回访，您签署的、来自那次随访的实验室报告显示，该受试者的hCG水平为2050.0mIU/mL。

于2015年4月29日收到的书面回复称，血清hCG结果并没有被作为异常结果标示出来，该受试者也没有报告有怀孕的症状，该受试者还说明，正使用含杀精子剂和海绵的避孕套。您还说明，实验室现在已经同意标示所有升高的血清hCG结果，把升高的结果放到单独一列，用红色打印。

您的回复是不充分的，因为您的纠正措施计划不够详细。具体而言，实验室报告上血清hCG参考范围清楚地显示，任何高于5.2 mIU/mL的值均提示怀孕，您还是入组了受试者1214，但您没有提供实验室拟采用新规程的细节，以及您及您的同事将采取的具体步骤，以确保实验室报告、合格受试者的入组得到适当的审查。没有这些信息，我们不能确认您的纠正措施计划是否足以防止将来发生类似的违规情况。

我们关注的重点是，您未能充分地审查该研究的入组标准，该标准是经专门设计，旨在最大程度减少对入组受试者的可预见的伤害，使收集到的数据保持可解释性。不合格受试者的入组引起我们极大的担忧：在您的研究机构对入组的受试者的保护是否充分？在您的研究机构收集的数据可靠性如何？

本警告信的目的并非是罗列您在试验药物临床研究中存在的所有缺陷。确保遵循法律和FDA相关法规的每一项要求是您的职责，您应当解决这些缺陷，并建立规程，以确保任何正在进行或将来进行的研究均符合FDA的法规。

自收到这封信的15个工作日内，您应当书面告知本办公室为预防将来发生类似违规情况而采取的措施。如果不能充分、迅速地解释上述违规问题，可能导致我们在不再通知的情况下采取监管措施。如果您认为您已经遵循了FDA的法规要求，请陈述理由，并提供所有支持资料，以供我们参考。

附：英文原文

Gregory J. Tracey, M.D.

WARNING LETTER

DEC 16, 2015

CERTIFIED MAIL
RETURN RECEIPT REQUESTED

Ref: 16-HFD-45-10-01

Gregory J. Tracey, M.D.
315 Park Avenue
Hoboken, NJ 07030

Dear Dr. Tracey:

This Warning Letter informs you of objectionable conditions observed during the U.S. Food and Drug Administration

(FDA) inspection conducted at your clinical site between March 25 and April 15, 2015. Ms. Jonee J. Mearns and Ms. Byungja E. Marciante, representing FDA, reviewed your conduct of the following clinical investigations:

- Protocol (b)(4), "(b)(4)," and
- Protocol (b)(4), "(b)(4)."

This inspection is a part of FDA's Bioresearch Monitoring Program, which includes inspections designed to evaluate the conduct of FDA-regulated research to ensure that the data are scientifically valid and accurate, and to help ensure that the rights, safety, and welfare of the human subjects of those studies have been protected.

At the conclusion of the inspection, Ms. Mearns and Ms. Marciante presented and discussed with you Form FDA 483, Inspectional Observations. We acknowledge receipt of your April 29, 2015, written response to the Form FDA 483.

From our review of the FDA Establishment Inspection Report, the documents submitted with that report, and your written response dated April 29, 2015, we conclude that you did not adhere to the applicable statutory requirements and FDA regulations governing the conduct of clinical investigations. We wish to emphasize the following:

You failed to ensure that the investigation was conducted according to the investigational plan [21 CFR 312.60].

As a clinical investigator, you are required to ensure that your clinical investigations are conducted in accordance with the investigational plan. The investigational plan for Protocol (b)(4) requires that you verify that study subjects meet all eligibility criteria, and, in particular, that you not include subjects with a positive serum pregnancy test at screening or at check-in. You failed to adhere to these requirements.

Protocol (b)(4) specifies that subjects with a positive serum pregnancy test at screening or at check-in will not be included in the trial, and requires that you or your designee verify that subjects meet all eligibility criteria at screening and at check-in. You failed to adhere to these requirements when you enrolled into the study Subject 1214, a 22-year-old female of childbearing potential, with positive serum pregnancy tests at screening and at check-in. Specifically:

- Screening laboratory report: On December 4, 2014, Subject 1214's screening laboratory report showed clearly that the subject's serum human chorionic gonadotropin (hCG) level was 70.8 mIU/mL. That value was significantly above the reference hCG level that indicates pregnancy. You signed that laboratory report on December 4, 2015, indicating that you had reviewed the information in the report.
- Rescreening laboratory report: On December 19, 2014, Subject 1214's rescreening laboratory report showed clearly that the subject's serum hCG level was 34,833.0 mIU/mL. That value continued to be significantly above the reference hCG level that indicates pregnancy. You signed that laboratory report on December 22, 2014, indicating that you had reviewed the information in the report.
- Screening eligibility checklist: On January 2, 2015, despite these elevated serum hCG levels, you signed Subject 1214's screening eligibility checklist and indicated that Subject 1214 was eligible for study participation. That screening eligibility checklist shows the box checked "No" for whether the subject had a positive serum pregnancy test at screening or at check-in (that is, a serum hCG level above the reference level). However, your determination that Subject 1214 was eligible for study participation was contrary to the protocol, because the laboratory reports that you had signed indicated that Subject 1214 had a positive serum pregnancy test both at screening and at rescreening.
- Check-in laboratory report: On January 4, 2015, Subject 1214's check-in laboratory report showed clearly that the subject's serum hCG was 135,828.0 mIU/mL. Again, that value continued to be significantly above the reference hCG level that indicates pregnancy. You signed that laboratory report on January 5, 2015, indicating that you had reviewed the information in the report.
- Study Day 1 inclusion/exclusion summary: On January 5, 2015, you signed a statement that you had reviewed the subject's inclusion/exclusion criteria and source documentation for the study; that you acknowledged having reviewed those records in order to determine the subject's eligibility to receive study drug; and that you had determined that the subject was eligible to receive study drug. However, as noted above, your determination that Subject 1214 was eligible to receive study drug was contrary to the protocol, because the records that you had signed indicated that Subject 1214 had a positive serum pregnancy test at screening, at rescreening, and at check-in.

As a result, on January 5, 2015 (Study Day 1), the subject received two oral (b)(4) doses of (b)(4). On January 6 through January 8, 2015 (Study Days 2 through 4), the subject received one (b)(4) capsule daily.

The subject did not return to the clinic and was discontinued from the study on January 9, 2015. On January 22,

2015, the subject completed the early withdrawal/follow-up visit, and the laboratory report from that visit, which you signed, indicated that the subject's serum hCG level was 2050.0 mIU/mL.

We acknowledge your April 29, 2015, written response that serum hCG results were not flagged as being abnormal; that the subject did not report symptoms of pregnancy; and that the subject reported using condoms with spermicide and sponges. You stated that the laboratory has now agreed to flag all elevated serum hCG results, and to place elevated results in a separate column, printed in red ink.

Your response is inadequate because your corrective action plan is not sufficiently detailed. Specifically, you enrolled Subject 1214 despite the reference range for serum hCG on the laboratory reports clearly stating that any values above 5.2 mIU/mL are indicative of pregnancy, but you did not provide details regarding the laboratory's plan to use new procedures, or specifics on the steps that you and your colleagues will take to ensure the appropriate review of the laboratory's reports and the enrollment of eligible subjects. Without this information, we are unable to determine whether your corrective action plan is adequate to prevent similar violations in the future.

We emphasize our concern that you failed to fully evaluate the eligibility criteria for the study that were specifically designed to minimize foreseeable harm to enrolled subjects, and to maintain the interpretability of collected data. The enrollment of ineligible subjects raises significant concerns about the adequacy of the protection of study subjects enrolled at your site, and also raises concerns about the integrity of the data collected at your site.

This letter is not intended to be an all-inclusive list of deficiencies with your clinical study of an investigational drug. It is your responsibility to ensure adherence to each requirement of the law and relevant FDA regulations. You should address these deficiencies and establish procedures to ensure that any ongoing or future studies will be in compliance with FDA regulations.

Within fifteen (15) working days of your receipt of this letter, you should notify this office in writing of the actions you have taken to prevent similar violations in the future. Failure to address the violations noted above adequately and promptly may result in regulatory action without further notice. If you believe you have complied with FDA regulations, include your reasoning and any supporting information for our consideration.

If you have any questions, please contact Douglas Pham at 301-796-1955; FAX 301-847-8748. Your written response and any pertinent documentation should be addressed to:

Douglas Pham, Pharm.D., J.D.
Branch Chief (Acting)
Compliance Enforcement Branch
Division of Enforcement and Postmarketing Safety
Office of Scientific Investigations
Office of Compliance
Center for Drug Evaluation and Research
U.S. Food and Drug Administration
Building 51, Room 5348
10903 New Hampshire Avenue
Silver Spring, Maryland 20993

Sincerely yours,

{See appended electronic signature page}

David Burrow, Pharm.D., J.D.
Director (Acting)
Office of Scientific Investigations
Office of Compliance
Center for Drug Evaluation and Research
U.S. Food and Drug Administration

第65封　给Thomas S. Tooma医学博士的警告信

2015年11月2日

参考号：16-HFD-45-10-02

尊敬的Tooma博士：

2015年6月29日至7月17日，Diane C. Van Leeuwen女士和Vickie L. Anderson女士代表FDA，在贵临床研究机构，对您作为申办者-研究者所开展的试验药物为0.1%和0.25%核黄素滴眼液的临床研究进行了审查（在光强度为18mW/cm^{2}的眼圆锥角膜或扩张中进行光化学诱导胶原交联反应的安全性和有效性研究）。这封警告信特告知您现场检查中发现的违规情况。

本次现场检查是FDA的生物研究监查项目的一部分。该项目通过设定的检查方法，对FDA所监管的研究的实施情况进行评估，以确认研究数据在科学上是有效和准确的，并帮助确保这些研究中受试者的权益、安全和福利得到了保护。

在现场检查结束时，Leeuwen女士和Anderson女士向您出示并讨论了FDA483表，即现场检查所发现的问题。您2015年8月4日对该FDA483表的书面回复已收悉。

经对现场检查报告、该报告的附件，以及您2015年8月4日的书面回复进行审查，我们认为，您没有遵循适用的法律要求和监管临床研究实施的FDA法规。我们想强调以下几点：

1. 未能根据21 CFR 312.2（a）的要求对开展新药临床研究提交IND申请［21 CFR 312.20（a），（b）和312.40（a），（b）］

在相关条文里，联邦食品药品和化妆品法案（以下简称FD&C法案）中将药物定义为：“用于诊断、治疗、缓解、治疗或预防疾病的物品”和“非食品类的用于影响人体或其他动物的结构和功能的物品”［21 U.S.C. 321（G）］。

您研究了0.1%和0.25%的核黄素滴眼液，与紫外线A（UVA）-诱导交联的角膜胶原结合使用，用于圆锥角膜或扩张治疗的有效性。所以，因为滴眼液用于治疗圆锥角膜或扩张，根据FD&C法案对药物的定义，核黄素滴眼液属于药物。

一项新药合法化上市，按照FD&C法案 505［21U.S.C.355］的规定，申办者必须获得新药申请或者简略新药申请的批准。研究性新药申请（IND）是指申办者获得豁免这一要求来提供试验的途径［21U.S.C.355（I）］。FDA法规要求申办者开展人体药物临床研究前必须提交新药申请，除非该临床研究符合IND豁免条款。

如果以下所有豁免条款都得到满足，一个上市的药物能够豁免IND要求：

- 该药品在美国合法化上市；
- 该项研究不是为了作为向FDA汇报一项完整规范的研究，并且没有意图去使用这项研究去支持在药物标签上的任何显著变化；
- 对于一个合法化上市的处方药而言，该研究不打算支持药物广告中的显著变化；
- 该研究不涉及给药途径、剂量水平、患者人群使用或其他能够明显增加与药品使用有关的风险（或降低风险的可接受性）的因素；
- 该研究的执行符合21 CFR 56中规定的机构处理审查的要求以及21 CFR 50中规定的知情同意的要求，并且该研究的执行符合21 CFR 312.7中对于研究药物推广的规定；
- 当21 CFR 320.31中的标准得到满足，计划进行人体生物利用度和生物等效性的研究的人不需要递交IND申请。

您的研究药物——核黄素滴眼液，在美国不属于合法上市药物，也不符合IND豁免要求。所以，在临床研究中使用核黄素滴眼液之前，您必须向FDA递交IND申请，并且具有21 CFR 312.40下有效的IND。

FDA的记录显示，在开展属于本次检查的研究，即核黄素滴眼液的临床研究之前，您未向FDA递交IND申请。我们注意到您的记录显示，您在至少7个不同的试验场所入组了受试者（从2012年9月开始），使用UVA光学仪器加上0.1%或0.25%的核黄素滴眼液。

2015年8月4日，在FDA 483表的书面回复中，您说，出于人道主义或同情心的目的，为受试者提供了外科手术，并将方案和知情同意书提交伦理委员会。您说，伦理委员会、核黄素滴眼液的经销商以及其他您交谈过的眼科医生都没有告诉您，做这项研究必须有IND。但是，您承认应该联系FDA询问是否需要IND。同时您承诺，在今后，没有和FDA讨论以及足够的调查之前，您将永远不会进行临床研究。

您的答复不够充分，因为您还未针对这项被检查的研究向FDA提交IND申请。此外，作为这项研究的申办者，您必须在发起研究和入组受试者之前提交IND，并保证IND有效。

2. 您未能确保对临床研究进行适当的监查［21 CFR 312.50 和 312.56（a）］

FDA法规要求申办者确保对临床研究进行适当的监控，并保证其临床研究者按照IND中的研究计划和方案进行研究。我们的调查发现，您没有对在研项目做好适当的监控。被检查研究的相关记录表明，您没有对项目进行适当的监控。

在您2015年8月4日对FDA483表的书面回复中，您承认，您依靠外科医生去遵循方案进行试验，并且对于这项研究，您没有一个监查员。此外，您承认没有意识到这些是作为发起人需要承担的职责。

就目前的研究而言，您表示将聘请一个有经验的监查员，以确保"所有试验场所的流程和方案得到足够的监控，所有收集的数据，所有知情同意的过程都遵循相关要求等。"您也声明，在将来，会聘请一个有经验的监查员，以确保所有的研究程序都是符合规范的。

您的书面回复是不充分的，因为您没有提供监查计划，例如何时您将聘请一个有经验的监查员。因此，我们无法确定您的建议计划是否足以防止将来类似的违规行为再次发生。另外，根据21 CFR 312.52的描述，发起人只能将监管项目的责任授权给合同研究组织（CRO），而且这种责任的授权必须以书面形式予以描述。

3. 您未能保存对药物处置的完整记录，包括受试者使用药物的日期、数量、使用情况［21 CFR 312.62（a）］

作为一名临床研究者，您必须要保存足够的药物处置记录，包括受试者使用药物日期，数量和使用情况。您没有遵守这一要求。具体来说，您未能保留在七个研究场所任何接受角膜横链接治疗和一个或两个眼睛接受核黄素滴眼液受试者的任何药物使用记录。

在2015年8月4日对FDA 483表的书面回复中，您提及您没有意识到您需要保留药物的处置记录。您表示，在将来，您将保留核黄素滴眼液的药物处置记录。

您的书面回复是不充分的，因为您没有解决为了目前研究，或作为一个研究者在未来研究中，将如何保留药物处置记录的问题。因此，我们无法确定将来是否不会再发生类似的违规行为。

本警告信并非是罗列您在试验药物临床研究中存在的所有缺陷。确保遵循法律和相关FDA法规的每一项要求是您的职责，您应当解决这些缺陷，并建立规程，以确保任何正在进行或将来进行的研究均符合FDA的法规。

自收到这封信的15个工作日内，您应当书面告知本办公室为预防将来发生类似违规情况而采取的措施。如果不能充分、迅速地解释上述违规问题，可能导致我们在不再通知的情况下采取监管措施。如果您认为您已经遵循了FDA的法规要求，请陈述理由，并提供所有支持资料，以供我们参考。

附：英文原文

Thomas S. Tooma, M.D.

WARNING LETTER

Nov 02, 2015

CERTIFIED MAIL
RETURN RECEIPT REQUESTED
November 2, 2015

Ref: 16-HFD-45-10-02

Thomas S. Tooma, M.D.
NVISION Laser Eye Centers
3501 Jamboree Road, Suite 1100
Newport Beach, California 92660-2956

Dear Dr. Tooma:

This Warning Letter informs you of objectionable conditions observed during the U.S. Food and Drug Administration (FDA) inspection conducted at your clinical site between June 29 and July 17, 2015. Ms. Diane C. Van Leeuwen and Ms. Vickie L. Anderson, representing FDA, reviewed your conduct as the sponsor- investigator of a clinical investigation ("Study of the Safety and Effectiveness of Photochemically Induced Collagen Cross-Linking at an Irradiance of 18 mW/cm^2 in Eyes with Keratoconus or Ectasia") for the investigational drug riboflavin ophthalmic solution (0.1% and 0.25%).

This inspection is a part of the FDA's Bioresearch Monitoring Program, which includes inspections designed to evaluate the conduct of FDA-regulated research to ensure that the data are scientifically valid and accurate, and to help ensure that the rights, safety, and welfare of the human subjects of those studies have been protected.

At the conclusion of the inspection, Ms. Van Leeuwen and Ms. Anderson presented and discussed with you Form FDA 483, Inspectional Observations. We acknowledge receipt of your August 4, 2015, written response to the Form FDA 483.

From our review of the FDA Establishment Inspection Report, the documents submitted with that report, and your August 4, 2015, written response, we conclude that you did not adhere to the applicable statutory requirements and FDA regulations governing the conduct of clinical investigations. We wish to emphasize the following:

1. You failed to submit an IND for the conduct of a clinical investigation with an investigational new drug that is subject to 21 CFR 312.2(a) [21 CFR 312.20(a), (b) and 312.40(a), (b)].

In relevant part, the Federal Food, Drug, and Cosmetic Act (FD&C Act) defines the term *drug* as "articles intended for use in the diagnosis, cure, mitigation, treatment, or prevention of disease" and "articles (other than food) intended to affect the structure or function of the body of man or other animals" [21 U.S.C. 321(g)].

You studied the efficacy of 0.1% and 0.25% riboflavin ophthalmic solutions, in combination with ultraviolet-A (UVA)-induced cross-linking of corneal collagen, for the treatment of keratoconus or ectasia. As a result, because the ophthalmic solution was intended for the treatment of keratoconus or ectasia, riboflavin ophthalmic solution meets the definition of a drug under the FD&C Act.

To market a new drug lawfully, a sponsor must obtain approval of a new drug application or an abbreviated new drug application under Section 505 of the FD&C Act [21 U.S.C. 355]. An Investigational New Drug application (IND) is the means by which a sponsor obtains an exemption from this requirement to distribute an investigational drug [21 U.S.C. 355(i)]. FDA regulations require a sponsor to submit an IND application before conducting a clinical investigation of a drug in human subjects, unless the clinical investigation qualifies for an IND exemption.

A marketed drug product is exempt from the IND requirements if all of the following exemption criteria are met:

The drug product is lawfully marketed in the United States;

- The investigation is not intended to be reported to FDA as a well-controlled study in support of a new indication for use, and there is no intent to use the investigation to support any other significant change in the labeling of the drug;
- In the case of a lawfully marketed prescription drug, the investigation is not intended to support a significant change in the advertising for the drug;
- The investigation does not involve a route of administration, dosage level, use in a patient population, or other factor that significantly increases the risks (or decreases the acceptability of the risks) associated with the use of the drug product;
- The investigation is conducted in compliance with the requirements for institutional review set forth in 21 CFR part 56 and with the requirements for informed consent set forth in 21 CFR part 50; and
- The investigation is conducted in compliance with the requirements of 21 CFR 312.7 regarding promotion of investigational drugs.

A person planning to conduct an in vivo bioavailability or bioequivalence study is not required to submit an IND when certain criteria under 21 CFR 320.31 are met.

Your investigational drug, riboflavin ophthalmic solution, is not a lawfully marketed drug product in the United States, nor is it exempt from IND requirements. As a result, before using riboflavin ophthalmic solution in a clinical investigation, you were required to submit an IND for the drug to FDA, and to have an IND that had gone into effect under 21 CFR 312.40.

FDA records indicate that you failed to submit an IND before conducting the investigation under the inspected study, a clinical investigation of riboflavin ophthalmic solution. We note that your records show human subjects were enrolled at a minimum of seven different sites, to participate in a clinical investigation (initiated in September 2012) with the UVA light device plus riboflavin ophthalmic solution 0.1% or 0.25%.

In the August 4, 2015, written response to the Form FDA 483, you indicated that you offered the surgical procedure for humanitarian/compassionate-use purposes, and that you submitted protocols and informed consent documents to an IRB. You stated that the IRB, the distributor of the riboflavin ophthalmic solution, and other ophthalmologists with whom you spoke did not inform you that an IND was required to conduct this study. You acknowledged, however, that you should have contacted FDA about whether an IND was required. You stated that in the future, you will never conduct a clinical study without adequate due diligence, including discussion with FDA.

Your response is inadequate because you have not yet submitted an IND application to FDA for the inspected study. In addition, as the sponsor of the inspected study, you were required to submit an IND and to have an IND that had gone into effect before initiating and enrolling human subjects into this study.

2. You failed to ensure proper monitoring of the clinical investigations [21 CFR 312.50 and 312.56(a)].

FDA regulations require that sponsors ensure proper monitoring of clinical investigations, and ensure that their clinical investigators conduct the investigations in accordance with the general investigational plan and protocols contained in the IND. Our investigation found that you failed to ensure proper monitoring of the inspected study. The records associated with the inspected study do not indicate that proper monitoring was performed.

In your August 4, 2015, written response to the Form FDA 483, you acknowledged that you depended on the surgeons to conduct the trial according to protocol, and that you did not have a monitor for this study. In addition, you acknowledged that you were not aware of all that was required of you as a sponsor.

You stated that for the current study, you will hire an experienced monitor to ensure that "all the procedures/protocol in all sites are adequately monitored, all data collected, all consent procedures are followed, etc." You also stated that in the future, you will hire an experienced monitor to ensure that all study procedures are precisely followed.

Your written response is inadequate because you did not provide your proposed monitoring plan, including a timeline for when the experienced monitor would be hired. As a result, we are unable to determine whether your proposed plan appears sufficient to prevent similar violations in the future. In addition, please note that a sponsor may transfer its obligation to monitor a study to a contract research organization only, and any such transfer of obligations must be described in writing [21 CFR 312.52].

3. You failed to maintain adequate records of the disposition of the drug, including dates, quantity, and use by subjects [21 CFR 312.62(a)].

As a clinical investigator, you are required to maintain adequate records of the disposition of the drug, including dates, quantity, and use by subjects. You failed to comply with this requirement. Specifically, you failed to maintain drug disposition records for any of the subjects at the seven study sites who underwent corneal cross-linking and received riboflavin ophthalmic solution in one or both eyes.

In the August 4, 2015, written response to the Form FDA 483, you stated that you were not aware that you needed to maintain records of the disposition of the drug. You indicated that in the future, you will maintain drug disposition records for riboflavin ophthalmic solution.

Your written response is inadequate because you did not address how you will maintain drug disposition records for the current study, or for future studies in which you serve as a clinical investigator. As a result, we are unable to determine whether similar violations will be prevented in the future.

This letter is not intended to be all-inclusive list of deficiencies with your clinical study of an investigational drug. It is your responsibility to ensure adherence to each requirement of the law and relevant FDA regulations. You should address these deficiencies and establish procedures to ensure that any ongoing or future studies will be in compliance with FDA regulations.

Within fifteen (15) working days of your receipt of this letter, you should notify this office in writing of the actions you have taken or will take to prevent similar violations in the future. Failure to explain the violations noted above adequately and promptly may result in regulatory action without further notice. If you believe that you have complied with FDA regulations, include your reasoning and any supporting information for our consideration.

If you have any questions, please contact Chrissy J. Cochran, Ph.D., at 301-796-5633; FAX 301-847-8748. Your written response and any pertinent documentation should be addressed to:

Chrissy J. Cochran, Ph.D.
Acting Division Director
Division of Enforcement and Postmarketing Safety
Office of Scientific Investigations
Office of Compliance
Center for Drug Evaluation and Research
Food and Drug Administration
Building 51, Room 5364
10903 New Hampshire Avenue
Silver Spring, MD 20993

Sincerely yours,

/S/

David C. Burrow, Pharm.D., J.D.
Acting Office Director
Office of Scientific Investigations
Office of Compliance
Center for Drug Evaluation and Research
Food and Drug Administration

第66封　给Michlin, Bernard A.医学博士的警告信

2015年7月13日

参考号：15-HFD-45-07-01

尊敬的Michlin博士：

2015年1月8日至1月23日，Allen Hall先生代表FDA，在您的临床研究场所，对您所开展的以下临床研究进行了审查：

试验方案（b）（4）[1]，“（b）（4）”，试验药物为（b）（4），申办者为（b）（4）。

试验方案（b）（4），“（b）（4）”，试验药物为（b）（4），申办者为（b）（4）。

这封警告信特告知您FDA现场检查中发现的违规情况。

本次现场检查是FDA的生物研究监查项目的一部分。该项目通过设定的检查方法，对FDA所监管的研究的实施情况进行评估，以确认研究数据在科学上是有效和准确的，并帮助确保这些研究中受试者的权益、安全和福利得到了保护。

在现场检查结束时，Allen Hall先生向您出示了FDA483表，即现场检查发现的问题，并与您进行了讨论。您2015年2月10日对该FDA483表的书面回复已收悉。

经对现场检查报告、该报告的附件，以及您2015年2月10日的书面回复进行审查，我们认为，您没有遵循适用的法律要求和监管临床研究实施的FDA法规。我们想强调以下几点：

您未能确保您的研究按照研究计划进行［21 CFR 312.60］

作为临床研究者，您必须确保您的临床研究按照研究计划进行。研究计划要求，筛选访视包括实验室安全性检查和尿液药物筛选。您没有遵循这些要求。具体而言：

a. 试验方案（b）（4）要求筛查访视包括受试者血液的安全性的实验室检查（包括病毒学、血液学和临床化学）。以下受试者的血液筛查样本没有被收集：

ⅰ. 受试者614005。

ⅱ. 受试者614009。

ⅲ. 受试者614015。

ⅳ. 受试者614016。

ⅴ. 受试者614017。

ⅵ. 受试者614019。

ⅶ. 受试者614022。

ⅷ. 受试者614023。

我们获知，您在2015年2月10日对以上a.条款中ⅰ，ⅱ和ⅲ项的书面回复中，您表示将定期使用有一个质量保证内部图表审查工具来确保研究所需的流程都已经完成。我们同样获知，您2015年2月10日对上述a.ⅵ.项书面回复中，您表示文档来源的标准操作规程（SOP）已被更新，包括做过的所有实验室检查的特定记录。但是，尽管在您回复中承诺了一些的纠正措施，但您没有特别针对未能收集方案要求的筛选血液样本的问题提出解决意见。

---

1 （b）（4）涉及商业秘密，根据法规内容不予公开。

您的回复不够充分，因为您没有向我们提供用来监管您进行的研究的标准操作规程的书面资料。此外，您没有提供任何您和您的工作人员有关在研方案和样本处理的培训内容的任何细节。没有这些信息，我们无法确认您的纠正措施计划是否能够在将来避免类似的违背情况再次发生。

我们发现，在给您的FDA 483表中，我们没有列出a条款中ⅳ、ⅴ、ⅶ和ⅷ项，因此，您对FDA 483表的书面回复没有涉及这些问题。

b. 试验方案（b）（4）要求在筛选和第1，2，3，4，5，15，22，29和36天进行尿液药物筛查，没有做尿液药物筛查的如下：

ⅰ. 受试者614011，在第1，2天没做尿液药物筛查。

ⅱ. 受试者614014，在筛查阶段没做尿液药物筛查。

ⅲ. 受试者614019，在第2～4，8，22或29天没做尿液药物筛查。

ⅳ. 受试者614020，在第1～4，8，15，22，29或36天没做尿液药物筛查。

ⅴ. 受试者614024，在第2，3天没做尿液药物筛查。

我们获知，您2015年2月10日对于以上b.ⅱ. 项的书面回复中表示您将定期进行核对，以确保研究所需的流程都已经完成。但是，您的回复没有特别针对未能实施方案要求的尿液药物筛查问题提出解决意见。

我们也发现，在您2015年2月10日对b.ⅲ. 项的书面回复中提到，当获知这些问题时，中断了受试者参加扩展研究［研究（b）（4）］。同时，您还更新了文档来源的标准操作规程（SOP），其中包含了所有做过实验室检查的特定记录。但是，我们注意到，尽管缺失尿液药物筛查，您还让受试者继续完成了研究，并且还将其纳入到了扩展研究中去。

您的回复不够充分，因为您没有向我们提供用来监管您开展的研究的标准操作规程的书面资料。此外，您没有提供任何您和您的工作人员有关在研方案和样本处理的培训的任何细节。没有这些信息，我们无法确认您的纠正措施是否能够在将来避免类似的违背情况再次发生。

我们承认，在给您的FDA 483表中我们没有列出b条款中ⅰ，ⅳ和ⅴ项，因此，您对FDA 483表的书面回复没有涉及这些问题。

未按照方案履行安全性的实验室筛选和尿液药物筛查这一点，危害了受试者的安全和福利，损害了在您的场所收集的研究数据的有效性和真实性。

本警告信的目的并非是罗列您在试验药物临床研究中存在的所有缺陷。确保遵循法律和相关FDA法规的每一项要求是您的职责，您应当解决这些缺陷，并建立规程，以确保任何正在进行或将来进行的研究均符合FDA的法规。

自收到这封信的15个工作日内，您应当书面告知本办公室为预防将来发生类似违规情况而采取的措施。如果不能充分、迅速地解释上述违规问题，可能导致我们在不再通知的情况下采取监管措施。如果您认为您已经遵循了FDA的法规要求，请陈述理由，并提供所有支持资料，以供我们参考。

附：英文原文

Michlin, Bernard A., M.D.

WARNING LETTER

JUL 13, 2015

CERTIFIED MAIL
RETURN RECEIPT REQUESTED

Ref: 15-HFD-45-07-01

Bernard A. Michlin, M.D.
6367 Alvarado Court, #200
San Diego, CA 92120

Dear Dr. Michlin:

This Warning Letter informs you of objectionable conditions observed during the U.S. Food and Drug Administration (FDA) inspection conducted at your clinical site between January 8 and January 23, 2015. Mr. Allen Hall, representing FDA, reviewed your conduct of the following clinical investigations:

- Protocol **(b)(4)**, "**(b)(4)**," of the investigational drug **(b)(4)**, performed for **(b)(4)**; and
- Protocol **(b)(4)**, "**(b)(4)**," of the investigational drug **(b)(4)**, performed for **(b)(4)**.

This inspection is a part of FDA's Bioresearch Monitoring Program, which includes inspections designed to evaluate the conduct of FDA-regulated research to ensure that the data are scientifically valid and accurate, and to help ensure that the rights, safety, and welfare of the human subjects of those studies have been protected.

At the conclusion of the inspection, Mr. Hall presented and discussed with you Form FDA 483, Inspectional Observations. We acknowledge receipt of your February 10, 2015, written response to the Form FDA 483.

From our review of the FDA Establishment Inspection Report, the documents submitted with that report, and your written response dated February 10, 2015, we conclude that you did not adhere to the applicable statutory requirements and FDA regulations governing the conduct of clinical investigations. We wish to emphasize the following:

You failed to ensure that the investigation was conducted according to the investigational plan [21 CFR 312.60].

As a clinical investigator, you are required to ensure that your clinical investigations are conducted in accordance with the investigational plan. The investigational plan requires that the screening visit include safety laboratory tests and urine drug screens. You failed to adhere to these requirements. Specifically:

a. Protocol **(b)(4)** requires the screening visit to include safety laboratory tests (including virology, hematology, and clinical chemistry) of the subjects' blood. Screening blood samples were not collected for the following subjects:

i. Subject 614005
ii. Subject 614009
iii. Subject 614015
iv. Subject 614016
v. Subject 614017
vi. Subject 614019
vii. Subject 614022
viii. Subject 614023

We acknowledge your February 10, 2015, written response to Items a.i., a.ii., and a.iii. above, in which you state that a Quality Assurance Internal Chart Review Tool will be used periodically to ensure that protocol-required procedures are being completed. We also acknowledge your February 10, 2015, written response to Item a.vi. above, in which you state that source documentation standard operating procedures (SOPs) were updated to include specific documentation of all laboratory tests performed. However, although you promised certain corrective measures in your response, you did not specifically address your failure to collect the protocol-specified screening blood samples.

Your response is inadequate because you did not provide documentation of the SOPs you will use for oversight of the studies you conduct. In addition, you did not provide any details of the in-service protocol and specimen-handling training for you and your staff. Without this information, we are unable to determine whether your corrective action plan is adequate to prevent similar violations in the future.

We recognize that Items a.ⅳ.,a.ⅴ., a.ⅶ., and a.ⅷ. above were not listed on the Form FDA 483 that was issued to you, and as a result, your written response to the Form FDA 483 does not address these issues.

b. Protocol **(b)(4)** requires that a urine drug screen be performed at screening and on Days 1, 2, 3, 4, 8, 15, 22, 29, and 36. Urine drug screens were not performed as follows:

ⅰ. For Subject 614011, no urine drug screens were performed on Days 1 or 2.

ⅱ. For Subject 614014, no urine drug screen was performed at screening.

ⅲ. For subject 614019, no urine drug screens were performed on Days 2-4, 8, 22, or 29.

ⅳ. For Subject 614020, no urine drug screens were performed on Days 1-4, 8, 15, 22, 29, or 36.

ⅴ. For Subject 614024, no urine drug screens were performed on Days 2 or 3.

We acknowledge your February 10, 2015, written response to Item b.ⅱ., in which you state that periodic checks will be performed to ensure that protocol-required procedures are being completed. However, your response did not specifically address your failure to perform these urine drug screens as the protocol required.

We also acknowledge your February 10, 2015, written response to Item b.ⅲ., in which you state that when these deficiencies were noted, the subject was discontinued from the extension study (Study **(b)(4)**), and that source documentation SOPs were updated to include specific documentation of all laboratory tests performed. However, we note that despite the deficient urine drug screens, you allowed the subject to complete the study; furthermore, you enrolled the subject in the extension study.

Your response is inadequate because you did not provide documentation of the SOPs you will use for oversight of the studies you conduct. In addition, you did not provide any details of the in-service protocol and specimen-handling training for you and your staff. Without this information, we are unable to determine whether your corrective action plan is adequate to prevent similar violations in the future.

We recognize that Items b.ⅰ., b.ⅳ. and b.ⅴ. above were not listed on the Form FDA 483 that was issued to you, and as a result, your written response to the Form FDA 483 does not address these issues.

Failure to perform screening safety laboratory tests and urine drug screens according to the protocol jeopardizes subject safety and welfare, and compromises the validity and integrity of the data collected at your site.

This letter is not intended to be an all-inclusive list of deficiencies with your clinical study of an investigational drug. It is your responsibility to ensure adherence to each requirement of the law and relevant FDA regulations. You should address these deficiencies and establish procedures to ensure that any ongoing or future studies will be in compliance with FDA regulations.

Within fifteen (15) working days of your receipt of this letter, you should notify this office in writing of the actions you have taken to prevent similar violations in the future. Failure to address the violations above adequately and promptly may result in regulatory action without further notice. If you believe that you have complied with FDA regulations, include your reasoning and any supporting information for our consideration.

If you have any questions, please contact Allen Lou at 301-796-5652; FAX 301-847-8748. Your written response and any pertinent documentation should be addressed to:

Allen Lou
Acting Branch Chief
Compliance Enforcement Branch
Division of Enforcement and Postmarketing Safety
Office of Scientific Investigations
Office of Compliance

Center for Drug Evaluation and Research
U.S. Food and Drug Administration
Building 51, Room 5260
10903 New Hampshire Avenue
Silver Spring, MD 20993

Sincerely yours,

{See appended electronic signature page}

Sean Y. Kassim, Ph.D.
Director
Office of Scientific Investigations
Office of Compliance
Center for Drug Evaluation and Research
U.S. Food and Drug Administration

This is a representation of an electronic record that was signed electronically and this page is the manifestation of the electronic signature.

/S/

SEAN Y KASSIM
07/13/2015

第 67 封　给 Gross, Howard M. 医学博士的警告信

2015年6月29日

参考号：15-HFD-45-06-02

尊敬的Gross博士：

2014年11月19日至2015年1月14日，Richard W. Berning先生代表FDA，在贵临床研究中心，对您所开展的以下临床研究进行了审查：

- 试验方案（b）（4）[1]，试验药物（b）（4），申办者（b）（4）；
- 试验方案（b）（4），试验药物（b）（4），申办者（b）（4）和（b）（4）。

这封警告信特告知您FDA现场检查中发现的违规情况。

本次现场检查是FDA的生物研究监查项目的一部分。该项目通过设定的检查方法，对FDA监管的研究的实施情况进行评估，以确认研究数据在科学上是有效和准确的，并帮助确保这些研究中受试者的权益、安全和福利得到了保护。

在现场检查结束时，Berning先生向您出示了FDA483表，即现场检查发现的问题，并与您进行了讨论。您2015年1月28日对该FDA483表的书面回复已收悉。

经对现场检查报告、该报告的附件，以及您2015年1月28日的书面回复进行审查，我们认为，您没有遵循适用的法律要求和监管临床研究实施及受试者保护的FDA法规。我们想强调以下几点：

1. 您未能确保按照研究计划进行研究［21 CFR 312.60］

作为临床研究者，您必须保证临床研究按研究计划进行。试验方案（b）（4）的研究计划要求您确保研究使受试者在入组前满足研究方案的入排标准。您没有遵守这些要求。具体而言：

a. 对于试验方案（b）（4）您未能确保研究受试者在入组前满足研究方案的入排标准。

i. 试验方案（b）（4）规定，对蛋白尿≥2+或尿蛋白肌酐比值≥0.5的受试者，应获取24小时尿蛋白，24小时尿蛋白的水平必须＜1g蛋白质才能入组。受试者2102的尿蛋白水平为37.1mg/dL，临床上被认为是2+的尿蛋白水平（＜100mg/dL），但没有进行24小时尿液检测。此受试者是2012年5月17日被随机进入临床研究。

ii. 试验方案（b）（4）规定，接受非甾体抗炎剂或其他抗血小板剂长期治疗，包括氯吡格雷治疗的受试者，将不能入组临床研究。受试者2100在2012年1月3日至3月2日期间服用过波立维（氯吡格雷）。但该受试者2012年2月6日被随机进入本临床研究。

在您2015年1月28日对上述1.a.中记录违规行为的书面回复中，您同意受试者2102和2100没有符合合格标准。您表示，作为您纠正措施计划的一部分，您制定了一个标准操作规程（SOP），“二次合格检查”，其中规定研究人员将在受试者入组前核查合格标准。

您的回复是不充分的，虽然您表示您的SOP“二次合格检查”已付诸实施，并且您的研究协调员也深知这个要求，但是您没有提供您的研究人员对这个SOP文件已进行充分培训的培训记录。如果没有这样的文件，我们无法确定您的纠正措施计划是否足以防止今后发生类似的违规行为。

每个临床研究的合格标准旨在优化收集的数据的可解释性，并尽量减少对入组受试者可预见的危害。不符合入排标准的受试者入组，将危及受试者的安全和福利，并引起对在贵研究中心所收集的研究数据的有效性和完整性的关注。特别让我们关注的是，在贵研究中心随机到试验方案（b）（4）的5名受试者中有2名受

1 (b) (4) 涉及商业秘密，根据法规内容不予公开。

试者被入组，尽管他们不符合临床研究的标准。

b. 试验方案（b）(4）规定，研究药物（b）(4）的给予需超过90（±10）分钟，且受试者给药后至少观察30分钟。在观察期之后，给予研究药物（b）(4）/安慰剂。任何输液相关的症状在给予研究药物（b）(4）/安慰剂之前一定要解决。

i. 您按相反的顺序给予了一名受试者研究药物。受试者006，在研究访视周期4~7和10~12中先给予了研究药物（b）(4）/安慰剂输注后再给予研究药物（b）(4）输注。

不遵守研究方案中规定的给药顺序有可能影响数据完整性和受试者的安全和福利。

ii. 您对所有入组的受试者在以下的研究访视中没有遵守在给予研究药物（b）(4）/安慰剂治疗前所要求的30分钟观察期。

（1）受试者001：周期1和周期2。

（2）受试者：003。

a. 周期2~7和周期9~14。

b. 周期8：没有观察期；在研究药物（b）(4）输注结束前1分钟给予研究药物（b）(4）/安慰剂。

（3）受试者006：周期2和周期3。

（4）受试者007：周期10~14。

在2015年1月28日对上述1.b.记录的违规行为的书面回复中，您确认受试者006有5个治疗周期的研究药物给药顺序与方案相反。您也证实4名受试者的多次治疗周期中没有遵循方案中要求的观察期。您表示作为您纠正错误的一部分，您培训了研究人员，在开始给予研究药物前审查研究方案顺序，并和输液护士一起审查输液要求。

您的回复是不充分的，因为它不包含足够的细节。具体来说，目前还不清楚研究人员和输液的护士是否在试验启动前就方案要求进行了充分的培训，或仅在每个受试者给药前进行了培训。因此，我们无法确定您的纠正措施是否足以预防今后发生类似的违规行为。

不能遵守方案中的给药要求，包括相反的给药顺序和没有方案中的特别观察期，这些都严重危及受试者的安全和福利，并引起了对在您的研究中心收集的试验数据的有效性和完整性的关注。

c. 试验方案（b）(4）要求在基线筛查、在周期4，8和9-X、在总结访视时及30天后续随访期做凝血功能实验室检查。根据方案（b）(4)，凝血功能检查包括凝血酶原时间（PT或INR）和部分凝血活酶时间（PTT）。您对5名接受试验药物治疗的受试者中的4名受试者，在以下指定的时间间隔中没有做凝血功能实验室检查：

i. 受试者2100：周期4和周期8~17。

ii. 受试者2102：周期4。

iii. 受试者2104：周期4，8和周期13~17。

Ⅳ. 受试者2105：周期1，4，8~15，17，19，20，22和周期23。

d. 试验方案（b）(4）要求在筛选期、在蒽环类抗生素治疗期间、在周期1~5，9和18周期的第1天前的3天内，以及在治疗结束时安全随访期做肝功能检查。试验方案（b）(4）中肝功能检查包括碱性磷酸酶ALP、ASAT、ALAT、LDH，以及总胆固醇、直接和间接胆红素。您所有入组的受试者在以下指定的时间间隔中没有做所有或部分肝功能检查。

i. 受试者001：筛选期和周期1，2：直接胆红素和间接胆红素。

ii. 受试者003：（1）周期1：所有肝功能。

（2）周期2~5，9，18：直接胆红素和间接胆红素。

（3）周期3：ASAT，ALAT和ALP。

（4）周期2，4，9：LDH。

iii. 受试者006：（1）周期6, 9：所有肝功能。

（2）周期1，2，4，5：直接胆红素和间接胆红素。

（3）周期2：LDH。

ⅳ. 受试者007：筛查期和周期2～5：直接胆红素和间接胆红素。

e. 试验方案（b）（4）要求在筛查期、在蒽环类抗生素治疗期间、在周期1～9，13和18周期的第1天前的3日内及在治疗结束时安全随访期做生化检查。试验方案（b）（4）中生化实验室检查包括血清肌酐、尿素氮（BUN）和电解质（磷、钙、镁、钠、钾和氯）。您入组的4名受试者中有3名受试者在以下指定的时间间隔中没有做所有或部分生化实验室检查。

ⅰ. 受试者003：（1）周期1，7：全部生化检查。

（2）周期3：血肌酐，血液尿素氮，钙、氯、钠、钾。

（3）周期4，6，8：磷。

（4）周期6，8：镁。

ⅱ. 受试者006：（1）周期9：所有生化检查。

（2）周期2，5，6：磷。

ⅲ. 受试者007：（1）周期2，8，9：磷。

（2）周期8：镁。

在2015年1月28日对上述1.c、1.d.和1.e.记录的违规书面回复中，您确认入组方案（b）（4）和（b）（4）的临床研究的受试者遗漏了研究方案要求的实验室检查。您表示，作为纠正措施的一部分，您已经增加了“临床试验链接”到贵临床现场的电子医疗记录（EMR）上，给研究人员提供研究信息。您进一步表示，您将与研究人员审查访问研究信息的程序和遵循研究日程表的重要性。

您的回复是不充分的，因为您没有提供充分的证明，使我们评估用于在任何未来临床研究中纠正措施计划的适合性。还不清楚如何增加一个“临床试验链接”到贵临床现场的EMR上，以确保在贵临床现场进行的研究满足研究方案的要求。您没有提供任何纠正措施计划的细节来防止将来发生类似的违规行为，也没有提供实施额外措施和程序计划的足够细节，以应对检查结果。没有这些细节，我们无法确定您的纠正措施是否足以预防今后发生类似的违规行为。

如上详述，您没有按照试验计划进行研究。具体来说，入组了不符合入排标准的受试者；没有按给药方案的要求使用研究药物；还有未执行方案要求的实验室检查，这些都危及受试者的安全和福利，并引起了对在贵临床现场收集的数据的有效性和完整性的关注。

2. 您未能保存对研究中使用试验药物或对照组的受试者的所有研究观察结果和其他相关数据的足够及准确的病历［21 CFR 312.62（b）］

作为临床研究者，您必须准备和保存对研究中使用试验药物或对照组的受试者的所有研究观察结果和其他相关数据的足够及准确的病历。对于试验方案（b）（4），这些病历包括了记录严重不良事件的原始文件。在试验方案（b）（4）中，严重不良事件被定义为需要住院治疗的不良事件。您未能保存这些研究记录的足够和准确的病历。

具体来说，一个电话记录显示，2012年6月6日，您的研究协调员注意到受试者001已经住院。然而，病程记录显示研究协调员于2012年6月13日才被通知受试者001住院。对这一矛盾之处没有书面解释。

这一点令我们特别关注，因为试验方案（b）（4）要求您意识到严重不良事件后，24小时内报告给申办者。申办者于2012年6月15日得到这起严重不良事件的通知，但是由于您在事件日期上的出入，我们不能评估您是否遵循了这个方案的要求。

我们承认，从书面文字看，这种违规行为没有包括在您收到的FDA 483表中。

您没有保存足够和准确的病历记录，包括上述提到的与严重不良事件相关文档上日期的偏差，引起了对在您的临床现场收集的试验数据的有效性和完整性的关注。

本警告信的目的并非是罗列您在试验药物临床研究中存在的所有缺陷。确保遵循法律和相关FDA法规的每一项要求是您的职责，您应当解决这些缺陷，并建立规程，以确保任何正在进行或将来进行的研究均符合FDA法规。

自收到这封信的15个工作日内，您应当书面告知本办公室为预防将来发生类似违规情况而采取的措施。如果不能充分、迅速地解释上述违规问题，可能导致我们在不再通知的情况下采取监管措施。如果您认为您已经遵循了FDA的法规要求，请陈述理由，并提供所有支持资料，以供我们参考。

附：英文原文

Gross, Howard M. M.D.

WARNING LETTER

Jun 29, 2015

CERTIFIED MAIL
RETURN RECEIPT REQUESTED

Ref: 15-HFD-45-06-02

Howard M. Gross, M.D.
Dayton Clinical Oncology Program
3123 Research Boulevard
Suite 150
Dayton, OH 45240

Dear Dr. Gross:

This Warning Letter informs you of objectionable conditions observed during the U.S. Food and Drug Administration (FDA) inspection conducted at your clinical site between November 19, 2014, and January 14, 2015. Mr. Richard W. Berning, representing FDA, reviewed your conduct of the following clinical investigations:

- Protocol (b)(4) of the investigational drug (b)(4), performed for (b)(4); and
- Protocol (b)(4) of the investigational drug (b)(4), performed for (b)(4). and (b)(4).

This inspection is a part of FDA's Bioresearch Monitoring Program, which includes inspections designed to evaluate the conduct of FDA-regulated research to ensure that the data are scientifically valid and accurate, and to help ensure that the rights, safety, and welfare of the human subjects of those studies have been protected.

At the conclusion of the inspection, Mr. Berning presented and discussed with you Form FDA 483, Inspectional Observations. We acknowledge receipt of your January 28, 2015, written response to the Form FDA 483.

From our review of the FDA Establishment Inspection Report, the documents submitted with that report, and your written response dated January 28, 2015, we conclude that you did not adhere to the applicable statutory requirements and FDA regulations governing the conduct of clinical investigations and the protection of human subjects. We wish to emphasize the following:

1. You failed to ensure that the investigation was conducted according to the investigational plan [21 CFR 312.60].

As a clinical investigator, you are required to ensure that your clinical investigations are conducted in accordance with the investigational plan. The investigational plan for Protocol (b)(4) required you to ensure that study subjects met the protocol inclusion and exclusion criteria before their enrollment. You failed to adhere to these requirements. Specifically:

a. For Protocol (b)(4), you failed to ensure that study subjects met the protocol inclusion and exclusion criteria before their enrollment.

i. Protocol (b)(4) specified that for subjects with proteinuria ≥ 2+ or urine protein creatinine ratio ≥0.5, a 24-hour urine protein should be obtained and the level must be <1 gram of protein in 24-hour urine to be eligible for enrollment. Subject 2102 had a protein level of 37.1 mg/dL, which is clinically considered 2+ protein (≤100 mg/dL). However, a 24-hour urine test was not performed. This subject was randomized into the clinical investigation on May 17, 2012.

ii. Protocol (b)(4) specified that subjects receiving chronic therapy with nonsteroidal antiinflammatory agents or other antiplatelet agents, including clopidogrel, will not be enrolled into the clinical investigation. Subject 2100 was taking Plavix (clopidogrel) between January 3, 2012, and March 2, 2012. However, this subject was randomized into this clinical investigation on February 6, 2012.

In your January 28, 2015, written response to the violations noted in Item 1.a., you agreed that Subjects 2102 and 2100 did not meet the eligibility criteria. You indicated that as part of your corrective action plan, you developed a standard operating procedure (SOP), "Second Eligibility Check," which specifies that study staff will verify that eligibility criteria are met prior to enrollment.

Your response is inadequate because, although you stated that your SOP "Second Eligibility Check" has been put into effect and that your research coordinators are well aware of this requirement, you failed to provide documentation that your research staff have been adequately trained in this SOP. Without such documentation, we are unable to determine whether your corrective action plan appears sufficient to prevent similar violations in the future.

The eligibility criteria for each clinical investigation are designed to optimize interpretability of collected data and to minimize foreseeable harm to enrolled subjects. Enrollment of subjects who do not meet the eligibility criteria jeopardizes subject safety and welfare, and raises concern about the validity and integrity of the data collected at your site. Particularly concerning to us is that two of the five subjects randomized into Protocol (b)(4) at your site were enrolled despite their being ineligible for the clinical investigation.

b. Protocol (b)(4) specified that (b)(4) will be administered over 90 (±10) minutes, and that subjects will be observed post-administration for at least 30 minutes. After this observation period, (b)(4)/placebo will be administered. Any infusion-related symptoms must have resolved before the administration of (b) (4)/placebo.

i. You administered the study drugs in reverse order for one subject. For Subject 006, (b) (4)/placebo infusion was followed by (b)(4) infusion at the following study visits: Cycles 4, 7, and 10-12.

Failure to follow the protocol-specified order of study drug administration has the potential to affect both data integrity and subjects' safety and welfare.

ii. You failed to adhere to the required 30-minute observation period before administering (b)(4)/placebo for all subjects enrolled in this clinical investigation at the following study visits:

1. For Subject 001:
   Cycles 1 and 2
2. For Subject 003:
   a. Cycles 2-7 and 9-14
   b. Cycle 8: No observation period was performed; (b)(4)/placebo was administered one minute before the (b)(4) infusion was stopped.
3. For Subject 006: Cycles 2 and 3
4. For Subject 007: Cycles 10-14

In your January 28, 2015, written response to the violations noted in Item 1.b. above, you confirmed that the order of administration of study drugs was reversed for five of Subject 006's treatment cycles. You also confirmed that observation periods were not followed for multiple treatment cycles for four subjects. You indicated that as part of your corrective action plan, you trained study staff to review protocol orders and infusion requirements with infusion nurses before starting study drug administration.

Your response is inadequate because it does not contain sufficient detail. Specifically, it is unclear whether study staff and infusion nurses would be adequately trained on protocol requirements before initiating the study, or only before study drug administration for each subject. As a result, we are unable to determine whether your corrective action appears sufficient to prevent similar violations in the future.

Failure to adhere to protocol requirements for study drug administration, including reversing the order of administration of study drugs and failure to follow the protocol-specified observation period, compromises subject safety and welfare significantly, and raises concerns about the validity and integrity of the data collected at your site.

Protocol (b)(4) required coagulation profile laboratory tests to be performed at baseline; at Cycles 4, 8, and 9-x; at the summary visit; and at the 30-day follow-up visit. For Protocol (b)(4), the coagulation profile included prothrombin time (PT or INR) and partial thromboplastin time (PTT). You failed to perform coagulation profile laboratory tests for four of the five subjects that received study drug at the following specified intervals:

i. For Subject 2100: Cycles 4 and 8-17

ii. For Subject 2102: Cycle 4

iii. For Subject 2104: Cycles 4, 8, and 13-17

iv. For Subject 2105: Cycles 1,4, 8-15, 17, 19, 20, 22, and 23

d. Protocol (b)(4) required that liver function tests be performed at screening; during the anthracyclines treatment period; within 3 days prior to Day 1 of Cycles 1-5, 9, and 18; and at safety follow-up at the end of treatment. For Protocol (b)(4), the liver function tests include ALP; ASAT; ALAT; LDH; and total, direct, and indirect bilirubin. You failed to perform all or certain liver function tests for all of the subjects enrolled at the following specified intervals:

i. For Subject 001, at screening and Cycles 1 and 2: direct and indirect bilirubin

ii. For Subject 003:

1. At Cycle 1: all liver function tests
2. At Cycles 2-5, 9, and 18: direct and indirect bilirubin
3. At Cycle 3: ASAT, ALAT, and ALP
4. At Cycles 2, 4, and 9: LDH

iii. For Subject 006:

1. At Cycles 6 and 9: all liver function tests
2. At Cycles 1, 2, 4, and 5: direct and indirect bilirubin
3. At Cycle 2: LDH

iv. For Subject 007, at screening and Cycles 2-5: direct and indirect bilirubin

e. Protocol (b)(4) required that biochemistry laboratory tests be performed at screening; during the anthracyclines treatment period; within 3 days prior to Day 1 of Treatment Cycles 1-9, 13, and 18; and at safety follow-up at the end of treatment. For Protocol (b)(4), biochemistry laboratory tests included serum creatinine, blood urea nitrogen (BUN), and electrolytes (phosphorus, calcium, magnesium, sodium, potassium, and chloride). You failed to perform all or certain biochemistry laboratory tests for three of the four subjects enrolled at the following specified intervals:

i. For Subject 003:

1. At Cycles 1 and 7: all biochemistry laboratory tests
2. At Cycle 3: serum creatinine, BUN, calcium, chloride, sodium, and potassium
3. At 3.Cycles 4, 6, and 8: phosphorus
4. At Cycles 6 and 8: magnesium

ii. For Subject 006:

1. At Cycle 9: all biochemistry laboratory tests
2. At Cycles 2, 5, and 6: phosphorus

iii. For Subject 007:

1. At Cycles 2, 8, and 9: phosphorus
2. At Cycle 8: magnesium

In your January 28, 2015, written response to the violations noted in Items 1.c., 1.d., and 1.e. above, you confirmed that protocol-required laboratory tests were missed for subjects enrolled in the clinical investigations for Protocols (b)(4) and (b)(4). You indicated that as a part of your corrective action plan, you have added a "clinical trials link" to your site's electronic medical record (EMR) to provide access to study information for study staff. You further indicated that you will review with study staff the process of accessing study information and the importance of following the study calendar.

Your response is inadequate because you did not provide sufficient information to enable us to evaluate the adequacy of your corrective action plan for use in any future clinical research that you may conduct. It is unclear how adding a "clinical trials link" to your site's EMR will ensure that protocol requirements will be met for studies conducted at your site. You did not provide any details of a corrective action plan to prevent similar violations from occurring in the future, nor have you provided sufficient details regarding your plan to implement additional measures and procedures to address the inspection findings. Without these details, we are unable to determine whether your corrective action plan appears sufficient to prevent similar violations in the future.

As detailed above, you failed to conduct the investigation in accordance with the investigational plan. Specifically, your enrollment of subjects who do not meet eligibility criteria; your failure to adhere to protocol requirements for study drug administration; and your failure to perform protocol-required laboratory tests jeopardize subject safety and welfare, and raise concerns about the validity and integrity of the data collected at your site.

2. You failed to maintain adequate and accurate case histories that record all observations and other data pertinent to the investigation on each individual administered the investigational drug or employed as a control in the investigation [21 CFR 312.62(b)].

As a clinical investigator, you are required to prepare and maintain adequate and accurate case histories that record all observations and other data pertinent to the investigation on each individual administered the investigational drug or employed as a control in the investigation. For Protocol (b)(4), these case histories include source documents recording serious adverse events. For Protocol (b)(4), a serious adverse event was defined as an adverse event requiring inpatient hospitalization. You failed to maintain adequate and accurate case histories with respect to these study records.

Specifically, a telephone record shows that on June 6, 2012, your study coordinator was made aware that Subject 001 had been hospitalized. However, a progress note shows that the study coordinator was notified on June 13, 2012, of Subject 001's hospitalization. There is no documented explanation for this discrepancy.

This is particularly concerning to us because Protocol (b)(4) required that serious adverse events be reported to the sponsor within 24 hours of your becoming aware of the event. The sponsor was notified of this serious adverse event on June 15, 2012. However, because of the discrepancy in the date of your awareness of the event, we were unable to evaluate whether you adhered to this protocol requirement.

We acknowledge that this violation, as written, was not included on the Form FDA 483 that you received.

Your failure to maintain adequate and accurate case histories, including the aforementioned discrepancies in the dates on documentation related to serious adverse events, raises concerns about the validity and integrity of data captured at your site.

This letter is not intended to be an all-inclusive list of deficiencies with your clinical study of an investigational drug. It is your responsibility to ensure adherence to each requirement of the law and relevant FDA regulations. You should address these deficiencies and establish procedures to ensure that any ongoing or future studies will be in compliance with FDA regulations.

Within fifteen (15) working days of your receipt of this letter, you should notify this office in writing of the actions you have taken to prevent similar violations in the future. Failure to address the violations noted above adequately and promptly may result in regulatory action without further notice. If you believe you have complied with FDA regulations, include your reasoning and any supporting information for our consideration.

If you have any questions, please contact Allen Lou at 301-796-5652; FAX 301-847-8748. Your written response and any pertinent documentation should be addressed to:

Allen Lou
Acting Branch Chief
Compliance Enforcement Branch
Division of Enforcement and Postmarketing Safety
Office of Scientific Investigations
Office of Compliance
Center for Drug Evaluation and Research
U.S. Food and Drug Administration

Building 51, Room 5260
10903 New Hampshire Avenue
Silver Spring, MD 20993

Sincerely yours,

{See appended electronic signature page}

Sean Y. Kassim, Ph.D.
Director
Office of Scientific Investigations
Office of Compliance
Center for Drug Evaluation and Research
U.S. Food and Drug Administration

This is a representation of an electronic record that was signed electronically and this page is the manifestation of the electronic signature.

--/S/

SEAN Y KASSIM
06/29/2015

第68封　给Binh Bui-Nguyen医学博士的警告信

2015年5月4日

参考号：15-HFD-45-05-01

尊敬的Bui博士：

2014年9月17日至2014年9月19日，Barbara D. Wright女士和Ni A. Khin医学博士代表FDA，在贵临床研究中心，对您所开展的试验药物为（b）（4）[1]，申办者为（b）（4）的以下临床研究进行了审查：

- 试验方案（b）（4），“（b）（4）”；
- 试验方案（b）（4），“（b）（4）”。

这封警告信特告知您FDA现场检查中发现的违规情况。

本次现场检查是FDA的生物研究监查项目的一部分。该项目通过设定的检查方法，对FDA监管研究的实施情况进行评估，以确认研究数据在科学上是有效和准确的，并帮助确保这些研究中受试者的权益、安全和福利得到了保护。

在现场检查结束时，Wright女士和Khin医生向您出示了FDA483表，即现场检查发现的问题，并与您进行了讨论。您2014年10月2日对该FDA483表的书面回复已收悉。

经对现场检查报告、该报告的附件，以及您2014年10月2日的书面回复进行审查，我们认为，您没有遵循适用的法律要求和监管临床研究实施的FDA法规。我们想强调以下几点：

您未能确保研究按照研究计划进行［21 CFR 312.60］

作为临床试验研究者，您必须确保研究按研究计划进行。试验方案（b）（4）的研究计划要求有关血液学实验室检查、生化［包括甲状腺刺激激素（TSH）］和尿常规在预定的时间点进行，并且严重不良事件（SAE）需在指定的时间内报告。同样，对于试验方案（b）（4）的研究计划也要求与血液学相关的实验室检查在预定的时间点进行，并且，严重不良事件（SAE）需在指定的时间内报告。对于这两个临床试验，如果受试者经历某些列举的不良事件，包括肾衰竭，应遵循治疗方案调整的规定。您没有遵守这些方案要求。这种方案违背的例子包括，但不限于以下：

1. 试验方案（b）（4）和（b）（4）规定法国的受试者在筛选时需进行血液学实验室检查：基线，第1，2，3，4，5，6，7，8，10，12周和此后每4周，直到和包括研究结束/最后访视

两个方案中的血液学实验室检查包括血细胞比容和血红蛋白、红细胞计数、白细胞总计数，包括嗜中性粒细胞、淋巴细胞、单核细胞、嗜酸性粒细胞和嗜碱性粒细胞，血小板计数，凝血酶原时间，部分凝血酶原时间和国际标准化比。这些血液学实验室检查是研究中的安全评估项目，因为它们被用于监测药物（b）（4）相关的不良事件，如中性粒细胞减少，受试者将根据其严重程度调整剂量或者停药。不能及时诊断中性粒细胞减少，将使受试者增加严重感染和败血症的风险。因此，方案要求的血液学实验室检查漏检，将危及受试者的安全。具体而言：

a. 试验方案（b）（4）中的受试者033-008-03第20周的血液学实验室检查未做。

b. 试验方案（b）（4）中的受试者033-008-04第5，6，7周的血液学实验室检查未做。

c. 试验方案（b）（4）中的受试者033-008-05第20周的血液学实验室检查未做。

d. 试验方案（b）（4）中的受试者1302第1周的血液学实验室检查未做。

1 (b)(4) 涉及商业秘密，根据法规内容不予公开。

2014年10月2日对FDA 483表的书面回复中，您表示这些漏做的实验室检查主要是因为受试者的依从性差。您表明每次访视都会给受试者开实验室检查的医嘱。您提到解决受试者依从性差的纠正措施包括电话通知受试者和临床访视期间口头提醒。

您的答复是不充分的，因为您没有提供关于纠正措施计划的充分细节。您没有提供您努力解决受试者依从性差问题的原始记录文件（例如，电话或临床访问期间口头提醒）。如果没有记录这些细节，我们无法确定您的纠正措施计划是否足以防止今后再发生类似的违规行为。

我们承认，在上面1.a. 项提到的调查结果（受试者033-008-03）未包括在您收到的FDA 483表中，因此您的书面回复并没有解决这一问题。

2. 试验方案（b）（4）要求在筛选期在基线，第4、8、12、16和24周，以及此后每12周进行尿试纸检测，直至研究结束/最后访问。尿试纸检测包括红细胞、白细胞和尿蛋白的检测。如果试验上检测到尿蛋白≥ 30mg/dL时则需收集24小时尿液检测蛋白质含量。在这项研究中，尿试纸检测是用于监测研究药物（b）（4）相关的肾功能障碍的安全评估。研究方案要求，基于受试者显示在试纸上试验测量被暂停尿蛋白≥ 30mg/dL的次数和24小时尿蛋白＞ 1.5g /24小时的确认，研究药物（b）（4）剂量被暂停减量或停药。因此，方案要求的尿试纸监测的漏检将危及受试者的安全，因为受试者可能患与药物（b）（4）相关的肾脏疾病。具体而言：

a. 受试者033-008-06第8周的尿试纸检测未做。

b. 受试者033-008-02第36周的24小时尿液收集未做。这个受试者尿试纸检测尿蛋白是30mg/dL。2014年10月2日对FDA 483表的书面回复中，您表明受试者033-008-02第36周有出血迹象，尿蛋白30mg/dL是由于术后长期导尿引起的泌尿系统感染。在您的书面回复中也表明未做的实验室检查主要是因为受试者依从性差。您指出每次访视都会给受试者实验室检查的医嘱。您解释说，针对受试者依从性差的纠正措施，包括电话通知受试者和临床访视期的口头提醒。

您的回复是不充分的，虽然受试者033-008-02尿液中有血，但是根据方案，受试者也在其尿液中有一个蛋白水平，需要收集24小时尿液。您没有提交关于应对24小时尿液收集漏做的纠正措施计划。此外，您没有提供您努力解决受试者依从性差问题的原始记录文件（例如，电话或临床访问期间口头提醒）。如果没有记录这些细节，我们无法确定您的纠正措施计划是否足以防止今后再发生类似的违规行为。

我们承认，在上面2.a.项提到的调查结果（受试者033-008-06）未包括在您收到的FDA 483表中，因此您的书面回复并没有解决这一问题。

3. 试验方案（b）（4）要求在检测TSH基线水平，在第24周，此后每24周，直至并包括试验结束/最后访视时检测TSH。TSH是这项研究中的安全评估项目。具体而言：

a. 受试者033-008-02第48和72周TSH检测未做。

b. 受试者033-008-03第24周TSH检测未做。

c. 受试者033-008-04试验结束时TSH检测未做。

2014年10月2日在对FDA 483表的书面回复中，您表示未做的实验室检查主要是因为受试者依从性差。您表明每次访视都会给受试者实验室检查的医嘱。您解释说，针对受试者依从性差的纠正措施包括电话通知受试者和临床访视期的口头提醒。

您的回复是不充分的，因为您没有提供关于纠正措施计划细节。您没有提供您努力解决受试者依从性差问题的原始记录文件（例如，电话或临床访问期间口头提醒）。如果没有记录这些细节，我们无法确定您的纠正措施计划是否足以防止今后再发生类似的违规行为。

我们承认在上面提到的3.a.项调查结果（受试者033-008-02）和3.b.项调查结果（受试者033-008-03）未包括在您收到的FDA 483表中，因此您的书面回复并没有解决这一问题。

4. 试验方案（b）（4）要求，如果发生以下三个事件之一需要调整（b）（4）治疗：

- 尿试纸上蛋白≥30mg/dL，24小时尿蛋白＞1.5g/24h证实。
- 肌酐清除率＜50mL/min（Cockcroft-Gault公式）。

● 尿素＞2倍正常值上限。

如果发生上述三个事件之一时，研究方案要求研究药物（b）（4）被暂停，直至升高的水平恢复至基线，然后研究药物（b）（4）在相同的剂量重新开始。如果上述三个事件之一第二次发生，研究药物（b）（4）将被暂停，直至升高的水平恢复至基线，然后研究药物（b）（4）的剂量以减少1.5mg/（kg·d）（即新的剂量是6mg/（kg·d））重新开始。如果上面提到的三个事件之一第三次发生，研究药物（b）（4）将被永久停止。不遵守上述的治疗方案修改规则将危及受试者的安全，受试者可能发展为（b）（4）相关的肾脏疾病。

2013年1月16日，方案（b）（4）中的受试者1313的肌酐基线水平是0.5mg/dL。2013年2月27日，该受试者的肌酐清除率为49.7mL/min（Cockcroft-Gault公式）；因此，方案要求（b）（4）治疗被暂停，直至肾功能恢复到基线水平。然而并没有这样做。于2013年3月13日，受试者的肌酐水平增加到1.6mg/dL，表明肾功能恶化。2013年3月18日上午，给予受试者（b）（4）终剂量，当天受试者因疾病进展停止试验。

在您2014年10月2日对FDA 483表的书面回复中，您指出受试者2级肾功能不全与“体液潴留，主要有腹水及下腔静脉受压和肿瘤的发展。”相关。您还表示“这一肾功能不全是没有威胁的”，并表示为了受试者的最佳利益，“持续忽略肾功能不全”是医学选择。

您的回复是不够的，因为肾功能不全的病因不是遵守方案中对肾脏疾病调整治疗方案的一个因素，您没有提供一个纠正措施计划来解决这个问题。没有描述您将如何遵守方案中对肾脏疾病调整治疗方案的纠正措施计划，我们无法确定未来是否可以预防类似的方案违规行为。

5. 试验方案（b）（4）和（b）（4）要求严重不良事件（SAE），无论是否与研究药物相关，都要以SAE表报告，并将在下一工作日结束前[方案（b）（4）]或在事件发生或研究者知晓的24小时内[方案（b）（4）]将表传真至申办者，即使事件与治疗不相关。在研究开始前计划的手术和其他侵入性操作不需要SAE报告。

试验方案（b）（4）和（b）（4）定义了SAE为：任何剂量导致死亡的意外医学事件；危及生命；需要住院治疗或延长住院时间；导致持续或显著残疾/无工作能力；先天性异常/出生缺陷；或可能危及受试者的健康其他重要的医学状况或可能需要干预的不良医学事件。

在方案规定的时间内没有报告给申办者的SAE实例包括，但不限于以下：

a. 在试验方案（b）（4）中，受试者033-008-05从2013年10月3日到10月10日经历了Ⅲ级皮肤毒性，您的授权研究人员在2013年10月10日病程记录中记录了受试者皮肤毒性。但贵研究中心直到2013年11月21日才把皮肤毒性以SAE表报告给申办者。

b. 在试验方案（b）（4）中，受试者1302住院并接受因为3级贫血来自（b）（6）的输血。您的授权研究人员在日期为（b）（6）的病程记录中记录了受试者住院。但贵研究中心直到2010年8月26日才把住院以SAE表报告给申办者。

c. 在试验方案（b）（4）中，受试者1311因膝关节炎并发静脉炎而在（b）（6）进行手术。您在2013年3月15日病程记录中记录了受试者手术。但贵研究中心直到2013年4月10日才把住院以SAE表报告给申办者。在您对FDA483表的回复中，您说明这手术未在研究开始前计划。因此，手术应该已根据方案要求的时间以SAE表报告。

在您2014年10月2日对FDA 483表中关于受试者1302和1311的书面回复中，您表示没有及时报告严重不良事件发生的事件数量有限，且被质疑的严重不良事件是与研究药物治疗不相关的事件。

尽管您随后和申办者讨论了受试者1302的贫血问题，并试图收集有关受试者1311手术的更多详细信息，但这些严重不良事件必须在方案规定时间内报告，且不论是否与研究药物有关它们都将被报告。此外，在初步SAE报告提交后，应提交后续SAE报告，附加受试者1311的手术信息。您的回复是不充分的，因为您没有提供一个纠正措施计划解决您将如何遵守方案规定的 SAE报告要求。如果没有纠正措施计划，我们无法确定是否将来可以预防类似的方案违规行为。

我们承认在上面提到5.a. 项调查结果（受试者033-008-05）未包括在您收到的FDA 483表中，因此您的书面回复并没有解决这一问题。

如上详述，您未能按照试验方案进行这两个临床研究。具体来说，您未能进行方案要求的评估；您没有遵守肾脏疾病的调整治疗规则；您没有在方案规定时间内将严重不良反应（SAE）报告给申办者，这些错误危害了受试者的安全，并且损害贵试验现场获得的试验数据的有效性和完整性。

本警告信的目的并非是罗列您在试验药物临床研究中存在的所有缺陷。确保遵循法律和相关FDA法规的每一项要求是您的职责，您应当解决这些缺陷，并建立规程以确保任何正在进行或将来进行的研究均符合FDA的法规。

自收到这封信的15个工作日内，您应当书面告知本办公室为预防将来发生类似违规情况而采取的措施。如果不能充分、迅速地解释上述违规问题，可能导致我们在不再通知的情况下采取监管措施。如果您认为您已经遵循了FDA的法规要求，请陈述理由，并提供所有支持资料，以供我们参考。

附：英文原文

Binh Bui-Nguyen, M. D.

WARNING LETTER

May 4, 2015

CERTIFIED MAIL
RETURN RECEIPT REQUESTED

Ref: 15-HFD-45-05-01

Binh Bui Nguyen, M.D.
Institut Bergonié
229 cours de l'Argonne – CS 61283
33076 Bordeaux Cédex
France

Dear Dr. Bui:

This Warning Letter informs you of objectionable conditions observed during the U.S. Food and Drug Administration (FDA) inspection conducted at your clinical site between September 17 and September 19, 2014. Ms. Barbara D. Wright and Ni A. Khin, M.D., representing FDA, reviewed your conduct of the following clinical investigations of the investigational drug (b)(4), performed for (b)(4):

- Protocol (b)(4), "(b)(4)"
- Protocol (b)(4), "(b)(4)"

This inspection is a part of FDA's Bioresearch Monitoring Program, which includes inspections designed to evaluate the conduct of FDA-regulated research to ensure that the data are scientifically valid and accurate, and to help ensure that the rights, safety, and welfare of the human subjects of those studies have been protected.

At the conclusion of the inspection, Ms. Wright and Dr. Khin presented and discussed with you Form FDA 483, Inspectional Observations. We acknowledge receipt of your October 2, 2014, written response to the Form FDA 483.

From our review of the FDA Establishment Inspection Report, the documents submitted with that report, and your written response dated October 2, 2014, we conclude that you did not adhere to the applicable statutory requirements and FDA regulations governing the conduct of clinical investigations. We wish to emphasize the following:

You failed to ensure that the investigation was conducted according to the investigational plan [21 CFR 312.60].

As a clinical investigator, you are required to ensure that investigations are conducted in accordance with the investigational plan. The investigational plan for Protocol (b)(4) required that laboratory tests related to hematology, biochemistry [including thyroid stimulating hormone (TSH)], and urinalysis be performed at scheduled time points, and that serious adverse events (SAEs) be reported within a specified time frame. Similarly, the investigational plan for Protocol (b)(4) required that laboratory tests related to hematology be performed at scheduled time points, and that SAEs be reported within a specified time frame. For both trials, treatment modification rules were required to be followed if subjects experienced certain enumerated adverse events, including renal failure. You failed to adhere to these protocol requirements. Examples of this failure include, but are not limited to, the following:

1. Protocols (b)(4) and (b)(4) require that subjects in France undergo hematologic laboratory tests at Screening; Baseline; Weeks 1, 2, 3, 4, 5, 6, 7, 8, 10, and 12; and every four weeks thereafter, up to and including the End of Study/Final Visit.

The hematologic laboratory tests for both protocols include hematocrit and hemoglobin; red blood cell count; total and differential white blood cell counts, including neutrophils, lymphocytes, monocytes, eosinophils, and basophils; platelet count; prothrombin time; partial thromboplastin time; and international normalized ratio. These hematologic laboratory tests are safety assessments in the studies, because they are used to monitor for (b)(4)-related adverse events such as neutropenia, for which subjects will have their doses interrupted or discontinued, depending on its severity. Failure to diagnose neutropenia in a timely manner places subjects at increased risk of developing serious infections and sepsis. Therefore, missed protocol-required hematologic laboratory tests compromise subject safety. Specifically:

a. Subject 033-008-03 in Protocol (b)(4) missed hematologic laboratory tests at Week 20.

b. Subject 033-008-04 in Protocol (b)(4) missed hematologic laboratory tests at Weeks 5, 6, and 7.

c. Subject 033-008-05 in Protocol (b)(4) missed hematologic laboratory tests at Week 20.

d. Subject 1302 in Protocol (b)(4) missed hematologic laboratory tests at Week 1.

In your October 2, 2014, written response to the Form FDA 483, you indicated that these missed laboratory tests were mainly due to subject noncompliance. You stated that orders for laboratory tests were given to the subjects at each visit. You noted that corrective measures to address subject noncompliance taken at the time included phone calls to subjects and oral reminders during the following clinical visit.

Your response is inadequate because you have not provided sufficient details about your corrective action plan. You have not provided adequate documentation of your efforts to address subject noncompliance (e.g., phone calls, oral reminders during the following clinical visit) in the source records. Without those details in the records, we are unable to determine whether your corrective action plan is adequate to prevent similar violations in the future.

We acknowledge that the finding noted in Item 1.a above (Subject 033-008-03) was not included on the Form FDA 483 you received, and that therefore, your written response does not address this finding.

2. Protocol (b)(4) requires that a urine dipstick test be performed at Screening; Baseline; Weeks 4, 8, 12, 16, and 24; and every 12 weeks thereafter, up to and including the End of Study/Final Visit. The urine dipstick test includes measurement of blood, leukocytes, and protein. A 24-hour urine collection to measure protein is performed if protein ≥30 mg/dL is detected on the dipstick. In this study, the urine dipstick test is a safety assessment that is used to monitor for (b)(4)-related renal disorders, and the study protocol requires that a subject's (b)(4) dose be interrupted, reduced, or discontinued, based on the number of times a subject experiences protein ≥30 mg/dL on the dipstick and confirmed by 24-hour urinary protein >1.5 g/24 hours. Therefore, missed protocol-required urine dipstick tests compromise subject safety, because subjects can develop (b)(4)-related renal disorders. Specifically:

a. Subject 033-008-06 missed the urine dipstick test at Week 8.

b. Subject 033-008-02 missed the 24-hour urine collection at Week 36. This subject's protein on the urine dipstick measured 30 mg/dL.

In your October 2, 2014, written response to the Form FDA 483, you indicated that the Week 36 urine protein of 30 mg/dL for Subject 033-008-02 showed traces of blood due to a urinary infection from prolonged urethral catheterization following surgery. You also indicated in your written response that missed laboratory tests were mainly due to subject noncompliance. You stated that orders for laboratory tests were given to the subjects at each visit. You noted that corrective measures taken at the time to address subject noncompliance included phone calls to subjects and oral reminders during the following clinical visit.

Your response is inadequate because, although Subject 033-008-02 had blood in the urine, the subject also had a level of protein in the urine that required a 24-hour urine collection, according to the protocol. You have not submitted a corrective action plan to address missed 24-hour urine collections. In addition, you have not provided adequate documentation of your efforts to address subject noncompliance (e.g., phone calls, oral reminders during the following clinical visit) in the source records. Without those details in the records, we are unable to determine whether your corrective action plan is adequate to prevent similar violations in the future.

We acknowledge that the finding noted in Item 2.a above (Subject 033-008-06) was not included on the Form FDA 483 you received, and that therefore, your written response does not address this finding.

3. Protocol (b)(4) requires that TSH be performed at Baseline, Week 24, and every 24 weeks thereafter, up to and including the End of Study/Final Visit. TSH is a safety assessment in the study. Specifically:

a. Subject 033-008-02 missed TSH collection at Weeks 48 and 72.

b. Subject 033-008-03 missed TSH collection at Week 24.

c. Subject 033-008-04 missed TSH collection at End of Study.

In your October 2, 2014, written response to the Form FDA 483, you indicated that missed laboratory tests were mainly due to subject noncompliance. You stated that orders for laboratory tests were given to the subjects at each visit. You noted that corrective measures taken at the time to address subject noncompliance included phone calls to subjects and oral reminders during the following clinical visit.

Your response is inadequate because you have not provided sufficient details about your corrective action plan. You have not provided adequate documentation of your efforts to address subject noncompliance (e.g., phone calls, oral reminders during the following clinical visit) in the source records. Without those details in the records, we are unable to determine whether your corrective action plan is adequate to prevent similar violations in the future.

We acknowledge that the findings noted in Items 3.a (Subject 033-008-02) and 3.b (Subject 033-008-03) above were not included on the Form FDA 483 you received, and that therefore, your written response does not address these findings.

4. Protocol (b)(4) requires that (b)(4) treatment be altered if one of the following three events occurs:

- Protein ≥30 mg/dL on the urine dipstick, confirmed by 24-hour protein >1.5 g/24 hours.
- Creatinine clearance <50 mL/min (Cockcroft and Gault formula).
- Urea >2 times the upper limit of normal.

If one of the three events noted above occurs, the study protocol requires that (b)(4) be interrupted until the noted level returns to baseline, and (b)(4) will then be restarted at the same dose. If one of the three events noted above occurs a second time, (b)(4) will be interrupted until the noted level returns to baseline, and (b)(4) will then restarted with a dose reduction of 1.5 mg/kg/day (i.e., the new dose will be 6 mg/kg/day). If one of the three events noted above occurs a third time, (b)(4) will be permanently discontinued. Failure to adhere to the treatment modification rules noted above compromises subject safety, because subjects can develop (b)(4)-related renal disorders.

On January 16, 2013, Subject 1313 in Protocol (b)(4) had a baseline creatinine level of 0.5 mg/dL. This subject's creatinine clearance on February 27, 2013, was 49.7 mL/min (Cockcroft and Gault formula); therefore, the protocol required that (b)(4) treatment be interrupted until a return to baseline renal function. This action was not taken, however. On March 13, 2013, the subject's creatinine level had increased to 1.6 mg/dL, indicating worsening renal function. The subject's final dose of (b)(4) was given on the morning of March 18, 2013, and the subject was discontinued from the study on the same day due to progressive disease.

In your October 2, 2014, written response to the Form FDA 483, you indicated that the subject's grade 2 renal insufficiency was "considered related to a major fluid retention, mainly with ascites and inferior vena cava compression, related to tumor evolution." You also indicated that "this functional renal deficiency was considered non-threatening," and that "continuation despite renal functional dysfunction was a medical choice" in the subject's best interest.

Your response is inadequate because the cause of renal insufficiency is not a factor in adhering to the protocol's treatment modification rules for renal disorders, and you have not provided a corrective action plan to address this issue. Without a corrective action plan describing how you will adhere to protocol specified treatment modification rules for renal disorders, we are unable to determine whether similar violations will be prevented in the future.

5. Protocols (b)(4) and (b)(4) require that SAEs, whether they are considered related to study drug or not, will be reported on an SAE form and will be faxed to the sponsor by the end of the next working day (Protocol (b)(4)) or within 24 hours (Protocol (b)(4)) of occurrence or investigator's knowledge of the event, even if the event does not appear to be treatment-related. SAE reporting is not required for surgeries and other invasive procedures planned before the start of the study.

Protocols (b)(4) and (b)(4) define an SAE as any untoward medical occurrence that at any dose results in death; is life-threatening; requires inpatient hospitalization or prolongation of existing hospitalization; results in persistent or significant disability/incapacity; is a congenital anomaly/birth defect; or is another important medical condition that may jeopardize the subject's health or may require intervention to prevent one of the preceding outcomes.

Examples of SAEs that were not reported to the sponsor within the protocol-required time frames include, but are not limited to, the following:

a. Subject 033-008-05 in Protocol (b)(4) experienced grade Ⅲ skin toxicity from October 3 to October 10, 2013. Your sub-investigator noted the subject's skin toxicity in a progress note dated October 10, 2013. However, your site did not report the skin toxicity to the sponsor on a SAE form until November 21, 2013.

b. Subject 1302 in Protocol (b)(4) was hospitalized and received blood transfusions for grade 3 anemia from (b)(6). Your sub-investigator noted the subject's hospitalization in a progress note dated (b) (6). However, your site did not report the hospitalization to the sponsor on a SAE form until August 26, 2010.

c. Subject 1311 in Protocol (b)(4) had surgery on (b)(6), for knee arthritis complicated by an episode of phlebitis. You noted the subject's surgery in a progress note dated March 15, 2013. However, your site did not report the hospitalization to the sponsor on an SAE form until April 10, 2013. In your response to the FDA Form 483, you state that this surgery was not planned before the start of the study. Therefore, the surgery should have been reported as an SAE form according to the protocol-specified time frame (i.e., within 24 hours).

In your October 2, 2014, written response to the Form FDA 483 concerning Subjects 1302 and 1311, you indicated that the failure to report SAEs in a timely manner occurred in a limited number of cases, and the SAEs in question were not events related to study drug treatment.

While you subsequently discussed Subject 1302's anemia with the sponsor and attempted to gather more details about Subject 1311's surgery, these SAEs were required to be reported within the protocol-specified time frames, and they were to be reported regardless of relationship to study drug. Also, a follow-up SAE report could have been submitted with additional information about Subject 1311's surgery after the initial SAE report was submitted. Your response is inadequate because you have not provided a corrective action plan addressing how you will adhere to protocol-specified SAE reporting requirements. Without a corrective action plan, we are unable to determine whether similar violations will be prevented in the future.

We acknowledge that the finding noted in Item 5.a above (Subject 033-008-05) was not included on the Form FDA 483 you received, and that therefore, your written response does not address this finding.

As detailed above, you failed to conduct these two investigations in accordance with the investigational plans. Specifically, you failed to perform protocol-required assessments; you failed to adhere to treatment modification rules for renal disorders; and you failed to report SAEs to the sponsor within protocol-specified time frames. These failures jeopardized subject safety and compromised the validity and integrity of data captured at your site.

This letter is not intended to be an all-inclusive list of deficiencies with your clinical study of an investigational drug. It is your responsibility to ensure adherence to each requirement of the law and relevant FDA regulations. You should address these deficiencies and establish procedures to ensure that any ongoing or future studies will be in compliance with FDA regulations.

Within fifteen (15) working days of your receipt of this letter, you should notify this office in writing of the actions

you have taken to prevent similar violations in the future. Failure to address the violations noted above adequately and promptly may result in regulatory action without further notice. If you believe you have complied with FDA regulations, include your reasoning and any supporting information for our consideration.

If you have any questions, please contact Khin M. U, M.D., at 301-796-1156; Fax 301-847-8748. Your written response and any pertinent documentation should be addressed to:

Khin M. U, M.D.
Acting Branch Chief
Compliance Enforcement Branch
Division of Enforcement and Postmarketing Safety
Office of Scientific Investigations
Office of Compliance
Center for Drug Evaluation and Research
U.S. Food and Drug Administration
Building 51, Room 5210
10903 New Hampshire Avenue
Silver Spring, MD 20993

Sincerely yours,

{See appended electronic signature page}

Sean Y. Kassim, Ph.D.
Director
Office of Scientific Investigations
Office of Compliance
Center for Drug Evaluation and Research
U.S. Food and Drug Administration

第 69 封　给 Taber, Louise A. 医学博士的警告信

2014年10月9日

参考号：14-HFD-45-10-01

尊敬的Taber博士：

2014年7月7日至18日，Sonia R. Peterson女士代表FDA，在您的临床研究场所，对您所开展的试验药物为重酒石酸氢可酮，申办者为Purdue Pharma L.P公司的以下临床研究进行了审查：

- 试验方案HYD3002，“一项多中心，随机，双盲，与安慰剂对照的开放研究以评估在中度至重度慢性腰痛受试者中酒石酸氢可酮（HYD）片剂20～120mg，每日一次的有效性和安全性。”
- 试验方案HYD3003，“一项开放、多中心研究，以评估在中-重度慢性非恶性和非神经病理性疼痛受试者中酒石酸氢可酮（HYD）片剂20～120mg，每日一次的长期安全性。”。

这封警告信特告知您现场检查中发现的违规情况。

本次现场检查是FDA的生物研究监查项目的一部分。该项目通过设定的检查方法，对FDA所监管的相关研究的实施情况进行评估，以确认研究数据在科学上是有效和准确的，并确保这些研究中受试者的权益、安全和福利得到了保护。

在现场检查结束时，Peterson女士向您出示了FDA483表，即现场检查发现的问题，并与您进行了讨论。您2014年8月1日对该FDA483表的书面回复已收悉。

经对现场检查报告、该报告的附件，以及您2014年8月1日的书面回复进行审查，我们认为，您没有遵循适用的法律要求和监管临床研究实施的FDA法规。我们想强调以下几点：

1. 您未能保存对研究中使用试验药物或对照组的受试者的所有研究观察结果和其他相关数据的足够及准确的病历［21 CFR 312.62（b）］

作为临床研究者，您必须准备和保存记录在该研究中每个给予研究药物或作为对照组的个体的研究相关的所有观察和其他数据的足够及准确的病历，包括所有观察数据及与试验相关的其他数据。方案HYD3003中病历包括气导纯音听力检测报告。对这些报告您没有保存足够和准确的病历。

具体而言，在现场检查期间，审查了19名受试者的记录，对其中4名受试者，代表这些受试者的报告的气导纯音听力检测报告是其他受试者的原始报告。在听力检测报告中，原始的受试者鉴认代码和访视日期被黑色标记笔涂黑，并且随后在这些报告中添加手写的受试者鉴认代码和与原始的受试者鉴认代码不一致的访视日期。

a. 受试者3045003，代表该受视者的访视2（2011年8月31日）和访视3（2011年9月22日）的报告的听力测试报告是其他受试者原始的，模糊的听力测试报告。

i. 2011年8月31日访视2的听力测试报告是受试者3045026的原始报告。值得注意的是，录入受试者3045003的电子病例报告表（eCRF）的访试2的听力测试结果与受试者3045026 eCRF的访视2的结果完全一致。

ii. 2011年9月22日访视3的听力检测报告是受试者3045040的原始报告。值得注意的是，录入受试者3045003的电子病例报告表（eCRF）的访视3的听力结果与受试者3045040 eCRF的访视2的结果完全一致。

b. 受试者3045005，代表该受试者的访视2（2011年9月6日）和访视3（2011年9月21日）的报告的听力测试报告是其他受试者的原始的、模糊的听力测试报告。

i. 2011年9月6日访视2的听力检测报告是受试者3045012的原始报告。值得注意的是，录入受试者

3045005的eCRF的访视2的听力测试报告结果与受试者3045012 eCRF中的访视3的结果完全一致。

ⅱ. 2011年9月21日访视3的听力检测报告是受试者3045016的原始报告。值得注意的是，录入受试者3045005的eCRF的访视3的听力测试结果与受试者3045016 eCRF中的访视2的结果完全一致。

c. 受试者3045011，代表该受试者的访视2（2011年9月20日）和访视3（2011年10月13日）的听力测试报告是其他受试者的原始的、模糊的听力测试报告。

ⅰ. 2011年9月20日访视2的听力检测报告是受试者3045012的原始报告。值得注意的是，录入受试者3045011的eCRF的访视2的听力测试结果与受试者3045012的eCRF中的访视3的结果完全一致，除了受试者3045011的电子病例报告表中包含一个抄写错误。

ⅱ. 2011年10月13日访视3的听力检测报告是受试者3045015的原始报告。值得注意的是，录入受试者30450011的eCRF访视3的听力测试结果与受试者3045015的访视2的结果完全一致。

d. 受试者3045013，代表该受试者的访视2（2011年9月21日）和访视3（2011年10月7日）的报告的听力测试报告是其他受试者的原始的、模糊的听力测试报告。

ⅰ. 2011年9月21日访视2的听力检测报告是受试者3045026的原始报告。值得注意的是，录入受试者3045013的eCRF的访视2的听力测试结果与受试者3045026 eCRF的访视2的结果完全一致。

ⅱ. 2011年10月7日访视3的听力检测报告是受试者3045026的原始报告。值得注意的是，录入受试者30450013的eCRF的访视3的听力测试结果与受试者的3045026 eCRF访视2结果完全一致。

2014年8月1日您对FDA 483表的书面回复中，您表明CRO现场监查员指示您的研究协调员（CRC）模糊受试者鉴认信息。此外，您承认您的研究协调员在抄录受试者信息中出现了错误。您表示在抄录受试者信息中所犯错误不是故意的，并且只涉及在您的研究中心为方案HYD3003所产生所有听力图的5%。

您还指出，在适用情况下您已经制定了额外的措施和程序，以应对检查结果。

您的回复是不够的，因为您没有提供足够的信息，以使我们能够评估您在未来的临床研究的纠正措施计划的可行性。您没有提供纠正措施计划的任何细节，以防止在将来发生类似的违规行为，也没有就您的纠正措施计划，提供实施额外的措施和程序的细节，以应对检查结果。如果没有这些细节，我们都无法确定您的纠正措施计划是否足以防止今后发生类似的方案违规情况。

您未能保存与听力检查报告有关的足够和准确的病历，引起了对在您的试验场所收集的数据的有效性和完整性的关注。

2. 您未能确保按照研究计划进行研究［21 CFR 312.60］

作为一个临床研究者，您必须确保您的临床研究按照研究计划进行。方案HYD3002的研究计划要求纯音气导听力检测在有资格入组研究的双盲随机阶段的受试者的访视3（随机访问）前的5天内进行。值得注意的是，听力测试是这项研究中一个重要的安全评估项。

您没有遵守这些要求。具体来说，您在以下受试者随机分组前没有进行纯音气导听力测试：

a. 受试者2033030在2012年9月6日随机入组，而直到2012年10月4日随机分组后约28天才进行听力测试。

b. 受试者2033034在2012年9月18日随机入组，而直到2012年10月11日随机分组后约23天才进行听力测试。

c. 受试者2033037在2012年8月29日随机入组，但没有进行听力测试。

d. 受试者2033038在2012年8月31日随机入组，而直到2012年10月2日随机分组后约32天才进行听力测试。

e. 受试者2033043在2012年9月12日随机入组，而直到2012年10月2日随机分组后约20天才进行听力测试。

f. 受试者2033044在2012年9月24日随机入组，而直到2012年11月5日随机分组后约42天才进行听力测试。

g. 受试者2033053在2012年8月28日随机入组，而直到2012年10月4日随机分组后约37天才进行听力测试。

在2014年8月1日对FDA 483表的书面回复中，您承认一些受试者在访视3没有按方案要求进行听力测试。您指出这个方案的程序在对原始文件修订后不再作为有关录入项。您还承认您忽略了此方案规定，该错误导致丢失了6%的您在试验场所为方案HYD3002所产生的所有听力图。您指出在适用情况下，您已经制定了额外的措施和程序以应对检查结果。您还指出在过去的几年中，您已经亲自审阅了“涵盖所有方案程序的原始文件的草案”，您也已经指定了一个内部质量监督协调员参照方案来审查原始文档。

您的回复是不够的，因为您的纠正措施计划不够详细。例如，目前还不清楚为什么您会有草案形式的原始文件，以及这些草案是否仅仅是获取研究信息的草案模板。因此，我们无法确定您的纠正措施是否能防止今后发生类似的方案违背情况。

您未能在受试者随机分组前没有进行听力测试，这种错误会危害受试者的安全和福利。尤其值得关注的是，对于方案HYD3002，审查了16名入组受试者的研究记录，其中有7名受试者在随机分组前没有进行用来评估受试者安全性的听力测试。

本警告信的目的并非是罗列您在试验药物临床研究中存在的所有缺陷。确保遵循法律和FDA相关法规的每一项要求是您的职责，您应当解决这些缺陷，并建立规程，以确保任何正在进行或将来进行的研究均符合FDA的法规。

自收到这封信的15个工作日内，您应当书面告知本办公室为预防将来发生类似违规情况而采取的措施。如果不能充分、迅速地解释上述违规问题，可能导致我们在不再通知的情况下采取监管措施。如果您认为您已经遵循了FDA的法规要求，请陈述理由，并提供所有支持资料，以供我们参考。

附：英文原文

Taber, Louise A., M D.

WARNING LETTER

OCT 09, 2014

CERTIFIED MAIL
RETURN RECEIPT REQUESTED

Ref: 14-HFD-45-10-01

Louise A. Taber, M.D.
2525 W. Greenway Road, Suite 114
Phoenix, AZ 85023-4226

Dear Dr. Taber:

This Warning Letter informs you of objectionable conditions observed during the U.S. Food and Drug Administration (FDA) inspection conducted at your clinical site between July 7 and July 18, 2014. Ms. Sonia R. Peterson, representing FDA, reviewed your conduct of the following clinical investigations of the investigational drug hydrocodone bitartrate, performed for Purdue Pharma L.P.:

- Protocol HYD3002, “A Multicenter, Randomized, Double-Blind, Placebo-Controlled Study with an Open-LabelRun-in to Assess the Efficacy and Safety of Hydrocodone Bitartrate (HYD) Tablets 20 to120 mg Once Daily in Subjects with Moderate to Severe Chronic Low Back Pain”; and
- Protocol HYD3003, “An Open-Label, Multicenter Study to Assess the Long-Term Safety of Hydrocodone Bitartrate (HYD) Tablets 20 to 120mg Once Daily in Subjects with Moderate to Severe Chronic Nonmalignant and Nonneuropathic Pain.”

This inspection is a part of FDA’s Bioresearch Monitoring Program, which includes inspections designed to evaluate the conduct of FDA-regulated research to ensure that the data are scientifically valid and accurate, and to help ensure that the rights, safety, and welfare of the human subjects of those studies have been protected.

At the conclusion of the inspection, Ms. Peterson presented and discussed with you Form FDA 483,

Inspectional Observations. We acknowledge receipt of your August 1, 2014, written response to the Form FDA 483. From our review of the FDA Establishment Inspection Report, the documents submitted with that report, and your written response dated August 1, 2014, we conclude that you did not adhere to the applicable statutory requirements and FDA regulations governing the conduct of clinical investigations. We wish to emphasize the following:

1. You failed to maintain adequate and accurate case histories that record all observations and other data pertinent to the investigation on each individual administered the investigational drug or employed as a control in the investigation [21 CFR 312.62(b)].

As a clinical investigator, you are required to prepare and maintain adequate and accurate case histories that record all observations and other data pertinent to the investigation on each individual administered the investigational drug or employed as a control in the investigation. Case histories for Protocol HYD3003 included pure-toneair-conduction audiometry reports. You failed to maintain adequate and accurate case histories with respect to these reports.

Specifically, for 4 of the 19 subjects whose records were reviewed during the inspection, pure-toneairconduction audiometry reports that were represented as reports for these subjects were originally reports for other subjects. The original subject identification numbers and visit dates on audiometry reports were obscured with black marks, and handwritten subject identification numbers and visit dates that do not correspond with the original subject identification numbers were subsequently added to these reports.

a. For Subject 3045003, audiometry reports that were represented as reports for this subject at Visit 2(August 31, 2011) and Visit 3 (September 22, 2011) are obscured audiometry reports that were originally for other subjects.

i. The audiometry report for Visit 2 (August 31, 2011) was originally a report for Subject 3045026.Also of note, the audiometry results entered into Subject 3045003's electronic case report form (eCRF) for Visit 2 are identical to the results in Subject 3045026's eCRF for Visit 2.

ii. The audiometry report for Visit 3 (September 22, 2011) was originally a report for Subject3045040. Also of note, the audiometry results entered into Subject 3045003's eCRF for Visit 3 are identical to the results in Subject 3045040's eCRF for Visit 2.

b. For Subject 3045005, audiometry reports that were represented as reports for this subject at Visit 2(September 6, 2011) and Visit 3 (September 21, 2011) are obscured audiometry reports that were originally for other subjects.

i. The audiometry report for Visit 2 (September 6, 2011) was originally a report for Subject 3045012.Also of note, the audiometry results entered into Subject 3045005's eCRF for Visit 2 are identical to the results in Subject 3045012's eCRF for Visit 3.

ii. The audiometry report for Visit 3 (September 21, 2011) was originally a report for Subject3045016. Also of note, the audiometry results entered into Subject 3045005's eCRF for Visit 3 are identical to the results in Subject 3045016's eCRF for Visit 2.

c. For Subject 3045011, audiometry reports that were represented as reports for this subject at Visit 2(September 20, 2011) and Visit 3 (October 13, 2011) are obscured audiometry reports that were originally for other subjects.

i. The audiometry report for Visit 2 (September 20, 2011) was originally a report for Subject3045012. Also of note, the audiometry results entered into Subject 3045011's eCRF for Visit 2 are identical to the results in Subject 3045012's eCRF for Visit 3, except that Subject 3045011's eCRF contains a transcription error.

ii. The audiometry report for Visit 3 (October 13, 2011) was originally a report for Subject 3045015.Also of note, the audiometry results entered into Subject 3045011's eCRF for Visit 3 are identical to the audiometry report results for Subject 3045015 for Visit 2.

d. For Subject 3045013, audiometry reports that were represented as reports for this subject at Visit 2(September 21, 2011) and Visit 3 (October 7, 2011) are obscured audiometry reports that were originally for other subjects.

i. The audiometry report for Visit 2 (September 21, 2011) was originally a report for Subject3045026. Also of note, the audiometry results entered into Subject 3045013's eCRF for Visit 2 are identical to the results in Subject 3045026's eCRF for Visit 2.

ii. The audiometry report for Visit 3 (October 7, 2011) was originally a report for Subject 3045026.Also of note, the audiometry results entered into Subject 3045013's eCRF for Visit 3 are identical to the results in Subject 3045026's eCRF for Visit 2.

In your August 1, 2014, written response to the Form FDA 483, you indicated that (b)(4), the clinical research organization (CRO) site monitor, instructed your study coordinator to obscure identifying subject information. In addition, you acknowledged that your study coordinator made errors in transcribing the subject information. You indicated that the errors in transcribing the subject information were not intentional and involved only 5% of all audiograms that your site generated for Protocol HYD3003.

You further indicated that, where applicable, you have instituted additional measures and procedures to address the inspection findings.

Your response is inadequate, because you did not provide sufficient information to enable us to evaluate the adequacy of your corrective action plans for use in any future clinical research that you may conduct. You did not provide any details of a corrective action plan to prevent similar violations from occurring in the future, nor have you provided sufficient details regarding your plan to implement additional measures and procedures to address the inspection findings. Without these details, we are unable to determine whether your corrective action plan appears sufficient to prevent similar violations in the future.

Your failure to maintain adequate and accurate case histories with respect to audiology reports raises concerns about the validity and integrity of the data captured at your site.

2. You failed to ensure that the investigation was conducted according to the investigational plan [21 CFR 312.60].

As a clinical investigator, you are required to ensure that your clinical studies are conducted in accordance with the investigational plan. The investigational plan for Protocol HYD3002 required that pure-tone air-conduction audiometry testing be performed within the 5 days before Visit 3 (randomization visit) for subjects who were eligible for randomization in the double-blind phase of the study. Of note, audiometry testing was an important safety assessment in this study.

You failed to adhere to these requirements. Specifically, you did not perform pure-tone air-conduction audiometry tests before randomization of the following subjects:

a. Subject 2033030 was randomized on September 6, 2012; however, audiometry testing was not performed until October 4, 2012, approximately 28 days after randomization.

b. Subject 2033034 was randomized on September 18, 2012; however, audiometry testing was not performed until October 11, 2012, approximately 23 days after randomization.

c. Subject 2033037 was randomized on August 29, 2012; however, no audiometry testing was performed.

d. Subject 2033038 was randomized on August 31, 2012; however, audiometry testing was not performed until October 2, 2012, approximately 32 days after randomization.

e. Subject 2033043 was randomized on September 12, 2012; however, audiometry testing was not performed until October 2, 2012, approximately 20 days after randomization.

f. Subject 2033044 was randomized on September 24, 2012; however, audiometry testing was not performed until November 5, 2012, approximately 42 days after randomization.

g. Subject 2033053 was randomized on August 28, 2012; however, audiometry testing was not performed until October 4, 2012, approximately 37 days after randomization.

In your August 1, 2014, written response to the Form FDA 483, you acknowledged that some subjects did not have audiometry testing at Visit 3, as required by the protocol. You noted that this protocol procedure was omitted as an entry on revisions to source documents. You also acknowledged that you overlooked this protocol requirement, and that error resulted in missed audiograms for 6% of all audiograms that your site generated for Protocol HYD3002. You indicated that, where applicable, you have instituted additional measures and procedures to address the inspection findings. You further indicated that for the last several years, you have personally reviewed "drafts of source documents for inclusion of all protocol procedures," and you have also designated an in-house quality assurance coordinator to review source documents against the protocol.

Your response is inadequate because your corrective action plan is insufficiently detailed. For example, it is unclear why you would have source documents in draft form, and whether these drafts are instead draft templates for capturing study information. As a result, we are unable to determine whether your corrective action appears sufficient to prevent similar violations in the future.

You failed to conduct audiometry tests before subject randomization, and this failure jeopardized subject safety and welfare. Of particular concern is the fact that, for Protocol HYD3002, audiometry tests that were used to assess the safety of subjects were not performed before randomization for 7 of the 16 enrolled subjects whose study records were reviewed.

This letter is not intended to be an all-inclusive list of deficiencies with your clinical study of an investigational drug. It is your responsibility to ensure adherence to each requirement of the law and relevant FDA regulations. You should address these deficiencies and establish procedures to ensure that any ongoing or future studies will be in compliance with FDA regulations.

Within fifteen (15) working days of your receipt of this letter, you should notify this office in writing of the actions you have taken to prevent similar violations in the future. Failure to address the violations noted above adequately and promptly may result in regulatory action without further notice. If you believe that you have complied with FDA regulations, include your reasoning and any supporting information for our consideration.

If you have any questions, please contact Constance Cullity, M.D., M.P.H., at 301-796-3397; FAX 301-8478748. Your written response and any pertinent documentation should be addressed to:

Constance Cullity, M.D., M.P.H.
Branch Chief
Good Clinical Practice Enforcement Branch
Division of Good Clinical Practice Compliance
Office of Scientific Investigations
Office of Compliance
Center for Drug Evaluation and Research
U.S. Food and Drug Administration
Building 51, Room 5354
10903 New Hampshire Avenue
Silver Spring, MD 20993

Sincerely yours,

{See appended electronic signature page}

Sean Y. Kassim, Ph.D.
Director
Office of Scientific Investigations
Office of Compliance
Center for Drug Evaluation and Research
U.S. Food and Drug Administration

第 70 封　给 Aqua, Keith A. 医学博士的警告信

2014年9月2日

参考号：14-HFD-45-08-02

尊敬的Aqua博士：

2014年2月3日至3月17日，Colleen Aspinwall女士代表FDA，在贵临床研究中心，对您所开展的以下临床试验：试验方案（b）（4）[1]，“（b）（4）”和试验方案（b）（4），“（b）（4）”进行了现场检查。这封警告信特告知您现场检查中发现的违规情况。

本次现场检查是FDA的生物研究监查项目的一部分。该项目通过设定的检查方法，对FDA监管的研究的实施情况进行评估，以确认研究数据在科学上是有效和准确的，并帮助确保这些研究中受试者的权益、安全和福利得到了保护。

在现场检查结束时，Aspinwall女士向您出示了FDA483表，即现场检查发现的问题，并与您进行了讨论。您2014年3月24日对该FDA483表的书面回复已收悉。

经对现场检查报告、该报告的附件，以及您2014年3月24日的书面回复进行审查，我们认为，您没有遵循适用的法律要求和监管临床研究实施的FDA法规。我们想强调以下几点：

您未确保按照研究计划进行［21 CFR 312.60］

作为一名临床研究者，您必须确保按照研究计划实施临床研究。试验方案（b）（4），“（b）（4）”和试验方案（b）（4），“（b）（4）”的研究计划，要求受试者自行记录所有疼痛评估，并完成某些实验室评估，但您未能遵守方案的这些要求，具体而言：

a. 试验方案（b）（4）和（b）（4），要求在研究期间，受试者自己记录所有疼痛强度评分和疼痛缓解评估。然而，入组试验方案（b）（4）的20名受试者的疼痛强度评分是由贵研究中心研究人员记录，而非受试者记录，试验方案（b）（4）的3名受试者的疼痛强度评分。值得注意的是，两项研究的主要疗效终点评价都是基于受试者自己记录的疼痛强度评分。

在您2014年3月24日的书面回复中，您声明“疼痛强度评分由研究人员记录在患者日志卡中”。您指出合同研究组织（CRO）指示研究人员去问患者的疼痛评分，然后帮患者记录于日志中。另外，您指出“在手术后即刻状态下，由受试者自我记录评估到日志卡中您认为是不可能的。”

我们确认您已针对上面1.a.项中提到的检查发现的问题采取纠正措施。您在您的书面回复中指出，与其他纠正措施一起，您已经建立了严格遵守试验方案的措施，您将会解释并书面记录任何方案偏离。

然而，您的回复是不充分的，因为未包含足够的细节。具体而言，您未提供您将如何完成您的纠正措施计划的细节，没有这些细节，我们不能判定您的纠正措施是否足以预防将来类似违规情况的发生。

b. 试验方案（b）（4）和“（b）（4）”要求您在筛选期和研究终止时（或终止后24小时内）均需获得受试者在当地实验室的丙氨酸氨基转移酶（ALT）和天冬氨酸氨基转移酶（AST）、总胆红素、肌酐和血尿素氮的检查结果。这些实验室的值被用来确定由手术引起的肾脏或肝脏损伤的受试者，无论这些损伤是先前存在的还是急性发生的。

i. 审查了试验方案（b）（4）中的13位受试者的记录，对于其中8 位受试者，您未获得研究结束时要求的部分或全部实验室结果。具体而言对受试者15907、15911、15912和 15917，您未获得ALT、AST和胆红素结

1 (b) (4) 涉及商业秘密，根据法规内容不予公开。

果；对编号为15901、15902、15903和15904的受试者，您未获得任何要求的实验室结果。

ii. 对试验方案（b）(4）的3位受试者中2位受试者（受试者53-903和53-904），在筛选或研究结束时，您均未获得AST、ALT和胆红素的结果。

在您2014年3月24日对上面1.b. 项提到的检查发现的书面回复中，您指出，即使下了医嘱，研究结束时的实验室检测也常常未被执行，并认为研究方案依从性难以保持。

我们确认，关于上面1.b. 项提到的检查发现，您计划在将来采取的纠正措施。您在您的书面回复中指出，与其他纠正措施一起，您将采取一切措施，确保研究义务得到满足，在整个试验期间，所有的实验室检查都将按照研究方案要求进行；同时您个人也会审查所有研究的实验室结果，确保这些结果被及时获得并记录。

您的回复是不充分的，因为未包含足够的细节。具体而言，您未提供您将如何完成您的纠正措施计划的细节，没有这些细节，我们不能确定您的纠正措施是否足以预防将来类似违规情况的发生。

本警告信的目的并非是罗列您在试验药物临床研究中存在的所有缺陷。确保遵循法律和相关FDA法规的每一项要求是您的职责，您应当解决这些缺陷，并建立规程，以确保任何正在进行或将来进行的研究均符合FDA的法规。

自收到这封信的15个工作日内，您应当书面告知本办公室为预防将来发生类似违规情况而采取的措施。如果不能充分、迅速地解释上述违规问题，可能导致我们在不再通知的情况下采取监管措施。如果您认为您已经遵循了FDA的法规要求，请陈述理由，并提供所有支持资料，以供我们参考。

附：英文原文

Aqua, Keith A. M.D.

WARNING LETTER

SEP 02, 2014

CERTIFIED MAIL
RETURN RECEIPT REQUESTED

Ref: 14-HFD-45-08-02

Keith A. Aqua, M.D.
8188 Jog Road, Suite 204
Boynton Beach, FL 33472

Dear Dr. Aqua:

This Warning Letter informs you of objectionable conditions observed during the U.S. Food and Drug Administration (FDA) inspection conducted at your clinical site between February 3 and March 17,2014. Ms. Colleen Aspinwall, representing FDA, reviewed your conduct of the following clinical investigations of the investigational drug (b)(4), (b)(4) performed for (b)(4):

- Protocol (b)(4), “(b)(4)”; and
- Protocol (b)(4), “(b)(4).”

This inspection is a part of FDA’s Bioresearch Monitoring Program, which includes inspections designed to evaluate the conduct of FDA-regulated research to ensure that the data are scientifically valid and accurate, and to help ensure that the rights, safety, and welfare of the human subjects of those studies have been protected.

At the conclusion of the inspection, Ms. Aspinwall presented and discussed with you Form FDA 483, Inspectional

Observations. We acknowledge receipt of your March 24, 2014, written response to the Form FDA 483.

From our review of the FDA Establishment Inspection Report, the documents submitted with that report, and your written response dated March 24, 2014, we conclude that you did not adhere to the applicable statutory requirements and FDA regulations governing the conduct of clinical investigations. We wish to emphasize the following:

1. You failed to ensure that the investigation was conducted according to the investigational plan [21 CFR 312.60].

As a clinical investigator, you are required to ensure that your clinical studies are conducted in accordance with the investigational plan. The investigational plan for Protocols (b)(4) and (b)(4) required that subjects self-record all pain assessments and have certain laboratory assessments completed. You failed to adhere to these requirements. Specifically:

a. Protocols (b)(4) and (b)(4) required that during the study period, subjects self-record all scores for pain-intensity and pain-relief assessments. However, site staff, rather than the subjects, recorded pain-intensity scores for the 20 subjects enrolled in Protocol (b)(4) and for the 3 subjects enrolled in Protocol (b) (4). Of note, the primary efficacy endpoint for both studies was based on the pain-intensity scores that the subjects self-recorded.

In your March 24, 2014, written response, you stated, "The pain intensity scores were recorded by the study staff in the diary." You indicated that the contract research organization (CRO) instructed site staff to "ask the patient the pain scores and then to record them in the diary for the patient." In addition, you indicated that in the immediate postoperative setting, you felt it was impossible for subjects to self-record assessments into a workbook.

We acknowledge the corrective actions that you have taken regarding the findings noted in Item 1.a. above. You indicated in your written response that, along with other corrective actions, you have instituted strict adherence to the protocol, and that you will seek justification and written documentation for any protocol deviation.

Your response is inadequate because it does not contain sufficient detail. Specifically, you did not provide details regarding how you will implement your corrective action plan. Without those details, we are unable to determine whether your corrective action is adequate to prevent similar violations in the future.

b. Protocols (b)(4) and (b)(4) required that you obtain subjects' local laboratory results for alanine aminotransferase (ALT) and aspartate aminotransferase (AST), total bilirubin, creatinine, and blood urea nitrogen, both at screening and at study termination (or within 24 hours after termination). These laboratory values were to be used to identify subjects with surgically induced renal or hepatic impairment, whether pre-existing or acute.

i. For 8 of the 13 subjects whose records were reviewed for Protocol (b)(4), you failed to obtain some or all of the laboratory results that were required at the end of the study. Specifically, for Subjects 15-907,15-911,15-912,and 15-917,you did not obtain results for ALT, AST, and total bilirubin; and for Subjects 15-901,15-902,15-903,and 15-904,you did not obtain any of these required laboratory results.

ii. For 2 of the 3 subjects enrolled in Protocol (b)(4) (Subjects 53-903 and 53-904),you failed to obtain results for AST, ALT, and bilirubin, either at screening or at the end of the study.

In your March 24, 2014, written response to the findings noted in Item 1.b. above, you indicated that many times, end-of-study laboratory tests were not performed even when ordered, and that protocol compliance was difficult to maintain.

We acknowledge the corrective actions that you plan to take in the future regarding the findings noted in Item 1.b. above. You indicated in your written response that, along with other corrective actions, you will take every measure to ensure that study obligations will be met; that all labs will be drawn throughout trials in accordance with the protocols; and that you personally will review all study laboratory results and ensure that these are obtained and documented in a timely fashion.

Your response is inadequate because it does not contain sufficient detail. Specifically, you did not provide details regarding how you will implement your corrective action plan. Without those details, we are unable to determine whether your corrective action is adequate to prevent similar violations in the future.

This letter is not intended to be an all-inclusive list of deficiencies with your clinical study of an investigational drug. It is your responsibility to ensure adherence to each requirement of the law and relevant FDA regulations. You should address these deficiencies and establish procedures to ensure that any ongoing or future studies will be in compliance with FDA regulations.

Within fifteen (15) working days of your receipt of this letter, you should notify this office in writing of the actions you have taken to prevent similar violations in the future. Failure to address the violations noted above adequately and promptly may result in regulatory action without further notice. If you believe you have complied with FDA regulations, include your reasoning and any supporting information for our consideration.

If you have any questions, please contact Constance Cullity, M.D., M.P.H., at 301-796-3397;FAX 301-847-8748. Your written response and any pertinent documentation should be addressed to:

Constance Cullity, M.D., M.P.H.
Branch Chief
Good Clinical Practice Enforcement Branch
Division of Good Clinical Practice Compliance
Office of Scientific Investigations
Office of Compliance
Center for Drug Evaluation and Research
U.S. Food and Drug Administration
Building 51, Room 5354
10903 New Hampshire Avenue
Silver Spring, MD 20993

Sincerely yours,

{See appended electronic signature page}

Sean Y. Kassim, Ph.D.
Acting Director
Office of Scientific Investigations
Office of Compliance
Center for Drug Evaluation and Research
U.S. Food and Drug Administration

第71封　给Wise, John M. 医学博士的警告信

2014年8月12日

参考号：14-HFD-45-08-01

尊敬的Wise博士：

2014年3月24日至3月28日，Mark W. Babbitt先生代表FDA，在贵临床研究中心，对您所开展的试验药物为帕拉米韦（BCX1812），申办者为BioCryst制药公司的以下临床研究进行了审查：

- 试验方案BCX1812-211，"一项Ⅱ期、多中心、随机、双盲、安慰剂对照研究，旨在评估对患有无并发症的急性流感的受试者肌内注射帕拉米韦的有效性和安全性"；
- 试验方案BCX1812-212，"一项Ⅱ期、多中心、随机、安慰剂对照研究，旨在评估对患有无并发症的急性流感的受试者肌内注射帕拉米韦600mg的有效性和安全性"；
- 试验方案BCX1812-311，"一项Ⅲ期、多中心、随机、双盲、安慰剂对照研究，旨在评估对患有无并发症的急性流感的受试者肌内注射帕拉米韦的有效性和安全性"；

这封警告信特告知您现场检查中发现的违规情况。

本次现场检查是FDA的生物研究监查项目的一部分。该目通过设定的检查方法，对FDA监管研究的实施情况进行评估，以确认研究数据在科学上是有效和准确的，并确保这些研究中受试者的权益、安全和福利得到了保护。

在现场检查结束时，检查员Babbitt向您出示了FDA483表，即现场检查发现的问题，并与您进行了讨论。

经对FDA现场检查报告、该报告的附件进行审查，我们认为，您没有遵循适用法律要求和监管临床研究实施的FDA法规。我们想强调以下几点：

您未能按照21 CFR 312的要求保留相关记录至该研究药物及研究的适应症上市申请获批之日起2年；或者，如果未提出上市申请或者该适应症的申请未获批准，则相应记录需保存至研究终止后2年［21 CFR 312.62（c）］

作为临床研究者，您必须保存药物处置记录，包括日期、数量和受试者使用记录，并保存完整、准确的病历，病历需记录此研究中每位给予试验药物或作为对照药物的受试者的所有观察结果和其他数据。您必须保存这些记录，为期两年，针对该药物及经过研究的适应症的药物上市申请被批准起；或者，如果上市申请未被提交或者该适应症的申请未被批准，则这些记录需保留至研究终止且FDA被通知后2年。

您未遵守这些要求，具体而言，对于方案编号为BCX1812-211和BCX1812-311：

- 您未保存药物处置记录，包括日期、数量和受试者使用记录。
- 您未保存足够的和准确的病历，包括签署姓名和日期的知情同意书、病例报告表和所有支持数据。

您必须保存这两项试验的研究记录，因为针对研究中适应症的新药申请（NDA）已经被提交，并且在您丢弃研究记录之前，该申请还没有定论（即是批准还是不批准）

检查期间，您声明试验方案BCX1812-211和 BCX1812-311的所有原始研究记录均于2014年1月24日用碎纸机销毁。您声明您的研究协调员"误将包括试验方案BCX1812-211和 BCX1812-311的研究文件在内的资料与准备销毁的业务文件一起交给了一家移动销毁公司……"

另外，您声明BioCryst制药公司2014年2月11日通知他们公司已向FDA提交了新药申请，而且此次提交包括试验方案BCX1812-211的数据。您进一步声明，您和您的员工从2001年以来一直参与了临床研究，因此非常了解保存记录的监管要求。

在现场检查期间，您声明：

“我们研究中心所有与试验方案BCX1812-211有关的研究记录与原始数据均已被销毁，包括但不限于：签署的知情同意书、受试者日志卡、筛选结果记录、相关访视额外研究的评估记录和实验室检查结果。这些数据是无法恢复的，也是无法供审查的。因为研究记录被销毁，所以此次检查中，FDA检查员既不能核实试验方案BCX1812-211的研究数据，也不能判定签署的知情同意书的存在。”

现场检查中，您的研究协调员提供给检查员Babbitt一份由您签署的生效日期为2008年10月30日的为了研究记录保存的标准操作规程（SOP）的复印件。我们担忧这个SOP没有足够的细节以预防将来研究中发生类似的违规情况。值得注意的是，基于现场检查中您提供的描述，被销毁的研究记录文件盒上标记了识别研究的相关信息，如申办者名称、研究的时间范围、受试者数量和方案号。但您的为了研究记录保存的SOP并未规定将来如何确保被适当标记的研究记录文件盒不被错误的销毁。

未按FDA法规要求保存研究记录明显损害了数据的有效性和完整性。因为您未保存试验方案BCX1812-211 和 BCX1812-311的药物管理记录和病历，所以我们认为在支持研究或上市申请中贵研究中心产生的这两项试验的数据是不可靠的。

本警告信的目的并非是罗列您在试验药物临床研究中存在的所有缺陷。确保遵循法律和相关FDA法规的每一项要求是您的职责，您应当解决这些缺陷，并建立规程，以确保任何正在进行或将来进行的研究均符合FDA的法规。

自收到这封信的15个工作日内，您应当书面告知本办公室为预防将来发生类似违规情况而采取的措施。在您的书面回复中，您应该描述您已采取的预防措施，确保将来符合与研究者记录和记录保存相关的监管要求（21 CFR 312.62）。如果不能充分、迅速地解释上述违规问题，可能导致我们在不再通知的情况下采取监管措施。如果您认为您已经遵循了FDA的法规要求，请陈述理由，并提供所有支持资料，以供我们参考。

附：英文原文

Wise, John M. M.D.

WARNING LETTER

AUG 12, 2014

CERTIFIED MAIL
RETURN RECEIPT REQUESTED

Ref: 14-HFD-45-08-01

John M. Wise, M.D.
Bozeman Urgent Care Center
1006 West Main Street
Bozeman, MT 59715

Dear Dr. Wise:

This Warning Letter informs you of objectionable conditions observed during the U.S. Food and Drug Administration (FDA) inspection conducted at your clinical site between March 24 and 28, 2014. Mark W. Babbitt,representing FDA, reviewed your conduct of the following clinical investigations of the investigational drug peramivir (BCX-1812), performed for BioCryst Pharmaceuticals, Inc. :

- Protocol BCX1812-211,“A Phase Ⅱ, Multicenter, Randomized, Double-Mask,Placebo Controlled Study to Evaluate the Efficacy and Safety of Intramuscular Peramivir in Subjects With Uncomplicated Acute Influenza”;
- Protocol BCX1812-212,“A Phase Ⅱ, Multicenter, Randomized, Placebo-Controlled Study To Evaluate The Efficacy and Safety Of Intramuscular Peramivir 600 mg In Subjects With Uncomplicated Acute Influenza”; and
- Protocol BCX1812-311,“A Phase 3 Multicenter, Randomized, Double-Blind, Placebo-Controlled Study to Evaluate the Efficacy and Safety of Intramuscular Peramivir in Subjects With Uncomplicated Acute Influenza.”

This inspection is a part of FDA’s Bioresearch Monitoring Program, which includes inspections designed to evaluate the conduct of FDA-regulated research to ensure that the data are scientifically valid and accurate, and to help ensure that the rights, safety, and welfare of the human subjects of those studies have been protected.

At the conclusion of the inspection, Investigator Babbitt presented and discussed with you Form FDA 483, Inspectional Observations.

From our review of the FDA Establishment Inspection Report, the documents submitted with that report, we conclude that you did not adhere to the applicable statutory requirements and FDA regulations governing the conduct of clinical investigations. We wish to emphasize the following:

You failed to retain records required to be maintained under 21 CFR Part 312 for a period of two years following the date a marketing application is approved for the drug for the indication for which the drug is being investigated; or, if no application is filed or if the application is not approved for such indication, until two years after the investigation is discontinued [21 CFR 312.62(c)].

As a clinical investigator, you are required to retain records of the disposition of the drug, including dates, quantity, and use by subjects, and to retain adequate and accurate case histories that record all observations and other data pertinent to the investigation on each individual administered the investigational drug or employed as a control in the investigation. You are required to retain these records for a period of two years following the date a marketing application is approved for the drug for the indication for which it is being investigated; or, if no application is to be filed or the application is not approved for such indication, until two years after the investigation is discontinued and FDA is notified.

You failed to adhere to these requirements. Specifically, for Protocols BCX1812-211 and BCX1812-311:

- You failed to retain records of the disposition of the drug, including dates, quantity, and use by subjects.
- You failed to retain adequate and accurate case histories, including signed and dated informed consent forms, case report forms, and all supporting data.

You were required to retain the study records for both protocols because a New Drug Application (NDA) had been filed for the indication under study, and the application had not yet been decided on (that is, approved or not approved) before you discarded the study records.

During the inspection, you stated that all original study records related to Protocols BCX1812-211 and BCX1812-311 were shredded on January 24, 2014. You stated that your study coordinator “mistakenly included the study files for BCX1812-211 and BCX1812-311, along with business documents intended for shredding, and provided them to a mobile shredding company ....”

In addition, you indicated that BioCryst notified you on February 11, 2014, that the company had filed an NDA with the FDA and had included the data from Protocol BCX1812-211 in this submission. You further stated that you and your staff were “well aware of regulatory record retention requirements having been involved in clinical research since 2001.”

During the inspection, you stated:

“ All study related records and source data pertaining to protocol BCX1812-211 at our site were shredded, including, but not limited to: signed informed consent forms, subject diary cards, records of screening results, documentation of assessments at additional study related visits, and laboratory test results. This data is not retrievable and was not available for inspection. Due to the destroyed study records, [the FDA investigator] was not able to verify the study data for protocol BCX1812-211, or the existence of signed informed consent forms during the inspection.”

During the inspection, your study coordinator provided Investigator Babbitt with a copy of a Standard Operating Procedure (SOP), signed by you and with an effective date of October 30, 2008, for study record-retention. We are concerned that this SOP appears to be insufficiently detailed to prevent similar violations in future studies. Of note, based on the description you provided during the inspection, the boxes of study records that were shredded were labeled with pertinent identifying study information, such as sponsor, date range of the study, subject numbers, and protocol number. Your SOP for study-record retention does not address how you will ensure that boxes of study records that are appropriately labeled will not be shredded erroneously in the future.

Failure to retain study records as required by FDA regulations compromises the validity and integrity of data significantly. Because you failed to retain drug accountability records and case histories for both studies, we consider the data generated at your site for Protocols BCX1812-211 and BCX1812-311 unreliable in support of a research or marketing application.

This letter is not intended to be an all-inclusive list of deficiencies with your clinical study of an investigational drug. It is your responsibility to ensure adherence to each requirement of the law and relevant FDA regulations. You should address these deficiencies and establish procedures to ensure that any ongoing or future studies will be in compliance with FDA regulations.

Within fifteen (15) working days of your receipt of this letter, you should notify this office in writing of the actions you have taken to prevent similar violations in the future. In your response, you should describe the preventive actions you have taken to ensure future compliance with regulatory requirements related to investigator record keeping and record retention (21 CFR 312.62). Failure to address the violations noted above adequately and promptly may result in regulatory action without further notice. If you believe you have complied with FDA regulations, include your reasoning and any supporting information for our consideration.

If you have any questions, please contact Constance Cullity, M.D., M.P.H., at 301-796-3397;FAX 301-847-8748. Your written response and any pertinent documentation should be addressed to:

Constance Cullity, M.D., M.P.H.
Branch Chief
Good Clinical Practice Enforcement Branch
Division of Good Clinical Practice Compliance
Office of Scientific Investigations
Office of Compliance
Center for Drug Evaluation and Research
U.S. Food and Drug Administration
Building 51, Room 5354
10903 New Hampshire Avenue
Silver Spring, MD 20993

Sincerely yours,

{See appended electronic signature page}

Sean Y. Kassim, Ph.D.
Acting Director
Office of Scientific Investigations
Office of Compliance
Center for Drug Evaluation and Research
U.S. Food and Drug Administration

第 72 封　给 Alzohalli, Opada 医学博士的警告信

2014年7月17日

参考号：14-HFD-45-03-01

尊敬的Alzohaili博士：

2013年7月18日至8月14日，L'Oreal F. Walker女士代表FDA，在贵临床研究机构对您所开展的试验药物为阿必鲁肽，申办者为Glaxo Smith Kline的以下临床研究进行了审查：

- 试验方案GLP108486，“在2型糖尿病受试者中进行的一项随机、开放、阳性对照、平行组、多中心研究，以确定阿必鲁肽和甘精胰岛素联合用药与甘精胰岛素和餐前赖脯胰岛素联合用药相比的安全性和有效性”。
- 试验方案GLP114179，“在2型糖尿病受试者中进行的一项随机、开放、平行组、多中心研究，以确定阿必鲁肽与利拉鲁肽相比的有效性和安全性”；
- 试验方案GLP112753，“在2型糖尿病受试者中进行的一项随机、双盲、安慰剂及阳性对照、平行组、多中心研究，以确定阿必鲁肽和二甲双胍联合用药与二甲双胍和西他列汀联合用药、二甲双胍和格列美脲联合用药以及二甲双胍和安慰剂联合用药相比的有效性和安全性”；
- 试验方案GLP112754，“在2型糖尿病受试者中进行的一项随机、开放、平行组、多中心研究，以确定阿必鲁肽和胰岛素相比的有效性和长期用药的安全性”；
- 试验方案GLP112755，“在2型糖尿病受试者中进行的一项随机、双盲、安慰剂对照、平行组、多中心研究，以确定阿必鲁肽和吡格列酮联合用药、同时联用或不用二甲双胍的有效性和安全性”；
- 试验方案GLP112756，“在2型糖尿病受试者中进行的一项随机、双盲、安慰剂对照、平行组、多中心研究，以确定两种剂量水平阿必鲁肽与安慰剂相比的有效性和安全性”；
- 试验方案GLP112757，“在2型糖尿病受试者中进行的一项随机、双盲、安慰剂和阳性对照、平行组、多中心研究，以确定阿必鲁肽、二甲双胍、格列美脲联合用药与二甲双胍、格列美脲、安慰剂联合用药以及二甲双胍、格列美脲、吡格列酮联合用药相比的有效性和安全性”。

这封警告信特告知您现场检查中发现的违规情况。

本次现场检查是FDA的生物研究监查项目的一部分。该项目通过设定的检查方法，对FDA所监管的相关研究的实施情况进行评估，以确认研究数据在科学上是有效和准确的，并帮助确保这些研究中受试者的权益、安全和福利得到了保护。

在现场检查结束时，Walker女士向您出示了FDA483表，即现场检查发现的问题，并与您进行了讨论。您2013年9月2日对该FDA483表的书面回复已收悉。

经对现场检查报告、该报告的附件，以及您2013年9月2日的书面回复进行审查，我们认为您没有遵循适用的法律要求和监管临床研究实施的FDA法规。我们想强调以下几点：

1. 您未能保护在您的监护下的受试者的权益、安全和福利［21 CFR 312.60］

作为临床研究者，您必须保护在您的监护下的受试者的权益、安全和福利。

a. 您未能确保有持续性高血糖的糖尿病受试者能够得到及时的抢救治疗，从而防止不受控制的高血糖引起的并发症，具体而言：

ⅰ. 试验方案GLP112756规定，第9次访视（第4周）后但是在第12次访视（试验第12周）前，单次空腹血糖测定（FPG）≥250mg/dL，并且在7天内抽取第2份血样经中心实验室检测确定无误的受试者，必须接受高

血糖急救。

受试者001 2009年5月15日（第8周）的FPG为261mg/dL，2009年5月19日（第9周）的FPG为304mg/dL。因此按照试验方案，该受试者应该接受高血糖急救。然而，研究记录显示，直到2009年6月10日（大约3周以后）急救药物都没有被下医嘱，受试者直到2009年7月10日才接受药物治疗。

在2013年9月2日对FDA483表的书面回复中，您指出对受试者001高血糖急救的延迟是由于受试者的不顺从。您提出，您曾多次联系受试者001，告知他开始采用急救药物治疗的重要性，但是该受试者不服从您的指令，直到2009年6月10日才去您的研究中心，那时候才下了急救药物治疗的医嘱。但是，据说该名受试者直到2009年7月10日才配药或开始急救药物治疗。

作为纠正措施，您提出在和医疗监查员进行沟通后，贵研究中心对遵循方案规定和受试者及时滴注治疗的重要性进行了再教育。

您的答复不够充分，因为您没有提供与受试者001进行联系、试图使他服从指令方面的记录。此外，您未能提供纠正措施计划的充分细节资料，使我们能够确定您的纠正措施是否足以防止将来发生类似违规的情况。

ⅱ. 试验方案GLP108486 4.6部分规定，在第4周及以后和第8周之前，受试者如果HbA1c＞9.0%且比基线降低＜0.5%，将有资格获得高血糖急救。

受试者004在2009年12月11日的基线HbA1c为7.8%，2010年1月8日（第4周）时HbA1c为9.4%。因此，2010年1月8日受试者004符合高血糖急救标准，但是该受试者直到2010年1月29日（3周后）才获得急救药物治疗。

在2013年9月2日对FDA483表的书面回复中，您指出受试者004急救药物治疗的延迟是由于您对试验方案的误解，以及您考虑到其他试验方案中有这种要求，想当然地以为急救前HbA1c水平需要得到确认。此外，您认为文件的缺少是发生上述违规情况的主要原因，作为一项纠正措施，您的研究中心将在受试者的原始文件和备忘录文件中记录所有与研究有关的数据。

您的答复不够充分，因为您没有提供纠正措施计划的任何细节，以确保您和您的员工在试验方案要求方面得到足够的培训，防止将来的违规；您也没有提供计划去记录所需研究数据方面的足够细节。没有这些细节，我们无法确定您的纠正措施是否足以防止将来发生类似违规的情况。

我们提醒您，作为临床研究者，您有责任确保您和您的研究人员在研究启动之前理解方案的要求。

b. 您未能确保在您监护下的受试者的安全和福利，因为您未能确保受试者获得了正确剂量的试验药物。具体而言：

ⅰ. 试验方案GLP112756中受试者005在2011年9月28日（第16周）、第24次访视时接收了一次未计划的替代试验药物，通过笔给药。但是，您的研究协调员把错误的笔分给了受试者。研究协调员在交互式语音应答系统（IVRS）中提出要一只替换笔的要求，本来是给入组同一个试验方案的受试者006的，但是研究协调员却把那支笔分给了受试者005。

ⅱ. 2009年10月29日，试验方案GLP112757中的受试者007收到并使用了2039854号试验药物笔，而那支笔是分配给入组不同的试验方案（试验方案GLP112755）中的受试者001的。

在对FDA483表的书面回复中，您承认受试者收到了错误的试验药物笔，并且指出您和您的研究人员对上述违规情况负全部责任。

作为纠正措施，您表示您开展了新的方法来防止将来类似的违规情况再次发生，包括要求两名研究协调员对任何分配给受试者的药物进行确认。

您所描述的纠正措施，如果恰当地执行，应该足以防止将来发生类似的违规情况。

您未能确保受试者收到正确剂量的试验药物，未能确保受试者在持续高血糖时获得及时的急救药物治疗，这引起对在贵研究中心对上述研究中招募的受试者的保护的极大关注。

2. 您未能确保按照研究计划进行研究［21 CFR 312.60］

作为一名临床研究者，您必须确保临床研究遵照研究计划进行。试验方案GLP112753、GLP112754、GLP112755、GLP112756和GLP112757的试验计划要求有持续性高血糖的随机的受试者获得试验药物剂量调整或者高血糖急救。此外，有资格获得急救药物治疗的受试者应该回到研究中心进行急救访视，内容包括疗效和实验室评价。您未能遵循这些要求，具体而言：

a. 试验方案GLP112754规定，如果受试者被分配阿必鲁肽治疗，并且存在持续的高血糖，可能有剂量调整的资格，规定如下：

治疗时间间隔	剂量滴注
大于等于12周和小于24周	HbA1c＞7.0%且从基线下降≤0.5%
大于等于24周和小于143周	HbA1c＞7.0%

试验方案还规定，试验场所在收到提示需要进行剂量调整的实验室结果的确认后2周内，要联系受试者并安排一次回访。

ⅰ. 对于受试者006，您在收到实验室结果的2周内未能调整阿必鲁肽剂量。受试者006 2009年11月9日（第24周）HbA1c为8.4%，然而您直到2009年12月23日，也就是延迟超过1个月，才调整了阿必鲁肽剂量。

在2013年9月2日对FDA483表的书面回复中，您指出剂量调整延迟之所以发生，是因为尽管研究中心人员已经发出指令，但是受试者不服从。但是您没有提供任何文件，表明在2周的时间段内您或者您的工作人员尝试联系受试者来安排一次剂量调整的回访。

ⅱ. 对于受试者007，您收到实验室结果2周内未能调整阿必鲁肽剂量。受试者007 2009年7月2日的基线HbA1c为8.3%，2009年10月19日（第16周）的HbA1c为7.8%（HbA1c下降≤0.5%）。但是，您直到2009年12月28日才调整了阿必鲁肽剂量，差不多推迟了两个月。

在对FDA483表的书面回复中，您指出您推迟了受试者007的药物剂量是因为考虑到低血糖的风险以及HbA1c水平下降的趋势。您还指出，关于受试者的安全，如何进行要由您来裁量。作为一个纠正措施，您提到经过与医疗监查员的沟通后，您的研究人员经过了再教育，内容是遵循试验方案的重要性，具体而言，是对需要剂量调整的受试者及时进行处置。

您的答复不够充分，因为您没有提供对受试者血糖水平进行评估的任何记录。您的答复还不够充分，因为您没有提供相关细节：您的纠正措施将如何实施或者您如何确保您和您的研究人员会遵循试验方案，重点在确保有资格的受试者在方案规定的窗口内获得剂量调整的步骤。没有这些细节内容，我们无法确定您的纠正措施是否足以防止将来发生类似的违规情况。

b. 试验方案GLP112755规定，“有资格获得急救的受试者应该返回试验场所进行急救访视，其中包括功效评价。实验室评价应该包括安全性实验室检查（例如化学和全血细胞计数）（原文如此），以及HbA1c”。

试验方案GLP112755入组的受试者005和003，在2009年8月11日和2010年1月26日的急救访视中，您未能进行实验室评价。

在2013年9月2日的书面回复中，您承认在急救访视中对受试者005和003的实验室评价没有进行。您提出这些违规情况之所以发生，是因为您和您的研究人员误解和/或忽视了试验方案中急救访视实验室评价的部分。作为一项纠正措施计划，您指出您的研究中心接受了多次培训会议，内容是关于试验方案和完成所有试验方案要求的规程的重要性。

您的答复不够充分，因为您没有提供纠正措施计划的任何文件，包括您和您的研究人员接受试验方案要求方面培训的细节。没有这些细节内容，我们无法确定您的纠正措施是否足以防止将来发生类似的违规情况。

c. 试验方案GLP112753规定，当受试者返回进行滴注/急救访视时，需要返还在以前访视时分发的药物。试验方案还规定在下次计划给药时间，受试者将得到指示领取新的药物。

受试者005有资格进行剂量调整，并在2009年11月18日收到了增加剂量的试验药物，您未能收回他所有未使用的药物。我们进一步注意到受试者005在2009年12月9日的给药剂量不准确。

在2013年9月2日对FDA483表的书面回复中，您承认之所以发生未能从受试者005收回所有未使用药物的情况，是因为您的研究协调员犯了错，因为要处理大量的、用于在贵研究中心进行的多个临床研究的试验药物。您提出受试者005得到指示，在去领取已经调整过剂量的笔时，把旧的笔还给贵研究中心。但是，据说这名受试者没有归还旧的笔，这就导致他不经意间使用了旧的笔，而没有使用新近发放的笔。

作为纠正措施，您在书面回复中表示您开展了新的方法防止类似事件发生，包括要求两名研究协调员对任何分配给受试者的药物进行确认。

您关于违规情况怎样发生的答复不够充分，因为在贵研究中心，确保受试者005获得正确的试验药物笔是您作为临床研究者的责任，而不是受试者的责任。

您所陈述的纠正措施，如果恰当地执行，应该足以防止将来发生类似的违规情况。

您不遵循试验方案要求的行为，使受试者的安全和福利受到危害，也令人关注在贵研究中心获得的数据的有效性和完整性。

3. 您未能保存对研究中使用试验药物或对照组的受试者的所有研究观察结果和其他相关数据的足够及准确的病历［21 CFR 312.62（b）］

作为一名临床研究者，您必须准备和保存对研究中使用试验药物或对照组的受试者的所有研究观察结果和其他相关数据的足够及准确的病历。病历包括例如体检表等原始文件。对于受试者的体检表，您未能保持完整和准确的病历。关于您是否在必需的访视中完成必需的体检（包括眼底镜检查），研究记录出现了出入。下面是一些例子，包括但不限于这些：

试验方案GLP108486中入组的受试者011，第17次访视/治疗结束原始文件工作表中关于眼底镜检查出现了不一致。这份文件最初记录眼底镜检查在2011年1月11日进行，但是代表已经做过检查的“是”被删掉了，在删除内容旁边加了一个“未做过”的标注。2011年6月2日，“未做过”被删掉，“错误”这个词出现在删除上面。这份文件还包括另外一个后期修改，标注日期是2011年6月2日，是关于眼底镜检查结果的。此外，该文件含有未标明日期的改动，“视力和眼底镜检查已经做过，但没有记录——记录缺失”。

因为对原始记录工作表改动的情形，我们无法确定是否在2011年1月11日或者2011年6月2日做过眼底镜检查。

在2013年9月2日对FDA483表的书面回复中，您承认研究记录中所有的不一致都直接归因于您不良的记录习惯。您指出未能正确地记录眼底镜检查结果是因为体检表中没有包含记录眼底镜检查结果的部分。此外，您认为错漏的评价是由于试验方案的混乱；眼底镜检查并不是每一次访视时都要求，有些眼底镜检查无意中漏掉了，而有些是没有要求做反而做了。

作为一项纠正措施，您表明您修正了原始记录表，已按照试验方案要求，在要求的访视日期里面包含体检和眼底镜检查结果。您还表示，研究中心工作人员进行了关于适当的原始记录和GCP的再教育。此外，您提出从今以后，您要在受试者进行访视时亲自记录所有需要的评价，避免进行后期修改。

您的答复不够充分，因为您没有提供修正过的原始文件或者对工作人员进行关于正确记录培训方面的文件。没有这些细节内容，我们无法确定您的纠正措施是否足以防止将来发生类似的违规情况。

作为一名临床研究者，您有责任确保记录在受试者记录中的数据是准确无误的。未能保留完整和准确的病历，削弱了贵研究中心获取的数据的真实性和完整性。

本警告信的目的并非是罗列您在试验药物临床研究中存在的所有缺陷。确保遵循法律和相关FDA法规的每一项要求是您的职责，您应当解决这些缺陷，并建立规程，以确保任何正在进行或将来进行的研究均符合FDA的法规。

自收到这封信的15个工作日内，您应当书面告知本办公室为预防将来发生类似违规情况而采取的措施。如果不能充分、迅速地解释上述违规问题，可能导致我们在不再通知的情况下采取监管措施。如果您认为您已经遵循了FDA的法规要求，请陈述理由，并提供所有支持资料，以供我们参考。

附：英文原文

Alzohalli, Opada M.D.

WARNING LETTER

JUL 17, 2014

CERTIFIED MAIL
RETURN RECEIPT REQUESTED

Ref: 14-HFD-45-03-01

Opada Alzohaili, M.D.
1331 Monroe Street, Suite 100
Dearborn, MI 48124

Dear Dr. Alzohaili:

This Warning Letter informs you of objectionable conditions observed during the U.S. Food and Drug Administration (FDA) inspection conducted at your clinical site between July 18 and August 14, 2013. Ms. L'Oreal F. Walker, representing FDA, reviewed your conduct of the following clinical investigations of the investigational drug Albiglutide, performed for GlaxoSmithKline:

- Protocol GLP108486, "A Randomized, Open-Label, Active-Controlled, Parallel-Group, Multicenter Study to Determine the Safety and Efficacy of Albiglutide Administered in Combination With Insulin Glargine as Compared With the Combination of Insulin Glargine and Preprandial Lispro Insulin in Subjects With Type 2 Diabetes Mellitus";
- Protocol GLP114179, "A Randomized, Open-Label, Parallel-Group, Multicenter Study to Determine the Efficacy and Safety of Albiglutide as Compared With Liraglutide in Subjects With Type 2 Diabetes Mellitus";
- Protocol GLP112753, "A Randomized, Double-Blind, Placebo and Active-Controlled, Parallel-Group, Multicenter Study to Determine the Efficacy and Safety of Albiglutide When Used in Combination with Metformin Compared With Metformin Plus Sitagliptin, Metformin Plus Glimepiride, and Metformin Plus Placebo in Subjects with Type 2 Diabetes Mellitus";
- Protocol GLP112754, "A Randomized, Open-Label, Parallel-Group, Multicenter Study to Determine the Efficacy and Long-Term Safety of Albiglutide Compared With Insulin in Subjects With Type 2 Diabetes Mellitus";
- Protocol GLP112755, "A Randomized, Double-Blind, Placebo-Controlled, Parallel-Group, Multicenter Study to Determine the Efficacy and Safety of Albiglutide When Used in Combination With Pioglitazone With or Without Metformin in Subjects With Type 2 Diabetes Mellitus";
- Protocol GLP112756, "A Randomized, Double-Blind, Placebo-Controlled, Parallel-Group, Multicenter Study to Determine the Efficacy and Safety of Two-Dose Levels of Albiglutide Compared With Placebo in Subjects With Type 2 Diabetes Mellitus"; and
- Protocol GLP112757, "A Randomized, Double-Blind, Placebo- and Active-Controlled, Parallel-Group, Multicenter Study to Determine the Efficacy and Safety of Albiglutide Administered in Combination With Metformin and Glimepiride Compared With Metformin Plus Glimepiride and Placebo and With Metformin Plus Glimepiride and Pioglitazone in Subjects With Type 2 Diabetes Mellitus."

This inspection is a part of FDA's Bioresearch Monitoring Program, which includes inspections designed to evaluate the conduct of FDA-regulated research to ensure that the data are scientifically valid and accurate, and to help ensure that the rights, safety, and welfare of the human subjects of those studies have been protected.

At the conclusion of the inspection, Ms. Walker presented and discussed with you Form FDA 483, Inspectional Observations. We acknowledge receipt of your September 2, 2013, written response to the Form FDA 483.

From our review of the FDA establishment inspection report, the documents submitted with that report, and your

September 2, 2013, written response, we conclude that you did not adhere to the applicable statutory requirements and FDA regulations governing the conduct of clinical investigations and the protection of human subjects. We wish to emphasize the following:

1. You failed to protect the rights, safety, and welfare of subjects under your care [21 CFR 312.60].

As a clinical investigator, you are required to protect the rights, safety, and welfare of subjects under your care.

a. You failed to ensure that diabetic subjects who are experiencing persistent hyperglycemia will receive a timely rescue treatment in order to prevent complications of uncontrolled hyperglycemia. Specifically:

i. Protocol GLP112756 states that after Visit 9 (Week 4) but before Visit 12 (Week 12), subjects who have a single fasting plasma glucose (FPG) $\geqslant$ 250 mg/dL that is confirmed by a second sample drawn within 7 days and analyzed by the central laboratory, are to receive hyperglycemia rescue.

Subject 001 had an FPG of 261 mg/dL at Week 8 on May 15, 2009, and an FPG of 304 mg/dL at Week 9 on May 19, 2009. According to the protocol, therefore, the subject should have received hyperglycemia rescue. However, study records show that the rescue medication was not prescribed until June 10, 2009 (approximately three weeks later), and the subject did not receive the medication until July 10, 2009.

In your September 2, 2013, written response to the Form FDA 483, you indicated that the delay in Subject 001's hyperglycemia rescue was due to the subject's noncompliance. You noted that on several occasions, you contacted Subject 001 and informed the subject of the importance of initiation of a rescue medication, but that the subject did not comply with your instructions and did not come to your study site until June 10, 2009, at which time a prescription for rescue medication was provided. However, the subject reportedly did not fill the prescription or start the rescue medication until July 10, 2009.

As a corrective action, you indicated that after you communicated with the medical monitor, your site was re-educated on the importance of following protocol procedures and being timely in the titration of subjects.

Your response is inadequate because you have not provided documentation regarding your communications with Subject 001 and your attempts to bring the subject into compliance. In addition, you have not provided sufficient details about your corrective action plan to enable us to determine whether your corrective action appears sufficient to prevent similar violations in the future.

ii. Section 4.6 of Protocol GLP108486 states that subjects would qualify for hyperglycemia rescue if HbA1c $>$ 9.0% and $<$ 0.5% decrease from Baseline, at $\geqslant$ Week 4 and $<$ Week 8.

Subject 004 had a Baseline HbA1c of 7.8% on December 11, 2009, and a Week 4 HbA1c of 9.4% on January 8, 2010. Therefore, Subject 004 met hyperglycemia rescue criteria on January 8, 2010, but the subject was not provided rescue medication until January 29, 2010 (three weeks later).

In your September 2, 2013, written response to the Form FDA 483, you indicated that Subject 004 had a delay in rescue medication due to your misunderstanding of the protocol and your assumption that HbA1c needed to be confirmed prior to rescue, given that other protocols contained this requirement. In addition, you indicated that your lack of documentation was the primary cause of the violations mentioned above, and that as a corrective action, your site will document all study-related data in the subjects' source documents and memos-to-file.

Your response is inadequate because you have not provided any details of a corrective action plan to ensure adequate training for you and your staff on protocol requirements to prevent future violations, and you have not provided sufficient details regarding your plan to document the required study data. Without these details, we are unable to determine whether your corrective action appears sufficient to prevent similar violations in the future.

We remind you that, as the clinical investigator, you are responsible for ensuring that you and your study staff personnel understand the protocol requirements prior to initiating the study.

b. You failed to ensure the safety and welfare of those under your care by failing to ensure that subjects received the correct dose of investigational drug. Specifically:

i. Subject 005 in Protocol GLP112756 was to receive an unscheduled replacement investigational drug, administered via a pen, at Visit 24/Week 16 on September 28, 2011. However, your study coordinator dispensed the wrong pen to the subject. The study coordinator placed a request into the Interactive Voice Response System (IVRS) for a replacement pen that was intended for Subject 006 enrolled in the same protocol, but the coordinator dispensed that pen to Subject 005.

ii. On October 29, 2009, Subject 007 in Protocol GLP112757 received and used the investigational drug pen #2039854 that was assigned to Subject 001 enrolled in a different protocol (Protocol GLP112755).

In your written response to the Form FDA 483, you acknowledged that subjects received the wrong investigational drug pens and indicated that you and your staff take full responsibility for the protocol violations noted above.

As a corrective action, you indicated that you developed new methods to prevent recurrence of similar violations in the future, including a requirement to have two study coordinators verify any assigned medication to subjects.

Your corrective action as described, if properly carried out, appears adequate to prevent similar violations in the future.

Your failure to ensure that subjects receive the correct dose of investigational drug, and that subjects received timely rescue medication during persistent hyperglycemia, raises significant concerns about the protection of study subjects enrolled at your site in the studies mentioned above.

2. You failed to ensure that the investigation was conducted according to the investigational plan [21 CFR 312.60].

As a clinical investigator, you are required to ensure that your clinical studies are conducted in accordance with the investigational plan. The investigational plan for Protocols GLP112753, GLP112754, GLP112755, GLP112756, and GLP112757 required that randomized subjects with persistent hyperglycemia receive either a dose adjustment of study drug or hyperglycemia rescue. In addition, subjects who qualify for rescue medication should return to the study site for a rescue visit, which includes efficacy and laboratory assessments. You failed to adhere to these requirements. Specifically:

a. Protocol GLP112754 states that subjects may qualify for dose adjustments if they are assigned to Albiglutide treatment and experience persistent hyperglycemia, as defined below.

Time Interval on Treatment	Dose Titration
≥ Week 12 and < Week 24	HbA1c > 7.0% with ≤ 0.5% reduction from Baseline
≥ Week 24 and < Week 143	HbA1c > 7.0%

The protocol also states that the site will contact the subject and schedule a return visit within 2 weeks from the time the site received confirmation of the laboratory results indicating a needed dose adjustment.

i. You failed to adjust the dose of Albiglutide within 2 weeks of receiving the laboratory results for Subject 006. Subject 006 had an HbA1c of 8.4% at Week 24 on November 9, 2009. However, you did not adjust the dose of Albiglutide until December 23, 2009, which is a delay of over 1 month.

In your September 2, 2013, written response to the Form FDA 483, you indicated that the delay in dose adjustment occurred due to the subject's noncompliance, despite site staff instructions. However, you have not provided any documentation of your or your staff's attempts to contact the subject to schedule a return visit for dose adjustment within the 2-week time frame.

ii. You failed to adjust the dose of Albiglutide within 2 weeks of receiving the laboratory results for Subject 007. Subject 007 had a baseline HbA1c of 8.3% on July 2, 2009, and a Week 16 HbA1c of 7.8% (≤ 0.5% reduction in HbA1c) on October 19, 2009. However, you did not adjust the dose of Albiglutide until December 28, 2009, which is a delay of almost 2 months.

In your written response to the Form FDA 483, you indicated that you delayed dose adjustments for Subjects 007 due to your concerns about the risk of hypoglycemia and the downward trend of HbA1c. You also indicated that with respect to subject safety, it was left to your discretion on how to proceed. As a corrective action, you indicated that after you communicated with the medical monitor, your study staff personnel were re-educated on the significance of adherence to the protocol, specifically with regard to timely management of subjects who require dose adjustment.

Your response is inadequate because you have not provided any documentation of your evaluation of the subjects' blood glucose levels. Your response is also inadequate because you have not provided details regarding how your corrective actions will be implemented or how you will ensure that you and your staff will follow the investigational plan, focusing on the steps to ensure that eligible subjects receive a dose adjustment within the protocol-specified window. Without these details, we are unable to determine whether your corrective actions appear sufficient to prevent similar violations in the future.

b. Protocol GLP112755 states, "Subjects who qualify for rescue should return to the study center for a rescue visit, which includes efficacy assessments. The laboratory assessments should include safety laboratory test (e.g. chemistry and complete blood count) [*sic*] and HbA1c."

For Subjects 005 and 003 enrolled in Protocol GLP112755, you failed to perform laboratory assessments at rescue visits on August 11, 2009, and January 26, 2010, respectively.

In your September 2, 2013, written response, you acknowledged that laboratory assessments for Subjects 005 and 003 were not performed at the rescue visits. You indicated that these protocol violations occurred because you and your study staff misunderstood and/or overlooked the rescue visit laboratory assessment section of the protocol. As a corrective action plan, you indicated that your site has received numerous training sessions on the protocol and on the significance of completing all protocol-required procedures.

Your response is inadequate because you have not provided any documentation of your corrective action plan, including the details of any training you and your staff received on protocol requirements. Without these details, we are unable to determine whether your corrective actions appear sufficient to prevent similar violations in the future.

c. Protocol GLP 112753 states that subjects are to return medication dispensed at their prior visits when returning for titration/rescue visits. The protocol also states that the subjects will be instructed to take their new medication at their next scheduled dosing time.

You failed to collect all unused medication from Subject 005, who qualified for a dose adjustment and received an increased dose of the investigational drug on November 18, 2009. We note further that Subject 005 was administered the incorrect dose of medication on December 9, 2009.

In your September 2, 2013, written response to the Form FDA 483, you acknowledged that the failure to collect all unused medication from Subject 005 occurred due to your study coordinator's mistake, and due to handling a large number of investigational drugs for multiple clinical studies conducted at your site. You indicated that Subject 005 was instructed to return the old pens to your study site when coming in to receive the dose-adjusted pens. However, the subject reportedly did not return the old pens, which resulted in the inadvertent use of an old pen instead of the more recently dispensed pen.

As a corrective action, you indicated in your written response that you developed new methods of organization to prevent such occurrences, including a requirement to have two study coordinators verify any medication assigned to subjects.

Your response regarding how the violation occurred is inadequate, because it was your responsibility as the clinical investigator, and not the subject's, to ensure that Subject 005 received the correct investigational drug pen at your site.

Your described corrective action, if properly carried out, appears adequate to prevent similar violations in the future.

Failure to follow the protocol requirements jeopardizes subject safety and welfare, and raises concerns about the validity and integrity of the data collected at your site.

3. You failed to maintain adequate and accurate case histories that record all observations and other data pertinent to the investigation on each individual administered the investigational drug or employed as a control in the investigation [21 CFR 312.62(b)].

As a clinical investigator, you are required to prepare and maintain adequate and accurate case histories that record all observations and other data pertinent to the investigation on each individual administered the investigational drug or employed as a control in the investigation. Case histories include source documents such as physical exam worksheets. You have failed to maintain adequate and accurate case histories with respect to subjects' physical examinations. Study records show discrepancies with regard to whether you completed required physical exams, including fundoscopy exams, at the required visits. Examples of this failure include, but are not limited to, the following:

For Subject 011 enrolled in Protocol GLP108486, the Source Document Worksheet for Visit 17/End of Treatment contains discrepancies regarding the fundoscopy exam. This document originally noted that the fundoscopy exam was performed on January 11, 2011, but the entry of "yes" for the performance of the exam was crossed out, and a notation of "Not Performed" was added next to the cross-out. On June 2, 2011, the words "Not Performed" were crossed out, with the word "Error" entered above that cross-out. The document also contains another late entry, dated June 2, 2011, with fundoscopy exam findings. In addition, the document contains the undated entry, "visual acuity and fundoscopy were done but not documented – Missed on Documentation."

Because of the way corrections were made to this Source Document Worksheet, we are unable to determine whether the fundoscopy exam was performed on January 11, 2011, or June 2, 2011.

In your September 2, 2013, written response for the Form FDA 483, you acknowledged that all discrepancies in the study records were directly related to your poor documentation practices. You stated that you failed to document the fundoscopy exam properly because the physical exam worksheets did not contain a section to capture fundoscopy exams. In addition, you indicated that missed assessments were due to a confusion of the protocols; the fundoscopy exams were not required for every visit, and some were inadvertently missed, while others were captured when they were not required.

As a corrective action, you indicated that you revised source documents to include the physical and fundoscopy exams on the required visit dates, as required by the protocol. You also indicated that site staff were re-educated on proper source documentation and on Good Clinical Practices. In addition, you indicated that moving forward, you would document all required assessments in your own writing at the time of subjects' visits to avoid late entries.

Your response is inadequate because you did not provide documentation of the revised source documents or of site staff training regarding proper documentation. Without these details, we are unable to determine whether your corrective action appears sufficient to prevent similar violations in the future.

As the clinical investigator, you are responsible for ensuring that data recorded on subjects' records are accurate. By failing to maintain adequate and accurate case histories, you have compromised the validity and integrity of data captured at your site.

This letter is not intended to be an all-inclusive list of deficiencies with your clinical study of an investigational drug. It is your responsibility to ensure adherence to each requirement of the law and relevant FDA regulations. You should address these deficiencies and establish procedures to ensure that any ongoing or future studies will be in compliance with FDA regulations.

Within fifteen (15) working days of your receipt of this letter, you should notify this office in writing of the actions you have taken to prevent similar violations in the future. Failure to address the violations noted above adequately and promptly may result in regulatory action without further notice. If you believe you have complied with FDA regulations, include your reasoning and any supporting information for our consideration.

If you have any questions, please contact Constance Cullity, M.D., M.P.H., at 301-796-3397; FAX 301-847-8748. Your written response and any pertinent documentation should be addressed to:

Constance Cullity, M.D., M.P.H.
Branch Chief
Good Clinical Practice Enforcement Branch
Division of Good Clinical Practice Compliance
Office of Scientific Investigations
Office of Compliance
Center for Drug Evaluation and Research
Food and Drug Administration
Building 51, Room 5354
10903 New Hampshire Avenue
Silver Spring, MD 20993

Sincerely yours,

{See appended electronic signature page}

Sean Y. Kassim, Ph.D.
Acting Director
Office of Scientific Investigations
Office of Compliance
Center for Drug Evaluation and Research
Food and Drug Administration

第 73 封　给 Weiner, Gilbert R. 的警告信

2014年7月14日

参考号：14-HFD-45-07-01

尊敬的Weiner博士：

2013年9月23日至11月25日，Brunilda Torres女士和Craig Garmendia先生代表FDA，在您的临床研究机构，对您所开展的以下临床研究：试验方案（b）（4）[1]，“（b）（4）”，试验药物为（b）（4），申办者为（b）（4）［被（b）（4）购买］，在原Cetero Research公司临床业务部下属的位于迈阿密花园市的临床试验机构进行了审查。这封警告信特告知您现场检查中发现的违规情况。

我们注意到从2009年5月5日签署FDA1572表开始到2010年4月12日，您一直担任试验方案（b）（4）的临床研究者。这次检查中发现的违规情况就发生在您担任临床研究者期间。

本次现场检查是FDA的生物研究监查项目的一部分。该项目通过设定的检查方法，对FDA监管研究的实施情况进行评估，以确认研究数据在科学上是有效和准确的，并帮助确保这些研究中受试者的权益、安全和福利得到了保护。

在现场检查结束时，Torres女士和Garmendia先生向您出示了FDA483表，即现场检查发现的问题，并与您进行了讨论。您2013年12月3日对该FDA483表的书面回复已收悉。

经对现场检查报告、该报告的附件，以及您2013年12月3日的书面回复进行审查，我们认为，您没有遵循适用的法律要求和监管临床研究实施的FDA法规。我们想强调以下几点：

1. 您未能确保按照研究计划进行研究［21 CFR 312.60］

作为临床研究者，您必须确保临床研究按照研究计划进行。试验方案（b）（4）研究计划要求：完成过敏反应评价表；评价不良事件的研究者不参与受试者给药；受试者不能是研究工作人员的家属；在第1天服用安慰剂后、第8天双盲试验药物给药前，出现任何过敏反应的体征或症状的受试者要终止参加。您未能遵循这些要求，具体而言：

a. 试验方案要求，所有的受试者在第1天获得一个单盲的安慰剂剂量，并在第1天和第2天评估对安慰剂存在过敏反应的体征和/或症状。此外，试验方案要求这些评估要记录在每个受试者的过敏反应评价表上。在这次检查期间，我们审查了129名随机受试者中55名受试者的研究记录，发现在第1天和第2天没有一名受试者完成了过敏反应评价表。例如，受试者031、032、047、256、262和271都没有第1天和第2天完成过敏反应评价表，而这是试验方案要求的。

在2013年12月3日的书面回复中，您声称您没有查看研究记录的权限，因而不能审查相关的信息来解释为什么55名受试者都没有完成过敏反应评价。您还提出，您想不起来哪些评价没有进行。但是，2013年11月20日，您和研究者们会面，对检查结果进行了初步讨论。在那次会议上，（b）（4），（b）（4）全球临床顺应性副主任，提出给您研究记录的复印件，而您拒绝了。

您的答复不够充分，因为在回复中未包含您作为一名临床研究者准备采取的、防止将来发生类似违规情况的任何纠正措施。

b. 试验方案要求，在每个给药日（即第1、8、36和78天）和给药次日（即第2、9、37和79天）对每一个受试者的过敏反应评价表必须完成。对检查到的每一名受试者，您都没有完成给药次日的过敏反应评价表。

1 （b）（4）涉及商业秘密，根据法规内容不予公开。

在2013年12月3日的书面回复中，您指出从给药到受试者退出日过敏反应评价一直在进行，过敏反应评价表在服药后第一个小时后填写；评价表填写后发生的任何不良反应作为不良事件处理；您还指出对于受试者的退出，您或您的授权研究者询问并检查受试者，以排除任何可能的过敏反应。

您的答复不够充分，因为您没有解释为什么在服药次日过敏反应评价表没有完成，也没有包含您作为一名临床研究者已经采取的防止将来发生类似违规情况的纠正措施。

c. 试验方案规定，受试者如果是研究人员或研究人员的家属，要被排除在外，不能参加研究。一份标注2010年6月20日的试验方案偏差表显示，受试者037是某位研究人员的表兄弟，受试者004是某位研究人员的儿子。

在2013年12月3日的书面回复中，您提出，您不能审查纳入排除标准的信息，您不能回忆起关于研究人员亲属的入组问题。您的回复不够充分，因为您没有提出纠正措施计划，以防止将来类似违规情况的发生。

您未能遵从试验方案（包括例如未能完成过敏反应评价表），使受试者的安全和福利受到危害，也使得在贵研究中心收集到的数据的完整性受到削弱。

2. 您未能保存对研究中使用试验药物或对照组的受试者的所有观察结果和其他相关数据的足够及准确的病历［21 CFR 312.62（b）］

作为一个临床研究者，您必须准备和保存对研究中使用试验药物或对照组的受试者的所有观察结果和其他相关数据的足够及准确性的病历。试验方案（b）（4）的病历包括过敏反应评价表，遥测和心电图。您未能保持足够多和准确的病历。具体而言：

a. 过敏反应的体征和症状没有记录在下面几名受试者的过敏反应评价表中：

i. 受试者032，心动过速，过敏反应的一种体征，报告在第36天的不良事件表中，但是没有报告在第36天的过敏反应评价表中。

ii. 受试者057，恶心，过敏反应的一种症状，报告在第8天的不良事件表中，但是没有报告在第8天的过敏反应评价表中。

iii. 受试者227，心动过速被报告在第78天的不良事件表中，但是没有报告在第78天的过敏反应评价表中。

在2013年12月3日的书面回复中，您指出出现心动过速的受试者在用药之前就有这种体征，而且他们的心率后来恢复到正常。但是，您没有提供相关文件来表明受试者032和227在用药前就已经出现心动过速，您也没有解释为什么恶心症状没有记录在受试者057过敏反应评价表上。您的回复还不够充分，您没有提出纠正措施计划，以防止将来发生类似违规情况。

b. 与列出的受试者的给药阶段相关的记录显示，下列受试者过敏反应评价表完成、但是评价表缺失如下：

i. 受试者002，第2阶段（第1周）和第4阶段（第11周）；

ii. 受试者004，第2阶段（第1周）；

iii. 受试者013，第1、2、3阶段（分别是第0、1、5周）；

iv. 受试者014，第1阶段（第0周）和第2阶段（第1周）；

v. 受试者015，第1阶段（第0周）和第2阶段（第1周）；

vi. 受试者021，第1阶段（第0周）；

vii. 受试者031，第2阶段（第1周）；

viii. 受试者201，第2阶段（第1周）；

ix. 受试者210，第2阶段（第1周）和第3阶段（第5周）；

x. 受试者213，第1阶段（第0周）和第2阶段（第1周）；

xi. 受试者214，第1阶段（第0周）和第2阶段（第1周）；

xii. 受试者215，第1阶段（第0周）和第2阶段（第1周）。

在2013年12月3日的书面回复中，您指出因为您没有查看研究记录的权限，所以您不能审查上述的发现。

您还指出“在一些患者中进行过敏反应评价，而仅在另一些患者中进行部分评价或者不进行评价不太合理”。您的答复不够充分，因为您没有对缺失的研究记录做出解释，也没有提出纠正措施计划以预防将来类似违规情况的发生。

c. 研究记录包含过敏反应评价表，该表经过签名和注明日期但是没有包含关于过敏反应体征和症状的受试者的身份证明或其他信息。例如，第36和78天的研究记录中含有您签署了姓名和日期的过敏反应评价表，但是没有其他的信息。还有，受试者210第36天的过敏反应评价表上有您签署的姓名和日期，但是竟然是空白的。

2013年9月9日，您给申办者发了一封电子邮件，解释说由于受试者数量太多，您“在表格填写之前”已经在空白表上签字并盖章。

在2013年12月3日的书面回复中，您指出您会给大量过敏反应评价表盖章，您本应该在已经签字但未使用的表上画一条线，草签并标注日期。您还提出您计划在将来的临床试验中避免这种类型的操作。请注意，我们希望以后您在FDA监管下的研究中不在空白表上预先签字。

d. 遥感记录缺失：在检查过程中，在对研究记录中包含遥感记录的情况进行审查的38名受试者中，至少有27名是缺失的。

e. 受试者004和201的心电图记录是缺失的。

我们承认上述2.d. 和2.e. 项并没有列在发给您的FDA483表中，因此，您对FDA483表的书面回复并没有解决这些违规情况。

您未能保留足够和准确的病历，包括未能记录过敏反应的体征和症状，未能保持遥感记录和心电图记录，使贵研究中心获得的数据的有效性和完整性被削弱，也引起对贵研究中心招募的研究受试者的保护的充分关注。

本警告信的目的并非是罗列您在试验药物临床研究中存在的所有缺陷。确保遵循法律和相关FDA法规的每一项要求是您的职责，您应当解决这些缺陷，并建立规程，以确保任何正在进行或将来进行的研究均符合FDA的法规。

自收到这封信的15个工作日内，您应当书面告知本办公室为预防将来发生类似违规情况而采取的措施。如果不能充分、迅速地解释上述违规问题，可能导致我们在不再通知的情况下采取监管措施。如果您认为您已经遵循了FDA的法规要求，请陈述理由，并提供所有支持资料，以供我们参考。

附：英文原文

Weiner, Gilbert R.

WARNING LETTER

JUL 14, 2014

CERTIFIED MAIL
RETURN RECEIPT REQUESTED

Ref: 14-HFD-45-07-01

Gilbert A. Weiner, D.O.
(b)(6) [*home address*]

Dear Dr. Weiner:

This Warning Letter informs you of objectionable conditions observed during the U.S. Food and Drug Administration (FDA) inspection conducted at your clinical site between September 23 and November 25, 2013. Ms. Brunilda Torres and Mr. Craig Garmendia, representing FDA, reviewed your conduct of a clinical investigation (Protocol **(b)(4)**, "**(b)(4)**") of the investigational drug **(b)(4)** (Sponsor: **(b)(4)**, which was purchased by **(b)(4)**), performed at the Miami Gardens clinical testing facility under the former Clinical Operations Division of Cetero Research.

We note that you served as the clinical investigator for Protocol **(b)(4)** from May 5, 2009, when you signed the Form FDA 1572, until April 12, 2010. The violations observed during the inspection occurred during the time that you were the clinical investigator.

This inspection is a part of FDA's Bioresearch Monitoring Program, which includes inspections designed to evaluate the conduct of FDA-regulated research to ensure that the data are scientifically valid and accurate, and to help ensure that the rights, safety, and welfare of the human subjects of those studies have been protected.

At the conclusion of the inspection, Ms. Torres and Mr. Garmendia presented and discussed with you Form FDA 483, Inspectional Observations. We acknowledge receipt of your December 3, 2013, written response to the Form FDA 483.

From our review of the FDA Establishment Inspection Report, the documents submitted with that report, and your written response dated December 3, 2013, we conclude that you did not adhere to the applicable statutory requirements and FDA regulations governing the conduct of clinical investigations. We wish to emphasize the following:

1. You failed to ensure that the investigation was conducted according to the investigational plan [21 CFR 312.60].

As a clinical investigator, you are required to ensure that your clinical studies are conducted in accordance with the investigational plan. The investigational plan for Protocol **(b)(4)** requires that hypersensitivity assessment forms be completed; that the investigator who evaluates adverse events not be involved in subject dosing; that subjects not be family members of study staff personnel; and that subject participation be terminated for any signs or symptoms of hypersensitivity after dosing of placebo on Day 1, but prior to dosing of double-blind trial medication on Day 8. You failed to adhere to these requirements. Specifically:

a. The protocol requires that all subjects receive a single-blind placebo dose on Day 1 and be evaluated for signs and/or symptoms of hypersensitivity to placebo on Days 1 and 2. In addition, the protocol requires that these evaluations be documented on each subject's hypersensitivity assessment form. During the inspection, we reviewed study records for 55 of the 129 randomized subjects and found that none had hypersensitivity assessment forms completed on Days 1 and 2. For example, Subjects 031, 032, 047, 256, 262, and 271 did not have hypersensitivity assessment forms completed on Days 1 and 2, as required by the protocol.

In your December 3, 2013, written response, you stated you did not have access to the study records and that you were therefore unable to review the information to explain why hypersensitivity assessments were not done for any of these 55 subjects. You also indicated that you did not recall that any of the assessments were not performed. However, on November 20, 2013, you met with the investigators to have a preliminary discussion of the inspection findings. During that meeting, **(b)(4)**, Associate Director of Global Clinical Compliance for **(b)(4)**, offered you copies of the study records, which you declined.

Your response is inadequate because you did not include any corrective actions that you, as a clinical investigator, have taken to prevent similar violations in the future.

b. The protocol requires that hypersensitivity assessment forms be completed on each dosing day (i.e., Days 1, 8, 36, and 78) and on the day following the dosing day (i.e., Days 2, 9, 37, and 79) for each subject. For each subject examined, you failed to complete the hypersensitivity assessment forms for the day following the dosing day.

In your December 3, 2013, written response, you indicated that hypersensitivity assessments were continuously performed from the dosing until the day of discharge; that the hypersensitivity assessment forms were filled out after the first hour post-dose; and that any adverse reaction occurring after the form was filled out was captured as an adverse event. You also noted that upon subjects' discharge, you or your subinvestigator questioned and examined subjects to rule out any possible hypersensitivity reaction.

Your response is inadequate because you did not explain why the hypersensitivity assessment forms were not completed on the days following dosing days, and because you did not include any corrective actions that you, as a clinical investigator, have taken to prevent similar violations in the future.

c. The protocol provides that " subjects who are part of the study staff personnel or family members of the study staff personnel" will be excluded from entry into the study. A Protocol Deviation Form dated June 20, 2010, indicated that Subject 037 was the cousin of a study staff member, and that Subject 004 was the son of a study staff member.

In your December 3, 2013, written response, you indicated that you were not able to review the inclusion/exclusion criteria information and that you did not recall issues regarding enrollment of relatives. Your response is inadequate because you did not provide a corrective action plan to prevent the recurrence of similar violations in the future.

Your failure to adhere to the investigational plan, including, for example, failure to complete hypersensitivity assessment forms, jeopardizes subject safety and welfare, and compromises integrity of the data collected at your site.

2. You failed to maintain adequate and accurate case histories that record all observations and other data pertinent to the investigation on each individual administered the investigational drug or employed as a control in the investigation [21 CFR 312.62(b)].

As a clinical investigator, you are required to prepare and maintain adequate and accurate case histories that record all observations and other data pertinent to the investigation on each individual administered the investigational drug or employed as a control in the investigation. Case histories for Protocol **(b)(4)** include the hypersensitivity assessment forms, telemetry, and electrocardiograms. You have failed to maintain adequate and accurate case histories. Specifically:

a. Signs and symptoms of hypersensitivity were not recorded on the hypersensitivity assessment forms for the following subjects:

i. For Subject 032, tachycardia, a sign of hypersensitivity, was reported on the adverse event form for Day 36, but was not reported on the hypersensitivity assessment form for Day 36.

ii. For Subject 057, nausea, a symptom of hypersensitivity, was reported on the adverse event form for Day 8, but was not reported on the hypersensitivity assessment form for Day 8.

iii. For Subject 227, tachycardia was reported on the adverse event form for Day 78, but was not reported on the hypersensitivity assessment form for Day 78.

In your December 3, 2013, written response, you indicated that subjects who experienced some tachycardia manifested this sign prior to dosing, and that their heart rates later returned to normal. However, you did not provide documentation to show that Subjects 032 and 227 experienced tachycardia prior to dosing, and you did not explain why nausea was not documented in the hypersensitivity assessment form for Subject 057. Your response is also inadequate because you have not provided a corrective action plan to prevent the recurrence of similar violations in the future.

b. Records corresponding to the listed subjects' dosing periods indicated that hypersensitivity assessment forms were completed, but those forms were missing, as follows:

i. Subject 002 – Periods 2 (Week1) and 4 (Week 11)
ii. Subject 004 – Period 2 (Week 1)
iii. Subject 013 – Periods 1, 2, and 3 (Weeks 0, 1, and 5, respectively)
iv. Subject 014 – Periods 1 (Week 0) and 2 (Week 1)
v. Subject 015 – Periods 1 (Week 0) and 2 (Week 1)
vi. Subject 021 – Period 1 (Week 0)
vii. Subject 031 – Period 2 (Week 1)
viii. Subject 201 – Period 2 (Week 1)
ix. Subject 210 – Periods 2 (Week 1) and 3 (Week 5)
x. Subject 213 – Periods 1 (Week 0) and 2 (Week 1)
xi. Subject 214 – Periods 1 (Week 0) and 2 (Week 1)
xii. Subject 215 – Periods 1 (Week 0) and 2 (Week 1)

In your December 3, 2013, written response, you indicated that you were unable to review the above findings because you did not have access to the study records. You also indicated that it "does not appear logical to conduct the [hypersensitivity] assessments on some of the patients and only part or none on others." Your response is inadequate because you did not provide an explanation for the missing study records, and because you did not provide a corrective action plan to prevent the recurrence of similar violations in the future.

c. Study records contained hypersensitivity assessment forms that were signed and dated but that did not contain any subject identification or any other information with regard to hypersensitivity signs and symptoms. For example, study records contained hypersensitivity assessment forms with your dated signature but no other information for Days 36 and 78. In addition, for Subject 210, the hypersensitivity assessment form for Day 36 contained your dated signature but was otherwise blank.

On September 9, 2013, you sent an e-mail to the sponsor noting that due to the large number of subjects, you signed and stamped the blank forms "just prior to filling them out."

In your December 3, 2013, written response, you indicated that you would stamp a block of hypersensitivity forms and indicated that you should have drawn a line across the signed, unused forms and initialed and dated them. You also stated that you plan to avoid this type of practice in future clinical trials. Please note, we expect that you will not pre-sign blank forms in FDA-regulated studies in the future.

d. Telemetry records were missing for at least 27 of the 38 subjects whose records were reviewed for inclusion of this record during the inspection.

e. Electrocardiograms were missing for Subjects 004 and 201.

We acknowledge that Items 2.d. and 2.e. above were not listed on the Form FDA 483 that was issued to you and, therefore, your written response to the Form FDA 483 did not address these violations.

Your failure to maintain adequate and accurate case histories, including the failure to record signs and symptoms of hypersensitivity and the failure to maintain telemetry records and electrocardiograms, compromises the validity and integrity of data captured at your site and raises concern about the adequacy of your protection of study subjects enrolled at your site.

This letter is not intended to be an all-inclusive list of deficiencies with your clinical study of an investigational drug. It is your responsibility to ensure adherence to each requirement of the law and relevant FDA regulations. You should address these deficiencies and establish procedures to ensure that any ongoing or future studies will be in compliance with FDA regulations.

Within fifteen (15) working days of your receipt of this letter, you should notify this office in writing of the actions you have taken to prevent similar violations in the future. Failure to address the violations noted above adequately and promptly may result in regulatory action without further notice. If you believe you have complied with FDA regulations, include your reasoning and any supporting information for our consideration.

If you have any questions, please contact Constance Cullity, M.D., M.P.H., at 301-796-3397; FAX 301-847-8748. Your written response and any pertinent documentation should be addressed to:

Constance Cullity, M.D., M.P.H.
Branch Chief
Good Clinical Practice Enforcement Branch
Division of Good Clinical Practice Compliance
Office of Scientific Investigations
Office of Compliance
Center for Drug Evaluation and Research
U.S. Food and Drug Administration
Building 51, Room 5354
10903 New Hampshire Avenue
Silver Spring, MD 20993

Sincerely yours,

{See appended electronic signature page}

Sean Y. Kassim, Ph.D.
Acting Director
Office of Scientific Investigations
Office of Compliance
Center for Drug Evaluation and Research
U.S. Food and Drug Administration

第74封　给Fandino, Ana J.的警告信

2014年4月30日

参考号：14-HFD-45-12-01

尊敬的Fandino博士：

2013年5月6日至5月22日，Craig A. Garmendia女士代表FDA，在贵临床研究机构，对您所开展的以下临床研究进行了审查：

- 试验方案（b）（4）[1]，“（b）（4），”试验药物为（b）（4），进行（b）（4）；
- 试验方案（b）（4），“（b）（4），”试验药物为（b）（4），进行（b）（4）。

这封警告信特告知您现场检查中发现的违规情况。

本次现场检查是FDA的生物研究监查项目的一部分。该项目通过设定的检查方法，对FDA监管的研究的实施情况进行评估，以确认研究数据在科学上是有效和准确的，并帮助确保这些研究中受试者的权益、安全和福利得到了保护。

在现场检查结束时，Garmendia女士向您出示了FDA483表，即现场检查发现的问题，并与您进行了讨论。您2013年6月3日对该FDA483表的书面回复已收悉。

经对现场检查报告、该报告的附件，以及您2013年6月3日的书面回复进行审查，我们认为，您没有遵循适用的法律要求和监管临床研究实施及受试者保护的FDA法规。我们想强调以下几点：

1. 您未能亲自进行临床研究或对研究进行监管［21 CFR 312.60］

当您为上述临床试验签署研究者声明（FDA1572表）时，您承诺在贵研究中心承担临床研究者职责。您作为临床研究者的总体职责包括确保临床试验按照签署的研究者声明、研究计划和适用的法规来实施，保护在您的监护下的受试者的权益、安全和福利，确保研究中药品的监管［21CFR 312.60］。签署FDA1572表意味着，您明确承诺亲自执行临床试验或对授权他人操作的部分进行监管。您可以将特定研究职责授权给合适的人来操作，但作为临床研究者您不能把总体职责授权给他人。我们的核查表明，对研究职责授权的人员未能进行充分的监管来确保临床试验按照签署的研究者声明、研究计划和适用的法规来实施，并且保护受试者的权益、安全和福利。

具体而言，您未能充分地监管您授权了研究职责的人员。您未能充分监管上述所指的试验的执行导致了很多这封信中提及的违规行为。这些违规行为包括且不限于，在试验方案（b）（4）和（b）（4）中入组了不合格的受试者，没有采取足够的预防措施来防止研究药物（b）（4），一种Ⅱ级管制药物被偷窃和转移。如果您进行了充分监管，可以避免很多此类违规行为的发生。

在您2013年6月3日对FDA483表的书面回复中，您解释了一个导致违背方案的可能原因是正确监管的缺失，这是由于临床研究者经验缺乏或不足，以及对不合格研究者的授权监管的不足。您也提及您加强了对临床研究的监管，您和您的员工重新进行了培训，您们实施了新的标准操作规程，包括职责授权、研究者和助理研究者的职责、研究者审阅必要研究资料、原始资料和病例报告表的填写、药剂操作、药品转移规章。

由于您的纠正措施计划不足以预防未来类似违规行为的发生，您的书面回复是不充分的。具体而言，我们发现您的标准操作规程是不完善的，您没有提供您和您的员工进行培训的细节。

您的题为“主要研究者和助理研究者职责”的SOP没有提及您个人如何来确保对试验流程、试验协调员

1 (b) (4) 涉及商业秘密，根据法规内容不予公开。

的行为以及您和您的研究委员的方案培训的足够监管。另外，您的SOP列举了一些临床研究者的职责，并且表明这不是一个详尽的职责清单。然而，请注意作为临床研究者，您应该遵循所有适用的法规开展工作，而不仅仅是列入您的SOP中的那些职责。

关于您和您的员工进行的培训，您没有提供与培训有关的细节。由于没有这个培训细节，我们无法判断培训是否能够帮助预防未来发生类似的违规情况。

作为临床研究者，最基本的职责就是确保这些试验正确地进行，依从FDA法规，保护试验受试者的权益、安全和福利，确保试验数据的准确性。您对临床试验缺乏监督和管理引起对在您研究中心参与上述试验受试者是否能得到充分保护的严重关注，同时也引起对在贵研究中心产生的数据准确性关注。

2. 您未能确保按照研究计划进行研究［21 CFR 312.60］

作为临床研究者，您必须确保临床试验按照研究计划来进行。试验方案（b）（4）和（b）（4）的研究计划要求您确保受试者在参加试验之前符合所有合格标准。您没有遵循这些要求。具体而言：

a. 试验方案（b）（4）要求受试者在参加试验前的5年内，经专业医生依照美国糖尿病协会指导原则诊断为（b）（4）。

受试者016、018、020和022（入组10个受试者中的4个）在同意参加试验方案（b）（4）时诊断为（b）（4）的时间已超过5年，因此，是不符合研究入组标准的。

i. 受试者016在2012年3月23日同意参加试验方案（b）（4），在2012年4月24日随机进入试验，然而，研究记录显示其在2001年就诊断为（b）（4）。

ii. 受试者018在2012年4月2日同意参加试验方案（b）（4），在2012年4月26日随机进入试验，然而，研究记录显示其在2005年就诊断为（b）（4）。

iii. 受试者020在2012年4月5日同意参加试验方案（b）（4），在2012年4月27日随机进入试验，然而，研究记录显示其在2003年就诊断为（b）（4）。

iv. 受试者022在2012年4月10日同意参加试验方案（b）（4），在2012年4月30日随机进入试验，然而，研究记录显示其在2005年就诊断为（b）（4）。

综上所述，受试者016、018、020、022代表了您入组的10例中的4例。10例中4例不合适的入组引起了对您是否能足够保护您中心受试者的严重关注，也引起对贵研究中心试验（b）（4）数据准确性的关注。

b. 试验方案（b）（4）要求新的受试者［定义为之前未用（b）（4）治疗过］正接受一个稳定治疗方案，这个稳定治疗方案是指在筛选非肿瘤相关疼痛之前每天口服吗啡30～1000mg或同等剂量的一个或多个阿片类药物治疗至少4周以上，并且预估在整个试验阶段随着疾病进展不需要调整阿片类药物的剂量。受试者030和014是作为新受试者入组的，但不符合方案关于阿片类药物治疗的要求。

i. 受试者030：受试者030在入组时的阿片类治疗方案是每天服用120mg可待因，每6小时以复方产品的形式服用一次（300mg对乙酰氨基酚，30mg可待因）。然而，为了符合方案规定的等同于每日口服30mg吗啡的最小剂量，受试者应该每天服用300mg可待因。受试者030在2011年9月15日随机进入试验，参与试验直到2012年8月10日。

在2011年10月6日，贵研究中心通知伦理委员会这个方案违背，解释说发生原因是对该受试者的吗啡同等剂量换算错误。然而，在发现这个错误后，您继续让受试者030参加试验直到2012年8月10日，为受试者随机后的11个月和汇报伦理方案违背后的10个月。

ii. 受试者014：受试者014在入组时阿片类药物的治疗方案是每日100mg曲马多。然而，为了符合方案规定的等同于每日口服30mg吗啡的最小剂量，受试者需要每日服用135mg曲马多。受试者014在2011年8月12日随机进入试验，参与试验直到2012年6月22日。

在2012年8月17日，受试者随机入组后大概1年时，您为这个受试者曲马多剂量写了个备忘录。在这个备忘录中，您指出一个前任协调员为了使受试者看上去符合试验，篡改了曲马多剂量，从每日一次改为每日4次。2012年8月29日，您修改了受试者014的合格性检查列表，指出受试者不符合方案规定的阿片类药物治疗方案。

您的试验记录表明受试者014尽管不符合合格标准，但还是入组了（b）（4）试验近1年。

您在2013年6月3日对上述项2.中提到的方案违背的书面回复中，您表示试验的开展没有被自始至终的正确跟进或监管。另外，您承认您未能在筛选和随机入组访视时有效的审查合格标准来确保受试者有资格参与试验。您也提及您加强了，例如对临床研究的监管，您和您的员工重新进行了培训，实施了新的标准操作规程，包括职责授权、研究者和助理研究者的职责、研究者审阅必要研究资料、原始资料和病例报告表的填写。

由于您的纠正措施计划不足以预防未来类似违规情况的发生，您的书面回复是不充分的。具体而言，我们发现您的标准操作规程（SOPs）是不完善的，另外，您没有提供您和您的员工进行培训的细节。由于没有这个培训细节，我们无法判断培训是否能够帮助预防未来发生类似的违规情况。

标题为“职责授权、执行和完成试验活动”的SOP没有考虑到试验特殊的要求而预先设置了授权，这点引起我们的关注。一个试验方案可能包含很多和这个SOP不符合的关于职责授权、执行和完成试验活动的要求。我们不确定当您的SOP和试验方案要求或指示冲突时，您如何符合您自己的SOP和试验方案。

我们对标题为“原始资料和病例报告表的填写”的SOP包含的下述内容有疑虑：

- 委派的试验协调员将在或大致在试验被伦理委员会批准的时候开始草拟试验的原始文件。
- 委派的试验协调员将是原始文件和病例报告表的主要作者，研究者的职责是质量保证审查员和编辑。

我们不清楚试验协调员在或大致在试验被伦理委员会批准的时候开始草拟试验的何种原始文件。试验特定的行为，包括原始文件的撰写，一般不能在伦理批准之前进行。

我们对这个情况也有疑虑，就是试验协调员将是原始文件和病例报告表的主要作者，研究者的职责是审查员和编辑。把所有试验的原始文件和病例报告表的作者这个职责交给试验协调员，也导致了关注您对试验的监管是否足够。您没有先考虑每个试验的特性和要求，再决定范围，就把这些职责都授予试验协调员，我们认为这点是不能接受的，即便可以，什么样的试验协调员是合格的，可以成为所有原始文件和病例报告表的第一作者。

我们进一步关注的是，当基于方案修订，原始文件和病例报告表需要修订时，SOP没有指出谁负责确认这些文件的修订是适当的、准确的、完整的。

关于您提供的病例报告表样本，我们不知道这个病例报告表样本的目的和您打算什么时候使用它。我们担忧您使用不是试验特定的病例报告表，有可能给未来的试验造成错误。

我们强调我们的关注，这就是您没有充分评估受试者的合格标准，这些合格标准是为每个试验专门设计的，有利于最优化对收集数据的解释，并且最小化对入组的受试者的可预期伤害。入组了不合格受试者会危害受试者的安全和福利，我们对您中心收集的数据的有效性和完整性产生关注。我们特别关注这个方案（b）（4）入组的10例受试者中4个不合格的病例。

3. 您未能采取合适的预防措施来防止按《特殊管制物质法》管理的试验药物被盗窃或非法转移［21 CFR 312.69］

作为临床研究者，在处理受《特殊管制物质法》监管的临床试验用药时，您必须采取足够的预防措施来防止药品被偷窃或转移至非法分销渠道。这些预防措施包括把临床试验用药储存在带锁的、构造牢固的柜子，或者其他带锁、构造牢固的地方，接触的权限是受限的。试验方案（b）（4）的临床试验用药由于结构与脱氧吗啡酮类似，被美国禁毒署定义为Ⅱ级管控物质。您未能采取足够的预防措施来防止（b）（4）被偷窃或转移。具体而言，您没有把（b）（4）存放在安全带锁的场所。相反，您把临床试验用药放在没有锁的不安全房间。迈阿密警方的一份报告指出在2011年11月3日大约有900片（b）（4）从贵研究中心被偷走。

您在2013年6月3日书面回复了上述第三条违背情况，您坦陈（b）（4）在贵研究中心的被窃是“由于缺乏严格的安全监控和措施”。您表示将采取以下措施来预防未来发生类似的违规情况：

- 2个新标准操作规程：
  - 药房运营（版本1，日期2012年3月16日）；

  - ○ 药品转移政策（版本1，日期2012年3月16日）。
- 使用新的监控摄像机和在通向药房的走廊和药房内部安装报警系统。
- 把药品转移到更安全的位置。
- 使用带锁的柜子系统来存放定义为管制物质的临床试验用药。
- 只给予授权的员工权限，来接触定义为管制物质的临床试验用药。
- 更换药房的门锁，把新钥匙只给予授权的员工。

由于您没有提供关于药房运营和药品转移预防措施的新的标准操作规程复印件，您的回复是不充分的。因此，我们无法判断您的纠正措施是否足够充分来防止类似违规情况的再发生。

本警告信的目的并非是罗列您在试验药物临床研究中存在的所有缺陷。确保遵循法律和相关FDA法规的每一项要求是您的职责，您应当解决这些缺陷，并建立规程，以确保任何正在进行或将来进行的研究均符合FDA的法规。

自收到这封信的15个工作日内，您应当书面告知本办公室为预防将来发生类似违规情况而采取的措施。如果不能充分、迅速地解释上述违规问题，可能导致我们在不再通知的情况下采取监管措施。如果您认为您已经遵循了FDA的法规要求，请陈述理由，并提供所有支持资料，以供我们参考。

附：英文原文

Fandino, Ana J. M.D.

WARNING LETTER

APR 30，2014

CERTIFIED MAIL
RETURN RECEIPT REQUESTED

Ref: 14HFD451201

Ana J. Fandino, M.D.
10281 SW 72nd Street
Suite 101
Miami, FL 33173

Dear Dr. Fandino:

This Warning Letter informs you of objectionable conditions observed during the U.S. Food and Drug Administration (FDA) inspection conducted at your clinical site between May 6 and May 22, 2013. Mr. Craig A. Garmendia, representing the FDA, reviewed your conduct of the following clinical investigations:

Protocol (b)(4), “(b)(4),” of the investigational drug (b)(4), performed for (b)(4).

Protocol (b)(4), “(b)(4),” of the investigational drug (b)(4), performed for (b)(4).

This inspection is a part of FDA’s Bioresearch Monitoring Program, which includes inspections designed to evaluate the conduct of FDA regulated research to ensure that the data are scientifically valid and accurate, and to help ensure that the rights, safety, and welfare of the human subjects of those studies have been protected.

At the conclusion of the inspection, Mr. Garmendia presented and discussed with you Form FDA 483, Inspectional Observations. We acknowledge receipt of your June 3, 2013 written response to the Form FDA 483.

From our review of the establishment inspection report, the documents submitted with that report, and your June

3, 2013 written response, we conclude that you did not adhere to the applicable statutory requirements and FDA regulations governing the conduct of clinical investigations and the protection of human subjects. We wish to emphasize the following:

1. You failed to personally conduct or supervise the clinical investigations [21 CFR312.60].

When you signed the Statement of Investigator (Form FDA 1572) for the above-referenced clinical trials, you agreed to take on the responsibilities of a clinical investigator at your site. Your general responsibilities as a clinical investigator include ensuring that the clinical trials are conducted according to the signed investigator statement, the investigational plan, and applicable regulations; protecting the rights, safety, and welfare of subjects under your care; and ensuring control of drugs under investigation [21 CFR 312.60]. By signing Form FDA 1572, you specifically agreed to personally conduct the clinical trial or to supervise those aspects of the trial that you did not personally conduct. While you may delegate certain study tasks to individuals qualified to perform them, as a clinical investigator you may not delegate your general responsibilities. Our investigation indicates that your supervision of personnel to whom you delegated study tasks was not adequate to ensure that the clinical trials were conducted according to the signed investigator statement, the investigational plan and applicable regulations, and in a manner that protects the rights, safety, and welfare of human subjects.

Specifically, you failed to adequately supervise individuals to whom you delegated study tasks. Your failure to adequately supervise the conduct of the studies referenced above led to many of the violations noted in this letter. These violations include, but are not limited to, enrollment of ineligible subjects in Protocols (b)(4) and (b)(4) and failure to take adequate precautions to prevent theft or diversion of the investigational drug (b)(4), a Schedule Ⅱ controlled substance. Had you provided adequate oversight, you may have been able to prevent many of these violations from occurring.

In your June 3, 2013 written response to the Form FDA 483, you explained that one probable cause of the protocol violations was lack of proper supervision due to lack of or limited clinical investigator experience and supervision in delegating responsibilities to unqualified staff. You also noted that you increased your supervision of clinical research, that you and your staff were retrained, and that you implemented new standard operating procedures about delegation of responsibilities, investigator and sub-investigator responsibilities, investigator review of essential study documents, source document and case report form creation, pharmacy operations and pharmacy diversion policy.

Your written response is inadequate because your corrective action plan is not sufficient to prevent similar violations in the future. Specifically, we find your Standard Operating Procedures (SOPs) insufficient and note that you did not provide details regarding the training that you and your staff underwent.

Your SOP titled "Principal Investigator and Sub-Investigator Responsibilites" does not address how you personally will ensure adequate oversight of study procedures, activities of study coordinators and protocol training for you and your study staff. In addition, your SOP lists some responsibilities of a clinical investigator, and states that it is not an all-inclusive list. However, please note that you are responsible for compliance with all regulations applicable to your conduct as a clinical investigator, not just those which are listed as responsibilities in your SOP.

Regarding the training that you and your staff underwent, you did not provide details regarding the training. Without having the details of this training, we are unable to determine whether it appears adequate to help prevent similar violations in the future.

As the clinical investigator, it was your ultimate responsibility to ensure that these studies were conducted properly and in compliance with FDA regulations to protect the rights, safety, and welfare of study subjects and ensure the integrity of study data. Your lack of supervision and oversight over the clinical studies raises significant concerns about the adequacy of your protection of study subjects enrolled at your site in the studies mentioned above, and also raises concerns about the integrity of the data generated at your site.

2. You failed to ensure that the investigation was conducted according to the investigational plan [21 CFR 312.60].

As a clinical investigator, you are required to ensure that your clinical studies are conducted in accordance with the investigational plans. The investigational plans for Protocols (b)(4) and (b)(4) required you to ensure that subjects met all eligibility criteria prior to the subjects' participation in the studies. You failed to adhere to these requirements. Specifically:

a. Protocol (b)(4) requires subjects to have (b)(4) diagnosed by a medical professional, in accordance with the American Diabetes Association guidelines, and within 5 years prior to consenting to participate in this study.

Subjects 016, 018, 020 and 022 (4 of the 10 subjects who you enrolled) were diagnosed with (b)(4) more than 5 years before they consented to participate in Protocol (b)(4) and, thus, were ineligible for the study.

i. Subject 016 consented to participate in Protocol (b)(4) on March 23, 2012, and was randomized into the study on April 24, 2012. However, study records show that Subject 016 was diagnosed with (b)(4) in 2001.

ii. Subject 018 consented to participate in Protocol (b)(4) on April 2, 2012, and was randomized into the study on April 26, 2012. However, study records show that Subject 018 was diagnosed with (b)(4) in 2005.

iii. Subject 020 consented to participate in Protocol (b)(4) on April 5, 2012, and was randomized into the study on April 27, 2012. However, study records show that Subject 020 was diagnosed with (b)(4) in 2003.

iv. Subject 022 consented to participate in Protocol (b)(4) on April 10, 2012, and was randomized into the study on April 30, 2012. However, study records show that Subject 022 was diagnosed with (b)(4) in 2005.

As noted above, Subjects 016, 018, 020 and 022 represent 4 of the 10 subjects who you enrolled. Your inappropriate enrollment of 4 out of 10 subjects in this study raises significant concerns about the adequacy of your protection of study subjects enrolled at your site and also raises concerns about the integrity of the data generated at your site for Protocol (b)(4).

b. Protocol (b)(4) requires that new subjects (defined as subjects not previously treated with (b)(4)) be on a stable regimen of 30 to 1000 mg oral morphine daily or an equivalent analgesic dose of one or more listed opioid therapies for at least 4 weeks before screening for non-cancer-related pain with no anticipated change in opioid dose requirement over the proposed study period as a result of disease progression. Subjects 030 and 014, who were enrolled as new subjects, were not on an opioid regimen that complied with this protocol requirement.

i. Subject 030: Subject 030's opioid regimen at enrollment was 120 mg of codeine daily, taken in the form of a combination product (300 mg acetaminophen and 30 mg codeine) every 6 hours. However, the subject needed to be taking 300 mg codeine daily to meet the protocol-required minimum equivalent of 30 mg oral morphine daily. Subject 030 was randomized into the study on September 15, 2011, and remained in the study until August 10, 2012.

On October 6, 2011, your site notified your Institutional Review Board (IRB) of this protocol violation and explained that it happened because the morphine-equivalent conversion dose for this subject was miscalculated. Yet, after finding the error, you continued Subject 030 in this study until August 10, 2012, 11 months after the subject was randomized and 10 months after reporting the violation to the IRB.

ii. Subject 014: Subject 014's opioid regimen at enrollment was 100 mg of Tramadol daily. However, the subject needed to be taking 135 mg of Tramadol daily to meet the protocol-required minimum equivalent of 30 mg oral morphine daily. Subject 014 was randomized into the study on August 12, 2011, and remained in the study until June 22, 2012.

On August 17, 2012, approximately one year after Subject 014 was randomized into Protocol (b) (4), you prepared a Memo to File regarding the subject's Tramadol dosing. In this memo, you indicated that a previous study coordinator falsified the Tramadol dosing frequency from once daily to 4 times daily to make the subject appear eligible for the study. On August 29, 2012, you amended Subject 014's Eligibility Checklist to reflect that the subject did not meet the study requirement regarding opioid regimen.

Your study records show that Subject 014 remained enrolled for nearly a year in Protocol (b)(4) even though the subject did not meet eligibility requirements for the study.

In your June 3, 2013 written response to the violations noted in Item 2 above, you stated that the studies were conducted without proper follow-through or supervision. In addition, you acknowledged your failure to review eligibility criteria effectively at screening and at randomization visits to ensure that subjects were eligible for study participation. You also noted that you have, for example, increased your supervision of clinical research, that you and your staff were retrained, and that you implemented new standard operating procedures about delegation of responsibilities, investigator and sub-investigator responsibilities, investigator review of essential study documents, and source document and case report form creation.

Your written response is inadequate because your corrective action plan is not sufficient to prevent similar violations in the future. Specifically, we find your Standard Operating Procedures (SOPs) insufficient. In addition, you have not provided details regarding the training that you and your staff underwent. Without having the details of this training, we are unable to determine whether it appears adequate to help prevent similar violations in the future.

Your SOP titled "Delegation of Responsibilities, Conduct and Completion of Study Activities" is of concern to us because it appears to have delegations pre-set without regard to study-specific requirements. A study protocol may contain requirements regarding delegation of responsibilities, conduct, and completed study activities that are not aligned with this SOP. We are uncertain how you would meet the requirements of your own SOP and study protocols when your SOP conflicts with directions or requirements contained in study protocols.

Your SOP titled "Sources [sic] Document/Case Report Form Creation" notes the following, which is of concern to us:

- The assigned study coordinator will start drafting study source documents at or about the time the study is approved by the Institutional Review Board
- The assigned study coordinator will be the primary author of source documents and Case Report Forms, with the investigator's role being that of Quality Assurance Reviewer and Editor

We are unclear on what type of source documents you would have a study coordinator start drafting at or about the time a study is approved by an IRB. Study specific activities, including creation of source documents, generally cannot be undertaken until after IRB approval of the study.

We are also concerned with the statement that a study coordinator will be the primary author of source documents and Case Report Forms, with your role being that of reviewer and editor. Placing responsibility on a study coordinator for authorship of all source documents and Case Report Forms in all studies raises concern about the adequacy of your oversight of studies. We do not find it acceptable for you to assign these responsibilities to study coordinators without first considering the specifics and requirements of each study that you undertake and determining the extent, if any, to which the study coordinator is qualified to be the primary author of all source documents and Case Report Forms.

We are further concerned that, where revisions to source documents or Case Report Forms may be required based on a protocol amendment, the SOP does not indicate who is responsible for ensuring that any document revisions are appropriate, accurate, and complete.

With respect to the sample Case Report Form that you provided, we are unable to determine the purpose of this sample Case Report Form and when you plan to use it. We are concerned that you may introduce error into future studies by using Case Report Forms that are not study-specific.

We emphasize our concern that you failed to fully evaluate eligibility criteria for subjects that were designed specifically for each research study to optimize interpretability of collected data and minimize foreseeable harm to enrolled subjects. Enrollment of subjects who do not meet eligibility criteria jeopardizes subject safety and welfare and raises concern about the validity and integrity of the data collected at your site. We are particularly concerned that 4 of the 10 subjects in Protocol (b)(4) were enrolled despite being ineligible for the study.

3. You failed to take adequate precautions to prevent theft or diversion of an investigational drug that is subject to the Controlled Substances Act [21 CFR 312.69].

As a clinical investigator, when handling an investigational drug that is subject to the Controlled Substances Act, you are required to take adequate precautions to prevent theft or diversion of the substance into illegal channels of distribution. These precautions include the storage of the investigational drug in a securely locked, substantially constructed cabinet, or other securely locked, substantially constructed enclosure, access to which is limited. The investigational drug for Protocol (b)(4), (b)(4), is classified by the U.S. Drug Enforcement Administration as a Schedule Ⅱ controlled substance based on structural relatedness to noroxymorphone. You failed to take adequate precautions to prevent theft or diversion of (b)(4). Specifically, you failed to store (b)(4) in a securely locked enclosure. Rather, you stored the investigational drug in an unlocked and unsecured room. A police report from the City of Miami Police Department indicates that approximately 900 (b)(4) tablets were stolen from your site on November 3, 2011.

In your June 3, 2013 written response to the violation noted in Item 3 above, you acknowledged that the theft of (b)(4) at your site was "due to the lack of stringent security monitoring and measures." You indicated that, to prevent similar violations in the future, you implemented the following:

- Two new standard operating procedures:
  - Pharmacy Operations (Version 1, dated March 16, 2012)
  - Pharmacy Diversion Policy (Version 1, dated March 16, 2012)
- Use of new surveillance cameras and an alarm system in hallways leading to and inside the pharmacy
- Moving the pharmacy to a more secure location
- Use of a locked cabinet system for storing investigational drugs classified as controlled substances
- Limiting access to these investigational drugs classified as controlled substances to designated employees
- Changing pharmacy door locks and reassigning new keys to designated employees only

Your response is inadequate because you failed to provide a copy of the new standard operating procedures about pharmacy operations and pharmacy diversion prevention policy. As a result, we are unable to determine whether your corrective actions appear sufficient to prevent a recurrence of similar violations.

This letter is not intended to be an all-inclusive list of deficiencies with your clinical studies of investigational drugs. It is your responsibility to ensure adherence to each requirement of the law and relevant FDA regulations. You should address these deficiencies and establish procedures to ensure that any ongoing or future studies will be in compliance with FDA regulations.

Within fifteen (15) working days of your receipt of this letter, you should notify this office in writing of the actions you have taken to prevent similar violations in the future. Failure to address the violations noted above adequately and promptly may result in regulatory action without further notice. If you believe you have complied with FDA regulations, include your reasoning and any supporting information for our consideration.

If you have any questions, please contact Constance Cullity, M.D., M.P.H., at 3017963397; FAX 3018478748. Your written response and any pertinent documentation should be addressed to:

Constance Cullity, M.D., M.P.H.
Branch Chief
Good Clinical Practice Enforcement Branch
Division of Good Clinical Practice Compliance
Office of Scientific Investigations
Office of Compliance
Center for Drug Evaluation and Research
Food and Drug Administration
Building 51, Room 5354
10903 New Hampshire Avenue
Silver Spring, MD 20993

Sincerely yours,

{See appended electronic signature page}

Sean Y. Kassim, Ph.D.
Acting Director
Office of Scientific Investigations
Office of Compliance
Center for Drug Evaluation and Research
Food and Drug Administration

第75封　给Sewell, Michele医学博士的警告信

2014年4月30日

参考号：14-HFD-45-04-03

尊敬的Sewell博士：

2013年6月17日至2013年8月19日，Nicole Bell女士和Vanessa coulter女士代表FDA，在您的临床研究机构，对您所开展的申办者为葛兰素史克公司，试验药物为注射用阿必鲁肽（albiglutide）的以下临床研究进行了审查：

- 试验方案 GLP112754，“一项随机、开放、平行组别、多中心试验，比较阿必鲁肽和胰岛素在2型糖尿病受试者中的有效性和长期安全性”；
- 试验方案GLP112757，“一项随机、双盲、安慰剂和活性药物对照、平行组别、多中心试验，比较阿必鲁肽联合二甲双胍和格列美脲、二甲双胍和格列美脲和安慰剂，二甲双胍和格列美脲和匹格列酮，在2型糖尿病受试者中的有效性和安全性”。

这封警告信特告知您现场检查中发现的违规情况。

本次现场检查是FDA的生物研究监查项目的一部分。该项目通过设定的检查方法，对FDA监管的研究的实施情况进行评估，以确认研究数据在科学上是有效和准确的，并帮助确保这些研究中受试者的权益、安全和福利得到了保护。

在现场检查结束时，Bell女士和Coulter女士向您出示并讨论了FDA483表，即现场检查发现的问题。在2013年9月5日，FDA发给了您FDA483表，修订版1，日期为2013年9月5日。您2013年9月12日对该FDA483表和FDA483表修订版1的书面回复已收悉。

经对现场检查报告、该报告的附件，以及您2013年9月12日的书面回复进行审查，我们认为，您没有遵循适用的法律要求和监管临床研究实施及受试者保护的FDA法规。我们想强调以下几点：

1. 您未能确保按照研究计划进行研究［21 CFR 312.60］

作为临床研究者，您必须确保临床研究按照研究计划进行。试验方案GLP112757的研究计划包括与合格性确认、筛选前磺酰脲类的使用、药代动力学（PK）血样的采集，以及增加药物剂量的标准相关的一些要求。

试验方案GLP112754的研究计划包括与严重不良事件（SAE）的报告、在特定研究访视时的特殊评估和流程相关的一些要求。这两个试验方案都要求试验访视在特定时间段内进行。您没有遵守这些要求。具体而言：

a. 受试者1398757001，试验方案GLP112757：

i. 试验方案GLP112757规定受试者在筛选前接受磺酰脲类治疗至少3个月，这个磺酰脲类治疗相当于至少4mg格列美脲。方案指出4mg格列美脲和5mg格列本脲一天2次是对等的。

2009年8月19日，受试者1398757001在筛选时每天服用5mg格列本脲（方案规定剂量的一半），不符合试验方案GLP112757。这个受试者的合并用药记录在2009年9月的某个时间（筛选后）从5mg每天一次变成5mg每天2次，受试者在2010年1月6日随机入组。剂量的纠正应该在筛选前至少3个月发生，而不是在筛选后。

2013年9月12日，您在书面回复FDA483表中提及经过额外审阅，发现自己没有正确的记录格列美脲剂量。您也提及作为纠正措施，您的研究人员将接受或已经接受了额外培训来确保依从方案。

由于没有充分的纠正计划的细节，您的回复是不充分的。您没有提供关于您的研究人员培训的任何细节或文件。您没有提及作为临床研究者您自己采取了什么纠正措施来确保方案的依从。没有这些细节，我们无

法判断您的纠正措施是否能够预防未来发生类似的违规。

ⅱ. 试验方案GLP112757规定有血红蛋白病的受试者不能参加试验，因为这会影响血红蛋白A1c的测定。

受试者1398757001对于试验方案112757是不合格的，在2009年8月19日筛选时，实验室结果显示“在血红蛋白A1c检测时发现明显的血红蛋白异常”。在2010年2月3日第4周访视时，实验室结果也显示同样的血红蛋白显著异常，复测也如此。在2011年4月22日的访视后实验室结果中实验人员注意到存在与镰刀型红细胞痕迹（杂合子）一致的血红蛋白形状和浓集，提示临床和血液学的相关性。

在您2013年9月12日书面回复FDA483表时，您表示以您的专业观点来看这个受试者不应该因为少量镰刀型红细胞而被排除，所以在筛选时没有备注。另外，您声明“我认为，在当时，基于（b）（4）提供的精确测定的方法学，虽然有些证据，但没有确切证据来说明HbA1c不能用来精确监测葡萄糖”。

您的回复是不合适的，因为试验方案GLP112757要求排除患有可能会影响HbAc1测定的血红蛋白病的受试者。镰刀型红细胞就是这种被排除的血红蛋白病。

ⅲ. 试验方案GLP112757规定所有研究访视发生不超过±3天，访视7（第一周）和访视8（基线）除外。方案注明受试者由于特殊情况（如假日、休假、个人紧急情况）无法在访视期内完成访视而延长访视期，不考虑为超出依从性。然而，方案特别规定最大访视期偏离的判断在于医学监查员的决定。

对于受试者1398757001，访视22（第65周）发生在超过方案允许的时间15天。方案对访视22的规定是在访视21（第52周）后的13周±3天。这个受试者的访视21是2011年1月7日，访视22发生在大概15周之后，为2011年4月26日。没有证据说明这是一个异常事件还是在医学监查员判定的最大时间窗内。

在2013年9月12日书面回复FDA483表时，您没有提供这个受试者访视延迟的解释。可是，您确认这个时间安排问题的发生。您表示您采取了纠正措施，作为纠正措施的一部分，您每周和研究人员以及临床工作人员开会。您也申明您有关于评估的标准操作规程（SOP），您和您的研究人员重新培训了这个SOP。

由于您没有提供异常事件的证明文件，或与医学监查员讨论来决定最大访视期偏离的证明文件，您的回复是不充分的。另外，您没有提供纠正措施计划的足够细节，您没有提供关于评估的标准操作规程的复印件，您表示您已经制定这个文件，您和您的员工重新培训过，您也没提供这个培训的细节。没有这些细节，我们无法判断您的纠正措施是否能充分预防未来类似违规情况的发生。

b. 受试者1398757002，试验方案GLP112757：

ⅰ. 试验方案GLP112757规定受试者要在筛选前至少3个月每天服用1500mg二甲双胍。然而，如果在随机前至少8周剂量已经稳定，方案允许入组有记录的二甲双胍最大耐受剂量不足每天1500mg的受试者。

尽管受试者1398757002没有在筛选前至少3个月每天服用1500mg二甲双胍，也不是在随机前至少8周剂量稳定，有记录的二甲双胍最大耐受剂量不足1500mg/d，但这个受试者入组了试验。合并用药记录显示在2009年8月20日（筛选前4天），受试者1398757002每日2次服用二甲双胍500mg（1000mg/d），这个比规定的剂量少500mg。在2009年8月21日，剂量被增加到二甲双胍1000mg一天两次（2000mg/d）。这个剂量的增加并不能使得该患者成为合格的入组受试者，因为受试者没有在筛选前至少3个月服用二甲双胍1500mg/d。然而，受试者1398757002在2009年8月24日，也就是3天后进行了筛选。此外，您没有提供证明文件来表明受试者在随机前至少8周剂量稳定，有记录的二甲双胍最大耐受剂量不足1500mg/d。

在2013年9月12日您书面回复FDA483表时，您声称这个受试者最大耐受剂量是二甲双胍1000mg（每天）。在您的书面回复中，您也提及您采取了纠正措施来确保及时进行方案规定的评估。由于您没有提供文件来支持您声称的受试者最大耐受剂量是二甲双胍1000mg/d，您的回复也是不充分的。值得注意的是，试验记录显示在2009年8月21日受试者的二甲双胍剂量增加到1000mg每天2次，共2000mg/d，没有文件记录显示受试者不能耐受这个剂量。

因为没有关于纠正措施的充分细节，您的回复也是不充分的。具体而言，您没有提供关于评估的标准操作规程的复印件，您表示开始执行这个文件，您和您的员工重新培训过，您也没提供这个培训的细节。没有这些细节，我们无法判断您的纠正措施是否能充分预防未来类似违规情况的发生。

ⅱ. 试验方案GLP112757只允许当受试者符合剂量增加的标准时，您可以增加试验药物的剂量。方案规定只有当受试者在第4周时单次空腹血糖在250mg/dL以上，7天内重新抽血，中心实验室检查确认，并且受试者的HbA1c水平和基线相比不变或上升，可以给受试者增加剂量。您没有遵守这个要求。具体而言：

尽管受试者1398757002没有符合试验方案关于剂量增加的标准，其在2009年12月3日增加了试验药物的剂量。这个受试者在2009年11月17日，第4周访视时空腹血糖是144mg/dL。除了低于要求水平的空腹血糖，您未能提供这个值在7天内被中心实验室复查的结果所确认的证据。因此，受试者1398757002在2009年12月3日不应该增加剂量。

在2013年9月12日您书面回复FDA483表时，您承认一些试验方案规定的流程、体格检查、实验室检查、心电图（ECGs）没有在合适的时间范围内进行。您声称您采取了纠正措施来确保试验评估在未来不会遗漏。您提到作为纠正措施的一部分，您请您的研究人员参与您与临床人员的周会，您每周和研究人员开会来了解受试者状态报告。另外，您说您和您的研究人员重新培训了关于试验评估的SOP。

由于您没有提供关于纠正措施的充分的细节，您的回复是不充分的。具体而言，您没有提供关于评估的标准操作规程的复印件，您表示这个文件已经制定，您和您的员工重新培训过，您也没提供这个培训的细节。没有这些细节，我们无法判断您的纠正措施是否足以预防未来类似违规情况的发生。

ⅲ. 试验方案GLP112757规定在第28周，受试者应在服药后至少2天采集PK血样。您没有遵守这些要求。具体而言：

在2010年5月4日（访视18/第28周），受试者1398757002服用了药包号为221065的研究药物，同时采集了他的PK血样。

在2013年9月12日您书面回复FDA483表时，您承认这些评估没有根据试验方案来进行，您指出您已采取纠正措施来确保未来试验评估不会被错过。您还提及作为纠正措施的一部分，您每周和研究团队开会，研究团队重新培训了关于试验评估的SOP。

由于您没有提供关于纠正措施的充分细节，您的回复是不充分的。具体而言，您没有提供关于评估的标准操作规程的复印件，您表示这个文件已经制定，您和您的员工重新培训过，您也没提供这个培训的细节。没有这些细节，我们无法判断您的纠正措施是否足以预防未来类似违规情况的发生。

c. 受试者13987574002，试验方案GLP112754：

ⅰ. 试验方案GLP112754规定所有SAEs应该在24小时内报告给申办者。方案定义严重不良事件为任何可导致死亡、危害生命、需要住院或延长住院时间、致残、致畸/出生缺陷，或其他临床研究者判断为严重的医学事件（如该事件需要医学或手术干预来防止上述结果）的意外医学发生。您没有遵守这些要求。具体而言：

受试者1398754002经历了不稳定型心绞痛的SAE导致根据（b）（6）的住院。然而，这个SAE直到2011年6月11日，大概15个月后才报告给申办者。

在2013年9月12日，您书面回复FDA483表时，您提出这个受试者在2010年5次不同的访视时没有告诉试验协调员住院的事情。您声称这个住院是在您中心为了另一个事件收到并审阅了受试者的医学记录后，于2011年6月9日发现的。

您的回复是不充分的，因为在受试者的与因为不稳定型心绞痛的（b）（6）入院的医院记录底部的打印条，提示这个记录的复印件发给了您。您既没有充分的解释受试者1398754002的SAE报告的失误，也没有解释在未来如何改正这个失误。

ⅱ. 试验方案GLP112754（原始版本日期2008年12月8日）要求所有研究访视的治疗窗为±3天。这个试验方案的修订1（日期2009年8月6日）规定了所有访视具有相同的时间窗，访视6（基线）除外，其治疗窗为±6天。方案注明受试者由于特殊情况（如假日、休假、个人紧急情况）无法在访视期内完成访视而延长访视期，不考虑为超出依从性。然而，最大访视期背离的判断在于医学监查员的决定。

受试者1398754002有多次研究访视显著超出了方案规定的时间范围。

访视/周	实际访视日期	超过时间/距离预期时间范围(允许的范围)
访视6/第0周	9/25/2009	超期15天（±6天）
访视16/第28周	5/17/2010	超期28天（±3天）
访视17/第36周	6/19/2010	提前20天（±3天）
访视18/第48周	8/24/2010	提前15天（±3天）

在2013年9月12日，您书面回复FDA483表时，您提到试验方案GLP112754对超窗访视的特殊说明（原始版本日期2008年12月8日）："所有研究访视的治疗窗为±3天。受试者由于特殊情况（如假日、休假、个人紧急情况）无法在±3天的访视期内完成访视而延长访视期，不考虑为超出依从性。然而，最大访视期背离的判断在于医学监查员的决定"。

由于您没有解释为什么这个受试者上面提到的访视有这么显著的延迟，您没有提供任何特殊情况或您与医学监查员讨论每个事件来决定最大访视期背离的任何记录，您的回复同样是不充分的，因为您没有提供纠正措施计划预防未来类似违规情况的重复发生。

d. 受试者1398754001，试验方案112754：

i. 试验方案112754规定您在访视1（筛选）时要进行全面的体格检查。您没有遵循这个要求。具体而言：

您没有在访视1（筛选）时对受试者1398754001（在FDA483表上误写成受试者1398764001）进行全面的体格检查。

在2013年9月12日，您书面回复FDA483表时，您承认研究人员没有在筛选时进行规定的体格检查。您表示访视1的体格检查在访视2时已经完成，这个是在判断合格性的其他程序进行之前，遗漏的体格检查被记录在"DVE报告"上。另外，您指出在2011年，访视事件流程图提供给了您的研究人员，来确保未来试验的评估不会被遗漏。

您的回复是不充分的，因为您没有提供任何受试者在访视2进行体格检查的记录，也没有您提供给研究人员的访视事件流程图，您也没有提供员工收到的流程图的使用说明细节。没有这些细节，我们无法判断您的纠正措施是否足以防止未来发生类似违规情况。

ii. 试验方案112754要求您在访视23（第104周）时获得一式三联的心电图和一份血样用于血液和化学检测。

受试者1398754001（在FDA483表上错误写成受试者1398764001）在访视23（第104周）没有一式三联的心电图记录和实验室检查。虽然受试者的试验记录解释了为什么心电图和抽血在这次访视没有进行，但没有证据说明这些操作在晚些时候进行了。

在2013年9月12日，您书面回复FDA483表时，您承认一些实验室检查和心电图没有按照试验方案规定的时间内进行。您也提到您采取了纠正措施来确保未来研究评估不会被遗漏。您提及作为纠正措施的一部分，您请您的研究人员参加与您与临床人员的周会，您每周和研究人员开会。您和您的研究人员重新培训了关于试验评估的SOP。在2011年，访视事件流程图提供给了您的研究人员，来确保未来试验的评估不会被遗漏。

由于您没有提供关于纠正措施的充分细节，您的回复是不充分的。您没有提供关于评估的标准操作规程的复印件，您表示这个文件已经制定，您和您的员工重新培训过，您没提供这个培训的细节。您也没有提供给研究委员的访视事件流程图，您没有提供关于员工收到的流程图的使用说明细节。没有这些细节，我们无法判断您的纠正措施是否能充分预防未来类似违背的发生。

根据上述情况，您没有按照研究计划来进行研究。具体而言，入组了不合格的受试者，没有及时报告严重不良事件给申办者，没有依从方案规定的剂量增加，没有进行方案规定的评估和流程，以及没有在方案特定的时间范围内进行研究访视会危害受试者安全和数据的准确性。另外，没有采集药代动力学检测的血样会引起对您中心数据的有效性和完整性的关注。

2. 您未能保存对研究中使用试验药物或对照组的受试者的所有观察结果和其他相关数据的足够和准确的病历［21 CFR 312.62（b）］

作为临床研究者，您必须准备和保存研究中使用试验药物或对照组的受试者的所有观察结果和其他相关数据足够和准确的病历。病历包括发生的不良事件的记录。您没有保存这些记录的足够和准确的病历。这些失误的例子包括，但不限于以下内容：

a. 试验方案GLP112754，受试者1398754002在访视14/第20周（2010年2月12日）时的实验室结果显示血红蛋白、红细胞压积、红细胞计数水平下降。实验室结果一开始标记为“无临床显著意义”，签字时间是2010年2月9日。但是，在2012年12月12日，这个判断改为了“临床诊断相关”，额外的注释说明了受试者临床上严重贫血，对这个在差不多3年后做出的修改没有解释。

在2013年9月12日，您书面回复FDA483表时，您提到经过更详细审阅方案中不良事件的定义，您更改了对于受试者1398754002血常规的专业判断，您把其贫血记录改为有显著临床意义。

由于您没有记录在3年后把贫血的临床意义进行修改的理由，您的回复是不充分的。没有您的判断依据，这些文件不足以获得受试者足够的和准确的病历。另外，您没有提供纠正措施计划来预防未来类似违规情况的重复发生。

b. 除了上述的不良事件，受试者1398754002还发生了其他不良事件，这些被记录在不良事件表中，如记忆缺失、咳嗽、贫血和右下肢疼痛。在不良事件表中这些不良事件一开始在“与药物相关性”上标记为“是”。但是，在3年后，即2013年2月13日，同样的不良事件把“与药物相关性”改为“否”，这些修改也没有解释。

在2013年9月12日，您书面回复FDA483表时，您提到对不良事件表中贫血的修改只是由于录入错误。您针对这个修改的回复是不充分的，因为您没有解释录入错误和更改记号的关系。另外，因为您没有记录在不良事件发生大概3年后，您更改其他不良事件（上面提及的特别例子）与临床试验药物关系的理由，您的回复是不充分的。没有您的判断依据，这些文件不足以获得受试者完整和准确的病历。另外，您的回复是不充分的，因为您没有提供纠正措施计划来预防未来类似违规情况的重复发生。

您没有保存完整和准确的病历，包括没有记录不良事件分类改变的理由及不良事件与临床试验用药关系的判断，这会危害受试者安全和福利，削弱了在贵研究中心获取的数据的真实性和完整性。

3. 您未能保存足够的包括日期、数量和受试者使用情况的药品处置记录［21 CFR 312.62（a）］

作为临床研究者，您必须保存足够的包括日期、数量和受试者使用情况的药品处置记录。根据试验方案GLP112757，试验药物的处置应该记录在药物计数表上，表明阿必鲁肽/对应的安慰剂，格列美脲，以及吡格列酮/对应的安慰剂发放和/或给予受试者的数量；研究受试者归还的数量；从申办者收到和归还的数量，如适用。您没有保留足够的文件记录。这些失误的例子包括，但不限于以下内容：

a. 对于受试者1398757001，试验药物处置标签和研究物资库存记录显示受试者在2010年7月28日接受了2剂注射：药包号2459470，在上午10点注射，药包号2144353，在1个小时后，也就是上午11点注射。

另外，试验药物处置标签显示受试者在2011年8月3日上午10点接受了2剂注射（药包号2359363和2565372）。研究物资库存记录不包括这两个药包的给药时间和日期。

b. 受试者1398757002

i. 研究物资库存记录显示药包2592361在2010年11月21日给过药，但病例报告表显示药包是在2011年1月21日给过药。

ii. 研究物资库存记录显示药包2305273在2010年3月9日给过药，而且在此之前的2010年3月6日被退回到研究中心。但病例报告表没有记录药包的给药日期，而显示这个药包没有被退回到研究中心。

iii. 2010年7月13日上午10:02分发生的一次注射，在试验药物处置标签和研究物资库存记录上有出入。标签显示受试者2010年7月13日接受了药包2306486的给药，但库存记录显示这一天受试者接受的是药包2276486的给药。库存记录显示药包2306486的给药发生在2010年8月24日。

另外，试验药物处置标签显示受试者在2011年5月10日上午10:26接受了药包号2133370的注射，6分钟后，即10:32接受了药包号2425379的注射。研究物资库存记录不包括这两个药包的给药时间和日期。

在2013年9月12日，您书面回复FDA483表时，您承认试验药物处置标签和研究物资库存记录的差异。您把这些差异归因为以下几点：

- 研究协调员记录信息时出现失误；
- 研究协调员把信息在表格里放错位置；
- 试验药物的给药信息记录在申办者表格和试验药物处置标签不匹配；
- 受试者接受注射和注射器退回研究中心间隔了很长时间，导致受试者很难回忆起相关信息；
- 受试者错误填写试验药物处置标签或者根本不填；
- 研究协调员无法在受试者离开研究中心之前验证试验药物处置标签的准确性，导致准确信息缺失；

您提到您认识到需要解决在准确记录临床试验用药处置情况方面的缺陷，而且您明白准确足够的记录每个受试者使用试验药物的重要性。您说过贵研究中心在试验药物取用和记录上被重新培训过，您也给我们提供了这次培训记录表格的复印件。我们相信您和您的员工接受的培训足够避免再次发生类似违规。

您没有保留足够的和准确的药物计数记录会危害受试者安全和福利，并影响在贵研究中心获取的数据的真实性和完整性。

本警告信的目的并非是罗列您在试验药物临床研究中存在的所有缺陷。确保遵循法律和相关FDA法规的每一项要求是您的职责，您应当解决这些缺陷，并建立规程，以确保任何正在进行或将来进行的研究均符合FDA的法规。

自收到这封信的15个工作日内，您应当书面告知本办公室为预防将来发生类似违规情况而采取的措施。如果不能充分、迅速地解释上述违规问题，可能导致我们在不再通知的情况下采取监管措施。如果您认为您已经遵循了FDA的法规要求，请陈述理由，并提供所有支持资料，以供我们参考。

附：英文原文

Sewell, Michele M.D.

WARNING LETTER

APR 30, 2014

CERTIFIED MAIL
RETURN RECEIPT REQUESTED

Ref: 14-HFD-45-04-03

Michele A. Sewell, M.D.
Stonecrest Pediatric and Adult Medicine
8225 Mall Parkway, Suite 250
Lithonia, GA 30058

Dear Dr. Sewell:

This Warning Letter informs you of objectionable conditions observed during the U.S. Food and Drug Administration

(FDA) inspection conducted at your clinical site between June 17 and August 19, 2013. Ms. Nicole Bell and Ms. Vanessa Coulter, representing FDA, reviewed your conduct of the following clinical investigations of the investigational drug albiglutide, performed for GlaxoSmithKline:

- Protocol GLP112754, "A Randomized, Open-Label, Parallel-Group, Multicenter Study to Determine the Efficacy and Long-Term Safety of Albiglutide Compared With Insulin in Subjects With Type 2 Diabetes Mellitus"; and
- Protocol GLP112757, "A Randomized, Double-Blind, Placebo-and Active-Controlled, Parallel-Group, Multicenter Study to Determine the Efficacy and Safety of Albiglutide Administered in Combination With Metformin and Glimepiride Compared With Metformin Plus Glimepiride and Placebo and With Metformin Plus Glimepiride and Pioglitazone in Subjects With Type 2 Diabetes Mellitus."

This inspection is a part of FDA's Bioresearch Monitoring Program, which includes inspections designed to evaluate the conduct of FDA-regulated research to ensure that the data are scientifically valid and accurate, and to help ensure that the rights, safety, and welfare of the human subjects of those studies have been protected.

At the conclusion of the inspection, Ms. Bell and Ms. Coulter presented and discussed with you Form FDA 483, Inspectional Observations. On September 5, 2013, FDA sent you Form FDA 483, Amendment 1, dated September 5, 2013. We acknowledge receipt of your September 12, 2013, written response to both the Form FDA 483 and the Form 483, Amendment 1.

From our review of the FDA Establishment Inspection Report, the documents submitted with that report, and your written response dated September 12, 2013, we conclude that you did not adhere to the applicable statutory requirements and FDA regulations governing the conduct of clinical investigations. We wish to emphasize the following:

1. You failed to ensure that the investigation was conducted according to the investigational plan [21 CFR 312.60].

As a clinical investigator, you are required to ensure that your clinical studies are conducted in accordance with the investigational plan. The investigational plan for Protocol GLP112757 includes certain requirements related to eligibility confirmation, sulfonylurea dosing prior to screening, and pharmacokinetic (PK) blood draws, as well as criteria for increasing study-drug dose. The investigational plan for Protocol GLP112754 includes certain requirements related to Serious Adverse Event (SAE) reporting and the performance of specific assessments and procedures at certain study visits. Both protocols require that study visits occur within specified time frames. You failed to adhere to these requirements. Specifically:

a. Subject 1398757001, Protocol GLP112757:

i. Protocol GLP112757 requires that subjects receive a sulfonylurea dose that is equivalent to at least 4 mg glimepiride for at least three months prior to screening. The protocol indicates that 4 mg glimepiride is equivalent to 5 mg glyburide dosed twice daily.

Subject 1398757001 was ineligible for Protocol GLP112757 at screening on August 19, 2009, while on glyburide 5 mg daily (half of the protocol-required dose). The medication log for this subject indicates that the dose of 5 mg once daily was changed to 5 mg twice daily sometime in September 2009 (after screening), and the subject was randomized on January 6, 2010. The dose correction should have occurred at least three months before, and not after, screening.

In your September 12, 2013, written response to the Form FDA 483, you indicated that after additional review, you found that you did not have proper documentation of the required dosage of glimepiride. You also indicated that, as corrective action, your study staff would receive or had received additional training to ensure protocol compliance.

Your response is inadequate because it is not sufficiently detailed with respect to your corrective action plan. You have not provided any details or documentation regarding the training of your study staff, and you have not indicated what corrective action you personally have taken, as clinical investigator, to ensure your own compliance with study protocols. Without those details, we are unable to determine whether your corrective action is adequate to prevent similar violations in the future.

ii. Protocol GLP112757 requires that subjects who have a hemoglobinopathy that may affect determination of hemoglobin A1c (HbA1c) not be enrolled in the study.

Subject 1398757001 was ineligible for Protocol GLP 112757 at screening on August 19, 2009, with an "apparent hemoglobin variant observed during analysis of hemoglobin A1c" noted in the laboratory results. The same apparent hemoglobin variant was also observed and verified by repeat analysis in the laboratory results following the Week-4 visit on February 3, 2010. In the laboratory results following the April 22, 2011, visit, laboratory personnel noted that a hemoglobin pattern and concentration consistent with sickle-cell trait (heterozygous) was found, and suggested a clinical and hematologic correlation.

In your September 12, 2013, written response to the Form FDA 483, you indicate that no notation was made at screening because it was your professional opinion that the subject should not be excluded because of sicklecell trait. In addition, you stated, "I felt, at the time, that there was some evidence but no definitive evidence that HbA1c could not be used for accurate glucose monitoring based on the methodology employed for accurate measurement by (b)(4)."

Your response is inadequate because Protocol GLP112757 requires exclusion of subjects who have hemoglobinopathies that may affect HbA1c determinations. Sickle-cell trait is one such exclusionary hemoglobinopathy.

iii. Protocol GLP112757 requires that all study visits occur within ±3 days, with the exception of Visit 7 (Week-1) and Visit 8 (Baseline). The protocol notes that subjects would not be considered out of compliance if visit windows extend because of extraordinary events that make it impossible for subjects to complete a visit within the visit window (e.g., holidays, vacations, personal emergencies). However, the protocol specifies that determination of the maximum visit window deviation is at the discretion of the medical monitor.

For Subject 1398757001, Visit 22 (Week 65) took place 15 days past the protocol-allowed time frame. The protocol required that Visit 22 occur 13 weeks after Visit 21 (Week 52), ±3 days. This subject's Visit 21 occurred on January 7, 2011, and Visit 22 occurred approximately 15 weeks later, on April 26, 2011. There is no evidence of an extraordinary event or of a determination by the medical monitor.

In your September 12, 2013, written response to the Form FDA 483, you did not provide any explanation for the delay in this subject's visit. However, you did acknowledge that problems with scheduling occurred. You noted that you have taken corrective action and that, as part of that corrective action, you hold weekly meetings with study staff and include the study staff in your weekly meetings with clinic staff. You also stated that you have Standard Operating Procedures (SOPs) on assessments, and that you, as well as the study staff, were retrained on this SOP.

Your response is inadequate because you have not provided documentation of any extraordinary events, or of any discussion with the medical monitor to determine maximum visit-window deviation in this case. In addition, you have not provided sufficient details about your corrective action plan. You have not provided a copy of the SOP on assessments, which you indicated that you have in place and on which you and your staff have been retrained, nor have you provided any details about that training. Without those details, we are unable to determine whether your corrective action is adequate to prevent similar violations in the future.

b. Subject 1398757002, Protocol GLP112757:

i. Protocol GLP112757 requires that subjects receive at least 1500 mg metformin daily for at least three months prior to screening; however, the protocol allows enrollment of subjects with a documented maximum tolerated dose of less than 1500 mg metformin daily, if the dose has been stable for at least eight weeks before randomization.

Subject 1398757002 was enrolled in the study despite the subject's not having received at least 1500 mg metformin daily for at least three months prior to screening, and despite the subject's not having received a documented maximum tolerated dose of less than 1500 mg daily that was stable for at least eight weeks before randomization. The concomitant medication study records show that as of August 20, 2009 (four days prior to screening), Subject 1398757002 was taking 500 mg metformin twice daily (1000 mg daily), which is 500 mg less than the requisite dose. On August 21, 2009, the dose was increased to 1000 mg metformin twice daily (2000 mg daily). This increase in the dose of metformin did not make the subject eligible for the study because the subject was not receiving at least 1500 mg metformin for a minimum of three months prior to screening. Nevertheless, Subject 1398757002 was screened for the study three days later, on August 24, 2009. Furthermore, you provided no documentation to indicate that the subject had a stable, maximum tolerated dose of less than 1500 mg metformin daily for at least eight weeks prior to randomization.

In your September 12, 2013, written response to the Form FDA 483, you stated that the subject's maximum tolerated dose was 1000 mg metformin (daily). In your written response, you also described corrective action that you have taken to ensure that protocol-required assessments are done in a timely manner. Your response is inadequate because you provided no documentation to support your statement that the subject's maximum tolerated dose was 1000 mg metformin daily. Of note, study records show that the subject's metformin dose was increased to 1000 mg twice daily on August 21, 2009, for a total daily dose of 2000 mg, and we have no documentation that the subject could not tolerate that dose.

Your response is also inadequate because it is not sufficiently detailed with respect to your corrective actions. Specifically, you have not provided a copy of the SOP on assessments, which you indicated that you have in place and on which your staff has been trained, nor have you provided any details about that training. Without those details, we are unable to determine whether your corrective action is adequate to prevent similar violations in the future.

ii. Protocol GLP112757 permits you to increase the dose of study drug only when the subject meets the protocol criteria for a dose increase. The protocol requires that a subject receive a dose increase at Week 4 only if the subject has a single fasting plasma glucose of at least 250 mg/dL, as confirmed by a second sample drawn within 7 days and analyzed by the central laboratory, and if the subject's HbA1c level is unchanged or increased from baseline. You failed to adhere to this requirement. Specifically:

Subject 1398757002 received an increased dose of study drug on December 3, 2009, even though the subject did not meet the protocol criteria for a dose increase. This subject had a fasting plasma glucose of 144 mg/dL at Week 4 on November 17, 2009. In addition to having a fasting plasma glucose below the required level, you provided no evidence that this level was confirmed by a second sample drawn within 7 days and analyzed by the central laboratory. Therefore, Subject 1398757002 should not have received a dose increase on December 3, 2009.

In your September 12, 2013, written response to the Form FDA 483, you acknowledged that several required protocol procedures, physical examinations, lab assessments, and electrocardiograms (ECGs) were not done within the appropriate time frames. You indicated that you have taken corrective action to ensure that study assessments are not missed in the future. You noted that as part of that corrective action, you include your research staff in your weekly meetings with clinic staff, and you hold weekly meetings with research staff to get subject status reports. In addition, you note that you and your study staff were retrained on the SOPs for study assessments.

Your response is inadequate because you have not provided sufficient details about your corrective action plan. Specifically, you have not provided a copy of the SOP on assessments, which you indicated that you have in place and on which you and your staff have been retrained, nor have you provided any details about that training. Without those details, we are unable to determine whether your corrective action is adequate to prevent similar violations in the future.

iii. Protocol GLP112757 requires that for Week 28, subjects have their PK blood samples taken at least 2 days after they receive a dose of study drug. You failed to adhere to these requirements. Specifically:

Study drug container #2201065 was administered to Subject 1398757002 on May 4, 2010 (Visit 18/Week 28), and the subject's PK blood sample was taken at the same visit.

In your September 12, 2013, written response to the Form FDA 483, you acknowledged that the assessments were not performed as required by the protocol, and you indicated that you have taken corrective action to ensure that study assessments are not missed in the future. You also noted that as part of that corrective action, you hold weekly meetings with study staff, and study staff were retrained on SOPs for study assessments.

Your response is inadequate because you have not provided sufficient details about the corrective action plan. Specifically, you have not provided a copy of the SOP on assessments, which you indicated that you have in place and on which your staff has been trained, nor have you provided any details about that training. Without those details, we are unable to determine whether your corrective action is adequate to prevent similar violations in the future.

c. Subject 1398754002, Protocol GLP112754:

i. Protocol GLP112754 requires that you report all SAEs to the sponsor within 24 hours. The Protocol defines SAEs as any untoward medical occurrence that results in death; is life threatening; requires hospitalization or prolongation of existing hospitalization; results in disability/incapacity; is a congenital anomaly/birth defect; or other medical event that, in the medical judgment of the clinical investigator, should be considered serious (such as an event that may require medical or surgical intervention to prevent one of the previously listed outcomes). You failed to adhere to this requirement. Specifically:

Subject 1398754002 experienced the SAE of unstable angina that resulted in hospitalization on (b)(6). However, this SAE was not reported to the sponsor until June 9, 2011, approximately 15 months later.

In your September 12, 2013, written response to the Form FDA 483, you indicated that the subject did not disclose the hospitalization to the study coordinator during five separate visits in 2010. You stated that the hospitalization was discovered on June 9, 2011, after your site received and reviewed the subject's medical records for a separate incident.

Your response is inadequate because a printed note at the bottom of the hospital record related to the subject's (b)(6), admission for unstable angina indicates that a copy of this record was sent to you. You have not adequately explained your failure to report the SAE experienced by Subject 1398754002, nor have you explained how you will correct this failure in the future.

ii.Protocol GLP112754 (original version dated December 8, 2008) requires that all study visits have a treatment window of ±3 days. Amendment 1 (dated August 6, 2009) of this protocol requires the same time frame for all study visits, with the exception of Visit 6 (Baseline), which will have a treatment window of ±6 days. The protocol notes that subjects will not be considered out of compliance if visit windows extend because of extraordinary events that make it impossible for subjects to complete a visit within the visit window (e.g., holidays, vacations, personal emergencies). However, determination of the maximum visit window deviation is at the discretion of the medical monitor.

Subject 1398754002 had multiple study visits that took place significantly outside of the protocol-specified time frames.

Visit/Wk	Date of Actual Visit	Days Past/Early Relative to the Expected Time Frame (Allowed Range)
Visit 6/Wk 0	9/25/2009	15 days past due (±6 days)
Visit 16/Wk 28	5/17/2010	28 days past due (±3 days)
Visit 17/Wk 36	6/19/2010	20 days early (±3 days)
Visit 18/Wk 48	8/24/2010	15 days early (±3 days)

In your September 12, 2013, written response to the Form FDA 483, you referred to Protocol GLP112754's specifications for out-of-window visits (original version dated December 8, 2008): "All study visits will have a treatment window of ±3 days. Subjects will not be out of compliance if visit windows extend because of extraordinary events that make it impossible for subjects to complete a visit window within the ±3 day window (e.g., holidays, vacations, personal emergencies). However, determination of the maximum visit window deviation is at the discretion of the medical monitor."

Your response is inadequate because you have not explained why there were significant delays in the subjects' visits noted above, and you have not provided documentation of any extraordinary events, or of any discussion with the medical monitor to determine maximum visit-window deviations in each of these cases. Your response is also inadequate because you have not provided a corrective action plan to prevent the recurrence of similar violations in the future.

d. Subject 1398754001, Protocol 112754:

i. Protocol 112754 requires that you perform a complete physical examination at Visit 1 (Screening). You failed to adhere to this requirement. Specifically:

You failed to perform a complete physical examination on Subject 1398754001 (written incorrectly on Form FDA 483 as Subject 1398764001) at Visit 1 (Screening).

In your September 12, 2013, written response to the Form FDA 483, you acknowledged that your study staff failed to perform the required physical examination at screening. You indicated that the Visit1 physical examination was completed at Visit 2, before other study procedures were done to determine the subject's eligibility, and that the missed physical examination was listed on a "DVE report." In addition, you indicated that in 2011 your study staff were provided with and instructed on a flow chart of visit events to ensure that assessments for this study are not missed in the future.

Your response is inadequate because you have not provided any documentation of the subject's physical examination at Visit 2, or the flow chart of visit events that you provided to study staff, and you have not provided any details about how the staff were instructed on the use of the flow chart. Without those details, we are unable to determine whether your corrective action is adequate to prevent similar violations in the future.

ii. Protocol 112754 requires that you obtain triplicate ECGs and a blood sample for hematology and chemistry assessments at Visit 23 (Week 104).

Subject 1398754001 (written incorrectly on Form FDA 483 as Subject 1398764001) did not have triplicate ECG recordings or laboratory assessments at Visit 23 (Week 104). Although the subject's study records document why the ECGs and blood draw could not be performed at this visit, there is no evidence that they were performed at a later date.

In your September 12, 2013, written response to the Form FDA 483, you acknowledged that several laboratory assessments and ECGs were not performed according to the time frames required by the protocol. You also noted that you have taken corrective action to ensure that study assessments are not missed in the future. You noted that as part of that corrective action, you include your research staff in your weekly meetings with clinic staff, and you hold weekly meetings with research staff. You and your study staff were also retrained on an SOP for study assessments, and in 2011 your study staff were provided with and instructed on a flow chart of visit events to ensure that assessments for this study are not missed in the future.

Your response is inadequate because you have not provided sufficient details about your corrective action plan. You have not provided a copy of the SOP on assessments, which you indicated that you have in place and on which you and your staff have been retrained, and you have not provided any details about that training. You also have not provided the flow chart of visit events that you provided to study staff, and you have not provided any details about how the staff were instructed on the use of the flow chart. Without those details, we are unable to determine whether your corrective action is adequate to prevent similar violations in the future.

As detailed above, you failed to conduct the investigation in accordance with the investigational plan. Specifically, enrollment of subjects who do not meet eligibility criteria, failure to report SAEs to the sponsor promptly, failure to adhere to protocol restrictions related to dose increases, failure to perform protocol-required assessments and procedures, and failure to conduct study visits within the protocol-specified time frames jeopardize subject safety and data integrity. In addition, failure to obtain blood samples for PK testing raises concern about the validity and integrity of the data collected at your site.

2. You failed to maintain adequate and accurate case histories that record all observations and other data pertinent to the investigation on each individual administered the investigational drug or employed as a control in the investigation. [21 CFR 312.62(b)].

As a clinical investigator, you are required to prepare and maintain adequate and accurate case histories that record all observations and other data pertinent to the investigation on each individual administered the investigational drug or employed as a control in the investigation. Case histories include records of adverse events that occur. You have failed to maintain adequate and accurate case histories with respect to these records. Examples of this failure include, but are not limited to, the following:

a. For Protocol GLP112754, laboratory results for Subject 1398754002 at Visit 14/Week 20 (February 12, 2010) showed decreased hemoglobin, hematocrit, and red blood cell count levels. The lab results were initially marked as "not clinically significant," with a signature dated February 19, 2010. However, on December 12, 2012, this determination was changed to "clinically relevant" with an additional notation that the subject had clinically significant anemia, without an explanation for the change made almost three years later.

In your September 12, 2013, written response to the Form FDA 483, you indicated that upon more detailed review of the protocol's definition of an adverse event, you changed your professional judgment regarding Subject 1398754002's hematology report, and you documented the subject's anemia as clinically significant.

Your response is inadequate because you have failed to document your rationale for the changes you made in the clinical significance of anemia nearly three years after the anemia was noted. Without the inclusion of your rationale, these documents are inadequate to capture the adequate and accurate case history of this subject. In addition, you have not provided a corrective action plan to prevent the recurrence of similar violations in the future.

b. In addition to the adverse event noted above, Subject 1398754002 experienced other adverse events that were recorded in the Adverse Event Log, such as memory loss, cough, anemia, and pain in the right lower extremity. These adverse events were originally marked as "Yes" for "Possible IP relationship" in the Adverse Event Log. However, the same adverse events were changed to "No" for "Possible IP relationship" three years later, on February 13, 2013, without an explanation for the change.

In your September 12, 2013, written response to the Form FDA 483, you note that the change made in the Adverse Event Log for anemia was due to entry error only. Your response with regard to this change is inadequate because you failed to explain the relationship between the entry error and the changed notation. In addition, your response was inadequate because you failed to document your rationale for the changes you made in the relationship of other adverse events (specific examples provided above) to the study drug, nearly three years after the adverse events were noted. Without the inclusion of your rationale, these documents are inadequate to capture the adequate and accurate case history of this subject. In addition, your response is inadequate because you have not provided a corrective action plan to prevent the recurrence of similar violations in the future.

Your failure to maintain adequate and accurate case histories, including the failure to document a rationale for changes in adverse event classification and in the assessment of adverse events' relationship to the study drug, jeopardizes subject safety and welfare and compromises the validity and integrity of data captured at your site.

3. You failed to maintain adequate records of the disposition of the drug, including dates, quantity, and use by subjects [21 CFR 312.62(a)].

As a clinical investigator, you are required to maintain adequate records of the disposition of the drug, including dates, quantity, and use by subjects. According to Protocol GLP112757, the disposition of the investigational drug should be recorded in product accountability documents stating the amounts of albiglutide/matching placebo, glimepiride, and pioglitazone/matching placebo dispensed and/or administered to study subjects; the amounts returned by study subjects; and the amounts received from and returned to the sponsor, when applicable. You did not adequately maintain records of these documents. Examples of this failure include, but are not limited to, the following:

a. For Subject 1398757001, the study-drug disposition label and the Investigational Supplies Inventory Log show that the subject received two injections on July 28, 2010: Container #2459470, administered at 10:00 a.m., and Container #2144353, administered one hour later, at 11:00 a.m.

In addition, study-drug disposition labels show that this subject received two injections (Containers #2359363 and #2565372) on August 3, 2011, at 10:00 a.m. The Investigational Supplies Inventory Log does not contain the dates and times of study-drug administration for either of these containers.

b. For Subject 1398757002:

i. The Investigational Supplies Inventory Log notes that Container #2592361 was administered on November 21, 2010, but the case report form notes that this container was administered on January 21, 2011.

ii. The Investigational Supplies Inventory Log notes that Container #2305273 was administered on March 9, 2010, and was returned to the site at an earlier date, on March 6, 2010. The case report form has no recording for the date of study-drug administration and indicates that this container was not returned to the site.

iii. The study-drug disposition label and the Investigational Supplies Inventory Log contain discrepancies regarding the injection received on July 13, 2010, at 10:02 a.m. The label indicates that the subject was administered Container #2306486 on July 13, 2010, but the log indicates that the subject was administered Container #2276486 on that date. The log indicates that Container #2306486 was administered on August 24, 2010, instead.

In addition, the study-drug disposition label shows that this subject was administered Container #2133370 on May 10, 2011, at 10:26 a.m., and was administered Container #2425379 six minutes later, at 10:32 a.m. The Investigational Supplies Inventory Log does not contain the dates and times of study-drug administration for either of these containers.

In your September 12, 2013, written response to the Form FDA 483, you acknowledged the presence of discrepancies between the recordings on the returned study-drug disposition labels and the logs. You attributed the discrepancies to the following:

- Study coordinator's error in recording the information;
- Study coordinator's putting information in the wrong section of a form;
- Mismatch between the sponsor forms and study-drug disposition labels with regard to the recording of the study-drug administration information;
- Long lapse in time between subjects' injection/dose and return of the injection pens to the site, resulting in the subjects' having difficulty in recalling the information;
- Subjects' filling out study-drug disposition labels improperly or not at all; and
- Study coordinator's failing to verify the accuracy of study-drug disposition labels before subjects left the site, resulting in lack of accurate information.

You stated that you recognized a need to address deficiencies in accurate recording of investigational drug disposition, and that you understood the importance of accurate and complete documentation of the use of study drug by each subject. You indicated that your site was retrained on study-drug handling and recording, and you provided us with a copy of the forms that documented this training. We believe that the training you and your staff received should be adequate to prevent a recurrence of similar violations.

Your failure to maintain adequate and accurate drug accountability records jeopardizes subject safety and welfare, and compromises the validity and integrity of the data at your site.

This letter is not intended to be an all-inclusive list of deficiencies with your clinical study of an investigational drug. It is your responsibility to ensure adherence to each requirement of the law and relevant FDA regulations. You should address these deficiencies and establish procedures to ensure that any ongoing or future studies will be in compliance with FDA regulations.

Within fifteen (15) working days of your receipt of this letter, you should notify this office in writing of the actions you have taken to prevent similar violations in the future. Failure to address the violations noted above adequately and promptly may result in regulatory action without further notice. If you believe you have complied with FDA regulations, include your reasoning and any supporting information for our consideration.

If you have any questions, please contact Constance Cullity, M.D., M.P.H., at 3017963397; FAX 3018478748. Your written response and any pertinent documentation should be addressed to:

Constance Cullity, M.D., M.P.H.
Branch Chief
Good Clinical Practice Enforcement Branch
Division of Good Clinical Practice Compliance
Office of Scientific Investigations
Office of Compliance
Center for Drug Evaluation and Research
U.S. Food and Drug Administration
Building 51, Room 5354
10903 New Hampshire Avenue
Silver Spring, MD 20993

Sincerely yours,

{See appended electronic signature page}

Sean Y. Kassim, Ph.D.
Acting Director
Office of Scientific Investigations

Office of Compliance
Center for Drug Evaluation and Research
U.S. Food and Drug Administration
This is a representation of an electronic record that was signed electronically and this page is the manifestation of the electronic signature.

/S/

SEAN Y KASSIM
04/30/2014

第76封　给Birhiray, Ruemu的警告信

2014年4月28日

参考号：14-HFD-45-04-0

尊敬的Birhiray博士：

2013年8月12日至9月5日，AndreaD.Swingle女士代表FDA，在您的临床研究中心，对您所开展的试验药物为（b）（4）[1]，申办者为（b）（4）的以下临床研究进行了审查：试验方案（b）（4）和（b）（4），试验方案（b）（4）。这封警告信特告知您现场检查中发现的违规情况研究。

本次现场检查是FDA的生物研究监查项目的一部分。该项目通过设定的检查方法，对FDA所监管的研究的实施情况进行评估，以确认研究数据在科学上是有效和准确的，并帮助确保这些研究中受试者的权益、安全和福利得到了保护。

在现场检查结束时，Swingle女士向您出示了FDA483表，即现场检查发现的问题，并与您进行了讨论。您2013年9月22日对该FDA483表的书面回复已收悉。

经对现场检查报告、该报告的附件，以及您2013年9月22日的书面回复进行审查，我们认为，您没有遵循适用的法律要求和监管临床研究实施及受试者保护的FDA法规。我们想强调以下几点：

1．您未能确保按照研究计划进行研究［21 CFR 312.60］

作为临床研究者，您必须确保临床研究按照试验计划进行。值得注意的是试验方案“（b）（4）”是关于“（b）（4）”的研究，研究药物“（b）（4）”对骨矿化和吸收有很显著的影响，并且这三个试验药物都是通过肾脏排泄的。因此，监测肌酐、镁和磷水平进而决定是否维持或者调整试验药物的剂量，对于保护受试者的安全性很重要。

试验方案（b）（4）试验计划要求您：①根据试验药物相关的不良事件来维持或者调整研究药物的剂量；②依照特定流程报告不良事件。此外，试验方案（b）（4）和（b）（4）要求您在特定的时间进行一些试验流程，例如体格检查、骨扫描和特定的实验室检查。您没有遵循这些要求，具体而言：

a. 试验方案（b）（4）要求，当受试者的肌酐水平较正常基线值上升0.5mg/dL或者较异常基线值上升1mg/dL，并且大于研究机构的正常值上限，就要停止受试者的研究用药，直到血清中肌酐水平降到基线值的10%以内。

受试者222626，被随机到治疗组2（氯膦酸盐组），符合停止氯膦酸盐剂量的标准，然而，该受试者在符合标准后继续接受超过一年的氯膦酸盐的治疗。受试者222626在2010年1月28日基线期的血清肌酐值为0.9mg/dL（在研究机构的正常值上限之内）。但是，在2011年1月11日该受试者的血清肌酐值升高到1.7mg/dL，这个比研究机构的正常值上限（1.0mg/dL）多0.5mg/dL，这种异常持续了10个多月。该受试者的血清肌酐值在2011年3月29日是1.6mg/dL；在2011年6月21日依然是1.6mg/dL；在2011年9月13日是1.8mg/dL；在2011年11月29日是1.98mg/dL。对受试者222626，直到2012年1月14日，您在应该停止研究用药长达一年多的时间内，都没能给该受试者停药。

b. 试验方案（b）（4）特别要求对于发生在随机到治疗2组或者3组（分别是氯膦酸盐组和伊班膦酸盐组）的受试者上的严重不良事件，要快速报告。除此之外，试验方案要求您用第四版的不良事件常用术语评定标准来判断严重不良事件的类别和严重性级别，试验方案也要求您通过不良事件快速报告系统（AdEERS系

1（b）（4）涉及商业秘密，根据法规内容不予公开。

统）在10个日历日内上报加速入院（或延长住院时间）的任何3级不良事件，无论是何种原因和是否预期。方案还要求您在获知事件的24小时内通过AdEERS系统报告任何下颌骨坏死不论级别、原因或是否预期。

您没能通过AdEERS系统报告以下的严重不良事件：

1）受试者214199，随机到治疗组3（伊班膦酸盐组ibandronate），在“（b）（4）”因社区获得性肺炎住院，CT检查发现有双侧肺部浸润。该受试者接受静脉滴注抗生素，左氧氟沙星治疗肺炎。根据不良事件常用术语评定标准对肺部感染的临床描述，肺炎如果需要用静脉滴注抗生素治疗，那么它的严重程度应该是3级。您没有通过AdEERS系统报告受试者214199因3级肺部感染导致的住院。

2）受试者214835，随机到治疗组3（伊班膦酸盐组），在2010年4月6号诊断为下颌骨坏死，然而您没有通过AdEERS系统报告受试者214835的下颌骨坏死事件。

c. 试验方案（b）（4）要求在第2个月研究访视执行以下的研究流程：体格检查、体重测量、体力状态评估、毒性标记和实验室检查（血清肌酐、钙、磷、镁、白蛋白、电解质类、肝功检测和全血细胞计数/分类/血小板计数）。

您没有完成以下受试者第2个月的研究访视：213854，214200，214393，214835，221968，222241，222626 和222698。

d. 试验方案（b）（4）要求您在第2，4，6，9，12，15，21，24，27，30，33 和36个月的研究访视时，进行镁、磷和全血细胞计数的检测。您没有在特定的访视中进行以下实验室检查：

受试者编号	未做的实验室检查	未做这些检测的研究访视（月）
213854	镁和磷	4，6 和9
214199	镁和磷	2，4，6 和21
214200	镁和磷	9和15
214393	镁和磷	4，6，9 和12
214632	镁和磷	2，4，6，9，12，24，27，30，33和36
214835	镁和磷	4，6 和9
217799	镁，磷和全血细胞计数	2，4和6
222242	镁和磷	2，4和6
222453	镁和磷	2

e. 试验方案（b）（4）要求您在第4个月研究访视时进行以下的实验室检测：

血清肌酐、钙、磷、镁｜白蛋白、电解质类、肝功检测和全血细胞计数/分类/血小板计数。

您未能在第4个月研究访视时对受试者222698做任何方案要求的实验室检测。

f. 试验方案（b）（4）要求您在筛查和第5个月研究访视时进行血清肌酐检测。

您没能在筛查时对以下受试者进行方案要求血清肌酐检测：

213854，214200，214632和221819。另外，您没能在第5个月研究访视时对受试者214853进行血清肌酐检查。

g. 试验方案（b）（4）要求在首次给药的72小时前要进行研究前的妊娠检查。

您没能对受试者221968做这项检查，该受试者在入组时年龄为31岁。

h. 试验方案（b）（4）要求在治疗研究访视结束时进行骨扫描。

您没能在治疗研究访视结束时对受试者214632进行骨扫描。

i. 试验方案（b）（4）要求在化疗的第7个周期之前进行血清肌酐实验室检测。

您没能在化疗的第7个周期之前对受试者81053082进行血清肌酐实验室检测。

在您2013年9月22号的针对上述项1中提及的发现的书面回复中，您表明您目前没有进行临床研究，也没有积极的招募受试者参加任何临床研究。您提到如果您继续进行临床研究，您会任命指定的行政和研究人员来协调您的临床研究，同时记录责任分工，进行常规的每周内部监查，实施新的电子医疗记录系统，并使用一个流程图/表来监控实验室检查结果。

您的回复是不充分的，因为您没有提供足够的信息，使我们能够评估，如果这个纠正措施计划应用到您未来的临床研究中，您的纠正措施计划是充分的。例如，您没有提供有关您如何实施纠正计划的详细信息，以预防方案违规情况的发生。另外，您也没有提供任何细节，这个纠正措施计划如何去确保您和您的员工得到充分的关于方案要求的培训，从而阻止方案违背的进一步发生。因此，我们无法评估上面列出的纠正措施是否足够可以防止类似的情况发生。

您没有执行方案要求的研究程序，包括不良事件的报告、体格检查和实验室检查，这危害了受试者的安全和福利。特别关注的是，对试验方案（b）(4)，在其记录被审查了的16名入组受试者当中有10名受试者，在所有的研究访视时都没有进行评估血清肌酐、镁和/或磷的实验室检测。如上提到的，试验方案（b）(4)是关于双磷酸盐化合物的研究，这个研究对骨矿化和吸收有很显著的影响，因而，监测肌酐、镁和磷对于保护受试者的安全性很重要。

2. 您未能保存研究中使用试验药物的受试者或对照受试者的所有观察结果和其他相关数据的足够和准确的病历［21 CFR 312.62（b）］

作为临床研究者，您必须准备和保存研究中使用试验药物的受试者或对照受试者的所有观察结果和其他相关数据的足够和准确的病历。对试验方案（b）(4)，病历包括签名和注明日期的知情同意书，以及研究登记表格。您没能保存足够且正确的这些文件，具体而言：

a. 试验方案（b）(4)的知情同意书中有6个关于受试者是否愿意参加未来可选择性研究的问题，需要受试者选择一个"是"或"否"来回答。您没能在研究登记表格中详细、准确地记录受试者是否同意参加未来可选择性研究。具体而言：

1）受试者214199没有对这6个关于参加可选择的未来研究的意愿的问题提供"是"或"否"的回答，然而在研究登记表格上记录了对这6个问题的每一个"是"的回答的显示该受试者已经回答了所有这些问题。

2）受试者214632没有对这6个关于参加可选择的未来研究的意愿的问题提供"是"或"否"的回答，然而在研究登记表格上记录了对这6个问题的每一个"是"的回答的显示该受试者已经回答了所有这些问题

b. 试验方案（b）(4)受试者810493082的一份知情同意书显示该受试者愿意参加未来可选择性研究，然后在另外一份相同的知情同意书中记录的是该受试者不愿意参加未来可选择性研究。没有书面文件解释这种不一致性，也没有记录表明这份知情同意书是什么时候或者被谁修改的。

在您2013年9月22日针对上述项2提及的发现问题的书面回复中，您表示您目前没有进行临床研究，也没有积极地推荐患者参加任何临床试验。您提及如果您继续进行临床研究，您会任命指定的行政和研究人员来协调您的临床研究，同时记录责任分工，进行常规的每周内部监查，实施新的电子医疗记录系统，并使用一个流程图/表来监控实验室检查结果。

您的回复是不充分的，因为您没有提供足够的信息使我们能够评估，如果这个纠正措施应用到您未来的任何临床研究中，您的纠正措施计划是足够的。例如，您没有提供如何实施这个纠正措施去预防方案违规情况的详细信息。另外，您也没有提供这个纠正措施计划的任何细节去确保您和您的员工关于方案要求得到充分的培训，从而阻止方案违背的进一步发生。因此，我们无法评估上面列出的纠正措施计划是否足以防止类似情况的发生。

您没能正确地记录知情同意，引起我们对受试者权益在您医院得到保护的程度的担忧。

本警告信的目的并非是罗列您在试验药物临床研究中存在的所有缺陷。确保遵循法律和相关FDA法规的每一项要求是您的职责，您应当解决这些缺陷，并建立规程，以确保任何正在进行或将来进行的研究均符合FDA的法规。

自收到这封信的15个工作日内，您应当书面告知本办公室为预防将来发生类似违规情况而采取的措施。如果不能充分、迅速地解释上述违规问题，可能导致我们在不再通知的情况下采用监管措施。如果您认为您已经遵循了FDA的法规要求，请陈述理由，并提供所有支持资料，以供我们参考。

附：英文原文

Birhiray, Ruemu

WARNING LETTER

APR 28, 2014

CERTIFIED MAIL
RETURN RECEIPT REQUESTED

Ref:14-HFD-45-04-0

Ruemu E. Birhiray, M.D.
8301 Harcourt Road, Suite 200
Indianapolis, IN 46260

Dear Dr. Birhiray:

This Warning Letter informs you of objectionable conditions observed during the U.S. Food and Drug Administration (FDA) inspection conducted at your clinical site between August 12 and September 5, 2013. Ms. Andrea D. Swingle, representing FDA, reviewed your conduct of the following clinical investigations:

- Protocol (b)(4) and
- (b)(4) Protocol (b)(4) of the investigational drug (b)(4) performed for (b)(4).

This inspection is a part of FDA's Bioresearch Monitoring Program, which includes inspections designed to evaluate the conduct of FDA-regulated research to ensure that the data are scientifically valid and accurate, and to help ensure that the rights, safety, and welfare of the human subjects of those studies have been protected.

At the conclusion of the inspection, Ms. Swingle presented and discussed with you Form FDA 483, Inspectional Observations. We acknowledge receipt of your September 22, 2013, written response to the Form FDA 483.

From our review of the FDA establishment inspection report, the documents submitted with that report, and your September 22, 2013, written response, we conclude that you did not adhere to the applicable statutory requirements and FDA regulations governing the conduct of clinical investigations. We wish to emphasize the following:

1. You failed to ensure that the investigations were conducted according to the investigational plan [21 CFR 312.60].

As a clinical investigator, you are required to ensure that your clinical studies are conducted in accordance with the investigational plan. Of note, Protocol (b)(4) is a study of (b)(4) which have significant effects on bone mineralization and resorption, and these three drugs are excreted through the kidneys. Therefore, monitoring the levels of creatinine, magnesium, and phosphate is important to determine whether to hold or adjust the dose of study drug to protect subject safety.

The investigational plan for Protocol (b)(4) required that you (1) hold or adjust the dose of the investigational drug in managing specific drug-related adverse events, and (2) follow specific procedures for reporting adverse events. In addition, Protocols (b)(4) and (b)(4) required that you perform certain study procedures, such as physical examinations, bone scans, and specified laboratory tests, at specific times. You failed to adhere to these requirements. Specifically:

a. Protocol (b)(4) requires that you stop dosing of (b)(4) in subjects with an increase of 0.5 mg/dL from a normal baseline creatinine that is greater than the institutional upper limit of normal (IULN), or any increase of at least 1 mg/dL from an abnormal baseline creatinine that is greater than the IULN, until serum creatinine returns to within 10% of baseline.

Subject 222626, who was randomized to Treatment Arm 2 (clodronate), met this protocol criterion for stopping the dosing of clodronate, and yet the subject continued to receive clodronate for more than one year after meeting the criterion. Serum creatinine for Subject 222626 was 0.9 mg/dL (within the institutional upper limit of normal) at baseline on January 28, 2010. However, the subject's serum creatinine increased to 1.7 mg/dL on January 11, 2011, and remained more than 0.5 mg/dL above the institutional upper limit of normal (1.0 mg/dL) for over 10 months. The subject had creatinine levels of 1.6 mg/dL on March 29, 2011; 1.6 mg/dL on June 21, 2011; 1.8 mg/dL on September 13, 2011; and 1.98 mg/dL on November 29, 2011. For Subject 222626, you failed to stop dosing of clodronate until January 24, 2012, more than one year after you should have done so.

b. Protocol (b)(4) specifies requirements for expedited reporting of serious adverse events for subjects randomized to Treatment Arms 2 or 3 (clodronate or ibandronate, respectively). In addition, the protocol requires that you utilize the Common Terminology Criteria for Adverse Events (CTCAE), Version 4.0, in determining the classification and severity (grade) of serious adverse events. The protocol also requires you to report any Grade 3 adverse event precipitating hospitalization (or prolonging hospitalization) within 10 calendar days via the Adverse Event Expedited Reporting System (AdEERS), regardless of attribution or expectedness. The protocol also requires you to report any osteonecrosis of the jaw, regardless of grade, attribution, or expectedness, within 24 hours of event recognition, via AdEERS.

You failed to report the following serious adverse events via AdEERS:

i) Subject 214199, who was randomized to Treatment Arm 3 (ibandronate), was hospitalized on (b)(4), for community-acquired pneumonia (CAP) with bilateral pulmonary infiltrates observed on Computed Tomography (CT) scan. The subject was treated for CAP with an intravenous (IV) antibiotic, Levaquin. Based on CTCAE clinical descriptions of lung infection, a lung infection indicating the use of IV antibiotic intervention meets the criterion for a Grade-3 severity. You failed to report a Grade-3 lung infection precipitated by hospitalization via AdEERS for Subject 214199.

ii) Subject 214835, who was randomized to Treatment Arm 3 (ibandronate), developed osteonecrosis of the jaw on April 6, 2010. You failed to report osteonecrosis of the jaw via AdEERS for Subject 214835.

c. Protocol (b)(4) requires you to perform the following study procedures at the Month-2 study visits: a physical examination, weight measurement, an evaluation of performance status, toxicity notation, and laboratory tests (serum creatinine, calcium, phosphate, magnesium, albumin, electrolytes, liver-function tests, and CBC/differential/platelets).

You failed to conduct Month-2 study visits for the following subjects: 213854, 214200, 214393, 214835, 221968, 222241, 222626, and 222698.

d. Protocol (b)(4) requires that you perform magnesium, phosphate, and complete blood count (CBC) laboratory tests at Months 2, 4, 6, 9, 12, 15, 21, 24, 27, 30, 33, and 36 study visits. You failed to conduct the following laboratory tests at the specified intervals:

Subject ID	Laboratory tests not performed	Study month(s) when these tests were not performed
213854	Magnesium and phosphate	4, 6, and 9
214199	Magnesium and phosphate	2, 4, 6, and 21
214200	Magnesium and phosphate	9 and 15
214393	Magnesium and phosphate	4, 6, 9, and 12
214632	Magnesium and phosphate	2, 4, 6, 9, 12, 24, 27, 30, 33, and 36
214835	Magnesium and phosphate	4, 6, and 9
217799	Magnesium, phosphate, and CBC	2, 4, and 6
222242	Magnesium and phosphate	2, 4, and 6
222456	Magnesium and phosphate	2

e. Protocol (b)(4) requires that you perform the following laboratory tests at the Month-4 study visits: serum creatinine, calcium, phosphate, magnesium, albumin, electrolytes, liver-function tests, and CBC/differential/platelets. You failed to perform any of the required laboratory tests at the Month-4 study visit for Subject 222698.

f. Protocol (b)(4) requires that you perform serum creatinine tests at screening and at Month-5 study visits.

You failed to perform the required serum creatinine tests at screening for the following subjects: 213854,

214200, 214632, and 221819. In addition, you failed to perform a serum creatinine for Subject 214835 at the Month-5 study visit.

g. Protocol (b)(4) requires that you perform a pre-study pregnancy test within 72 hours prior to initiation of study drug.

You failed to perform pre-study pregnancy testing for Subject 221968, who was 31 years of age at enrollment.

h. Protocol (b)(4) requires that you perform a bone scan at the end-of-treatment study visit.

You failed to perform a bone scan at the end-of-treatment study visit for Subject 214632.

i. Protocol (b)(4) requires that you perform a serum creatinine laboratory test prior to Cycle 7 of chemotherapy.

You failed to perform a serum creatinine laboratory test prior to Cycle 7 of chemotherapy for Subject 81053082.

In your September 22, 2013, written response to the findings noted in Item 1 above, you stated that you are not currently conducting clinical research or actively recruiting subjects to any studies. You noted that, had you continued to conduct clinical research, you would have appointed designated administrative and research staff to coordinate your clinical studies, to document delegation of responsibilities, to conduct routine weekly internal monitoring, to implement a new electronic medical record system, and to use a table/flowchart to monitor laboratory results.

Your response is inadequate because you did not provide sufficient information to enable us to evaluate the adequacy of your corrective action plans for use in any future clinical research that you may conduct. For example, you did not provide details regarding how you will implement your corrective action plan to prevent protocol violations. In addition, you did not provide any details of a corrective action plan to ensure adequate training for you and your staff on protocol requirements, to prevent future violations. As a result, we are unable to evaluate whether the corrective actions outlined above are adequate to prevent the occurrence of similar violations in the future.

Failure to perform protocol-required study procedures, including adverse event reporting and the performance of physical examinations and laboratory tests, jeopardizes subject safety and welfare. Of particular concern is the fact that, for Protocol (b)(4), laboratory tests to evaluate serum creatinine, magnesium, and/or phosphate were not done at all study visits for 10 of the 16 enrolled subjects whose records were reviewed. As mentioned above, Protocol (b)(4) is a study of bisphosphonate compounds, which have significant effects on bone mineralization and resorption; therefore, monitoring the levels of creatinine, magnesium, and phosphate is important to protect subject safety.

2. You failed to maintain adequate and accurate case histories that record all observations and other data pertinent to the investigation on each individual administered the investigational drug or employed as a control in the investigation [21 CFR 312.62(b)].

As a clinical investigator, you are required to prepare and maintain adequate and accurate case histories that record all observations and other data pertinent to the investigation on each individual administered the investigational drug or employed as a control in the investigation. For Protocols (b)(4) and (b)(4), case histories include signed and dated informed consent documents and study registration forms. You have failed to maintain adequate and accurate case histories with respect to these documents. Specifically:

a. The informed consent document for Protocol (b)(4) requires a “yes” or “no” response to six questions regarding subjects’ consent to participate in optional research studies in the future. You failed to record subjects’ consent to these optional studies adequately and accurately on the subjects’ study registration forms. Specifically:

i) Subject 214199 did not provide a “yes” or “no” response to any of the six questions regarding consent to participate in optional future studies; however, a “yes” response to each of the six questions was recorded on the subject’s registration form, indicating that the subject had provided a response to all of these questions.

ii) Subject 214632 did not provide a “yes” or “no” response to three of the six questions regarding consent to participate in optional future studies; however, a “yes” response to all six questions was recorded on the subject’s registration form, indicating that the subject had provided a response to all of these questions.

b. For Protocol (b)(4), one copy of the informed consent document for Subject 810493082 shows that the subject consented to optional future research; however, another copy of the same informed consent document shows that the subject did not consent to optional future research. There is no documented explanation for this discrepancy, and no documentation of when this informed consent document was amended or by whom.

In your September 22, 2013, written response to the findings noted in Item 2 above, you stated that you are not currently conducting clinical research or actively recruiting subjects to any studies. You noted that, had you continued to conduct clinical research, you would have appointed designated administrative and research staff to coordinate your clinical studies, to document delegation of responsibilities, to conduct routine weekly internal monitoring, to implement a new electronic medical record system, and to use a table/flowchart to monitor laboratory results.

Your response is inadequate because you did not provide sufficient information to enable us to evaluate the adequacy of your corrective action plans for use in any future clinical research that you may conduct. For example, you did not provide details regarding how you will implement your corrective action plan to prevent protocol violations. In addition, you did not provide any details of a corrective action plan to ensure adequate training for you and your staff on protocol requirements, to prevent future violations; and you have not provided sufficient details regarding your plan to document required study data adequately. As a result, we are unable to evaluate whether the corrective actions outlined above are adequate to prevent the occurrence of similar violations in the future.

Your failure to document informed consent properly, raises concerns about the extent to which subjects' rights were protected at your site.

This letter is not intended to be an all-inclusive list of deficiencies with your clinical study of an investigational drug. It is your responsibility to ensure adherence to each requirement of the law and relevant FDA regulations. You should address these deficiencies and establish procedures to ensure that any ongoing or future studies will be in compliance with FDA regulations.

Within fifteen (15) working days of your receipt of this letter, you should notify this office in writing of the actions you have taken to prevent similar violations in the future. Failure to address the violations noted above adequately and promptly may result in regulatory action without further notice. If you believe you have complied with FDA regulations, include your reasoning and any supporting information for our consideration.

If you have any questions, please contact Constance Cullity, M.D., M.P.H., at 301-796-3397; FAX 301-847-8748. Your written response and any pertinent documentation should be addressed to:

Constance Cullity, M.D., M.P.H.
Branch Chief
Good Clinical Practice Enforcement Branch
Division of Good Clinical Practice Compliance
Office of Scientific Investigations
Office of Compliance
Center for Drug Evaluation and Research
Food and Drug Administration
Building 51, Room 5354
10903 New Hampshire Avenue
Silver Spring, MD 20993

Sincerely yours,

{See appended electronic signature page}

Sean Y. Kassim, Ph.D.
Acting Director
Office of Scientific Investigations
Office of Compliance
Center for Drug Evaluation and Research
Food and Drug Administration

第 77 封　给 Zimmermann, Ralf C. 的警告信

2014年2月21日

参考号：14-HFD-45-02-02

尊敬的Zimmermann博士：

2013年6月5日至25日，Thomas Hansen先生代表FDA，在您的临床研究机构，对您所开展的以下临床试验进行了审查：

试验方案（b）（4）[1]，"（b）（4）"，试验药物为（b）（4），申办者为（b）（4）。

试验方案（b）（4），"（b）（4）"，试验药物为（b）（4），申办者为（b）（4）。

这封警告信特告知您现场检查中发现的违规情况。

本次现场检查是FDA的生物研究监查项目的一部分。该项目通过设定的检查方法，对FDA所监管的相关研究的实施情况进行评估，以确认研究数据从科学上来说是有效和准确的，并帮助确保这些研究中受试者的权益、安全和福利得到了保护。

在现场检查结束时，Thomas Hansen先生，向您出示了FDA483表，即现场检查发现的问题，并与您进行了讨论。您2013年7月11日对该FDA483表的书面回复已收悉。

经对现场检查报告、该报告的附件，以及您2013年7月11日提交的书面回复进行审查，我们认为，您没有遵循临适用的法律要求和监管临床研究及受试者保护的FDA法规。我们想强调以下几点：

1．您未能亲自进行临床研究或对研究进行监督［21 CFR 312.60］

当您签署研究者声明（FDA 1572表）时，您同意承担贵研究中心临床研究者的职责。作为临床研究者，您的总体职责包括确保临床研究按照签署的研究者声明、研究计划和适用的法规执行，同时要保护在您的监护下受试者的权益、安全和福利，也要确保研究药品的管控（21 CFR 312.60）。通过签署FDA 1572 表，您明确承诺亲自执行临床试验或对授权他人操作的部分进行监管。尽管您可以将一些研究任务授权给有资质的人去做，但是您不可以把总体职责授权给他人。我们的检查表明，您对您授权的研究人员的监督不足以确保临床研究按照签署的研究者声明、研究计划和适用的法规执行，同时也不能保护受试者的权益、安全和福利。

具体而言，对于试验方案（b）（4），您没能充分监督您授权的研究人员，也没能充分监督试验方案（b）（4）的执行，这导致了这份信中提到的很多的违规行为。这些违规行为包括但不限于，当哥伦比亚大学医学中心伦理委员会对该研究的批件已经失效时，还入组受试者到这个研究；没有获得入组受试者50人中28个人的知情同意书；在获得知情同意前，对10个受试者随机分组并发放研究药物。

在您的2013年7月11日书面回复中，您承认您"没有提供足够的监督或者适当的授权实施临床研究的责任。"您也承认您的责任是确保伦理委员会批准的方案被遵循，同时表示您"授权了这个责任却没有进行适当的监督。"

作为临床研究者，为了保护参加研究受试者的权益、安全和福利以及数据完整性，您的主要责任是确保研究正确执行并符合FDA的法规要求。您缺乏对试验方案（b）（4）的监督和监管，使得我们很担心入组到试验方案（b）（4）中的受试者权益在贵研究中心得到保护的程度和试验方案（b）（4）数据的完整性。

2. 您未能按照 21 CFR 50 的要求获取知情同意［21 CFR 312.60 和 21 CFR 50.20］

作为研究者，您的责任是根据21 CFR 50的要求获取知情同意书。FDA法规的21 CFR 第50部分声明，除

---

1 （b）（4）涉及商业秘密，根据法规内容不予公开。

了21 CFR 50.23和21 CFR 50.24规定的情况之外，如果没有获得受试者的合法有效的知情同意或者受试者法定授权代表的同意，研究者不能在人身上，开展法规规定的临床研究。您未能获得合法有效的知情同意，总体而言：

a. 在入组试验方案（b）（4）的50个受试者中，以下28个受试者的知情同意书没有获得：受试者C1，C4~C7，C9~C12，C17，C19，C20，C22，C26，C28，C30，C31，C33，C34，C37~C42，C45，A3和A5。

b. 您入组了10个受试者到试验方案（b）（4），在他们签署知情同意书之前，给他们发放了临床试验用药具体信息如下。

受试者	第一次发放临床试验用药的时间	第一次签署知情同意书的时间
C15	2010年9月15日	2010年12月10日
C16	2010年9月15日	2010年9月22日
C21	2010年11月28日	2010年12月17日
C24	2010年12月17日	2010年12月23日
C25	2010年12月20日	2010年12月28日
C32	2011年5月19日	2011年6月16日
C36	2011年1月26日	2011年2月9日
C43	2011年4月7日	2011年4月26日
C44	2011年5月10日	2011年5月27日
C47	2011年4月29日	2011年5月26日

在2013年7月11日对FDA 483表格的书面回复（3~4页）中，您承认您没能获得2a 部分列出的28个受试者的知情同意书，并给上述项2b列出的另外10名受试者签署知情同意书之前发放了研究用药。另外，在您的回复中，您声称“您承认对授权参加招募和获取知情同意书的研究人员没有提供指导和监管，您将承担全部责任”。

我们接受您在书面回复中总结的哥伦比亚大学医学中心伦理委员会和妇产科所采取的措施。2011年8月19号，在发现严重的违规操作和对受试者有潜在的风险后，哥伦比亚大学医学中心伦理委员会和妇产科决定暂停本研究，妇产科内部对现有的研究记录进行了稽查，同时在伦理委员会的指导下，通知了所有50个受试者有关在获取知情同意和研究程序中的违规操作。

我们也接受您以下的纠正措施计划：

- 重新教育参加试验方案（b）（4）的研究者；
- 所有的研究必须进行部门审批，这样可以使适当的保障措施和监查可以启动；
- 科室要建立制度，规定每一个研究者启动的FDA监管研究，都要分配一个协调员；
- 科室质量保证部门的研究监查员，在每个季度进行临床研究的绩效监查；
- 使用一个知情同意书的清单来协助记录知情同意的过程

关于上述项2所列出的问题，您的书面回复是不够的。我们担心的是大多数的纠正措施看起来都是哥伦比亚大学医学中心的行为，并没有反映出您个人所采取的纠正措施。需要您注意的是，作为研究者，您要担负起最终的职责，确保依据21 CFR 50规定去获取知情同意书。

对于您计划使用知情同意书的清单来确保知情的过程被正确的记录，我们也是担心的。这个清单没有包含获取知情同意书的时间，因此无法获知受试者参加临床研究前是否获得充分的知情。另外，这个清单中知情同意的部分是从“Rascal”系统打印的，我们要求您说明一下这个系统，因为它涉及研究数据的跟踪记录，例如知情同意。

您没能在受试者参加试验前获得知情同意书，这危害到了受试者的安全性和福利，因为您这样做是没有给受试者一个机会去评估他们参加临床研究的风险和受益。

3. 您未能确保按照研究计划进行研究［21 CFR 312.60］

作为临床研究者，您必须确保临床研究按照临床研究计划实施。试验方案“（b）（4）”的临床研究计划要求您根据受试者分配的治疗组发放方案特殊规定剂量的研究药物，并获得研究相关的实验室检查结果。您没有遵循这些要求。这些不遵循的例子包括，但不限于以下内容：

试验方案“（b）（4）”包含两个研究组：（1）“传统的”“（b）（4）”治疗组和（2）阶梯治疗组。“传统的”治疗组要求受试者在第一个月经周期的第5~9天接受5天的研究药物“（b）（4）”的治疗，剂量是50mg/d。如果受试者在第一个月经周期没有发生阳性反应（即卵泡的直径至少要达到17mm），那么根据方案要求在第二个月经周期，研究药物的剂量要增加到100mg。如果受试者在第二个月经周期没有发生阳性反应，方案要求在第三个月经周期，研究药物的剂就要增加到150mg。在阶梯治疗组要求受试者接受相同的起始剂量的“（b）（4）”（例如，从50mg，100mg或者150mg开始）去诱发阳性反应，但是不必等到下一个月经周期，可以在比较短的时间内将研究药物的剂量从50mg提高到100mg，或者从100mg提到到150mg。

对于试验方案“（b）（4）”，有4个受试者的药物剂量不是根据他们特殊研究分组（标准剂量组或者阶梯剂量组）给予的，具体而言：

a. 受试者C4在2010年10月10号入组到方案“（b）（4）”，被分配到传统组也就是标准治疗组。该受试者的剂量表显示，受试者C4在第一个周期和第二个周期分别接受了50mg和100mg剂量的研究药物“（b）（4）”。然而在第三个周期，受试者依旧接受了5天，剂量为100mg/d的研究药物的治疗，而不是按照方案要求的将剂量提高到150mg/d。医疗记录的备注显示，受试者在接受50mg剂量的研究药物时出现了阳性反应，不需要进一步的评估。但是这个备注不能被药物剂量表上的信息支持。

在您对FDA483表的书面回复中，您表示受试者C4在接受5天，剂量为50mg的研究药物后出现了阳性反应，出现了一个排卵前卵泡，因此退出了研究。您的回复是不充分的，因为它缺乏支持性的书面文件和为什么剂量表和您的医疗记录备注以及回复是矛盾的解释。

b. 受试者C6在2010年12月17日入组试验方案（b）（4）临床研究，被分配到“阶梯”治疗组。该受试者的剂量表显示，受试者C6分别在2011年1月11日至15日和2011年3月31日至4月6日接受了50mg的研究药物“（b）（4）”，然后，在2011年4月7日至14日，接受了75mg的研究药物，而不是按照研究方案要求阶梯剂量。对受试者C6的医疗记录的备注显示该受试者，C6在接受50mg剂量的研究药物“（b）（4）”时出现了阳性反应并怀孕了。但是医疗记录里的备注和药物剂量表上的信息是互相矛盾的。

在您对FDA483表的书面回复中，您表示受试者C6在接受5天、剂量为50mg的研究药物“（b）（4）”后出现了阳性反应，出现了一个排卵前卵泡，因此退出了研究。您的回复是不充分的，因为它缺乏支持性的书面文件和为什么剂量表和您的回复是矛盾的解释。

c. 受试者C19在2010年12月13日入组到方案“（b）（4）”，被分配到“阶梯”治疗组。该受试者的剂量表显示，受试者C19在2010年12月13日至17日和2011年2月15日至19日接受了每天25mg的研究药物“（b）（4）”，而不是按照方案要求的阶梯式的剂量。医疗记录的备注显示C19在每一个周期接受的都是50mg剂量的研究药物“（b）（4）”。但是医疗记录里的备注和药物剂量表上的信息是互相矛盾的。

在您对FDA483表的书面回复中，您说受试者C19在接受5天、剂量为50mg的研究药物后出现了过激反应退出了研究；她要求在下一个周期里降低剂量。您的回复是不充分的，因为它缺乏支持性的书面文件和对为什么剂量表和医疗记录备注与您的回复是矛盾的解释。

d. 受试者C35在2011年1月21号入组到方案“（b）（4）”，被分配到“传统”也就是“标准”治疗组。该受试者的剂量表显示，受试者C35在第一个周期、第二个周期和第三个周期接受了持续5天、每天100mg研究药物“（b）（4）”，而不是按照研究方案要求的，在第一个治疗周期以50mg治疗剂量开始，第二个周期和第三个周期分别调整到100mg和150mg。医疗记录里的备注显示，受试者在第一个治疗周期接受了50mg的研究药物，随后进行了3个每月100mg研究药物的治疗周期。

在您对FDA483表的书面回复中，您指出受试者C35在接受5天、剂量为50mg的研究药物“(b)(4)”后出现了延迟反应，因此在下一个周期提高剂量到100mg。提高剂量后受试者有了正常反应，继而退出了研究。您的回复是不充分的，因为它缺乏支持性的书面文件和对为什么剂量表和您的医疗记录备注以及回复是矛盾的解释。

在2013年7月11日，您书面回复了FDA483表，您声称“我同意不是所有受试者的给药都是按照伦理委员会批准的方案特定的剂量标准，这导致了方案违背”。您还解释到：“审阅了受试者的病历后，发现大多数的受试者接受了标准的临床治疗，而没有严格遵循伦理委员会批准的方案里规定的剂量和时间表。”

在您的书面回复中，您也承认您的责任是确保按照伦理委员会批准的方案进行研究，也认为您要对“这些不足负责”。同时您阐述到，您“将来会监督和监查方案违背，并相应地把这些违背汇报给伦理委员会和申办者”。

您的回复是不充分的，因为您没有提供关于您纠正措施计划的详细内容。例如，您没能提供怎样执行计划去监督和监查方案违背情况的细节。没有这些细节，我们没有办法判定您的纠正措施计划是否能避免将来类似违规情况的发生。

没有按照方案里规定的剂量和时间表给受试者发放研究药物危害到了您试验场所数据的有效性和完整性。

4. 您未能确保符合 21 CFR 56 要求的 IRB 负责对拟进行的临床研究进行初始审查、跟踪审查和批准［21 CFR 312.66］

作为一个研究者，您应该确保伦理委员会遵循21 CFR56的要求审阅及批准递交的临床研究。您未能做到这一点。

具体而言，试验方案(b)(4)的伦理批件在2011年3月30日至6月3日是失效的。然而在此期间，您入组了6个受试者(C42-C47)并发放了研究用药。

在2013年7月11日，您书面回复了FDA483表，您承认您“您没能确保获得伦理委员会的持续批准”并“在伦理批件失效的期间入组并治疗受试者”。在回复中，您也写到了您将会采取的纠正措施，包括您将对伦理委员会的持续批准进行监查并且确保没有获得伦理委员会批准或IRB批准文件过期期间，不进行试验相关的流程。

您关于没有伦理委员会批准就进行研究流程的回复是不充分的。例如，您没有提供关于您将怎样对伦理委员会的持续批准进行监查并且确保没有获得伦理委员会批准或IRB批准文件过期期间，不进行试验相关的流程。没有这些细节，我们没有办法判定您的纠正措施计划是否能避免将来类似违规情况的发生。

您没能确保获得伦理委员会对本研究持续的审阅和批准，这妨碍了伦理委员会审阅您递交的研究申请并决定这个申请是否充分的能力。

本警告信的目的并非是罗列您在试验药物临床研究中存在的所有缺陷。确保遵循法律和相关FDA法规的要求是您的职责，您应当解决这些缺陷，并建立规程，以确保任何正在进行或将来进行的研究均符合FDA的法规。

自收到这封信的15个工作日内，您应当书面告知本办公室为预防将来发生类似违规情况而采取的措施。如果不能充分、迅速地解释上述违规问题，可能导致我们在不再通知的情况下采取监管措施。如果您认为您已经遵循了FDA的法规要求，请陈述理由，并提供所有支持资料以供我们参考。

附：英文原文

Zimmermann, Ralf C.

WARNING LETTER

FEB 21, 2014

CERTIFIED MAIL
RETURN RECEIPT REQUESTED

14-HFD-45-02-02

Ralf Zimmerman, M.D.
Columbia University Medical Center
622 West 168th Street, PH 18
New York, New York 10032

Dear Dr. Zimmerman:

This Warning Letter informs you of objectionable conditions observed during the U.S. Food and Drug Administration (FDA) inspection conducted at your clinical site between June 5 and 25, 2013. Mr. Thomas Hansen, representing the FDA, reviewed your conduct of the following clinical investigations:

Protocol (b)(4), "(b)(4)," of the investigation drug (b)(4), performed for Dr. (b)(4)

Protocol (b)(4), "(b)(4)," of the investigational drug (b)(4), performed for (b)(4)

This inspection is a part of FDA's Bioresearch Monitoring Program, which includes inspections designed to evaluate the conduct of FDA-regulated research to ensure that the data are scientifically valid and accurate, and to help ensure that the rights, safety, and welfare of the human subjects of those studies have been protected.

At the conclusion of the inspection, Mr. Hansen presented and discussed with you Form FDA 483, Inspectional Observations. We acknowledge receipt of your July 11, 2013 written response to the Form FDA 483.

From our review of the FDA Establishment Inspection Report, the documents submitted with that report, and your July 11, 2013 written response, we conclude that you did not adhere to the applicable statutory requirements and FDA regulations governing the conduct of clinical investigations and the protection of human subjects. We wish to emphasize the following:

1. You failed to personally conduct or supervise the clinical investigations [21 CFR 312.60].

When you signed the Statement of Investigator (Form FDA 1572) for the above-referenced clinical trials, you agreed to take on the responsibilities of a clinical investigator at your site. Your general responsibilities as a clinical investigator include ensuring that the clinical trials are conducted according to the signed investigator statement, the investigational plan, and applicable regulations; protecting the rights, safety, and welfare of subjects under your care; and ensuring control of drugs under investigation [21 CFR 312.60]. By signing Form FDA 1572, you specifically agreed to personally conduct the clinical trial or to supervise those aspects of the trial that you did not personally conduct. While you may delegate certain study tasks to individuals qualified to perform them, as a clinical investigator you may not delegate your general responsibilities. Our investigation indicates that your supervision of personnel to whom you delegated study tasks was not adequate to ensure that the clinical trial was conducted according to the signed investigator statement, the investigational plan, and applicable regulations, and in a manner that protects the rights, safety, and welfare of human subjects.

Specifically, for Protocol (b)(4), you failed to supervise adequately the individuals to whom you delegated study tasks. Your failure to supervise adequately the conduct of Protocol (b)(4) led to many of the violations noted in this letter. These violations include, but are not limited to, enrollment of subjects into the protocol when approval by the Columbia University Medical Center (CUMC) Institutional Review Board (IRB) had lapsed; failure to obtain informed consent from 28 of 50 enrolled subjects; and randomization and administration of investigational drug to 10 subjects before obtaining their informed consent to participate in the study.

In your July 11, 2013 written response, you acknowledged that you "did not provide adequate supervision or delegate the responsibilities of conducting the study appropriately." You also acknowledged that it was your responsibility to ensure that the IRB-approved protocol was followed, and you stated that you "delegated this responsibility without providing the proper oversight."

As the clinical investigator, it was your ultimate responsibility to ensure that the studies were conducted properly and in compliance with FDA regulations in order to protect the rights, safety, and welfare of study subjects and to ensure the integrity of the study data. Your lack of supervision and oversight over Protocol (b)(4) raises significant concerns about the adequacy of your protection of study subjects enrolled at your site in the studies mentioned above and also raises data integrity concerns generated for Protocol (b)(4).

2. You failed to obtain informed consent in accordance with the provisions of 21 CFR part 50 [21 CFR 312.60 and 21 CFR 50.20].

As a clinical investigator, it is your responsibility to obtain informed consent in accordance with 21 CFR part 50. FDA's regulations at 21 CFR 50.20 state that, except as provided in 21 CFR 50.23 and 21 CFR 50.24, no investigator may involve a human being as a subject in research covered by the regulations unless the investigator has obtained the legally effective informed consent of the subject or the subject's legally authorized representative. You failed to obtain legally effective informed consent. Specifically:

a. You failed to obtain informed consent from the following 28 of 50 subjects who were enrolled in Protocol (b)(4): Subjects C1, C4 through C7, C9 through C12, C17, C19, C20, C22, C26, C28, C30, C31, C33, C34, C37 through C42, C45, A3, and A5.

b. You enrolled 10 subjects into Protocol (b)(4) and gave them investigational drug before each signed the informed consent document. These subjects are listed in the Table below.

Subject	Date Subject first given investigational drug	Date Subject first signed the Informed Consent Document
C15	September 15, 2010	December 10, 2010
C16	September 15, 2010	September 22, 2010
C21	November 28, 2010	December 17, 2010
C24	December 17, 2010	December 23, 2010
C25	December 20, 2010	December 28, 2010
C32	May 19, 2011	June 16, 2011
C36	January 26, 2011	February 9, 2011
C43	April 7, 2011	April 26, 2011
C44	May 10, 2011	May 27, 2011
C47	April 29, 2011	May 26, 2011

In your July 11, 2013 written response to the Form FDA 483 [pages 3-4] you agreed that you failed to obtain consent from the 28 subjects listed in Item 2.a. above and that you gave investigational drug to the additional 10 enrolled subjects listed in item 2.b. above, prior to subjects signing the informed consent document. In addition, in that written response you stated, "I acknowledge and take full responsibility for not providing the instruction and oversight of the research staff delegated to recruiting and obtaining informed consent."

We acknowledge you summarized, in the written response, actions that the Columbia University Medical Center Institutional Review Board (CUMC IRB) and the Department of Obstetrics and Gynecology (Department) have taken. You indicated that after serious noncompliance and the potential risk to subjects was discovered, on August 19, 2011, the CUMC IRB and the Department suspended Protocol (b)(4), the Department performed an audit of all available study records and, at the direction of the IRB, all 50 subjects were notified of the violations in the consent process and study procedures.

We also acknowledge your corrective action plan that includes the following:

Re-education of investigators involved in Protocol (b)(4);

Mandatory Department approval of all research so that appropriate safeguards and monitoring can be initiated;
Establishment of a Department requirement for assigning a research coordinator to each investigator-initiated FDA regulated research study;
Performance of quarterly monitoring by the Department Quality Assurance (QA) Research Monitor, and;
Use of an Informed Consent Process Checklist to assist in the documentation of the consent process.

Your written response is inadequate as it relates to the findings noted in Item 2 above. We are concerned that the majority of the corrective actions appear to represent actions taken by Columbia University Medical Center and do not reflect corrective actions that you personally have taken. Please note that, as the clinical investigator, you are ultimately responsible for ensuring that informed consent is obtained in accordance with 21 CFR part 50.

We are also concerned about your plans to use the Informed Consent Process Checklist to ensure that the consent process is documented appropriately. This checklist does not address the timing of consent and, therefore, does not appear adequate to acquire informed consent prior to a subject's participation in clinical research. In addition, the checklist refers to consent forms printed from "Rascal." We request clarification on the "Rascal" system as it relates to study data tracking, such as informed consent.

Your failure to obtain informed consent prior to involving subjects in research jeopardizes the safety and welfare of subjects by denying them an opportunity to assess the risks and benefits of their participation in the clinical investigation.

3. You failed to ensure that the investigation was conducted according to the investigational plan [21 CFR 312.60].

As a clinical investigator, you are required to ensure that your clinical studies are conducted in accordance with the investigational plan. The investigational plan for Protocol (b)(4) required you to administer the protocol-specified dose of investigational drug to each subject according to their assigned study arm, and to obtain study-related laboratory tests. You failed to adhere to these requirements. Examples of this failure include but are not limited to the following:

Protocol (b)(4) contained two study arms: (1) a "traditional" (b)(4) treatment arm, and (2) a "stair-step" arm. The "traditional" treatment arm required that the subject receive 50 mg of (b)(4) daily for 5 days on Day 5 - 9 of the first menstrual cycle during the study. If the subject did not develop a positive response (i.e., follicles of at least 17 mm in size) after the first menstrual cycle, the protocol required that the dose be increased to 100 mg on the second menstrual cycle. If the subject did not develop a positive response after the second cycle, the protocol required that the dose be increased to 150 mg on the third cycle. The "stair-step" arm required that the subject receive the same dosing of (b)(4) (50 mg to 150 mg) in an attempt to induce a positive response, but in a shorter timeframe and without having to wait for the next menstrual cycle before increasing the (b)(4) dose from 50 mg to 100 mg or from 100 mg to 150 mg.

For Protocol (b)(4), four subjects were not dosed according to their protocol-specified study arm (standard dosing or stair-step dosing). Specifically:

a. Subject C4 was enrolled in Protocol (b)(4) on October 10, 2010, and assigned to the "traditional" or "standard" dosing arm. The subject's dosing log shows that Subject C4 received the protocol-required (b)(4) dose of 50 mg and 100 mg during Cycles 1 and 2, respectively. However, the dosing log shows that for Cycle 3, the subject again received 100 mg daily for 5 days rather than 150 mg daily for 5 days as required by the protocol. The Progress Note Addendum for Subject C4 states that the subject responded to 50 mg of (b)(4) and no further assessment was needed, but this statement is not supported by the dosing log.

In your written response to the Form FDA 483, you indicate that Subject C4 received 50 mg daily for 5 days, responded with the development of one preovulatory follicle, and then exited the study. Your response is inadequate because it lacks supporting documentation and an explanation as to why the dosing records described above conflict with the Progress Note Addendum and your response.

b. Subject C6 was enrolled in Protocol (b)(4) on December 17, 2010, and assigned to the "stair-step" dosing arm. The subject's dosing log shows that Subject C6 received (b)(4) 50 mg daily from January 11 to 15, 2011, and from March 31 to April 6, 2011, and then received 75 mg daily from April 7 to 14, 2011, rather than the protocol-required stair-step dosing. The Progress Note Addendum for Subject C6 states that the subject responded to 50 mg of (b)(4) and became pregnant. The Progress Note Addendum conflicts with the dosing log.

In your written response to the Form FDA 483, you indicate that Subject C6 received 50 mg of (b)(4) for 5 days, responded with the development of a preovulatory follicle, and exited the study. Your response is inadequate because it lacks supporting documentation and an explanation as to why the subject's dosing log conflicts with your response.

c. Subject C19 was enrolled in Protocol (b)(4) on December 13, 2010 and assigned to the "stair-step" dosing arm. The subject's dosing log shows that Subject C19 received (b)(4) 25 mg daily from December 13 to 17, 2010, and from February 15 to 19, 2011, rather than the protocol-required stair-step dosing. The Progress Note Addendum notes the subject received 50 mg of (b)(4) for each cycle. The Progress Note Addendum conflicts with the dosing log.

In your written response to the Form FDA 483, you state that Subject C19 "had a hyper-response to 50 mg for 5 days and exited the study; she required a dose decrease with her next cycle." Your response is inadequate because it lacks supporting documentation and an explanation as to why the subject's dosing log and Progress Note Addendum conflict with your response.

d. Subject C35 was enrolled in Protocol (b)(4) on January 21, 2011 and assigned to the "traditional" or "standard" dosing arm. According to the subject's dosing log, Subject C35 received (b)(4) 100 mg daily for 5 days during Cycles 1, 2, and 3 rather starting with the protocol-required dose of 50 mg in Cycle 1 and progressing to 100 mg and 150 mg in Cycles 2 and 3, respectively. The Progress Note Addendum indicates the subject's first treatment cycle was for 50 mg, followed monthly by three 100 mg cycles.

In your written response to the Form FDA 483, you indicate that Subject C35 received (b)(4) 50 mg for 5 days, had a delayed response, had a dose increase to (b)(4) 100 mg at the next cycle, and then achieved a normal response and exited the study. Your response is inadequate because it lacks supporting documentation and an explanation as to why the subject's dosing log conflicts with your response as well as the Progress Note Addendum.

In your July 11, 2013 written response to the Form FDA 483, you stated, "I agree that the IRB-approved protocol-specific dosing regimens were not followed for all subjects, resulting in protocol violations." You further explained that, "A review of subjects' charts noted that many of the subjects were treated according to clinical standards, instead of adhering to the strict dose and schedule in the IRB-approved protocol."

In your written response, you also acknowledged your responsibility to ensure that the IRB-approved study protocol is followed and acknowledged that you were "responsible for these errors." You also stated that you "will supervise and monitor for protocol violations and report to the IRB and the sponsor, accordingly."

Your written response is inadequate because you failed to provide sufficient details with respect to your corrective action plan. For example, you did not provide details regarding how you will carry out your plan to supervise and monitor protocol violations. Without having these details, we are unable to determine whether your corrective action appears sufficient to prevent similar violations in the future.

Failure to administer investigational drug to subjects according to the protocol-required dosing schedule compromises the validity and integrity of data generated at your site for Protocol (b)(4).

4. You failed to assure that an IRB that complies with the requirements set forth in part 56 was responsible for the initial and continuing review and approval of the proposed clinical study [21 CFR 312.66].

As a clinical investigator, you are required to assure that an IRB that complies with 21 CFR part 56 reviews and approves a proposed clinical investigation. You failed to assure that an IRB that complies with 21 CFR part 56 reviewed and approved a proposed clinical study.

Specifically, IRB approval to conduct Protocol (b)(4) lapsed from March 30 to June 3, 2011. During this lapsed period, you enrolled six subjects (Subjects C42 through C47) into this protocol and gave them the investigational drug.

In your July 11, 2013 written response to the Form FDA 483, you acknowledged that you "failed to ensure that continuing IRB approval was maintained" and that "subjects were enrolled and treated during a lapse in IRB approval." In that response, you also described corrective actions that you will take, including monitoring the protocol for continuing IRB approval and ensuring that no study-related procedures are performed without IRB approval or during a period in which IRB approval has lapsed.

Your response is inadequate with respect to the conduct of study activities without IRB approval. Specifically, you did not provide details regarding how you will ensure that you will monitor protocols for continuing IRB approval or how you will ensure that no study-related procedures are performed without IRB approval or during a period in which IRB approval has lapsed. Without having these details, we are unable to determine whether your corrective action appears sufficient to prevent similar violations in the future.

Your failure to ensure continuing IRB review and approval of Protocol (b)(4) impeded the IRB's ability to review your application to conduct Protocol (b)(4) and make a determination regarding the adequacy of that application.

This letter is not intended to be an all-inclusive list of deficiencies with your clinical study of an investigational drug. It is your responsibility to ensure adherence to each requirement of the law and relevant FDA regulations. You should address these deficiencies and establish procedures to ensure that any ongoing or future studies will comply with FDA regulations.

Within fifteen (15) working days of your receipt of this letter, you should notify this office in writing of the actions you have taken to prevent similar violations in the future. Failure to address the violations noted above adequately and promptly may result in regulatory action without further notice. If you believe you have complied with FDA regulations, include your reasoning and any supporting information for our consideration.

If you have any questions, please contact Constance Cullity, M.D., M.P.H., at 301-796-3397; FAX 301-847-8748. Your written response and any pertinent documentation should be addressed to:

Constance Cullity, M.D., M.P.H.
Branch Chief
Good Clinical Practice Enforcement Branch
Division of Good Clinical Practice Compliance
Office of Scientific Investigations
Office of Compliance
Center for Drug Evaluation and Research
Food and Drug Administration
Building 51, Room 5354
10903 New Hampshire Avenue
Silver Spring, MD 20993

Sincerely yours,

{See appended electronic signature page}

Thomas N. Moreno, M.S.
Acting Director
Office of Scientific Investigations
Office of Compliance
Center for Drug Evaluation and Research
Food and Drug Administration

This is a representation of an electronic record that was signed electronically and this page is the manifestation of the electronic signature.

/S/

THOMAS N MORENO
02/21/2014

第78封　给Burzynski, Stanislaw R. 医学博士的警告信

2013年12月3日

参考号：13-HFD-45-11-04

尊敬的Burzynski博士：

2013年1月7日至3月15日，Joel Martinez先生、Hugh McClure先生和Cynthia Kleppinger博士代表FDA，在贵临床研究机构，对您为Burzynski Research Institute的试验药物抗瘤酮A10和AS2开展的以下临床研究以及对这两种药物的慈善供药物情况进行了审查。这封警告信特告知您现场检查中发现的违规情况。

- 试验方案 BT-09，"抗瘤酮A10和AS2-1治疗脑肿瘤患者的Ⅱ期研究"。
- 试验方案 BT-10，"抗瘤酮A10和AS2-1治疗儿童脑肿瘤患者的Ⅱ期研究"。
- 试验方案 BT-21，"抗瘤酮A10和AS2-1治疗成人原发性恶性脑肿瘤患者的Ⅱ期研究"。
- 试验方案 BT-22，"抗瘤酮A10和AS2-1治疗儿童原发性恶性脑肿瘤患者的Ⅱ期研究"。
- 试验方案 AD-02，"抗瘤酮A10和AS2-1治疗肾上腺肿瘤患者的Ⅱ期研究"。

本次现场检查是FDA的生物研究监查项目一部分。该项目通过设定的检查方法，对FDA所监管的研究的实施情况进行评估，以确认研究数据在科学上是有效和准确的，并帮助确保这些研究中受试者的权益、安全和福利得到了保护。

在现场检查结束时，Martinez先生、McClure先生和Kleppinger博士向您出示了FDA483表，即现场检查发现的问题，并与您进行了讨论。您2013年4月5日对该FDA483表的书面回复和2013年5月15日对FDA483表的进展更新的回复已收悉。

经对现场检查报告、该报告的附件，以及您2013年4月5日的书面回复进行审查，我们认为，您没有遵循适用的法律要求和监管临床研究实施及受试者保护的FDA法规。我们想强调以下几点：

1. 您未能确保按照研究计划进行研究［21 CFR 312.60］

作为临床研究者，您必须确保按照研究计划进行临床研究。试验方案BT-09、BT-10和BT-21的研究计划要求您根据受试者肿瘤对药物的反应来分类治疗反应，并向申办者报告不良事件。正确分类治疗反应对于决定肿瘤是否对药物治疗有反应非常重要。报告不良反应对于降低受试者的风险也很重要，而且能保证申办者收集到试验药物完整、正确的安全性数据。您未能按照研究计划实施试验方案BT-09、BT-10和BT-21，具体表现为：

a. 试验方案BT-09、BT-10和BT-21定义了每个可能的治疗反应（完全缓解，部分缓解，疾病稳定和疾病进展），并包括临床研究者应使用的标准将受试者的治疗反应分为其中的一种。此次现场检查审查了27位受试者的治疗分类，其中9位的分类是错误的。具体而言：

ⅰ. 对于完全缓解的分类，试验方案BT-09、BT-10和BT-21要求：①所有的对比增强神经影像检查，以及辅助放射检查显示肿瘤完全消失持续至少4周；②受试者未使用皮质类固醇治疗。

您错误地将以下受试者分类为完全缓解：

（1）试验方案BT-10：受试者006389和013660所有的神经影像检查显示，未达到对比增强的肿瘤完全消失持续至少4周的标准，但研究者错误地将其分类为完全缓解。

a）受试者006389病例报告表肿瘤测量页和您提供的截至2013年1月7日入组试验方案BT-10受试者清单均确认该受试者达到完全缓解。但病例报告表肿瘤测量页显示：没有任何神经影像学研究显示的对比增强肿瘤

完全消失持续至少达到4周。因此该受试者未达到完全缓解的标准。

b）对于受试者013660，病例报告表肿瘤测量页和您提供的截至2013年1月7日入组试验方案BT-10受试者清单均确认该受试者达到完全缓解。但病例报告表肿瘤测量页显示：没有神经影像研究显示的对比增强肿瘤完全消失持续至少4周。因此该受试者未达到完全缓解的标准。

（2）试验方案BT-09：对于受试者007197，病例报告表肿瘤测量页显示，根据2001年7月25日、2001年9月11日，和2001年11月8日的MRI检查结果，所有对比增强的肿瘤均完全消失至少4周。但病例报告表皮质类固醇页及肿瘤血液流程表显示，该受试者于2001年7月25日和2001年9月11日接受MRI检查当天，以及这些MRI检查期间，直至2001年11月8日MRI检查前一周，都在接受皮质类固醇治疗，因此该受试者未达到完全缓解的标准。

（3）试验方案BT-21：对于受试者009990，病例报告表肿瘤测量页显示，根据正电子发射断层扫描（PET）结果，疾病达到完全缓解。但病例报告表皮质类固醇报告页显示，该受试者在接受PET扫描当天及期间（检查日期为2005年1月4日、2月4日、6月14日和8月16日）均接受了皮质类固醇治疗。因此该受试者未达到完全缓解的标准。

ⅱ. 对于部分缓解的分类，试验方案BT-09要求：①与基线比较增强肿瘤垂直直径乘积的总和减少50%以上并持续至少4周；②任何病变大小未同时增长，无新病变出现；③皮质类固醇剂量稳定或减少。

您错误地将受试者008765分类为部分缓解。受试者008765病例报告表肿瘤测量页显示，根据2003年5月1日放射学检查报告，该受试者被分类为部分缓解。尽管2003年5月1日的放射学检查报告显示，肿瘤缩小大于50%，但从2002年11月1日（基线MRI）以来无MRI检查，而2003年5月1日的放射学检查报告显示，肿瘤缩小大于50%并持续至少4周，并且2003年4月29日的放射学报告（MRI检查日期2003年4月21日）实际显示肿瘤增大。因此，该受试者不符合部分缓解的标准。

ⅲ. 对于疾病稳定的分类，试验方案BT-10要求：①与基线比较增强肿瘤最大垂直直径乘积的总和减少不足50%（大于或小于）；②持续至少12周；③皮质类固醇剂量稳定或减少。

您错误地将以下受试者分类为疾病稳定：

（1）试验方案BT-10：受试者012184，012206和012252的皮质类固醇剂量未稳定或减少，因此将他们分类为疾病稳定是错误的。受试者011373不符合肿瘤大小减少不足50%且持续至少12周的标准，皮质类固醇剂量未稳定或减少，因此不符合疾病稳定的标准。

a）受试者012184病例报告表肿瘤测量页显示，根据2009年1月7日、4月20日、6月18日和7月24日的MRI检查，该受试者肿瘤大小和基线相比减少不足50%，且保持了至少12周。但是，病例报告表皮质类固醇报告页显示，该受试者皮质类固醇剂量未稳定或减少。因此该受试者不符合疾病稳定期的标准。

b）受试者012206病例报告表肿瘤测量页显示，根据2009年1月15日、5月6日的MRI检查，该受试者肿瘤大小和基线值相比减少不足50%，且保持了至少12周。但是，病例报告表皮质类固醇报告页显示，该受试者皮质类固醇剂量不稳定或减少。因此该受试者不符合疾病稳定的标准。

c）受试者012252病例报告表肿瘤测量页显示，根据2009年4月20日、8月7日的MRI检查，该受试者肿瘤大小和基线值相比减少不足50%，且保持了至少12周。但是，病例报告表皮质类固醇报告页显示该受试者皮质类固醇剂量未稳定或减少。因此，该受试者不符合疾病稳定的标准。

d）受试者0111373病例报告表肿瘤测量页显示，该受试者肿瘤大小和基线值相比减少不足50%，且保持了至少12周。另外，病例报告表皮质类固醇报告页显示受试者皮质类固醇剂量未稳定或减少。

受试者011373病例报告表肿瘤测量页显示，基线MRI检查的日期为2007年4月12日，受试者于2007年4月13日开始接受试验药物的治疗，并于2007年5月18日、7月6日、7月19日分别接受了MRI检查。病例报告表肿瘤测量页记录为该受试者肿瘤大小减少不足50%，并从2007年5月18日持续至7月19日；然而，2007年7月19日以后无MRI 或PET检查，因此无证据表明肿瘤减小持续至少12周。并且病例报告表皮质类固醇报告页显示受试者皮质类固醇剂量不稳定或减少。因此该受试者不符合疾病稳定的标准。

您于2013年4月5日对以上问题的书面回复中声明“我们遵循的‘停用皮质类固醇药物的定义’为继续使用最低剂量以维持神经稳定性，维持舒适性及功能性”。您的回复还同时引用神经肿瘤工作组的建议：当患者使用生理替代剂量的皮质类固醇时可以定义为完全及部分缓解。并且，回复中还指出申办者已修改方案草案BT-09、BT-10及BT-21并准备递交伦理委员会，对目前方案中“停用皮质类固醇”进行符合操作常规的解释，您还指出申办者将修改方案以保证和原来允许使用皮质类固醇激素的用意一致。

另外，您在书面回复中指出您保存有上述受试者013660，009990，008765，012184，012206，012252和011373相应的完全缓解、部分缓解和疾病稳定（如适用）的原始评估。您还指出，除了受试者009990和011373外，您将根据申办者修订的肿瘤评价标准维持对其他受试者原来的评价，而非受试者在被评估时所使用方案中的肿瘤评价标准。对于受试者009990，您指出基于申办者提出的修订的肿瘤评价标准和中心影像审阅意见，其建议为代谢完全缓解，您维持评价结果为完全缓解。对于受试者011373，您指出该受试者连续两次增强MRI丢失，根据相应MRI肿瘤非增强部分定义为疾病稳定。

您关于以上部分的回复内容不充分。方案要求特别考虑皮质类固醇的使用。另外，您声明您遵循的“停用皮质类固醇患者”的定义未列在上述任一方案中。

我们承认维持生理水平的皮质类固醇剂量是恰当的，尽管方案要求完全缓解的受试者应该完全停用皮质类固醇。然而，以上所列受试者全都使用了皮质类固醇，而且远远超出维持生理水平的剂量。具体为这些受试者使用地卡特隆（地塞米松，一种皮质类固醇）的剂量为4~16mg/d不等，而等同生理水平的地卡特隆用量为0.25~0.75mg/d。

同时，试验方案要求受试者‘停用皮质类固醇’仅适用于完全缓解的评价。您的书面回复没有提及您错误地将那些未处于皮质类固醇剂量稳定或减少的受试者分类为疾病稳定。而且，您的书面回复没有提及以上提到的受试者011373缺乏疾病稳定持续12周的检查结果而被错误地评价为疾病稳定。最后，您的书面回复不够充分，因为您未承诺如何更正研究记录中错误的治疗反应分类。请注意对研究记录的所有更正必须遵循法规21CFR312.62（b）和（c）以保存足够、准确的病历。

未按试验方案规定进行肿瘤反应评价会损害受试者的安全、权益以及质疑贵试验现场数据的有效性和可靠性。

b. 试验方案BT-10要求临床研究者向申办者报告任何不良事件。您未遵循该要求。具体表现在，受试者023612经历了不良事件，见下表，这些不良事件没有向申办者报告。

表 未向申办者报告的受试者023612 的不良事件

不良事件日期	不良事件
2012年7月21日	手术部位皮疹
2012年8月6日	发热
2012年8月10日	虚弱和疲乏
2012年8月28日	恶心，疲乏和眩晕
2012年9月14日	关节痛
2012年9月22日	恶心和呕吐
2012年11月27日	右踝关节扭伤

您于2013年4月5日的书面回复中承认您未向申办者汇报以上不良事件，并声明“研究人员已采取纠正措施”。

由于您未提供关于纠正措施的细节，以致我们无法判断纠正措施是否足以预防将来类似违规情况的再次发生，因此您的书面回复不够充分。

2. 您未能保护在您的监护下的受试者的权益、安全和福利［21 CFR 312.60 和 21 CFR 312.305（c）（1）］

作为临床研究者，您必须在您的监护下保护受试者及慈善供药患者的权益、安全和福利。该要求包括采取合适的预防措施确保受试者和慈善供药患者没有过量服用试验药物。您没有采取合适的预防措施来保护受试者和慈善供药患者，以避免他们过量服用试验药物。举例如下，但不限于：

记载抗瘤酮过量的研究记录显示，入组试验方案BT-09、BT-10和AD-02的受试者和慈善供药患者服用抗瘤酮过量。在这些研究记录中确认经过药物过量的受试者和慈善供药患者中，以下患者有过多次药物过量：

a. 试验方案 BT-10：受试者 012184，013660和021539及慈善供药患者 019813。

i. 受试者 012184 于2009年1月18日和2月26日药物过量。

ii. 受试者 013660 于2010年4月25日和7月19日药物过量。

iii. 受试者 021539 于2012年7月12日和10月29日药物过量。

iv. 受试者 019813 于2011年4月5日、4月30日和5月5日，2012年2月19日药物过量。

b. 试验方案 AD-02：受试者008809于 2008年10月5日和2006年12月13日药物过量。

我们确认除了受试者019813，其他上述所列受试者没有列入您收到的FDA483表附件中，因此您的书面回复未针对上述问题做解释。但是，FDA483表包括了受试者019813以及其他药物过量的案例，您在书面回复中均对此予以了解释。

具体而言，您于2013年4月5日的书面回复中声明："报告药物过量和确保对每例事件都进行认真随访的培训……我们审阅了视察发现中的案例，确认所有受试者/看护人在每例事件发生后被重新培训"，您还声明您将立即开始进行以下工作。

- 对研究人员进行额外强化培训：关于抗肿瘤药物给药，以及如何迅速处理并记录偶发性药物过量的事件。
- 每月和看护人联系以强化培训。

您以上的书面回复不够充分。根据您的声明，您确保在每次事件发生后对所有患者/看护人再次培训，事实上以上所列患者有过不止一次的药物过量，这显示您提供的再次培训并不足以预防药物过量事件重复发生。

关于计划采取的措施对研究人员进行额外培训以及每月联系看护人再次培训，您未提供详细的内容来帮助我们判断培训是否足以预防将来类似情况再次发生。

您未采取合适的预防措施来避免受试者和慈善供药患者使用试验药物过量，据此我们对您如何保护贵研究中心入组的受试者有很大的顾虑，同时对保护使用试验药物抗瘤酮A10和AS2的慈善供药患者也有很大顾虑。

3. 您未能按照21 CFR 50的要求获得知情同意［21 CFR 312.60，21 CFR 50.25（b）（3）和21 CFR 50.27（b）（1）］

作为临床研究者，您必须遵循法规21 CFR 50获得受试者知情同意。除了有限的一些特殊情况不适用外，知情同意必须使用含有法规21CFR 50.25关于知情同意书基本内容的书面知情文件。研究者必须在签署知情同意书之前给予受试者或者受试者法律认可的代理人合适的机会阅读书面知情同意书（包括所有必需的基本内容）。由于您在研究BT-10和BT-22中使用的知情同意书未包含所有知情同意必需的基本内容，因此您没有按照法规21CFR 50的要求获取知情同意。

具体而言，知情同意书没有包含法规21 CFR 50.25（b）（3）对于受试者参加研究而产生的额外费用的声明。治疗费用协议仅在同意参加临床研究后才提供给受试者。

您于2013年4月5日针对该发现所做的书面回复中，承认"［a］治疗费用协议仅在签署知情同意文件之后提供给患者。"另外，您指出"［a］签署知情同意文件和提供治疗费用协议之间的间隔可能为数小时、数天，或者数周"。作为纠正措施，您提议通过修改知情同意文件的措辞来解决关于缺少受试者因参加研究而产生额外费用的描述缺陷。

由于修改知情同意文件措辞主要集中于使用试验药物是否产生费用；对于可能产生的额外费用仅作了笼统的描述；由受试者自己负责询问是否有增加的费用，而不是提供给受试者关于参加研究可能产生的具体的额外费用，因此这个回复并不充分。相比之下，治疗费用协议包含了受试者因参加研究而产生的额外费用。知情同意文件本身必须包括受试者因参加研究而产生额外费用的信息。

获取知情同意之前未向受试者说明额外费用，这就否定了受试者有关于他们参加临床研究的知情决定的机会。

4. 您未能遵守所有扩大药物使用时关于保存准确的病历与312.62一致地保留记录的要求［21 CFR 312.305（c）（4）和21 CFR 312.62（b）（c）］

作为临床研究者，您必须按照21 CFR 312.62 的要求对所有慈善供药患者保存准确的病历和保留记录。法规21 CFR 312.62（b）要求您维护每例接受试验药物或者对照组治疗的患者所有观察记录，以及其他与研究相关的数据的病历。法规21 CFR 312.62（c）要求您保存21CFR 312规定的记录至研究药物上市后2年；如果没有递交新药申请或者适应症未被批准，则记录应保留至研究终止后2年，且通知FDA。

您未维护和保留慈善供药患者的准确病历。具体表现在，您未维护和保留患者022378的准确病历，该患者是单一患者试验方案（单个慈善供药患者）的患者，也称为试验方案BT-10的特殊例外。

针对缺陷a（b）（6），FDA肿瘤产品组2（DOP2）要求申办者，Burzynski研究所（BRI）向其提供患者022387病历复印件。

对于（b）（6），BRI向DOP2提供了患者022387的以下记录：

- （b）（6）体格检查的病例报告表页“体格检查-基线”；
- 病例报告表页“基线随访-肿瘤治疗前”；
- 病例报告表页“基线随访-病理史”；
- 病例报告表页“不良事件”。

现场检查时提供的患者022387文件中未包括以上BRI向FDA递交的关于（b）（6）的记录。但在现场检查过程中，您提供了该患者的其他病例报告表，文件名称、随访日期和以上文件一致，但是内容和BRI递交FDA的不一样，有以下显著的差异。

（b）（6）；

（b）（6）；

（b）（6）。

我们确认向您发出的FDA483表没有包括这个缺陷，因此您的书面回复未就此问题做出解释。

请解释为何您在试验场所显示患者022387的病例报告表和Burzynski研究所递交FDA肿瘤产品组2的病例报告表不一致。未维护和保留准确的病历让我们关注患者安全和数据的可靠性，以及对于贵研究中心入组的慈善供药患者是否有适当的保护。

本警告信的目的并非是罗列您在药物临床研究中存在的所有缺陷。确保遵循法律和相关FDA法规的每一项要求是您的职责，您应当解决所这些缺陷，并建立规程，以确保任何正在进行或将来进行的研究均符合FDA的法规。

自收到这封信的15个工作日内，您应当书面告知本公室您为预防将来发生类似违规情况而采取的措施。如果不能充分、快速地解释上述违规问题，可能导致我们在不再通知的情况下采取监管措施。如果您认为您已经遵循了FDA的法规要求，请陈述理由，并提供所有支持资料，以供我们参考。

---

1. 完全缓解的分类不能反映出是否该缓解会持续并超越治疗反应分类的时间点。也就是说，一名正确分类为完全缓解的受试者后期可能会出现肿瘤复发。

2. 我们注意到受试者005297与以前治疗的受试者是不一致的。该受试者肿瘤测量CRF显示，基于1997年8月11日和1997年10月2日的MRIs检查，所有对比增强的肿瘤完全消失至少4周。但病例报告表皮质类固醇页及肿瘤血液流程表显示该受试者于1997年8月11日和1997年8月11日至1997年10月2日期间（包括1997年10月2日）接受MRI检查，都在接受皮质类固醇治疗，因此该受试者未达到完全缓解的标准。对于受试者005297，您指出您提出过再进行独立的影像审阅，以确认正确的反应分类，并声称在收到后将会将信息转发给FDA。我们注意到直至写这封信时，FDA未收到这方面的信息。

3. 我们注意到，受试者是否根据方案规定的标准进行合适分类为疾病稳定的问题与FDA是否接受疾病稳定率数据作为有效性要求的基础问题是不同的。

4. 我们注意到，上述提到的2个例子与以前试验方案BT-10和试验方案BT-22（疾病稳定的分类与方案10相同）中治疗的受试者是一致的。对于试验方案BT-10的受试者005974肿瘤测量CRF显示，基于1999年1月12日和1999年4月6日的MRIs检查，肿瘤大小与基线值比变化小于50%，该状态维持至少12周。但病例报告表显示，该受试者皮质类固醇既没有维持稳定剂量，也没有减小剂量，因此不满足疾病稳定的标准。在您2013年4月5日的书面回复中，您声称您根据申办者提出的肿瘤评估标准的变更对受试者005974进行了重新分类，分类为疾病进展。试验方案BT-22中的受试者004240，肿瘤测量CRF显示，在1996年2月21日进行了基线MRI检查，于1996年3月6日开始服用研究药物，在1996年4月10日、6月26日和7月31日又进行了MRI检查。肿瘤测量CRF记录肿瘤大小与基线值比变化小于50%，仅从1996年4月10日维持至5月22日，小于12周。因此，该受试者不满足疾病稳定的标准。在您2013年4月5日的书面回复中，您声称对于该受试者您根据申办者提出的肿瘤评估标准的变更维持原来的评估。然而，您没有提及疾病稳定的不正确分类原因是不足12周维持期。

5. 我们注意到，试验方案BT-09、BT-10和BT-21已经结束。您的书面回复中也指出申办者已经准备递交给IRB的试验方案BT-22的修订草案。BT-22也结束了。

6. 我们注意到，在您2013年4月5日的书面回复中，您也指出根据申办者提出的肿瘤评估标准的变更维持受试者007197完全缓解的原始评估。

7. 我们注意到，基于2013年4月5日的书面回复，用于试验方案BT-09的知情同意书也没有包含这些信息，仅在受试者签署知情同意书后介绍了计费协议。

最后更新：10/05/2015

注意：如果您需要以不同的文件格式获取信息，请参照U.S. FDA操作指南。

10903 New Hampshire Avenue
Silver Spring, MD 20993
Ph. 1888INFOFDA
(18884636332)

附：英文原文

Burzynski, Stanislaw R. M.D.

WARNING LETTER

DEC 3, 2013

CERTIFIED MAIL
RETURN RECEIPT REQUESTED

Ref: 13-HFD-45-11-04

Stanislaw R. Burzynski, M.D., Ph.D.
9432 Katy Road
Houston, TX 770556349

Dear Dr. Burzynski:

This Warning Letter informs you of objectionable conditions observed during the U.S. Food and Drug Administration (FDA) inspection conducted at your clinical site between January 7, 2013, and March 15, 2013. Mr. Joel Martinez, Mr. Hugh McClure, and Dr. Cynthia Kleppinger, representing the FDA, reviewed your conduct of the following clinical investigations of the investigational drugs Antineoplastons A10 and AS2, performed for Burzynski Research Institute, as well as your expanded access use of the investigational drugs Antineoplastons A10 and AS2:

- Protocol BT-09, "Phase Ⅱ Study of Antineoplastons A1 0 and AS2-1 in Patients with Brain Tumors";
- Protocol BT-10, "Phase Ⅱ Study of Antineoplastons A1 0 and AS2-1 in Children with Brain Tumors";
- Protocol BT-21, "Phase Ⅱ Study of Antineoplastons A10 and AS2-1 in Adults with Primary Malignant Brain Tumors";
- Protocol BT-22, "Phase Ⅱ Study of Antineoplastons A10 and AS2-1 in Children with Primary Malignant Brain Tumors"; and
- Protocol AD-02, "Phase Ⅱ Study of Antineoplastons A10 and AS2-1 in Patients with Carcinoma of the Adrenal Gland."

This inspection is a part of FDA's Bioresearch Monitoring Program, which includes inspections designed to evaluate the conduct of FDA regulated research to ensure that the data are scientifically valid and accurate, and to help ensure that the rights, safety, and welfare of the human subjects of those studies have been protected.

At the conclusion of the inspection, Mr. Martinez, Mr. McClure, and Dr. Kleppinger presented and discussed with you Form FDA 483, Inspectional Observations. We acknowledge receipt of your April 5, 2013, written response to the Form FDA 483. We also acknowledge receipt of a progress update from you, dated May 15, 2013, regarding your response to the Form FDA 483.

From our review of the FDA establishment inspection report, the documents submitted with that report, and your April 5, 2013, written response, we conclude that you did not adhere to the applicable statutory requirements and FDA regulations governing the conduct of clinical investigations and the protection of human subjects. We wish to emphasize the following:

1. You failed to ensure that the investigation was conducted according to the investigational plan [21 CFR 312.60].

As a clinical investigator, you are required to ensure that your clinical studies are conducted in accordance with the investigational plans. The investigational plans for Protocols BT-09, BT-10, and BT-21 require that you assign therapeutic responses based on how the subjects' tumors respond to the study drug, and that you report adverse events to the sponsor. Correct assignment of therapeutic responses is important to determine the extent, if any, to which the tumors respond to the study drug. Reporting of adverse events is important to minimize risk to subjects and to ensure that the sponsor has complete and accurate data regarding the safety of the study drug. You failed to ensure that Protocols BT-09, BT-10, and BT-21 were conducted according to the investigational plans. Specifically:

a. Protocols BT-09, BT-10, and BT-21 define each possible therapeutic response (Complete Response, Partial Response, Stable Disease, and Progressive Disease), and include specific criteria you must use to classify a subject as having one of those responses. You assigned therapeutic responses incorrectly for 9 of the 27 subjects whose therapeutic response classifications were reviewed during the inspection. Specifically:

ⅰ. For a classification of Complete Response[1], Protocols BT-09, BT-10, and BT-21 required: (1) complete disappearance of all contrast enhancing tumor on neuroimaging studies, and ancillary radiographic studies if appropriate, for a minimum duration of four weeks; and (2) that the subject be off corticosteroids.

You incorrectly classified the following subjects as having a Complete Response:

1. Protocol BT-10: Subjects 006389 and 013660 did not have complete disappearance of all contrast enhancing tumor for at least four weeks and, therefore, were incorrectly classified as having a Complete Response.

a. For Subject 006389, both the Tumor Measurements Case Report Form (CRF) and the list that you provided us of subjects enrolled in Protocol BT-10 as of January 7, 2013, identify this subject as having a Complete Response. However, the Tumor Measurements CRF shows that none of the neuroimaging studies showed complete disappearance of contrast enhancing tumor for at least four weeks. Therefore, the subject did not meet the criteria for Complete Response.

b. For Subject 013660, both the Tumor Measurements CRF and the list that you provided us of subjects enrolled in Protocol BT-10 as of January 7, 2013, identify this subject as having a Complete Response. However, the Tumor Measurements CRF shows that none of the neuroimaging studies showed complete disappearance of contrast enhancing tumor for at least four weeks. Therefore, the subject did not meet the criteria for Complete Response.

2. Protocol BT-09: For Subject 007197, the Tumor Measurements CRF indicates, based on Magnetic Resonance Imaging (MRI) taken on July 25, 2001; September 11, 2001; and November 8, 2001, complete disappearance of all contrast enhancing tumor for a minimum duration of four weeks. However, the Steroids Report CRF and the Oncology Hematology Flow Sheet show that the subject was on corticosteroids preceding the July 25, 2001 and September 11, 2001 MRIs; during the period between these MRIs; and up to one week prior to the November 8, 2001 MRI. Therefore, the subject did not meet the criteria for Complete Response.[2]

3. Protocol BT-21: For Subject 009990, the Tumor Measurements CRF shows that the subject was classified as having a Complete Response based on Positron Emission Tomography (PET) scan results. However, the Steroids Report CRF shows that the subject was on corticosteroids preceding all of the relevant PET scan dates (January 4, February 4, June 14, and August 16, 2005), as well as during the period between these PET scans. Therefore, the subject did not meet the criteria for Complete Response.

ii. For a classification of Partial Response, Protocol BT-09 required: (1) that subjects have more than 50% reduction in the sum of the products of the greatest perpendicular diameters of contrast enhancing tumors, compared to the corresponding baseline evaluation, for at least four weeks; (2) that no simultaneous increase in size of any lesion or the appearance of new lesions may occur; and (3) that subjects be on a stable or decreasing dose of corticosteroids.

You incorrectly classified Subject 008765 as having a Partial Response. For Subject 008765, the Tumor Measurements CRF shows that the subject was classified as having a Partial Response based on a radiology report dated May 1, 2003. Although the May 1, 2003 radiology report shows a tumor reduction of greater than 50%, there are no MRIs between November 1, 2002 (baseline MRI) and the May 1, 2003 radiology report that show that the tumor reduction of greater than 50% was maintained for at least four weeks during that time period. Further, the April 29, 2003 radiology report (for the April 21, 2003 MRI) actually shows an increase in tumor size. Therefore, the subject did not meet the criteria for Partial Response.

iii. For a classification of Stable Disease[3], Protocol BT10 required: (1) that subjects have less than 50% change (either greater or smaller) in the sum of the products of the perpendicular diameters of the enhancing tumor compared to the baseline evaluation; (2) that this state be maintained for a minimum of 12 weeks; and (3) that the corticosteroid dose is stable or decreasing.

You incorrectly classified the following subjects as having Stable Disease[4]:

1. Protocol BT-10: Subjects 012184, 012206, and 012252 were not on stable or decreasing doses of corticosteroids and, therefore, were incorrectly classified as having Stable Disease. Subject 011373 did not have a less than 50% change in tumor size maintained for at least 12 weeks and was not on either a stable or decreasing dose of corticosteroids and, therefore, did not meet the criteria for Stable Disease.

a. For Subject 012184, the Tumor Measurements CRF indicates, based on MRIs taken on January 7, April 20, June 18, and July 24, 2009, that the subject had a less than 50% change in tumor size compared to baseline, and that this state was maintained for a minimum of 12 weeks. However, the Steroids Report CRF shows that the subject was not on either a stable or decreasing dose of corticosteroids. Therefore, the subject did not meet the criteria for Stable Disease.

b. For Subject 012206, the Tumor Measurements CRF indicates, based on MRIs taken on January 15 and May 6, 2009, that the subject had a less than 50% change in tumor size compared to baseline, and that this state was maintained for a minimum of 12 weeks. However, the Steroids Report CRF shows that the subject was not on either a stable or decreasing dose of corticosteroids. Therefore, the subject did not meet the criteria for Stable Disease.

c. For Subject 012252, the Tumor Measurements CRF indicates, based on MRIs taken on April 20 and August 7, 2009, that the subject had a less than 50% change in tumor size compared to baseline, and that this state was maintained for a minimum of 12 weeks. However, the Steroids Report CRF shows that the subject was not on either a stable or decreasing dose of corticosteroids. Therefore, the subject did not meet the criteria for Stable Disease.

d. For Subject 011373, the Tumor Measurements CRF shows that the subject did not have a less than 50% change in tumor size, compared to baseline, maintained for at least 12 weeks. In addition, the Steroids Report CRF shows that the subject was not on either a stable or decreasing dose of corticosteroids. The Tumor Measurements CRF shows that Subject 011373 had a baseline MRI taken on April 12, 2007. The subject began receiving investigational drug on April 13, 2007, and had additional MRIs taken on May 18, July 6, and July 19, 2007.

The Tumor Measurements CRF documents that a change of less than 50% in tumor size, compared to baseline, was maintained from May 18 through July 19, 2007; however, there are no confirmatory MRIs or PET scans after July 19, 2007, and there is therefore no evidence that the reduction was maintained for a minimum of 12 weeks. In addition, the Steroids Report CRF shows that the subject was not on either a stable or decreasing dose of corticosteroids. Therefore, the subject did not meet the criteria for Stable Disease.

In your April 5, 2013 written response to the findings noted above, you stated that " the definition of a 'patient off corticosteroids' that we follow is one who continues on the lowest dosage necessary for neurologic stability and is maintained at their level of comfort and function." In your response, you also cited the Neuro-Oncology Working Group recommendations that complete and partial responses can be determined when a patient is on physiologic replacement doses of corticosteroids. Further, you indicated that draft amendments for Protocols BT-09, BT-10, and BT-21 have been prepared by the sponsor for submission to the Institutional Review Board (IRB), to "correct the practical interpretation of 'off steroids' as currently specified in our protocols," and you stated that the sponsor will amend the protocols to concur with the original intent of allowing steroids[5].

In addition, you indicated in your written response that you are retaining the original assessments of Complete Response, Partial Response, and Stable Disease (as applicable) for Subjects 013660, 009990, 008765, 012184, 012206, 012252, and 011373 listed above. You indicated that, with the exception of Subjects 009990 and 011373, you are maintaining the original assessment for all of these subjects based on the sponsor's proposed changes to the tumor assessment criteria, that is, not based on the tumor assessment criteria as included in the protocols at the time the relevant subjects were evaluated.[6] For Subject 009990, you indicated that you were maintaining the assessment as a Complete Response based on the sponsor's proposed changes to the tumor assessment criteria and based on central radiology review, which suggested a Complete Response metabolically. For Subject 011373, you indicated that two consecutive MRIs of the subject using enhancement were unavailable, and that the subject was classified as having Stable Disease based upon the nonenhancement portion of the tumor for the corresponding MRIs.

Your responses noted in the preceding paragraphs are inadequate. The protocols required specific consideration of corticosteroid use. In addition, the definition of "a patient off corticosteroids" that you stated you followed, was not included in any of the protocols listed above.

We acknowledge that the use of corticosteroids to maintain physiologic levels may be appropriate, despite protocol wording requiring that subjects be off corticosteroids completely for a Complete Response. However, for all of the subjects listed above as having been classified as a Complete Response despite being on corticosteroids, their corticosteroid doses were well beyond those needed to maintain physiologic levels. Specifically, these subjects were on doses of Decadron (dexamethasone, a corticosteroid) that ranged from 4 mg/day to 16 mg/day, while the physiologicreplacement equivalent of Decadron is in the range of 0.25 mg/day to 0.75 mg/day.

Also, the protocols' requirement that a subject be "off corticosteroids" applies only to the Complete Response assessment. Your written response does not address your incorrect classifications of Stable Disease in cases where subjects were not on stable or decreasing doses of corticosteroids. Further, your written response does not address the incorrect classification of Stable Disease that resulted from lack of a 12week maintenance period for Subject 011373, as described above. Lastly, your written response is inadequate because you have not included a commitment to correct the study records that contain these incorrect response classifications. Please note that all corrections to study records must be done in accordance with the requirements of 21 CFR 312.62(b) and (c) to maintain and retain adequate and accurate case histories.

Failure to assess tumor response in accordance with the protocol requirements jeopardizes subject safety and welfare and raises concern about the validity and integrity of the data collected at your site.

Protocol BT-10 requires the clinical investigator to report any adverse events to the sponsor. You failed to adhere to this requirement. Specifically, Subject 023612 experienced adverse events, noted in Table 1, that were not reported to the sponsor.

Table 1. Adverse Events for Subject 023612 Not Reported to the Sponsor

Date of Adverse Event	Adverse Events
July 21, 2012	Rash at surgical site
August 6, 2012	Fever
August 10, 2012	Weakness and fatigue
August 28, 2012	Nausea, fatigue, and dizziness
September 14, 2012	Arthralgias
September 22, 2012	Nausea and vomiting
November 27, 2012	Rightankle sprain

In your April 5, 2013 written response, you acknowledged that you did not report the adverse events listed above to the sponsor and stated, "Corrective action has been undertaken with staff."

Your written response is not adequate because you have not provided details regarding the corrective action, to enable us to determine whether that corrective action appears adequate to prevent similar violations from occurring in the future.

2. You failed to protect the rights, safety, and welfare of subjects under your care [21 CFR 312.60 and 21 CFR 312.305(c)(1)].

As a clinical investigator, you are required to protect the rights, safety, and welfare of subjects and expanded access patients under your care. This requirement includes, among other things, the responsibility to take adequate precautions to ensure that subjects and expanded access patients are not overdosed with the investigational drug. You failed to protect the safety and welfare of subjects and expanded access patients under your care by failing to take adequate precautions to ensure that these individuals were not overdosed. Examples of your failure include but are not limited to the following:

Study records documenting Antineoplaston overdoses show that expanded access patients and subjects in Protocols BT09, BT10, and AD02 had overdoses. Of those subjects and expanded access patients identified in study records as having experienced overdoses, the following individuals experienced multiple overdoses:

a. Protocol BT10: Subjects 012184, 013660, and 021539, and Expanded Access Patient 019813

i. Subject 012184 was overdosed on January18 and February 26, 2009.

ii. Subject 013660 was overdosed on April 25 and July 19, 2010.

iii. Subject 021539 was overdosed on July 12 and October 29, 2012.

iv. Patient 019813 was overdosed on April 5, April 30, and May 5, 2011, and on February 19, 2012.

b. Protocol AD02: Subject 008809 was overdosed on December 13, 2006, and on October 5, 2008.

We recognize that with the exception of Patient 019813, the specific subjects listed above were not included in the related subpart of the Form FDA 483 that you received and, therefore, your written response did not address the specific instances noted above. However, the Form FDA 483 did include Patient 019813, as well as other examples of overdoses, and you addressed those examples in your written response.

Specifically, in your April 5, 2013 written response, you state, "Overdose reports and the training that ensues following each event are carefully followed up upon [*sic*]....We reviewed the cases cited in the inspectional observations and ascertained that all the patients/caregivers were retrained following each event." You also note that effective immediately, you are instituting the following:

- Additional reinforcement training of staff regarding antineoplaston administration and how to handle and document accidental overdosing in an expedited manner.
- Monthly contacts with all caregivers to reinforce the training.

Your written response noted above is not adequate. With respect to your statement that you ascertained that all patients/caregivers were retrained following each event, the fact that the individuals listed above experienced more than one overdose indicates that any retraining that was provided was not adequate to prevent repeat overdosing.

With respect to your planned action to institute additional reinforcement training of staff and monthly contacts with all caregivers to reinforce their training, you have not provided details to enable us to determine whether that training appears sufficient to prevent similar violations from occurring in the future.

Your failure to take adequate precautions to ensure that subjects and expanded access patients were not overdosed with investigational drug raises significant concerns about your protection of study subjects enrolled at your site in the studies mentioned above, as well as concerns about your protection of expanded access patients whom you treated with the investigational drugs Antineoplastons A10 and AS2.

3. You failed to obtain informed consent in accordance with the provisions of 21 CFR part 50 [21 CFR 312.60, 21 CFR 50.25(b)(3), and 21 CFR 50.27(b)(1)].

As a clinical investigator, you are required to obtain informed consent in accordance with 21 CFR part 50. Except in limited circumstances not applicable here, informed consent requires the use of a written consent document that embodies the elements of informed consent required by 21 CFR 50.25. An investigator shall give either the subject or the subject's legally authorized representative an adequate opportunity to read the written consent document (including all required elements) before it is signed. You failed to obtain informed consent in accordance with 21 CFR part 50 because the informed consent documents that you used for Protocols BT10 and BT22 did not contain all of the required elements of informed consent.

Specifically, the informed consent forms did not contain a statement regarding any additional costs to the subject that may result from participating in the research, as required by 21 CFR 50.25(b) (3). Research subjects were presented with a billing agreement only after they had already consented to participate in clinical research.[7]

In your April 5, 2013 written response to this observation, you acknowledged that "a treatment billing agreement is only presented to the patient… after the ICD is signed." In addition, you stated that "a times, days or weeks may elapse between signing the ICD and presenting the treatment billing agreement." As a corrective action, you proposed amended wording to informed consent documents to address the lack of a statement regarding additional costs to the subject that may result from participating in the research.

Your proposed amended wording is not adequate because it focuses primarily on whether there is a charge for the investigational agent; contains only general statements regarding the possibility of additional costs; and puts the responsibility on the subject to inquire about any expected added costs, rather than providing the subject with specific additional costs that may result from participation in the research. In contrast, the treatment billing agreement identifies the specific additional costs the subject will be expected to pay as a result of participating in the research. The informed consent document itself must include the information about the additional costs to the subject that may result from his or her participation in the research.

Failure to provide subjects with information regarding any additional costs prior to obtaining informed consent denies subjects the opportunity to make an informed decision regarding their participation in the clinical investigation.

4. You failed to adhere to requirements for all expanded access uses with respect to maintaining accurate case histories and retaining records in a manner consistent with 21 CFR 312.62 [21 CFR 312.305(c)(4) and 21 CFR 312.62(b) and (c)].

As a clinical investigator, in all cases of expanded access, you are responsible for maintaining accurate case histories and retaining records in a manner consistent with the requirements of 21 CFR 312.62. The regulation at 21 CFR 312.62(b) requires that you maintain accurate case histories that record all observations and other data pertinent to the investigation on each individual administered the investigational drug or employed as a control in the investigation. The regulation at 21 CFR 312.62(c) requires that you retain records required to be maintained under 21 CFR part 312 for a period of two years following the date a marketing application is approved for the drug for the indication for which it is being investigated; or if no application is to be filed or if the application is not approved for such indication, until two years after the investigation is discontinued and FDA is notified.

You have failed to maintain and retain accurate case histories as required in all cases of expanded access. Specifically, you failed to maintain and retain accurate case histories for Patient 022387, whom you treated under a Single Patient Protocol (individual patient expanded access), also referred to as a Special Protocol Exception, to Protocol BT10.

In response to a (b)(6), FDA's Division of Oncology Products 2 (DOP 2) requested that the sponsor, Burzynski Research Institute (BRI), provide DOP 2 with copies of the records for Patient 022387.

On (b)(6), BRI provided DOP 2 with copies of the following records for Patient 022387:

- Case Report Form titled "Physical Exam – Baseline," for physical examination conducted on (b) (6)
- Case Report Form titled "Baseline Visit – Prior Cancer Treatment History"
- Case Report Form titled "Baseline Visit – Pathology History"
- Case Report Form titled "Adverse Events"

The records BRI submitted to FDA on (b)(6), were not in the files that you provided regarding Patient 022387 during the inspection. However, during the inspection, you provided other Case Report Forms for this patient, with the same titles and for the same visit date as noted above, but containing information that differed from that which BRI submitted to FDA. Notable differences are contained in the following tables.

(b)(6)

(b)(6)

(b)(6)

We recognize that the Form FDA 483 issued to you does not include this as an observation and, therefore, your written response did not address this issue.

Please explain why the Case Report Forms at your site for Patient 022387 differed from the Case Report Forms that Burzynski Research Institute submitted to FDA's Division of Oncology Products 2.

Failure to maintain and retain accurate case histories raises concerns about subject safety and data integrity, as well as concerns about the adequacy of safeguards in place at your site to protect patients being treated under expanded access.

This letter is not intended to be an all-inclusive list of deficiencies with your clinical study of an investigational drug. It is your responsibility to ensure adherence to each requirement of the law and relevant FDA regulations. You should address these deficiencies and establish procedures to ensure that any ongoing or future studies will be in compliance with FDA regulations.

Within fifteen (15) working days of your receipt of this letter, you should notify this office in writing of the actions you have taken to prevent similar violations in the future. Failure to address the violations noted above adequately and promptly may result in regulatory action without further notice. If you believe you have complied with FDA regulations, include your reasoning and any supporting information for our consideration.

If you have any questions, please contact Constance Cullity, M.D., M.P.H., at 3017963397;
FAX 3018478748.

Your written response and any pertinent documentation should be addressed to:

Constance Cullity, M.D., M.P.H.
Branch Chief
Good Clinical Practice Enforcement Branch
Division of Good Clinical Practice Compliance
Office of Scientific Investigations
Office of Compliance
Center for Drug Evaluation and Research
Food and Drug Administration
Building 51, Room 5354
10903 New Hampshire Avenue
Silver Spring, MD 20993

Sincerely yours,

{See appended electronic signature page}

Thomas N. Moreno, M.S.
Acting Director
Office of Scientific Investigations
Office of Compliance
Center for Drug Evaluation and Research
Food and Drug Administration
This is a representation of an electronic record that was signed electronically and this page is the manifestation of the electronic signature.
12/03/2013

1 A classification of Complete Response does not reflect whether the response continued beyond the point in time at which the therapeutic response classification was made. That is, it is possible that a subject who is correctly classified as having a Complete Response could have tumor return later.

2 We note that this is consistent with a previously treated subject, Subject 005297. The Tumor Measurements CRF for that subject indicates, based on MRIs taken on August 11, 1997, and October 2, 1997, complete disappearance of all contrast-enhancing tumor for a minimum duration of four weeks. However, the Steroids Report CRF and Oncology Hematology Flow Sheet show that the subject was on corticosteroids preceding the August 11, 1997 MRI and during the period between August 11, 1997, and the October 2, 1997 MRI (including on October 2, 1997). Therefore, Subject 005297 did not meet the criteria for Complete Response. For Subject 005297, you indicated that you had requested a second independent radiology review to confirm the correct response, and stated that you would forward this information to FDA after receipt. We note that as of the date of this letter, FDA has not received this information from you.

3 We note that the question of whether subjects were appropriately classified as having Stable Disease under protocol-specific criteria is distinct from the question of whether FDA would accept data on Stable Disease rates as the basis of an efficacy claim.

4 We note that the examples cited above are consistent with two previously treated subjects from Protocol BT10 and Protocol BT22 (which had the same criteria as Protocol BT10 regarding classification of Stable Disease). For Subject 005974 in Protocol BT10, the Tumor Measurements CRF indicates, based on MRIs taken on January 12, 1999, and April 6, 1999, that the subject had less than 50% change in tumor size compared to baseline, and that this state was maintained for a minimum of 12 weeks. However, the Steroids Report CRF shows that the subject was not on either a stable or a decreasing dose of corticosteroids. Therefore, the subject did not meet the criteria for Stable Disease. In your April 5, 2013 written response, you stated that you were reclassifying Subject 005974 as Progressive Disease, based on the sponsor' s proposed changes to the tumor assessment criteria. For Subject 004240 in Protocol BT22, the Tumor Measurements CRF shows that the subject had a baseline MRI taken on February 21, 1996. The subject began receiving investigational drug on March 6, 1996, and had additional MRIs taken on April 10, May 22, June 26, and July 31, 1996. The Tumor Measurements CRF documents that a change of less than 50% in tumor size, compared to baseline, was maintained only from April 10 through May 22, 1996, which is less than 12 weeks. Therefore, the subject did not meet the criteria for Stable Disease. In your April 5, 2013 written response, you stated that you were retaining the original assessment for this subject, based on the sponsor's proposed changes to the tumor assessment criteria. However, your response for this subject did not address the incorrect classification of Stable Disease that resulted from lack of a 12week maintenance period.

5 We note that Protocols BT09, BT10, and BT21 are closed. Your written response also indicated that the sponsor has prepared draft amendments for Protocol BT22 for submission to the IRB. BT22 is also closed.

6 We note that in your April 5, 2013 written response, you also indicated that you are maintaining the original assessment of Complete Response for Subject 007197, based on the sponsor' s proposed changes to the tumor assessment criteria.

7 We note that, based on your April 5, 2013 written response, the informed consent forms used for Protocol BT09 also did not contain this information, and subjects were only presented with a billing agreement after they had signed the informed consent forms.

Page Last Updated: 10/05/2015
Note: If you need help accessing information in different file formats, see Instructions for
U.S. Food and Drug Administration
10903 New Hampshire Avenue
Silver Spring, MD 20993
Ph. 1888INFOFDA
(18884636332)

第79封　给Velmahos, George C.医学博士的警告信

2013年11月29日

参考号：CBER-14-01

尊敬的Velmahos博士：

这封信特告知您2013年7月25日FDA现场检查的结果。一名FDA检查员与您的员工会面，审查了您实施的名为（b）（4）的临床研究的情况。本次现场检查是FDA生物研究监查项目的一部分，该项目通过设定的检查方法，审查试验药物相关研究的实施情况。

现场检查结束时，检查员向您出示并讨论了FDA483表，即现场检查发现的问题。我们收到并审查了您日期为2013年8月2日的对FDA 483表的回复信。

基于对FDA获得的证据进行的评估，我们认为您违反了发布在美国联邦法规（CFR）第21篇312部分、对正确实施与试验用新药有关的临床研究进行监管的规定。（法规内容详见http://www.gpoaccess.gov/cfr/index.html）。以下列出的每个违规项均指出了CFR中的相应条款。

1. 您未能确保按照签署的研究者声明、研究计划、适用法规来进行研究，未能保护在您的监护下的受试者的权益、安全和福利［21 CFR 312.60］

A.（b）（4）

受试者	给药剂量	结果
（b）（6）	（b）（4）	（b）（4）
（b）（6）	（b）（4）	（b）（4）
（b）（6）	（b）（4）	（b）（4）
（b）（6）	（b）（4）	（b）（4）

由于您把错误的剂量给予了上表每一个受试者，因此您未能确保研究遵照研究计划开展。您的回复函没有对给药剂量错误提供解释。对此请给予书面回复。

B.（b）（4）

i.（b）（4）

ii.（b）（4）

您的回复函未就（b）（4）在随机化前即已开具处方的原因进行解释。请对此予以书面回复。

C. 从受试者（b）（6）获得知情同意的医生未列在签署的FDA1572表中。

您的回复函称您将每六个月检查一次相关研究人员名单，并将用授权表清单以检查所有参与研究的人员情况。我们接受您的纠正措施计划并提醒您请及时更新FDA 1572表，以准确反映研究人员的变动情况。

D. 根据研究方案11.1的规定，原始文档资料不充分，因此您未按照研究计划开展研究。对于原始数据和记录，方案11.1要求“每位入组的受试者，研究者应在原始记录中写明该受试者参与了此项研究……研究者应在受试者文件中记录以下常规文档中没有的特别数据：研究识别码［（b）（4）］、试验中的受试者人数、受试药的详细信息（包括数量、批号、给药日期）、试验中发生的任何AE、当地实验室检验结果、提前出组时间和原因。”我们检查发现，受试者原始记录中并没有包含方案11.1规定的记录。

在您的回复函中，您承认对原始记录的收集可能并不理想。为改进原始数据的收集而采取的纠正措施包括但不仅限于：对现有项目进行检查；对参与研究的人员进行指导，确保原始数据的获得以支持CRF录入；每周例会均向研究人员重复提醒知情同意过程、研究药物（b）(4)、给药、出组和长期随访所需的原始记录；同时进行额外的培训。如果上述措施得以认真执行，您的纠正措施是可以被认可的。

2. 您未能做到只给予在研究者亲自监督或在研究者下属的助理研究者监督下的受试者研究药物［21 CFR 312.61］

未列在已签署的FDA 1572表（该表列出了协助进行试验的授权研究者）或机构职责分工表中的研究者向受试者开具了受试药（b）(4)的处方。这些人员向（b）(4)受试者开具了受试药处方。

在检查中，您解释说主治医师不写处方，处方由外科住院医师出具。此种操作模式对“仅在研究者亲自监督或对研究者负责的授权研究者亲自监督下受试者才能给药”的要求而言是错误的。

您的回复函未解释为何未列在已签署的FDA 1572表或机构职责分工表中的研究者给受试者开具受试药（b）(4)的处方。对此请给予书面解释。

3. 您未能保存对研究中使用药物或对照组的受试者的所有观察结果和其他相关数据的足够及准确的病历［21 CFR 312.62（b）］

A. CRFs中多处支持性数据和记录缺失或不匹配。特别是对于（b）(4)受试者，其体重或者未记录在原始记录中，或者与CRFs中的记录不匹配。

在检查中，您解释说急诊科无床秤，因此受试者体重是估计的，或是受试者自己提供，或者没有记录。在您的回复函中称2013年4月对患者的体重和身高进行了常规检查和记录，而且您将确保将来对需要按体重给药的受试者进行体重测定和记录。如果上述措施得以认真执行，您的纠正措施是可以被认可的。

B. 原始记录不完整，未能充分而准确地记录受试者的病史。

i. 包括大部分受试者的（b）(4)次数、关键体征和体重等原始数据，来自于CRF文件夹中的活页纸上。这些数据不能溯源，同时也不完整。您的回复函未能对上述支持性数据不完整进行解释。请对此予以书面回复。

ii. 检查发现原始记录不能充分说明受试者已被通知和/或计划完成方案要求的第21天、3个月和6个月的随访，导致不能获得且记录不良事件。

在您的回复函中，您承认6个月的长期随访（患者离开医院后）与方案要求不一致。尽管如此，您解释说您估计主要的不良事件不会被遗漏，因为您们的临床操作系统是封闭的，患者的医疗护理提供者几乎均在此系统内，患者返回就医时也几乎只能遇到该系统中的医生。您估计发生严重不良事件的受试者将会在您的医院系统内进行治疗，因此此类不良事件您会被通知到或者可能参与对这些受试者的治疗。

在您的回复函中，您承认对原始记录的收集可能并不是理想的。改进原始记录收集的纠正措施包括但并不限于：对目前项目进行检查；对参与研究的人员进行指导，确保原始数据的获得以支持CRF录入；每周例会均向研究人员重复提醒知情同意过程、研究药物（b）(4)、给药、出组和长期随访所需的原始记录；同时进行额外的培训。如果上述措施得以认真执行，您的纠正措施是可以被认可的。

4. 您未能按 21 CFR 50 的要求，获得每位接受药物治疗的受试者的知情同意［21 CFR 312.60］

A. 检查期间未提供文件证明已获得受试者（b）(6)的知情同意。

在您的回复函中您承认缺失了受试者（b）(6)的知情同意。您已实行了新的流程去记录知情同意过程，并确认签字文件被恰当地归档。如果上述措施得以认真执行，您的纠正措施是可以被认可的。

B. 采用过期的知情同意书来获得受试者（b）(6)的知情同意。受试者（b）(6)在2010年6月3日签署了知情同意书，其版本在2010年5月28日即已过期。受试者（b）(6)在2010年7月29日签署的知情同意书，其版本在2010年5月28日即已过期。

在您的回复函中，您称已审阅了所有正在使用的知情同意书，以保证其均为现行有效的版本，同时，您创建了相应的检查表以确保正在使用的知情同意书均为现行的版本。如果上述措施得以认真执行，您的纠正措施是可以被认可的。

本警告信的目的非是罗列您在试验药物的临床研究中存在的所有缺陷。确保遵循法律和FDA相关法规的每一项要求是您的职责。

在您的回复函中，您提供了针对检查发现问题的纠正措施。我们在此要求您请提供本信中所要求的其他信息。

自收到这封信的15个工作日内，请提供书面文件，为了纠正这些违规并防止现在或者将来在您作为临床研究者的研究中类似违规情况的再次发生，您将采取的措施。需要特别注意的是，请提供此信中要求的另外信息。未能对本警告信进行回复并采取适当的纠正措施，可能导致FDA在不再通知的情况下采取出监管措施。比如，FDA可根据21 CFR 312.70启动吊销您资格的程序。如果您不认为您存在FDA要求的违规，请陈述理由，并提供所有支持资料，以供我们参考。

附：英文原文

Velmahos, George C. M.D., Ph.D

WARNING LETTER

NOV 29, 2013

CBER-14-01

Dear Dr. Velmahos:

This letter describes the results of a Food and Drug Administration (FDA) inspection that concluded on July 25, 2013. An FDA investigator met with your staff to review your conduct of a clinical study entitled **(b)(4)**. The FDA conducted this inspection under the Bioresearch Monitoring Program,which includes inspections designed to review the conduct of research involving investigational drugs.

At the end of the inspection a Form FDA 483, Inspectional Observations, was issued and discussed with you. We received and reviewed your letter dated August 2, 2013 ("Response Letter") in response to the Form FDA 483.

Based on our evaluation of the evidence obtained by the FDA, we have determined that you violated regulations governing the proper conduct of clinical studies involving investigational new drugs, as published in Title 21, Code of Federal Regulations (CFR) Part 312 (available athttp://www.gpoaccess.gov/cfr/index.html). The applicable provisions of the CFR are cited for each violation listed below.

1. You failed to ensure that the investigation was conducted according to the signed investigator statement, the investigational plan, and the applicable regulations, and to protect the rights, safety, and welfare of subjects under your care. [21 CFR § 312.60].

A.**(b)(4)**

Subject	Dose	Outcome
(b)(6)	(b)(4)	(b)(4)
(b)(6)	(b)(4)	(b)(4)
(b)(6)	(b)(4)	(b)(4)
(b)(6)	(b)(4)	(b)(4)

By administering an incorrect dose to each of the patients above, you failed to ensure that the investigation was conducted according to the investigative plan. Your Response Letter did not provide an explanation for the incorrect dose administration. Please provide a written response.

B. **(b)(4)**

i. **(b)(4)**

ii. **(b)(4)**

Your Response Letter did not explain why **(b)(4)** was ordered prior to randomization. Please provide a written response.

C. Informed consent was obtained from Subjects **(b)(6)** by physicians not included on the signed Form FDA 1572.

Your Response Letter explained that you will conduct a review of study-related personnel every six months and that Delegation of Authority Logs will be used as a master list of staff to track personnel involvement. We accept your explanation and remind you that the Form FDA 1572 should be promptly updated to accurately reflect all changes to study personnel.

D. You failed to comply with the investigational plan in that source documentation was inadequate according to protocol section 11.1. Protocol section 11.1, Source Data and Records, requires that "For each subject enrolled, the investigator will indicate in the source record(s) that the subject participates in this study...The investigator will record the following specific data which are not part of routine documentation in the patient's file: study identification code ((b)(4)), patient number in the study, investigational drug details (including amount and batch number, dates of administration), any AE occurring during course of the study, laboratory test results obtained locally, time and reason for premature withdrawal, if appropriate." The inspection revealed that subject source records did not include documentation of the study as required by protocol section 11.1.

In your Response Letter, you acknowledge that the collection of source documentation may not have been optimal. Corrective actions implemented to improve collection of source documentation include, but are not limited to, a review of current projects; instructions to staff to ensure that source documentation is available to support CRF entries; repeated announcements at weekly meetings regarding source documentation of the informed consent process, study drug **(b)(4)**, dosing, termination, and long term follow-up; and additional training. Your corrective actions are acceptable if they are properly implemented.

2. You failed to administer the drug only to subjects under the investigator's personal supervision or under the supervision of a subinvestigator responsible to the investigator. [21 C.F.R. § 312.61].

Personnel not included on the signed Form FDA 1572, which lists subinvestigators who will assist in the conduct of the investigation, or on the Site Responsibility Log issued orders for **(b)(4)** of the study drug to study subjects. These personnel ordered study drugs for **(b)(4)** subjects.

During the inspection, you explained that the Attending Physician does not write orders. You explained that orders are written by surgical residents. This practice constitutes a failure to administer a study drug only to subjects under the investigator's personal supervision or under the supervision of a subinvestigator responsible to the investigator.

Your Response Letter did not explain why personnel not included on the signed Form FDA 1572 or the Site Responsibility Log issued orders for **(b)(4)** of the study drug to study subjects. Please provide a written response.

3. You failed to prepare and maintain adequate and accurate case histories that recorded all observations and other data pertinent to the investigation on each individual administered the investigational drug. Case histories include case report forms and supporting data. [21 CFR § 312.62(b)].

A. Supporting data and documentation were missing from or did not match CRFs in numerous instances. In particular, subject weight either was not recorded in source documentation or did not match the subject weight recorded in the CRF for **(b)(4)** subjects.

During the inspection, you explained that there were no bed scales in the Emergency Department and, as a result, subject weight was estimated, self-reported, or not recorded. Your Response Letter explains that routine recording of patient weight and height was implemented in April 2013, and that, in the future, you will ensure documentation of weight for weight-based dosing studies. Your corrective actions are acceptable if they are properly implemented.

B. Source documentation was inadequate to capture adequate and accurate case histories for subjects.

i. Source data, including (b)(4) times, vital signs, and weight for the majority of subjects, was captured on loose leaf paper maintained in the CRF binder. This source data was unattributable and incomplete. Your Response Letter failed to provide an explanation for this incomplete supporting data. Please provide a written response.

ii. The inspection revealed that source documentation was inadequate to show that subjects were contacted and/or scheduled to complete the protocol-required 21 day, 3 month and 6 month follow-up visit, resulting in failure to capture and document adverse events.

In your Response Letter, you acknowledge that long-term follow-up (after the patient's discharge from the hospital) to six months was inconsistent. Although follow-up was inconsistent, you explain that you expect that no major adverse events were missed because your clinical operations system is a closed one, in that patient care providers refer almost exclusively within the system and patients return almost exclusively to physicians within the system. You expect that subjects experiencing serious adverse events would be managed within your hospital system, and that you would have been notified of the adverse events or possibly involved in the care of these subjects.

In your Response Letter, you acknowledge that the collection of source documentation may not have been optimal. Corrective actions implemented overall to improve collection of source documentation include, but are not limited to, a review of current projects; instructions to staff to ensure that source documentation is available to support CRF entries; repeated announcements at weekly meetings regarding source documentation of the informed consent process, study drug **(b)(4)**, dosing, termination, and long term follow-up; and additional training. Your corrective actions are acceptable if they are properly implemented.

4. You failed to obtain the informed consent of each human subject to whom the drug was administered in accordance with the provisions of 21 CFR Part 50. [21 CFR § 312.60].

A. No documentation was located during the inspection to show that informed consent was obtained from Subject **(b)(6)**

In your Response Letter, you acknowledge that the informed consent for Subject **(b)(6)** is missing. You implemented new procedures to document the informed consent process and verify that the signed documents are properly filed, The corrective actions described in your Response Letter are acceptable if they are properly implemented.

B. An outdated informed consent document was used to obtain informed consent from Subjects **(b)(6)**. Subject **(b)(6)** signed a version of the consent form on June 3, 2010, that had expired on May 28, 2010. Subject **(b)(6)** signed a version of the consent form on July 29, 2010, that had expired on May 28, 2010.

In your Response Letter, you explain that you have reviewed all informed consent forms currently in use to ensure that all are current, and that you developed checklists to confirm that the current forms are being used. Your corrective actions are acceptable if they are properly implemented.

This letter is not intended to be an all -inclusive list of deficiencies with your clinical study of this investigational product. It is your responsibility to ensure adherence to each requirement of the law and relevant regulations.

In your Response Letter, you describe corrective actions implemented to address the inspectional findings. We request that you provide the additional information requested in this letter.

Within fifteen (15) business days of receipt of this letter, please provide such written documentation of the actions you will take to correct these violations and prevent the recurrence of similar violations in current and future studies for which you are the clinical investigator. Specifically, please provide the additional information requested in this letter. Failure to respond to this letter and to take appropriate corrective action could result in FDA taking regulatory action without further notice to you. For instance, FDA could initiate disqualification proceedings against you in accordance with 21 CFR 312.70. If you do not believe you are in violation of FDA requirements, include your reasoning and any supporting information for our consideration.

Please send your written response to:
Christine Drabick
Division of Inspections and Surveillance (HFM-664)
Office of Compliance and Biologics Quality

Center for Biologics Evaluation and Research
1401 Rockville Pike, Suite 200N
Rockville, Maryland 20852-1488
Telephone: 301-827-6323

We also request that you send a copy of your response to the FDA District Office listed below.

Sincerely,

/S/

Mary A. Malarkey, Director
Office of Compliance and Biologics Quality
Center for Biologics Evaluation and Research

Cc: CAPT Mutahar Shamsi, District Director
Food and Drug Administration
One Montvale Avenue, Fourth Floor
Stoneham, Massachusetts, 02180

第80封　给Agnes E. Ubani的警告信

2013年11月21日

参考号：13-HFD-45-11-02

尊敬的Ubani博士：

2013年5月29日至6月6日，Gene R. Gunn先生代表FDA，在贵临床研究机构，对您所开展的以下临床研究进行了审查。这封警告信特告知您现场检查中发现的违规情况。

- 试验方案1245.25，为Boehringer Ingelheim制药公司试验药物恩格列净进行的“比较心血管风险增加的2型糖尿病患者接受 BI 10773（10mg，20mg每日一次口服给药）和常规治疗的国际多中心、随机、平行分组、双盲、心血管安全性研究”。
- 试验方案H9X-MC-GBDN，为Eli Lilly公司的试验药物LY2189265进行的“通过动态血压监测仪评价LY2189265对2型糖尿病患者的血压和心率的疗效”。

本次现场检查是FDA的生物研究监查项目的一部分。该项目通过设定的检查方法，对FDA所监管研究的实施情况进行评估，以确认研究数据在科学上是有效和准确的，并帮助确保这些研究中受试者的权益、安全和福利得到了保护。

在现场检查结束时，Gunn先生向您出示了FDA483表，即现场检查发现的问题，并与您进行了讨论。您2013年6月28日对该FDA483表的书面回复已收悉。

经对现场检查报告、该报告的附件，以及您2013年6月28日的书面回复进行审查，我们认为，您没有遵循适用的法律要求和监管临床研究实施的FDA法规。我们想强调以下几点：

1. 您未能确保按照研究计划进行研究［21 CFR 312.60］

作为一名临床研究者，您必须确保临床研究按照研究计划进行。方案1245.25的研究计划要求排除符合排除标准和不符合入组标准的受试者。您未遵循这些要求。具体为：

a.试验方案1245.25要求排除入组前5年内有肿瘤病史（基底细胞癌除外）和/或有肿瘤治疗史的受试者。受试者58823和58827入组前5年内有肿瘤病史（分别是前列腺癌和黑色素瘤）。

b. 试验方案1245.25要求所有受试者都有“心血管高危因素”，定义为至少以下一项：

i. 确认的心肌梗死病史（知情同意前2个月以上）；

ii. 有多血管冠状动脉病变的证据，2支或以上主要冠状动脉，无论是否有再血管化的状态（疾病影响到左主冠状动脉被认为是2支血管病变）；

iii. 有单血管冠状动脉疾病的证据。

○ 存在显著的狭窄，即随后未成功再血管化的患者影像学显示一条主动脉管腔直径狭窄超过至少50%（通过冠状动脉血管造影或多层螺旋CT血管造影测评）；

○ 和至少以下一项（1或2）：

（1）无创性应激试验阳性，经以下任一条确认

- 无完全性左束支阻滞，无Wolff-Parkinson-White综合征，或无起搏心率的受试者运动负荷试验阳性；
- 负荷超声心动图结果阳性，显示局部收缩期室壁运动异常；
- 核素闪烁扫描试验结果阳性，显示应激诱导缺血，例如，既往心肌灌注显像时出现短暂灌注缺损。

（2）或者受试者入组前12个月内出院诊断为不稳定型心绞痛

iv. 最后一次不稳定型心绞痛发生在知情同意2个月前，有以上定义的冠状动脉多支血管病变或单支血管病变

Ⅴ. 有缺血或出血性卒中（知情同意前2个月以上）

ⅵ. 有任一外周动脉疾病（有或无症状）的证明：既往肢体血管造影，支架植入或旁路手术；或既往由于循环功能不全所致截肢/足；或血管造影证明至少一侧肢体有显著（＞50%）的外周动脉收缩；或者无创性检查发现至少一侧肢体有显著（＞50%或者报告为血液动力学显著异常）的外周动脉狭窄；或者至少一侧肢体踝臂指数＜0.9。

入组试验方案1245.25的受试者58828没有以上所述的心血管高危因素。该受试者有不稳定型心绞痛病史，以及无创性应激试验阳性，但是没有入组标准中要求的冠状动脉多血管或单血管疾病证据。受试者的主要冠状血管腔（右冠状动脉）狭窄约20%，但是入组标准要求狭窄达到50%及以上。另外，病历记录提示受试者可能患有心肌缺血而不是心肌梗死。基于上述入组标准，该受试者不符合入组排除标准，因此不能入组。

在您2013年6月28日对上述发现1.a.和1.b.的书面回复中您指出，您已建立纠正措施计划，以避免再次发生类似违规。您指出只有收集受试者所有的病历，并按照方案入组排除标准审阅后才能筛选受试者。您未提供如何实施纠正措施的具体计划，因此您的回复是不充分的。对于如何确保随机前收集受试者病历，以及如何保证您和您的团队按照方案的入组排除标准审阅这些记录，您未提供具体的计划。没有这些具体计划，我们无法判断您采取的纠正措施是否足以预防将来类似违规情况的发生。

c. 试验方案1245.25要求排除安慰剂筛选期禁食过夜后血糖＞240mg/dL（＞13.3mmol/L），且经第二次测量确认（非同一天）的未控制的高血糖患者。

受试者58832尽管有符合上述条件的未控制的高血糖仍然入组试验方案1245.25。受试者58832在安慰剂筛选期2012年1月23日的空腹血糖值为246mg/dL，随后在2012年1月24日变为261mg/dL。

在您2013年6月28日对上述1.c.的书面回复中，您表示您不再授权直接或间接影响受试者资格的相关评估，只有研究者能审阅受试者的日记卡，而不是研究协调员。您的回复对预防将来发生类似违规情况是充分的。

受试者58823，58827，58828和58832代表50%入组在方案1245.25中的受试者。因此，您入组的一半受试者对研究来说是不合格的。入组不符合合格标准的受试者会危害他们的安全和福利，而且引起对在贵研究中心收集数据的有效性和可靠性的关注。

2. 您未能保存研究中使用试验药物或对照组的受试者的所有观察结果和其他与研究相关的个体数据的足够及准确的病历［21 CFR 312.62（b）］

作为临床研究者，您必须准备和保存研究中使用试验药物或对照组的受试者的所有观察结果和其他与研究相关的个体数据的足够和准确的病历，您未能保存足够的关于试验方案1245.25研究文件上签名日期的病历。具体为：

a. 受试者58823，您于2012年7月11日收到访视8的实验室检查结果，但是您在实验报告的签名的日期是2012年6月12日。

b. 受试者58836，访视4的实验室报告日期为2012年4月12日，但您在实验室报告的签名日期是2012年3月21日。

在您2013年6月28日对上述条目2.的书面回复中，您指出："实验室报告将会被迅速修正并及时记录"。由于该回复没有明确您如何修正实验室报告，因此回复是不充分的。没有您修正实验室报告计划的细节，我们无法确定您采取的纠正措施是否足以预防将来类似违规情况的发生。

您未能保存足够和准确的关于署名日期的病历，引起我们关注在贵研究场所收集数据的有效性和可靠性。

本警告信的目的并非是罗列您在试验药物临床研究中存在的所有缺陷。确保遵循法律和FDA相关法规的每一项要求是您的职责，您应当解释这些缺陷，并建立规程，以确保任何正在进行或将来进行的研究均符合FDA法规的。

自收到这封信的15个工作日内，您应当书面告知本办公室为预防将来发生类似违规情况而采取的措施。如果不能充分、迅速地解释上述违规问题，可能导致我们在不再通知的情况下采取监管措施。

附：英文原文

Agnes E. Ubani, M.D.

WARNING LETTER

NOV 21, 2013

CERTIFIED MAIL
RETURN RECEIPT REQUESTED

Ref: 13-HFD-45-11-02

Agnes Ubani, M.D.
Windsor Medical Clinic
11434 N 53 rd Street
Tampa, FL 33617-2216

Dear Dr. Ubani:

This Warning Letter informs you of objectionable conditions observed during the U.S. Food and Drug Administration (FDA) inspection conducted at your clinical site between May 29 and June 6, 2013. Mr. Gene R. Gunn, representing the FDA, reviewed your conduct of the following clinical investigations:

- Protocol 1245.25,"A Phase Ⅲ, multicenter, international, randomized, parallel group, double blind cardiovascular safety study of BI 10773 (10 mg and 25 mg administered orally once daily) compared to usual care in Type 2 diabetes mellitus patients with increased cardiovascular risk," of the investigational drug empagliflozin, performed for Boehringer Ingelheim Pharmaceuticals, Inc.
- Protocol H9X-MC-GBDN, "The Effect of LY2189265 on Blood Pressure and Heart Rate, as Assessed by Ambulatory Blood Pressure Monitoring, in Patients with Type 2 Diabetes Mellitus," of the investigational drug LY2189265, performed for Eli Lilly and Company.

This inspection is a part of FDA's Bioresearch Monitoring Program, which includes inspections designed to evaluate the conduct of FDA-regulated research to ensure that the data are scientifically valid and accurate, and to help ensure that the rights, safety, and welfare of the human subjects of those studies have been protected.

At the conclusion of the inspection, Mr. Gunn presented and discussed with you Form FDA 483, Inspectional Observations. We acknowledge receipt of your June 28, 2013 written response to the Form FDA 483.

From our review of the FDA establishment inspection report, the documents submitted with that report and your June 28, 2013 written response, we conclude that you did not adhere to the applicable statutory requirements and FDA regulations governing the conduct of clinical investigations. We wish to emphasize the following:

1. You failed to ensure that the investigation was conducted according to the investigational plan [21 CFR 312.60].

As a clinical investigator, you are required to ensure that your clinical studies are conducted in accordance with the investigational plan. The investigational plan for Protocol 1245.25 requires you to exclude subjects who meet the exclusion criteria and who do not meet the inclusion criteria. You failed to adhere to these requirements. Specifically:

a. Protocol 1245.25 requires that you exclude subjects who have a history of cancer (except for basal cell carcinoma) and/or treatment for cancer within the last five years prior to enrollment.

Subjects 58823 and 58827 were enrolled in the study with a history of cancer (prostate cancer and melanoma, respectively) within the last five years prior to enrollment.

b. Protocol 1245.25 requires all subjects to have "high cardiovascular risk," which is defined as at least one of the following:

ⅰ. Confirmed history of myocardial infarction (>2 months prior to informed consent)

ii. Evidence of multi-vessel coronary artery disease, in 2 or more major coronary arteries, irrespective of the revascularization status (disease affecting the left main coronary artery is considered as a 2 vessel disease)

iii. Evidence of a single-vessel coronary artery disease with:

- The presence of a significant stenosis, i.e., the imaging evidence of at least 50% narrowing of the luminal diameter of one major coronary artery in subjects not subsequently successfully revascularized (measured during a coronary angiography or a multisliced computed tomography angiography)
- And at least one of the following (either 1 or 2):

1. A positive non-invasive stress test, confirmed by either:
   - A positive exercise tolerance test in subjects without a complete left bundle branch block, Wolff Parkinson White syndrome, or paced ventricular rhythm, or
   - A positive stress echocardiography showing regional systolic wall motion abnormalities, or
   - A positive scintigraphic test showing stressinduced is chemia, i.e., the development of transient perfusion defects during myocardial perfusion imaging
2. Or subject discharged from hospital with a documented diagnosis of unstable angina within 12 months prior to selection

iv. Last episode of unstable angina >2 months prior to informed consent with confirmed evidence of coronary multivessel or single vessel disease as defined above

v. History of ischemic or hemorrhagic stroke (>2 months prior to informed consent)

vi. Presence of peripheral artery disease (symptomatic or not) documented by either: previous limb angiography, stenting or by pass surgery; or previous limb or foot amputation due to circulatory insufficiency; or angiographic evidence of significant (>50%) peripheral artery stenosis in at least one limb; or evidence from a non-invasive measurement of significant (>50% or as reported as hemodynamically significant) peripheral artery stenosis in at least one limb; or ankle brachial index of <0.9 in at least one limb

Subject 58828 was enrolled in Protocol 1245.25 without having high cardiovascular risk as defined above. This subject had a history of unstable angina and a positive non-invasive stress test, but did not have confirmed evidence of coronary multivessel or single vessel disease, as defined in the inclusion criteria. The subject had an approximately 20% narrowing of the lumen of a major coronary vessel (right coronary artery), but the inclusion criteria required a 50% or greater narrowing. In addition, records indicate that the subject had a defect suggestive of myocardial is chemia rather than confirmation of a myocardial infarction. Based on inclusion criteria outlined above, this subject was ineligible and should not have been enrolled.

In your June 28, 2013 written response to the findings noted in Items 1.a and 1.b above, you indicate that you have established corrective action plans to prevent these violations from reoccurring. You state that subjects will be screened only after all medical records have been received and reviewed against protocol inclusion and exclusion criteria. Your response is inadequate because you have not provided details regarding how your corrective actions will be implemented. You have not provided details regarding how you will ensure that medical records are received prior to randomization, and how you will ensure that you and your staff review those records against protocol inclusion and exclusion criteria. Without these details, we are unable to determine whether your corrective actions appear sufficient to prevent similar violations from occurring in the future.

c. Protocol 1245.25 requires that you exclude subjects who have uncontrolled hyperglycemia with a glucose level of >240 mg/dL (>13.3 mmol/L) after an overnight fast during the placebo run-in and confirmed by a second measurement (not on the same day).

Subject 58832 was enrolled in the study, despite having uncontrolled hyperglycemia that met the conditions described above. Subject 58832 had a fasting blood glucose level of 246 mg/dL on January 23, 2012, during the placebo run-in period, followed by a reading of 261 mg/dl on January 24, 2012.

In your June 28, 2013 written response to the finding noted in Item 1.c above, you indicate that you will no longer delegate assessments that have direct or indirect bearing on subject eligibility and that subject diary reviews will be done by the investigator and not the study coordinator. Your response appears adequate to prevent similar violations from occurring in the future.

Subjects 58823, 58827, 58828 and 58832 represent 50% of the subjects who you enrolled in Protocol 1245.25. Thus, one-half of the subjects you enrolled were not eligible for the study. Enrollment of subjects who do not meet eligibility criteria jeopardizes subject safety and welfare and raises concern about the validity and integrity of the data collected at your site.

2. You failed to maintain adequate and accurate case histories that record all observations and other data pertinent to the investigation on each individual administered the investigational drug or employed as a control in the investigation [21 CFR 312.62(b)].

As a clinical investigator, you are required to prepare and maintain adequate and accurate case histories that record all observations and other data pertinent to the investigation on each individual administered the investigational drug or employed as a control in the investigation. You have failed to maintain adequate and accurate case histories with respect to signature dates on study documents for Protocol 1245.25. Specifically:

a. For Subject 58823, you received Visit 8 laboratory results on July 11, 2012. However, your signature on the laboratory report is dated June 12, 2012.

b. For Subject 58836, the Visit 4 laboratory report is dated April 21, 2012. However, your signature on the laboratory report is dated March 21, 2012.

In your June 28, 2013 written response to the finding noted in Item 2 above, you state that "Laboratory reports will be promptly revised and documented in a timely manner." Your response is inadequate because it is unclear what you intend to do with respect to revising laboratory reports. Without details regarding your plans to revise laboratory reports, we are unable to determine whether your corrective actions appear sufficient to prevent similar violations from occurring in the future.

Your failure to maintain adequate and accurate case histories with respect to signature dates raises concerns about the validity and integrity of data captured at your site.

This letter is not intended to be an all-inclusive list of deficiencies with your clinical study of an investigational drug. It is your responsibility to ensure adherence to each requirement of the law and relevant FDA regulations. You should address these deficiencies and establish procedures to ensure that any ongoing or future studies will be in compliance with FDA regulations.

Within fifteen (15) working days of your receipt of this letter, you should notify this office in writing of the actions you have taken to prevent similar violations in the future. Failure to address the violations noted above adequately and promptly may result in regulatory action without further notice.

If you have any questions, please contact Constance Cullity, M.D., M.P.H., at 301-796-3397; FAX 301-847-8748.

Your written response and any pertinent documentation should be addressed to:

Constance Cullity, M.D., M.P.H.
Branch Chief
Good Clinical Practice Enforcement Branch
Division of Good Clinical Practice Compliance
Office of Scientific Investigations
Office of Compliance
Center for Drug Evaluation and Research
Food and Drug Administration
Building 51, Room 5354
10903 New Hampshire Avenue
Silver Spring, MD 20993

Sincerely yours,

{See appended electronic signature page}

Thomas N. Moreno, M.S.
Acting Director

Office of Scientific Investigations
Office of Compliance
Center for Drug Evaluation and Research
Food and Drug Administration

第81封　给Samudrala, Sreedhar的警告信

2013年11月19日

参考号：13-HFD-45-11-01

尊敬的Samudrala博士：

2013年3月12日至3月28日，Laura Staples女士和Bonnie Pierson女士代表FDA，在贵临床研究中心，对您所开展的以下临床研究进行了审查。这封警告信特告知您现场检查中发现的违规情况。

- 试验方案HZC113782，“一项比较100/25 mcg 氟替卡松糠酸盐/维兰特罗吸入粉与安慰剂对患有中度慢性阻塞性肺病（COPD）和存在心血管疾病史或存在提高风险的受试者的生存有效性的临床疗效研究”，试验药物是葛兰素史克的氟替卡松糠酸盐。
- 试验方案（b）(4)，“（b）(4)”，试验药物是（b）(4）公司的（b）(4）的一部分。

本次现场检查是FDA的生物研究监查项目的一部分。该项目通过设定的检查方法，对FDA所监管的相关研究的实施情况进行评估，以确认研究数据在科学上是有效和准确的，并帮助确保这些研究中受试者的权益、安全和福利得到保护。

在现场检查结束时，检查员Staples和Pierson向您出示了FDA483表，即现场检查发现的问题，并与您进行了讨论。您2013年4月15日对该FDA483表的书面回复已收悉。

经对FDA现场检查报告、该报告的附件，以及您2013年4月15日的书面回复进行审查，我们认为，您没有遵循适用的法律要求和监管临床研究实施的FDA法规。我们想强调以下几点：

您未能确保按照研究计划进行研究［21 CFR 312.60］

作为一名临床研究者，您应该确保您的临床研究按照研究计划进行。试验方案HZC113782的研究计划要求您入组符合特定入组标准的受试者。您未能遵守这些要求。具体而言：

a. 试验方案HZC113783要求入组受试者在筛选（第一次访视）时使用舒瑞宁/舒喘灵后每秒用力呼气量（FEV1）与用力肺活量（FVC）的比值≤0.70。但是，在贵试验场所入组的31名受试者中，有11人未符合该入组标准，如下表1所示。

表1　在筛选时使用舒瑞宁/舒喘灵后FEV_1/FVC比值＞ 0.70的入组受试者

受试者编号	筛选访视日期	FEV1/FVC比值
300172	2011年5月25日	0. 79（最佳值）
300173	2011年5月25日	0. 77（最佳值）
300212	2011年6月6日	0. 87（最佳值）
300214	2011年6月6日	0. 80（最佳值）
300256	2011年6月14日	0. 80（最佳值）
300283	2011年6月20日	0. 77（最佳值）
300342	2011年6月28日	0. 80（最佳值）
300422	2011年7月14日	0. 74（最佳值）
300448	2011年7月12日	0. 80（最佳值）
300566	2011年7月26日	0. 75（最佳值）
300643	2011年8月3日	0. 75（最佳值）

b. 试验方案HZC113783要求入组受试者在筛选（第一次访视）时使用舒瑞宁/舒喘灵后FEV_1与按照国家健康和营养检查调查（NHANES）3参考方程计算的预期正常值的比率≥50%且≤70%。但在贵试验场所入组的31名受试者中，有4人未符合该入组标准，如下表2所示。

表2 在筛选时使用舒瑞宁/舒喘灵后FEV1与预期正常值比率FVC比值不在≥50%且≤70%范围内的入组受试者

受试者编号	筛选访视日期	FEV_1与预期正常值比率
300167	2011年5月24日	46%
300212	2011年6月6日	74%
300214	2011年6月6日	73%
300335	2011年6月26日	78%

c. 试验方案HZC113783要求入组正在接受下列疾病中任意两种疾病治疗的60岁或60岁以上的受试者：高胆固醇血症、高血压、糖尿病或周围血管疾病。受试者300296入组时73岁，未接受任何上述疾病的治疗。受试者300555入组时63岁，只在接受周围性血管疾病的治疗。

在您的书面回复中，您表明以下纠正措施计划："研究者在受试者随机前必须签署一份文件，指出受试者是否符合入组/排除标准。所有研究者和研究辅助人员已经接受再培训。已购买新的肺活量计，取代研究中不足的肺活量计。"

您的回复是不充分的，因为您的纠正措施计划不够详细。您没有提供关于研究者必须签署文件的细节，并且您没有提交该文件的复印件。您也没有提供进行再培训的细节或记录。没有这些信息，我们无法评估以上纠正措施是否足以防止将来这类违规情况的发生。

入组不符合标准的受试者会危害受试者的安全和福利，并损害了在贵研究中心收集的数据的真实性和完整性。

本警告信的目的并非是罗列试验药物临床研究中存在的所有缺陷。确保遵循法律和FDA相关法规的每一项要求是您的职责，您应当解决这些缺陷，并建立规程，以确保任何正在进行或将来进行的研究均符合FDA的法规。

自收到这封信的15个工作日内，您应当书面告知本办公室为预防将来发生类似违规情况而采取的措施。如果不能充分、迅速地解释上述违规问题，可能导致我们在不再通知的情况下采取监管措施。

附：英文原文

Samudrala, Sreedhar

WARNING LETTER

NOV 19, 2013

CERTIFIED MAIL
RETURN RECEIPT REQUESTED

Ref: 13-HFD-45-11-01

Sreedhar Samudrala, M.D.
377 Riverside Drive, Suite 202
Franklin, TN 37064

Dear Dr. Samudrala:

This Warning Letter informs you of objectionable conditions observed during the U.S. Food and Drug Administration (FDA) inspection conducted at your clinical site between March 12 and March 28, 2013. Ms. Laura Staples and Ms. Bonnie Pierson, representing the FDA, reviewed your conduct of the following clinical investigations:

- Protocol HZC113782,"A Clinical Outcomes Study to Compare the Effect of Fluticasone Furoate/Vilanterol Inhalation Powder 100/25 mcg with Placebo on Survival in Subjects with Moderate Chronic Obstructive Pulmonary Disease (COPD) and a History of or at Increased Risk fo Cardiovascular Disease", of the investigational drug fluticasone furoate, performed for GlaxoSmith Kline
- Protocol (b)(4), "(b)(4)", of the investigational drug (b)(4), performed for (b)(4).

This inspection is a part of FDA's Bioresearch Monitoring Program, which includes inspections designed to evaluate the conduct of FDA-regulated research to ensure that the data are scientifically valid and accurate, and to help ensure that the rights, safety, and welfare of the human subjects of those studie have been protected.

At the conclusion of the inspection, Investigators Staples and Pierson presented and discussed with you Form FDA 483, Inspectional Observations. We acknowledge receipt of your April 15, 2013, written response to the Form FDA 483.

From our review of the FDA establishment inspection report, the documents submitted with that report and your April 15, 2013 written response, we conclude that you did not adhere to the applicable statutory requirements and FDA regulations governing the conduct of clinical investigations. We wish to emphasize the following:

You failed to ensure that the investigation was conducted according to the investigational plan [21 CFR 312.60].

As a clinical investigator, you are required to ensure that your clinical studies are conducted in accordance with the investigational plan. The investigational plan for Protocol HZC113782 requires that you enroll subjects who meet specific inclusion criteria. You failed to adhere to these requirements. Specifically:

a. Protocol HZC113783 requires enrolled subjects to have a measured post-albuterol/salbutamol Forced Expiratory Volume in One Second (FEV1)/Forced Vital Capacity (FVC) ratio of ≤0.70 at screening (Visit 1). However, 11 of 31 subjects enrolled at your site did not meet this enrollment criterion, as shown in Table 1 below.

Table 1 Enrolled subjects with post-albuterol/salbutamol FEV1/FVC ratios > 0.70 at screening

Subject #	Screening Visit Date	FEV1/FVC Ratios
300172	May 25, 2011	0. 79 (best value)
300173	May 25, 2011	0. 77 (best value)
300212	June 6, 2011	0. 87 (best value)
300214	June 6, 2011	0. 80 (best value)
300256	June 14, 2011	0. 80 (best value)
300283	June 20, 2011	0. 77 (best value)
300342	June 28, 2011	0. 80 (best value)
300422	July 14, 2011	0. 74 (best value)
300448	July 12, 2011	0. 80 (best value)
300566	July 26, 2011	0. 75 (best value)
300643	August 3, 2011	0. 75 (best value)

b. Protocol HZC113783 requires enrolled subjects to have a measured post-albuterol/salbutamol FEV1 ≥50% and ≤0.70% of predicted normal values calculated using the National Health and Nutrition Examination Survey (NHANES) Ⅲ reference equations at screening (Visit 1). However, 4 of 31 subjects enrolled at your site did not meet this enrollment criterion, as shown in Table 2 below.

Table 2 Enrolled subjects without a post-albuterol/salbutamol $FEV_1 \geqslant 50\%$ and $\leqslant 70\%$ of predicted normal value at screening

Subject	Screening Visit Date	FEV_1 Percentage(s) of Predicted Normal Value
300167	May 24, 2011	46%
300212	June 6, 2011	74%
300214	June 6, 2011	73%
300335	June 26, 2011	78%

c. Protocol #HZC113783 requires enrolled subjects 60 years of age or older to be under treatment for any 2 of the following conditions: hypercholesterolemia, hypertension, diabetes mellitus, or peripheral vascular disease. Subject 300296 was 73 years of age at enrollment and was not being treated for any of the conditions listed above. In addition, Subject 300555 was 63 years of age at enrollment and was being treated for peripheral vascular disease only.

In your written response, you indicate that you have the following corrective action plan: "Investigator are required to sign a document prior to randomization that states that whether [sic] Inclusion/Exclusion Criteria have been met. All Investigators and study staff personnel were re- educated. A new spirometer was purchased to replace the spirometer that was inadequate for this study."

Your response is inadequate because it is insufficiently detailed with respect to your corrective action plan. You have not provided details regarding the document that investigators are required to sign, and you have not submitted a copy of that document. You also have not provided details or documentation regarding the re-education that took place. Without this information, we cannot assess whether these corrective actions are adequate to prevent future occurrences of this type of violation.

Enrollment of subjects who do not meet eligibility criteria may jeopardize subject safety and welfare and raises concerns about the validity and integrity of the data collected at your site.

This letter is not intended to be an all-inclusive list of deficiencies with your clinical study of an investigational drug. It is your responsibility to ensure adherence to each requirement of the law and relevant FDA regulations. You should address these deficiencies and establish procedures to ensure that any ongoing or future studies will be in compliance with FDA regulations.

Within fifteen (15) working days of your receipt of this letter, you should notify this office in writing of the actions you have taken to prevent similar violations in the future. Failure to address the violations noted above adequately and promptly may result in regulatory action without further notice.

If you have any questions, please contact Constance Cullity, M.D., M.P.H., at 301-796-3397;FAX 301- 847-8748. Your written response and any pertinent documentation should be addressed to:

Constance Cullity, M.D., M.P.H. Branch Chief
Good Clinical Practice Enforcement Branch Division of Good Clinical Practice Compliance Office of Scientific Investigations
Office of Compliance
Center for Drug Evaluation and Research
Food and Drug Administration
Building 51, Room 5354 10903 New Hampshire Avenue Silver Spring, MD 20993

Sincerely yours,

{See appended electronic signature page}

Thomas N. Moreno, M.S. Acting Director
Office of Scientific Investigations Office of Compliance
Center for Drug Evaluation and Research Food and Drug Administration

第 82 封　给 Sirakoff, Dimitri 的警告信

2013年9月12日

参考号：13-HFD-45-08-03

尊敬的Sirakoff博士：

2013年1月9日至2月6日，Yvette M. LaCour-Davis女士代表FDA，在贵临床研究机构，对您所开展的以下临床研究进行了审查。这封警告信特告知您现场检查中发现的违规情况。

- 试验方案1VIT09031，“一项研究静脉麦芽糖羧基铁（FCM）对缺血性贫血患者的有效性和安全性的多中心、随机、阳性对照研究，”试验药物是麦芽糖羧基铁，申办者为Luitpold制药股份有限公司。
- 试验方案（b）（4）[1]，“（b）（4）”，试验药物是（b）（4），申办者为（b）（4）。

本次现场检查是FDA的生物研究监查项目的一部分。该项目通过设定的检查方法，对FDA所监管的相关研究的实施情况进行评估，以确认研究数据在科学上是有效和准确的，并帮助确保这些研究中受试者的权益、安全和福利得到保护。

在现场检查结束时，LaCour-Davis女士向您出示了FDA483表，即现场检查发现的问题，并与您进行了讨论。您2013年4月10日针对该FDA483表的书面回复已收悉。

经对现场检查报告、该报告的附件，以及您2013年4月10日的书面回复进行审查，我们认为，您没有遵循适用的法律要求和监管临床研究实施的FDA法规。我们想强调以下几点：

您未能确保按照研究计划进行研究［21 CFR 312.60］

作为一名临床研究者，您必须确保您的临床研究按照研究计划进行。方案1VIT09031和（b）（4）的研究计划要求您确保受试者在随机入组前符合所有入组和排除标准。此外，方案1VIT09031要求您确保随机队列2、D组的受试者接受静脉铁剂的标准治疗。您未能遵守这些方案要求。具体而言：

1. 在1VIT09031和（b）（4）研究中，您未能确保研究受试者在随机入组之前符合方案入组和排除标准。

a. 试验方案（b）（4）的第三条入组标准，要求受试者“必须在过去的12个月内有根据美国风湿病学会标准（附件1）诊断，并由X射线（Kellgren-Lawrence X射线等级≥2）确认的髋关节OA（骨关节炎）”。方案附录1指出：“方案对髋关节OA的诊断要求是存在髋关节疼痛，X射线存在骨赘，并且ESR（红细胞沉降率）＜20mm/h或X射线关节空间缩小。”附录1进一步指出，X射线存在骨赘是按照Kellgren-Lawrence X射线等级≥2的方案要求。

i. 受试者1107~1057入组试验方案（b）（4）的即使受试者不符合第三条入组标准。2009年10月7日该受试者的放射学报告显示，其在2009年9月29日的右髋关节X射线的放射和医生意见：“关节间隔轻度减小，无骨赘形成的证据。”根据此放射学报告，该受试者没有资格入组试验方案（b）（4）。但是，该受试者随机进入2009年10月26日的试验方案。

2010年7月22日，在受试者1107~1057随机入组后大约9个月时，您在其放射学报告和筛选访视研究记录中，增加了一条后期加入的备注，指出在随机入组前已经观察到关节间隙变窄和骨赘，从而使该受试者看上去符合入组标准。但是，您未能提供解释性文件来支持您的后期加入的结论即受试者1107~1057符合入组标准的。

ii. 进入（b）（4）研究的受试者1107~1062不满足第三条入组标准。2009年9月22日该受试者的放射学报

1 （b）（4）涉及商业秘密，根据法规内容不予公开。

告显示其在2009年9月18日的右髋关节X射线的放射科医生意见："有髋骨轻度轴向关节间隙减小的证据，无骨赘形成。"根据此放射学报告，该受试者不符合（b）（4）研究的入组标准。但是，该受试者于2009年10月30日进入研究。

2010年7月22日，在该受试者入组后大约9个月时，您在其筛选访视研究记录中，增加了一条后期加的备注，指出在随机入组前已经观察到关节间隙变窄和骨赘，从而使该受试者看上去符合入组标准。但是，您未能提供解释性文件来支持您的后期加入的结论，即受试者1107~1062在随机前符合入组标准。

ⅲ. 进入（b）（4）研究的受试者1107~1060不满足第三条入组标准。2009年10月7日该受试者的放射学报告显示，其在2009年10月1日的左髋关节X射线结果："关节空间轻微丧失，无证据表明骨赘形成。"根据此放射学报告，该受试者不满足（b）（4）研究的入组标准。但是，该受试者于2009年10月29日进入研究。

ⅳ. 进入（b）（4）研究的受试者1107~1045不满足第三条入组标准。2009年9月10日该受试者的放射学报告显示，其在2009年9月4日的右髋关节X射线结果："关节空间轻微丧失，无证据表明骨赘形成。"根据此放射学报告，该受试者不满足（b）（4）研究的入组标准。但是，该受试者于2009年10月1日进入研究。

2010年7月22日，即该受试者入组后大约9个月时，您在其筛选访视研究记录和放射学报告中，延迟增加了一条记录，指出在入组前已经观察到关节缩小和骨赘，从而使该受试者看上去满足入组标准。但是，您未能提供支持该受试者满足入组标准的延迟性记录的解释记录。

在您2013年4月10日对上述1.a.中违规情况的书面回复中，您指出对于这四名受试者，您在放射科医生评估之前对X射线片进行了最初评估，这些受试者都存在关节空间缩小。您也指出，您理解Kellgren-Lawrence等级2是观察到明确的骨赘或者可能的关节空间缩小（关节宽度丧失小于50%）。但是，我们注意到，Kellgren-Lawrence评分等级2需要明确的骨赘和关节空间缩小同时存在。我们进一步注意到，方案对髋关节OA的诊断要求是X射线片存在骨赘，并且存在髋关节疼痛，同时红细胞沉降率＜ 20mm/h或X射线关节空间缩小。

在您的书面回复中，您进一步指出，在您"24年的临床实践和审阅放射学片的经历中"，您"从未看到过Kellgren-Lawrence放射学评估等级的结果。"我们强调，使用Kellgren-Lawrence分级系统是决定受试者入组标准的方案要求，您未能遵守这个要求。

您的回复不充分，因为您未能提供支持受试者（1107~1045，1107~1057，1107~1060和1107~1062）符合入组标准的延迟进入的解释记录。此外，您没有提交防止这类违规情况在将来再次发生的纠正措施。

b. 试验方案（b）（4）的第六条入组标准，要求受试者在基线访视时，髋部的西安大略和麦克迈斯特大学骨关节炎指数（WOMAC）疼痛分量数字评定量表（NRS）指数≥5。此外，试验方案（b）（4）第9.2章节（有效性分析），指定从基线到第16周访视时，WOMAC疼痛分量的变化是方案要求的三个联合主要终点之一。

ⅰ. 受试者1107~1045于2009年10月1日进入研究，比2009年10月2日，即评估入组标准的基线访视（第一天）提前一天。该受试者不符合第六条入组标准。在基线访视时，其WOMAC疼痛指数为4.0。该受试者不符合入组标准，但是进入了研究。

在您2013年4月10日针对上述1.b.ⅰ.中违规情况的书面回复中，您指出该违规情况出于您的研究协调员对WOMAC疼痛分量的计算错误，您同时承认您忽略了这个错误。此外，您指出您的研究协调员和其他研究人员已经重新接受了WOMAC疼痛分量和研究方案的培训。

您的回复不充分。虽然您指出研究协调员和您的团队已经重新接受了WOMAC培训，您没有提交该培训的记录。因此我们无法评估该培训是否足以防止这类违规情况在将来再次发生。

ⅱ. 受试者1107~1053不符合第六条入组标准，但是进入了（b）（4）研究。在2009年10月1日基线访视（第一天）时，该受试者的WOMAC疼痛指数为2.2。第六条入组标准要求WOMAC疼痛指数分数≥5。该受试者不符合入组标准，但是于2009年10月1日进入研究。

我们确认上述违规情况没有被记录在您收到的FDA 483表中。

c. 试验方案（b）（4）的第九条入组标准，要求受试者在基线的全球骨关节炎患者评价为“一般”“差”或者“很差”。此外，试验方案（b）（4）第9.2章节（有效性分析），指定从基线到第16周访视时，全球骨关节炎患者评价的变化是方案要求的三个联合主要终点之一。

受试者1107~1053不符合第九条入组标准，但是进入了（b）（4）研究。在2009年10月1日基线访视（第一天）时，该受试者的全球骨关节炎患者评价为“好”。该受试者不符合入组标准，但是于2009年10月1日进入研究。

在您2013年4月10日针对上述1.c.中违规情况的书面回复中，您确认了受试者1107~1053不符合第九条入组标准。（我们注意到，在您的回复中，您错误地使用了受试者编号1107~1055，但是使用了受试者1107~1053的姓名首字母缩写。）

您对此违规情况的书面回复是不充分。虽然您指出您和您的研究协调员已经重新接受了WOMAC培训，您没有提交针对入组不符合入组标准（在基线的全球骨关节炎患者评价为“一般”、“差”或者“很差”）的受试者的纠正措施。

d. 方案1VIT09031的第三条入组标准，要求受试者“在第一次筛选时铁蛋白≤100ng/ml，或者在TSAT（转铁蛋白饱和度）≤30%时铁蛋白≤300ng/ml。”

受试者21903不符合第三条入组标准，但是于2010年7月31日进入1VIT09031研究。该受试者的血液样本于2010年7月16日筛选访视时采集。2010年7月18日的实验室报告表明，其TSAT为33%，铁蛋白为881.4ng/ml，明显高于方案所允许的最大值100mg/ml。因此该受试者不符合方案1VIT09031的入组标准。

在您2013年4月10日针对上述1.d.中违规情况的书面回复中，您指出入组该受试者没有违规，因为在收到中心实验室结果之前，受试者按照方案进入研究；当您收到中心实验室结果时，您认为该受试者情况稳定，可以继续参加研究。您进一步指出，您持续紧密地监测该受试者，认为您的临床判断是正确的。此外，您指出申办者审阅了该受试者的记录，允许其入组并继续参加研究。

您的回复不充分，因为方案1VIT09031不允许只通过临床研究者的判断入组不符合入组标准（包括第三条入组标准）的受试者。此外，您没有提交给我们关于申办者和伦理委员会同意入组该受试者的记录。

每个临床研究的入组标准是为了对受试者优化所收集数据的解释，并将对入组受试者可预见的危害降到最低。入组不符合入组标准的受试者将危害其安全和福利，引起对在贵试验现场所收集数据的有效性和完整性的担忧。特别引起我们注意的是，在贵试验现场入组（b）（4）研究的13名受试者中，有5人不符合入组标准。

2. 在1VIT09031研究中，您未能遵守方案要求，即进入队列2、D组的受试者由研究医生决定接受“静脉标准治疗（其他静脉铁）”，所有研究药物和静脉铁标准治疗（包括蔗糖铁注射液USP和右旋糖酐铁注射液USP）由申办者提供。

研究记录显示，受试者21639被分配到队列2、D组，因此应该接受静脉铁标准治疗。但是其于第0天（2010年6月8日）和第7天（2010年6月15日）接受了研究药物FCM。

在您2013年4月10日针对上述2.中违规情况的书面回复中，您指出让随机队列2、D组的受试者使用研究药物FCM不是方案偏离，因为临床研究者可以根据判断决定治疗分配。此外，您陈述，“因此根据我的临床判断，我决定让该患者进入研究药物D组，使用FCM。”您进一步正确地指出，D组受试者可以根据研究者判断接受额外的静脉铁剂。

您的回复不充分，因为在队列2、D组的受试者，方案只允许其使用“静脉标准治疗（其他静脉铁）”。虽然方案允许向D组受试者提供额外的静脉铁剂，方案不允许向D组受试者提供试验药物FCM。

不遵守方案要求的治疗分配和规则，将对数据完整性存在潜在的负面影响。

本警告信的目的并非是罗列您在试验药物临床研究中存在的所有缺陷。确保遵循法律和FDA相关法规的每一项要求是您的职责，您应当解决这些缺陷，并建立规程，以确保任何正在进行或将来进行的研究均符合FDA的法规。

自收到这封信的15个工作日内，您应当书面告知本办公室为预防将来发生类似违规情况而采取的措施。如果不能充分、迅速地解释上述违规问题，可能导致我们在不再通知的情况下采取监管措施。

附：英文原文

Sirakoff, Dimitri

WARNING LETTER

SEP 12, 2013

CERTIFIED MAIL
RETURN RECEIPT REQUESTED

Ref: 13-HFD-45-08-03

Dimitri Sirakoff, D.O.
1206 E. 17th Street, Suite 204
Santa Ana, CA 92701

Dear Dr. Sirakoff:

This Warning Letter informs you of objectionable conditions observed during the U.S. Food and Drug Administration (FDA) inspection conducted at your clinical site between January 9 and February 6, 2013. Ms. Yvette M. LaCour-Davis, representing the FDA, reviewed your conduct of the following clinical investigations:

- Protocol 1VIT09031, titled "A Multicenter, Randomized, Active Controlled Study to Investigate the Efficacy and Safety of Intravenous Ferric Carboxymaltose (FCM) in Patients with Iron Deficiency Anemia (IDA)," of the investigational drug ferric carboxymaltose, performed for Luitpold Pharmaceuticals, Inc.
- Protocol (b)(4), titled "(b)(4)," of the investigational drug (b)(4), performed for (b)(4).

This inspection is a part of FDA's Bioresearch Monitoring Program, which includes inspections designed to evaluate the conduct of FDA-regulated research to ensure that the data are scientifically valid and accurate, and to help ensure that the rights, safety, and welfare of the human subjects of those studie have been protected.

At the conclusion of the inspection, Ms. LaCour-Davis presented and discussed with you Form FDA 483, Inspectional Observations. We acknowledge receipt of your April 10, 2013, written response to the Form FDA 483.

From our review of the FDA establishment inspection report, the documents submitted with that report and your April 10, 2013, written response, we conclude that you did not adhere to the applicable statutory requirements and FDA regulations governing the conduct of clinical investigations. We wish t emphasize the following:

You failed to ensure that the investigation was conducted according to the investigational plan [21 CFR 312.60].

As a clinical investigator, you are required to ensure that your clinical studies are conducted in accordance with the investigational plan. The investigational plans for Protocols 1VIT09031 and (b)(4) required you to ensure that subjects met all inclusion and exclusion criteria prior to randomization. In addition, Protocol 1VIT09031 required you to ensure that subjects who were randomized to Cohort 2, Group D, received intravenous (iv) iron standard of care. You failed to adhere to these protocol requirements. Specifically:

1. For Protocols 1VIT09031 and (b)(4), you failed to ensure that study subjects met the protocol inclusion and exclusion criteria prior to subject randomization.

a. Protocol (b)(4), Inclusion Criterion # 3, specifies that subjects "must have a diagnosis of OA [osteoarthritis] of the hip based on American College of Rheumatology criteria (Appendix 1) with x-ray confirmation (a Kellgren-Lawrence x-ray grade of ≥ 2)" taken within the last 12 months. Appendix 1 of the protocol notes that the "protocol-defined requirement for diagnosis of OA of the Hip [*sic*] will be the presence of hip pain, presence of osteophytes on x-ray and either an ESR [erythrocyte sedimentation rate] < 20 mm/hour OR joint space narrowing on x-ray." Appendix 1 further notes that the presence of osteophytes on X ray is a protocol requirement, defined by a Kellgren-Lawrence X-ray grade of ≥ 2.

i. Subject 1107-1057 was enrolled into Protocol **(b)(4)** even though the subject did not meet Inclusion Criterion # 3.The October 7, 2009, radiology report for this subject's right hip X rays, taken September 29, 2009, states the radiologist's impressions: "Mild superior loss of joint space. No evidence of osteophyte formation." Based on this radiology report, Subject 1107-1057 was not eligible for enrollment into Protocol **(b)(4)**. Nevertheless, this subject was randomized into this protocol on October 26, 2009.

On July 22, 2010, approximately nine months after Subject 1107-1057's randomization, yo added a late entry note both on this subject's radiology report and on the Screening Visit study record, indicating that joint narrowing and osteophytes had been observed prior to randomization, thus making the subject appear to have been eligible for the study. However, you failed to provide explanatory documentation to support your late entries' conclusion that Subject 1107-1057 was eligible prior to randomization.

ii. Subject 1107-1062 was enrolled into Protocol **(b)(4)** even though the subject did not meet Inclusion Criterion # 3. The September 22, 2009, radiology report for this subject's right hip x-rays, which were taken on September 18, 2009, states the radiologist's impressions: "Evidence of mild axial joint space loss at the hip. No osteophyte formation." Based on this radiology report, Subject 1107-1062 was not eligible for enrollment into Protocol **(b)(4)**. Nevertheless, this subject was randomized into this protocol on October 30, 2009.

On July 22, 2010, approximately nine months after Subject 1107-1062's randomization, yo added a late entry note on this subject's Screening Visit study record, indicating that joint space narrowing and osteophytes had been noted prior to randomization, thus making the subject appear to have been eligible for the study. However, you failed to provide explanatory documentation to support your late entry's conclusion that Subject 1107-1062 was eligible prior to the randomization.

iii. Subject 1107-1060 was enrolled into Protocol **(b)(4)** even though the subject did not meet Inclusion Criterion # 3. The October 7, 2009, radiology report for this subject's left hip X rays, which were taken on October 1, 2009, states the radiologist's
impressions: "Minimal superior femoral joint space loss. No evidence of osteophyte formation." Based on this radiology report, Subject 1107-1060 was not eligible for enrollment into Protocol **(b)(4)**. Nevertheless, this subject was randomized into this protocol on October 29, 2009.

iv. Subject 1107-1045 was enrolled into Protocol (b)(4) even though the subject did not meet Inclusion Criterion # 3. The September 10, 2009, radiology report for this subject's left hip X rays, which were taken on September 4, 2009, states the radiologist's impressions: "Minimal medial joint space loss. No hip osteophytes." Based on this radiology report, Subject 1107-1045 was not eligible for enrollment into Protocol **(b)(4)**. Nevertheless, this subject was randomized into this protocol on October 1, 2009.

On July 22, 2010, approximately nine months after Subject 1107-1045's randomization,you added a late entry noteon this subject's Screening Visit source record and radiology report.

These late entries indicated that you re-examined Subject 1107-1045's X ray prior to randomization and noted joint narrowing and osteophytes, thus making the subject appear to have been eligible for the study. However, you failed to provide explanatory documentation to support your late entries' conclusion that Subject 1107-1045 was eligible prior to the randomization.

In your April 10, 2013, written response to the violations noted in Item 1.a. above, you indicated that for all four subjects listed above, you initially evaluated the X rays prior to referring them to the radiologist for review, and that joint space narrowing was present in all subjects. You also indicated that you understood a Kellgren-Lawrence Grade of 2 to be either observation of a definite osteophyte o possible narrowing of joint space that was less than 50% loss of joint space width. However, we note that the Kellgren-Lawrence Grading Scale Grade 2 classification required both definite osteophytes and definite narrowing of joint space. We further note that the protocol-defined criteria for the diagnosis of OA of the hip required the presence of osteophytes on X ray, in addition to the presence of hip pain an either an erythrocyte sedimen-tation rate ＜ 20 mm/hour or joint space narrowing on X ray.

In your written response, you further noted that in your "24 years of clinical practice and reading radiographs" you have "never received radiology results with the Kellgren-Lawrence radiological assessment grades." We emphasize that the use of the Kellgren-Lawrence grading system was a protocol requirement for determination of subject eligibility, and that you failed to follow this requirement.

Your response is inadequate because you have not provided explanatory documentation to support you late entries' conclusions that these four subjects (1107-1045, 1107-1057, 1107-1060, and 1107-1062) were eligible for the study prior to randomization. Your response is also inadequate because you have not submitted a corrective action plan that, if properly carried out, would prevent the recurrence of thi type of violation in the future.

b. Protocol (b)(4), Inclusion Criterion # 6, required that subjects have a Western Ontario and McMaster Universities Osteoarthritis Index (WOMAC) pain subscale Numeric Rating Scale (NRS) score ⩾ 5 in the index hip at the Baseline Visit. In addition, Protocol (b)(4), Section 9.2., Efficacy Analysis, specifies that change from Baseline to Week 16 in the WOMAC pain subscale is one of three co-primary endpoints of the protocol.

ⅰ.Subject 1107-1045 was randomized on October 1, 2009, one day prior to evaluation of eligibility criteria pertinent to the Baseline Visit (Day 1) on October 2, 2009. As a result, Subject 1107-1045 was enrolled into Protocol (b)(4) when the subject did not meet Inclusion Criterion # 6. At the Baseline Visit (Day 1) on October 2, 2009, Subject 1107- 1045's WOMAC pain score was 4.0. This subject was randomized even though the subject was not eligible for the study.

In your April 10, 2013, written response to the violation noted in Item 1.b.i. above, you attribute the violation to your study coordinator's miscalculation of the WOMAC pain subscale;you also acknowledged that you overlooked this error. In addition, you indicated that your study coordinator and other study staff members were retrained on both the WOMAC pain subscale and the study protocol.

Your response is inadequate because, although you stated that the study coordinator and your team were retrained on the WOMAC, you have submitted no documentation of that training. As a result, we are unable to evaluate whether the training was adequate to prevent occurrence of thi and similar violations in the future.

ⅱ. Subject 1107-1053 was enrolled into Protocol (b)(4) even though the subject did not meet Inclusion Criterion # 6. At the Baseline Visit (Day 1) on October 1, 2009, Subject 1107-1053's WOMAC pain score was 2.2. Inclusion Criterion # 6 requires a WOMAC pain score ⩾ 5. You randomized this subject on October 1, 2009, despite the fact that the subject was not eligible for the study.

We acknowledge that this violation, as written, was not included on the Form FDA 483 that you received.

c. Protocol (b)(4), Inclusion Criterion # 9, required the Patient Global Assessment of Osteoarthritis for each subject to be "fair," "poor," or "very poor" at Baseline. In addition, Section 9.2. (Efficacy Analysis) of the protocol indicates that a change from Baseline to Week 16 in the Patient Global Assessment of Osteoarthritis is one of the three co-primary efficacy endpoints of the study.

Subject 1107-1053 was enrolled into Protocol (b)(4) even though the subject did not meet Inclusion Criterion # 9. At the Baseline Visit (Day 1) on October 1, 2009, Subject 1107-1053 checked the Patient Global Assessment of Osteoarthritis as "Good," thereby making the subject ineligible for the study. This subject was randomized on October 1, 2009, despite the fact that th subject was not eligible for the study.

In your April 10, 2013, written response to the violation noted in Item 1.c. above, you appear to have acknowledged that Subject 1107-1053 did not meet Inclusion Criterion # 9. (We note that in your response to this violation, you incorrectly noted the subject number as 1107-1055, but you associated that number with the same subject initials as those for Subject 1107-1053.)

Your written response to this violation is inadequate because, although you noted that you and your study coordinator were retrained on the WOMAC, you failed to address the violation of enrolling a subject who did not meet the eligibility requirement of a "fair," "poor," or "very poor" score on the Patient Global Assessment of Osteoarthritis scale at Baseline.

d. Protocol 1VIT09031, Inclusion Criterion # 3, required that subjects have "Screen 1 ferritin ⩽ 100 ng/ml or ⩽ 300 when TSAT [transferrin saturation] is ≤ 30%."

Subject 21903 was randomized into Protocol 1VIT09031 on July 31, 2010, even though the subject failed to meet Inclusion Criterion # 3. Subject 21903's blood sample was collected during the screenin visit on July 16, 2010. The laboratory report dated July 18, 2010, indicates that this subject had a screening TSAT of 33% and a screening ferritin value of 881.4 ng/ml, which is significantly higher than the protocol-allowed maximum value of 100 ng/ml. Therefore, Subject 21903 was not eligible for Protocol 1VIT09031.

In your April 10, 2013, written response to the violation noted in Item 1.d. above, you indicated that n deviation occurred with reference to randomizing this subject because the subject was randomized per protocol prior to receiving central lab results;and that, when you received the central lab results, you felt that the subject was stable enough to continue with the study. You further noted that you monitore the subject closely and felt that your clinical judgment was correct. Further, you indicated that the sponsor reviewed this subject's records and allowed the subject to enroll and to continue in the study.

Your response is inadequate in that Protocol 1VIT09031 does not allow enrollment of subjects based solely on the clinical investigator's judgment when the subject does not meet required inclusion criteria, including Inclusion Criterion #3. In addition, you did not provide us with documentation of sponsor and IRB approval to enroll this subject prior to your doing so.

The eligibility criteria for each clinical investigation are designed to optimize interpretability of collecte data and to minimize foreseeable harm to enrolled subjects. Enrollment of subjects who do not meet the eligibility criteria jeopardizes subject safety and welfare and raises concern about the validity and integrity of the data collected at your site. Particularly concerning to us is the fact that five of the thirteen subjects enrolled into Protocol (b)(4) at your site were ineligible for enrollment into the protocol.

2. For Protocol 1VIT09031, you failed to adhere to the requirement that subjects randomized to Cohort 2, Group D, receive "IV standard of care (other IV iron) as determined by the study site physician" and that all study medication and IV iron standard of care (including iron sucrose injection USP and iron dextran injection USP) be provided by the sponsor.

Study records show that Subject 21639 was assigned to Cohort 2, Group D, and therefore should have received IV iron standard of care, but instead received study drug, FCM, on Day 0 (June 8, 2010) and Day 7 (June 15, 2010).

In your April 10, 2013, written response to the violation noted in Item 2 above, you indicated that administering study drug, FCM, to subjects in Cohort 2, Group D, was not a protocol deviation because treatment assignment was at the discretion of the clinical investigator. In addition, you stated, "Therefore, per my clinical judgment, I chose to randomize the patient on the study medications Group D, medication FCM (Ferris [*sic*] Carboxymaltose)." Further, you noted correctly that subjects in Group D may receive additional IV iron at the discretion of the investigator.

Your response is inadequate because for subjects in Cohort 2, Group D, the protocol allows you to assign subjects only to an "IV standard of care (other IV iron)." Although the protocol does allow you to provide additional IV iron to subjects in Group D, the protocol does not allow you to give the investigational drug, FCM, to a subject assigned to Group D.

Failure to follow the protocol-specified treatment assignment and regimen has the potential to affect data integrity negatively.

This letter is not intended to be an all-inclusive list of deficiencies with your clinical study of an investigational drug. It is your responsibility to ensure adherence to each requirement of the law and relevant FDA regulations. You should address these deficiencies and establish procedures to ensure tha any ongoing or future studies will be in compliance with FDA regulations.

Within fifteen (15) working days of your receipt of this letter, you should notify this office in writing of the actions you have taken to prevent similar violations in the future. Failure to address the violations noted above adequately and promptly may result in regulatory action without further notice.

If you have any questions, please contact Constance Cullity, M.D., M.P.H., at 301-796-3397; FAX 301- 847-8748. Your written response and any pertinent documentation should be addressed to:

Constance Cullity, M.D., M.P.H. Branch Chief
Good Clinical Practice Enforcement Branch Division of Good Clinical Practice Compliance Office of Scientific Investigations
Office of Compliance
Center for Drug Evaluation and Research
Food and Drug Administration
Building 51, Room 5354 10903 New Hampshire Avenue Silver Spring, MD 20993

Sincerely yours,

{See appended electronic signature page}

Thomas N. Moreno, M.S. Acting Director
Office of Scientific Investigations Office of Compliance
Center for Drug Evaluation and Research
Food and Drug Administration

第 83 封　给 Nassim, Omid 医学博士的警告信

2013年9月3日

参考号：13-HFD-45-08-04

尊敬的Nassim博士：

2012年10月12日至12月5日，YvetteLaCour-Davis女士代表FDA，在贵临床研究中心，对您所开展的申办者为勃林格-英格翰制药公司，试验药物为BI10773（empagliflozin）的以下临床研究进行了审查。这封警告信特告知您现场检查中发现的违规情况。

- 试验方案1245.23“一项在二甲双胍或二甲双胍伴有磺酰脲类药物治疗仍未能有效控制胰高血糖素的2型糖尿病患者中每日单次口服BI10773（10mg,25mg）超过24周的Ⅲ期、随机、双盲、安慰剂对照、平行分组的有效性和安全性研究”；
- 试验方案1245.25“一项在心血管风险升高的2型糖尿病患者中使用BI10773（每日单次口服10mg和25mg）和常规治疗比较的Ⅲ期、国际多中心、随机、平行、双盲的心血管安全性研究”。

本次现场检查是FDA的生物研究监查项目的一部分。该项目通过设定的检查方法，对FDA所监管的相关研究的实施情况进行评估，以确认研究数据在科学上是有效和准确的，并帮助确保这些研究中受试者的权益、安全和福利得到了保护。

在现场检查结束时，LaCour-Davis女士向您出示了FDA483表，即现场检查发现的问题，并与您进行了讨论。您2012年12月24日对该FDA483表的书面回复已收悉。

经对现场检查报告、该报告的附件，以及您2012年12月24日的书面回复进行审查，我们认为，您没有遵循适用的法律要求和监管临床研究实施的FDA法规。我们想强调以下几点：

1. 您未能确保按照研究计划进行研究［21 CFR 312.60］

作为一名临床研究者，您必须确保您的临床研究按照研究计划进行。试验方案1245.25的研究计划要求您排除符合排除标准及不符合入组标准的受试者。您未能遵守这些要求。具体而言：

试验方案1245.25的研究计划要求所有受试者伴有心血管高风险。符合这个要求，受试者必须在筛选和入组前伴有至少一种以下高风险情况：

- 心肌梗死病史（知情同意前两个月以上）；
- 不稳定型心绞痛（知情同意前两个月以上）记录有多支冠脉血管疾病（血管造影片显示至少两根冠状主动脉）或正应力检测（ST段压低≥2mm或心肌灌注闪烁显像阳性）；
- 知情同意两个月前多支冠状动脉介入治疗（PCI）；
- 知情同意四年前多支冠状动脉旁路治疗（CABG）或伴有术后复发心绞痛；
- 缺血性或出血性脑卒中病史（知情同意两个月前）；
- 外周动脉闭塞性疾病［既往下肢搭桥手术或经皮腔内血管成形术；既往因循环功能不全进行的下肢或足部切除术；血管造影或成像（例如超声、核磁共振）发现明显血管狭窄（＞50%下肢主动脉）］。

我们发现这个列表并没有包括下面所列受试者所记录的心脏情况：短暂性脑缺血发作（TIA）、深部静脉血栓形成或既往未进行手术或血管造影或成像未发现血管明显狭窄（超过50%）。

贵试验现场11名受试者中5名没有符合心血管高风险方案要求被随机入组试验方案1245.25。

a. 受试者56782：于2010年12月10日的筛选访视，仅记录心血管情况短暂性脑缺血发作，受试者未在入

组及治疗随机过程中被排除。

b. 受试者56784：于2010年12月14日的筛选访视，心血管情况记录有短暂性脑缺血发作和既往未进行手术或血管造影术或成像未发现明显下肢主动脉血管狭窄的左下肢外周动脉疾病。受试者未在入组治疗随机过程中被排除。

c. 受试者56791：于2011年1月5日的筛选访视，心血管情况仅记录短暂性脑缺血发作，受试者未在治疗随机过程中被排除[1]。

d. 受试者56799：于2011年1月5日[2]的筛选访视记录，心血管情况仅记录短暂性脑缺血发作，受试者未在治疗随机过程中被排除。

e. 受试者56795：于2011年1月6日的筛选访视心血管情况仅记录腿部的深部静脉血栓形成，受试者未在治疗随机过程中被排除。

在您2012年12月24日对于以上1.a.至1.e.违规的书面回复中，确认受试者并未按照方案1245.25规定的心血管高风险标准进行入组。您的回复是不充分的，因为您并未提供充分信息，让FDA对您的纠正措施计划是否适当进行评估。尽管在您的书面回复中也表明将遵守方案的入组/排除标准，但您并未提供任何具体信息描述您如何避免类似违规在未来重复发生的措施。

入组不符合入组标准的受试者危害到受试者的安全和福利，引起对贵研究中心所采集的数据的准确性和完整性的担忧。

2. 您未能在实施研究的变更前，获得伦理委员会的批准［21 CFR 312.66］

作为一名临床研究者，您必须获得伦理委员会对于研究变更的批准，除非是必须消除对受试者明显的直接危害这一例外情况。您未获得伦理委员会对于不属于消除对受试者明显的直接危害内容的变更信息的批准。具体而言：

贵试验现场在获得伦理批准之前实施了方案1245.25于2011年12月29日的修订3（版本4）的变更内容。方案1245.25版本4中包含多处变更，包括对于入组标准的明显变更。这些变更包括3.3.2重新定义患者心血管风险合格条件，包括单支血管病变和未接受过手术介入治疗的外周心血管疾病的入组标准修订。这些修订相对于方案1245.25版本1明显扩增了入组标准。未见任何记录显示方案1245.25版本4获得伦理委员会批准。方案1245.25的新版本不能实施，除非获得伦理委员会的批准。在实施方案1245.25版本4的这些修订（因与消除对受试者明显的直接危害无关，故这些不符合伦理委员会批准的豁免情况）前未见伦理委员会批准记录，您未能符合21 CFR 312.66的要求。

在您2012年12月24日对上述第2条违规的书面回复中，您说明“对于方案1245.25的修订于2011年12月29日被伦理委员会批准，监查员未将该情况告知该研究中心”。我们理解为研究监查员未能告知研究人员关于伦理委员会批准方案1245.25新版本的信息。然而，确保在实施任何变更前获得伦理委员会对变更内容的批准是您作为研究者的职责（而不是监查员的职责）。另外，您的回复是不充分的，因为您未能提供关于伦理委员会的批准的任何证据或纠正措施计划，以预防类似违规情况在未来再次发生。

您未能在对研究变更之前获得伦理委员会的批准，这妨碍了伦理委员会对于入组到您的临床研究中受试者的持续的安全性作出有根据的决定。

本警告信的目的并非是罗列您在试验药物临床研究中存在的所有缺陷。确保遵循法律和相关FDA法规的每一项要求是您的职责，您应当解决这些缺陷，并建立规程，以确保任何正在进行或将来进行的研究均符合FDA的法规。

自收到这封信的15个工作日内，您应当书面告知本办公室为预防将来发生类似违规情况而采取的措施。如果不能充分、快速地解释上述违规问题，可能导致我们在不再通知的情况下采取监管措施。

1　我们注意到在筛选过程记录中有一个后来手写的备注，日期为2011年6月2日，声称该受试者实际上从2003年以来确实有缺血性发作病史，但是，符合入组标准的这种情况，在随机时却没有被记录。

2　另外的相关文件表明，这个日期实际上本来应该是2011年1月7日。

附：英文原文

Nassim, Omid M.D.

WARNING LETTER

SEP 03, 2013

CERTIFIED MAIL
RETURN RECEIPT REQUESTED

Ref: No.13-HFD-45-08-04

Omid Nassim,M.D.
Alia Clinical Research, Inc.
2620 Zoe Avenue
Huntington Park, CA 90255

Dear Dr. Nassim:

This Warning Letter informs you of objectionable conditions observed during the U.S. Food and Drug Administration (FDA) inspection conducted at your clinical site between October 12 and December 5, 2012. Ms. Yvette LaCour-Davis, representing the FDA, reviewed your conduct of the following clinical investigations of the investigational drug BI 10773 (empagliflozin), performed for Boehringer Ingelheim Pharmaceuticals (BI):

- Protocol 1245.23, "A phase Ⅲ randomized, double-blind, placebo-controlled, parallel group, efficacy and safety study of BI 10773 (10 mg, 25 mg) administered orally, once daily over 24 weeks in patients with type 2 diabetes mellitus with insufficient glycaemic control despite treatment with metformin alone or metformin in combination with a sulfonylurea (Pro00005609)"; and Protocol 1245.25, "A Phase Ⅲ multicenter, international, randomized, parallel group, double blind cardiovascular safety study of BI 10773 (10 mg and 25 mg administered orally once a daily) compared to usual care in type 2 diabetes mellitus patients with increased cardiovascular risk."

This inspection is a part of FDA's Bioresearch Monitoring Program, which includes inspections designed to evaluate the conduct of FDA-regulated research to ensure that the data are scientifically valid and accurate, and to help ensure that the rights, safety, and welfare of the human subjects of those studies have been protected.

At the conclusion of the inspection, Ms. LaCour-Davis presented and discussed with you Form FDA 483, Inspectional Observations. We acknowledge receipt of your December 24, 2012, written response to the Form FDA 483.

From our review of the FDA establishment inspection report, the documents submitted with that report, and your December 24, 2012, written response, we conclude that you did not adhere to the applicable statutory requirements and FDA regulations governing the conduct of clinical investigations. We wish to emphasize the following:

1. You failed to ensure that the investigation was conducted according to the investigational plan [21 CFR 312.60].

As a clinical investigator, you are required to ensure that your clinical studies are conducted in accordance with the investigational plan. The investigational plan for Protocol 1245.25 required you to exclude subjects who met the exclusion criteria and who did not meet the inclusion criteria. You failed to adhere to this requirement. Specifically:

The investigational plan for Protocol 1245.25 required all subjects to be at "high cardiovascular risk." To meet this requirement, subjects must have at least one of the following high-risk conditions prior to screening and enrollment:

- History of myocardial infarction (＞2 months prior to informed consent);
- Unstable angina (＞2 months prior to informed consent) with documented multivessel coronary disease (of at least two major coronary arteries in angiogram) or positive stress test (ST segment depression ⩾ 2 mm or a positive nuclear perfusion scintigram);

- Multivessel Percutaneous Coronary Intervention (PCI) > 2 months prior to informed consent;
- Multivessel Coronary Artery By-pass Grafting (CABG) > 4 years prior to informed consent or with recurrent angina following surgery;
- History of ischemic or hemorrhagic stroke (> 2 months prior to informed consent); or
- Peripheral occlusive arterial disease (previous limb bypass surgery or percutaneous transluminal angioplasty; previous limb or foot amputation due to circulatory insufficiency; angiographic or imaging detected (for example: ultrasound, MRI) significant vessel stenosis (> 50% stenosis of major limb arteries).

We note that this list does not include transient ischemic attack (TIA), deep venous thrombosis, or peripheral arterial disease without previous surgery or significant vessel stenosis (greater than 50%) detected by angiography or imaging, which were the cardiac-related conditions documented for the subjects described below.

Five of eleven subjects at your site were randomized into Protocol 1245.25 without having met the protocol requirement for being at high cardiovascular risk.

a. Subject 56782: At the December 10, 2010, screening visit, the only cardiovascular condition documented was transient is chemic attack. This subject was not excluded from enrollment and treatment randomization.

b. Subject 56784: At the December 14, 2010, screening visit, the only cardiovascular conditions documented were transient is chemic attack and transient peripheral arterial disease of the left limb without past surgery or confirmation of significant vessel stenosis detected by angiography or imaging. This subject was not excluded from treatment randomization.

c. Subject 56791: At the January 5, 2011, screening visit, the only documented cardiovascularcondition was transient ischemic attack. This subject was not excluded from treatment randomization. [1]

d. Subject 56799: On the screening narrative, dated January 5, 2011 [2], the only cardiovascular condition documented was transient ischemic attack. This subject was not excluded from treatment randomization.

e. Subject 56795: At the January 6, 2011, screening visit, the only cardiovascular condition documented was deep venous thrombosis of the leg. This subject was not excluded from treatment randomization.

In your December 24, 2012, written response to the violations noted in Items 1.a through 1.e. above, you acknowledged that the subjects described were enrolled into Protocol 1245.25 without meeting protocol specified criteria for being at high cardiovascular risk. Your response is inadequate because you have not provided sufficient information to enable FDA to evaluate the adequacy of your corrective action plan. Although you stated in your written response that you will follow protocol inclusion/exclusion eligibility criteria, you did not provide any details describing how you plan to prevent recurrence of similar violations in the future.

Enrollment of subjects who do not meet eligibility criteria jeopardizes subject safety and welfare, and raises concern about the validity and integrity of the data collected at your site.

2. You failed to obtain Institutional Review Board (IRB) approval for changes in the research prior to implementing the changes [21 CFR 312.66].

As a clinical investigator, you are required to obtain IRB approval for any changes in the research, except where necessary to eliminate apparent immediate hazards to human subjects. You failed to obtain IRB approval for changes in the research that were not related to the elimination of apparent immediate hazards to subjects. Specifically:

Your site implemented changes contained in Protocol 1245.25, Revision 3 (Version 4), dated December 29, 2011, before you received IRB approval for this version of the protocol. Protocol 1245.25, Version 4 contains multiple changes, including significant changes to the inclusion criteria. These changes include revisions to Section 3.3.2 of the inclusion criteria that redefine patients' cardiovascular eligibility risk factors to include patients with single-vessel disease and peripheral artery disease who have not undergone any corrective surgical intervention. These revisions are a significant expansion of the inclusion criteria from those in Version 1 of Protocol 1245.25. There is no documentation to show that the amendments to Protocol 1245.25, Version 4 were ever approved by the IRB. This newer version of Protocol 1245.25 should not be used unless IRB approval has been received. Without documentation of IRB approval for these revisions (which do not qualify for an exception from IRB approval, as they are unrelated to the elimination of apparent immediate hazards to human subjects) in Version 4 of Protocol 1245.25 prior to implementation, you have failed to meet the requirements of 21 C.F.R. § 312.66.

In your December 24, 2012, written response to the violation noted in Item 2 above, you said, “The monitor failed to inform and educate the site about the amendment to the Protocol #1245.25, revision 03, dated 29 Dec 2011 was approved [sic] by the IRB.” We interpret this to mean that the study monitor failed to inform the staff of IRB approval of a new version of Protocol 1245.25. However, it is your responsibility as the investigator (not the monitor’s responsibility) to ensure that the IRB has approved any changes in the research prior to implementing those changes. In addition, your response is inadequate because you failed to provide evidence of IRB approval or a corrective action plan to prevent recurrence of similar violations in the future.

Your failure to obtain IRB approval for research changes prior to implementing those changes prevented the IRB from making an informed determination regarding the continued safety of the subjects enrolled in your investigational research.

This letter is not intended to be an all-inclusive list of deficiencies with your clinical study of an investigational drug. It is your responsibility to ensure adherence to each requirement of the law and relevant FDA regulations. You should address these deficiencies and establish procedures to ensure that any ongoing or future studies will be in compliance with FDA regulations.

Within fifteen (15) working days of your receipt of this letter, you should notify this office in writing of the actions you have taken to prevent similar violations in the future. Failure to address the violations noted above adequately and promptly may result in regulatory action without further notice.

If you have any questions, please contact Constance Cullity, M.D., M.P.H., at 301-796-3397; FAX 301-8478748. Your written response and any pertinent documentation should be addressed to:

Constance Cullity, M.D., M.P.H.
Branch Chief
Good Clinical Practice Enforcement Branch
Division of Good Clinical Practice Compliance
Office of Scientific Investigations
Office of Compliance
Center for Drug Evaluation and Research
Food and Drug Administration
Building 51, Room 5354
10903 New Hampshire Avenue
Silver Spring, MD 20993

Sincerely yours,

{See appended electronic signature page}

Thomas N. Moreno, M.S.
Acting Director
Office of Scientific Investigations
Office of Compliance
Center for Drug Evaluation and Research
Food and Drug Administration

1 We note in the screening narrative that there is a later handwritten note, dated June 2, 2011, stating that the subject actually did have a history of ischemic stroke from 2003. However, this condition, which meets the inclusion criteria, was not documented at the time of randomization.

2 The other related documents suggest that this date actually may have been January 7, 2011.

第84封　给Janet K. Tillisch医学博士的警告信

2013年6月20日

参考号：CBER-13-03

尊敬的Tillisch博士：

这封信特告知您2013年4月9日结束的FDA现场检查的结果。FDA检查员与您会面，审查了您在以下临床研究中的实施情况：

（b）（4）;

（b）（4）。

FDA生物研究监查项目之下的这次现场检查，通过设定的检查方法，审查试验药物相关研究的实施情况。

现场检查结束时，检查员向您出示并讨论了FDA 483表，即现场检查发现的问题。我们收到并审查了您日期为2013年4月24日对FDA 483表的回复。

我们认为您违反了美国联邦法规（CFR）第21篇第312部分对正确实施与试验用新药有关的临床研究进行监管的规定（详见http://www.gpoaccess.gov/cfr/index.html）。以下列出的每个违规项均指出了CFR中的相应条款。

1. 您未能履行研究者的总体职责［21 CFR 312.60和312.50］

研究者有责任确保试验根据已签署的研究者声明、研究计划和适用的法规开展；保护在研究者的照料下的受试者的权益、安全和福利，负责对试验药物的管理。当您在2011年5月16日就上述临床研究签署研究者声明（FDA 1572表）时，您明确同意亲自进行此项临床试验或对试验中您不能亲自开展的部分进行监督。在您可能将某些研究任务授权给有资格的人进行时，应对此授权人进行充分的监督。您有责任对研究人员进行监管并审查研究人员的工作，以确保遵守研究计划和程序。

但我们检查发现，您将（b）（4）研究访视和完成访视记录，包括CRFs，均授权给了现场管理组织（SMO）进行。无证据证明您对您授权给（b）（4）的研究活动进行了充分的监督和审查。如下所述，您未能对（b）（4）的研究记录进行合理而认真的审查，包括您不能保证在试验进行过程中有权限能获得试验相关的原始文档。监管的缺失和未能亲自参与试验，导致不能确保试验在遵守已签署的研究者声明、研究计划和相应法规的情况下进行。

A. 已获得的信息表明，在试验开展过程中，您没有权限获得某些原始记录（电子日志或e-日志），在日志中受试者记录与受试者的病历相关的AE信息和其他观察到的信息。由此，您将受试者置于危险之中，因为您不能及时审查和评估AEs，判断其严重程度及其与研究药物的关系，并采取任何必要的医学干预措施。此外，如下述第2点所述，您未能保证AEs按方案要求记录在CRFs中。

您的回复函称您已获配了电子日志的密码。请解释您何时收到进入电子日志的授权，何时您可对电子日志进行审查。

B. 如下述第3点所述，多种研究记录不完善或缺失，包括CRFs。

回复函中您解释说（b）（4）管理临床试验的关键部分，包括临床研究的协调及记录保存。您进一步解释说（b）（4）突然在2012年8月关闭了试验，并未向您提供其管理的研究的任何文档或信息。如上所述，当您把某些研究任务授权给有资格的其他人进行时，应对此种授权进行充分的监督。而您作为研究者，应合理而认真地审查研究记录，此种记录保存的缺陷对您来说是显而易见的。

2. 您未能确保按照签署的研究者声明、研究计划、适用法规进行研究，以保护在您的监护下的受试者的权益、安全和福利［21 CFR 312.60］

A. 下述不良事件记录在受试者电子日志中，但是并未按照研究（b）（4）方案9.12.2的要求，在CRFs的不良事件表中报告。

ⅰ.（b）（4），（b）（6）。

ⅱ.（b）（4），（b）（6）。

ⅲ.（b）（4），（b）（6）。

ⅳ.（b）（4），（b）（6）。

B. 研究（b）（4）方案7.8要求必须尽可能确定为何受试者未返回进行必要的访视，同时要求将受试者未返回进行必要访视的原因或从研究脱落的详细信息以及脱落日期记录在CRF的研究结果页面上。但下述两例受试者未符合上述要求。

ⅰ.（b）（4），（b）（6）。

ⅱ.（b）（4），（b）（6）。

在回复函中对此您未予以解释。请就此提供书面回复。

3. 您未记录和保持受试者的足够和准确的病历，包括记录每位受试者给予受试药后试验相关的所有观察情况和其他数据，以及CRF和支持性数据［21 CFR 312.62（b）］

A.（b）（4），（b）（6）

在回复函中您对此未予以解释。就此请提供书面回复。

B. 检查中发现下述记录的保存有问题：

研究（b）（4）

ⅰ.（b）（4），（b）（6）。

ⅱ.（b）（4），（b）（6）。

ⅲ.（b）（4），（b）（6）。

在回复函中您对此未予以解释，就此请提供书面回复。

研究（b）（4）

ⅳ.（b）（4），（b）（6）。

ⅴ.（b）（4），（b）（6）。

a.（b）（4），（b）（6）。

b.（b）（4），（b）（6）。

在回复函中您对此未予以解释，就此请提供书面回复。

ⅵ.（b）（4），（b）（6）。

a.（b）（4），（b）（6）。

b.（b）（4），（b）（6）。

c.（b）（4），（b）（6）。

您在回复函中未就第ⅵ项a和b予以解释。第ⅵ项c未列在FDA 483表中。请对第ⅵ项a~c提供书面回复。

研究（b）（4）

ⅶ. 多个CRFs使用错误的表头，填写了另一研究中心的研究者姓名。

您在回复函中承认确实某些CRFs的表头有误。您解释说在（b）（4）通知试验关闭后，Essentia Health人员在随后对该试验进行内部审查时对这些表头作了改正。您进一步解释说，由于Essentia Health人员更正表头时未签署日期、时间或姓名首字母，而且这些更正的人员联系不到。

本警告信的目的并非是罗列您在试验疫苗的临床研究中存在的所有缺陷。确保遵循法律和相关法规的每一项要求是您的职责。

在您的回复函中，您描述了针对（b）（4）关闭以及试验操作的常规采取的纠正措施。我们还要求您提供此信中要求的其他信息。

自收到这封信的15个工作日内，请提供书面文件告知您为预防当前和将来再次发生类似违规情况已经采取的措施。如果未回复此信，不能采取适当的纠正措施，可能导致我们在不再通知的情况下采取监管措施。比如，FDA可根据21 CFR 312.70启动吊销您的资格的程序。如果您不认为您违反了FDA的法规要求，请陈述您的理由，并提供所有支持资料，以供我们参考。

附：英文原文

Janet K. Tillisch, M.D.

WARNING LETTER

JUN 20, 2013

Ref: CBER-13-03

Janet K. Tillisch, M.D.
1702 South University Drive
Fargo, North Dakota 58103

Dear Dr. Tillisch:

This letter describes the results of a Food and Drug Administration (FDA) inspection that concluded on April 9, 2013. The FDA investigators met with you to review your conduct of the following clinical studies:

(b)(4)

(b)(4)

The FDA conducted this inspection under the Bioresearch Monitoring Program, which includes inspections designed to review the conduct of research involving investigational drugs.

At the end of the inspection a Form FDA 483, Inspectional Observations, was issued and discussed with you. We received and reviewed your letter dated April 24, 2013 ("Response Letter"), in response to the Form FDA 483.

We have determined that you violated regulations governing the proper conduct of clinical studies involving investigational new drugs, as published in Title 21, Code of Federal Regulations (CFR) Part 312 (available at http://www.gpoaccess.gov/cfr/index.html). The applicable provisions of the CFR are cited for each violation listed below.

1. You failed to fulfill the general responsibilities of an investigator. [21 CFR § 312.60 and Part 50].

An investigator is responsible for ensuring that an investigation is conducted according to the signed investigator statement, the investigational plan, and applicable regulations; for protecting the rights, safety, and welfare of subjects under the investigator's care; and, for the control of drugs under investigation. When you signed the investigator statement (Form FDA 1572) for the above-referenced clinical investigations on May 16, 2011, you specifically agreed to personally conduct the clinical studies or to supervise those aspects of the studies that you did not personally conduct. While you may delegate certain study tasks to individuals qualified to perform them, such delegation requires adequate supervision of those to whom you delegate authority. You are responsible for the oversight of study personnel and for reviewing the work of study personnel to ensure that they follow the investigational plan and procedures.

Our investigation indicates that you delegated to the Site Management Organization (SMO), **(b)(4)** the conduct of the study visits and the completion of study records for such visits, including Case Report Forms (CRFs). There is no evidence that you adequately oversaw and reviewed the study activities you delegated to **(b)(4)**. As described below, it appears that you failed to review study records generated by **(b)(4)** with reasonable care, including by failing to ensure that you had access to certain source documents while the studies were ongoing. Your lack of supervision and personal involvement resulted in failure to ensure that the study was conducted according to the signed investigator statement, the investigational plan, and applicable regulations.

A. Based on the available information, it appears that, while the studies were ongoing, you did not have access to certain source records ("electronic diaries" or "e-diaries") in which subjects recorded adverse event information and other observations pertinent to the subject's case history. As a result, you placed subjects at risk because you did not promptly review and evaluate adverse events to determine their seriousness and relationship to the investigational product, and to perform any necessary medical intervention. In addition, as described below in item 2, you failed to ensure that adverse events were recorded in CRFs as required by the protocol.

In your Response Letter you explain that you were issued a password to access the e-diaries. Please explain when you received access to the e-diaries and when the e-diaries were accessible to you for review.

B. As described below in item 3, multiple study records, including CRFs, were incomplete or missing.

In your Response Letter you explain that **(b)(4)** managed key aspects of your clinical trials, including clinical study coordination and recordkeeping. You further explain that **(b)(4)** abruptly closed in August 2012 and did not provide you with documentation or information for any of the trials they managed. As noted above, while you may delegate certain study tasks to individuals qualified to perform them, such delegation requires adequate supervision. Had you, as the clinical investigator, reviewed the study records with reasonable care, these recordkeeping deficiencies would have been obvious to you.

2. You failed to ensure that the investigation was conducted according to the signed investigator statement, the investigational plan, and the applicable regulations in order to protect the rights, safety, and welfare of subjects under your care. [21 CFR § 312.60].

A. The following adverse events were recorded in the subjects' e-diaries but were not reported in the Adverse Event Log of the CRFs as required by section 9.12.2 of the protocol for Study **(b)(4)**

i. **(b)(4), (b)(6)**

ii. **(b)(4), (b)(6)**

iii. **(b)(4), (b)(6)**

iv. **(b)(4), (b)(6)**

B. Section 7.8 of the protocol for Study **(b)(4)** requires that an effort must be made to determine why subjects failed to return for the necessary visits and that information detailing why a subject fails to return for the necessary visits or is discontinued from the study, as well as the date of withdrawal, will be recorded on the study outcome CFR. This requirement was not met for the following two subjects:

i. **(b)(4), (b)(6)**

ii. **(b)(4), (b)(6)**

In your Response Letter you did not address these findings. Please provide a written response.

3. You failed to prepare and maintain adequate and accurate case histories recording all observations and other data pertinent to the investigation on each individual administered the investigational drug, including case report forms and supporting data. [21 CFR § 312.62(b)].

A. **(b)(4), (b)(6)**

In your Response Letter you did not address this finding. Please provide a written response.

B. The following recordkeeping deficiencies were observed during the inspection:

STUDY **(b)(4)**

i. **(b)(4), (b)(6)**

ii. **(b)(4), (b)(6)**

iii. **(b)(4), (b)(6)**

In your Response Letter you did not address these findings. Please provide a written response.

STUDY **(b)(4)**

iv. **(b)(4), (b)(6)**

v. **(b)(4), (b)(6)**

a.**(b)(4), (b)(6)**

b.**(b)(4), (b)(6)**

In your Response Letter you did not address this finding. Please provide a written response.

vi. **(b)(4), (b)(6)**

a.**(b)(4), (b)(6)**

b.**(b)(4), (b)(6)**

c.**(b)(4), (b)(6)**

Items vi. a. and b. were not addressed in your Response Letter. Item vi. c. was not on the Form FDA 483. Please provide a written response to items vi. a-c.

STUDIES **(b)(4)**

vii. Multiple CRFs contained an incorrect header showing the name and site number of another investigator.

In your Response Letter you acknowledge that certain CRFs had incorrect headers. You explain that the headers were later corrected by Essentia Health staff during the internal review of the study, after notification of the **(b)(4)** closure. You further explain that the headers corrected by Essentia Health staff were not dated, timed, or initialed and the staff who made the corrections are no longer available to be contacted.

This letter is not intended to be an allinclusive list of deficiencies with your clinical studies of investigational vaccines. It is your responsibility to ensure adherence to each requirement of the law and relevant regulations.

In your Response Letter you describe corrective actions to address both the **(b)(4)** closure and the conduct of research studies in general. We request that you provide the additional information requested in this letter.

Within fifteen (15) business days of receipt of this letter, please provide written documentation of the actions you will take to correct these violations and prevent the recurrence of similar violations in current and future studies for which you are the clinical investigator. Failure to respond to this letter and to take appropriate corrective action could result in FDA taking regulatory action without further notice to you. For instance, FDA could initiate disqualification proceedings against you in accordance with 21 CFR 312.70. If you do not believe you are in violation of FDA requirements, include your reasoning and any supporting information for our consideration.

Please send your written response to:

Christine Drabick
Division of Inspections and Surveillance (HFM-664)
Office of Compliance and Biologics Quality
Center for Biologics Evaluation and Research
1401 Rockville Pike, Suite 200N
Rockville, Maryland 20852-1488
Telephone: 301-827-6323

We also request that you send a copy of your response to the FDA District Office listed below.

Sincerely,

/S/

Mary A. Malarkey, Director
Office of Compliance and Biologics Quality
Center for Biologics Evaluation and Research
Cc: Michael Dutcher, District Director

Food and Drug Administration
250 Marquette Avenue, Suite 600
Minneapolis, Minnesota 55401

第 85 封　给 Doft, Bernard H. 医学博士的警告信

2013年6月12日

参考号：13-HFD-45-05-01

尊敬的Doft博士：

2012年9月17日至9月28日，Erica Nicoll女士代表FDA，在贵临床研究机构，对您所开展的试验药物为血管抑制剂（兰尼单抗），申办者为基因泰克公司的试验方案FVF4579，"一项观察黄斑下新生血管性老年性黄斑变性的患者每月注射或者按需要注射0.5mg及2.0mg的血管抑制剂的有效性和安全性的Ⅲ期、双盲、多中心、随机、阳性治疗对照研究"进行了现场检查。这封警告信特告知您现场检查中发现的违规情况。

本次现场检查是FDA的生物研究监查项目的一部分。该项目通过设定的检查方法，对FDA监管的相关研究的实施情况进行评估，以确认研究数据在科学上是有效和准确的，并帮助确保这些研究中受试者的权益、安全和福利得到了保护。

在现场检查结束时，Nicoll女士向您出示了FDA483表，即现场检查发现的问题，并与您进行了讨论。您2012年10月8日对该FDA483表的书面回复已收悉。

经对现场检查报告、该报告的附件，以及您2012年10月8日的书面回复进行审查，我们认为，您没有遵循适用的法律要求和监管临床研究实施及受试者保护的FDA法规。我们想强调以下几点：

1. 您未能确保按照研究计划进行研究［21 CFR 312.60］

作为一名临床研究者，您必须确保您的临床研究按照研究计划进行。研究计划要求您遵循试验方案（例如仅入组符合入组标准的受试者，由具备资质的人员进行视敏度检测，确保视敏度检测由对研究眼保持盲态的人员进行）。您未能遵守这些要求。具体而言：

a. 试验方案4.1.2"入组标准"部分要求受试者使用糖尿病视网膜病变早期治疗研究（EDTRS）量表评价的最佳矫正视敏度（BCVA）在20/40~20/320（斯内伦当量）之间。两名不符合入组标准的受试者入组研究。受试者704201在第0天时最佳矫正视敏度为20/32及受试者704220在筛选时最佳矫正视敏度为20/400。

b. 试验方案附录G规定"最佳矫正视敏度必须由试验场所经过培训且有资格的人员进行测量"。在14例中有5名受试者（受试者704201、704202、704203、704204和704205）的最佳矫正视敏度由不具备资格的人员测量。具体而言，受试者704201有3次访视发生这种情况；受试者704202有3次访视；受试者704203有2次访视；受试者704204有3次访视；受试者704205有3次访视。

c. 试验方案4.2.2部分规定"对于研究眼保持盲态的视敏度检查人员将实施折射、视敏度评估及低亮度测试等非直接患者医疗护理任务"。您的视敏度检查人员在共计35次方案违背情况中对9名受试者（受试者编号704201、704202、704203、704204、704205、704206、704207、704208、704209）进行了眼内压检测并未对研究眼保持盲态。

我们确认您于2012年10月8日的书面回复中声明您已执行了14号SOP"预筛、筛选及随机流程"、23号SOP"确认研究人员资质"、24号SOP"筛选失败患者"及25号SOP"受试者随访流程"。如果恰当地贯彻执行这些SOP，将防止类似违背在未来重复发生。然而，确认试验方案FVF4579按照研究计划操作是您作为临床研究者的职责，包括确认仅入组符合入组标准的受试者、由具备资质的人员进行视敏度检测、确保视敏度检测由研究眼保持盲态的人员进行。

入组不符合筛选标准及由未确认资格及未完全保持盲态的检查人员检测视敏度，将引起对于您的试验场

所收集的数据正确性及完整性的关注。

2. 您未能保存研究中使用试验药物或对照组的受试者的所有研究观察结果和其他相关数据的足够及准确的病历［21 CFR 312.62（b）］

作为一名临床研究者，您必须准备并保存研究中使用试验药物或对照组的受试者的所有研究观察结果和其他相关数据的足够及准确的病历。对于试验方案FVF4579，病历包括基因泰克视敏度工作表。您未能保存足够和准确的病历，因为未确保在基因泰克视敏度工作表上列明的检测人员与受试者病历一致。

此次现场检查显示，10例记录于基因泰克视敏度工作表的视敏度检测人员不是记录于受试者病历中操作检测的人员。在本研究中心共计23名受试者中5名出现违背（22%）。具体而言：

- 受试者704201：2份基因泰克视敏度工作表未能准确确认谁操作视敏度检测。
- 受试者704202：2份基因泰克视敏度工作表未能准确确认谁操作视敏度检测。
- 受试者704203：1份基因泰克视敏度工作表未能准确确认谁操作视敏度检测。
- 受试者704204：3份基因泰克视敏度工作表未能准确确认谁操作视敏度检测。
- 受试者704205：2份基因泰克视敏度工作表未能准确确认谁操作视敏度检测。

我们确认您2012年10月8日的回复中声明的您实施了26号SOP“原始文件的准备”。如果恰当地贯彻执行这个SOP将避免类似违背在未来重复发生。然而，准备并保存足够及准确的病历记录与每个给予研究药物或作为对照的个体的研究相关的所有观察结果和其他数据是您作为一名临床研究者的职责。

您未能保存足够及准确的病历，包括未能确保研究人员的姓名及签名准确记录于基因泰克视敏度工作表，将引起对于您中心采集的数据的准确性、可靠性和完整性的关注。

3. 您未能按 21 CFR 50 的要求获得知情同意［21 CFR 312.60，21 CFR 50.20］

作为一名临床研究者，按照21 CFR 50的规定获得知情同意是您的职责。美国食品药品监督管理局的21 CFR 50.20说明除21 CFR 50.23及21 CFR 50.24条款之外，研究者在获得受试者或受试者法定代表的合法有效的知情同意之前，不可以让受试者参与研究。您未能获得合法有效的知情同意。

具体而言，两名受试者（受试者10461和10620）在签署知情同意书之前已开始执行试验流程（即最佳矫正视敏度、眼内压、眼成像、荧光素血管造影、光学相干层析成像、扩瞳或实验室样本采集）。受试者10461于2010年3月18日签署知情同意书，但自2009年12月开始执行筛选流程（最佳矫正视敏度、眼内压、荧光素血管造影、光学相干层析成像和扩瞳）。

受试者10620于2010年1月28日签署知情同意书，但在签署知情同意书当天之前已开始执行筛选流程，包括最佳矫正视敏度及扩瞳。另外，我们发现，受试者10620似乎无法阅读知情同意书，因为知情同意书是在受试者扩瞳之后提供给受试者。

我们确认您于2012年10月8日的书面回复中说明您执行了几个流程，包括8号SOP“知情同意”和27号SOP“口头知情同意”及知情同意书预警系统。如果恰当地贯彻执行这些流程将避免类似的违规在未来重复发生。然而，按照21 CFR 50的规定，获得知情同意是您作为一名临床研究者的职责。您未能按照21 CFR 50的规定在受试者进入研究之前获得知情同意，将引起对于您的试验场所入组受试者的保护的质疑。

本警告信的目的并非是罗列您在试验药物临床研究中存在的所有缺陷。确保遵循法律和相关FDA法规的每一项要求是您的职责，您应当解决这些缺陷，并建立规程，以确保任何正在进行或将来进行的研究均符合FDA的法规。

自收到这封信的15个工作日内，您应当书面告知本办公室为预防将来发生类似违规情况而采取的措施。如果不能充分、迅速地解释上述违规问题，可能导致我们在不再通知的情况下采取监管措施。如果您确信您于2012年10月08日的对于FDA483表格的书面回复，充分说明了您在未来为避免类似违规而采取的措施，请在15个工作日内与我们联系。您对此封信的回复可参考10月8日的书面回复。

附：英文原文

Doft, Bernard H. M.D.

WARNING LETTER

Jun 12, 2013

CERTIFIED MAIL
RETURN RECEIPT REQUESTED

Ref: 13-HFD-45-05-01

Bernard H. Doft, M.D.
3501 Forbes Ave. Suite 500
Pittsburgh, PA 15213-3327

Dear Dr. Doft:

This Warning Letter informs you of objectionable conditions observed during the U.S. Food and Drug Administration (FDA) inspection conducted at your clinical site between September 17, 2012, and September 28, 2012. Ms. Erica Nicoll, representing the FDA, reviewed your conduct of a clinical investigation (Protocol FVF4579), titled “A Phase Ⅲ, Double-Masked, Multicenter, Randomized, Active Treatment-Controlled Study of the Efficacy and Safety of 0.5 mg and 2.0 mg Ranibizumab Administered Monthly or on an As-Needed Basis (PRN) in Patients with Subfoveal NeovascularAge-Related Macular Degeneration”, of the investigational drug, ranibizumab (Lucentis®), performed for Genentech, Inc.

This inspection is a part of FDA’s Bioresearch Monitoring Program, which includes inspections designed to evaluate the conduct of FDA-regulated research to ensure that the data are scientifically valid and accurate, and to help ensure that the rights, safety, and welfare of the human subjects of those studies have been protected.

At the conclusion of the inspection, Ms. Nicoll presented and discussed with you Form FDA 483,Inspectional Observations. We acknowledge receipt of your October 8, 2012 written response to the Form FDA 483.

From our review of the FDA’s Establishment Inspection Report, the documents submitted with that report, and your October 8, 2012 written response, we conclude that you did not adhere to the applicable statutory requirements and FDA regulations governing the conduct of clinical investigations and the protection of human subjects. We wish to emphasize the following:

1. You failed to ensure that the investigation was conducted according to the investigational plan [21 CFR 312.60].

As a clinical investigator, you are required to ensure that your clinical studies are conducted in accordance with the investigational plan. The investigational plan requires that you ensure adherence to protocol (e.g., enrolling only subjects who meet the eligibility criteria, using certified personnel for visual acuity (VA) testing, and ensuring that VA testing was performed by personnel properly masked to the study eye). You failed to adhere to these requirements.

Specifically:

a. Protocol Section 4.1.2 “Inclusion Criteria” requires the subject to have a Best Corrected Visual Acuity (BCVA), using Early Treatment Diabetic Retinopathy Study (EDTRS) charts, of 20/40−20/320 (Snellen equivalent). Two subjects who did not meet this inclusion criterion were included in the study. Subject #704201 had a BCVA of 20/32 at Day 0 and Subject # 704220 had a BCVA of 20/400 at screening.

b. Protocol Appendix G states that the “Best corrected visual acuity (BCVA) will be measured by trained and certified personnel at the study sites". BCVA was measured by uncertified personnel in 5 subjects (Subjects 704201, 704202, 704203, 704204 and 704205) in 14 instances.

Specifically, this occurred for Subject# 704201 on 3 visits; Subject# 704202 on 3 visits; Subject# 704203 on 2 visits; Subject# 704204 on 3 visits; and Subject# 704205 on 3 visits.

c. Protocol Section 4.2.2 states “the VA examiner will be masked to the patient’s study eye and will conduct refraction, VA assessments, and low luminance testing . . . No other direct patient care tasks can be performed by the VA examiner”. Your VA examiners measured the intraocular pressure (IOP), without being masked to the study eye, in nine subjects (Subject# 704201, 704202, 704203, 704204, 704205, 704206, 704207, 704208, and 704209) for a total of 35 documented protocol violations.

We acknowledge that, in your October 8, 2012 written response to the Form FDA 483, you stated that you have implemented Standard Operating Procedure (SOP) # 14 “Prescreening, Screening, and Randomization Procedures,” SOP # 23 “Certification of Research Personnel,” SOP # 24 “Screen Failure Patients,” and SOP # 25 “Subject Visit Procedure.” If properly implemented and executed, these SOPs appear adequate to prevent recurrence of similar violations in the future. However, it was your responsibility as the clinical investigator to ensure that Protocol FVF4579 was conducted in accordance with the investigational plan, including ensuring that only subjects that met eligibility criteria were enrolled, that subjects had BCVA measurements performed by certified personnel, and that VA measurements were made by personnel properly masked to the study eye.

Enrollment of subjects who do not meet eligibility criteria and failure to ensure that certified and properly masked evaluators measured VAraise concern about the validity and integrity of the data collected at your site.

2. You failed to maintain adequate and accurate case histories that record all observations and other data pertinent to the investigation on each individual administered the investigational drug or employed as a control in the investigation [21 CFR 312.62(b)].

As a clinical investigator, you are required to prepare and maintain adequate and accurate case histories that record all observations and other data pertinent to the investigation on each individual administered the investigational drug or employed as a control in the investigation. For Protocol FVF4579, case histories include the Genentech Visual Acuity Worksheets. You have failed to maintain adequate and accurate case histories by failing to ensure that Genentech Visual Acuity Worksheets accurately listed the person who conducted exams as documented in subjects’ medical charts.

Our inspection revealed 10 examples in which the VA Examiner listed in the Genentech Visual Acuity (VA) Worksheets was not the person conducting the exams as documented in the subjects’ medical charts. These violations occurred in 5 of the 23 total subjects (22%) at this site. Specifically:

- Subject # 704201: 2 Genentech VA Worksheets did not accurately identify who conducted the VA exams.
- Subject # 704202: 2 Genentech VA Worksheets did not accurately identify who conducted the VA exams.
- Subject # 704203: 1 Genentech VA Worksheet did not accurately identify who conducted the VA exams.
- Subject # 704204: 3 Genentech VA Worksheets did not accurately identify who conducted the VA exams.
- Subject # 704205: 2 Genentech VA Worksheets did not accurately identify who conducted the VA exams

We acknowledge that, in your October 8, 2012 written response, you stated that you have implemented SOP # 26 “Preparation of Source Documents.” If properly implemented and executed, this SOP appears adequate to prevent recurrence of similar violations in the future. However, as the clinical investigator, it was your responsibility to prepare and maintain adequate and accurate case histories that record all observations and other data pertinent to the investigation on each individual administered the investigational drug or employed as a control in the investigation.

Your failure to maintain adequate and accurate case histories, including the failure to ensure that the names and signatures of study personnel were accurately recorded on the Genentech VA Worksheets, raises concerns about the validity, reliability, and integrity of data captured at your site.

3. You failed to obtain informed consent in accordance with the provisions of 21 CFR par 50 [21 CFR 312.60, 21 CFR 50.20].

As a clinical investigator, it is your responsibility to obtain informed consent in accordance with 21 CFR Part 50. FDA regulations at 21 CFR 50.20 state that except as provided in 21 CFR 50.23 and 21 CFR 50.24, no investigator may involve a human being as a subject in research covered by the regulations unless the investigator has obtained the legally effective informed consent of the subject or the subject’s legally authorized representative. You failed to obtain legally effective informed consent.

Specifically, two subjects (Subject #10461 and #10620) underwent study procedures (i.e., BCVA, IOP, ocular imaging, fluorescein angiograms, optical coherence tomography, eye dilation, or the collection o laboratory examples) prior to signing the informed consent form. Subject #10461 signed the informed consent form on 03/18/2010, but underwent screening procedures (BCVA, IOP, fluorescein angiograms, optical coherence tomography and dilation of the eyes) in December 2009.

Subject #10620 signed the informed consent form on 01/28/2010, but underwent screening procedures including BCVA and dilation of the eyes, prior to signing the consent form on the same day. Additionally, we note that it appears as if subject #10620 could not read the informed consent form, because the form was provided to the subject after the subject's eyes were dilated.

We acknowledge that, in your October 8, 2012 written response, you stated that you have implemented several procedures including SOP # 8 "Informed Consent" and SOP # 27 "Oral Informed Consent" as well as a consent form alert system. If properly implemented and executed, these procedures appear adequate to prevent recurrence of similar violations in the future. However, as the clinical investigator, it was your responsibility to obtain informed consent in accordance with 21 CFR Part 50. Your failure to obtain informed consent in accordance with 21 CFR Part 50 prior to involving subjects in research raises concerns about your protection of study subjects enrolled at your site.

This letter is not intended to be an all-inclusive list of deficiencies with your clinical study of an investigational drug. It is your responsibility to ensure adherence to each requirement of the law and relevant FDA regulations. You should address these deficiencies and establish procedures to ensure that any ongoing or future studies will be in compliance with FDA regulations.

Within fifteen (15) working days of your receipt of this letter, you should notify this office in writing of the actions you have taken to prevent similar violations in the future. Failure to address the violations noted above adequately and promptly may result in regulatory action without further notice. If you believe that your written response to the Form FDA 483 dated October 8, 2012, fully explains the actions you have taken to prevent similar violations in the future, please communicate that to us in writing within fifteen (15) business days. You may reference the written response dated October 8, 2012, in your response to this letter.

If you have any questions, please contact Susan Thompson, M.D., at 301-796-0823; FAX 301-847-8748. Your written response and any pertinent documentation should be addressed to:

Susan Thompson, M.D.
Acting Branch Chief
Good Clinical Practice Assessment Branch
Division of Good Clinical Practice Compliance
Office of Scientific Investigations
Office of Compliance
Center for Drug Evaluation and Research
Food and Drug Administration
Building 51, Room 5350
10903 New Hampshire Avenue
Silver Spring, MD 20993

Sincerely yours,

{See appended electronic signature page}

Thomas N. Moreno, M.S.
Acting Director
Office of Scientific Investigations
Office of Compliance
Center for Drug Evaluation and Research
Food and Drug Administration

第 86 封　给 Frazer, Henry A. 博士的警告信

2013年6月5日

参考号：13-HFD-45-05-02

尊敬的Frazer博士：

2012年9月24日至10月3日，Kimberly Dutzek女士代表FDA，在贵临床研究中心，对您所开展的以下临床研究进行了审查：

试验方案（b）（4）[1]，“（b）（4）”，试验药物为（b）（4），申办者为（b）（4）；

试验方案（b）（4），“（b）（4）”，试验药物为（b）（4），申办者为（b）（4）。

这封警告信特告知您现场检查中发现的违规情况。

本次现场检查是FDA的生物研究监查项目的一部分。该项目通过设定的检查方法，对FDA监管的相关研究的实施情况进行评估，以确认研究数据在科学上是有效和准确的，并帮助确保这些研究中受试者的权益、安全和福利得到了保护。

在现场检查结束时，Dutzek女士向您出示了FDA483表，即现场检查发现的问题，并与您进行了讨论。您2012年10月3日对该FDA483表的书面回复已收悉。

经对现场检查报告、该报告的附件，以及您2012年10月3日的书面回复进行审查，我们认为，您没有遵循适用的法律要求和监管临床研究实施的FDA法规。我们想强调以下几点：

1. 您未能确保按照研究计划进行研究［21 CFR 312.60］

作为一名临床研究者，您必须保证您的临床研究按照研究计划进行。您未能遵循这些要求，具体来说：

a. 试验方案（b）（4）要求您在V2访视的时候，在做手术之前发放一个手持式的电子设备（LogPad）给受试者，并且受试者在这个LogPad中记录在研究过程中的疼痛评估。在2011年3月4日，您没有在受试者09-006V2访视的时候发放这个LogPad，因为受试者使用了镇静剂并且带着呼吸机。此外，受试者09-006的五次疼痛评估是由研究协调员录入到LogPad，而不是受试者本人。在现场检查过程中，研究协调员指出，当时受试者无法给出疼痛分数，她是使用了受试者的登陆密码输入的受试者疼痛评估。

在您2012年10月3日的书面回复中，您承认当时没有在手术前将LogPad发给受试者09-006。您提到，在手术之后受试者带着呼吸机，使用了镇静剂，无法通过LogPad或者其他方式进行疼痛评估。

在您的书面回复中，您指出您的研究协调员是基于从研究护士或受研究受试者处得到的信息直接在LogPad中进行的录入。您指出，研究协调员录入的疼痛分数是：“基于研究护士对患者疼痛级别的猜测（原文如此），证据（原文如此）是患者的抽搐和脸上痛苦的表情。”您还表明：“有时受试者不愿意完成疼痛数值或者不清楚如何在日志或LogPad中记录，（研究协调员）询问了受试者疼痛值并将数值录入日志中，然后写上了患者的姓名缩写”。

您指出，当您获知这个操作之后，贵试验现场已经入组了八名受试者，并且所有人均已完成试验。您同时指出，监查员质疑了疼痛值的有效性。

您的回复是不充分的。虽然您解释了违规是怎么发生的，但是您未能提供防止类似的违规情况将来再次发生的纠正措施计划。

根据您的书面回复，我们关注您的研究协调员可能也在其他受试者的LogPad中不恰当地录入了数据。

---

1 （b）（4）涉及商业秘密，根据法规内容不予公开。

我们要求您书面告知我们，哪些疼痛评估数据不是直接从受试者处获得的，除了受试者外还有哪些人在LogPads中录入了受试者疼痛评估的数据；以及您打算如何防止以后再次发生类似的违规情况。

由于未能确保按照方案的要求仅由受试者录入疼痛评估的数据，在贵试验现场采集的数据其有效性和可靠性均受到了损害。

b. 试验方案（b）（4）要求受试者的身体状况为美国麻醉医师协会（ASA）规定的1~3等级，Q-Tc间期小于450毫秒，以符合入组资格。受试者09-006不符合这些入组标准。2011年3月4日手术当天，受试者09-006的ASA的身体状况等级为4，这是定义为有严重的全身性疾病且有生命威胁的患者。此外，受试者09-006手术当天的Q-Tc间期为453毫秒。因此，受试者09-006不符合试验方案（b）（4）的入组标准。

在您2012年10月3日的书面回复中，您未能对上述条目1.b.的内容进行回复。另外，您未能提供纠正措施计划来防止类似的违规将来再次发生。

入组不符合标准的受试者是对受试者安全和福利的危害，并且引发了我们对在贵试验现场采集数据的有效性和可靠性的关注。

c. 试验方案（b）（4）要求从第0天到完成试验期间禁止使用止痛药扑热息痛和盐酸羟考酮。

i. 2010年12月16日到18日，受试者31-003接受了止痛药扑热息痛的多次给药。

ii. 2011年3月4日到14日期间，受试者09-005接受了止痛药（盐酸羟考酮）的多次给药。

在您2012年10月3日的书面回复中，您未能对上述条目1.c.进行回复。另外，您未能提供纠正措施计划来防止类似的违背将来再次发生。

您在研究过程中未能防止对禁用的止痛药的管理和使用，阻止了对研究药物单独使用的治疗效果的评估，对数据的可靠性造成了损害。

2. 您未能保存研究中使用试验药物或对照组的受试者的所有研究观察结果和其他相关数据的足够及准确的病历［21 CFR 312.62（b）］

作为一名研究者，您必须准备和保存对研究中使用试验药物或对照组的受试者的所有研究观察结果和其他相关数据的足够及准确的病历。对试验方案（b）（4），病历包含录入到LogPad的数据。您未能足够、准确地保存病历，具体来说：

试验方案（b）（4）要求受试者在研究过程中将疼痛评估的情况记录在LogPad中。对受试者09-006，LogPad中包含据称是受试者本人所做并录入的评估情况，然而，有五次疼痛评估是由研究协调员录入的，并且反映的是研究协调员或者研究护士的评估，而不是受试者本人的评估。

在现场检查过程中，您的研究协调员指出，当受试者无法提供疼痛数值的时候，她使用了受试者的登陆号码并且在LogPad中录入了受试者的疼痛评估分数。在您2012年10月3日的书面回复中，您提到，在手术之后受试者戴着呼吸机，使用了镇静剂，无法通过LogPad或者其他方式进行疼痛评估。

在您的书面回复中，您还指出研究协调员是基于从研究护士或研究受试者处得到的信息直接在LogPad中进行的录入。您指出研究协调员录入的疼痛分数是“基于研究护士对患者疼痛级别的猜测（原文如此），证据（原文如此）是患者的抽搐和脸上痛苦的表情。”您还表明“有时受试者不愿意完成疼痛数值或者不清楚如何在日志或LogPad中记录，（研究协调员）询问了受试者疼痛值并将数值录入日志中，然后写上了患者的姓名缩写”。

您指出，当您获知这个操作之后，贵试验现场已经入组了八名受试者，并且所有人均已完成试验。您同时指出，监查员质疑了疼痛值的有效性。

您的回复是不充分的。虽然您解释了违规是怎么发生的，但是您没有提供任何信息来降低这些违背对数据的完整性、可靠性和有效性造成的严重影响。此外，您未能提供纠正措施计划来防止类似的违规情况将来再次发生。

基于您的回复，我们关注除了受试者09-006的记录外，其他受试者的记录也可能包含来源于LogPad的不准确的数据。我们要求您通过书面形式通知我们，哪些疼痛评估数据不是直接从受试者处获得的，除了受试者外还有哪些人在LogPads中录入了受试者疼痛评估的数据；以及您打算如何防止以后再次发生类似的违背。

因您未能完整和准确地维护疼痛评估从而导致未能保存足够及准确的病历，对在贵研究中心获取数据的有效性和可靠性造成了损害。

附：英文原文

Frazer, Henry A. Pharm D.

WARNING LETTER

JUN 05, 2013

CERTIFIED MAIL
RETURN RECEIPT REQUESTED

Ref: 13-HFD-45-05-02

Henry A. Frazer, Pharm.D.
1758 Park Place, Suite 200
Montgomery, AL 36106-1134

Dear Dr. Frazer:

This Warning Letter informs you of objectionable conditions observed during the U.S. Food and Drug Administration (FDA) inspection conducted at your clinical site between September 24 and October 3, 2012. Ms. Kimberly Dutzek, representing FDA, reviewed your conduct of the following clinical investigations:

- Protocol (b)(4), "(b)(4)," of the investigational drug (b)(4), performed for (b)(4)
- Protocol (b)(4), "(b)(4)," of the investigational drug (b)(4), performed for (b)(4).

This inspection is a part of FDA's Bioresearch Monitoring Program, which includes inspections designed to evaluate the conduct of FDA-regulated research to ensure that the data are scientifically valid and accurate, and to help ensure that the rights, safety, and welfare of the human subjects involved in those studies have been protected.

At the conclusion of the inspection, Ms. Dutzek presented and discussed with you Form FDA 483, Inspectional Observations. We acknowledge receipt of your October 3, 2012, written response.

From our review of the establishment inspection report, the documents submitted with that report, and your October 3, 2012, written response, we conclude that you did not adhere to the applicable statutor requirements and FDA regulations governing the conduct of clinical investigations. We wish to emphasize the following:

1. You failed to ensure that the investigation was conducted according to the investigational plan [21 CFR 312.60].

As a clinical investigator, you are required to ensure that your clinical studies are conducted in accordance with the investigational plan. You failed to adhere to these requirements. Specifically:

a. Protocol (b)(4) required that you dispense a handheld electronic device (LogPad) to subjects at Visit 2, prior to surgery, and that the subjects record their pain assessments in the LogPad during the study. You did not dispense a LogPad to Subject 09-006 at Visit 2 on March 4, 2011, because the subject was sedated and on a ventilator. In addition, five pain assessments for Subject 09-006 were entered into the LogPad by the study coordinator, rather than by the subject. During the inspection, your study coordinator indicated that she used the subject's login code and entered the subject's pain assessment scores into the LogPad when the subject was unable to provide a pain score.

In your October 3, 2012, written response, you acknowledged that the LogPad was not dispensed to Subject 09-

006 prior to surgery. You noted that after surgery, the subject was put on a "vent" (ventilator), was sedated, and was unable to participate in the evaluation of pain, via the LogPad or otherwise.

In your written response, you indicated that your study coordinator entered data directly into the LogPad, based on information she received either from the nursing staff or from study subjects. You indicated that your study coordinator entered pain scores "based on the staff nurses [sic] educated guess as to the pain level when the patient was obviously in pain as evidence of [sic] the patient's tossing and painful expressions on the patient's face." You also stated that "at times when the patient was either unwilling to complete the pain score or too disoriented to write into the diary or use the LogPad, [your study coordinator] asked the patient what her pain score was and entered that value onto the diary and added the patient's initials."

You indicated that by the time you became aware of this practice, your site had enrolled 8 subjects into the study, and all of them had completed the trial. You also indicated that the monitors challenged the validity of the pain data.

Your response is inadequate. Although you explained how the violation occurred, you failed to provide a corrective action plan to prevent recurrence of similar violations in the future.

Based on your written response, we have concerns that your study coordinator may have inappropriately entered data into the LogPad for other subjects, as well. We request that you inform us, in writing, of the extent to which pain assessment data were not obtained directly from the subjects; the extent to which anyone other than the subjects entered pain assessment data into LogPads; and how you intend to prevent the recurrence of similar violations in the future.

By failing to ensure that pain assessment data were entered only by the subjects, as required by the protocol, you compromised the validity and integrity of data collected at your site.

b. Protocol (b)(4) required that subjects have an American Society of Anesthesiologists (ASA) Physical Status Classification of 1 to 3 and a QTc interval shorter than 450 milliseconds in order to be eligible for enrollment. Subject 09-006 did not meet these inclusion criteria. On March 4, 2011, the day of surgery, Subject 09-006 had an ASA Physical Status Classification of 4, which is defined as a patient with a severe systemic disease that is a constant threat to life. In addition, Subject 09-006 had a QTc interval of 453 milliseconds on the day of surgery. Consequently, Subject 09-006 was ineligible for Protocol (b)(4).

In your October 3, 2012, written response, you failed to respond to Item 1.b. above. In addition, you failed to provide a corrective action plan to prevent recurrence of similar violations in the future.

Enrollment of subjects who do not meet eligibility criteria jeopardizes subject safety and welfare, and raises concerns about the validity and integrity of the data collected at your site.

c. Protocol (b)(4) prohibited the use of pain medications Percocet and Oxycontin (oxycodone hydrochloride) from Day 0 through completion of the trial.

1. From December 16 to December 18, 2010, Subject 31-003 received multiple doses of Percocet.
2. From March 4 to March 14, 2011, Subject 09-005 received multiple doses of oxycodone.

In your October 3, 2012, written response, you failed to respond to Item 1.c. above. In addition, you failed to provide a corrective action plan to prevent recurrence of similar violations in the future.

Your failure to prevent the administration and use of prohibited pain medications during the study compromised data integrity by prohibiting an evaluation of the therapeutic benefit of the study drug alone.

2. You failed to prepare and maintain adequate and accurate case histories that record all observations and other data pertinent to the investigation on each individual administered the investigational drug or employed as a control in the investigation [21 CFR 312.62(b)].

As a clinical investigator, you are required to prepare and maintain adequate and accurate case histories that record all observations and other data pertinent to the investigation on each individual administered the investigational drug or employed as a control in the investigation. For Protocol (b) (4), case histories include the data entered into the LogPads. You have failed to maintain adequate an accurate case histories. Specifically:

Protocol (b)(4) required that the subjects record their pain assessments in the LogPad during the study. For Subject 09-006, the LogPad contained assessments purportedly made and entered by the subject; however, five pain assessments were entered by the study coordinator and reflect the study coordinator's or nursing staff's assessments, rather than the subject's assessments.

During the inspection, your study coordinator indicated that she used the subject's login code and entered the subject's pain-assessment scores into the LogPad when the subject was unable to provide pain score. In your October 3, 2012, written response, you noted that after surgery, the subject was put on a "vent" (ventilator), was sedated, and was unable to participate in the evaluation of pain, via the LogPad or otherwise.

In your written response, you also indicated that your study coordinator entered data directly into the LogPads, based on information received either from the nursing staff or from study subjects. You indicated that your study coordinator entered pain scores "based on the staff nurses [sic] educated guess as to the pain level when the patient was obviously in pain as evidence of [sic] the patient's tossing and painful expressions on the patient's face." You also stated that "at times when the patient was either unwilling to complete the pain score or too disoriented to write into the diary or use the LogPad, [your study coordinator] asked the patient what her pain score was and entered that value onto the diary and added the patient's initials."

You indicated that by the time you became aware of this practice, your site had enrolled 8 subjects int the study, and all of them had completed the trial. You also indicated that the monitors challenged the validity of the pain data.

Your response is inadequate. Although you explained how the violation occurred, you did not provide any information that would mitigate the violation's significant impact on data integrity, reliability, and validity. In addition, you failed to provide a corrective action plan to prevent recurrence of similar violations in the future.

Based on your written response, we have concerns that, in addition to Subject 09-006's records, other subjects' records may contain inaccurate data from the LogPads. We request that you inform us, in writing, of the extent to which subjects' records contain pain-assessment data that were not obtained directly from the subjects; the extent to which anyone other than the subjects entered pain-assessmen data into LogPads; and how you intend to prevent the recurrence of similar violations in the future.

Your failure to maintain adequate and accurate case histories by failing to maintain adequate and accurate pain assessments compromised the validity and integrity of data captured at your site.

If you have any questions, please contact Constance Cullity, M.D., M.P.H., at 301-796-3397; FAX 301- 847-8748. Your written response and any pertinent documentation should be addressed to:

Constance Cullity,
M. D., M.P.H. Branch Chief
Good Clinical Practice Enforcement Branch
Division of Good Clinical Practice Compliance
Office of Scientific Investigations
Office of Compliance
Center for Drug Evaluation and Research
Food and Drug Administration
Building 51, Room 5354
10903 New Hampshire Avenue
Silver Spring, MD 20993

Sincerely yours,

{See appended electronic signature page}

Thomas N. Moreno, M.S.
Acting Director
Office of Scientific Investigations
Office of Compliance
Center for Drug Evaluation and Research
Food and Drug Administration

第 87 封　给 Joseph-Vempilly, Jose 医学博士的警告信

2013年5月14日

参考号：13-HFD-45-05-01

尊敬的Joseph-Vempilly博士：

2012年9月13日至10月11日，Gulshan Anand博士代表FDA，在贵临床研究中心，对您所开展的申办者为葛兰素史克，试验药物为糠酸氟替卡松/GW642444M 吸入性粉末的临床研究进行了审查。这封警告信特告知您现场检查中发现的违规情况。试验方案HZA106837为“一项长期、随机、双盲、平行分组研究，评估糠酸氟替卡松/GW642444M 吸入性粉末每日一次和糠酸氟替卡松吸入性粉末每日一次在哮喘患者中的应用”。

本次现场检查是FDA的生物研究监查项目的一部分。该项目通过设定的检查方法，对由FDA监管的相关研究的实施情况进行评估，以确认研究数据在科学上是有效和准确的，并帮助确保这些研究中受试者的权益、安全和福利得到了保护。

在现场检查结束时，Anand博士向您出示了FDA483表，即现场检查发现的问题，并与您进行了讨论。您2012年10月16日对该FDA483表的书面回复已收悉。

经对现场检查报告、该报告的附件，以及您2012年10月16日的书面回复进行审查，我们认为，您没有遵循适用的法律要求和监管临床研究实施的FDA法规。我们想特强调以下几点：

1. 您未能确保按照研究计划进行研究［21 CFR 312.60］

作为一名临床研究者，您必须保证您的临床研究按照研究计划进行。您未能遵循这些要求，具体来说：

a. 方案要求受试者在V1访视之前至少提前12周使用批准剂量的吸入性皮质类固醇激素，在V1访视之前至少提前四周使用固定剂量的吸入性皮质类固醇激素。受试者在V1访视和V2访视之间改变哮喘药物的（不含在V1访视时提供的沙丁胺醇/沙丁胺醇吸入型喷雾）将不得进入随机。

i. 受试者00621在V1访视时中断了吸入性皮质类固醇激素（哮喘药物），在V1访视和V2访视期间也未提供吸入性皮质类固醇激素的处方。这名受试者并未被排除随机。

ii. 受试者00624在V1访视之前就停止使用了吸入性皮质类固醇激素。这名受试者并未被排除随机。

iii. 受试者00625在V1访视的时候中断了吸入性皮质类固醇激素，而且在V1和V2访视期间没有给予吸入性皮质类固醇的处方。这名受试者并未被排除随机。

iv. 受试者00626在V1访视之前的一天就停止使用了吸入性皮质类固醇。这名受试者并未被排除随机。

b. 研究方案规定受试者从V1访视开始禁止使用白三烯类拮抗剂。但受试者00638在V1访视之后继续使用了白三烯类拮抗剂。

入组不符合标准的受试者，并且未能保证停止使用方案规定的禁止用药是对受试者安全和福利的危害，由此引发了对在贵试验现场采集数据的有效性和可靠性的关注。

2. 您未能保存研究中使用试验药物或对照组的受试者的所有研究观察结果和其他相关数据的足够及准确的病历［21 CFR 312.62（b）］

作为一名研究者，您必须准备和保存研究中使用试验药物或对照组的受试者的所有研究观察结果和其他相关数据的足够及准确的病历。试验方案HZA106837的病历包含需要在研究的每次访视时记录的血压、脉搏以及体温。关于这些检测指标，您未能保存足够和准确的病历，具体来说：

a. 受试者00621的血压读数、脉搏和体温并未检测，但是却被记录。2011年7月18日的病程记录中阐述了受试者对每次访视没有进行血压、脉搏和体温检测的声明。

b. 受试者00623的血压并未检测，但是却被记录。2011年7月14日的病程记录中阐述了受试者对每次访视没有进行血压检测的声明。

c. 受试者00628的血压读数、脉搏和体温并未检测，但是却被记录。2011年7月15日的病程记录中阐述了受试者对每次访视没有进行血压、脉搏和体温检测的声明。

除了以上的例子，我们没有办法判断对上述受试者的生命体征（如血压、脉搏和体温）进行伪造的程度。然而，在您2012年10月16日的书面回复中，您承认了在上述受试者的病例报告表中录入了生命体征的数据，而其实这些数据并未采集。

因为未能维护适当和准确的病历，具体而言，未能确保记录数据的准确性，您对本试验场所采集数据的有效性和可靠性造成了损害。

我们已收到您在2012年10月16日的书面回复，报告中表明您在2011年7月获知这些发现的时候已经立即将这些向申办者和伦理委员会进行了汇报。我们也收到了您关于询问了所有受试者生命体征测量情况的声明。

我们承认在您2012年10月16日的书面报告中，下列纠正措施计划解决了上述第一条和第二条的违规行为。

- 伪造数据的研究协调员已经被停职；
- 所有研究者和工作人员必须证实他们在进行研究的时候已经阅读并且会遵守部门的标准操作规程；
- 部门会对所有新的研究协调人员进行全面的、标准化的培训和能力评估；
- 医学部研究经理和工作人员会进行持续的内部研究项目监查；
- 所有研究相关的入组标准将会在部门周会上进行审查，而且研究者需要签署资格清单；
- 研究团队将被要求取得强制性的继续教育。

您的回复不充分，因为您没有提供足够的信息能让我们评估您的纠正措施计划的适用性。具体来说，您没有提供您已实施了纠正措施的记录。另外，您的回复并不充分，因为您只提到了您部门需要采取的措施。您未能包含任何您作为临床研究者需要采取的措施，来防止类似的违规行为将来再次发生。

附：英文原文

Joseph-Vempilly, Jose, M.D.

WARNING LETTER

MAY 14, 2013

CERTIFIED MAIL
RETURN RECEIPT REQUESTED

Ref: 13-HFD-45-05-01

Jose Joseph-Vempilly, M.D.
155 N. Fresno Street
Fresno, CA 701-2302

Dear Dr. Joseph-Vempilly:

This Warning Letter informs you of objectionable conditions observed during the U.S. Food and Drug Administration (FDA) inspection conducted at your clinical site between September 13 and October 11, 2012. Gulshan Anand, Ph.D., representing the FDA, reviewed your conduct of a clinical investigation (Protocol HZA106837, "A Long-term, Randomized, Double-blind Parallel Group Study of Fluticasone furoate/GW642444M Inhalation Powder Once Daily and Fluticasone Furoate Inhalation Powder Once- Daily in Subjects with Asthma") of the investigational drug Fluticasone furoate/GW642444M Inhalation Powder, performed for GlaxoSmithKline.

This inspection is a part of FDA's Bioresearch Monitoring Program, which includes inspections designed to evaluate the conduct of FDA regulated research to ensure that the data are scientifically valid and accurate, and to help ensure that the rights, safety, and welfare of the human subjects of those studies have been protected.

At the conclusion of the inspection, Dr. Anand presented and discussed with you Form FDA 483, Inspectional Observations. We acknowledge receipt of your October 16, 2012, written response to the Form FDA 483.

From our review of the establishment inspection report, the documents submitted with that report, and your October 16, 2012, written response, we conclude that you did not adhere to the applicable statutory requirements and FDA regulations governing the conduct of clinical investigations. We wish to emphasize the following:

1. You failed to ensure that the investigation was conducted according to the investigational plan [21 CFR 312.60].

As a clinical investigator, you are required to ensure that your clinical studies are conducted in accordance with the investigational plan. You failed to adhere to these requirements. Specifically:

a. The investigational plan requires that subjects be using an approved dose of an inhaled corticosteroid for at least 12 weeks preceding Visit 1, and a stable dose for at least 4 weeks preceding Visit 1. Subjects with changes in asthma medication occurring between Visits 1 and 2 (excluding albuterol/salbutamol inhalation aerosol provided at Visit 1) were to be excluded from treatment randomization.

i. Subject 00621 was taken off an inhaled corticosteroid (asthma medication) at Visit 1 and was not given a prescription for an inhaled corticosteroid during the period between Visits 1 and 2. This subject was not excluded from treatment randomization.

ii. Subject 00624 stopped using an inhaled corticosteroid before Visit 1. This subject was not excluded from treatment randomization.

iii. Subject 00625 was taken off an inhaled corticosteroid at Visit 1 and was not given a prescription for an inhaled corticosteroid during the period between Visits 1 and 2. This subject was not excluded from treatment randomization.

iv. Subject 00626 stopped using an inhaled corticosteroid one day prior to Visit 1.This subject was not excluded from treatment randomization.

b. The investigational plan prohibits subjects from using leukotriene antagonists starting at Visit 1. However, Subject 00638 continued to use a leukotriene antagonist after Visit 1.

Enrollment of subjects who do not meet eligibility criteria, and failure to ensure discontinuation of prohibited medications as required by the protocol, jeopardize subject safety and welfare and raise concerns about the validity and integrity of the data collected at your site.

2. You failed to maintain adequate and accurate case histories that record all observations and other data pertinent to the investigation on each individual administered the investigational drug or employed as a control in the investigation [21 CFR 312.62(b)].

As a clinical investigator, you are required to prepare and maintain adequate and accurate case histories that record all observations and other data pertinent to the investigation on each individual administered the investigational drug or employed as a control in the investigation. Case histories for Protocol HZA106837 include records of blood pressure, pulse rate, and body temperature that were required to be taken at every visit during the study. You have failed to maintain adequate and accurate case histories with respect to these measurements. Specifically:

a. Blood-pressure readings, pulse rates, and body temperatures were recorded for Subject 00621 when these measurements were not taken. A July 18, 2011, progress note documents that the subject stated that blood pressure, pulse rate, and temperature were not taken at every visit.
b. Blood-pressure readings were recorded for Subject 00623 when these measurements were not taken. A July 14, 2011, progress note documents that the subject reported that blood pressure was not measured at every visit.
c. Blood-pressure readings, pulse rates, and body temperatures were recorded for Subject 00628 when these measurements were not taken. A July 15, 2011, progress note documents that the subject stated that these measurements were not taken at every visit.

Other than the examples above, we are unable to determine the extent to which the above-mentioned subjects' vital signs (i.e., blood pressure, pulse rate, and body temperature) were falsified. However, in your October 16, 2012, written response, you acknowledged that data for vital signs were entered into the case report forms for the above-mentioned subjects when such data had not been collected.

By failing to maintain adequate and accurate case histories, and specifically, by failing to ensure that the data recorded were accurate, you have compromised the validity and integrity of data captured at your site.

We acknowledge your October 16, 2012, written response that indicates that you promptly reported these findings to the sponsor and IRB when you became aware of them in July 2011. We also acknowledge your statement that you contacted all other subjects to inquire about the performance of vital sign measurements.

We acknowledge the following corrective action plan that is noted in your October 16, 2012, written response and that addresses the violations in Items 1 and 2 above:

- The research coordinator who falsified data was terminated;
- All investigators and staff must attest that they have read and will adhere to the department's Standard Operation Procedures when conducting research;
- The department will conduct comprehensive standardized training and competency validation for all new research coordinators;
- The Department of Medicine research manager and staff will perform continuous internal monitoring of studies;
- Study-specific enrollment criteria for all studies will be reviewed at weekly department research meetings, and investigators will be required to sign eligibility checklists; and
- Research teams will be required to obtain mandatory continuing education.

Your response is inadequate because you have not provided sufficient information to enable us to evaluate the adequacy of your corrective action plans. Specifically, you have not provided documentation of the corrective actions that you have implemented. In addition, your response is inadequate because you have only referenced actions that your department is taking, and you have failed to include any corrective actions that you, as a clinical investigator, are implementing to prevent similar violations in the future.

If you have any questions, please contact Constance Cullity, M.D., M.P.H., at 3017963397;FAX 3018478748.Your written response and any pertinent documentation should be addressed to:

Constance Cullity,
M. D., M.P.H. Branch Chief
Good Clinical Practice Enforcement Branch
Division of Good Clinical Practice Compliance
Office of Scientific Investigations
Office of Compliance
Center for Drug Evaluation and Research
Food and Drug Administration
Building 51, Room 5354
10903 New Hampshire Avenue
Silver Spring, MD 20993

Sincerely yours,

{See appended electronic signature page}

Thomas N. Moreno, M.S.
Acting Office Director
Office of Scientific Investigations
Office of Compliance
Center for Drug Evaluation and Research
Food and Drug Administration

第 88 封　给 Boyce, Steven W. 医学博士的警告信

2012年9月28日

参考号：12-HFD-45-09-02

尊敬的Boyce博士：

2011年8月24日至9月15日，Krista Flores女士代表FDA，在您的临床研究机构，对您所开展的以下临床研究进行审查：试验方案（b）(4)[1]，标题为（b）(4)，试验药物（b）(4)，申办者为（b）(4)。这封警告信特告知您现场检查中发现的违规情况。

本次现场检查是FDA的生物研究监查项目的一部分。该项目通过设定的检查方法，对FDA监管的相关研究的实施情况进行评估，以确认研究数据在科学上是有效和准确的，并帮助确保这些研究中受试者的权益、安全和福利得到了保护。

在现场检查结束时，Flores女士向您出示了FDA483表，即现场检查发现的问题，并与您进行了讨论。您2011年10月5日对该FDA483表的书面回复已收悉。

经对现场检查报告、该报告的附件，以及您2011年10月5日的书面回复进行审查，我们认为，您没有遵循适用的法律要求和监管临床研究实施的FDA法规。我们想强调以下几点：

1. 您未能确保符合 56 部分所列要求伦理委员会负责对拟进行的临床研究进行初始审查、跟踪审查及批准［21 CFR 312.66］

作为临床研究者，您必须确保伦理委员会按照21CFR第56部分的要求，对拟进行的临床研究进行审查和批准。您未能确保伦理委员会按照21CFR第56部分的要求，对拟进行的临床研究进行审查和批准，具体来说：

伦理委员会对上述临床研究的批准期限截止至2010年5月11日。以下五位受试者于伦理委员会批准期限之外于贵研究中心入组：

a. 受试者23/015852，2010年5月19日入组；

b. 受试者24/001699，2010年5月23日入组；

c. 受试者25/015964，2010年6月23日入组；

d. 受试者26/001970，2010年7月5日入组；

e. 受试者27/016052，2010年7月26日入组。

在您对FDA483表的书面回复中，表明方案与更新的知情同意书于2010年4月7日递交伦理委员会审批；在其回复中，伦理委员会提出了批复要求。具体而言，您提到的，伦理委员会的回复函中要求，在伦理委员会批准前，授权研究者需要完成更新的GCP培训并签署利益冲突声明。您进一步提及，您的研究协调员被授权了确保伦理委员会的要求得以实施，并获得伦理委员会的批准的职责。您指出此次未获得伦理委员会批准是此协调员的责任，您直至上述5位受试者入组后才知道本临床研究的伦理委员会批准已逾期。

我们知道您已提供了一个纠正措施计划，计划包括：将研究的过期/更新日期放置在您的个人日历中；确认看到实际的伦理委员会批件及批准的知情同意；用临床研究助理会议的形式来询问研究助理对文件及流程是否有疑问；每个临床研究配备2名协调员。

由于您未提供确保获得伦理委员会审批的流程文件，您的回复是不完整的。没有此流程信息，我们无法

1 （b）(4) 涉及商业秘密，根据法规内容不予公开。

对您的纠正措施的潜在使用进行评估，无法确认此措施是否可以阻止类似的违规情况将来再发生。此外，确保符合21CFR第56部分的要求的伦理委员会负责对试验方案（b）(4）进行初始和跟踪审查及批准，是您作为临床研究者的责任。请知悉，虽然您表明当前的雇主在密切监视着伦理委员会批准的到期日期，但是，确保伦理委员会审批仍然是您作为临床研究者的职责。

您未能确保伦理委员会对试验方案（b）(4）的批准，已影响贵研究中心的受试者权益和福利。

2. 您未能保存研究中使用试验药物或对照组的受试者的所有研究观察结果和其他相关数据的足够及准确的病历［21 CFR 312.62（b）］

作为一名临床研究者，您必须准备和保存研究中使用试验药物或对照组的受试者的所有研究观察结果和其他相关数据的足够和准确的病历。病历应包含带有签名及日期的知情同意书。您未能保存完整准确地记录病历，使用了不能准确表明伦理委员会已批准的知情同意书。具体而言：

在伦理委员会批准逾期后入组的5位受试者知情同意书上（受试者23/015852，24/001699，25/015964/，26/001970及27/016052），发现了误反映文件已被伦理委员会批准的印章。此知情同意书上的印章错误显示了伦理委员会的批准日期（2010年5月11日）以及到期日期（2011年5月9日）。

根据您2011年9月15日的证词显示，您直至2010年8月30日才意识到伦理委员会的批件于2010年5月11日到期；并且在2010年9月9日，由贵研究中心经理告知，您的研究协调员从办公用品商店购买了定制的印章，用来敲盖伦理委员会批件过期后入组的5位受试者的知情同意书。

在您对FDA483表的书面回复中提及，上述行为是“居心不良员工的过分行为”。我们知道您的书面回复提供了一个纠正措施计划，计划包括：将研究的过期/更新日期放置在您的个人日历中；所有研究在确认看到实际的伦理委员会批件及批准的知情同意之后再入组受试者；使用临床研究助理会议的形式来询问研究助理对文件及流程是否有疑问；每个临床研究配备2名协调员。

由于您未提供对研究的日常监管流程文件，您的回复并不完整。我们无法对您纠正措施的潜在使用进行评估，无法确认此措施是否可以预防将来类似的违规情况再发生。此外，作为临床研究者，对试验方案（b）(4）的病历进行足够及准确的记录和保存，是您的职责。请知悉，虽然您当前的雇主使用了内部流程来帮助确保更新知情同意书的使用，但是，作为临床研究者，充分准确的记录和维护病历资料，仍然是您的职责。

您未能准备和保存足够和准确的病历，因为您的研究的病历包含不准确地表明已批准状态的知情同意书信息。以此，并如后述内容提及，您可能在签署知情同意书的过程中，就伦理委员会的审批状态误导受试者（23/015852，24/001699，25/015964/，26/001970和27/016052）影响了贵研究中心受试者权益保护的充分性。

3. 您未能确保按照研究计划进行研究［21 CFR 312.60］

作为临床研究者，您应该确保您的临床研究按照研究计划进行。试验方案（b）(4）的研究计划要求，除了其他原因外，术后应随访，并在指定时间记录心电图。您未遵守此要求，具体如下：

a. 方案要求术后28天的办公室随访，必须发生于服用研究药物的28个完整天之后。在现场检查过程中，审阅的9位受试者的术后28天评估中，有6位（20/001483，23/015852，24/001699，25/015964，26/001970和27/016052）的术后28天评估未进行或早于服药后的完整28天进行。

b. 方案要求在术后24小时，96小时和出院时分别记录标准12导联心电图。在现场检查过程中审阅的9位受试者心电图记录中，7位受试者（17/015693，18/001401，21/015769，23/015852，25/015964，26/001970和27/016052）未在相关要求时间点内进行心电图记录。

在您对FDA483表的书面回复中，您认同上述项目3a中描述的发现项，其与受试者20/001483，23/015852，24/001699和25/015964相关。对于遗漏的心电图记录（上述项目3b发现项），在您的书面回复中表明，遗漏的原因为医院工作人员与研究协调员未按照方案要求，在相应的时间获取心电图记录。

我们知道您提供了纠正措施计划，以避免类似的违背在日后再次发生。作为您的纠正措施计划的一部分，您表明您将继续确保医院和研究工作人员意识到依从研究流程的重要性，并且在适当时候，您将对发现的不依从行为进行书面报告。并且，您的回复中显示，您的当前雇主用了内部的方案偏离报告流程，协调员必须向监查团队报告偏离，提交给伦理委员会。

由于您未能提供您实施研究时的监管流程文件，您的回复不完整。我们无法对您纠正措施的潜在使用进行评估，无法确认此措施是否可以阻止将来类似的违背再发生。此外，作为临床研究者，您是确保试验方案（b）（4）按照研究计划执行的最终负责人。

您未能确保试验方案（b）（4）按照研究计划进行，影响了贵研究中心受试者权益、安全和福利的保护以及试验数据的可靠性和完整性。需要关注的是，在服用研究药物不足完整28天情况下获取的术后28天评估数据，可能影响评价主要疗效终点，包括全因性死亡、非致命性卒中，或者发生在术中或术后（术后28天随访发现）需要机械支持的严重左心室功能不全的首次发生。并且，9位进行心脏手术的受试者中，7位受试者的心电图缺失，为重大安全问题，进一步影响了贵研究中心所收集数据的可靠性和完整性。

4. 您未能按照 21 CFR 50 的要求获得知情同意［21 CFR 312.60，21 CFR 50.27］

作为一名临床研究者，您的职责是按照21 CFR 50要求获取知情同意。除了21CFR 56.109（c）的要求外，知情同意过程应使用伦理委员会批准的知情同意书记录，由受试者或受试者法定代表人在知情的同时签署姓名及日期。您未能恰当地记录知情同意过程。具体来说：

受试者26/001970签名的知情同意书未签署日期。

而且，如上文所述，伦理委员会批准期限之后入组的5位受试者（受试者23/015852，24/001699，25/015964/，26/001970及27/016052）所使用的知情同意书未被伦理委员会批准，并且盖有不正确地表明知情同意书已被伦理委员会批准的印章。

在您对FDA483表的书面回复中，您承认受试者26/001970的知情同意书没有签署日期。作为纠正措施，您表明您会向您的研究人员强调按照要求进行文件日期签署的重要性。另外，您说会有另外一位研究人员来检查知情同意书的完整性。在您的书面回复中，您也提供了与未被伦理委员会批准的知情同意书使用问题相关的纠正措施，包括：将研究的过期/更新日期放置在您的个人日历中；所有研究在确认看到实际的伦理委员会批件及批准的知情同意之后再进行受试者入组；采用临床研究助理会议的形式来询问研究助理对文件及流程是否有疑问；每个临床研究配备2名协调员。

由于您未能提供您实施研究时的监管流程文件，或对研究工作人员进行新流程的培训，您的回复并不完整。没有这些相关信息，我们无法对您纠正措施的潜在使用进行评估，无法确认此措施是否可以阻止将来类似的违背再发生。此外，作为临床研究者，按照21 CFR 50要求，获取知情同意，您是这项职责的最终负责人。值得注意的是，使用错误显示伦理委员会批复信息的知情同意书，在知情同意书签署过程中，针对伦理委员会审批状态，可能误导受试者23/015852，24/001699，25/015964/，26/001970及27/016052。

您未能按照21CFR50的要求，在受试者进入研究前对其进行知情同意，对上述研究在贵研究中心入组的研究受试者的保护，影响重大。

本警告信的目的并非是罗列您在试验药物临床研究中存在的所有缺陷。确保遵循法律和相关FDA法规的每一项要求是您的职责，您应当解决这些缺陷，并建立规程，以确保任何正在进行或将来进行的研究均符合FDA的法规。

自收到这封信的15个工作日内，您应当书面告知本办公室为预防将来发生类似违规情况而采取的措施。如果不能充分、迅速地解释上述违规问题，可能导致我们在不再通知的情况下采取监管措施。

附：英文原文

Boyce, Steven W. M. D.

WARNING LETTER

SEP 28, 2012

CERTIFIED MAIL
RETURN RECEIPT REQUESTED

Ref: 12-HFD-45-09-02

Steven W. Boyce, M.D.
Washington Hospital Center
110 Irving Street NW/1E-03
Washington, DC 20010

Dear Dr. Boyce:

This Warning Letter informs you of objectionable conditions observed during the U.S. Food and Drug Administration (FDA) inspection conducted at your clinical site between August 24 and September 15, 2011, by Krista Flores, representing the FDA, to review your conduct of a clinical investigation [Protocol **(b)(4)** entitled **(b)(4)** of the investigational drug **(b)(4)** performed for **(b)(4)**

This inspection is a part of FDA's Bioresearch Monitoring Program, which includes inspections designed to evaluate the conduct of FDA-regulated research to ensure that the data are scientifically valid and accurate, and to help ensure that the rights, safety, and welfare of the human subjects of those studies have been protected.

At the conclusion of the inspection, Ms. Flores presented and discussed with you Form FDA 483, Inspectional Observations. We acknowledge receipt of your October 5, 2011, written response to the Form FDA 483.

From our review of the establishment inspection report, the documents submitted with that report, and your October 5, 2011, written response, we conclude that you did not adhere to the applicable statutory requirements and FDA regulations governing the conduct of clinical investigations. We wish to emphasize the following:

1. You failed to assure that an Institutional Review Board (IRB) that complies with the requirements set forth in part 56 was responsible for the initial and continuing review and approval of the proposed clinical study [21 CFR 312.66].

As a clinical investigator, you are required to assure that an IRB that complies with 21 CFR part 56 reviews and approves a proposed clinical investigation. You failed to assure that an IRB that complies with 21 CFR part 56 reviewed and approved a proposed clinical study. Specifically:

IRB approval expired on May 11, 2010, for the above-mentioned clinical investigation. The following five subjects were enrolled at your site after IRB approval had expired:

a. Subject 23/015852 was enrolled on May 19, 2010;

b. Subject 24/001699 was enrolled on May 23, 2010;

c. Subject 25/015964 was enrolled on June 23, 2010;

d. Subject 26/001970 was enrolled on July 5, 2010; and

e. Subject 27/016052 was enrolled on July 26, 2010.

In your written response to the Form FDA 483, you note that the protocol and revised informed consent document were submitted to the IRB on April 7, 2010, for continuing review approval; and that, in response, the IRB communicated stipulations required to be met prior to IRB approval. Specifically, you noted that the IRB's letter stipulated that subinvestigators needed to complete updated training in Good Clinical Practice (GCP) and to sign a conflict of interest statement before IRB approval could be granted. You further note that your study coordinator was delegated the responsibility of ensuring that the IRB's stipulations were addressed, and that IRB approval was obtained. You indicate that your failure to obtain IRB approval was the result of the actions of your study coordinator, and that you were not aware that IRB approval of your clinical investigation had expired until after all five of the above listed subjects were enrolled.

We acknowledge that you have provided a corrective action plan that includes placing expiration/renewal dates for studies on your personal calendar; seeing the actual IRB approval letter and approved informed consent; using a clinical research associate meeting form to inquire if the clinical research associate has any concerns about documents or processes; and conducting a clinical study with two coordinators.

Your response is incomplete because you have not provided documentation of procedures to ensure that IRB review and approval are obtained. Without this information, we cannot conduct an informed evaluation of the potential use of your corrective actions to prevent the recurrence of this type of violation in the future. Moreover, it was your responsibility as a clinical investigator to ensure that an IRB that complied with 21 CFR part 56 was responsible for the initial and continuing review and approval of Protocol **(b)(4)**. Please note that, although you indicate that your current employer closely monitors protocols nearing expiration of IRB approval, it remains your responsibility as a clinical investigator to ensure IRB review and approval.

Your failure to ensure IRB approval of Protocol **(b)(4)** raises concerns about the extent to which subjects' rights and welfare were protected at your site.

2. You failed to maintain adequate and accurate case histories that record all observations and other data pertinent to the investigation on each individual administered the investigational drug or employed as a control in the investigation [21 CFR 312.62(b)].

As a clinical investigator, you are required to prepare and maintain adequate and accurate case histories that record all observations and other data pertinent to the investigation on each individual administered the investigational drug or employed as a control in the investigation. Case histories include the signed and dated consent forms. You have failed to maintain adequate and accurate case histories by using informed consent forms that inaccurately indicated they had been approved by the IRB. Specifically:

Informed consent forms for the five subjects enrolled at your site after IRB approval for your study had expired (Subjects 23/015852, 24/001699, 25/015964, 26/001970, and 27/016052) were found to have stamps on the documents inaccurately indicating that they had been approved by the IRB. The stamps on these informed consent forms inaccurately showed an IRB approval date of May 11, 2010, and an IRB approval expiration date of May 9, 2011.

According to your September 15, 2011, affidavit, you were not aware until August 30, 2010, that IRB approval had expired on May 11, 2010, and you were informed by your site manager on September 9, 2010, that your study coordinator had purchased a custom-made stamp at Office Depot, which he had used to stamp the informed consent documents that were used to enroll five subjects after the study's IRB expiration date.

In your written response to the Form FDA 483, you indicate that the above finding was the "egregious act of one rogue employee." We acknowledge that your written response provided a corrective action plan that includes placing expiration/renewal dates for studies on your personal calendar; seeing the actual IRB approval letter and approved informed consent prior to enrolling subjects in any study; using a clinical research associate meeting form to inquire if the clinical research associate has any concerns about documents or processes; and conducting a clinical study with two coordinators.

Your response is incomplete because you have not provided documentation of procedures for regulatory oversight of studies that you conduct. Without this information, we cannot conduct an informed evaluation of the potential use of your corrective actions to prevent the recurrence of this type of violation in the future. Moreover, it was your responsibility as a clinical investigator to prepare and maintain adequate and accurate case histories for Protocol **(b)(4)**. Please note that, although you indicate that your current employer has internal processes for helping to ensure that updated informed consent documents are used, it remains your responsibility as a clinical investigator to prepare and maintain adequate and accurate case histories.

You failed to prepare and maintain adequate and accurate case histories because the case histories for your study included informed consent documents that inaccurately indicated they had been approved by the IRB. By doing so, as also noted below, you may have caused Subjects 23/015852, 24/001699, 25/015964, 26/001970, and 27/016052 to be misled regarding the status of IRB approval of the informed consent documents they were signing, thus raising concerns about the adequacy of human subject protections at your site.

3. You failed to ensure that the investigation was conducted according to the investigational plan [21 CFR 312.60].

As a clinical investigator, you are required to ensure that your clinical studies are conducted in accordance with the investigational plan. The investigational plan for Protocol **(b)(4)** requires, among other things, that postoperative day (POD) visits occur and electrocardiograms (ECGs) be recorded at specified times. You failed to adhere to these requirements. Specifically:

a. The protocol requires that the office visit on POD 28 occur no earlier than 28 full days after study drug administration. For six subjects (20/001483, 23/015852, 24/001699, 25/015964, 26/001970, and 27/016052) out of the nine subjects whose POD 28 assessments were reviewed during the inspection, POD 28 assessments either were not performed or were performed earlier than 28 full days after study drug administration.

b. The protocol requires that standard 12-lead ECGs be recorded at 24 hours and 96 hours after completion of surgery and at discharge. For seven subjects (17/015693, 18/001401, 21/015769, 23/015852, 25/015964, 26/001970, and 27/016052) out of the nine subjects whose ECG records were reviewed during the inspection, ECGs were not performed at certain required times.

In your written response to the Form FDA 483, you concur with the findings noted in Item 3a. above, as they relate to Subjects 20/001483, 23/015852, 24/001699, and 25/015964. Regarding the missing ECGs (see the findings in Item 3b. above), you state in your written response that the reason why ECGs were missing is that hospital staff and the study coordinator did not obtain ECGs as required by the protocol.

We acknowledge that you have provided a corrective action plan to prevent future recurrence of similar violations. As part of your corrective action plan, you state that you will continue to ensure that hospital and research staff are aware of the importance of following study procedures, and that you will escalate findings of noncompliance to a written report when appropriate. Furthermore, in your response, you state that your current employer has an internal process for reporting protocol deviations, and that coordinators must report deviations to the regulatory team for submission to the IRB.

Your response is incomplete because you have not provided documentation of procedures that you will use for oversight of studies that you conduct. Without this information, we cannot conduct an informed evaluation of the potential use of your corrective actions to prevent the recurrence of this type of violation in the future. Moreover, as the clinical investigator, you were ultimately responsible for ensuring that Protocol **(b)(4)** was conducted according to the investigational plan.

Your failure to ensure that Protocol **(b)(4)** was conducted according to the investigational plan, raises concerns about the extent to which the rights, safety, and welfare of subjects were protected, and about the validity and integrity of the data at your site. Of note, obtaining data for the POD 28 assessment prior to 28 full days after study drug administration may have affected the primary efficacy endpoint of first occurrence of the composite of all-cause death, nonfatal stroke, or need for mechanical support for severe left ventricular dysfunction (SLVD) occurring during and following **(b)(4)** surgery through POD 28. In addition, failure to obtain protocol-required ECGs in seven of the nine subjects undergoing cardiac surgery is a significant safety concern, and further raises concerns about the validity and integrity of the data collected at your site.

4. You failed to obtain informed consent in accordance with the provisions of 21 CFR part 50 [21 CFR 312.60, 21 CFR 50.27].

As a clinical investigator, it is your responsibility to obtain informed consent in accordance with 21 CFR part 50. Except as provided in 21 CFR 56.109(c), informed consent shall be documented by the use of a written consent form approved by the IRB and signed and dated by the subject or the subject's legally authorized representative at the time of consent. You failed to properly document informed consent. Specifically:

The informed consent form signed by Subject 26/001970 was not dated.

In addition, as noted above, the informed consent forms for the five subjects enrolled at your site after IRB approval for your study had expired (Subjects 23/015852, 24/001699, 25/015964, 26/001970, and 27/016052) were not approved by the IRB, and were found to have stamps on the documents inaccurately indicating that they had been approved by the IRB.

In your written response to the Form FDA 483, you acknowledge that the informed consent form for subject

26/001970 was not dated. As a corrective action, you state that you will emphasize to your research staff the importance of dating documents as required. Furthermore, you state that a second research staff person will inspect the informed consent forms for completeness. In your written response, you also provide corrective actions related to the use of informed consent documents that were not approved by the IRB, including placing expiration/renewal dates for studies on your personal calendar; seeing the actual IRB approval letter and approved informed consent prior to enrolling subjects in any study; using a clinical research associate meeting form to inquire if the clinical research associate has any concerns about documents or processes; and conducting a clinical study with two coordinators.

Your response is incomplete because you have not provided documentation of procedures that you will use for oversight of studies that you conduct, or of training that study staff have received on the new procedures. Without this information, we cannot conduct an informed evaluation of the potential use of your corrective actions to prevent the recurrence of this type of violation in the future. Moreover, as the clinical investigator, you were ultimately responsible for ensuring that informed consent was obtained in accordance with 21 CFR part 50. Of note, your use of informed consent forms that inaccurately indicated they had been approved by the IRB, may have caused Subjects 23/015852, 24/001699, 25/015964, 26/001970, and 27/016052 to be misled regarding the status of IRB approval of the informed consent documents they were signing.

Your failure to obtain informed consent in accordance with 21 CFR part 50 prior to involving subjects in research, raises significant concerns about your protection of study subjects enrolled at your site in the study mentioned above.

This letter is not intended to be an all-inclusive list of deficiencies with your clinical study of an investigational drug. It is your responsibility to ensure adherence to each requirement of the law and relevant FDA regulations. You should address these deficiencies and establish procedures to ensure that any ongoing or future studies will be in compliance with FDA regulations.

Within fifteen (15) working days of your receipt of this letter, you should notify this office in writing of the actions you have taken to prevent similar violations in the future. Failure to address the violations noted above adequately and promptly may result in regulatory action without further notice.

If you have any questions, please contact Constance Cullity, M.D., M.P.H., at 301-796- 3397; FAX 301-847-8748. Your written response and any pertinent documentation should be addressed to:

Constance Cullity, M.D., M.P.H.
Branch Chief
Good Clinical Practice Enforcement Branch
Division of Good Clinical Practice Compliance
Office of Scientific Investigations
Office of Compliance
Center for Drug Evaluation and Research
Food and Drug Administration
Building 51, Room 5354
10903 New Hampshire Avenue
Silver Spring, MD 20993

Sincerely yours,

/S/

Thomas N. Moreno, M.S.
Acting Office Director
Office of Scientific Investigations
Office of Compliance
Center for Drug Evaluation and Research
Food and Drug Administration

第89封　给Sanderlin, Damien医学博士的警告信

2012年7月27日

参考号：CBER-12-08

尊敬的Sanderlin博士：

本警告信特告知您2012年6月21日至7月18日FDA进行现场检查的结果。一名FDA检查员与您会面，并对您所实施的以下临床研究：试验方案 OQ-OTC-5，标题为"一项多中心临床试验，在未经培训的人群中实际使用OraQuick ADVANCE®HIV 1/2抗体检测以及计数器产品性能评价"进行了审查。此次现场检查是FDA的生物研究监查项目的一部分。该项目通过设定的检查方法，评估试验性医疗器械相关研究的实施情况。

在现场检查结束时，检查员向您出示并讨论了FDA483表，即现场检查发现的问题。基于FDA483表以及掌握的其他信息，我们的结论是：您违反了发布在美国联邦法规第21篇第812部分（21 CFR 812，法规详见http://www.gpoaccess.gov/cfr/index.html）、试验性医疗器械临床研究监管相关的法规，以下列出的每个违规项均指出了CFR中的相应条款。

您未能确保按照研究计划、签署的协议、适用的FDA法规及IRB或FDA批准的条件来进行研究，以保护在您的监护下的受试者的权益、安全和福利［21 CFR 812.100和812.110（b）］

试验方案Ⅲ.L部分要求临床研究者遵守联邦、州和地方政府关于新发现HIV阳性的实验室结果应向疾病控制与预防中心（CDC）报告的规定。在德州休斯顿，18个受试者采用FDA批准的方法由中心实验室确认HIV阳性，第一个受试者确证HIV阳性的时间为2010年12月，18个多月前。下面的表格为新诊断为HIV阳性的受试者清单和中心实验室报告HIV阳性结果的日期，还有第三次受试者随访的时间。根据试验方案，在第三次随访时查看受试者自测和实验室检测结果。所有这些受试者的随访时间至今均已超过1年。

受试者编号/组别	中心实验室HIV阳性结果研究者签署日期	第3次随访日期
（b）（6）	2010年12月23日	2010年12月23日
（b）（6）	2011年1月24日	2011年1月24日
（b）（6）	2011年2月21日	2011年2月21日
（b）（6）	2011年2月24日	2011年2月24日
（b）（6）	2011年3月17日	2011年3月17日
（b）（6）	2011年4月18日和5月6日	2011年4月18日
（b）（6）	2011年4月18日	2011年4月18日
（b）（6）	2011年4月18日	2011年4月18日
（b）（6）	2011年4月18日	2011年4月18日
（b）（6）	2011年6月27日	2011年6月27日
（b）（6）	2011年6月27日	2011年6月27日
（b）（6）	2011年6月27日	2011年6月27日
（b）（6）	2011年6月27日	2011年6月27日
（b）（6）	2011年6月27日	2011年6月27日
（b）（6）	2011年7月1日	2011年7月1日
（b）（6）	2011年7月1日	2011年7月1日
（b）（6）	2011年7月1日	2011年7月1日
（b）（6）	2011年7月18日	2011年7月18日

现场检查发现您未根据州政府的法规要求报告这些HIV阳性受试者的实验室结果，具体而言，德克萨斯行政法25篇、第1部分、第97章，F节，97.133条款），它要求任何来自人体的标本，经显微镜、培养、血清学或其他方法证实有HIV时，均要向德州政府上报相关信息。据德克萨斯州健康服务部的“技术援助公告：报告HIV快速测试结果追溯到 2010年3月，您是用std-27表（州健康服务部性传播疾病机密报告表）报告HIV阳性检测结果的，完成的表格应在收到阳性测试结果7天内寄到本地或地区卫生局。与您的工作人员在检查过程中告诉FDA的相反，疾病预防控制中心不接受来自个人的直接报告。而是由国家卫生部门，如德克萨斯州的卫生服务部，一旦在本州内收到HIV阳性的实验室结果，将使用电子HIV/AIDS报告系统向疾病预防控制中心报告该监测数据。

自收到这封信的15个工作日内，您应当提供书面材料，确认您向德克萨斯州卫生服务部报告了HIV实验室检查阳性的18名受试者的情况，一并提供您进行报告的日期。如果您没有向德克萨斯州卫生服务部报告部分或全部HIV实验室检查阳性的结果，请提供相关情况的细节。

请提供您作为临床研究者为预防当前或将来研究中再次发生类似违规情况，将要采取的具体措施。未能对本警告信进行回复并采取适当的纠正措施，可能导致我们在不再通知的情况下采取监管措施。

本警告信中列出的违规情况的严重性以及对公共卫生潜在的影响，使我们在对FDA483表中列出的所有违规情况进行全面审查之前就发出了这封警告信，因此，此信并没有列出所有的缺陷。我们将继续对在您的研究中心进行的两次近期检查（2012年3月27日至3月29日，以及本警告信第一段中提及的检查）中发现的问题进行审查。确保符合每一项法律及相关FDA法规的要求是您的职责。

附：英文原文

Sanderlin, Damien M.D.

WARNING LETTER

JUL 27, 2012

Ref: CBER-12-08

Damien B. Sanderlin, M.D.
Lone Star Clinical Research
8240 Antoine Street, Suite 107
Houston, Texas 77088

Dear Dr. Sanderlin:

This letter describes some of the results of a Food and Drug Administration (FDA, the Agency) inspection conducted between June 21, 2012, and July 18, 2012. The FDA investigator met with you to review your conduct of a clinical study entitled A Multi-Center, Actual Use Clinical Trial of the OraQuick ADVANCE® HIV 1/2 Antibody Test Over-the Counter Product Performance in Untrained Users, Protocol OQ-OTC-5. The FDA conducted this inspection under the agency's Bioresearch Monitoring Program, which includes inspections designed to review the conduct of research involving investigational devices.

At the end of the inspection, the FDA investigator met with you to discuss the items listed on the Form FDA 483, Inspectional Observations. Based on the Form FDA 483 and other information available to the Agency, we have determined that you violated regulations governing the proper conduct of clinical studies involving investigational devices, as published in Title 21, Code of Federal Regulations (CFR) Part 812, (available at http://www.gpoaccess.gov/cfr/index.html). The applicable provisions of the CFR are cited for the violation listed below.

You failed to ensure that the investigation was conducted according to the investigational plan, the signed agreement, applicable FDA regulations, and conditions of approval imposed by the Institutional Review Board (IRB) or FDA, this, in order to protect the rights, safety, and welfare of the subjects under your care. [21 CFR § 812.100 and 812.110(b)].

The Protocol's Study Design, Section Ⅲ.L, Follow-up for HIV Positive Test Results, requires the clinical investigator to "comply with all federal, state, and local regulations regarding the reporting of newly-identified HIV positive laboratory results to the Centers for Disease Control and Prevention (CDC)." Eighteen (18) study subjects in Houston, Texas were confirmed HIV positive using FDA-approved methods at the central laboratory, with the first subject being confirmed HIV positive in December 2010, more than 18 months ago. The table below identifies each newly-diagnosed HIV positive subject and the date you signed the central lab report form with a positive HIV test result. Also listed below is the date of Visit 3 for the subjects. According to the protocol, review of the subject's self test data and laboratory results occurred during Visit 3. All of these subject visits occurred more than one year ago.

Subject #/Initials	Date the central lab positive HIV test result form was signed by CI	Date of Visit 3
(b)(6)	12/23/2010	12/23/2010
(b)(6)	1/24/2011	1/24/2011
(b)(6)	2/21/2011	2/21/2011
(b)(6)	2/24/2011	2/24/2011
(b)(6)	4/18/2011 and 5/6/2011	4/18/2011
(b)(6)	4/18/2011	4/18/2011
(b)(6)	4/18/2011	4/18/2011
(b)(6)	4/18/2011	4/18/2011
(b)(6)	6/27/2011	6/27/2011
(b)(6)	6/27/2011	6/27/2011
(b)(6)	6/27/2011	6/27/2011
(b)(6)	6/27/2011	6/27/2011
(b)(6)	6/27/2011	6/27/2011
(b)(6)	7/1/2011	7/1/2011
(b)(6)	7/1/2011	7/1/2011
(b)(6)	7/1/2011	7/1/2011
(b)(6)	7/18/2011	7/18/2011

The inspection revealed no documentation that you had reported the subjects with HIV positive laboratory results in accordance with state requirements, specifically, the Texas Administrative Code Title 25, Part 1, Chapter 97, Subchapter F, Rule 97.133, which requires you to submit to the State of Texas information for any specimen derived from a human body that yields microscopic, cultural, serological or any other evidence of HIV. According to the Texas Department of State Health Services' "Technical Assistance Bulletin: Reporting Rapid HIV Test Results" dated March 2010, you are to report positive HIV test results on the Form STD-27 (Department of State Health Services Confidential Report of Sexually Transmitted Diseases Form), and the completed forms are to be sent to the local or regional health authority within seven days of receiving the positive test result. Contrary to what your staff told FDA during the inspection, the CDC does not accept direct reports from individuals. Instead, state health departments, such as the Texas Department of State Health Services, upon receipt of HIV positive laboratory results from within the state, report such surveillance data to the CDC using an electronic HIV/AIDS reporting system.

Within fifteen (15) business days of receipt of this letter, please provide written documentation to confirm that you reported the eighteen (18) subjects with HIV positive laboratory results to the Texas Department of State Health

Services, along with the dates on which you made these reports. If you did not report some or all of the HIV positive laboratory results to the Texas Department of State Health Services, please provide details regarding that information as well.

Please provide specific actions you will take to prevent the recurrence of similar violations in current and future studies for which you are the clinical investigator. Failure to respond to this letter and to take appropriate corrective action could result in FDA taking regulatory action without further notice to you.

The seriousness of the violation referenced in this letter, and its potential public health implications, has caused us to issue this letter prior to a complete review of all of the violations listed on the Form FDA 483 and, as a result, this letter is not intended to be an all-inclusive list of deficiencies. We are continuing to review information from the two recent inspections conducted at your site (March 27, 2012 through March 29, 2012 and the inspection noted in the first paragraph of this letter). It is your responsibility to ensure adherence to each requirement of the law and relevant FDA regulations.

Please send your written response to:

Janet White
Division of Inspections and Surveillance (HFM-664)
Office of Compliance and Biologics Quality
Center for Biologics Evaluation and Research
1401 Rockville Pike, Suite 200N
Rockville, Maryland 20852-1488
Telephone: 301-827-6323

We also request that you send a copy of your response to the FDA District Office listed below.

Sincerely,

/S/

Mary A. Malarkey, Director
Office of Compliance and Biologics Quality
Center for Biologics Evaluation and Research

Cc: District Director
Food and Drug Administration
4040 North Central Expressway, Suite 300
Dallas, Texas 75204
Texas Department of State Health Services
PO Box 149347 Austin, Texas 78714-9347

第 90 封　给 Houser, Elizabeth E. 医学博士的警告信

2012年5月25日

参考号：12-HFD-45-05-01

尊敬的Houser博士：

2010年12月6日至2011年1月6日，Robert Lorenz先生代表FDA，在您的临床研究机构，对您所开展的试验药物为氟班色林，申办者为勃林格殷格翰制药公司的以下临床研究进行了审查：

- 试验方案511.75，一项为期24周、随机、双盲、安慰剂对照，比较绝经前女性性欲减退的氟班色林每日50mg与氟班色林每日100mg安全性和有效性的试验；
- 试验方案511.84，一项为期12个月、开放、比较绝经前女性性欲减退的氟班色林每日50mg与氟班色林每日100mg安全性的试验。

这封警告信特告知您现场检查中发现的违规情况。

本次现场检查是FDA的生物研究监查项目的一部分。该项目通过设定的检查方法，对由FDA监管的相关研究的实施情况进行评估，以确认研究数据在科学上是有效和准确的，并帮助确保这些研究中受试者的权益、安全和福利得到了保护。

在现场检查结束时，Lorenz先生向您出示了FDA483表，即现场检查发现的问题，并与您进行了讨论。您2011年1月14日对该FDA483表的书面回复已收悉。

经对现场检查报告、该报告的附件，以及您2011年1月14日的书面回复进行审查，我们认为，您没有遵循适用的法律要求和监管临床研究实施的FDA法规。我们想强调以下几点：

1. 在提供给 FDA 或申办者的所需报告中，您反复或者故意地提交虚假信息［21 CFR 312.70.（a）］

作为试验方案511.84的临床研究者，您本应该进行以下（量表）评估并将评估结果报告至申办者：①临床疗效总评量表（CGI）中的病情严重程度；②CGI的疗效指数。FDA认为您在提供给申办者的这些所需量表评估结果中，存在虚假信息。具体而言：

试验方案511.84的受试者27881，记录显示以下评估由（b）（4）医生完成，她是您的助理研究者：①访视2，4，5，6和7时，完成临床疗效总评量表中的病情严重程度评估；②访视4，5，6和7时，完成临床疗效总评量表中的疗效指数评估。然而，根据（b）（4）医生确认，她并未（对受试者）进行过这些量表评估。研究协调员（b）（6）冒用（b）（4）医生的名字完成了量表的评估伪造了这些记录。

虽然此项违背未被列于FDA483表上，但是在现场检查过程中我们的现场检查员与您和（b）（4）医生就此违背进行了讨论。当时，您指出，试验方案511.84的研究协调员（b）（6）由与您签署合同的现场管理组织（SMO）提供，您在既往的研究中已多次使用该SMO。现场检查过程中，您未表明是否进行调查以确定（b）（6）（他声称量表评估由研究工作人员完成，实际上该工作人员并未进行评估）在其他研究中是否参与数据录入。

作为临床研究者，您必须确保所收集的研究受试者数据准确可靠，可用于任何研究终点的分析。当您签署研究者声明（FDA1572表）时，您已认可应保持足够、准确的记录，确保在开展试验药物的临床研究时，遵守FDA的法规要求；您已认可，您应确保所有参与研究的助理、同事以及雇员知晓其职责，以满足其所承担的职位要求。而且，您的签名不仅代表您确认您可以胜任进行临床研究，并且还是您的书面承

诺，表明您会遵守FDA的法规要求进行临床研究。使用虚假信息严重地损害了研究完整性，以及数据的可靠性和有效性。

2．您未能确保按照研究计划进行研究［21 CFR 312.60］

作为临床研究者，您必须确保您的临床研究按照研究计划进行。试验方案511.84的研究计划要求，在门诊随访时进行相关评估，CGIs中的病情严重程度和疗效由临床专家进行评估。此外，试验方案511.84和511.75禁止受试者使用某些药物，定义了每一个受试者的入组标准。您未能遵守这些要求。具体来说：

a. 试验方案511.84要求在门诊进行访视2（基线），4，5，6和7时，进行以下测试：血压和脉搏、体重、Beck自杀意念量表（BSS），女性性痛苦量表-修订版（FSDS-R），女性性功能指数量表（FSFI），任何不良事件和伴随疗法的评估。方案还要求，入排标准的评估在访视2（基线）时在门诊进行；CGI中的疗效指数与服药依从性的评估在访视4，5，6和7时在门诊进行；心电图和实验室检查在访视7时在门诊进行。此外，方案还要求CGI评估由临床专家（D.O.，M.D.、医学博士、临床心理学家、性治疗师、医师助理及执业护士进行。

受试者27881，访视2，4，5，6和7均在院外而非方案要求的门诊进行。并且，这些访视的CGI中的病情严重程度和疗效评估均由您的研究协调员完成。此研究协调员未持有任何可以完成此评估量表的资格认定证明，没有完成此量表评估的资格。

b. 试验方案511.84，6.2.1部分要求在第1周（访视1）完成实验室检测，包括催乳素水平。方案的这部分还要求所有具有重要临床意义的（由研究者判断）的实验室检测异常值，均应在每一位受试者入组前进行复测。

受试者27839，于2007年7月20日的访视2中入组研究给予试验药物，而此时其催乳素实验室检测结果还未获得。此受试者的催乳素检测结果报告日期为2007年7月26日，结果显示其催乳素水平为61ng/mL，贵研究中心认为其具重要临床意义。所以，受试者27839不符合入组标准，不应该被入组研究。

c. 试验方案511.84，10.3.1部分（禁忌药品列表）和试验方案511.84，10.1.1部分（禁忌药品列表）禁止（受试者）使用激素激受体动剂。受试者27884于2005年9月22日起，持续使用口服孕酮（激素激动剂），每日剂量为100mg。因此，受试者27884参加上述的两个研究不合适。

在您2011年1月14日对FDA483表的书面回复中，您表明您做了如下措施：与您的现场管理组织终止了合同，迅速向申办者报告了院外访视，对研究文件进行稽查，创建了新的入组标准操作规程（SOP），在您的回复之外增加了额外的计划在研究部门中执行。此外，您同意受试者27839与27884不应入组研究。

由于您未能提供在研究中心执行纠正措施的文件，我们认为您的回复不充分。没有足够的文件，我们无法判断您的纠正措施是否合适。您的回复中未包含您内部稽查的标准、新的受试者入组的标准操作规程、您的研究工作人员接受新标准操作规程的培训记录。并且，您未具体明确将要在您的研究部门中执行的额外计划是什么。

在您对这封信函的回复中，请提供您的纠正措施的相关文件。回复应包括您用来确认研究协调员（b）（6）未进行下列行为的稽查计划的复印件，以确认研究协调员（b）（6）并未：①进行了她并无资质的任何其他评估；②将她所做的评估记录冠以其他有资质却并未实际实施评估的人员名字；③实施其他未被批准的院外访视。

在您回复的陈述中，我们得知您已关闭您的研究部门，您“除了本文提及之处，仍有几个计划和措施将会在研究部门实施。由于部门关闭，一些项目无法完成和/或实施。”然而，请注意，解决本信函中涉及的问题仍然是您的责任。

受试者入组不符合入组标准、临床疗效总评量表的评估由不具有资质的人员完成、虚假地将临床疗效总评量表的病情严重程度和疗效评估结果冠名给授权研究者，极大地损害了贵研究中心受试者安全和福祉的保护，以及所收集数据的有效性和可靠性。

本警告信的目的并非是罗列您在试验药物临床研究中存在的所有缺陷。确保遵循法律和相关FDA法规的每一项要求是您的职责，您应当解决这些缺陷，并建立规程，以确保任何正在进行或将来进行的研究均符合

FDA的法规。

自收到这封信的15个工作日内，您应当书面告知本办公室为预防将来再次发生类似违规情况而采取的措施。如果不能充分、迅速地解释上述违规问题，可能导致我们在不再通知的情况下采取监管措施。如果您认为您已经遵循了FDA的法规要求，请陈述理由，并提供所有支持资料，以供我们参考。

附：英文原文

Houser, Elizabeth E. M.D.

WARNING LETTER

MAY 25, 2012

CERTIFIED MAIL
RETURN RECEIPT REQUESTED

Ref: 12-HFD-45-05-01

Elizabeth E. Houser, M.D
11410 Jollyville Road, Suite 1101
Austin, Texas 78705-1922

Dear Dr. Houser:

This Warning Letter informs you of objectionable conditions observed during the U.S. Food and Drug Administration (FDA) inspection conducted at your clinical site between December 6, 2010, and January 6, 2011, by Mr. Robert Lorenz, representing the FDA, to review your conduct of the following clinical investigations of the investigational drug flibanserin, performed for Boehringer Ingelheim Pharmaceuticals:

- Protocol #511.75, "A Twenty-Four Week, Randomized, Double-Blind, Placebo-Controlled, Safety and Efficacy Trial of Flibanserin 50 milligrams Daily and , with Up-Titration, 100 milligrams Daily in Premenopausal Women with Hypoactive Sexual Desire"; and
- Protocol #511.84, "A Twelve Month, Open-Label, Safety Trial of Flibanserin 50 milligrams to 100 milligrams Daily in Women with Hypoactive Sexual Desire Disorder."

This inspection is a part of FDA's Bioresearch Monitoring Program, which includes inspections designed to evaluate the conduct of FDA-regulated research to ensure that the data are scientifically valid and accurate, and to help ensure that the rights, safety, and welfare of the human subjects involved in those studies have been protected.

At the conclusion of the inspection, Mr. Lorenz presented and discussed with you Form FDA 483, Inspectional Observations. We acknowledge receipt of your January 14, 2011, written response to the Form FDA 483.

From our review of the establishment inspection report and the documents submitted with that report, and your January 14, 2011, written response, we conclude that you did not adhere to the applicable statutory requirements and FDA regulations governing the conduct of clinical investigations. We wish to emphasize the following:

1. You repeatedly or deliberately submitted to FDA or to the sponsor false information in any required report [21 CFR 312.70(a)].

As a clinical investigator for Protocol 511.84, you were required to conduct the following assessments and report these to the sponsor: (1) Clinical Global Impression (CGI) of Severity, and (2) CGI of Efficacy Index. FDA has concluded that as the clinical investigator for Protocol 511.84, you submitted false information to the sponsor through the submission of these required assessments. Specifically:

For Subject 27881 enrolled into Protocol 511.84, the records for the following assessments indicate that they were completed by Dr. **(b)(4)**, your sub-investigator: (1) CGI of Severity for Visits 2, 4, 5, 6, and 7; and (2) CGI of Efficacy Index for Visits 4, 5, 6, and 7. However, according to Dr. **(b)(4)**, she did not conduct these assessments. The study coordinator, **(b)(6)**, falsified these records by entering Dr. **(b)(4)**'s name as having completed the assessments. Although this violation was not listed on the Form FDA 483, our field investigator discussed this violation with you and Dr. **(b)(4)** during the inspection. At that time, you indicated that the site management organization (SMO) with which you contracted to assist in the conduct of Protocol 511.84 had provided you with study coordinator **(b)(6)**, and that you had used this SMO for numerous prior studies. During the inspection, you did not indicate whether you investigated to determine if any other studies you conducted contained entries from **(b)(6)**, purporting to be assessments conducted by study staff who did not actually conduct the assessments.

As the clinical investigator, it is your responsibility to ensure that the data collected from study subjects are accurate and can be relied upon in any analyses of the study endpoints. When you signed the Statement of the Investigator, Form FDA 1572, you agreed to maintain adequate and accurate records and to ensure that you will comply with FDA regulations related to the conduct of the clinical investigations of the investigational drugs; and you agreed to ensure that all associates, colleagues, and employees assisting in the conduct of the study are informed about their obligations in meeting their commitments. Furthermore, your signature constitutes both your affirmation that you are qualified to conduct the clinical investigation and your written commitment to abide by FDA regulations in the conduct of the clinical investigations. The use of falsified information significantly compromises the study integrity, as well as the reliability and validity of the data.

2. You failed to ensure that the investigation was conducted according to the investigational plan [21 CFR 312.60].

As a clinical investigator, you are required to ensure that your clinical studies are conducted in accordance with the investigational plan. The investigational plan for Protocol 511.84 requires that certain evaluations be performed at clinic visits, and that the CGIs of Severity and Efficacy be performed by a clinical expert. In addition, Protocols 511.84 and 511.75 both prohibit the use of certain medications by subjects and have defined inclusion criteria for each subject. You failed to adhere to these requirements. Specifically:

a. Protocol 511.84 required that the following evaluations be ***performed at the clinic***during Visits 2 (Baseline), 4, 5, 6, and 7: Blood pressure and pulse rate, weight, Beck Scale for Suicidal Ideation (BSS), Female Sexual Distress Scale – Revised (FSDS-R), Female Sexual Function Index (FSFI), and assessments for any adverse events and concomitant therapy. The protocol further required that assessment of inclusion/exclusion criteria was to be ***performed at the clinic*** at Visit 2 (Baseline); CGI of Efficacy Index and assessment of medication compliance were to be ***performed at the clinic*** during Visits 4, 5, 6, and 7; and an electrocardiogram (ECG) and laboratory tests were to be ***taken at the clinic*** during Visit 7. In addition, the protocol required that the CGI assessments be performed by an expert clinician who holds one of the following credentials: D.O., M.D., Clinical Ph.D. psychologist, sex therapist, Physician's Assistant or Nurse Practitioner.

For Subject 27881, Visits 2, 4, 5, 6, and 7 were conducted off-site instead of at the clinic, as required by the protocol. In addition, the CGIs of Severity and Efficacy for these visits were conducted by your study coordinator, who does not hold any of the required credentials and was therefore not qualified to conduct these assessments.

b. Protocol 511.84, Section 6.2.1 requires laboratory tests, including prolactin levels, at Week-1 (Visit 1). This section of the protocol further requires that all clinically significant (in the investigator's judgment) abnormal laboratory tests be repeated before any subject can be enrolled.

Subject 27839 was enrolled into the study and was provided with study drug at Visit 2 on July 20, 2007, before the prolactin laboratory results were available. The subject's prolactin result was provided in a laboratory report dated July 26, 2007, and was at a level (61 ng/mL) that you deemed clinically significant. As a result, Subject 27839 did not meet inclusion criteria and should not have been enrolled.

c. Protocol 511.84, Section 10.3.1 (List of Prohibited Medications) and Protocol 511.84, Section 10.1.1 (List of Prohibited Medications) prohibit the use of hormonal agonists. Subject 27884 was on a continuing dose of 100 mg/day Prometrium (a hormonal agonist) beginning September 22, 2005. Therefore, Subject 27884 was inappropriately enrolled into both studies.

In your January 14, 2011, written response to the Form FDA 483, you state that you have done the following: You terminated the services of your site management organization; promptly reported the off-site visits to the sponsor; conducted an audit of study files; created a new subject enrollment Standard Operating Procedure (SOP); and developed additional plans that were not included in your response, to be implemented in your research department. In addition, you agreed that Subjects 27839 and 27884 should not have been enrolled.

We find your response inadequate, because you failed to provide documentation of the corrective actions implemented at your clinical site. Without adequate documentation, we cannot assess whether or not the corrective actions are appropriate. You did not include in your response the criteria used in your internal audit, copies of your new SOP for subject enrollment, or training your study staff received on the new SOP. Further, you did not specifically identify what the additional plans developed by your research department were intended to address.

In your response to this letter, please provide documentation of your corrective actions. This response should include a copy of the audit plan you used to verify that study coordinator **(b)(6)** did not: (1) conduct any other assessments that she was not qualified to do; (2) attribute any such assessments to qualified persons who did not actually conduct the assessments; or (3) conduct additional unapproved off-site visits.

We acknowledge your statement in your response that you have closed your research department and that you "had several plans and actions to be taken in our Research Department that are not included in this letter. Due to department closure [,] several of these items were not completed and/or implemented." However, please note that it remains your responsibility to address the issues noted in this letter.

Enrollment of subjects who do not meet eligibility criteria, the conduct of CGIs by unqualified staff, and false attribution of CGIs of Severity and Efficacy to a sub- investigator jeopardize subject safety and welfare and raise concerns about the validity and integrity of the data collected at your site.

This letter is not intended to be an all-inclusive list of deficiencies with your clinical study of an investigational drug. It is your responsibility to ensure adherence to each requirement of the law and relevant FDA regulations. You should address these deficiencies and establish procedures to ensure that any ongoing or future studies will be in compliance with FDA regulations.

Within fifteen (15) working days of your receipt of this letter, you should notify this office in writing of the actions you have taken to prevent similar violations in the future. Failure to address the violations noted above adequately and promptly may result in regulatory action without further notice.

We acknowledge your assurance that you do not intend to perform clinical investigations (clinical trials) in the future. If you should change your mind about conducting clinical trials, please inform this office of your plans.

If you have any questions, please contact Constance Cullity, M.D., M.P.H., at 301-796-3397; FAX 301-847-8748. Your written response and any pertinent documentation should be addressed to:

Constance Cullity, M.D., M.P.H.
Branch Chief
Good Clinical Practice Enforcement Branch
Division of Good Clinical Practice Compliance
Office of Scientific Investigations
Office of Compliance
Center for Drug Evaluation and Research
Food and Drug Administration
Building 51, Room 5354
10903 New Hampshire Avenue
Silver Spring, MD 20993

Sincerely yours,

/S/

Leslie K. Ball, M.D. Acting Director
Office of Scientific Investigations
Office of Compliance
Center for Drug Evaluation and Research
Food and Drug Administration

第91封　给Tuller, Betty博士的警告信

2011年11月21日

参考号：12-HFD-45-11-01

尊敬的Tuller博士：

2011年1月18日至2月14日，Sean Creighton先生代表FDA，对您所开展的试验药物为（b）（4）[1]的临床研究进行了审查。已经批准在美国上市的药品的临床研究，如果其满足21 CFR 312.2（b）（1）的标准可免除法规 21CFR312要求的临床研究。但是，上述所列出的研究因为包含一种能显著增加该药物风险的给药途径或剂量水平，所以不符合免除临床研究的标准［21CFR312.2（b）（iii）］。因此，这些研究在21 CFR 第312部分［21 CFR 312.2（a）］的法规监管范围内，应该通过新药研究IND［21 CFR 312.20］申请来开展临床研究。您作为这些研究的临床研究者也被要求遵从21 CFR 312的法规要求。

在您进行这些研究的过程中，您的工作地址是：Florida Atlantic University，Center for Complex Systems and Brain Sciences，777 Glades Road，Boca Raton，FL 33431。

本次现场检查是FDA的生物研究监查项目的一部分。该项目通过设定的检查方法，对研究的实施情况进行评估，以确认研究数据在科学上是有效和准确的，并帮助确保这些研究中受试者的权益、安全和福利得到了保护。

经对现场检查报告、该报告的附件进行审查，我们认为，您没有遵循适用的法律要求和监管临床研究实施及受试者保护的FDA法规。

在现场检查结束时，Creighton先生向您出示了现场检查发现的问题，并与您进行了讨论。我们想强调以下几点：

1. 您未能按照21 CFR 50的要求规定获得知情同意［21 CFR 312.60］

作为研究者，您有责任按照21 CFR 50［21 CFR 312.60］的法规要求获得知情同意。法规21 CFR 50.25（a）项描述了获取知情同意必须提供给每个受试者的基本信息。但是，在上述5个关于（b）（4）和（b）（4）的研究中，其中的四个研究，您未能保证向受试者们提供法规21 CFR 50.25（a）项要求的所有基本信息。

具体来讲，用于这四个研究的知情同意中没有包含下列要求的信息：

a. 指明任何试验性质的程序 [CFR 50.25（a）1）]；

b. 告知合适的可选择程序或可能对受试者有利的治疗过程 [21 CFR 50.25（a）（4）]；

c. 声明FDA可能检查研究记录 [21 CFR 50.25（a）（5）]；

d. 解释是否有任何补贴，如发生伤害是否可以受到医疗救治，救治的组成内容，或者在哪里可以得到进一步的信息 [21 CFR 50.25（a）（6）]。

e. 描述对受试者任何能合理预见的风险或不适 [21 CFR 50.25（a）（2）]。

这些知情同意中写道"（b）（4）的风险主要是低血糖症"。但是，在现场检查中发现，在研究记录中的（b）（4）说明书上，还包括低钾血症等其他风险。未经治疗的低钾血症可能引起呼吸麻痹、心室性心律失常和死亡。（b）（4）使用（b）（4）后快速起效，因此（b）（4）疗法在用于有低钾血症风险的受试者时应该谨慎（例如，患者正在进行降血钾治疗，或者患者正在进行会造成血浆钾浓度变化的治疗），应该在应用（b）（4）过程中定期监测血钾浓度，以避免致死性低钾血症。

1 （b）（4）涉及商业秘密，根据法规内容不予公开。

您未能把这些能合理预见的引发低钾血症及并发症的风险告知受试者。这在给受试者的知情同意书中是一个非常严重的信息缺失，对受试者保护而言是一个重大隐患。

因为您未能把这些能合理预见的引发低钾血症和并发症的风险以及上述法规所要求的其他基本信息告知受试者，导致受试者没有机会评估自己参与这些临床研究的风险和受益。此外，因为您未能对这些参与您临床研究的受试者提供法律规定的受试者应该得到的信息，使这些受试者在决定是否参与这些研究的过程中无法基于这些必要信息来做出决定。这使得受试者们的权益，安全和福利受到了损害。

2. 您未能保存研究中使用研究药物或对照组的受试者的所有研究观察和其他相关数据的足够和准确的病历［21 CFR 312.62（b）］

作为临床研究者，您应该保存研究中使用研究药物或对照组的受试者的所有观察和其他相关的数据的足够和准确的病历，病历包括受试者的入组、参与试验过程中和试验结束的相关信息。但是，在检查过程中，您向检查员Creighton先生承认您没有记录受试者入组数、脱落数和完成试验数。因此您未能遵循21 CFR 312 62（b）的要求完整准确地记录和保存病历。

您未能保存足够和准确的病历，包括与受试者入组和完成试验研究的相关信息，导致记录无法准确区分试验受试者参与试验的情况。这引起了我们对受试者安全和数据可靠性的担忧，同时也影响了对临床研究终点的解释和研究有效性。

3. 您未能及时向IRB报告给受试者或他人带来风险的所有非预期事件［21 CFR 312.66］

作为临床研究者，您必须及时向IRB 报告所有非预期事件，包括涉及受试者风险的事件或其他事件［21 CFR 312.66］。我们在检查中发现，您收集了2004~2009年间，在上述5个临床研究中发生的不良事件的清单，其中包括一些导致受试者住院治疗的不良事件。但是，在我们检查期间您向Creighton先生表示，在您给IRB递交的所有文件中没有报告关于这些研究的不良事件。我们检查中进一步发现，没有任何记录表明，您曾经向IRB报告过这些记录在不良事件清单里的涉及受试者风险非预期事件。

您未能确保向IRB通报所有涉及受试者风险的非预期事件，导致我们对受试者的权益、安全和福利受到保护的程度有一定担忧。IRB在没有足够的涉及受试者风险的非预期事件清单的情况下，无法对研究中受试者的持续安全做出合理的判定。

本警告信的目的并非是罗列您在试验药物临床研究中存在的所有缺陷。确保遵循法律和相关FDA法规的每一项要求是您的职责，您应当解决这些缺陷，并建立规程，以确保任何正在进行或将来进行的研究均符合FDA的法规。

自收到这封信的15个工作日内，您应当书面告知本办公室为预防将来发生类似违规行为已经采取的措施。如果不能充分地、迅速地解释上述违规问题，可能导致我们在不再通知的情况下采取监管措施。

附：英文原文

Tuller, Betty Ph.D.

WARNING LETTER

NOV 21, 2011

UNITED PARCEL SERVICE (UPS)

Ref: 12-HFD-45-11-01

Betty Tuller, Ph.D.
(b)(6)

Dear Dr. Tuller:

Between January 18, 2011, and February 14, 2011, Mr. Sean Creighton, representing the U.S. Food and Drug Administration (FDA), conducted an investigation and met with you to review your conduct of the following clinical investigations of the investigational drug (b)(4):

(b)(4)

The clinical investigation of a drug product that is lawfully marketed in the United States is exempt from the requirements of Title 21, Code of Federal Regulations (CFR) Part 312 if the criteria in 21 CFR 312.2(b)(1) are met. However, the studies listed above do not meet these criteria because they involved a route of administration or dosage level that significantly increased the risks (or decreased the acceptability of the risks) associated with the use of this drug product [21 CFR 312.2(b)(iii)]. Therefore, these studies were subject to 21 CFR Part 312 [21 CFR 312.2(a)] and should have been conducted under an Investigational New Drug (IND) application [21 CFR 312.20]. As a result, your conduct as the clinical investigator for these studies was required to conform to the requirements in 21 CFR Part 312.

During the time you conducted these studies, you were working at the following address: Florida Atlantic University, Center for Complex Systems and Brain Sciences, 777 Glades Road, Boca Raton, FL 33431.

This inspection is a part of FDA's Bioresearch Monitoring Program, which includes inspections designed to evaluate the conduct of research and to help ensure that the rights, safety, and welfare of the human subjects of those studies have been protected.

From our review of the establishment inspection report and the documents submitted with that report, we conclude that you did not adhere to the applicable statutory requirements and FDA regulations governing the conduct of clinical investigations and the protection of human subjects.

We are aware that at the conclusion of the inspection, Mr. Creighton presented and discussed with you the inspectional findings. We wish to emphasize the following:

1. You failed to obtain informed consent in accordance with the provisions of 21 CFR Part 50 [21 CFR 312.60].

As the investigator, it was your responsibility to obtain informed consent in accordance with 21 CFR Part 50 [21 CFR 312.60]. 21 CFR 50.25(a) describes the basic information that must be provided to each subject when seeking informed consent. However for four of the five studies listed above (b)(4) and (b)(4), you failed to ensure that subjects were provided with all of the basic information required by 21 CFR 50.25(a).

Specifically, the informed consent documents used for these four studies failed to include the following required elements:

a. Identification of any procedures which are experimental [CFR 50.25(a)1)]

b. A disclosure of appropriate alternative procedures or courses of treatment that might be advantageous to the subject [21 CFR 50.25(a)(4)].

c. A statement noting the possibility that the Food and Drug Administration may inspect the records [21 CFR 50.25(a)(5)].

d. An explanation as to whether any compensation and an explanation as to whether any medical treatments are available if injury occurs; and, if so, what they consist of, or where further information may be obtained [21 CFR 50.25(a)(6)].

e. A description of any reasonably foreseeable risks or discomforts to the subject [21 CFR 50.25(a)(2)].

The informed consent documents for these studies indicate that "Risks from the (b)(4) are primarily hypoglycemia." However, according to the (b)(4) label found in study records at your site, the risks associated with the use of (b)(4) products also include, but are not limited to, hypokalemia. Untreated hypokalemia may cause respiratory paralysis, ventricular arrhythmia, and death. (b)(4) administered (b)(4) has a rapid onset of action. Therefore, this modality of (b)(4) therapy should be used with caution in subjects at risk for hypokalemia (e.g., patients using potassium-lowering medications and patients taking medications sensitive to serum potassium concentrations), and potassium should be monitored frequently when (b)(4) is administered (b)(4) to avoid fatal hypokalemia.

You failed to inform subjects of the reasonably foreseeable risk of developing hypokalemia and its complications. This is a critical omission in the information provided to subjects when seeking informed consent, and represents a significant human subject protection concern.

Your failure to inform subjects of the reasonably foreseeable risk of hypokalemia and its complications, along with your failure to inform subjects of the additional required elements of consent listed above, denied the subjects an opportunity to assess the risks and benefits of their participation in the clinical investigations. Additionally, by not providing the subjects under your care with the information they were entitled to receive to assist them in making an informed decision about whether to participate in the studies, you compromised the rights, safety, and welfare of those subjects.

2. You failed to maintain adequate and accurate case histories that record all observations and other data pertinent to the investigation on each individual administered the investigational drug or employed as a control in the investigation [21CFR 312.62(b)].

As the clinical investigator, you were required to prepare and maintain adequate and accurate case histories that record all observations and other data pertinent to the investigation on each individual administered the investigational drug or employed as a control in the investigation [21CFR 312.62(b)]. Case histories include information related to subject's enrollment and participation in, and completion of, the study. However, during the inspection, you indicated to

Mr. Creighton that you did not keep records of how many subjects were enrolled, how many subjects withdrew from the study, and how many subjects completed the study. As a result, it appears that you failed to maintain adequate and accurate case histories as required by 21 CFR 312.62(b).

Your failure to maintain adequate and accurate case histories, including information related to subject enrollment and completion of the study, impacts the ability to accurately characterize subject participation in your studies; raises concerns about subject safety and data integrity; and compromises the interpretation and validity of the investigational endpoints.

3. You failed to promptly report to the IRB all unanticipated problems involving risk to human subjects or others [21 CFR 312.66].

As the clinical investigator, you were required to promptly report to the IRB all unanticipated problems involving risk to human subjects or others [21 CFR 312.66]. Our investigation revealed that you collected lists of adverse events that occurred during the conduct of the five studies listed above, between 2004 and 2009, including some adverse events that resulted in hospitalization of subjects. However, during the course of our investigation, you indicated to Mr. Creighton that you reported there were "no adverse events" in these studies on all of your submissions to the IRB. Moreover, during our investigation, we did not find any records to indicate that you reported any of the unanticipated problems involving risk to human subjects, which were recorded on your lists of adverse events, to the responsible IRB.

Your failure to ensure that the IRB was notified of all unanticipated problems involving risk to subjects, raises concerns about the extent to which subjects' rights, safety, and welfare were protected. Without a complete listing of the unanticipated problems involving risks to the subjects, the IRB was unable to make an informed determination regarding the continued safety of the subjects enrolled in your investigations.

This letter is not intended to be an all-inclusive list of deficiencies with your clinical study of an investigational drug. It is your responsibility to ensure adherence to each requirement of the law and relevant FDA regulations. You should address these deficiencies and establish procedures to ensure that any ongoing or future studies will be in compliance with FDA regulations.

Within fifteen (15) working days of your receipt of this letter, you should notify this office in writing of the actions you have taken to prevent similar violations in the future. Failure to adequately and promptly explain the violations noted above may result in regulatory action without further notice.

If you have any questions, please contact Constance Cullity, M.D., M.P.H., at 3017963397;

FAX 3018478748.

Your written response and any pertinent documentation should be addressed to:

Constance Cullity (formerly Lewin), M.D., M.P.H.
Branch Chief
Good Clinical Practice Enforcement Branch
Division of Good Clinical Practice Compliance
Office of Scientific Investigations
Office of Compliance
Center for Drug Evaluation and Research
Food and Drug Administration
Building 51, Room 5354
10903 New Hampshire Avenue
Silver Spring, MD 20993

Sincerely yours,

/S/

/Leslie K. Ball, M.D./
Leslie K. Ball, M.D.
Acting Director
Office of Scientific Investigations
Office of Compliance
Center for Drug Evaluation and Research
Food and Drug Administration

第 92 封　给 Diaz, Leslie 医学博士的警告信

2011年11月4日

参考号：11-HFD-45-10-01

尊敬的Diaz博士：

2011年1月12日至2011年3月8日，Colleen Aspinwall女士代表 FDA 与您会面，对您所开展的以下临床研究进行了审查。这封警告信特告知您现场检查中发现的违规情况。

试验方案（b）(4）[1]，标题为“（b）(4),”试验药物为（b）(4)，申办者为（b）(4)。

试验方案（b）(4)，标题为“（b）(4),”试验药物为（b）(4)，申办者为（b）(4)。

本次现场检查是FDA的生物研究监查项目的一部分。该项目通过设定的检查方法，评估研究的实施情况，并帮助确保这些研究中受试者的权益、安全和福利得到了保护。

经对现场检查报告、该报告的附件，以及您2011年3月11日的书面回复进行审查，我们认为，您没有遵循适用的法律要求和监管临床研究实施的FDA法规。在现场检查结束时，Aspinwall女士向您出示了FDA 483表，即现场检查发现的问题，并与您进行了讨论。我们想强调以下几点：

1. 您未能亲自进行临床研究或对研究进行充分监督［21 CFR 312.60］

当您为上述临床研究签署研究者声明（FDA 1572表）时，您同意在您的研究中心承担临床研究者的职责。您的总体职责包括按照您签署的研究者声明、研究计划以及适用的法规进行；保护在您的照护下的受试者的权益、安全和福利；确保对试验药物的管理（21 CFR 312.60）。在签署的研究者声明中，特别说明您同意亲自实施研究或将对非您本人亲自实施的研究工作予以监管。尽管您可以将一些研究任务授权给有资质的人员完成，但作为临床研究者，您不能授权您的总体职责。我们的检查发现，您对研究的监督管理不足以确保研究按照签署的研究者声明、研究计划以及适用的法规而开展。您对研究的参与和监督管理的不充分，令人担心贵中心对入组该项研究的受试者的权益、安全和福利的保护以及数据的完整可靠。

在您2011年3月8日签署的书面陈述中，您声称尽管您的执业经历了数次所有权的变更，但您一直担任着上述研究的主要研究者，您充分知晓您对上述研究始终承担着最终的责任，以及您继续承担着对实施和监督这项研究的全部责任。

在您的书面陈述中，您承认不充分的监督管理下的一些重要问题，包括但不限于以下情况：

“我承认作为主要研究者，在这些临床试验中我缺乏参与和监督管理。”

“在查询研究文件时，我也发现了寄给我而我从未打开和（或）阅读的信函。这些信函来自监查员，申办者和伦理委员会，包括一些要求我终止临床试验的信函。”这些信函通知您，因为您未能提交跟踪审查报告，对方案的批准被暂停或终止；数次尝试都未能联系到您；或者您未能回复数次的沟通。

“我承认试验［（b）(4)］和（b）(4）的不良事件……没有按照研究方案的要求进行评估（分级）。”

“我也承认忽视了临床试验。我也没有对收到的和发出的邮件进行追踪。”

“2007年12月初，我的研究助理离开之后，所有的研究记录就结束了。”

“我不了解这些研究是怎样被监查的。”

我们希望再一次强调，作为临床研究者，为了保护研究受试者的权益、安全和福利以及确保数据的完整可靠，您承担最终的责任，以确保正确地开展研究并遵循FDA的法规。当将您书面陈述中的说明与以下所述的违规问题相结合时，显示您在开展临床研究中存在着系统性缺陷。因此，我们非常担心贵研究中心入组这些研究的受试者的权益、安全和福利，以及数据的完整可靠。

1 (b) (4) 涉及商业秘密，根据法规内容不予公开。

2. 您未能确保按照研究计划进行研究［21 CFR 312.60］

作为研究者，您被要求确保研究按照签署的研究者声明、研究计划以及适用的法规而进行。您未能按照研究计划实施试验方案（b）(4）和（b）(4）。包括但不限于以下所列举的情况。

a. 试验方案（b）(4）

i. 试验方案2.3部分详述此项研究将排除严重肾功能不全者。FDA现场检查期间，在您研究中心可见到的原始记录显示，受试者02145在2007年5月8日筛选后入组研究。然而，既往病史显示，该受试者在入组前持续存在慢性肾衰竭。因此，入组这名受试者违背了研究计划。

ii. 试验方案3.3.6部分和表3-1提供了评估不良事件（AE）的说明，并规定具有医师资质的研究者对所有不良事件的最强程度、严重性、持续时间、采取的措施，以及与研究药物的关系进行评估。在您的书面陈述中，您承认在试验方案（b）(4）中，记录在受试者病历夹中，包括临床症状的不良事件都没有按照方案要求进行评估和分级。例如，受试者02145和01323，不良事件记录在受试者的医疗评估的原始记录中，然而，这些不良事件都没有按照方案要求进行评估和分级。

iii. 试验方案3.3.5.1部分特别规定，对于入组这项研究的受试者，在停止治疗的14天之内，或根据方案要求，在确定的停止治疗后的安全性随访期间，发生的严重不良事件，包括因任何原因导致的死亡，无论是否与研究药物相关，必须在24小时之内报告申办者。

受试者00996于2007年3月2日被入组研究。记录显示在2007年5月至6月初，这名受试者仍在研期间，接受了心导管术，显示受试者发生了因三支冠状动脉闭塞而手术的严重不良事件。此外，我们注意到您在申办者的严重不良事件报告表上将此严重不良事件定为“有即刻生命危险”。然而，您没有根据方案的要求，在24小时之内报告，而是直到2007年7月30日您才报告了该严重不良事件。此外，您没有提供申办者严重不良事件报告表上要求的所有信息，报告该严重不良事件是否与研究药物相关。

b. 试验方案（b）(4）5.4.1部分特别规定受试者应在完成筛选评估，并经申办者或其指定人员确认符合入组标准后，获得试验用药［（b）(4）］。原始记录显示受试者214-002102在2007年6月27日分发获得了研究药物，几乎是在您获得申办者确认其符合合格标准即2007年7月9日的2周之前。因此，您未能遵循方案的要求，即在确认受试者入组后才予以研究药物。

综上所述，您未能确保根据研究计划开展研究，因为您入组了不符合合格标准的受试者，未能正确地评估不良事件，未能正确地报告严重不良事件，以及在确认受试者入组前即分发了研究药物。此外，在您签署的书面陈述中，您承认您未能充分地参与和监督这些研究的开展，没有记录确认受试者符合合格标准的流程，没有根据方案评估不良事件。

这些说明，与以上所述的违规问题相结合时，显示您在开展临床研究中存在着系统性缺陷。因此，我们非常担心贵中心入组这些研究的受试者的权益、安全和福利，以及贵中心的数据的完整可靠。

3. 您未能按照21 CFR 312.59的要求将未使用的药物归还给申办者，或提供对未使用的药物的处置情况［21 CFR 312.62（a）］

在我们的现场检查中，在您的研究中心发现了研究（b）(4）和（b）(4）中未归还的研究药物。在您的书面陈述中，您说在找寻研究文件记录时，您发现了一箱从未归还申办者的研究药物。这个箱子里包括了全满或半满的药瓶，还有一些空瓶子。

在您的研究中心发现的这些未归还的药物令人非常关注您对研究实施的监督以及研究药物的管理是否充分。在您的书面陈述中，您承认您对研究实施的参与和监督管理存在不足。这种总体上的缺乏监管，结合您未能管控好药物这一问题，削弱了我们对您给受试者分发药物合规性的信心。因此，我们非常担心贵研究中心纳入这些研究的受试者的权益、安全和福利，以及数据的完整可靠。

本警告信的目的并非是罗列您在药物临床研究中存在的所有缺陷。确保遵循法律和相关FDA法规的每一项要求是您的职责。

我们注意到在您的书面陈述中，您说明目前您未参与任何属于FDA监管的试验，并且在将来没有意愿再开展任何FDA监管的临床试验。尽管如此，确保遵循FDA法规仍是您的职责。因此，自收到这封信的15个工作日内，您应当书面告知本办公室为预防将来发生类似违规情况已经采取的措施。如果不能充分、快速地解释上述违规问题，可能导致我们在不再通知的情况下采取监管措施。此外，我们要求，将来如果您改变主意，决定要开展FDA监管的研究，您应立即将您有意愿做临床研究者的决定通知本办公室。

附：英文原文

Diaz, Leslie, M.D.

WARNING LETTER

Nov 4 , 2011

CERTIFIED MAIL
RETURN RECEIPT REQUESTED

Ref:11-HFD-45-10-01

Leslie E. Diaz, M.D.
Infectious Disease Associates of the Palm Beaches
840 U.S. Highway #1, Suite 120
North Palm Beach, FL 33408

Dear Dr. Diaz:

Between January 12, 2011, and March 8, 2011, Ms. Colleen Aspinwall, representing the U.S. Food and Drug Administration (FDA), conducted an investigation and met with you to review your conduct of the following clinical investigations:

Protocol (b)(4), titled "(b)(4)," of the investigational drug (b)(4), performed for (b)(4)

Protocol (b)(4), titled "(b)(4)," of the investigational drug (b)(4), performed for (b)(4)

This inspection is a part of FDA's Bioresearch Monitoring Program, which includes inspections designed to evaluate the conduct of research and to help ensure that the rights, safety, and welfare of the human subjects of those studies have been protected.

From our review of the establishment inspection report, the documents submitted with that report, and your written response dated March 11, 2011, we conclude that you did not adhere to the applicable statutory requirements and FDA regulations governing the conduct of clinical investigations. At the conclusion of the inspection, Ms. Aspinwall presented you with a Form FDA 483, Inspectional Observations, and discussed the observations listed on the form with you. We wish to emphasize the following:

1. You failed to personally conduct or adequately supervise the clinical investigations [21 CFR 312.60].

When you signed the investigator statements (Form FDA 1572) for the above-referenced clinical investigations, you agreed to take on the responsibilities of a clinical investigator at your site. Your general responsibilities include ensuring that the investigation is conducted according to the signed investigator statement, the investigational plan, and applicable regulations; protecting the rights, safety, and welfare of subjects under your care; and ensuring control of drugs under investigation (21 CFR 312.60). In the signed investigator agreement, you specifically agreed to personally conduct the clinical studies or to supervise those aspects of the studies that you did not personally conduct. While you may delegate certain study tasks to individuals qualified to perform them, as clinical investigator, you may not delegate your general responsibilities. Our investigation indicates that your supervision over the studies was not adequate to ensure that clinical trials were conducted according to the signed investigator statement, the investigational plan, and applicable regulations. This lack of adequate involvement in and oversight of the studies raises concerns regarding the protection of the rights, safety, and welfare of subjects enrolled into the studies and the integrity of the data from your site.

In a written affidavit signed by you on March 8, 2011, you stated that even though your practice went through multiple ownership changes, you always remained as the principal investigator for the above trials, you were fully aware that you always had the ultimate responsibility for these clinical trials, and you continued to take full responsibility for their conduct and oversight.

In your written affidavit, you acknowledged a number of significant instances of inadequate oversight and supervision, including but not limited to the following:

"I am admitting to the Agency that as a Clinical Investigator/Principal Investigator, I had a lack of involvement and oversight in the conduct of these clinical trials."

"In searching for study documentation, I also found letters that were sent to me that I had never opened and/or had seen before. These letters were from monitors, sponsors, and IRB's, including some of which involved the termination of my clinical studies." These letters informed you that approval of the audited protocols had been suspended or terminated, due to your failure to submit continuing review reports; inability to contact you after multiple attempts; or your failure to respond to multiple communications.

"I acknowledge that adverse experiences for [(b)(4)] and the (b)(4) trials … were not evaluated/graded as required by study protocols."

"I am also admitting to having ignored the clinical trials. I also did not keep track of the mail as far as what was coming in or going out."

"All study documentation ended in early December 2007 after my study coordinator left."

"I had no knowledge of how these studies were monitored."

We wish to emphasize again that as the clinical investigator, it was your ultimate responsibility to ensure that the studies were conducted properly and in compliance with FDA regulations, in order to protect the rights, safety, and welfare of study subjects and to ensure the integrity of the study data. The statements in your affidavit, when taken in conjunction with the violations described below, indicate systemic failures in your conduct of investigational research. As a result, we have significant concerns about the safety and welfare of subjects enrolled into these studies and the integrity of the data from your site.

2. You failed to ensure that the investigation was conducted according to the investigational plan [21 CFR 312.60].

As a clinical investigator, you are required to ensure that an investigation is conducted according to the signed investigator statement, the investigational plan, and applicable regulations. You have failed to conduct Protocols (b)(4) and (b)(4) according to the investigational plans. Examples of this failure include but are not limited to the following:

a. For Protocol (b)(4):

i. Protocol Section 2.3 specified that subjects with severe renal insufficiency were to be excluded from the study. Source records available at your clinical site during the FDA inspection showed that Subject 02145 was screened for enrollment into the study on May 8, 2007. However, the medical history showed that this subject had continuing chronic renal failure prior to enrollment. Thus, the enrollment of this subject into the study violated the investigational plan.

ii. Protocol Section 3.3.6 and Table 3-1 provided instructions for evaluating adverse events (AEs) and stated that an investigator who was a qualified physician was to evaluate all AEs with regard to maximum intensity, seriousness, duration, action taken, and relationship to test drug. In your written affidavit, you acknowledged that for Protocol (b)(4), AEs that included the clinical symptoms recorded in the subjects' charts were not evaluated or graded, as required by the protocol. For example, for Subjects 02145 and 01323, AEs were recorded in the subjects' medical evaluation source documents; however, these were not evaluated or graded according to protocol requirements.

iii. Protocol Section 3.3.5.1 specified that any serious adverse experience (SAE), including death due to any cause, that occurs to any subject entered into this study or within 14 days following cessation of treatment or within the established off-therapy follow-up period for safety as described in the protocol, whether or not related to the investigational product, must be reported to the sponsor within 24 hours.

Subject 00996 was enrolled into the study on March 2, 2007. Records show that between May and early June 2007, when the subject was still in the study, the subject underwent cardiac catheterization that revealed an SAE of triple-vessel coronary artery occlusive disease and required surgery. Also, we note that you characterized this SAE as "immediately life-threatening" on the sponsor's SAE reporting form. However, you did not report this SAE to the sponsor until July 30, 2007, which was beyond the 24-hour window specified by the protocol. In addition, you did not provide all of the information requested on the sponsor's SAE form, including whether the SAE was related to the study drug.

b. For Protocol (b)(4), Section 5.4.1 specified that the subject was to receive the investigational medication ((b)(4)) once eligibility was confirmed after completion of the screening form and evaluation by the sponsor or its designee. Source records indicate that Subject 214-002102 was dispensed study drug on June 27, 2007, nearly two weeks before you received confirmation of the subject's eligibility for enrollment by the sponsor or its designee on July 9, 2007. You therefore failed to follow the protocol requirements by dispensing investigational medication to a subject prior to confirming the subject's enrollment into the study.

To summarize, you have failed to ensure that the investigations were conducted in accordance with the investigational plan, because you enrolled ineligible subjects, failed to properly evaluate AEs, failed to properly report SAEs, and dispensed investigational medication to subjects prior to confirming their enrollment. Furthermore, in your signed affidavit, you acknowledge that you had a lack of involvement and oversight in the conduct of these clinical trials, did not document the process for confirming subject eligibility, and did not evaluate AEs according to the protocol. These statements, when taken in conjunction with the violations described above, indicate systemic failures in your conduct of investigational research. As a result, we have significant concerns about the safety and welfare of subjects enrolled into these studies and the integrity of the data from your site.

3. You did not return the unused supplies of the drug to the sponsor, or otherwise provide for disposition of the unused supplies of the drug under 21 CFR 312.59 [21 CFR 312.62(a)].

During our inspection, unreturned investigational drugs for both the (b)(4) and (b)(4) studies were found at your site. In your written affidavit, you stated that in searching for documentation for the audited studies, you found a box of study drug product which had never been returned to the sponsors. The box contained full, partially full, and empty bottles of study drug.

The identification of these unreturned investigational drugs at your site raises significant concerns regarding the adequacy of your oversight and control of investigational drugs. In your signed affidavit, you admit to a lack of involvement and oversight in the conduct of these clinical trials. This general lack of oversight, when taken in conjunction with your failure to maintain control of investigational drugs, serves to undermine the confidence we have in your drug dispensation to subjects. As a result, we have significant concerns about the safety and welfare of subjects enrolled into these studies and the integrity of the data from your site.

This letter is not intended to be an all-inclusive list of deficiencies with your clinical study of an investigational drug. It is your responsibility to ensure adherence to each requirement of the law and relevant FDA regulations.

We note that in your written affidavit, you state that you are currently not involved in any FDA-regulated trials and do not have any intentions of ever conducting an FDA-regulated clinical trial in the future. Nevertheless, it is your responsibility to ensure compliance with FDA regulations. Therefore, within fifteen (15) working days of your receipt of this letter, you should notify this office in writing of the actions you have taken to prevent similar violations in the future. Failure to adequately and promptly explain the violations noted above may result in regulatory action without further notice. Further, we request that, if your plans should change in the future and you should decide to begin conducting FDA-regulated research, you promptly notify this office of your intention to become a clinical investigator.

If you have any questions, please contact Constance Cullity, M.D., M.P.H., at 301-796-3397; FAX 301-847-8748.

Your written response and any pertinent documentation should be addressed to:

Constance Cullity (formerly Lewin), M.D., M.P.H.
Branch Chief
Good Clinical Practice Enforcement Branch
Division of Good Clinical Practice Compliance
Office of Scientific Investigations
Office of Compliance
Center for Drug Evaluation and Research
Food and Drug Administration
Building 51, Room 5354
10903 New Hampshire Avenue
Silver Spring, MD 20993

Sincerely yours,

/S/

Leslie K. Ball, M.D.
Acting Director
Office of Scientific Investigations
Office of Compliance
Center for Drug Evaluation and Research
Food and Drug Administration

第93封　给Teasley, Laura A.医学博士的警告信

2011年10月14日

参考号：11-HFD-45-09-03

尊敬的Teasley博士：

2010年7月26日至2010年8月24日，Thomas R.Beilke先生代表FDA，在您之前就职的诊所进行现场检查。在现场检查期间，Beilke先生与您会面，对您所开展的以下临床研究进行了审查：试验方案（b）（4）[1]，标题为“（b）（4）”，申办者为（b）（4）。2008年3月到2009年3月，您作为研究者开展了这项临床研究。

本次现场检查是FDA的生物研究监查项目的一部分。该项目通过设定的检查方法，评估研究的实施情况，并帮助确保这些研究中受试者的权益、安全和福利得到了保护。

经对现场检查报告、该报告的附件进行审查，我们认为，您没有遵循适用的法律要求和监管临床研究实施的FDA法规。我们想强调以下几点：

1. 您未能确保按照签署的研究者声明进行研究，您未能亲自进行临床研究或对研究进行监督［21 CFR 312.60］

当您签署上述研究的研究者声明（FDA 1572表）时，您同意在您的研究中心承担临床研究者的职责。作为临床研究者，您的总体职责包括确保临床试验按照签署的研究者声明、研究计划和适用的法规进行；保护在您的照护下的受试者的权益、安全和福利；确保对试验药物的管控（21 CFR 312.60）。在签署的研究者声明中，特别说明您同意亲自实施临床试验或将对非您本人亲自实施的临床试验工作予以监督和管理。尽管您可以将一些研究任务授权给有资质的人员完成，但是作为研究者，您不能授权总体的职责。我们的检查发现您对授权研究任务的人员的监督管理不足以确保试验方案（b）（4）是根据签署的研究者声明、研究计划和适用的法规而开展，不能确保方案实施的方式足以保护受试者的权益、安全和福利。

具体而言，试验方案（b）（4）［第一章，1.3（F）］（检查程序），以及第二章2.3.2（基线检查程序）要求，获得每个入组的受试者眼睛的眼底照片和光学相干层析技术（OCT）扫描，依此评估受试者是否符合入组标准，同时作为研究的基线检查。作为临床研究者，您将获得眼底照片和OCT扫描的职责授权给了研究协调员。

您的书面陈述中提到“依据我的专业观点，后期的扫描与基线时的OCT扫描不匹配。我也将基线扫描（上的眼底照片）和该受试者同一只眼在基线期附近另外拍摄的眼底照片进行了比较，发现它们也不能匹配。同一个受试者的同一只眼在不同的日期的眼底照片，其视网膜的血管样式应该完全匹配。”基于此，对于特定的眼睛，与OCT扫描分开拍摄的眼底照片，应该与OCT扫描上的眼底照片相匹配。

然而，我们发现某些受试者，基线时OCT扫描上的眼底照片与单独拍摄的眼底照片不匹配。因此，这显示有些研究受试者基线的OCT扫描被其他不知名的患者的OCT扫描所取代。在记录中发现的这种不一致，包括，但不限于：

a. 受试者0035，日期为2008年10月16日的OCT扫描上的眼底照片，与该患者2008年10月16日单独拍摄的眼底照片不匹配。

b. 受试者0015，日期为2008年8月13日的OCT扫描上的眼底照片，与该患者2008年8月14日单独拍摄的眼底照片不匹配。

1 （b）（4）涉及商业秘密，根据法规内容不予公开。

c. 受试者0015，日期为2008年8月13日的OCT扫描上的左眼眼底照片，与该患者2008年8月14日单独拍摄的左眼眼底照片不匹配。

基于上述记录的不一致，无法确定这些受试者符合这项研究的入组合格标准。

您在2010年8月19日的书面陈述中说，作为临床研究者的职责之一是有必要仔细检查每个受试者的OCT扫描。您在该书面陈述中承认“这种替代或篡改（OCT扫描和眼底照片）可能令那些受试者被不实地纳入研究”。您未能充分地监督那些被您授权承担研究任务的人员，导致了您研究记录的不一致，而且受试者的入组不符合合格标准。入组不符合合格标准的受试者令人担心贵研究中心对受试者的权益、安全和福利的保护程度，以及所获得的数据的可靠性与完整性。

2. 您未能确保按照研究计划进行研究［21 CFR 312.60］

试验方案（b）(4)（版本号：5.0，版本日期2008年3月24日）第二章2.2.2具体规定一项纳入标准是随机前8天内临床检查发现存在糖尿病黄斑水肿，并且OCT显示中央分支厚度≥250μm。然而，以下的OCT扫描偏离了中心位置：

a. 2008年6月5日，受试者0003左眼的OCT扫描；

b. 2008年12月4日，受试者0040右眼的OCT扫描。

这些偏离中心位置的数值可能令这两名受试者表面看来符合纳入标准，而实际并非如此。

您未能根据方案指定的要求完成OCT扫描，造成了可能入组不符合合格标准的受试者，这将严重地影响到贵研究中心获得的数据的可靠性和完整真实性。此外，入组可能不符合合格标准的受试者，以及未能正确地遵循研究相关流程，令人担心对受试者的权益、安全和福利的保护程度。

本警告信的目的并非是罗列您在试验药物临床研究中存在的所有缺陷。确保遵循法律和相关FDA法规的每一项要求是您的职责，您应当解决这些缺陷，并建立规程，以确保任何正在进行或将来进行的研究均符合FDA的法规。

自收到这封信的15个工作日内，您应当书面告知本办公室为预防将来发生类似违规情况而采取的措施。如果不能充分、迅速地解释上述违规问题，可能导致我们在不再通知的情况下采取监管措施。

附：英文原文

Teasley, Laura A. M.D.

WARNING LETTER

OCT 14, 2011

CERTIFIED MAIL
RETURN RECEIPT REQUESTED

Ref:11-HFD-45-09-03

Laura A. Teasley, M.D.
Loma Linda University Health Care
Faculty Medical Offices, Suite 1800
11370 Anderson Street
Loma Linda, CA 92354

Dear Dr. Teasley:

Between July 26 and August 24, 2010, Thomas R. Beilke, representing the U.S. Food and Drug Administration (FDA), conducted an investigation of your former practice. During the course of the inspection, Mr. Beilke met with you to review your conduct of a clinical investigation (Protocol (b)(4), titled "(b)(4)") performed for (b)(4). You were the investigator for this clinical investigation between March 2008 and March 2009.

This inspection is a part of FDA's Bioresearch Monitoring Program, which includes inspections designed to evaluate the conduct of research and to help ensure that the rights, safety, and welfare of the human subjects of those studies have been protected.

From our review of the establishment inspection report and the documents submitted with that report, we conclude that you did not adhere to the applicable statutory requirements and FDA regulations governing the conduct of clinical investigations. We wish to emphasize the following:

1. You failed to ensure that the investigation was conducted according to the signed investigator statement, in that you failed to personally conduct or supervise the clinical investigation [21 CFR 312.60].

When you signed the Statement of Investigator (Form FDA 1572) for the above-referenced clinical trial, you agreed to take on the responsibilities of a clinical investigator at your site. Your general responsibilities as a clinical investigator include ensuring that the clinical trial is conducted according to the signed investigator statement, the investigational plan, and applicable regulations; protecting the rights, safety, and welfare of subjects under your care; and ensuring control of drugs under investigation [21 CFR 312.60]. By signing Form FDA 1572, you specifically agreed to personally conduct the clinical trial or to supervise those aspects of the trial that you did not personally conduct. While you may delegate certain study tasks to individuals qualified to perform them, as a clinical investigator you may not delegate your general responsibilities. Our investigation indicates that your supervision of personnel to whom you delegated study tasks was not adequate to ensure that Protocol (b)(4) was conducted according to the signed investigator statement, the investigational plan, and applicable regulations, and in a manner that protects the rights, safety, and welfare of human subjects.

Specifically, Protocol (b)(4) [Chapter 1, Section 1.3(F) (Examination Procedures), and Chapter 2, Section 2.3.2 (Baseline Testing Procedures)] required that fundus photographs and optical coherence tomography (OCT) scans be obtained for each enrolled eye, both to assess subject eligibility and to serve as baseline measures for the study. As the clinical investigator, you delegated the responsibility for obtaining these fundus photographs and OCT scans to the study coordinator at your clinical site.

Your affidavit states, "It is my professional opinion that the later scans [...] do not match those OCT scans taken at baseline. I also compared the [fundus photographs on the] baseline scans with the fundus photographs taken of the respective subject's eyes approximately at baseline, and it appears that they do not match, either. Photographs that are taken of the same eye from the same subject on different dates should have retinal blood vessel patterns that match exactly." As such, it is expected that for any given eye, fundus photographs taken separately from the OCT scans should match the fundus photographs on the OCT scans.

However, it appears that for some subjects, the fundus photographs on the baseline OCT scans do not match the fundus photographs taken separately. Thus, it appears that some study subjects' baseline OCT scans have been substituted for other unknown patients' OCT scans. This inconsistency was found in records for subjects including, but not limited to, the following:

a. The fundus photograph on the OCT scan of Subject 0035's OD dated October 16, 2008, does not match the fundus photograph taken separately of Subject 0035's OD dated October 16, 2008.

b. The fundus photograph on the OCT scan of Subject 0015's OD dated August 13, 2008, does not match the fundus photograph taken separately of Subject 0015's OD dated August 14, 2008.

c. The fundus photograph on the OCT scan of Subject 0015's OS dated August 13, 2008, does not match the fundus photograph taken separately of Subject 0015's OS dated August 14, 2008.

As a result of these discrepancies in the records, it is not possible to ascertain if these subjects were eligible for enrollment in the study.

You indicate in your August 19, 2010, affidavit that one of your responsibilities as clinical investigator was to double-check the OCT scans necessary for each subject. You also acknowledged in your August 19, 2010, affidavit that "this substitution or manipulation [of the OCT scans and fundus photographs] may have allowed them [the subjects] to have been falsely qualified for the study." Your failure to adequately supervise the individuals to whom you delegated study tasks resulted in these discrepancies in your study records, as well as the enrollment of subjects who may not have met the eligibility criteria. Enrollment of subjects who may not meet eligibility criteria raises concerns about the extent to which subjects' rights, safety, and welfare were protected, and about the reliability and integrity of the data captured at your site.

2. You failed to ensure that the investigation was conducted according to the investigational plan [21 CFR 312.60].

Chapter 2, Section 2.2.2 of Protocol (b)(4)(Version 5.0, dated March 24, 2008) specified an inclusion criterion of diabetic macular edema present on clinical exam and central subfield thickness on optical coherence tomography (OCT) ⩾ 250 microns, within 8 days of randomization. However, the following OCT scans were taken off-center:

a. June 5, 2008, OCT scan of Subject 0003's OS; and

b. December 4, 2008, OCT scan of Subject 0040's OD.

These off-center readings made these two subjects appear eligible when they may not have been.

Your failure to ensure that OCT scans were obtained as specified by the protocol, which led to the enrollment of subjects who may not have met the eligibility criteria for the investigation, significantly undermines the reliability and integrity of the data captured at your site. In addition, enrollment of subjects who may not have met eligibility criteria, and failure to properly perform study-related procedures, raise concerns about the extent to which subjects' rights, safety, and welfare were protected.

This letter is not intended to be an all-inclusive list of deficiencies with your clinical study of an investigational drug. It is your responsibility to ensure adherence to each requirement of the law and relevant FDA regulations. You should address these deficiencies and establish procedures to ensure that any ongoing or future studies will be in compliance with FDA regulations.

Within fifteen (15) working days of your receipt of this letter, you should notify this office in writing of the actions you have taken to prevent similar violations in the future. Failure to adequately and promptly explain the violations noted above may result in regulatory action without further notice.

If you have any questions, please contact Constance Cullity, M.D., M.P.H., at 301-796-3397; FAX 301-847-8748. Your written response and any pertinent documentation should be addressed to:

Constance Cullity (formerly Lewin), M.D., M.P.H.
Branch Chief
Good Clinical Practice Enforcement Branch
Division of Good Clinical Practice Compliance
Office of Scientific Investigations
Office of Compliance
Center for Drug Evaluation and Research
Food and Drug Administration
Building 51, Room 5354
10903 New Hampshire Avenue
Silver Spring, MD 20993

Sincerely yours,

{See appended electronic signature page}

Leslie K. Ball, M.D.
Acting Office Director
Office of Scientific Investigations
Office of Compliance
Center for Drug Evaluation and Research

Food and Drug Administration

This is a representation of an electronic record that was signed electronically and this page is the manifestation of the electronic signature.

/S/

LESLIE K BALL

10/14/2011

第 94 封　给 Caton, John Jr. 医学博士的警告信

2011年8月26日

参考号：11-HFD-45-08-02

尊敬的Caton博士：

2010年8月2日至20日，Heika R. Tait先生代表FDA与您会面，对您所开展的试验药物为（b）（4）[1]，申办者为（b）（4）的以下临床研究进行了审查：试验方案（b）（4），标题为“（b）（4）”。

本次现场检查是FDA的生物研究监查项目的一部分。该项目通过设定的检查方法，评估研究的实施情况，并帮助确保这些研究中受试者的权益、安全和福利得到了保护。

经对现场检查报告、该报告的附件，以及您2010年9月10日的书面回复进行审查，我们认为，您没有遵循适用的法律要求和监管临床研究实施及受试者保护的FDA法规。我们知道在现场检查结束时，Heika R. Tait先生向您出示并讨论了FDA483表，即现场检查发现的问题。我们想强调以下几点：

1. 您未能确保按照研究计划进行研究［21 CFR 312.60］

您作为临床试验研究者的总体责任包括：确保按照签署的研究者声明、研究计划及适用的法规开展临床试验；保护您负责的受试者的权利、安全和利益；对研究药物进行管控［21CFR312.60］。不符合研究计划的内容举例如下，但不仅限于此：

a. 试验方案第3部分明确指出受试者被随机去接受（b）（4）或者（b）（4）。尽管受试者6002（作为该中心仅两名随机受试者中的一位）被随机分配至仅接受（b）（4）治疗，但根据2009年11月2日递交给机构伦理委员会（IRB）的报告，该受试者于2009年7月29日接受了（b）（4）和（b）（4）的联合用药。并且，根据2009年10月20日申办者给您的信函，对受试者6002注射后血样的分析显示其使用了两种药物。

b. 试验方案9.2部分具体规定，不良事件的记录必须包括但不限于研究者对如下方面属性的判定：对事件的描述（包括对事件的适当的详细描述），对与研究产品（IP）、化疗或者IP与化疗联合用药的相关性判定。在受试者6002的不良事件表中没有对这些属性判断的记录。

受试者随机不当以及缺乏不良事件判定导致对受试者权利、安全和利益保护存疑，并引起对该中心数据可靠性的顾虑。您的书面回复声明：以后您将在“美国肿瘤研究委员会指导的核对和平衡”下进行临床研究以确保类似违规不再发生，并引入新的药物清点标准操作规程（SOP）。无论如何，作为临床研究者，确保研究根据研究计划执行是您的职责，美国肿瘤研究委员会的政策、流程和活动不能抵消您作为临床研究者的责任。

2. 药物分发的记录包括日期、数量和受试者使用记录不全［21 CFR 312.62（a）］

a. 试验药物回收销毁表中记录4支试验药物（b）（4）丢失，但没有这些药物处置情况的记录。

b. 在检查过程中，研究人员告知检查员Tait试验药物保存在一个办公室，在给受试者分发药物时将转运至另一个房间，但没有记录表明这个试验药物的转运。

c. 方案要求试验药物的计数和准备记录应该保持更新，并记录分发药物的日期和数量等详细信息。检查显示没有任何有关分发试验药物（b）（4）和（b）（4）记录，每位受试者使用试验药物的日期和数量也没有记录。

药物处置记录不充分引起对受试者安全性和数据完整性的疑虑。我们获知，您的书面回复提及您一经获

1 （b）（4）涉及商业秘密，根据法规内容不予公开。

悉缺少药品计数记录以及丢失的药瓶，便已经对药房和临床研究SOP进行了评估和修订；在以后的研究中将在美国肿瘤研究会的规定下，采用电子药物计数系统。无论如何，作为临床研究者，保存药物处置的完整记录是您的职责，美国肿瘤研究会的政策、流程和活动不能抵消您作为临床研究者的责任。

3. 未能及时向 IRB 报告给受试者或其他人带来风险的所有非预期事件［21 CFR 312.66］

a. 受试者6002因双侧深静脉血栓和肺栓塞于（b）（4）住院，于（b）（4）出院。直到2009年11月2日，该住院事件才被报告给IRB.

b. 受试者6002于（b）（4）死亡。直到2009年11月4日，该死亡事件才被报告给伦理委员会（IRB）。

未能及时向IRB汇报给受试者带来风险的非预期问题，将削弱IRB对受试者的风险进行跟踪审查和评估的职能，会对受试者安全带来隐患。我们获知，您在书面回复中声明：以后将在美国肿瘤研究会的规定下进行研究。在美国肿瘤研究会的规定下，非预期的问题将报告给项目经理或者安全专家，再由他们报告给IRB。无论如何，向IRB及时报告研究中出现的给受试者带来风险的非预期问题是临床研究者的职责；美国肿瘤研究委员会的政策、流程和活动不能抵消您作为临床研究者的职责。

4. 您未能按 21 CFR 50 的要求获得知情同意［21 CFR 312.60］

根据21CFR50［21 CFR 312.60］条款，从每一位接受药物治疗的受试者处获得知情同意，这是作为临床研究者的总体职责。21 CFR 50.27要求知情同意应该使用被IRB批准过的书面知情同意书进行记录。但受试者6002在2009年7月10日签署的知情同意书模板未经过IRB批准。在知情同意书每一页的顶部有文字“于2008年10月2日修订，可批准模板，在中心使用前必须获得中心批准”。2009年5月12日的IRB对方案的批件证书上指示您，作为临床研究者，需“使用载有IRB‘批准’盖章的最新版本的知情同意书”。受试者6002签署的知情同意书上没有“批准”盖章，而是未获得IRB批准的同意书模板，表示受试者6002的知情同意过程未使用被IRB批准的书面知情同意书进行记录。

未按照21CFR第50条获得知情同意，会对受试者权利、安全和利益受保护的程度带来担忧您在提供的书面回复中声明，在以后的临床研究中，将会按照美国肿瘤研究会的规定及其提供的临床研究管理系统进行。美国肿瘤研究会提供的临床研究管理系统只允许研究人员为每一位受试者打印最新版本的知情同意书。您也声明所有临床研究协调员将只在需要时才为每个患者从系统中打印知情同意书，以确保使用的是最新版本。无论如何，确保按照21 CFR 50的条款获得知情同意是临床研究者的职责；美国肿瘤研究委员会的政策、流程和活动不能抵消您作为临床研究者的责任。

本警告信的目的并非是罗列您在药物临床研究中存在的所有缺陷。确保遵循法律和相关FDA法规的每一项要求是您的职责，您应当解决这些缺陷，并建立规程，以确保任何正在进行或将来进行的研究均符合FDA的法规。

自收到这封信的15个工作日内，您应当书面告知本办公室为预防将来发生类似违规情况而采取的措施。如果不能充分、快速地解释上述违规问题，可能导致我们在不再通知的情况下采取监管措施。

附：英文原文

Caton, John Jr., M.D.

WARNING LETTER

AUG 26, 2011

CERTIFIED MAIL
RETURN RECEIPT REQUESTED

Ref: 11-HFD-45-08-02

John Caton, Jr., M.D.
Willamette Valley Cancer Institute
3377 Riverbend Drive, Suite 500
Springfield, OR 97477-8802

Dear Dr. Caton:

Between August 2 and August 20, 2010, Heika R. Tait, representing the U.S. Food and Drug Administration (FDA), conducted an investigation and met with you to review your conduct of a clinical investigation (Protocol **(b)(4)**, titled "**(b)(4)**") of the investigational drugs **(b)(4)** and **(b)(4)** performed for **(b)(4)**.

This inspection is a part of FDA's Bioresearch Monitoring Program, which includes inspections designed to evaluate the conduct of research and to help ensure that the rights, safety, and welfare of the human subjects of those studies have been protected.

From our review of the establishment inspection report, the documents submitted with that report, and your September 10, 2010, written response to the Form FDA 483 ("written response"), we conclude that you did not adhere to the applicable statutory requirements and FDA regulations governing the conduct of clinical investigations and the protection of human subjects. We are aware that at the conclusion of the inspection, Heika R. Tait presented and discussed with you Form FDA 483, Inspectional Observations.

We wish to emphasize the following:

1. You failed to ensure that the investigation was conducted according to the investigational plan [21 CFR 312.60].

Your general responsibilities as a clinical investigator include ensuring that the clinical trial is conducted according to the signed investigator statement, the investigational plan, and applicable regulations; protecting the rights, safety, and welfare of subjects under your care; and ensuring control of drugs under investigation [21 CFR 312.60]. Examples of your failure to follow the investigational plan include, but are not limited to, the following:

a. Section 3 of the protocol specified that subjects be randomized to receive either **(b)(4)** or **(b)(4)**. However, according to your November 2, 2009, report to the Institutional Review Board (IRB), Subject 6002 received a combination of the investigational drugs **(b)(4)** and **(b)(4)** on July 29, 2009, even though this subject, one of only two enrolled at your site, was randomized to receive only **(b)(4)**. In addition, according to an October 20, 2009, letter from the sponsor addressed to you, analyses of post-infusion blood samples for Subject 6002 indicated the presence of both **(b)(4)** and **(b)(4)**.

b. Section 9.2 of the protocol specified that records of adverse events must have certain adverse event attributes assigned by the investigator, including, but not limited to, the following: event description (with detail appropriate to the event); and assessment of relatedness to investigational product (IP), chemotherapy, or the combination of IP and chemotherapy.

These attributes were not recorded in the adverse events log for Subject 6002.

Failure to randomize subjects properly and to capture adverse event attributes raises concerns about the extent to which subjects' rights, safety, and welfare were protected, and also raises concerns about the reliability of the data at your site. Your written response states generally that you will conduct research studies "under the umbrella of US Oncology Research going forward as there are checks and balances in place" to prevent a recurrence of the violations cited in this letter, and includes new Standard Operating Procedures (SOPs) for drug accountability. However, as the clinical investigator, it was your responsibility to ensure that the study was conducted in accordance with the investigational plan; and US Oncology Research's policies, procedures, and activities do not negate your responsibility as the clinical investigator.

2. You failed to maintain adequate records of the disposition of the drug, including dates, quantity, and use by subjects [21 CFR 312.62(a)].

a. The Return of Investigation Product for Destruction Form indicates that 4 vials of investigational product (**(b)(4)**) were missing. You have no records to account for the disposition of these vials.

b. During the inspection, you and your staff informed Investigator Tait that the investigational drugs were stored at one office, and were transported to another office, where the subjects received the drugs. However, there are no records to document this transfer of the investigational drugs.

c. The protocol required that an IP Accountability and Preparation Record be kept current, and that it contain specific information, including the dates and quantity of the investigational drug dispensed. It appears that you did not maintain any investigational drug accountability records with respect to the dispensing of **(b)(4)** and **(b)(4)**. The dates and quantity of investigational drug used for each subject were not documented.

Failure to maintain adequate drug disposition records raises concerns about subject safety and data integrity. We acknowledge that your written response states that upon your discovery of both the lack of drug accountability and the missing vials, pharmacy and research SOPs were evaluated and revised; and that future studies at your site will be conducted under the umbrella of US Oncology Research, which has an electronic drug accountability system. However, as the clinical investigator, it was your responsibility to ensure that adequate records of the disposition of the drug were maintained; and US Oncology Research's policies, procedures, and activities do not negate your responsibility as the clinical investigator.

3. You failed to promptly report to the IRB all unanticipated problems involving risk to human subjects or others [21 CFR 312.66].

a. Subject 6002 was admitted to the hospital for bilateral deep venous thrombosis (DVT) and pulmonary embolism on **(b)(4)** and was discharged on **(b)(4)**. You did not report this hospitalization to the IRB until 11/2/09.

b. Subject 6002 expired on **(b)(4)**, and you did not report this death to the IRB until 11/4/09.

Failure to report to the IRB unanticipated problems involving risks to subjects raises concerns about subject safety by undermining the IRB's role in continuing review and evaluating risks to subjects. We acknowledge that your written response states that future studies at your site will be conducted under the umbrella of US Oncology Research, and that with all US Oncology Research studies, unanticipated problems are reported to a project manager or safety specialist, who in turn reports the problem to the IRB. However, as the clinical investigator, it was your responsibility to ensure that unanticipated problems involving risks to human subjects or others were promptly reported to the IRB; and US Oncology Research's policies, procedures, and activities do not negate your responsibility as the clinical investigator.

4. You failed to obtain informed consent in accordance with the provisions of 21 CFR part 50 [21 CFR 312.60].

Your general responsibilities as a clinical investigator include obtaining the informed consent of each human subject to whom the drug is administered, in accordance with the provisions of 21 CFR part 50 [21 CFR 312.60]. 21 CFR 50.27 requires that informed consent be documented by the use of a written consent form approved by the IRB. However, on July 10, 2009, Subject 6002 signed an informed consent form that appears to be an informed consent template that was not approved by the IRB. At the top of each page of the form signed by Subject 6002, the form states, "Approvable Template MUST BE APPROVED FOR SITES BEFORE USE AS MODIFIED Oct 02, 2008." The IRB's May 12, 2009, Certificate of Approval for Protocol **(b)(4)** directed you, as the clinical investigator, to "use only the most current consent form bearing the IRB 'APPROVED' stamp." Because the informed consent form signed by Subject 6002 did not bear this "APPROVED" stamp, and instead indicated that it was a template form not yet approved by the IRB, it appears that Subject 6002's informed consent was not documented by the use of a written consent form approved by the IRB.

Failure to obtain informed consent in accordance with the provisions of 21 CFR part 50 raises concerns about the extent to which subjects' rights, safety, and welfare were protected. We acknowledge that your written response states that future studies at your site will be conducted under the umbrella of US Oncology Research, and that the Clinical Trials Management System provided by US Oncology Research studies will only allow staff to print the most current informed consent form. Your response also states that all Clinical Research Coordinators will only print the informed consent form as needed for each patient from the Clinical Trials Management System, to ensure that the most up-to-date informed consent form is used. However, as the clinical investigator, it was your responsibility to ensure that informed consent was obtained in accordance with the provisions of 21 CFR part 50; and US Oncology Research's policies, procedures, and activities do not negate your responsibility as the clinical investigator.

This letter is not intended to be an all-inclusive list of deficiencies with your clinical study of an investigational drug. It is your responsibility to ensure adherence to each requirement of the law and relevant FDA regulations. You should address these deficiencies and establish procedures to ensure that any ongoing or future studies will be in compliance with FDA regulations.

Within fifteen (15) working days of your receipt of this letter, you should notify this office in writing of the actions you have taken to prevent similar violations in the future.

Failure to adequately and promptly explain the violations noted above may result in regulatory action without further notice.

If you have any questions, please contact Constance Cullity, M.D., M.P.H., at 301-796-3397; FAX 301-847-8748. Your written response and any pertinent documentation should be addressed to:

Constance Cullity (formerly Lewin), M.D., M.P.H.
Branch Chief
Good Clinical Practice Enforcement Branch
Division of Good Clinical Practice Compliance
Office of Scientific Investigations
Office of Compliance
Center for Drug Evaluation and Research
Food and Drug Administration
Building 51, Room 5354
10903 New Hampshire Avenue
Silver Spring, MD 20993

Sincerely yours,

{See appended electronic signature page}

Leslie K. Ball, M.D.
Acting Office Director
Office of Scientific Investigations
Office of Compliance
Center for Drug Evaluation and Research
Food and Drug Administration

第95封　给Cohen, Yale医学博士的警告信

2011年8月12日

参考号：11-HFD-45-08-01

尊敬的Cohen博士：

2011年2月7日至2月11日，Barbara Wright女士和Teresa Navas女士代表FDA与您会面，对您所开展的试验药物为（b）（4）[1]，申办者为（b）（4）的临床试验进行了审查：试验方案（b）（4），标题为"（b）（4）"。这封警告信特告知您现场检查中发现的违规情况，要求您对于信中描述的违规情况马上采取纠正措施，其中有些是FDA于2009年10月8日给您的信中提及的问题的重复和延续。

本次现场检查是FDA的生物研究监查项目的一部分。该项目通过设定的检查方法，对研究的实施情况进行评估，以确认研究数据在科学上是有效和准确的，并帮助确保这些研究中受试者的权益、安全和福利得到了保护。

经对现场检查报告、该报告的附件，以及您2011年2月28日的书面回复进行审查，我们认为，您没有遵循适用法律的要求和监管临床研究实施的FDA法规。在现场检查结束时，Wright女士和Navas女士向您出示了FDA483表，即现场检查发现的问题，并与您进行了讨论。我们想强调以下几点：

1. 您未能确保按照研究计划开展研究［21 CFR 312.60］

研究者有责任确保按照已签署的研究者声明、研究计划和适用的法规来开展研究。研究方案第7部分详述了收集和报告不良事件和严重不良事件的步骤。具体而言，7.3.3部分（非严重不良事件）要求"对于发现的所有的非严重不良事件，都必须在病例报告表的非严重不良事件的页面中进行记录和描述。"此外，7.3.1部分（严重不良事件）要求"所有的严重不良事件，都必须在24小时之内进行报告。"我们检查发现，临床随诊或医院的报告中发现的几例不良事件和/或严重不良事件，既没有在病例报告表中记录也没有向申办者恰当地报告。您未能恰当地记录和报告的不良事件和或严重不良事件包括但不限于以下列举的情况：

受试者编号	日期	不良事件和/或严重不良事件
03461	2009年10月13日	呼吸急促
12285	2010年8月23日	支气管炎和病毒感染
12285	2010年6月26日	颈部疼痛/跌倒
12285	2010年5月28日	跌倒
14055	2010年9月15日	背部疼痛
16666	2011年1月15日	跌倒/头部损伤
20418	2010年12月1日	跛行和水肿

未报告不良事件会危及受试者的安全和福利，并且会损害对研究终点的解释和效力。

在2011年2月28日的书面回复中，您声称这些不良事件是急诊就诊时发现的，而在研究访视中，您和研究协调员询问过受试者是否有任何不良事件或住院，但受试者的回答是"没有"。您还称，您相信您需要改善和这些受试者面谈的方式以及在受试者访视前更好的准备病历资料。您声称，作为纠正措施，您已经报告了所有的不良事件。为了预防这一发现的重复出现，您提出：①在不良事件的面谈中，将向受试者询问急诊

1 （b）（4）涉及商业秘密，根据法规内容不予公开。

就诊、住院和任何其他主诉的信息；②在受试者访视之前，查阅受试者医院的急诊就诊记录；③应给医生办公室所有人员提供沟通研究受试者急诊就诊情况的专业培训。

您的回复是不充分的。FDA注意到，在2008年8月对您的试验场所的现场检查中已发现了晚报严重不良事件以及对不良事件和严重不良事件记录不准确的情况。在对FDA发现的回复中，您递交了承诺的纠正措施。具体而言，在2008年12月29日递交的对FDA2008年8月现场检查发现的回复中，您提供了更新的标准操作规程，并称所有研究人员都接受过对于更新规程相关的培训，并且您还声称这些规程将用于今后的研究。附件C“管理不良事件的流程”（即“不良事件报告”这个标准操作规程中的部分）的第一条“发现、评估和管理不良事件”指出，用以确保适当检查不良事件的步骤包括恰当检查“病历和病程记录等文件中记录的可能的不良事件”。您的试验场所似乎没有遵循该标准操作规程。此外，我们注意到，您的研究协调员告诉FDA检查员，声称她不知道您的试验场所有任何正在使用的书面的临床研究流程。

由于您尚未履行对2008年现场检查中发现问题承诺的纠正措施，我们对于您目前提出的纠正措施能否被妥善落实和执行以预防今后此类违规行为的重复出现引起关注。在对本警告信的回复中，请您提供您对试验场所人员关于用以预防此类违规行为在将来发生的流程的相关培训的记录。此外，请具体明确您在与受试者面谈过程中获得不良事件信息的机制，以及您描述的关于沟通研究受试者急诊就诊情况的专业培训的记录。此外，我们要求您提供能证实已经将上述不良事件和/或严重不良事件报告给了申办者的文件。我们希望提醒您，作为临床研究者，您有职责确保妥善收集和报告所有的不良事件和严重不良事件，即使它们来源于急诊就诊的信息。

2. 您未能保存研究中使用试验药物或对照组的受试者的所有观察和其他相关数据的足够及准确的病历［21 CFR 312.62（b）］

研究者必须保存研究中使用药物的受试者或对照组受试者的所有观察和其他相关数据的足够及准确的病历。

a. 根据方案，研究者在审阅了受试者的国际标准化比值（INR）的数值后对药物剂量做出最终决定。而您未能保存足够的、准确的病历来记录您在研究过程中对于给药剂量的决定。这一点包括但不限于下面列举的情况：

唯一记录受试者给药剂量的决定的文件是由研究协调员填写的未被签署过的“封皮页”。在查看了受试者03461、07600、12285、14055、16496、16666、20418和20544封皮页后，我们发现没有任何记录显示：您对研究药物剂量的维持、暂停或调整做出了指示，或您确认了研究协调员记录的关于用药剂量的决定与您的指示一致。

您和研究协调员均表示，您的试验场所传达药物剂量信息的流程是：研究协调员会将盲态的INR结果以口头或短信方式告诉您，然后您会告诉研究协调员是维持、暂停还是调整当前的剂量。研究协调员则会根据您的口头指示给出用药指导并根据需要订药。我们的检查显示，那些未被签署的封皮页是唯一记录受试者用药决定的文件。因此，无法确定研究协调员记录的药物剂量的决定与您的指示是一致的。

未保留足够的、准确的原始病历会损害对研究终点的解释和效力。

在您的书面回复中，您声称INR数值是研究协调员打电话告知您的，并且您对于剂量调整或是暂停用药的决定作出了口头指示。您还称，申办者提供的原始文件模板要求研究协调员对这种改变进行签署。然而，您提到这些改变事实上是由您做出的。为了预防这类发现的重复出现，您说会事后补充记录一下这个流程，并且您不再允许使用申办者提供的原始文件模板了。

您的回复不够充分，因为您对于不再使用申办者提供的原始文件模板的承诺并不能根本解决此违规行为或者确保有适当的纠正和预防措施。作为一名临床研究者，您有责任在临床试验过程中妥善地记录分发药物的剂量和给药，以确保采取了有效的方法来预防问题在将来重复出现。

此外，我们注意到，在我们2009年10月8日的警告信中曾提到过您没有准备和保存足够的、准确的原始病历来记录对每个个体的所有观察数据和其他研究相关数据［21 CFR 312.62（b）］。您在未署明日期的

（2009年12月10日收到的）书面回复中提到，您会“妥善记录所有的医疗决定，包括剂量计算和……妥善完成和保留所有的原始记录。我会亲自审阅有关医疗决定相关的原始记录，并亲自写审阅意见和签名。”您在对2009年10月8日FDA警告信的回复中承诺的纠正措施尚未实施。因此，我们对于您在2011年2月28日的回复中提出的纠正措施能否被妥善落实，并且能否预防今后此类违规行为的重复出现引起关注。

b. 要求研究者保留足够和准确的受试者的原始病历，也包括要求他们确保知情同意书得到妥善的签署。签字和署明日期的知情同意书的相关的记录必须充分和准确，必须包括获得知情同意过程中相关所有记录。

伦理委员会在日期为2010年11月1日的信中批准了如何对研究参与阶段相对不活跃或进行跟踪访视的受试者进行重新知情的流程。这个流程要求您的试验场所把纸质知情同意文件邮寄给受试者，并跟进一个电话来确保受试者收到并理解了该信函和更新的同意书。2010年11月1日的伦理委员会的信中还要求在原始记录中记录重新知情的过程。同时，当收到受试者签署的知情同意书的副本时，和受试者进行知情讨论的人需在更新的知情文件上签字并签日期，以表明已经在某个确定的日期通过电话讨论过同意书上的内容。然而，我们注意到，五位受试者（03461、12285、14055、16496和20418）的研究记录中没有关于电话知情同意过程的记录，并且在更新的知情同意文件上也没有注明在某个确定的日期通过电话讨论过知情同意书内容的记录。

3. 您未能在研究作出变更前获得伦理委员会的批准［21 CFR 312.66］

研究者必须在研究做出变更前获得伦理委员会的批准，包括变更研究者获得受试者知情同意的流程也需取得伦理委员会的事先批准。

如上文中提到的，伦理委员会在日期为2010年11月1日的信中批准了如何对研究参与阶段相对不活跃或进行跟踪访视的受试者进行重新知情的流程。这个流程要求您的试验场所把纸质知情同意文件邮寄给受试者并跟进一个电话来确保受试者收到并理解了该信函和更改的同意书。但是您把这个流程使用在了五位（03461、12285、14055、16496和20418）正处在研究活跃阶段并接受研究用药的受试者身上。您未能获得伦理委员的批准允许您使用邮件和电话对仍处于研究活跃参与阶段的受试者进行重新知情。

您在书面回复中未对于这一发现提出任何的纠正措施。因此，您的回复是不充分的。在您对本警告信的回复中，请包括预防此类违规行为在将来发生的纠正措施。

不能及时获得伦理委员会对研究活动变更的批准及不能妥善地记录试验受试者的知情同意，会危及参加临床研究的受试者的安全和福利。

本警告信的目的并非是罗列您在试验药物临床研究中存在的所有缺陷。确保遵循法律和相关FDA法规的每一项要求是您的职责，您应当解决这些缺陷，并建立规程，以确保任何正在进行或将来进行的研究均符合FDA的法规。

自收到这封信的15个工作日内，您应当书面告知本办公室为预防将来发生类似违规情况而采取的措施。如果不能充分、快速地解释上述违规问题，可能导致我们在不再通知的情况下采取监管措施。

附：英文原文

Cohen, Yale M.D.

WARNING LETTER

Aug 12, 2011.

CERTIFIED MAIL
RETURN RECEIPT REQUESTED

Ref:11-HFD-45-08-01

Yale Cohen,M.D
3702 Washington Street, Suite401
Hollywood, FL33021

Dear Dr. Cohen:

Between February 7 and February 11, 2011, Ms. Barbara Wright and Ms. Teresa Navas, representing the U.S. Food and Drug Administration (FDA), conducted an investigation and met with you to review your conduct of a clinical investigation (Protocol **(b)(4)**, titled "**(b)(4)**") of the investigational drug **(b)(4)**, performed for **(b)(4)**. This letter requests prompt corrective action to address the violations cited some of which are recurrences or continuations of observations noted in the letter FDA sent to you on October 8, 2009.

This inspection is a part of FDA's Bioresearch Monitoring Program, which includes inspections designed to evaluate the conduct of research and to help ensure that the rights, safety, and welfare of the human subjects of those studies have been protected.

From our review of the establishment inspection report, the documents submitted with that report, and your written response dated February 28, 2011, we conclude that you did not adhere to the applicable statutory requirements and FDA regulations governing the conduct of clinical investigations. At the conclusion of the inspection, Ms. Wright and Ms. Navas presented you with a Form FDA 483, Inspectional Observations, and discussed the observations listed on the form with you. We wish to emphasize the following:

1. You failed to ensure that the investigation was conducted according to the investigation a plan [21 CFR 312.60]

An investigator is responsible for ensuring that an investigation is conducted according to the signed investigator statement, the investigational plan, and applicable regulations. Section 7 of the protocol specifies procedures for collecting and reporting adverse events (AEs) and serious adverse events (SAEs). Specifically, Section 7.3.3, Nonserious Adverse Events, requires that " all identified nonserious AEs must be recorded and described on the appropriate nonserious AE page of the CFR." In addition, Section 7.3.1, Serious Adverse Events, requires that " all SAEs must be reported within 24 hours." Our investigation found several instances in which AEs and/or SAEs identified in either clinic visits or hospital reports, were neither documented in the CRFs no appropriately reported to the sponsor. Examples of AEs and/or SAEs which you failed to appropriately document and report include, but are not limited to, the following:

Subject#	Date	AEand/or SAE
03461	10/13/09	Shortness of Breath
12285	8/23/10	Bronchitis and Viral infection
12285	6/26/10	Neck Pain/Fall
12285	5/28/10	Fall
14055	9/15/10	Back Pain
16666	1/15/11	Fall/Head Injury
20418	12/1/10	Claudication & Edema

Failure to report adverse events jeopardizes subject safety and welfare and compromises the interpretation and validity of the investigational endpoints.

In your written response dated February 28, 2011, you state that the AEs identified were emergency room (ER) visits and that at study visits, you and the study coordinator asked subjects whether they had had any AEs or hospitalizations, and the subjects responded, "No." You further state that you believe the manner in which you interviewed these subjects and prepared charts prior to the subjects' visits needed to be improved. As a corrective action, you note that all the AEs have now been reported. To prevent the recurrence of this finding, you state that: (1) During the AE interview, information regarding ER visits, hospitalizations, and any other complaints would be requested; (2) prior to the subject's visit, chart preparation would also involve reviewing hospital records for ER visits; and (3) an inservice shall be provided to all physician's office staff to discuss communication of ER visits of research subjects.

Your response is inadequate. FDA notes that the inspection of your site in August 2008 identified findings related to delay in reporting of SAEs, and inaccuracies in documentation of AE and SAEs. In response to FDA's findings, you submitted written responses promising corrective actions. Specifically, in a December 29, 2008, written response to the FDA's August 2008 inspectional observations, you provided updated SOPs, stated that all research staff had been trained on them, and stated that they would be used for all future studies. In Attachment C, "Procedures for Managing Adverse Events," which is found in the SOP for "Adverse Event Reporting," Item #1, "Identification, assessment, and management of an adverse event," states that procedures to be utilized for ensuring that AEs are appropriately investigated include properly investigating "possible AEs documented in medical records, progress notes, etc." Your site does not appear to be following that SOP. In addition, we note that your study coordinator further informed FDA investigators that she was unaware of any active written clinical research procedures used at your site.

Given that you have not implemented the corrective actions promised in response to the August 2008 inspectional observations, we have concerns about whether the corrective actions that you have currently outlined will be properly implemented and executed in a manner that will prevent the recurrence of this and similar types of violations in the future. In your response to this letter please provide documentation of the training your staff has received on the procedures in place at your clinical site that are intended to prevent the recurrence of this type of violation in the future. In addition, please specifically identify the mechanisms by which you will be requesting information from the subjects during the AE interview, as well as documentation of the in-service you have described regarding communication of ER visits for research subjects. Further, we request that you provide documentation to verify that the AEs and/or SAEs noted above have been reported to the sponsor. We wish to remind you that as a clinical investigator, it is your responsibility to ensure that all AE and SAEs, even those AE and/or SAEs that were ER visits, are properly collected and reported.

2. You failed to prepare and maintain adequate and accurate case histories that record all observations and other data pertinent to the investigation on each individual administered the investigational drug or employed as a control in the investigation [21 CFR 312.62(b)].

An investigator is required to prepare and maintain adequate and accurate case histories that record all observations and other data pertinent to the investigation on each individual administered the investigational drug or employed as a control in the investigation.

a. According to the protocol, after reviewing a subject's international normalized ratio (INR value, the investigator was to make the final dosing decision. You failed to maintain adequate and accurate case histories that recorded your dosing decisions for the drugs administered during the course of this investigation. Examples of this failure include, but are not limited to, the following:

The only documentation of dosing decisions for subjects was the unsigned "face sheets" filled out by the study coordinator. Our review of the face sheets for Subjects 03461, 07600, 12285, 14055, 16496, 16666, 20418, and 20544 found no documentation that you ordered the study drug dose to be maintained, withheld, or adjusted, or that you confirmed that the drug dosing decisions recorded by the study coordinator were in line with your orders.

Both you and the study coordinator stated that your site's process for relaying dosage information was as follows: The study coordinator would communicate blinded INR results to you, either verbally or via text messages, and you would tell the study coordinator to maintain, withhold, or adjust the current dose. The study coordinator would then issue dosing instructions and order drug supplies as needed, according to your verbal orders. Our investigation found that these unsigned face sheets served as the only documentation of th dosing decisions for subjects. As a result, there was no way to confirm that the drug dosing decisions recorded by the study coordinator were in line with your orders.

Failure to maintain adequate and accurate case histories compromises the interpretation and validity of the investigational endpoints.

In your written response, you stated that the INR values are called in to the study coordinator, who notifies you, and that you provide verbal orders concerning dose adjustments or your decision to suspend doses. You further stated that the sponsor provided a source document template that had the study coordinator sign off on such changes; however, you stated that you actually performed the changes. To prevent the recurrence of this finding, you stated that you would document this process via a late entry and that you would no longer permit the use of sponsorprovided source document templates.

Your response is inadequate in that a promise that you will not use the sponsorprovided source document template does not address the cause of this violation or ensure appropriate corrective and preventive actions. As a clinical investigator, you are responsible for properly documenting the dosing and administration of drugs dispensed during the course of this clinical trial, and for ensuring that effective measures are implemented to prevent future reoccurrence.

In addition, we note that in our letter dated October 8, 2009, you had previously been cited for not preparing and maintaining adequate and accurate case histories that record all observations and other data pertinent to the investigation on each individual [21 CFR 312.62(b)]. In your undated written response (received on December 10, 2009), you stated that you would " properly document all medical decision making, including dose calculations, and … properly complete and maintain all source documentation. All source documentation relating to medical decisions making [sic]/dose changes will be personally reviewed by me as indicated by my personal comments and signature."

You have not implemented the corrective actions that you promised in your response to the October 8, 2009, letter from FDA. As a result, we have concerns about whether the corrective actions that you have currently identified in your February 28, 2011, response will be properly implemented and executed in a manner that will prevent the recurrence of these and similar types of violations in the future.

b. The requirement that an investigator maintain adequate and accurate case histories for subjects includes the requirement to ensure that informed consent forms are properly signed and dated. The records of the signed and dated informed consent forms must be adequate and accurate in the respect that they must contain all required documentation of the process through which informed consent was obtained.

In a letter dated November 1, 2010, the IRB approved a process for reconsenting of subjects who were not actively participating in the study or coming in for followup visits. This process required your site to mail the paper informed consent documents and to follow up with a telephone call to ensure that both the letter and the revised consent were received and understood. The IRB's November 1, 2010, letter further required that the re-consenting process be documented in the source records. Also, upon receipt of the signed copies from the subject, the person conducting the consent discussion was to sign and date the revised consent documents to indicate that the consent discussion was conducted via telephone on the identified date. However, we note that for five subjects (Subjects 03461, 12285, 14055, 16496, and 20418), there was no documentation found in the study records regarding the telephone consent process that was used, and no documentation on the revised consent documents to indicate that the consent discussion was conducted via telephone on an identified date.

3. You failed to obtain IRB approval before making changes in the research [21 CFR 312.66]

An investigator is required to obtain IRB approval before making changes in the research. The requirement for prior IRB approval includes changes in the process by which an investigator obtains informed consent of subjects.

As noted above, in a letter dated November 1, 2010, the IRB approved a process for reconsentin of subjects who were not actively participating in the study or coming in for followup visits. This process required your site to mail the paper informed consent documents and to follow up with a telephone call to ensure that both the letter and the revised consent were received and understood. However, you utilized this reconsenting process for five subjects

(Subjects 03461, 12285, 14055, 16496, and 20418) who were still actively participating in the study and receiving study drugs. You failed to obtain IRB approval for the use of the mail and telephone reconsenting process for subjects who were still actively participating in the clinical trial.

Your written response did not provide any corrective measures to prevent the recurrence of this finding. As a result, your response is inadequate. In your response to this letter, please include corrective actions that will prevent the recurrence of this and similar types of violations in the future.

Failure to promptly obtain IRB approval for changes in the research activity, and failure to properly document the informed consent of trial subjects, can compromise the safety and welfare of subjects enrolled in the clinical investigation.

This letter is not intended to be an all-inclusive list of deficiencies with your clinical study of an investigational drug. It is your responsibility to ensure adherence to each requirement of the law and relevant FDA regulations. You should address these deficiencies and establish procedures to ensure tha any ongoing or future studies will be in compliance with FDA regulations.

Within fifteen (15) working days of your receipt of this letter, you should notify this office in writing of the actions you have taken to prevent similar violations in the future. Failure to adequately and promptly explain the violations noted above may result in regulatory action without further notice.

If you have any questions, please contact Constance Cullity, M.D., M.P.H., at 301-796-339; FAX 301 847-8748. Your written response and any pertinent documentation should be addressed to:

Constance Cullity (formerly Lewin), M.D., M.P.H. Branch Chief
Good Clinical Practice Enforcement Branch Division of Good Clinical Practice Compliance Office of Scientific Investigations
Office of Compliance
Center for Drug Evaluation and Research
Food and Drug Administration
Building 51, Room 5354
10903 New Hampshire Avenue
Silver Spring, MD 20993

Sincerely yours,

{See appended electronic signature page}

Leslie K. Ball, M.D.
Acting Director
Office of Scientific Investigations
Office of Compliance
Center for Drug Evaluation and Research
Food and Drug Administration

第 96 封　给 Linda D. Bosserman 医学博士的警告信

2011年7月19日

参考号：11-HFD-45-07-01

尊敬的Bosserman博士：

2010年12月8日12月22日，Carla J. Lundi女士代表FDA与您会面，对您所开展的以下临床研究进行了审查：

试验方案（b）（4）[1]，试验药物为（b）（4），申办者为（b）（4）。

试验方案（b）（4），试验药物为（b）（4），申办者为（b）（4）。

试验方案（b）（4），试验药物为（b）（4），申办者为（b）（4）。

试验方案（b）（4），试验药物为（b）（4），申办者为（b）（4）。

本次现场检查是FDA的生物研究监查项目的一部分。该项目通过设定的检查方法，评估研究的实施情况，并帮助确保这些研究中受试者的权益、安全和福利得到了保护。

经对现场检查报告、该报告的附件，以及您2011年1月10日的书面回复进行审查，我们认为，您没有遵循适用的法律要求和监管临床研究实施的FDA法规。在现场检查结束时，Lundi女士向您出示了FDA483表，即现场检查发现的问题，并与您进行了讨论。我们想强调以下几点：

1. 您未能确保按照签署的研究者声明进行研究，您未能亲自进行临床研究或对研究进行监督［21 CFR 312.60］

当您签署上述提及的研究者声明（FDA1572表）时，您即同意在您的试验场所承担研究者的职责。您作为研究者的总体职责包括确保按照已签署的研究者声明、研究计划和适用的法规进行临床试验；保护在您的监护下临床受试者的权益、安全及福利；以及确保试验药物管控［21 CFR 312.60］。签署了FDA1572表，则表示您同意亲自实施临床试验或监督那些试验中您没有亲自实施的各方面。尽管您可以将某些研究任务授权给具有资质的人员去做，但作为临床研究者您不能授权总体职责。我们的调查表明您对您授权了职责的人员的监督管理并不足以确保方案“（b）（4）”和方案“（b）（4）”是按照已签署的研究者声明、研究计划和适用的法规来进行的，及在某种程度上保护了受试者的权益、安全及福利。

具体来说，我们发现您未能在方案“（b）（4）”和方案“（b）（4）”中充分监管一位研究协调员，而导致这些研究中出现下述问题，包括未能保存完整而准确的病历，未能按照方案要求来做评估。

我们发现，在您2011年1月10日对FDA483表的回复中，您提到是被授权了任务的研究协调员导致下述违规行为，承认她的过失并于2010年2月辞职。我们也了解您的回复中提及已经采取的纠正和预防措施，包括指派一名每周至少能有8小时，并至少每周能与研究协调员和数据管理员会面一次的临床研究总监来监督该研究。然而，您的回复并不充分，因为您并没有递交如2011年1月10日对FDA483表的回复中所提及的修订后的标准操作规程，或特别指出哪些变更如何预防将来再次发生此类违规。在您对此信的回复中，请提供这些文件。如果不能提供这些信息，当局将无法对您为预防这些违规再次发生的措施进行知情评价。而且，作为研究者，您的职责是确保方案“（b）（4）”和方案“（b）（4）”按照签署的研究者声明来实施，您疏于对研究协调员的监管导致了下述这些问题。

1 （b）（4）涉及商业秘密，根据法规内容不予公开。

2. 您未能保存研究中使用试验药物或对照组的受试者的所有研究观察结果和其他相关数据的足够及准确的病历［21 CFR 312.62（b）］

FDA法规规定，研究者必须准备、保存研究中使用试验药物或对照组的受试者的所有研究观察结果和其他相关数据的足够及准确的病历。病历包括病例报告表及其支持性数据。您未能保存足够而准确的病历的例子，包括但不限于以下：

a. 试验方案（b）（4）：

受试者107-380B的姓名和出生日期是手写在2009年12月18日的筛查心电图上的。然而，受试者107-380B并未在2009年12月18日接受心电图检查。您的记录显示您所提交的107-380B的心电图与另一研究中的受试者在2009年12月6日的完全相同。您在2011年1月10日对FDA483表的回复中承认了该矛盾。

您的记录显示受试者107-380B在2009年11月25日签署了知情同意书。然而，该同意书在接下来被修改以体现2009年12月14日的重新知情。您在2011年1月10日对FDA483表的回复中承认了该矛盾。我们同时发现，根据您在2011年1月10日对FDA483表的回复和2010年4月27日的您在咨询申办者监查员之后，文件备注，您解释了受试者107-380B在2010年2月24日进行跟踪访视，以及受试者在该日重新签署知情同意书。这些违背包括了试验方案（b）（4）中入组的三名受试者中的一名的记录。尽管研究协调员承认了该错误做法并从您的团队辞职，作为研究者您有确保实施临床研究的最终责任。您未能保存完整而准确的病历，这将潜在危害临床研究中收集的数据的可靠性。

b. 试验方案（b）（4）：

受试者089002的病历记录包含标注不同日期但却重复的记录。

具体来说，标注日期为2009年11月12日对入组标准和排除标准的审查来看，是标注日期为2009年11月5日的表格的复印件。两表唯一的不同是2009年11月12日的版本上的日期。根据您2011年1月10日对FDA483表的回复，出现该处不一致是因为入/排标准的检查表被用作“工作”文件，并且研究协调员被允许在研究记录中使用您的姓名印章。然而，根据21CFR312.62（b），作为研究者，您负有确保起草并维护充足而准确的记录的职责。试验方案（b）（4）记录中的不一致项是反映您未能维护充足准确的病历记录的另一个示例，并可能潜在地危害临床研究中采集的数据的可靠性。

我们承认在您于2011年1月10日对FDA483表的回复中，您描述了针对以上列明的违背的纠正和预防措施。它们包括：

- 对篡改数据事件的调查；
- 篡改数据的研究协调员辞职；
- 对该研究协调员参与的其他研究的稽查；
- 向UCLATORI研究网络的管理团队、申办者和伦理委员会通告关于您的调查、稽查、发现和纠正措施。
- 向您的研究团队提供临床试验标准操作规程（SOP）、GCP和受试者保护的培训，并更新您的与签署临床试验中入/排标准检查表、签署受试者实验室或诊断性研究有关的SOP。

然而，根据21 CFR 312.62（b），作为研究者，您负有确保起草并维护充足而准确的记录的职责。另外，您的回应并不充分，因为您并未提交您修改后的SOP，或特别指明这些对流程的修改将如何帮助避免此类违规以后再次发生。

如果不能提供这些信息，本办公室将无法对您为预防这些违规再次发生而采取的措施进行明智的评价。

具体而言，在您2011年1月10日对FDA483表的回复中声明您的SOP［2010年2月9日版（附件J）］记录了医生的签名印章将不再使用。但是，附在附件J的文件中看上去是一个备忘录文件而非SOP。而且，在您回复的第8页第8项中，您说您已经修改了关于签署临床试验受试者的实验室和诊断研究的SOP。然而，该SOP并未包含在您的回复当中，同时也不清楚该SOP与2010年2月9日的备忘录文件有何关联。由于这两项与研究文件的签署有关，您对此信的回复中须指明并恰当记录您回复中第8项中指出的SOP与2010年2月9日的备忘录文件之间的关联，并且须包含这些政策的文件。

您在2011年1月10日对FDA483表的回复中同样表明您现在已理解“所有的工作文件都应当从研究文件中剔除，因为他们不是源文件。然而，不论这些文件是被认为是“工作”文件或是“源”文件，该回复不能确保您将保存充足而准确的病历，记录与研究相关的所有发现和其他数据。您回复的第78页的第7项表明您在2010年6月制定了一项政策，即所有的入／排标准的检查表将由研究者完成和签署。在您对此信的回复中，请一并提交该政策文件，并解释该政策文件和新的SOP将如何预防类似违规的发生。

3. 您未能确保按照研究计划进行研究［21 CFR 312.60］

您作为临床研究者的总体职责包括确保按照所签署的研究者声明、研究计划以及适用法规来实施临床试验；保护在您的监护下的受试者权益、安全性以及福利；以及确保管控研究药物［21CFR312.60］。试验方案（b）（4）在第6.3章节和附件2“研究治疗期的检查”中列出了所要求的检查类型和时间点；您未能确保按照研究计划实施试验方案（b）（4），因为您未能确保试验方案（b）（4）中要求的所有检查均得以进行。一些您未能遵从研究计划的例证包括但不限于以下：

对受试者089002未做以下要求的检查：

（a）2009年11月18日（第一周期，第1天）循环肿瘤细胞、药物代谢动力学、药物基因组学；

（b）2009年12月9日（第二周期，第1天）生活质量FACTO量表及循环肿瘤细胞；

（c）2009年12月30日（第三周期，第1天）生活质量FACTO量表。

我们承认，在您2011年1月10日对FDA483表的回复中，您描述了已采取的纠正和预防措施以回应以上列出的违规。这些纠正措施包括：

- 雇佣额外的工作人员；
- 给所有研究人员提供临床试验标准操作规程、GCP和受试者保护的培训；
- 更新您的标准操作规程。

然而，作为临床研究者，您的职责是确保研究相关的流程按照方案要求来实施，不能执行研究相关步骤会潜在威胁受试者安全和福利，并且会威胁研究终点的解释和效力。尽管按照方案，以上列出的检查并非研究的主要终点，但必须把研究的实施和方案的依从性看作一个整体。将诊断为卵巢癌的受试者入组到研究中，表明采集循环肿瘤细胞、药物代谢动力学和药物基因组学的有效数据对于完整评估研究结果的价值。此外，试验方案（b）（4）规定，研究的次要终点是评估健康相关的生活质量，所以表明有效的生活质量数据的必要性。

此外，您的回复并不充分，因为您并没有递交您2011年1月10日对FDA483表的回复中提到的修改后的标准操作规程，或特别指出那些流程上的更改将如何预防此类违规将来再次发生。在您对此信的回复中，请您提供这些文件。如果不能提供这些信息，本办公室将无法对您为预防这些违规再次发生的措施进行明智的评估。

本警告信的目的并非是罗列您在试验药物临床研究中存在的所有缺陷。确保遵循法律和相关FDA法规的每一项要求是您的职责，您应当解决这些缺陷，并建立规程，以确保任何正在进行或将来进行的研究均符合FDA的法规。

自收到这封信的15个工作日内，您应当书面告知本办公室为预防将来再次发生类似违规情况而采取的措施。如果不能充分、迅速地解释上述违规问题，可能导致我们在不再通知的情况下采取监管措施。

附：英文原文

Linda D. Bosserman M.D.

WARNING LETTER

JUL 19, 2011

CERTIFIED MAIL
RETURN RECEIPT REQUESTED

Ref: 11-HFD-45-0701

Linda D. Bosserman, M.D.
Wilshire Oncology Medical Group, Inc.
1502 Arrow Highway
La Verne, CA 91750-5318

Dear Dr. Bosserman:

Between December 8 and December 22, 2010, Ms. Carla J. Lundi, representing the U.S. Food and Drug Administration (FDA), conducted an investigation and met with you to review your conduct of the following clinical investigations:

- Protocol (b)(4) of the investigational drug (b)(4), performed for (b)(4);
- Protocol (b)(4) of the investigational drug (b)(4), performed for (b)(4);
- Protocol (b)(4) of the investigational drug (b)(4), performed for (b)(4); and
- Protocol (b)(4) of the investigational drug (b)(4), performed for (b)(4).

This inspection is a part of FDA's Bioresearch Monitoring Program, which includes inspections designed to evaluate the conduct of research and to help ensure that the rights, safety, and welfare of the human subjects of those studies have been protected.

From our review of the establishment inspection report, the documents submitted with that report, and your January 10, 2011, written response to the Form FDA 483, we conclude that you did not adhere to the applicable statutory requirements and FDA regulations governing the conduct of clinical investigations. We are aware that at the conclusion of the inspection, Ms. Lundi presented and discussed the inspection observations on the Form FDA 483 with you. We wish to emphasize the following:

1. You failed to ensure that the investigation was conducted according to the signed investigator statement, in that you failed to personally conduct or supervise the clinical investigation [21 CFR 312.60].

When you signed the Statement of Investigator (Form FDA 1572) for the above referenced clinical trials, you agreed to take on the responsibilities of a clinical investigator at your site. Your general responsibilities as a clinical investigator include ensuring that the clinical trial is conducted according to the signed investigator statement, the investigational plan, and applicable regulations; protecting the rights, safety, and welfare of subjects under your care; and ensuring control of drugs under investigation [21 CFR 312.60]. By signing Form FDA 1572, you specifically agreed to personally conduct the clinical trial or to supervise those aspects of the trial that you did not personally conduct. While you may delegate certain study tasks to individuals qualified to perform them, as a clinical investigator you may not delegate your general responsibilities. Our investigation indicates that your supervision of personnel to whom you delegated study tasks was not adequate to ensure that Protocol (b)(4) and Protocol (b)(4) were conducted according to the signed investigator statement, the investigational plan, and applicable regulations, and in a manner that protects the rights, safety, and welfare of human subjects.

Specifically, we note that your failure to adequately supervise a study coordinator for Protocol (b)(4) and Protocol (b)(4) led to problems with the conduct of these investigations as described below, which included failure to maintain adequate and accurate case histories, and failure to conduct assessments required by the protocols.

We note that in your January 10, 2011, response to the Form FDA 483, you state that the study coordinator who was delegated the tasks that led to the violations cited below, admitted her wrong doing and resigned in February 2010. We also acknowledge that your response describes corrective and preventive actions that you have taken, including the appointment of a Director of Clinical Research with at least 8 hours per week designated to work on oversight of the clinical trials program, who will meet at least weekly with clinical trial coordinators and data managers. However, your response is inadequate because you have not submitted the revised standard operating procedures referenced in your January 10, 2011, response to the Form FDA 483, or specifically identified how changes in those procedures will serve to prevent the recurrence of this type of violation in the future. In your response to this letter, please provide this documentation. Without the submission of this information, the Agency is unable to undertake an informed evaluation of the potential use of your actions in preventing the recurrence of these violations. Moreover, as the investigator, it was your responsibility to ensure that Protocol (b)(4) and Protocol (b)(4) were conducted according to the signed investigator statements, and your failure to supervise your study coordinator led to the problems with these investigations described below.

2. You failed to maintain adequate and accurate case histories that record all observations and other data pertinent to the investigation on each individual administered the investigational drug or employed as a control in the investigation [21 CFR 312.62(b)].

FDA regulations state that an investigator is required to prepare and maintain adequate and accurate case histories that record all observations and other data pertinent to the investigation on each individual administered the investigational drug or employed as a control in the investigation. Case histories include the case report forms and supporting data. Examples of your failure to maintain adequate and accurate case histories include, but are not limited to, the following:

a. Protocol (b)(4):

- The name and date of birth for Subject 107-380B were handwritten on a screening electrocardiogram (ECG) dated December 18, 2009. However, Subject 107-380B did not receive an ECG on December 18, 2009. Your records indicate that the ECG submitted on behalf of Subject 107-380B is identical to the ECG performed on December 6, 2009, for a research subject enrolled in a different clinical trial. This discrepancy in your records was acknowledged in your January 10, 2011, response to the Form FDA 483.
- Your records indicate that Subject 107-380B signed the informed consent form on November 25, 2009. However, this form was subsequently altered to reflect a reconsent date of December 14, 2009. This discrepancy in your records was acknowledged in your January 10, 2011 response to the Form FDA 483. We also note that, according to your January 10, 2011, response to the Form FDA 483 and your April 27, 2010, Note to File, after consulting with the sponsor's monitor, you explained the error to Subject 107-380B during the subject's February 24, 2010, followup visit, and the subject resigned the informed consent form on that date.

These violations involve the records of one of the three subjects enrolled in Protocol (b)(4). Although the study coordinator admitted this wrongdoing and resigned from your practice, as the clinical investigator you maintain overall responsibility for the conduct of this clinical investigation. Your failure to maintain adequate and accurate case histories could potentially compromise the integrity of the data collected during the clinical investigation.

b. Protocol (b)(4):

- Case history records for Subject 089002 contain duplicate records with discrepant dates.
- Specifically, the Review of Inclusion & Exclusion Criteria form dated November 12, 2009, is a photocopy of the form dated November 5, 2009. The only difference between these two records is the altered date on the November 12, 2009, version.

According to your January 10, 2011, response to the Form FDA 483, this discrepancy occurred because inclusion/exclusion checklists were used as "working" documents, and the study coordinator was permitted to use your signature stamp on study records. However, it was your responsibility as the investigator to ensure that adequate and accurate records were prepared and maintained, as required by 21 CFR 312.62(b). The discrepancy in the study records for Protocol (b)(4) represents an additional example of your failure to maintain adequate and accurate case histories, and could potentially compromise the integrity of the data collected during the clinical investigation.

We acknowledge that in your January 10, 2011, response to the Form FDA 483, you described your corrective and preventive actions taken in response to the above listed violations. These actions include:

- the conduct of an investigation into the incidents of altered records;
- the resignation of the study coordinator who admitted to the alterations;
- the audit of the other clinical trials in which the study coordinator was involved;
- providing notice to the UCLATORI research network leadership, the study sponsor, and the IRB concerning your investigation, audit, findings, and corrective actions;
- providing training for your research staff on Standard Operating Procedures (SOPs) for clinical trials, Good Clinical Practices, and Human Subject Protection; and
- updating your SOPs with regard to signing inclusion/exclusion checklists and signing laboratory or diagnostic studies for subjects in clinical trials.

However, it was your responsibility as the investigator to ensure that adequate and accurate records were prepared and maintained, as required by 21 CFR 312.62(b). Furthermore, your response was inadequate in that you have not submitted your revised SOPs or specifically identified how changes in those procedures will serve to prevent the recurrence of these types of violations in the future. Without the submission of this information, the Agency is unable to undertake an informed evaluation of the potential use of your actions in preventing the recurrence of these violations.

Specifically, your January 10, 2011, response to the Form FDA 483 states that your "SOP dated 2/9/10 (Appendix J)" documents that physician signature stamps will no longer be used at your site. However, the document attached as Appendix J appears to be a Memo to File rather than an SOP. Furthermore, on page 8 of your response, in Item 8, you state that you have changed your SOPs with regard to signing off on laboratory and diagnostic studies for patients on clinical trials. However, this SOP has not been included in your response, and it is not clear how this SOP relates to the February 9, 2010, Memo to File. Because these two items are related to the signing of study records, your response to this letter should identify and appropriately document the relationship between the SOP identified in Item 8 of your response and the February 9, 2010, Memo to File, and should include documentation of these policies.

Your January 10, 2011, response to the Form FDA 483 also states that you now understand that all "working documents should have been pulled from the study documents , as they are not source documents." However, this response does not provide assurance that you will maintain adequate and accurate case histories that record all observations and other data pertinent to the investigation, whether the documents are considered "working" documents or "source" documents. Item 7 on pages 78 of your response states that you instituted a policy in June 2010 that all internal inclusion/exclusion checklists will be completed and signed by an investigator. In your response to this letter, please submit documentation of this policy, as well as an explanation of how this policy and the new SOPs prevent the occurrence of violations similar to those listed above.

3. You failed to ensure that the investigation was conducted according to the investigational plan [21 CFR 312.60].

Your general responsibilities as a clinical investigator include ensuring that the clinical trial is conducted according to the signed investigator statement, the investigational plan, and applicable regulations; protecting the rights, safety, and welfare of subjects under your care; and ensuring control of drugs under investigation [21 CFR 312.60]. Protocol (b)(4) outlines the types and timing of required assessments in Section 6.3 and Table 2, Assessments During Study Treatment. You failed to ensure that Protocol (b)(4) was conducted according to the investigational plan in that you failed to ensure that all assessments required by Protocol (b)(4) were performed. Examples of your failure to follow the investigational plan include, but are not limited to, the following:

The following required assessments were not performed for Subject 089002:

a. November 18, 2009 (Cycle 1, Day 1): Circulating tumor cells, pharmacokinetics, and pharmacogenomics;
b. December 9, 2009 (Cycle 2, Day 1): Quality of Life FACTO Questionnaire and circulating tumor cells; and
c. December 30, 2009 (Cycle 3, Day 1): Quality of Life FACTO Questionnaire.

We acknowledge that in your January 10, 2011, response to the Form FDA 483, you describe the corrective and preventive actions taken in response to the above listed violations. These corrective actions include:

- hiring additional staff;

- providing training for all your research staff on Standard Operating Procedures for clinical trials,
- Good Clinical Practices, and Human Subject Protection; and
- updating your Standard Operating Procedures.

However, as the clinical investigator, it was your responsibility to ensure that study related procedures were performed in accordance with the protocol requirements. Failure to perform study related procedures has the potential to jeopardize subject safety and welfare, and to compromise the interpretation and validity of the investigational endpoints. Although the assessments listed above are not the primary endpoints of the investigation according to the protocol, the conduct of the investigation and conformance to protocol must be taken as a whole. The inclusion of subjects who have been diagnosed with ovarian cancer in this study indicates that the collection of valid data on circulating tumor cells, pharmacokinetics, and pharmacogenomics is valuable for the complete evaluation of the study results. In addition, Protocol (b)(4) states that a secondary endpoint of the study is to assess health-related quality of life, thus indicating that valid quality of life data are necessary.

In addition, your response is inadequate in that you have not submitted the revised standard operating procedures referenced in your January 10, 2011, response to the Form FDA 483, or specifically identified how changes in those procedures will serve to prevent the recurrence of these types of violations in the future. In your response to this letter, please provide this documentation. Without the submission of this information, the Agency is unable to undertake an informed evaluation of the potential use of your actions in preventing the recurrence of these violations.

This letter is not intended to be an all-inclusive list of deficiencies with your clinical study of an investigational drug. It is your responsibility to ensure adherence to each requirement of the law and relevant FDA regulations. You should address these deficiencies and establish procedures to ensure that any ongoing or future studies will be in compliance with FDA regulations.

Within fifteen (15) working days of your receipt of this letter, you should notify this office in writing of the actions you have taken to prevent similar violations in the future. Failure to adequately and promptly explain the violations noted above may result in regulatory action without further notice.

If you have any questions, please contact Constance Cullity, M.D., M.P.H., at 301-796-3397; FAX 301-847-8748. Your written response and any pertinent documentation should be addressed to:

Constance Cullity (formerly Lewin), M.D., M.P.H.
Branch Chief
Good Clinical Practice Enforcement Branch
Division of Good Clinical Practice Compliance
Office of Scientific Investigations
Office of Compliance
Center for Drug Evaluation and Research
Food and Drug Administration
Building 51, Room 5354
10903 New Hampshire Avenue
Silver Spring, MD 20993

Sincerely yours,

/S/

Leslie K. Ball, M.D.
Director (Acting)
Office of Scientific Investigations
Office of Compliance
Center for Drug Evaluation and Research
Food and Drug Administration

第97封 给Michelson, Joseph B. 医学博士的警告信

2011年7月6日

参考号：11-HFD-45-06-01

尊敬的Michelson博士：

2010年7月26日至8月24日期间，Thomas R. Beilke先生代表FDA与您会面，并对您所实施的申办者为（b）（4）[1]的以下临床研究进行了现场审查：试验方案（b）（4），标题为“（b）（4）”。我们注意到您于2009年3月2日开始成为本研究的研究者，在此之前，本研究的研究者是由Laura A. Teasley医学博士担任的。

本次现场检查是FDA的生物研究监查项目的一部分。该项目通过设定的检查方法，评估研究的实施情况，并帮助确保这些研究中受试者的权益、安全和福利得到了保护。

经对现场检查报告、该报告的附件，以及您2010年9月8日的书面回复进行审查，我们认为，您没有遵循适用的法律要求和监管临床研究实施的FDA法规。在现场检查结束时，Beilke先生向您出示了FDA483表，即现场检查中发现的问题，并与您进行了讨论。我们想强调以下几点：

您未能确保按照研究计划进行该研究［21 CFR 312.60］

a. 试验方案（第5.0版，2008年3月24日）第2章，第2.2.2部分具体规定了一条入组标准为临床检查所见糖尿病黄斑水肿以及在随机后8日内的光学相干断层扫描（OCT）所见中心区范围厚度≥250μm，但以下受试者的OCT扫描是偏离中心的。因此，读取的数据使得受试者看上去合格而实际可能并非如此。

ⅰ）受试者0046（b）（6）的2009年5月20日的右眼；

ⅱ）受试者0042（b）（6）的2009年4月22日的左眼；

我们承认您在2010年9月8日对FDA483表的回复中描述的纠正措施，说您未来会采取措施并不再入组OCT扫描偏离中央的受试者。然而，不管纠正措施如何，作为研究者，您对实施研究并确保入组的所有受试者合格负有最终责任。

b. 试验方案（第5.0版，2008年3月24日）第3章第3.2部分规定所有研究的眼均需要接受（b）（4）和（b）（4）。研究中入组的18只眼中的6只并未接受（b）（4）。

具体如下：

ⅰ）受试者0044（b）（6）左眼于2009年5月7日接受（b）（4），以及2009年5月14日接受（b）（4），以得到总（b）（4）。

ⅱ）受试者0045（b）（6）右眼于2009年5月19日接受（b）（4），以及2009年6月2日接受（b）（4），以得到总（b）（4）。

ⅲ）受试者0045（b）（6）右眼于2009年5月20日接受（b）（4），以及2009年6月3日接受（b）（4），以得到总（b）（4）的总（b）（4）。

ⅳ）受试者0043（b）（6）右眼于2009年5月14日接受（b）（4），以及2009年5月20日接受（b）（4），以得到总（b）（4）。

ⅴ）受试者0041（b）（6）左眼于2009年2月26日接受（b）（4），以及2009年4月2日接受（b）（4），以得到总（b）（4）。

---

1 (b) (4) 涉及商业秘密，根据法规内容不予公开。

ⅵ）受试者0046（b）（6）右眼于2009年5月27日接受（b）（4），以及2009年6月3日接受（b）（4），以得到总（b）（4）。

我们承认您在2010年9月8日书面回复中声明，尽管在初次评估时您感到至少（b）（4）及额外的（b）（4）是可行的，而在治疗时，就无法按照方案要求进行额外的（b）（4）了。方案要求一定量的（b）（4）而且并未允许任何弹性。然而，您的书面回复并没有解释，也没有提供任何证据，证明您在意识到他们不能接受所要求的（b）（4）的数量之后将他们排除在研究之外。将这些受试者留在研究中，将损害数据可靠性。

本警告信的目的并非是罗列您在试验药物临床研究中存在的所有缺陷。确保遵循法律和相关FDA法规的每一项要求是您的职责，您应当解决这些缺陷，并建立规程以确保任何正在进行或将来进行的研究均符合FDA的法规。

自收到这封信的15个工作日内，您应当书面告知本办公室为预防将来发生类似违规情况而采取的措施。如果不能充分、迅速地解释上述违规问题，可能导致我们在不再通知的情况下采取监管措施。

附：英文原文

Michelson, Joseph B. M.D.

WARNING LETTER

JUL 6, 2011

CERTIFIED MAIL
RETURN RECEIPT REQUESTED

Ref: 11-HFD-45-06-01

Joseph B. Michelson, M.D.
11423 187th St., Suite 200
Artesia, CA 90701

Dear Dr. Michelson:

Between July 26 and August 24, 2010, Thomas R. Beilke, representing the U.S. Food and Drug Administration (FDA), conducted an investigation and met with you to review your conduct of a clinical investigation (Protocol (b)(4), entitled (b)(4)" performed for the (b)(4). We note that you became the clinical investigator responsible for the study on March 2, 2009, and that, prior to that time, Laura A. Teasley, M.D., was the clinical investigator responsible for the study.

This inspection is a part of the FDA's Bioresearch Monitoring Program, which includes inspections designed to evaluate the conduct of research and to help ensure that the rights, safety, and welfare of the human subjects of those studies have been protected.

From our review of the establishment inspection report and the documents submitted with that report and your written response dated September 8, 2010, we conclude that you did not adhere to the applicable statutory requirements and FDA regulations governing the conduct of clinical investigations.

We are aware that at the conclusion of the inspection, Mr. Beilke presented and discussed with you Form FDA 483, Inspectional Observations. We wish to emphasize the following:

You failed to ensure that the investigation was conducted according to the investigational plan [21 CFR 312.60].

a. Chapter 2, Section 2.2.2 of the protocol (Version 5.0, dated March 24, 2008) specified an inclusion criterion of diabetic macular edema present on clinical exam and central subfield thickness on optical coherence tomography (OCT) ≥ 250 microns, within 8 days of randomization. OCT scans were taken off center for the subjects identified below. Thus, readings taken made subjects appear eligible when they may not have been.

i) Subject 0046 (b)(6)'s OD eye dated May 20, 2009

ii) Subject 0042 (b)(6)'s OS eye dated April 22, 2009

We acknowledge the corrective actions described in your September 8, 2010, written response to Form FDA 483 that you will be taking to prevent inclusion of subjects with off centered OCT scans in the future. However, regardless of your corrective actions, as the clinical investigator, you were ultimately responsible for the conduct of this study and for ensuring that all subjects enrolled in the study were eligible.

b. Chapter 3, Section 3.2 of the protocol (Version 5.0, dated March 24, 2008) specified that all study eyes were to receive (b)(4) with (b)(4). Six of 18 eyes enrolled in the study did not receive (b)(4).

Specifically:

i) Subject 0044 (b)(6) received (b)(4) on May 7, 2009 and (b)(4) on May 14, 2009 for a total of (b)(4) to the OS eye.

ii) Subject 0045 (b)(6) received (b)(4) on May 19, 2009 and (b)(4) on June 2, 2009 for a total of (b)(4) to the OD eye.

iii) Subject 0045 (b)(6) received (b)(4) on May 20, 2009 and (b)(4) on June 3, 2009 for a total of (b)(4) total (b)(4) to the OD eye.

iv) Subject 0043 (b)(6) received (b)(4) on May 14, 2009 and (b)(4) on May 20, 2009 for a total of (b)(4) to the OD eye.

v) Subject 0041 (b)(6) received (b)(4) on February 26, 2009 and (b)(4) on April 2, 2009 for a total of (b)(4) to the OS eye.

vi) Subject 0046 (b)(6) received (b)(4) on May 27, 2009 and (b)(4) on June 3, 2009 for a total of (b)(4) to the OD eye.

We acknowledge your statement in your September 8, 2010, written response that, although at the initial evaluation, you felt that at least (b)(4) additional (b)(4) would be possible, at the time of treatment, it was not possible to place the additional (b)(4) as required by protocol. The protocol required a certain number of (b)(4) and did not allow flexibility. However, your written response did not explain nor did you provide any evidence that you removed these subjects from the study after realizing that they were unable to receive the required number of (b)(4). Keeping these subjects in the study compromised data integrity.

This letter is not intended to be an all-inclusive list of deficiencies with your clinical study of an investigational drug. It is your responsibility to ensure adherence to each requirement of the law and relevant FDA regulations. You should address these deficiencies and establish procedures to ensure that any ongoing or future studies will be in compliance with FDA regulations.

Within fifteen (15) working days of your receipt of this letter, you should notify this office in writing of the actions you have taken to prevent similar violations in the future.

Failure to adequately and promptly explain the violations noted above may result in regulatory action without further notice.

If you have any questions, please contact Constance Cullity, M.D., M.P.H., at 301-796-3397; FAX 301-847-8748. Your written response and any pertinent documentation should be addressed to:

Constance Cullity (formerly Lewin), M.D., M.P.H.
Branch Chief
Good Clinical Practice Enforcement Branch
Division of Good Clinical Practice Compliance
Office of Scientific Investigations
Office of Compliance
Center for Drug Evaluation and Research
Food and Drug Administration

Building 51, Room 5354
10903 New Hampshire Avenue
Silver Spring, MD 20993

Sincerely yours,

{See appended electronic signature page}

Leslie K. Ball, M.D.
Acting Office Director
Office of Scientific Investigations
Office of Compliance
Center for Drug Evaluation and Research
Food and Drug Administration

第 98 封　给 Horowitz, Jeffrey 医学博士的警告信

2011年3月21日

参考号：11-HFD-45-03-02

尊敬的Horowitz博士：

2010年8月16日至9月3日，Matthew Watson先生和Anthony Thomas先生代表FDA与您会面，对您所开展的试验药物为（b）（4）[1]，申办者为（b）（4）的以下临床研究进行了审查：试验方案（b）（4），标题为“（b）（4）”。

本次现场检查是FDA的生物研究监查项目的一部分。该项目通过设定的检查方法，评估研究的实施情况，并帮助确保这些研究中受试者的权益、安全和福利得到了保护。

经对现场检查报告、该报告的附件进行审查，我们认为，您没有遵循适用的法律要求和监管临床研究的实施及受试者保护的FDA法规。在现场检查结束时，Watson先生向您出示了FDA 483表，即现场检查发现的问题，并与您进行了讨论。我们想强调以下几点：

1. 您未能按照 21 CFR 312 的要求，保留记录直到研究终止且已通知 FDA 后 2 年［21 CFR 312.62（c）］

在2009年10月1日，申办者终止了您对试验方案（b）（4）的继续参与，FDA在2009年10月5日以书信的方式被告知您被停止继续参与试验方案（b）（4）的实施。如上所述，2010年8月16日至9月3日，Matthew Watson先生和Anthony Thomas先生代表FDA，和您一起对您所实施的临床试验方案（b）（4）进行了回顾和现场检查。现场检查发生在研究被终止和FDA被告知后的两年内，现场检查发现您对于以下的文件没有进行保存：

a. 电子病例报告表（eCRFs）：在FDA的现场检查中，您指出您的研究协调员使用申办者提供的手提电脑为每位受试者进行数据录入，而且在关闭研究中心的访问中，申办者的监查员回收了申办者提供的包括eCRF的手提电脑。在2010年9月14日您对FDA 483表的书面回复中，您进一步解释了申办者从未向您提供包含eCRF数据的光盘。然而，根据 21 CFR 312.62（c）的规定，这属于您的职责，即研究者需要在研究终止或在FDA被通知后的两年内保存eCRFs的副本。

b. 患者入组和进展表以及筛选/入组表格：在FDA的现场检查中，您的研究协调员从申办者处获取了这两份表的复印件，然而根据 21 CFR 312.62（c）的规定，这属于您的职责，即研究者需要在研究终止或在FDA被通知后的两年内保存这些表的副本。

我们认可您在书面回复中声明，和过去相比，您将会有意加强对于文件的监管。然而，您没有明确指出您会采取什么样的纠正措施来解决这些违规以及预防此类违规在未来的重复发生。

2. 您未能保存对研究中使用研究药物或对照组的受试者的所有研究观察结果和其他相关数据的足够及准确的病历［21 CFR 312.62（b）］

在参加试验方案（b）（4）的两个受试者中，FDA均发现病历不一致和不充分的情况，因此对您试验场所数据的可靠性引起严重关注。具体信息如下：

a. 研究流程表中记录了透析后的生命体征而不是透析前的生命体征。方案要求对生命体征的评估，包括体温、坐位血压和脉搏，应该在每次随访的透析前进行。在FDA的现场检查中，您的研究协调员指出她从透析中心的患者治疗记录中转录了生命体征的数据到研究流程表中，然后再把研究流程表中的数据转录到

1 （b）（4）涉及商业秘密，根据法规内容不予公开。

eCRF。但是经过对一些随访患者治疗记录和研究流程表的比对，发现您的研究协调员在某些访视的研究流程表中记录了透析后的生命体征，而没有按照方案的要求记录透析前的生命体征（请参照下表中的举例）。这些差异使得对您试验场所数据的可靠性产生了疑问，部分原因是因为您的研究协调员参照研究流程表的数据进行了eCRFs的数据录入。

受试者	随访#	患者治疗记录（透析前）	患者治疗记录（透析后）	研究流程表
00013[2]	清洗期第一周	坐位血压163/103 体温94.8°F 心率90	站位血压118/69 体温98.2°F 心率92	坐位血压118/69* 体温98.2°F 坐位脉搏92
	随访#9	坐位血压127/94 体温96.4°F 心率93	坐位血压106/91 体温98.3°F 心率99	坐位血压106/91 体温98.3°F 坐位脉搏99
00016	筛选期	坐位血压150/68 体温97.5°F 心率59	坐位血压129/87 体温97.4°F 心率80	坐位血压129/87 体温97.4°F—透析前97.5°F** 坐位脉搏80
	随访#5	坐位血压148/66 体温97.2°F 心率57	坐位血压164/87 体温97.4°F 心率58	坐位血压164/87 体温97.4°F 心率58

注：*受试者00013的清洗期第一周，显示研究协调员在研究流程表上记录了透析后站位血压。
**受试者00016的筛选随访，显示研究协调员在研究流程表上记录了透析前、后的体温。因为没有eCRF的副本，我们无法确定eCRF上记录的是透析前、后的体温的哪个数值。

b. 在上述1.b.的发现中所提及的患者入组和进展表以及筛选/入组表之间有差异。比如，患者入组和进展表显示受试者00013知情同意书的签署日期是2009年3月2日，但在筛选/入组表格上的日期是2009年2月23日。同样的受试者00016，知情同意书的签署日期是2009年3月9日，但在筛选/入组表格上的日期是2009年3月2日。

我们注意到，您在书面回复中强调了，和过去相比，您将会加强对于文件的监管。然而作为一名研究者，根据21 CFR 312.62（b）的要求准备和保存完整和准确的文件是您的职责。并且，您没有明确指出您会采取什么样的纠正措施来解决这些违规并预防此类违规在未来的重复发生。

3. 您没有确保按照研究计划进行研究［21 CFR 312.60］

试验方案的第七章列举了方案中所有要求的评估并具体指出了这些评估需要在什么时间进行。我们观察到您没有按照方案要求进行下列评估：

a. 对上述两位受试者，没有记录显示根据试验方案的要求进行了血压测定。试验方案中具体规定了每位受试者需要测量3次血压，以及每次随访以3次测量的平均值作为该受试者的血压。没有记录显示这两个受试者的随访中血压的测定是按照方案进行的。

b. 对于受试者00016：

i. 实验室报告显示在第4次和第8次随访时未按试验方案要求进行血常规检测结果的计算。

ii. 没有记录显示在第13次随访时按照试验方案的要求进行了实验室评估。

c. 对于受试者00013：

i. 没有记录显示在第1次随访（筛选）根据试验方案的要求进行了体检。

ii. 没有记录显示在第1次（筛选）和第4次随访时，根据试验方案的要求进行了实验室评估。

不进行研究相关的评估可能会损害受试者的权益、安全和福利，并损害您试验场所数据的可靠性。根据在现场检查时所有的文件记录，显示您没有确保根据试验方案进行这些评估。作为研究者，按照21 CFR 312.60的规定，您有职责确保研究按照研究计划来实施。

我们承认eCRFs有可能提供记录来证明您按照方案测量了血压；您对于受试者00016的第13次随访按照方案进行了实验室评估；以及您对于受试者00013的第1次随访完成了体检和第1次和第4次随访的实验室评估。但是，如上所解释的，您违背了21 CFR 312.62（c）的规定，您没能保存eCRFs的副本。并且，就eCRF没有提供文件证明这些评估已经按照方案实施的来说，这些差异提示，即使您按照方案进行了这些评估，您没能按照21 CFR 312.62（b）的要求来准备和保存充分和准确的病历记录。

4. 您未能保存足够的包括日期、数量、受试者的使用情况的药物处置记录［21 CFR 312.62（a）］

每次给受试者发药时，方案要求把药物的标签从外包装上撕掉然后粘贴到该受试者的药物标签表上。然而，受试者00013的药物标签表上没有下面两个药物的标签（药物随机号[3] 1010589和1020640），根据药物计数表，这两个药物在2009年5月22日发给了受试者。

我们注意到，您在书面回复中声明您“同意纸质的药物分发记录有不完善之处”但您相信“记录在eCRF会更好”。然而作为研究者，您有责任按照21 CFR 312.62（a）的规定保存充分的药物处置记录。如上所述，作为研究者，您有责任根据 21 CFR 312.62（c）的规定，在研究终止或在FDA被通知后的两年内保存eCRF的副本。此外，您在您的书面回复中没有明确指出您会采取什么样的措施来纠正这些违规并预防此类违规在未来的重复发生。

本警告信的目的并非是罗列您在试验药物临床研究中存在的所有缺陷。确保遵循法律和相关FDA法规的每一项要求是您的职责，您应当解决这些缺陷，并建立规程，以确保任何正在进行或将来进行的研究均符合FDA的法规。

自收到这封信的15个工作日内，您应当书面告知本办公室为预防将来发生类似违规情况而采取的措施。如果不能充分、迅速地解释上述违规问题，可能导致我们在不再通知的情况下采取监管措施。

附：英文原文

Horowitz, Jeffrey M.D.

WARNING LETTER

MAR 21, 2011

CERTIFIED MAIL
RETURN RECEIPT REQUESTED

Ref: 11-HFD-45-03-02

Jeffrey Horowitz, M.D.
1030 President Avenue, Room 304
Fall River Nephrology
Fall River, MA 02720-5923

Dear Dr. Horowitz:

Between August 16, 2010, and September 3, 2010, Mr. Matthew Watson and Mr. Anthony Thomas, representing the Food and Drug Administration (FDA), conducted an investigation and met with you to review your conduct of a clinical investigation (Protocol (b)(4), entitled “(b)(4)”) of the investigational drug (b)(4), performed for (b)(4).

This inspection is a part of FDA’s Bioresearch Monitoring Program, which includes inspections designed to evaluate the conduct of research and to help ensure that the rights, safety, and welfare of the human subjects of those studies have been protected.

From our review of the establishment inspection report, the documents submitted with that report, and your September 14, 2010, written response to the Form FDA 483, we conclude that you did not adhere to the applicable statutory requirements and FDA regulations governing the conduct of clinical investigations. We are aware that at the conclusion of the inspection, Mr. Watson presented and discussed with you Form FDA 483, Inspectional Observations. We wish to emphasize the following:

1. You failed to retain records required to be maintained under 21 CFR part 312 until 2 years after the investigation was discontinued and FDA was notified [21 CFR 312.62(c)].

On October 1, 2009, the sponsor discontinued your participation in Protocol (b)(4). FDA was notified in a letter dated October 5, 2009, that your participation in Protocol (b)(4) was discontinued. As explained above, between August 16, 2010, and September 3, 2010, Mr. Watson and Mr. Thomas, representing FDA, conducted an inspection and met with you to review your conduct of Protocol (b)(4). At the time of the inspection, which was less than two years after your investigation was discontinued and FDA was notified, the inspection revealed that you failed to retain the following records:

a. Electronic case report forms (eCRFs). During FDA's inspection, you stated that your study coordinator used a sponsor provided laptop to enter data into the eCRF for each subject. You also stated that during the closeout visit conducted by the sponsor's monitor, the monitor took the sponsor provided laptop computer containing the eCRFs. In your September 14, 2010, written response to Form FDA 483 (your written response), you further explained that the actual eCRF data disks were never obtained from the sponsor. However, it was your responsibility as the investigator to retain copies of the eCRFs for two years after the investigation was discontinued and FDA was notified [21 CFR 312.62(c)].

b. The Enrollment and Patient Status Log and the Screening/Enrollment Log. During FDA's inspection, your study coordinator obtained copies of these two logs from the sponsor. However, it was your responsibility as the investigator to retain copies of the logs for two years after the investigation was discontinued and FDA was notified [21 CFR 312.62(c)].

We acknowledge that in your written response you stated that you intend to "be more vigilant in documentation oversight than in the past." However, you did not specify the corrective actions you will take to address these violations or to prevent this type of violation from reoccurring in the future.

2. You failed to prepare and maintain adequate and accurate case histories that record all observations and other data pertinent to the investigation on each individual administered the investigational drug or employed as a control in the investigation [21 CFR 312.62(b)].

FDA found discrepancies and deficiencies in records for both of the subjects enrolled in Protocol (b)(4) which raises significant questions about the reliability of data at your site. Specifically:

a. The study flowsheets appear to document post-dialysis vital signs rather than pre-dialysis vital signs. The protocol required that vital sign assessments, including body temperature, sitting blood pressure and sitting pulse measurements, be performed pre-dialysis at every visit. During FDA's inspection, your study coordinator stated that she transcribed vital sign data from the dialysis center's Patient Treatment Records onto the study flowsheets, and then used the flowsheets to enter the data into the eCRFs. However, a comparison of the Patient Treatment Records and the flowsheets suggests that for some visits, your study coordinator recorded the post-dialysis vital sign data on the study flowsheets rather than the pre-dialysis vital sign data, as required by the protocol (see table below for examples). This discrepancy raises questions about the reliability of the data at your site, in part because the Study Coordinator used the flowsheets to enter data into the eCRFs.

Subject #	Visit #	Patient Treatment Record (pre-dialysis)	Patient Treatment Record (post-dialysis)	Study Flowsheet
00013[2]	Washout Week 1	Sitting Blood ressure (BP) 163/103 Body Temp 94.8°F Heart Rate (HR) 90	Standing BP 118/69 BodyTemp 8.2°F HR 92	Sitting BP 118/69* Body Temp98.2°F Sitting Pulse92
	Visit #9	Sitting BP 127/94 Body Temp 96.4°F HR 93	Sitting BP 106/91 Body Temp 98.3°F HR 99	Sitting BP 106/91 Body Temp 98.3°F Sitting Pulse 99
00016	Screening	Sitting BP 150/68 Body Temp 97.5°F HR 59	Sitting BP 129/87 Body Temp 97.4°F HR 80	Sitting BP 129/87 Body Temp 97.4°F--pre pre 97.5°F** Sitting Pulse 80
	Visit #5	Sitting BP 148/66 Body Temp 97.2°F HR 57	Sitting BP 164/87 Body Temp 97.4°F HR 58	Sitting BP 164/87 Body Temp 97.4°F HR 58

*For Subject 00013's Washout Week 1 visit, the study coordinator appears to have recorded the post-dialysis standing blood pressure measurement on the flowsheet.

**For Subject 00016's Screening visit, the study coordinator appears to have recorded both the pre- and post-dialysis body temperatures on the flowsheet. Without a copy of the eCRF, we cannot determine whether the pre- or post-dialysis temperature was recorded in this subject's eCRF.

b. There are discrepancies between the Enrollment and Patient Status Log and the Screening/Enrollment Log referenced in 1.b. above. For example, the Enrollment and Patient Status Log for Subject 00013 shows March 2, 2009, as the date of informed consent; however, the Screening/Enrollment Log shows February 23, 2009, as the date of consent. Likewise for Subject 00016, the Enrollment and Patient Status Log shows March 9, 2009, as the date of informed consent; however, the Screening/Enrollment Log shows March 2, 2009, as the date of consent.

We note that in your written response, you stated that you intend to "be more vigilant in documentation oversight than in the past." However, it was your responsibility as the investigator to ensure that adequate and accurate records were prepared and maintained as required by 21 CFR 312.62(b). Furthermore, you did not specify the corrective actions you will take to address these violations or to prevent this type of violation from reoccurring in the future.

3. You failed to ensure that the investigation was conducted according to the investigational plan [21 CFR 312.60].

Section 7 of the protocol lists all of the required assessments in the protocol, and specifies when those assessments were to be performed. It appears that the following protocol required assessments were not performed:

a. For both subjects, there was no documentation showing that the blood pressure measurements were taken in accordance with the protocol. The protocol specified that each subject's blood pressure should be measured three times, and the mean of those three measurements should be used as the subject's blood pressure measurement, at every visit. There was no documentation to show that subjects' blood pressures were measured in accordance with these protocol requirements at any of the subjects' visits.

b. For Subject 00016:

i. Laboratory Reports show that the protocol required hematology test results were not calculated at Visits 4 (Baseline) and 8.

ii. There was no documentation available to show that the protocol required laboratory evaluations were conducted at Visit 13.

c. For Subject 00013:

i. There was no documentation available to show that the protocol required physical examination was conducted at Visit 1 (Screening).

ii. There was no documentation available to show that the protocol required laboratory evaluations were conducted at Visits 1 (Screening) and 4.

Failure to perform study related assessments may jeopardize subjects' rights, safety, and welfare, and may compromise the reliability of the data at your site. Based on the documentation available at the time of the inspection, it appears that you did not ensure that these assessments were conducted in accordance with the protocol. It was your responsibility as the investigator to ensure that the investigation was conducted according to the investigational plan [21 CFR 312.60].

We acknowledge that it is possible that the eCRFs provide documentation that you measured blood pressure in accordance with the protocol, conducted the protocol required laboratory evaluations at Visit 13 for Subject 00016, and conducted the protocol required physical examination at Visit 1 and laboratory evaluations at Visits 1 and 4 for Subject 00013. However, as explained above, you failed to retain copies of the eCRFs in violation of 21 CFR 312.62(c). Moreover, to the extent that the eCRFs do not provide documentation that these assessments were conducted in accordance with the protocol, such deficiencies would suggest that, even if you conducted these assessments according to the protocol, you failed to prepare and maintain adequate and accurate case histories, as required by 21 CFR 312.62(b).

4. You failed to maintain adequate records of the disposition of the drug, including dates, quantity, and use by subjects [21 CFR 312.62(a)].

Each time the study drug was dispensed to a subject, the protocol required that the drug label be removed from the packaging and affixed to the Drug Label Form for that subject. However, the Drug Label Form for Subject 00013 did not include labels for the two drugs (medication randomization numbers[3] 1010589 and 1020640) that, according to the Drug Accountability Log, were dispensed to the subject on May 22, 2009.

We note that in your written response, you stated that you "agree that there was [sic] inadequate drug dispensing records in the paperwork," but that you believed "it was better documented in the eCRF." However, it was your responsibility as the investigator to maintain adequate records of the disposition of the drug [21 CFR 312.62(a)]. As explained above, it was also your responsibility as the investigator to retain copies of the eCRFs for two years after the investigation was discontinued and FDA was notified [21 CFR 312.62(c)]. In addition, in your written response, you did not specify any corrective actions that you will take to address these violations or to prevent this type of violation from reoccurring in the future.

This letter is not intended to be an all-inclusive list of deficiencies with your clinical study of an investigational drug. It is your responsibility to ensure adherence to each requirement of the law and relevant FDA regulations. You should address these deficiencies and establish procedures to ensure that any ongoing or future studies will be in compliance with FDA regulations.

Within fifteen (15) working days of your receipt of this letter, you should notify this office in writing of the actions you have taken to prevent similar violations in the future. Failure to adequately and promptly explain the violations noted above may result in regulatory action without further notice.

If you have any questions, please contact Constance Cullity, M.D., M.P.H., at 3017963397; FAX 3018478748. Your written response and any pertinent documentation should be addressed to:

Constance Cullity (formerly Lewin), M.D., M.P.H.
Branch Chief
Good Clinical Practice Branch I
Division of Scientific Investigations
Office of Compliance
Center for Drug Evaluation and Research
Food and Drug Administration
Building 51, Room 5354
10903 New Hampshire Avenue
Silver Spring, MD 20993

Sincerely yours,

{See appended electronic signature page}

Leslie K. Ball, M.D.

Director

Division of Scientific Investigations

Office of Compliance

Center for Drug Evaluation and Research

Food and Drug Administration

1 Mr. Thomas was present at the inspection from August 16, 2010, through August 20, 2010.

2 We note that on some of your study records, the number for this subject is recorded as “0013” instead of “00013.”

3 On the drug labels affixed to the Drug Label Form, the medication randomization number was referred to as the “Med. #.” On the Drug Accountability Log, this same number was referred to as the “Lot number.”

第 99 封　给 Zaiac, Martin N. 的警告信

2011年3月21日

参考号：11-HFD-45-03-0

尊敬的Zaiac博士：

2010年4月22日至7月14日，Dianiris Ayala女士代表FDA，与您会面，对您所开展的试验药物为（b）（4）[1]，申办者为（b）（4）的以下临床研究进行了审查：试验方案（b）（4），版本4.0，日期为2009年8月13日，标题为"（b）（4）"。

本次现场检查是FDA的生物研究监查项目的一部分。该项目通过设定的检查方法，评估研究的实施情况，并帮助确保这些研究中受试者的权益、安全和福利得到了保护。

经对现场检查报告、该报告的附件进行审查，我们认为，您没有遵循适用的法律要求和监管临床研究实施及受试者保护的FDA法规。在现场检查结束时，Dianiris Ayala女士向您出示了FDA483表，即现场检查发现的问题，并与您进行了讨论。您2010年8月5日对该FDA483表的回复已收悉，但是该回复是在现场检查结束后15个工作日后收到的。因此，根据2009年8月11日颁布的局长执行倡议的要求，虽然我们审阅了这些回复，但是并没有将对这些回复的讨论包括在这封警告信中。我们想强调以下几点：

1. 您未能亲自进行临床研究或对研究进行监督［21 CFR 312.60］

当您签署上述临床试验的研究者申明（FDA1572表）时，您同意在本试验场所履行作为临床研究者的职责。您作为临床研究者的总体职责包括：确保临床试验按照签署的研究者声明、研究计划和适用的法规进行；保护受到您医学照顾的受试者的权益、安全和福利；和确保对研究药物管控［21 CFR 312.60］。通过签署FDA1572表，您同意亲自开展本临床试验，或者对不是由您亲自执行的部分进行监管。尽管您可以将某些研究检查的任务授权给有资质的研究人员，但是作为临床研究者，您并不能将总体责任授权给别人。我们的检查发现，您对被授权进行研究任务的人员的监督是不充足的，没有能够确保本临床试验按照签署的研究者声明，研究计划和适用的法规进行，同时没有确保试验的开展保护了受试者的权利、安全和福利。

我们发现，由于您未履行对本研究充分监督的职责，导致了如下所述的和研究开展有关的严重问题，包括入组不符合合格标准的受试者，未按照安全监测流程对实验室异常值和Q-TcF间期进行监测，以及其他的违背。

2. 您未能进行研究或确保按照研究计划进行研究，未能保护在研究者监护下的受试者的权益、安全和福利［21 CFR 312.60］

试验方案7.5.3提到：

当任何受试者出现Q-Tc间期延长（使用Fridericia法校正），需遵循下列监测流程：

- 假如一名入组受试者的心电图记录到Q-TcF超过450毫秒，在30~60分钟内受试者需进行心电图复测。如果复测心电图仍然记录到一次Q-TcF高于450毫秒，需对合并用药进行确认，同时应邀请一名心脏病学专家来确认心电图机读值，考虑并决定 [sic] 随后的监测活动。
- 假如一名入组受试者的心电图记录到Q-TcF超过480毫秒，或者观察到受试者的Q-TcF间期比基线期时增加超过60毫秒，在30~60分钟内受试者需进行心电图复测。如果复测心电图仍然记录到一次Q-TcF高于480毫秒，或者相比基线期时增加超过60毫秒，需通过血样对受试者的电解质水平进行评估（必

1 (b) (4) 涉及商业秘密，根据法规内容不予公开。

须包括钾离子和镁离子）。任何异常值都应被纠正，需对合并用药进行确认，同时应邀请一名心脏病学专家来确认心电图机读值，并决定随后对受试者适当的监测活动。如果异常值被心脏病学专家确认，应停止对受试者的治疗，并且按照方案7.5.1的流程进行处置。需通知申办者，同时与项目的医师讨论这个案例。

- 假如一名入组受试者的心电图记录到Q-TcF超过500毫秒，受试者应入住有进行持续心电监护能力的远程监护或急诊室，直至受试者Q-TcF间期恢复正常。受试者在远程监护或急诊室中进行心电监护时，将遵循标准的医疗照顾流程，至少应包括心电监护、连续的12导联心电图和心脏病学专家会诊。如果异常值被急诊或远程监护室确认，应停止对受试者的治疗，并且按照方案7.5.1的流程进行处置。需通知申办者，同时与项目的医师讨论这个案例。

a. 正如在下述2.i.项中讨论的，受试者0270309在2009年7月16日进行了第36周的心电图检测，心电图机读值显示受试者Q-TcF间期为526毫秒。您没有按照方案的要求将受试者送往有进行持续心电监护能力的远程监护或急诊室直至Q-TcF恢复正常，您也没有对受试者进行心电监护或进行持续的12导联心电图检查，也没有请心脏病学专家进行会诊。

b. 受试者0270393在2009年4月27日进行了第36周的心电图检测，心电图机读值显示受试者Q-TcF间期为458毫秒。您没有按照方案的要求在30~60分钟内进行重复的心电图检测。此外，您在2009年5月8日收到并签署了送往您办公室的经确认的第36周心电图报告，而报告显示受试者的Q-TcF间期为509毫秒。您没有按照方案的要求将受试者送往有进行持续心电监护能力的远程监护或急诊室直至Q-TcF恢复正常，您也没有对受试者进行心电监护或进行持续的12导联心电图检查，也没有请心脏病学专家进行会诊。

c. 受试者02700419在2008年12月8日、2009年1月9日和2009年2月2日分别进行了第4、8和12周的心电图检测，心电图机读值显示Q-TcF间期分别为470毫秒、460毫秒和464毫秒。在这几次访视中，您都没有按照方案的要求在30~60分钟内进行重复心电图检测。

d. 试验方案7.3，合格标准第7条提到："筛选期时如果受试者的丙氨酸氨基转移酶（ALT），天冬氨酸氨基转移酶（AST），或总胆红素高于1.5倍正常值上限，该受试者不能入组……"。

受试者0270249在2008年9月22日进行筛选期实验室检查，检查结果为AST 63U/L，ALT 87U/L。这些检测值都大于1.5倍的实验室正常值上限——AST（41×1.5）61.5U/L和ALT（45×1.5）67.5U/L，因此这导致了该受试者不合格入组本临床研究。此外，该受试者在整个临床研究中都出现了AST和ALT值增高的现象，支持这一发现的证据为下列访视的实验室检查结果：基线期访视——2008年11月24日；第4周访视——2008年12月22日；第8周访视——2009年1月20日；第12周访视——2009年2月16日；第16周访视——2009年3月16日；第20周访视——2009年4月13日；第24周访视——2009年5月11日；第30周访视——2009年6月22日；第36周访视——2009年8月4日和最后第52周访视——2009年12月10日。

您没有按照方案的要求而入组了这个受试者。此外，您没有能够保护这个受试者的权益，安全和福利，同时在整个52周的试验周期中，保留该受试者在试验中是将受试者置于风险中的行为。

e. 试验方案7.5.4，临床实验室检测值提到："对于ALT和/或碱性磷酸酶和/或总胆红素超过正常值上限两倍的受试者，应对其密切监测，同时受试者应停止使用研究药物直至实验室检查值恢复到正常范围。应查实合并用药，同时评估可能引起肝功能异常的原因……"。

如下表所示，受试者0270436在2009年1月5日（第4周）时实验室检查值ALT为370，超过了正常值上限的两倍（45×2=90）；同时在2009年2月2日（第8周）时，ALT为144U/L。您没有按照方案的要求，将受试者置于风险中，因为受试者的记录并没有显示出您对其状态有密切的监测，并且记录显示您没有停止给受试者用药直至这些实验室异常值恢复到正常范围内。该受试者的ALT在整个试验过程中一直增高且从来没有恢复到正常范围内。

此外，该受试者本不应该被入组到临床研究中，因为其在基线期ALT偏高（＞67.5U/L）。方案9.1.2提到："以下评估和流程将在基线期时完成：入/排标准……"如果涉及上述提到的入组标准，该受试者本应该被排除在试验之外，因为ALT 67.5 U/L大于正常值上限的1.5倍。

周	日期	ALT值	药物编号
筛选	2008年10月16日	42	无
基线	2008年12月8日	80	20354
4	2009年1月5日	370	20697
8	2009年2月2日	144	20714
12	2009年3月2日	无记录	20783
16	2009年3月30日	82	22128
提前终止	2009年4月27日	74	无

f. 试验方案7.3，入组标准第2.d条要求，受试者必须具有皮肤真菌培养的阳性结果。

受试者0270532在随机和开始使用研究药物时，皮肤真菌培养的结果为阴性。您没有按照方案的要求，入组了一个不符合入组标准的受试者。

g. 试验方案9.1.1，筛选，提到“如果受试者没有在筛选后60天内随机，其所有的筛选期评估都必须重新检测。”

受试者0270249，0270253和0270281都未在筛选后60天内随机，并且筛选期的评估检查也没有复测。

i. 受试者0270249在2008年9月22日筛选。受试者在筛选期60天范围之外随机，且在2008年11月24日进行了基线期访视。

ii. 受试者0270253在2008年9月23日筛选。受试者在筛选期60天范围之外随机，且在2009年1月8日进行了基线期访视。

iii. 受试者0270281在2008年9月25日筛选。受试者在筛选期60天范围之外随机，且在2008年12月4日进行了基线期访视。

h. 试验方案11.5，安全性实验室检测，提到：“在用药后所有安全性实验室检测异常值，只要达到临床有意义的水平都必须重复检测至该异常值稳定。如果实验室异常值没有在合理的时间段恢复正常或者恢复到基线期水平，需找出原因并通知申办者。”

此外，试验方案7.4，排除标准中提到：

受试者如果出现下列情况或符合下列特质，将被排除在试验之外：

“10.受试者目前患有任何疾病或情况，也可以包括异常的实验室检测值和/或正在服用其他药物，经研究者判断这些疾病或症状或伴随用药，可能会影响到对研究产品的评估，或者将受试者置于不合理的风险中。

12.受试者患有可能影响到药物吸收的病史（比如胃切除术），不受控的糖尿病，有临床意义的周围性血管疾病或者末梢循环障碍，或者在筛选检查前30天内患有任何严重疾病。”

我们发现多个受试者在筛选期和/或在一次或多次研究访视中，出现不受控的糖尿病症状。您没能够按照方案的要求排除这些受试者以不让他们进入试验；同时在受试者的记录中也没有任何证据证明您按照方案第11.5的要求对这些异常值进行了复测直至其稳定。

i. 受试者0270292在筛选期和整个试验中，都出现了血糖和尿糖增高。

ii. 受试者0270360在筛选期和整个试验中，都出现了血糖和尿糖增高。

iii. 受试者0270281在筛选期和整个试验中，都出现了血糖和尿糖增高。

i.试验方案7.3，入组标准第5和第6条，提到：

“5. 性活跃、非哺乳期和具有生育能力的女性受试者，参与该研究时必须同意从接受方案分配的研究产品开始，直至接受最后一剂研究产品后60天出现的第一次月经，使用医学上认可的避孕措施。一个具有生育能力的女性定义为在生物学上具备怀孕的能力；包括围绝经期女性，定义为最后一次月经后两年内。避孕方法包括：

- 激素避孕，包括筛选前至少2个月内开始口服、注射和植入激素。如果激素避孕没有在筛选前至少2个月内开始使用，需加用一种非激素避孕的方法，直至激素避孕方法持续使用3个月。
- 两种非激素避孕的方法，包括子宫内避孕器或者适当的阻隔类避孕方法（包括男性或女性避孕套，薄膜，或子宫颈帽）。接受过绝育手术的受试者，包括输卵管结扎或伴侣的输精管切除术，必须使用一种非激素类避孕方法。阻隔类避孕法或输卵管结扎，加上杀精子药，是可以被接受的。

女性受试者目前非性活跃，或者不在哺乳期，必须同意使用医学上认可的避孕方法，以防受试者［sic］在试验过程中变为性活跃。

6. 具有生育能力的女性受试者，在入组阶段妊娠试验为阴性。”

此外，试验方案9.1，研究访视评估，要求妊娠试验需在如下访视点进行：筛选（尿样），基线期（血清和尿样），第12周（尿样），第24周（尿样），第36周（尿样），和第52周（尿样）。

另外，试验方案11.6，妊娠试验，提到：“对于具备生育能力的女性受试者，在下列访视时都需进行尿样妊娠试验：筛选，基线，第12/24/26和52周。此外，基线期时，所有女性受试者都要进行血清妊娠试验。在随机或者开始使用研究产品之前，必须收到一个阴性结果的尿妊娠试验。”这一信息同时在方案第3部分通过图表的形式表现了出来，研究流程图，表1，标题为“评估计划表——通用。”

我们发现，在受试者0270309参与研究的36周以来，您并没有记录受试者怀孕和怀孕的进展直至结束。我们承认您按照方案的要求在筛选、基线、第12周、第24周和第36周，进行了妊娠试验，同时这些检测的结果均为阴性。尽管如此，在体检时您并没有记录受试者的体重增加或者怀孕状腹部的存在，而是在筛选、第12周、第24周和第36周，体格检查您都报告为正常。因此，发育中的胎儿因为暴露在研究药物下可能会受到伤害。受试者在（b）（6）时死亡。我们在尸检报告中发现，受试者体重为316磅；但是，在多个研究访视的受试者研究记录中（包括她最后一次来院随访，第36周，2009年7月16日），她的体重为265磅。此外，尸检发现受试者子宫内存在正常发育的男性胎儿，基于体重和测量，该男性胎儿和平均足月胎儿基本一致。尸检报告提示，受试者的死因为围生期心肌病，同时肺炎、病态肥胖、药物滥用（可卡因代谢物的存在），也成为受试者死亡的附带原因。

我们发现在临床研究过程中，您没有充分地监督妊娠试验，体格检查和Q-TcF间期监测，这些都促成了受试者0270309在本临床研究中不恰当的持续参与和足月妊娠。

入组不符合入组标准的受试者和未进行研究相关的流程，这些行为危害到了受试者的安全和福祉，同时也危害到了研究终点的解读和有效性。

3. 您未能保存对研究中使用药物或对照组的受试者的所有研究观察结果和其他相关数据的足够及准确的病历［21 CFR 312.62（b）］

试验方案15.1，病例报告表，提到：“研究者应保存足够的和准确的病例报告表，并且记录所有的观察发现和其他相关的数据。应使用不褪色的水笔以整洁的清晰的方式填写病例报告表，以确保数据被准确地解读。”

a. 我们发现研究资料审阅后被签署的日期早于资料被传真到试验场所的日期，或者是早于报告提交的日期。举例如下：

i. 受试者0270281：受试者基线期心电图报告审阅后被签署时间为2008年12月7日，但是该报告出具日期为2008年12月8日。

ii. 受试者0270532：受试者筛选期心电图报告审阅后被签署时间为2009年2月2日，但是该报告出具日期为2009年2月3日。

iii. 受试者0270576：受试者真菌学结果审阅后被签署日期为2009年2月9日，但真菌学结果报告是在2009年2月10日通过传真的方式传递给试验场所。

b. 我们发现下列研究资料的签署日期早于其研究监查员提醒Zaiac医生审阅的日期：

i. 受试者0270145：在2009年4月21日，监查员指出Zaiac医生没有审阅和签署受试者第12周的心电图，同时没有评估第12周的实验室异常值。随后对这些文件的检查显示，这些文件签署的日期为试验场所接收到文件的日期，而不是在2009年4月21日监查员提醒Zaiac医生注意后的日期。

ii. 受试者0270174：在2008年11月19日，监查员指出Zaiac医生未签署筛选期心电图。随后对筛选期心电图的检查显示，心电图签署的日期为进行心电图检测的时间，而不是2008年11月19日监查员提醒Zaiac医生注意之后的日期。

未保存足够的和准确的原始记录（该记录包括全部观察发现和其他相关的数据），危害到了研究终点的解读和有效性。

4. 您未能按 21 CFR 50 的要求获得每位受试者的知情同意［21 CFR 312.60］

除了 21 CFR 50.23和50.24 所规定的情况，除非获取了受试者或其法律授权人在法律上被认为有效的知情同意，任何研究者不得在研究中入组受试者。

作为临床研究者，您有职责按照21CFR 50的要求获取知情同意。研究者只有在向潜在受试者或其代理人提供了足够的机会考虑是否参加并尽量减少对受试者的胁迫或不当影响的情况下向受试者获取知情同意。向受试者及其代理人提供的信息应该是他们可以理解的语言。

您未能对编号为0270354和0270174的受试者获取法律上有效的知情同意，但对他们开具了研究用药（b）（4）的处方。具体来说，编号为0270354的受试者在2008年8月7日签署的针对试验方案（b）（4）的知情同意书和编号为0270174的受试者在2009年10月13日签署的针对试验方案（b）（4）的知情同意书是用英语签署的，不像其他受试者签署的知情同意书是用西班牙语签署的。

不能获得充分的知情同意和减少对受试者可能的胁迫或不正当影响，因没有对受试者提供对参加研究的风险和获益进行评估的机会，从而损害入组受试者的安全和福利。

5. 您未能确保符合 56 部分所列要求的 IRB 负责对试验方案（b）（4）进行初始审查、跟踪审查和批准［21 CFR 312.66］

FDA 法规要求按照了21 CFR 56的要求获得伦理委员会的审查和批准，才能启动新药（IND）（21 CFR 312有关的）临床试验。研究者负责确保有合适的伦理委员会对试验方案（b）（4）进行首次和持续审阅和批准［21 CFR 312.66］。研究者也需要确保对试验的任何变化或未预期的问题中涉及对受试者或他人的风险快速向伦理委员会报告，并且研究者在未获得伦理委员会的批准前不会做任何改变，除非是必须消除对受试者的即刻危害。您违背了以上的要求，具体情况如下：

a. 您未能向伦理委员会报告申办者已经停止了您的研究。申办者在2009年12月停止了您的研究，但是您直到在FDA启动了此次核查后，在2010年4月30日时才通知了伦理委员会试验场所已关闭。我们注意到在核查的时候，您向检查员承认，您当时认为通知伦理委员会是申办者的责任。

b. 您未能报告伦理委员会有关受试者0270436和0270532的所有非预期的问题，其中涉及对他们的风险。具体来说，您知道受试者0270436 的HIV和肝炎指标在2009年4月呈现阳性，但您直到2009年9月才报告给伦理委员会。您也未能报告给伦理委员会受试者0270532在随机和服用药物时没有阳性的皮肤真菌培养结果。

您未能报告伦理委员会申办者已经停止了您的研究和一些非预期的问题其中涉及对受试者的风险，由此阻碍了伦理委员会对您进行试验方案（b）（4）申请的审查以及对您是否能够继续进行试验的充分性的判断。因此，您未能确保伦理委员会按照21 CFR 312.66的要求对试验方案（b）（4）进行持续性审阅［21 CFR 312.66］。

本警告信的目的并非是罗列您在试验药物临床研究中存在的所有缺陷。确保遵循法律和相关FDA法规的每一项要求是您的职责，您应当解决这些缺陷，并建立规程，以确保任何正在进行或将来进行的研究均符合FDA的法规。

自收到这封信的15个工作日内，您应当书面告知本办公室为预防将来发生类似违规情况而采取的措施。如果不能充分、迅速地解释上述违规问题，可能导致我们在不再通知的情况下采取监管措施。如果您认为您确信2010年8月5日对FDA483表书面回复充分解释了您所采取的预防将来类似违规的措施，请在15个工作日内告知我们。对本封信的回复您可以参考2010年8月5日的书面回复。

附：英文原文

Zaiac, Martin N.

WARNING LETTER

MAR 21, 2011

CERTIFIED MAIL
RETURN RECEIPT REQUESTED

Ref: 11-HFD-45-03-0

Dr. Martin Zaiac
Greater Miami Skin and Laser Center
4308 Alton Road, Suite 750
Miami Beach, FL 33140

Dear Dr. Zaiac:

Between April 22 and July 14, 2010, Ms. Dianiris Ayala, representing the Food and Drug Administration (FDA), conducted an investigation and met with you to review your conduct of a clinical investigation (Protocol (b)(4), Version 4.0, dated August 13, 2009, entitled "(b)(4)") of the investigational drug (b)(4), performed for (b)(4).

This inspection is a part of FDA's Bioresearch Monitoring Program, which includes inspections designed to evaluate the conduct of research and to help ensure that the rights, safety, and welfare of the human subjects of those studies have been protected.

From our review of the establishment inspection report and the documents submitted with that report, we conclude that you did not adhere to the applicable statutory requirements and FDA regulations governing the conduct of clinical investigations and the protection of human subjects. We are aware that at the conclusion of the inspection, Ms. Ayala presented and discussed with you Form FDA 483, Inspectional Observations. We acknowledge receipt of your August 5, 2010, response to Form FDA 483, but note that this response was received past the 15 working days from close of the inspection. Thus, while we have reviewed the response, we have not included a discussion of the response in this letter, as per the Commissioner's Enforcement Initiative announced on August 11, 2009. We wish to emphasize the following:

1. You failed to personally conduct or supervise the clinical investigation [21 CFR 312.60].

When you signed the Statement of Investigator (Form FDA 1572) for the above-referenced clinical trial, you agreed to take on the responsibilities of a clinical investigator at your site. Your general responsibilities as a clinical investigator include ensuring that the clinical trial is conducted according to the signed investigator statement, the investigational plan, and applicable regulations; protecting the rights, safety, and welfare of subjects under your care; and ensuring control of drugs under investigation [21 CFR 312.60]. By signing Form FDA 1572, you specifically agreed to personally conduct the clinical trial or to supervise those aspects of the trial that you did not personally conduct. While you may delegate certain study tasks to individuals qualified to perform them, as a clinical investigator you may not delegate your general responsibilities. Our investigation indicates that your supervision of personnel to whom you delegated study tasks was not adequate to ensure that the clinical trial was conducted according to the signed investigator statement, the investigational plan, and applicable regulations, and that these trials were conducted in a manner that protects the rights, safety, and welfare of human subjects.

We note that your failure to adequately supervise this study led to significant problems with the conduct of the study as mentioned below, which included enrollment of subjects who did not meet eligibility criteria, and failure to follow safety monitoring procedures with respect to abnormal laboratory values and QTcF intervals, among other violations.

2. You failed to conduct the studies or ensure they were conducted according to the investigational plan, and failed to protect the rights, safety, and welfare of subjects under the investigator's care [21 CFR 312.60].

Section 7.5.3 of the protocol states:

The following monitoring procedures should be followed for any subject who develops a QTc prolongation (Fridericia's correction will be used):

- If an ECG from an enrolled subject records a QTcF exceeding 450 ms, an ECG should be repeated within 30 to 60 minutes. If the repeat ECG also records a QTcF greater than 450 ms, concomitant medication should be verified and a cardiologist should be consulted to confirm the read out and consider to determine [sic] subsequent monitoring activities.
- If an ECG from an enrolled subject records a QTcF exceeding 480 ms, or if an increase in QTcF versus baseline exceeding 60 ms is observed, an ECG should be repeated within 30 to 60 minutes. If the repeat ECG also records a QTcF greater than 480 ms or a change versus baseline > 60 ms, levels of electrolytes (these must include potassium and magnesium) should be assessed from a blood sample. Any abnormalities should be corrected, concomitant medication should be verified, and a clinical cardiologist should be consulted to confirm the read out and determine proper subsequent monitoring activities. If the abnormalities are confirmed by the cardiologist, subjects will be discontinued from treatment and procedures in Section 7.5.1 should be followed. The sponsor must be notified and the case discussed with the Project Physician.
- If an ECG from an enrolled subject records a QTcF interval exceeding 500 ms, subjects should be admitted to a telemetry unit or an emergency unit with continuous ECG recording capabilities until normalization of the QTcF interval. During the subject's monitoring at the emergency or telemetry unit, standard practices for the unit will be followed including, at a minimum, electrolyte monitoring, serial 12-lead ECGs, and consultation with a clinical cardiologist. If the abnormalities are confirmed by the emergency or telemetry unit, subjects will be discontinued from treatment and procedures in Section 7.5.1 should be followed. The sponsor must be notified and the case discussed with the Project Physician.

a. As discussed in Item 2.i. below, Subject 0270309 had a Week 36 ECG conducted on July 16, 2009, that resulted in a QTcF value of 526 ms, according to the ECG machine readout. You failed to follow the protocol because you did not admit the subject to a telemetry unit or an emergency unit with continuous ECG recording capabilities until normalization of the QTcF interval, nor did you perform electrolyte monitoring or serial 12-lead ECGs, or obtain consultation with a clinical cardiologist.

b. Subject 0270393 had a Week 36 ECG conducted on April 27, 2009, that resulted in a QTcF value of 458 ms, according to the ECG machine readout. You failed to follow the protocol because you did not perform a repeat ECG within 30 to 60 minutes. Furthermore, when the confirmed ECG report of the Week 36 ECG was received by your office and signed by you on May 8, 2009, it stated that the QTcF was 509 ms. You failed to follow the protocol because you did not admit the subject to a telemetry unit or an emergency unit with continuous ECG recording capabilities until normalization of the QTcF interval, nor did you perform electrolyte monitoring or serial 12-lead ECGs, or obtain consultation with a clinical cardiologist.

c. Subject 02700419 had a Week 4 ECG conducted on December 8, 2008, that resulted in a QTcF value of 470 ms; a Week 8 ECG conducted on January 9, 2009, that resulted in a QTcF value of 460 ms; and a Week 12 ECG conducted on February 2, 2009, that resulted in a QTcF value of 464ms, according to the ECG machine readouts. You failed to follow the protocol because you did not perform a repeat ECG within 30 to 60 minutes at each of these visits.

d. Section 7.3 of the protocol, eligibility criterion number 7, states: "Subjects will not be enrolled if they have alanine aminotransferase (ALT), aspartate aminotransferase (AST), or total bilirubin values greater than 1.5 times the upper normal limit at screening…."

Subject 0270249 had screening labs performed on September 22, 2008, that reported an AST of 63 U/L and an ALT of 87 U/L. These values are greater than 1.5 times the upper normal limit values of AST (41 × 1.5) 61.5 U/L and ALT (45 × 1.5) 67.5 U/L, and therefore render the subject ineligible to enroll in the clinical investigation. Additionally, the subject continued to have elevated AST and ALT values throughout the clinical investigation, as evidenced by laboratory results from the baseline visit on November 24, 2008; the Week 4 visit on December 22, 2008; the Week 8 visit on January 20, 2009; the Week 12 visit on February 16, 2009; the Week 16 visit on March 16, 2009; the Week

20 visit on April 13, 2009; the Week 24 visit on May 11, 2009; the Week 30 visit on June 22, 2009; the Week 36 visit on August 4, 2009; and finally, the Week 52 visit on December 10, 2009.

You failed to follow the protocol by enrolling this subject in the clinical investigation. Furthermore, you failed to protect the rights, safety, and welfare of this subject and placed this subject at risk by maintaining this subject in the clinical investigation for the entire 52-week investigative period.

e. Section 7.5.4 of the protocol, Clinical Laboratory Test Values, states: "Subjects with ALT and/or alkaline phosphates and/or total bilirubin exceeding twice the upper normal limit should be closely monitored and not receive additional study drug until values are back in the normal range. Concomitant medication should be verified and possible causes of liver function abnormalities evaluated…."

As illustrated by the table below, Subject 0270436 had elevated laboratory test values exceeding twice the upper normal limit (45 × 2 = 90) on January 5, 2009 (Week 4), with an ALT of 370 U/L; and on February 2, 2009 (Week 8), with an ALT of 144 U/L. You did not follow the protocol and placed the subject at risk because the subject's record does not reflect that you closely monitored the situation, nor does the record indicate that you stopped study drug until the values were back in the normal range. The subject's ALT remained elevated throughout the study and never returned to the normal range.

Furthermore, this subject should not have been enrolled in the clinical investigation due to the elevated ALT at the baseline visit (> 67.5 U/L). Section 9.1.2 of the protocol states: "The following assessments and procedures will be performed at the baseline visit: inclusion/exclusion criteria…." If one refers to the inclusion criterion mentioned above, the subject would have been excluded because the ALT was > 1.5 times the upper normal limit of 67.5 U/L.

Week	Date	ALT Value	Medication Kit #
Screening	10/16/08	42	None
Baseline	12/8/08	80	20354
4	1/5/09	370	20697
8	2/2/09	144	20714
12	3/2/09	No record available	20783
16	3/30/09	82	22128
Early Withdrawal	4/27/09	74	None

f. Section 7.3 of the protocol, Inclusion Criteria, number 2.d., states that subjects must have " a positive dermatophyte culture."

Subject 0270532 did not have a positive dermatophyte culture at the time of randomization and administration of study drug. You failed to follow the protocol by enrolling this subject, who did not meet eligibility criteria.

g. Section 9.1.1 of the protocol, Screening, states that " if subject is not randomized within 60-days of screening, all screening assessments must be repeated."

Subjects 0270249, 0270253, and 0270281 were not randomized within the 60-days of screening, yet the screening assessments were not repeated.

i. Subject 0270249 was screened September 22, 2008. Subject was randomized outside the 60-day screening period and underwent the baseline visit on November 24, 2008.

ii. Subject 0270253 was screened September 23, 2008. Subject was randomized outside the 60-day screening period and underwent the baseline visit on January 8, 2009.

iii. Subject 0270281 was screened september 25, 2008. Subject was randomized outside the 60-day screening period and underwent the baseline visit on December 4, 2008.

h. Section 11.5 of the protocol, Safety Laboratory Determinations, states: "All safety laboratory tests with values that become abnormal to a clinically important degree after study product administration should be repeated until the values stabilize. If laboratory values do not return to normal or baseline within a reasonable period, the etiology should be identified and the sponsor notified."

In addition, Section 7.4 of the protocol, Exclusion Criteria, states:

Subjects with any of the following conditions or characteristics will be excluded from study enrollment:

10. Subject is currently suffering from any disease or condition, that could include abnormal laboratory tests, and/or who are currently using medication which in the opinion of the investigator may affect the evaluation of the study product or place the subject at undue risk.

12. Subject has a history of any condition that could possibly affect absorption of drug (e.g., gastrectomy), uncontrolled diabetes, clinically significant peripheral vascular disease or peripheral circulatory impairment, or has had any major illness within 30 days prior to screening examination.

We note that multiple subjects had uncontrolled diabetes at the time of screening and/or at one or more study visits. You did not follow the protocol because you did not exclude any of the subjects from enrollment; nor is there any evidence in the subjects' records that you repeated the abnormal values until stabilized, according to Section 11.5 of the protocol.

i. Subject 0270292 had elevated blood glucose values and urine glucose values at screening and throughout his participation in the study.

ii. Subject 0270360 had elevated blood glucose values and urine glucose values at screening and throughout his participation in the study.

iii. Subject 0270281 had elevated blood glucose values and urine glucose values at screening and throughout his participation in the study.

i. Section 7.3 of the protocol, Inclusion Criteria numbers 5 and 6, state:

5. Sexually active non-lactating females of childbearing potential participating in the study must agree to use a medically acceptable method of contraception while receiving protocol assigned product and up to the first menses 60 days following the last dose of study product. A woman of childbearing potential is defined as one who is biologically capable of becoming pregnant; including perimenopausal women who are less than 2 years from their last menses. Contraceptive methods include:

- Hormonal contraception, including oral, injectable, or implantable methods started at least 2 months prior to screening. If hormonal contraception was started less than 2 months prior to screening, then a form of non-hormonal contraception should be added until the third continuous month of hormonal contraception has been completed.
- Two forms of non-hormonal contraception, including intrauterine devices or properly used barrier methods (eg, male or female condoms, diaphragm, or cervical cap). Subjects with surgical sterilization, including tubal ligation or partner's vasectomy, must use a form of nonhormonal contraception. A barrier method or sterilization plus spermaticide are acceptable.

Women who are not currently sexually active or lactating must agree to use a medically accepted method of contraception should she [*sic*] become sexually active while participating in the study.

6. Women of childbearing potential must have a negative pregnancy test at enrollment.

Additionally, Section 9.1 of the protocol, Study Visit Assessments, outlines that pregnancy tests are to be obtained at Screening (urine), Baseline (serum and urine), Week 12 (urine), Week 24 (urine), Week 36 (urine), and at Week 52 (urine). Furthermore, Section 11.6 of the protocol, Pregnancy Testing, states: "A pregnancy test will be conducted on urine from female subjects of childbearing potential at screening, baseline, weeks 12, 24, 26, and 52 visits. In addition a serum pregnancy test will be performed on all female subjects at baseline. A negative urine pregnancy test result must be received before either randomization or administration of study product." This information is also graphically expressed in Section 3 of the protocol, Study Flowcharts, Table 1, labeled "Schedule of Assessments – General."

We note that during the 36 weeks that Subject 0270309 participated in the study, you did not document the presence of a pregnancy and its progression to term. We acknowledge that you performed the pregnancy tests as required by the protocol at screening, baseline, Week 12, Week 24, and Week 36 visits, and that those tests were negative. However, you did not document the subject's weight gain or the presence of a gravid abdomen at the time of her physical exams, which you reported as normal during study visits at screening, Week 12, Week 24, and Week 36, thereby exposing the developing fetus to harm from the investigational drug. The subject died on (b)(6). We note that in the autopsy, the subject was reported as weighing 316 pounds; however, in the subject's study records for multiple study visits, including her final visit (Week 36, dated July 16, 2009), she was reported as weighing 265 pounds. Additionally, the autopsy reported the presence of an intrauterine, normally developed, male fetus that was consistent with an average full-term fetus, based on weight and measurements. The autopsy reported the subject's cause of death as peripartum cardiomyopathy, with contributory causes of pneumonia, morbid obesity, and substance abuse (evidence of a cocaine metabolite).

We note that your failure to adequately supervise pregnancy tests, physical examinations, and QTcF monitoring procedures during the clinical investigation, contributed to the inappropriate continued participation of Subject 0270309 and her full-term fetus in the clinical investigation.

Enrollment of subjects who do not meet eligibility criteria and failure to perform study-related procedures jeopardize subject safety and welfare and compromise the interpretation and validity of the investigational endpoints.

3. You failed to maintain adequate and accurate case histories that record all observations and other data pertinent to the investigation on each individual administered the investigational drug or employed as a control in the investigation [21 CFR 312.62(b)].

Section 15.1 of the protocol, Case Report Forms, states: "The investigator is required to maintain adequate and accurate CRFs [Case Report Forms] and to record all observations and other data relevant to the clinical investigation. These forms are to be completed in a neat, legible manner with permanent ink to ensure accurate interpretation of data."

a. We note that study records were signed as having been reviewed on a date prior to the date they were faxed to the clinical site, or prior to the submission of the report. For example:

i. For Subject 0270281: The subject's baseline ECG report was signed as having been reviewed on December 7, 2008, when the record itself was dated December 8, 2008.

ii. For Subject 0270532: The subject's screening ECG was signed as having been reviewed on February 2, 2009, when the record itself was dated February 3, 2009.

iii. For Subject 0270576: The subject's mycology results were signed as having been reviewed on February 9, 2009, when the records were not received by facsimile until February 10, 2009.

b. We note that the following study records were signed as having been reviewed on a date prior to the date they were brought to Dr. Zaiac's attention during a study monitor's visit:

i. For Subject 0270145: On April 21, 2009, the study monitor pointed out that Dr. Zaiac had not reviewed and signed the Week 12 ECG and had not evaluated the Week 12 abnormal laboratory results. A subsequent review of these records disclosed that they had been signed using the date they were received at the site, instead of using a date after April 21, 2009, when the monitor had brought them to Dr. Zaiac's attention.

ii. For Subject 0270174: On November 19, 2008, the study monitor pointed out that Dr. Zaiac had not signed the screening ECG. A subsequent review of the screening ECG disclosed that it had been signed using the date it was conducted, instead of using a date after November 19, 2008, when the monitor had brought it to Dr. Zaiac's attention.

Failure to maintain adequate and accurate case histories that record all observations and other data pertinent to the investigation compromises the interpretation and validity of the investigational endpoints.

4. You failed to obtain informed consent of each subject in accordance with the provisions of 21 CFR part 50 [21 CFR 312.60].

Except as provided in 21 CFR 50.23 and 50.24, no investigator may involve a human being as a subject in research unless the investigator has obtained the legally effective informed consent of the subject or the subject's legally authorized representative [21 CFR 50.20].

As an investigator, it is your responsibility to obtain informed consent in accordance with 21 CFR part 50. An investigator shall seek such consent only under circumstances that provide the prospective subject or the representative sufficient opportunity to consider whether or not to participate and that minimize the possibility of coercion or undue influence. The information that is given to the subject or the representative shall be in language understandable to the subject or the representative.

You failed to obtain legally effective informed consent from Subjects 0270354 and 0270174, to whom you prescribed the investigational new drug, (b)(4). Specifically, the informed consent forms for Subject 0270354 that were dated

August 7, 2008, and the informed consent forms for Subject 0270174 that were dated October 13, 2009, for Protocol (b)(4) were written in English, unlike the other consent forms signed by these subjects, which were written in Spanish.

Failure to obtain adequate informed consent and to minimize the possibility of coercion or undue influence jeopardizes the safety and welfare of enrolled subjects by denying them an opportunity to assess the risks and benefits of their participation in the clinical investigation.

5. You failed to assure that an Institutional Review Board (IRB) that complies with the requirements set forth in part 56 was responsible for the initial and continuing review and approval of Protocol (b)(4) [21 CFR 312.66].

FDA regulations require that clinical investigations conducted under an IND (i.e., those subject to 21 CFR part 312) not be initiated unless that investigation has been reviewed and approved by an IRB meeting the requirements of 21 CFR Part 56. Clinical investigators are responsible for ensuring that an appropriate IRB conducts initial and continuing reviews of clinical investigations [21 CFR 312.66]. The investigator shall also ensure that he or she will promptly report to the IRB all changes in the research activity and all unanticipated problems involving risk to human subjects or others, and that he or she will not make any changes in the research without IRB approval, except where necessary to eliminate apparent immediate hazards to human subjects. You violated these requirements as described below:

a. You failed to report to the IRB that the clinical investigation was terminated at your site by the study sponsor. The sponsor terminated your site in December 2009, yet you did not notify the IRB of site closure until April 30, 2010, after the initiation of this FDA inspection. We note that at the time of the inspection, you admitted to the FDA investigator that you thought the sponsor was responsible for submitting the report to the IRB.

b. Your failed to report all unanticipated problems involving risk for Subjects 0270436 and 0270532. Specifically, you were aware that Subject 0270436 was positive for HIV and hepatitis in April 2009, yet you did not report that information to the IRB until September 2009. You also failed to report to the IRB that Subject 0270532 did not have a positive dermatophyte culture at the time of randomization and administration of study drug.

Your failure to ensure that the IRB was notified of the termination of your site by the sponsor, and your failure to report unanticipated problems involving risk to subjects, impeded the IRB's ability to review your application to conduct Protocol (b)(4), and to make a determination regarding the continued adequacy of that application. Therefore, you failed to ensure continuing IRB review of Protocol (b)(4), as required under 21 CFR 312.66.

This letter is not intended to be an all-inclusive list of deficiencies with your clinical study of an investigational drug. It is your responsibility to ensure adherence to each requirement of the law and relevant FDA regulations. You should address these deficiencies and establish procedures to ensure that any ongoing or future studies will be in compliance with FDA regulations.

Within fifteen (15) working days of your receipt of this letter, you should notify this office in writing of the actions you have taken to prevent similar violations in the future. Failure to adequately and promptly explain the violations noted above may result in regulatory action without further notice. If you believe that your written response to the Form FDA 483 dated August 5, 2010, fully explains the actions you have taken to prevent similar violations in the future, please communicate that to us in writing within fifteen (15) business days. You may reference the written response dated August 5, 2010, in your response to this letter.

If you have any questions, please contact Constance Cullity, M.D., M.P.H., at 301-796-3397; FAX 301-847-8748. Your written response and any pertinent documentation should be addressed to:

Constance Cullity (formerly Lewin), M.D., M.P.H.
Branch Chief
Good Clinical Practice Branch I
Division of Scientific Investigations
Office of Compliance
Center for Drug Evaluation and Research
Food and Drug Administration

Building 51, Room 5354
10903 New Hampshire Avenue
Silver Spring, MD 20993

Sincerely yours,

{See appended electronic signature page}

Leslie K. Ball, M.D.
Director
Division of Scientific Investigations
Office of Compliance
Center for Drug Evaluation and Research
Food and Drug Administration

第 100 封　给 Griffin, John 医学博士的警告信

2011年3月14日

参考号：11-HFD-45-02-01

尊敬的Griffin博士：

2010年5月12日至7月15日，Sherry Secrist女士代表FDA，并与您会面，对您所开展的以下临床研究进行了审查：

试验方案（b）(4）[1]，标题为（b）(4），试验药物为（b）(4），申办者为（b）(4)；

试验方案（b）(4），标题为（b）(4），试验药物为（b）(4），申办者为（b）(4)。

本次现场检查是FDA的生物研究监查项目的一部分。该项目通过设定的检查方法，评估研究的实施情况，并帮助确保这些研究中受试者的权益、安全和福利得到了保护。

经对现场检查报告及该报告的附件进行审查，我们认为，您没有遵循适用的法律要求和监管临床研究实施的FDA法规。在现场检查结束时，Secrist女士向您出示了FDA483表，即现场检查发现的问题，并与您进行了讨论。您2010年8月13日对该FDA483表的书面回复已收悉，但收到该回复的日期晚于核查结束后15天，因此尽管收到了回复，在此信函中我们未按2009年8月11日发布的“委员强制措施”，包含对此回复进行的讨论。

1. 您未能确保按照签署的研究者声明进行研究，因为您未能亲自进行临床研究或对研究和监督［21 CFR 312.60］

当您签署上面提到临床试验的“研究者声明”（FDA1572表）时，您同意承担作为贵中心临床研究者的职责。作为临床研究者，您的总体职责包括确保临床试验按照签署的研究者声明，研究计划和其他适用法规进行；通过医疗监护接受您保护受试者的权益、安全和福利；并确保研究药物的管控［21 CFR 312.60］。签署了FDA1572表，表明您明确同意亲自实施临床试验或监管您未亲自参加的临床试验内容。尽管您可以将一些研究工作授权给满足要求的其他人员进行，但作为临床研究者您不可以将您的总体职责授权给他人。我们的检查发现，您对您授权研究工作的全体人员的监管不足以确保临床研究按照签署的研究者协议、研究计划和其他适用法规进行和保护受试者的权益、安全和福利。

具体而言，您未能充分监管您授权的研究护士的工作。因您未能充分监管研究护士，造成了此信中列举的其他诸多违规行为。例如，研究护士不恰当地在试验方案（b）(4）相关的文件中完成了或签署了您的名字，如日期为2007年10月11日的FDA1572表，日期为2007年7月12日的保密声明，日期为2007年8月8日机密研究方案；试验方案（b）(4）相关的文件，包括一个日期为2008年1月14日的伦理委员会财务披露表，以及2份日期为2008年1月25日的向伦理委员会递交的严重不良事件报告表。另外，根据下述第2项，试验方案（b）(4）随机入组的4名受试者中的2名不符合方案规定的入组条件。如果您对研究进行了充分的监管，您将可以通过审阅研究文件发现研究相关的文件非您本人签署，以及2名受试者不符合入组条件。

我们注意到，根据您的多封与相关方面［（b）(4)，Sentara Virginia Beach综合医院（SVBGH）伦理委员会，(b）(4)（此方案的申办者），(b）(4)（此方案的申办者），(b）(4)］，日期为2008年2月22日、3月5日、3月9日、3月14日、3月17日、3月19日、3月26日、4月3日、5月19日、6月2日及6月5日的信函，您于2008年2月20日首次获知了一位研究护士不恰当签名的情况。您报告，您于2008年2月21日进行了一次内部调查，此研究护士对您的办公室经理承认她不恰当地在文件上签署了您的姓名。此次内部调查导致了当事研究护士被

1 (b) (4) 涉及商业秘密，根据法规内容不予公开。

解聘，并将其行为报告至国家护理委员会。您于2008年2月22日将研究护士及不恰当签字一事通知伦理委员会，并立即主动暂停了正在进行的研究的筛选和入组。

另外，我们注意到，根据您的多封与相关方面的信函，您报告了发生在2008年2月27日和28日的一次内部稽查，并与2008年3月3日收到了初步的稽查报告。您表明，一个纠正措施计划于2008年3月5日实施，其中包括重新对入组的患者进行知情同意，评估和更新原始文件，修改中心的研究标准操作规程，以及相关文件的重新递交。我们注意到由于申办者发现的与GCP相关的严重不合规事件，试验方案（b）（4）的申办者终止了贵中心参与试验。并且，由于GCP不合规事件，SVBGH伦理委员会无限期中止了对您参加的临床试验的批准，并暂停了全部您参加的临床试验的入组，直到伦理委员会能够确认此研究护士参与其他试验的程度并且确定此违规行为的严重程度。

在日期为2008年6月2日的关于试验方案（b）（4）的来往信函中，您记录，“我们承认，我们撰写的澄清信证明我们未获知或批准入组的4名患者……”我们注意到您未能充分监管这些临床研究导致了这些研究实施的重大问题，包括向伦理委员会和申办者递交的研究相关文件中不恰当的签名以及项目2所述的不符合入组条件的受试者。

我们认可您已经发现这个问题并且采取了一定的纠正措施。我们也认可通过您的纠正措施，您发现并提出了此研究护士参与的其他临床研究中存在的研究流程问题和数据问题。但是，我们发现您没有充分指出您未来将如何提高您对研究人员的监管。

2. 您未能进行研究或者确保按照研究计划进行研究［21 CFR 312.60］

a. 您未能确保您授权审阅合格标准的研究护士理解试验方案（b）（4）的入组标准。入组标准#2规定：

受试者必须有冠状动脉、脑部或周围血管系统动脉粥样硬化的证据或者病史，包括下述：

a）由推测的自发MI病史提示的CAD（入院治疗并最终诊断为MI，除外围手术期或明确的继发性MI，如由于严重贫血或高血压危症、脓毒症导致的肌钙蛋白升高引起）；MI病史≥2周，≤12个月；

b）由缺血性卒中病史证实的缺血性（推测血栓性）CVD（入院治疗并最终诊断为非出血性卒中）；缺血性卒中≥2周，≤12个月；

c）由间歇性跛行病史证实的PAD，并且

i. 踝肱指数（ABI）<0.85，或者

ii. 继发于缺血的四肢的截肢、外周旁路术，或外周血管成形术。

我们注意到受试者00272和00276入组了临床研究，尽管他们并不符合上述入组标准。我们注意到您在两个受试者的研究文件中放入了一份日期为2008年3月11日的“备忘录”，其中声明（节选）“…未经我审查和批准筛选数据随机入组。我审查了全部筛选数据；此患者不符合此研究入组标准。”

b. 试验方案（b）（4）5.7.1要求CK及CKMB“……血样在索引流程后2小时（+1小时）内采集，之后24小时内每8小时（+/– 1小时采集或直到患者出院……）”。您未能确保受试者301082002在出院前按照要求的时间点和次数完成血样采集。

入组不符合合格性标准的受试者以及不能按照试验方案要求进行研究相关操作，损害了受试者的安全和利益，也对研究终点的分析和有效性造成影响。

我们认可您采取了纠正措施，以确保您对受试者筛选数据的收集和受试者入组前进行合格性审查，并且方案要求的评估项目未来会按要求完成。

本警告信的目的并非是罗列您在试验药物临床研究中存在的所有缺陷。确保遵循法律和相关FDA法规的每一项要求是您的职责，您应当解决这些缺陷，并建立规程，以确保任何正在进行或将来进行的研究均符合FDA的法规。

自收到这封信的15个工作日内，您应当书面告知本办公室为预防将来发生类似违规情况而采取的措施。如果不能充分、迅速地解释上述违规问题，可能导致我们在不再通知的情况下采取监管措施。

如果您确信您2010年8月13日对FDA483的书面回复完整地解释了您为预防未来类似违规行为而采取的措

施，请于15个工作日内和我们对此进行沟通。您回复此信时可以参考日期为2010年8月13日的书面回复。

附：英文原文

Griffin, John M.D.

WARNING LETTER

March 14, 2011

CERTIFIED MAIL
RETURN RECEIPT REQUESTED

Ref: 11-HFD-45-02-01

John Griffin, M.D.
Cardiovascular Associates, Ltd.
1708 Old Donation Parkway
Virginia Beach, VA 23454

Dear Dr. Griffin:

Between May 12 and July 15, 2010, Ms. Sherry Secrist, representing the Food and Drug Administration (FDA), conducted an investigation and met with you to review your conduct of the following clinical investigations:

- Protocol **(b)(4)** , entitled "**(b)(4)**" of the investigational drug **(b)(4)**, performed for **(b)(4)**; and
- Protocol **(b)(4)**, entitled "**(b)(4)**" of the investigational drug **(b)(4)**, performed for **(b)(4)**.

This inspection is a part of FDA's Bioresearch Monitoring Program, which includes inspections designed to evaluate the conduct of research and to help ensure that the rights, safety, and welfare of the human subjects of those studies have been protected.

From our review of the establishment inspection report and the documents submitted with that report, we conclude that you did not adhere to the applicable statutory requirements and FDA regulations governing the conduct of clinical investigations. We are aware that at the conclusion of the inspection, Ms. Secrist presented and discussed with you Form FDA 483, Inspectional Observations. We acknowledge receipt of your August 13, 2010, response to Form FDA-483, but note that this response was received past the 15 working days from close of the inspection. Thus, while we have reviewed the response, we have not included a discussion of the response in this letter, as per the Commissioner's Enforcement Initiative announced August 11, 2009.

We wish to emphasize the following:

1. You failed to ensure that the investigation was conducted according to the signed investigator statement, in that you failed to personally conduct or supervise the clinical investigation [21 CFR 312.60].

When you signed the Statement of Investigator (Form FDA 1572) for the above-referenced clinical trials, you agreed to take on the responsibilities of a clinical investigator at your site. Your general responsibilities as a clinical investigator include ensuring that the clinical trial is conducted according to the signed investigator statement, the investigational plan, and applicable regulations; protecting the rights, safety, and welfare of subjects under your care; and ensuring control of drugs under investigation [21 CFR 312.60]. By signing Form FDA 1572, you specifically agreed to personally conduct the clinical trial or to supervise those aspects of the trial that you did not personally conduct. While you may delegate certain study tasks to individuals qualified to perform them, as a clinical investigator you may not delegate your general responsibilities. Our investigation indicates that your supervision of personnel to whom you delegated study tasks was not adequate to ensure that the clinical trial was conducted according to the signed investigator statement, the investigational plan, and applicable regulations, and that these trials were conducted in a manner that protects the rights, safety, and welfare of human subjects.

Specifically, you failed to adequately supervise the research nurse to whom you delegated tasks. Your failure to adequately supervise the research nurse caused many of the other violations listed in this letter. For example, your research nurse improperly completed or signed your name on documents related to Protocol **(b)(4)**, such as the Form FDA 1572 dated October 11, 2007, a nondisclosure agreement dated July 12, 2007, and the confidential study protocol dated August 8, 2007; and documents related to Protocol **(b)(4)** that include an IRB financial disclosure form dated January 14, 2008, two serious adverse event reports to the IRB dated January 25, 2008, and the signature and delegation form. Additionally, as noted in Item 2 below, two of four subjects randomized in Protocol **(b)(4)** did not meet eligibility criteria as required by the protocol. Had you provided adequate oversight, you would have observed from a review of the study documents that the signatures on the study-related documents were not yours and that the two randomized subjects were not eligible according to the protocol.

We note, according to your multiple letters to the various stakeholders [**(b)(4)**, Sentara Virginia Beach General Hospital (SVBGH) IRB, **(b)(4)** (sponsor of Protocol **(b)(4)**), **(b)(4)**(sponsor of Protocol **(b)(4)**), and **(b)(4)**] dated February 22, March 5, March 9, March 14 , March 17, March 19, March 26, April 3, May 19, June 2, and June 5, 2008, that you were first made aware of the situation regarding improper signatures by one of your research nurses on February 20, 2008. You reported that you conducted an internal investigation on February 21, 2008, in which the research nurse reportedly admitted to your office manager that she had improperly signed your name to documents. This internal investigation reportedly resulted in termination of employment of the responsible research nurse, as well as notification of her actions to thc State Board of Nursing. You notified the IRB on February 22, 2008, of the situation involving your research nurse and the inappropriate signatures, and you immediately voluntarily placed your active studies on hold to screening and enrollment.

Additionally, we note, according to your multiple letters to the various stakeholders, that you reported that an internal audit was conducted on February 27 and 28, 2008, and that you received preliminary audit results on March 3, 2008. You indicated that a corrective action plan was implemented on March 5, 2008, that included repeating the informed consented process of the enrolled subjects; evaluation and updating of source documentation; modification of your research Standard Operating Procedures; and resubmission of affected documents. We note that as a result of the sponsor's finding of serious noncompliance with respect to Good Clinical Practice (GCP), the sponsor for Protocol **(b)(4)** terminated your site. In addition, due to the GCP noncompliance, the SVBGH IRB suspended approval indefinitely and halted enrollment for all other studies in which you participated until the IRB could independently confirm the extent of involvement of the research nurse and verify the level of misconduct.

In your June 2, 2008, written correspondence to **(b)(4)**, you stated that "…we accept that the Memos to File we wrote indicate the lack of knowledge or approval of four patients enrolled …." We note that your failure to adequately supervise these studies led to significant problems with the conduct of the studies, including the submission of improper signatures on study-related documents to both the IRB and the sponsor, as well as the randomization of ineligible subjects in Protocol **(b)(4)**, as described in Item 2 below.

We acknowledge that you identified the problem and have established certain corrective actions. We also acknowledge that through your corrective actions, you identified and addressed the integrity of the investigational procedures and data in the other clinical investigations in which the terminated research nurse was involved. However, we find that you have not adequately addressed how you will improve your supervision of study staff in the future.

2. You failed to conduct the studies or ensure they were conducted according to the investigational plan [21 CFR 312.60].

a. You failed to ensure that the research nurse to whom you delegated the responsibility of reviewing the eligibility criteria understood the inclusion criteria for Protocol **(b)(4)**. Inclusion criterion #2 states:

Subject must have evidence or a history of atherosclerosis involving the coronary, cerebral, or peripheral vascular systems as follows:

b. CAD as indicated by a history of presumed spontaneous MI (hospitalized with final diagnosis of MI, excluding periprocedural or definite secondary MI [eg, due to profound anemia or hypertensive emergency, troponin increase in sepsis]) ≥2 weeks but ≤12 months prior

b. ischemic (presumed thrombotic) CVD as indicated by a history of ischemic stroke (hospitalized with final diagnosis of non hemorrhagic stroke) ≥2 weeks but ≤12 months prior

c. PAD as indicated by a history of intermittent claudication and

i. an ankle/brachial index (ABI) of <0.85, or

ii. amputation, peripheral bypass, or peripheral angioplasty of the extremities secondary to ischemia

We note that Subjects 00272 and 00276 were enrolled in the clinical investigation even though they did not satisfy the inclusion criterion noted above. We note that you placed a "Memo to File" dated March 11, 2008, in both subjects' study records that stated, in part, "…randomized to study without my review and approval of the screening data. I reviewed all screening data. The subject did not meet inclusion criteria for the trial."

b. Section 5.7.1 of Protocol **(b)(4)** requires that CK and CK-MB "…blood samples be taken 2 hours (+ 1 hour) after the index procedure, and then every 8 hours (+/- 1 hour) for the next 24 hours or until hospital discharge …." You failed to ensure that Subject 301082002 had the required timing of and number of post-procedural blood samples obtained prior to discharge.

Enrollment of subjects who do not meet eligibility criteria and failure to perform study-related procedures as outlined in the protocol, jeopardize subject safety and welfare, and compromise interpretation and validity of the investigational endpoints.

We acknowledge that you have established corrective actions to ensure that subject screening data collection and review for eligibility prior to enrollment, and the completion of protocol-required assessments, will occur in the future.

This letter is not intended to be an all-inclusive list of deficiencies with your clinical study of an investigational drug. It is your responsibility to ensure adherence to each requirement of the law and relevant FDA regulations. You should address these deficiencies and establish procedures to ensure that any ongoing or future studies will be in compliance with FDA regulations.

Within fifteen (15) working days of your receipt of this letter, you should notify this office in writing of the actions you have taken to prevent similar violations in the future. Failure to adequately and promptly explain the violations noted above may result in regulatory action without further notice. If you believe that your August 13, 2010, written response to the Form FDA 483 fully explains the actions you have taken to prevent similar violations in the future, please communicate that to us in writing within fifteen (15) business days. You may reference the written response dated August 13, 2010, in your response to this letter.

If you have any questions, please contact Constance Cullity, M.D., M.P.H., at 301-796-3397; FAX 301-847-8748. Your written response and any pertinent documentation should be addressed to:

Constance Cullity (formerly Lewin), M.D., M.P.H.
Branch Chief
Good Clinical Practice Branch I
Division of Scientific Investigations
Office of Compliance
Center for Drug Evaluation and Research
Food and Drug Administration
Building 51, Room 5354
10903 New Hampshire Avenue
Silver Spring, MD 20993

Sincerely yours,

{See appended electronic signature page}

Leslie K. Ball, M.D.
Director
Division of Scientific Investigations
Office of Compliance
Center for Drug Evaluation and Research
Food and Drug Administration

第 101 封　给 Thurmond-Anderle, Margaret E. 医学博士的警告信

2011年2月25日

参考号：11-HFD-45-02-05

尊敬的Thurmond-Anderle博士：

2010年8月17日至8月20日，Joel Martinez先生代表FDA，与您会面，对您所开展的试验药物为（b）（4）[1]，申办者为（b）（4）的以下临床研究进行了审查：

试验方案（b）（4），标题为“（b）（4）”；

试验方案（b）（4），标题为“（b）（4）”；

试验方案（b）（4），标题为“（b）（4）”。

本次现场检查是FDA的生物研究监查项目的一部分。该项目通过设定的检查方法，评估研究的实施情况，并帮助确保这些研究中受试者的权益、安全和福利得到了保护。

经对现场检查报告、该报告的附件，以及您2010年8月23日的书面回复进行审查，我们认为，您没有遵循适用的法律要求和监管临床研究实施的FDA法规。在现场检查结束时，Martinez先生向您出示了FDA483表，即现场检查发现的问题，并与您进行了讨论。我们想强调以下几点：

您未能进行研究或确保按照研究计划进行研究，未能保护受试者的权益、安全和福利［21 CFR 312.60］

试验方案（b）（4）要求药师或者合适的有资质的人员准备和提供含有200mg（6.7mL）试验药物或安慰剂的输液袋。我们的检查表明，您的办公室经理，不是一位药师，也似乎没有合适的资历准备输液袋，不正确地准备了大约1/10试验方案特别要求的剂量的试验药物或者安慰剂进行输液。您在2008年7月21日给申办者的反馈信函中承认了这个剂量错误，并解释该错误是由于使用了不正确尺寸的注射器导致的结果。很明显，您的办公室经理受注册护士指导，需要用一个1mL的注射器来达到更高精度的0.7mL的测量。然而，她（办公室经理）错误地使用了一个10mL的注射器代替1mL的注射器进行了所有的测量。您认识到了这个错误并向申办者承认，入组研究的一例受试者的研究结果受到了影响。

在您2010年8月23日的书面回复中，您概述了避免将来再次发生此类事件的纠正措施。然而，我们也注意到，在您的书面回复中，您没有充分证明您会采取预防措施来确保只有合适的有资质人员进行试验药物的准备工作。此外，我们要求您提供关于该剂量到处出现错误的额外信息。具体而言，您没有解释这一剂量错误是否延伸到了试验方案（b）（4）和（b）（4），这两个试验方案是由同一位办公室经理准备输液袋的；您也没有表述有多少受试者的药物剂量受此影响以及您没有提供这个错误发生的时间段。不正确的试验药物准备工作不仅使贵试验场所获得的数据之可靠性受到负面影响，也使得受试者的安全性受到了严重伤害。

本警告信的目的并非是罗列您在试验药物临床研究中存在的所有缺陷。确保遵循法律和相关FDA法规的每一项要求是您的职责，您应当解决这些缺陷，并建立规程，以确保任何正在进行或将来进行的研究均符合FDA的法规。

自收到这封信的15个工作日内，您应当书面告知本办公室为预防将来发生类似违规行为而采取的措施。如果不能充分、迅速地解释上述违规问题，可能导致我们在不再通知的情况下采取监管措施。

1 (b) (4) 涉及商业秘密，根据法规内容不予公开。

附：英文原文

Thurmond-Anderle, Margaret E. M.D.

WARNING LETTER

FEB 25, 2011

CERTIFIED MAIL
RETURN RECEIPT REQUESTED

Ref: 11-HFD-45-02-05

Margaret E. Thurmond-Anderle, M.D.
6701 Woodward Street
Amarillo, TX 79106

Dear Dr. Thurmond-Anderle:

Between August 17 and August 20, 2010, Mr. Joel Martinez, representing the Food and Drug Administration (FDA), conducted an investigation and met with you to review your conduct of the following clinical investigations of the investigational drug **(b)(4)** performed for **(b)(4)**.:

Protocol **(b)(4)**, entitled "**(b)(4)**";
Protocol **(b)(4)** entitled "**(b)(4)**"; and
Protocol **(b)(4)** entitled "**(b)(4)**."

This inspection is a part of FDA's Bioresearch Monitoring Program, which includes inspections designed to evaluate the conduct of research and to help ensure that the rights, safety, and welfare of the human subjects of those studies have been protected.

From our review of the establishment inspection report, the documents submitted with that report, and your written response dated August 23, 2010, we conclude that you did not adhere to the applicable statutory requirements and FDA regulations governing the conduct of clinical investigations. We are aware that at the conclusion of the inspection, Mr. Martinez presented and discussed with you Form FDA 483, Inspectional Observations. We wish to emphasize the following:

You failed to conduct the studies or ensure they were conducted according to the investigational plans, and to protect the rights, safety, and welfare of subjects [21 CFR 312.60].

Protocol **(b)(4)** required that a pharmacist or appropriately qualified person prepare and provide infusion bags containing 200 mg (6.7 mL) of study medication or placebo. Our investigation revealed that your office manager, who is not a pharmacist and does not appear to be appropriately qualified to prepare infusion bags, inaccurately prepared the study drug or placebo for infusion at approximately one-tenth of the protocol-specified dose. You acknowledged this dosage error in your correspondence to the sponsor dated July 21, 2008, in which you explained that the error resulted from the use of an inappropriately-sized syringe. Apparently, your office manager was instructed by the registered nurse to use a 1-mL syringe to achieve greater accuracy of the 0.7-mL measurement. However, she [the office manager] mistakenly used this 1-mL syringe, instead of a 10-mL syringe, for all measurements. You acknowledged the error and admitted to the sponsor that study results for the one subject enrolled into the study were impacted.

In your August 23, 2010, written response, you outlined corrective measures to prevent future recurrence of this finding. We note, however, that in your written response, you did not adequately address the preventive measures you would take to ensure that only appropriately qualified individuals are involved in the preparation of study drugs. In addition, we request that you provide additional information regarding the pervasiveness of the dosage error.

In particular, you did not explain whether the dosage error extended to Protocols **(b)(4)** and**(b)(4)**, for which the same office manager prepared study infusion bags; you did not say how many subjects' dosages were impacted; and you did not give the period of time over which the errors occurred. Inaccurate preparation of study drugs not only compromises the reliability of the data captured at your site, but could also significantly jeopardize subject safety.

This letter is not intended to be an all-inclusive list of deficiencies with your clinical study of an investigational drug. It is your responsibility to ensure adherence to each requirement of the law and relevant FDA regulations. You should address these deficiencies and establish procedures to ensure that any ongoing or future studies will be in compliance with FDA regulations.

Within fifteen (15) working days of your receipt of this letter, you should notify this office in writing of the actions you have taken to prevent similar violations in the future. Failure to adequately and promptly explain the violations noted above may result in regulatory action without further notice.

If you have any questions, please contact Constance Cullity, M.D., M.P.H., at 301-796-3397; FAX 301-847-8748.

Your written response and any pertinent documentation should be addressed to:

Constance Cullity (formerly Lewin), M.D., M.P.H.
Branch Chief
Good Clinical Practice Branch I
Division of Scientific Investigations
Office of Compliance
Center for Drug Evaluation and Research
Food and Drug Administration
Building 51, Room 5354
10903 New Hampshire Avenue
Silver Spring, MD 20993

Sincerely yours,

{See appended electronic signature page}

Leslie K. Ball, M.D.
Director
Division of Scientific Investigations
Office of Compliance
Center for Drug Evaluation and Research
Food and Drug Administration

第102封 给Simmons, John F.医学博士的警告信

2011年2月18日

参考号：11-HFD-45-02-02

尊敬的Simmons博士：

2010年7月26日至8月10日，Patricia Smith女士代表FDA，在您的临床研究场所，对您所开展的试验药物为（b）（4）[1]，申办者为（b）（4）的以下临床研究进行了现场检查：

试验方案（b）（4），标题为（b）（4）和（b）（4）；

试验方案（b）（4），标题为（b）（4）。

本次现场检查是FDA的生物研究监查项目的一部分。该项目通过设定的检查方法，对FDA所监管的相关研究的实施情况进行评估，以确保这些研究中受试者的权益、安全和福利得到了保护。

经对现场检查报告和该报告的附件，以及您2010年8月31日的书面回复进行审查。我们认为，您没有遵循适用的法律要求和监管临床研究实施及受试者保护的FDA法规。在现场检查结束时，Smith女士向您出示了FDA483表，即现场检查发现的问题，并与您进行了讨论。我们想强调以下几点：

1. 您未能亲自进行临床研究或者对研究进行监督［21 CFR 312.60］

当您签署上述提到的临床研究的研究者声明（FDA 1572表）时，您同意承担在您试验场所的研究者的职责。作为临床研究者，您的总体职责包括确保临床研究按照签署的研究者声明、研究计划及适用的法规进行；保护在您的监护下受试者的权益、安全及福利；确保研究药物得到管控［21 CFR 312.60］。通过签署FDA 1572表，您明确地同意了亲自进行临床研究试验，或者监督您不能亲自参与的内容。尽管您可以将一些研究任务授权给有资质的人员去完成，但作为临床研究者，您不能授权您的总体职责。我们检查显示，您对您授权相应工作的人员监督不够充分，以致无法确保临床研究按照签署的研究者声明、研究计划及适用的法规实施，并保护受试者的权益、安全及福利。

我们注意到，由于您未能充分监督这项研究，导致了以下研究实施过程中的严重问题，包括入组不符合入组标准的受试者和未能在方案规定的时间内完成与受试者安全和有效性终点有关的研究要求的流程。

2. 您未能进行研究或者确保按照签署的研究者声明、研究计划来进行研究，未能保护在您的监护下的受试者的权益、安全及福利［21 CFR 312.60］

作为临床研究者，您的职责包括确保研究按照签署的研究者声明、研究计划及适用的法规进行和保护受试者的权益、安全及福利。

a. 试验方案（b）（4），4.2.2，排除标准的第一段，在筛选期排除有禁止使用（b）（4）疗法症状的受试者。受试者140360013入组试验方案（b）（4）时，在受试者的病史中记录，对（b）（4）过敏。

b. 试验方案（b）（4），4.2.2，排除标准的第四段，在筛选期排除严重肾功能不全的受试者。其在方案中定义为肌酐清除率（CrCl）低于30mL/min。

i. 试验方案设计用来衡量肾功能的肌酐清除率筛查，在31位受试者中，有22位受试者未在筛选访视时进行测量。您应从方案中获知，研究药物（b）（4）有一部分是通过肾脏排泄的。

ii. 受试者140360015和受试者140360016入组了研究，但在筛选访视时其CrCl分别为29和21mL/min。

---

1 （b）（4）涉及商业秘密，根据法规内容不予公开。

c. 试验方案（b）（4），4.2.2，排除标准的第二段，在筛选期排除（b）（4）大于1.5的受试者。

ⅰ. 在31名入组的受试者中有21名，在筛选期没有获得用来评估（b）（4）的测试（b）（4）。

ⅱ. 入组试验的受试者140360019在筛选时（b）（4）为1.9 。

d. 试验方案（b）（4），4.5.7，之前和伴随的治疗，当伴随疾病（b）（4）的受试者入组试验，允许其每天使用一次总量不超过100mg的（b）（4）。根据受试者140360005、140360013及140360016病史记录，其在入组试验时每天服用（b）（4）325mg。受试者140360005、140360013有（b）（4）疾病记录在他们的病史里，以及受试者140360016的筛选记录显示，其无需使用超过2日的预防性使用（b）（4）。

关于上面记录的发现，入组试验的31名受试者中的5名，应当在筛选过程中剔除。另外，已经随机的另外23名受试者是否符合入组试验的条件仍不清楚。因为在筛选时，没有对其实施方案要求的肌酐清除率检查和/或没有在筛选时获得（b）（4）。因此，您对入组的5名不符合方案入组条件的受试者，以及没有实施方案要求的肌酐清除率检查和/或没有在筛选时获得（b）（4）的另外23名受试者的安全和福利造成了威胁。

e. 试验方案（b）（4）规定在访视第10天，在最后注射研究药物的24小时内，需要实施超声检查，以判断有效性。

在入组的31名受试者中，10名受试者在末次注射的24小时之外进行了超声检查，以及3名受试者在末次注射之前进行了超声检查。

入组不符合入组标准的受试者，以及没有实施研究相关流程危害了受试者的安全和福利，并危及了研究终点的阐释和有效性。

在您2010年8月31日的回复中，您承认大量的流程没有被恰当遵守。您宣称误解了方案的流程，以及没有从申办者得到任何指导和说明，直到试验开始。另外，您的回复，声明您已经开始实施纠正措施并且重新培训研究人员。我们认可您的回复。然而，我们担心您的回复不足以避免上述违背在未来再次发生。因为您未提供具体的纠正措施和再培训的细节。

3. 您未能及时地向 IRB 报告研究活动中所有的变更［21 CFR 312.66］

FDA法规要求试验研究者需要确保及时向IRB报告研究活动中的所有变化和所有对受试者等产生风险的意外情况。在IRB批准之前，研究中的任何改变都不被允许，除了在需要立即消除对受试者明显危害的情况下［21 CFR 312.66］。

您未能向IRB报告研究活动中的下列变化：

a. 您未能在2009年5月4日向IRB通知以下事实，试验方案（b）（4）的申办者依据贵试验场所的系统性违背,和研究监查员无法获得所有受试者的病史记录，暂时叫停贵试验场所入组。

b. 您未能在2009年8月18日向IRB通知以下事实，试验方案（b）（4）的申办者依据贵场所对临床研究规范的极不依从，通知您关闭试验场所。

c. 您未能在2009年7月16日向IRB通知以下事实，申办者已于2009年5月7日停止试验方案（b）（4）的入组。

在您2010年8月31日的回复中，您声明试验方案（b）（4）的申办者已经通知IRB关于暂停入组，以及停止您继续参与研究及试验场所的关闭。您的回复不可接受，因为您没有说明，作为试验的研究者，您需要立即将研究活动中所有变化报告给IRB的责任。而且，您未能说明您延期通知IRB停止入组的原因。

在您的回复中，您声明所有的问题都在发现和引起您的注意之后，立即进行了纠正。您的回复不够充分，因为您未能提供防止此类问题发生的纠正措施的细节。

未能立即将研究活动中的变化报告至IRB，危及了临床研究入组受试者的安全和福利。

4. 您未能按 21 CFR 50 的要求，获得知情同意［21 CFR 312.60］

除了21 CFR 50.23和21 CFR 50.24的规定之外，任何研究者都不能让个人作为受试者参与研究，除非研究者获得了受试者或者受试者法律认可代理人合法有效的知情同意［21 CFR 50.20］。

作为研究者，根据21 CFR第50部分，获取知情同意是您的责任。除了 21 CFR 56.109（c）的规定之外，知情同意需要通过使用IRB批准的书面的知情同意书记录，以及需要受试者或者受试者法律认可代理人在知情时签署姓名和日期。一份副本需要给予签署知情同意书的人［21 CFR 50.27（a）］。

您未能获得使用试验用新药（b）（4）的受试者1403060015合法有效的知情同意。尤其是，试验方案（b）（4）受试者1403060015的知情同意书是由他人签署。在现场检查期间，我们注意到，受试者1403060015在受试者知情同意文件和受试者研究日记上的签字和笔迹不一致。

在您2010年8月31日的回复中，您承认由于受试者手抖，其他人签署知情同意文件。然而，您未能确认或者记录这个人是受试者法律认可代理人。法规要求，知情同意由受试者或受试者法律认可代理人在进入研究前签署姓名和日期［21 CFR 50.20］。未能获得充足的知情同意，会使受试者失去评估参加临床研究的风险和收益的机会，并危及其安全和福利。

我们承认您的回复。然而，我们担心您的回复并不充分，因为您未能提出纠正措施以预防将来上述违规情况的再次发生。

本警告信的目的并非是罗列您在试验药物临床研究中存在的所有缺陷。确保遵循法律和相关FDA法规的每一项要求是您的职责，您应当解决这些缺陷，并建立规程，以确保任何正在进行或将来进行的研究均符合FDA的法规。

自收到这封信的15个工作日内，您应当书面告知本办公室为预防将来发生类似违规行为而采取的措施。如果不能充分、迅速地解释上述违规问题，可能导致我们在不再通知的情况下采取监管措施。

附：英文原文

Simmons, John F., M. D.

WARNING LETTER

Feb 18, 2011

CERTIFIED MAIL
RETURN RECEIPT REQUESTED

Ref: 11-HFD-45-02-02

John F. Simmons, M.D.
915 West Hospital Drive
Geneva, AL 36340-1645

Dear Dr. Simmons:

Between July 26 and August 10, 2010, Ms. Patricia Smith, representing the Food and Drug Administration (FDA), conducted an investigation and met with you to review your conduct of the following clinical investigations of the investigational drug **(b)(4)**, performed for **(b)(4)**:

- Protocol **(b)(4)** entitled **(b)(4)** and **(b)(4)**
- Protocol **(b)(4)** entitled **(b)(4)**

This inspection is a part of FDA's Bioresearch Monitoring Program, which includes inspections designed to evaluate the conduct of research and to help ensure that the rights, safety, and welfare of the human subjects of those studies have been protected.

From our review of the establishment inspection report, the documents submitted with that report, and your written response dated August 31, 2010, we conclude that you did not adhere to the applicable statutory requirements and FDA regulations governing the conduct of clinical investigations and the protection of human subjects. We are aware that at the conclusion of the inspection, Ms. Smith presented and discussed with you Form FDA 483, Inspectional Observations. We wish to emphasize the following:

1. You failed to personally conduct or supervise the clinical investigation [21 CFR 312.60].

When you signed the Statement of Investigator (Form FDA 1572) for the above-referenced clinical trials, you agreed to take on the responsibilities of a clinical investigator at your site. Your general responsibilities as a clinical investigator include ensuring that the clinical trial is conducted according to the signed investigator statement, the investigational plan, and applicable regulations; protecting the rights, safety, and welfare of subjects under your care; and ensuring control of drugs under investigation [21 CFR 312.60]. By signing the Form FDA 1572, you specifically agreed to personally conduct the clinical trial or to supervise those aspects of the trial that you did not personally conduct. While you may delegate certain study tasks to individuals qualified to perform them, as a clinical investigator, you may not delegate your general responsibilities. Our investigation indicates that your supervision of personnel to whom you delegated study tasks was not adequate to ensure that the clinical trial was conducted according to the signed investigator statement, the investigational plan, and applicable regulations, and that these trials were conducted in a manner that protects the rights, safety, and welfare of human subjects.

We note that your failure to adequately supervise this study led to significant problems with the conduct of the study as described below, including the enrollment of subjects who did not meet eligibility criteria and the failure to perform study-required procedures related both to subject safety and to the efficacy endpoints within the protocol time frames.

2. You failed to conduct the studies or ensure that they were conducted according to the signed investigator statement and the investigational plan, and to protect the rights, safety, and welfare of the subjects under your care [21 CFR 312.60].

As the clinical investigator, you are responsible for ensuring that the investigation was conducted according to the signed investigator statement, the investigational plan, and applicable regulations, and for protecting the rights, safety, and welfare of study subjects. Specifically:

a. Protocol **(b)(4)**, Section 4.2.2, Exclusion Criteria, Subsection 1, excludes subjects at screening with conditions that contraindicate the use of **(b)(4)** therapy with **(b)(4)**. Subject #140360013 was enrolled in protocol **(b)(4)** with a known allergy to **(b)(4)**, which was documented in the subject's medical history.

b. Protocol **(b)(4)**, Section 4.2.2, Exclusion Criteria, Subsection 4, excludes subjects at screening with severe renal insufficiency, which is defined in the protocol as a calculated creatinine clearance (CrCl) less than 30 mL/min.

i. Creatinine clearance screening, which is designed to measure kidney function, was not performed at the screening visit for 22 of the 31 subjects enrolled in the study. As you should be aware from the protocol, the investigational drug **(b)(4)** is excreted, in part, through the kidneys,

ii. Subjects #140360015 and 140360016 were enrolled into the study with screening CrCl values of 29 and 21 mL/min, respectively.

c. Protocol **(b)(4)**, Section 4.2.2, Exclusion Criteria, Subsection 2, excludes subjects at screening with an **(b)(4)** greater than 1.5.

i. An **(b)(4)**, which is designed to evaluate **(b)(4)**, was not obtained at the screening visit for 23 of the 31 subjects enrolled in the study.

ii. Subject #140360019 was enrolled into the study with a screening **(b)(4)** of 1.9.

d. Protocol **(b)(4)**, Section 4.5.7, Prior and Concomitant Therapy, permitted the concomitant use of **(b)(4)**in total daily doses not to exceed 100 mg when administered once daily in subjects with **(b)(4)** disease. Subjects #140360005, 140360013, and 140360016 were enrolled into the study with a 325 mg/day use of **(b)(4)** documented in their medical histories. Subjects #140360005 and 140360013 have **(b)(4)**disease documented in their medical histories, and the screening records for Subject #140360016 indicated that the subject did not require more than a 2-day prophylactic use of an **(b)(4)**.

With respect to the findings noted above, 5 of the 31 subjects you enrolled into the study should have been excluded during the screening process. In addition, it is unclear whether 23 additional subjects randomized were eligible for enrollment into the study, because you did not conduct the protocol-required creatinine clearance screening and/or did not obtain **(b)(4)** at screening for these subjects. Therefore, you jeopardized the safety and welfare of 5 subjects by enrolling them into a study for which they were ineligible, and another 23 subjects by not conducting required creatinine clearance screening and/or by not obtaining required screening **(b)(4)**.

e. Protocol **(b)(4)** stipulates that an ultrasonography to determine efficacy should be performed after the last parenteral dose of study medication, within 24 hours of its administration on visit Day 10.

Of the 31 subjects enrolled in the study, 10 subjects received the ultrasonography more than 24 hours after the last parenteral dose, and 3 subjects received the ultrasonography prior to receiving the last parenteral dose.

Enrollment of subjects who do not meet eligibility criteria and failure to perform study-related procedures jeopardize subject safety and welfare and compromise the interpretation and validity of the investigational endpoints.

In your response dated August 31, 2010, you acknowledge that a number of procedures were not appropriately followed. You alleged that you misinterpreted the protocol procedures and that you were not given any guidance or clarification from the sponsor until well into the study. In addition, your response concludes with the statement that you have initiated corrective action and retraining of staff. We acknowledge your response. However, we are concerned that the response is not adequate to prevent future recurrence of the violation noted above, because you failed to provide the details of your corrective actions and the staff retraining.

3. You failed to report promptly to the IRB all changes in the research activity [21 CFR 312.66].

FDA regulations require that the clinical investigator shall assure that they will promptly report to the IRB all changes in the research activity and all unanticipated problems involving risk to human subjects or others, and that they will not make any changes in the research without IRB approval, except where necessary to eliminate apparent immediate hazards to human subjects [21 CFR 312.66].

You failed to notify the IRBs of the following changes in the research activities:

a. You failed to inform the IRB that on May 4, 2009, the sponsor of Protocol **(b)(4)** placed your site on temporary recruitment hold, based on your site's systematic deviations and the inability of the study monitors to gain access to all subjects' medical histories.

b. You failed to inform the IRB that on August 18, 2009, the sponsor of Protocol **(b)(4)** notified you of their closure of your site due to significant noncompliance with good clinical practices.

c. You failed to notify the IRB until July 16, 2009, that enrollment of Protocol **(b)(4)** had been halted by the sponsor on May 7, 2009.

In your response dated August 31, 2010, you state that the sponsor of Protocol **(b)(4)** notified the IRB of the temporary recruitment hold and the termination of your participation in the study and the site closure. This response is unacceptable, because you did not address your responsibility as a clinical investigator to promptly report to the IRB all changes in research activity. Moreover, you failed to address your delay in notifying the IRB of Protocol **(b)(4)** enrollment halt at your site.

In your response, you state that all of the observed issues were corrected immediately once they were identified and brought to your attention. Your response is inadequate, because you failed to provide the details of the corrective action that would prevent such occurrences in the future.

Failure to promptly report changes in the research activity to the IRB compromises the safety and welfare of subjects enrolled in the clinical investigation.

4. You failed to obtain informed consent in accordance with the provisions of 21 CFR part 50 [21 CFR 312.60].

Except as provided in 21 CFR 50.23 and 21 CFR 50.24, no investigator may involve a human being as a subject in research unless the investigator has obtained the legally effective informed consent of the subject or the subject's legally authorized representative [21 CFR 50.20].

As an investigator, it is your responsibility to obtain informed consent in accordance with 21 CFR part 50. Except as provided in 21 CFR 56.109(c), informed consent shall be documented by the use of a written consent form approved by the IRB and signed and dated by the subject or the subject's legally authorized representative at the time of consent. A copy shall be given to the person signing the form [21 CFR 50.27(a)].

You failed to obtain legally effective informed consent from Subject #1403060015, who was prescribed the investigational new drug, **(b)(4)**. Specifically, the informed consent form for Subject #1403060015 in Protocol **(b)(4)** was signed by someone other than the subject. During the inspection, it was observed that both the handwriting and the signature of Subject #1403060015 were inconsistent between the subject's consent documents and the subject's study diary.

In your response dated August 31, 2010, you acknowledge that someone other than the subject signed the consent documents because the subject's hands were shaking. However, you failed to confirm or document that this person was the subject's legally authorized representative. The regulations require that informed consent be signed and dated by the subject or the subject's legal representative prior to the subject's involvement in the investigation [21 CFR 50.20]. Failure to obtain adequate informed consent jeopardizes the safety and welfare of enrolled subjects by denying them an opportunity to assess the risks and benefits of their participation in the clinical investigation.

We acknowledge your response. However, we are concerned that the response is inadequate, since you did not propose corrective actions to prevent future recurrence of the violation noted above.

This letter is not intended to be an all inclusive list of deficiencies with your clinical study of an investigational drug. It is your responsibility to ensure adherence to each requirement of the law and relevant FDA regulations. You should address these deficiencies and establish procedures to ensure that any ongoing or future studies will be in compliance with FDA regulations.

Within fifteen (15) working days of your receipt of this letter, you should notify this office in writing of the actions you have taken to prevent similar violations in the future. Failure to adequately and promptly explain the violations noted above may result in regulatory action without further notice.

If you have any questions, please contact Constance Cullity, M.D., M.P.H., at 301-796-3397; FAX 301-847-8748. Your written response and any pertinent documentation should be addressed to:

Constance Cullity (formerly Lewin), M.D., M.P.H.
Branch Chief
Good Clinical Practice Branch I
Division of Scientific Investigations
Office of Compliance
Center for Drug Evaluation and Research
Food and Drug Administration
Building 51, Room 5354
10903 New Hampshire Avenue
Silver Spring, MD 20993

Sincerely yours,

{See appended electronic signature page}

Leslie K. Ball, M.D.
Director
Division of Scientific Investigations
Office of Compliance
Center for Drug Evaluation and Research
Food and Drug Administration

第103封　给Mancha, Vaughn H. Jr.医学博士的警告信

2011年2月17日

参考号：11-HFD-45-02-03

尊敬的Mancha博士：

2010年9月7日至9月23日，Patricia Smith女士代表FDA进行了现场检查，并与您会面，对您所开展的以下临床研究进行了审查：[试验方案（b）（4）[1]，题为（b）（4）]，试验药物为（b）（4）（b）（4），申办者为（b）（4）。

本次现场检查是FDA的生物研究监查项目的一部分。该项目通过设定的检查方法，评估研究的实施情况，并帮助确保这些研究中受试者的权益、安全和福利得到了保护。

经对现场检查报告、该报告的附件，以及您2010年10月4日的书面回复进行审查，我们认为，您没有遵循适用的法律要求和监管临床研究实施的FDA法规。在现场检查结束时，Smith女士向您出示了FDA483表，即现场检查发现的问题，并与您进行了讨论。我们想强调以下几点：

1. 您未能确保按照研究计划进行研究［21 CFR 312.60］

a. 试验方案9.5.3.1.5，报告和记录严重不良事件（SAE），规定："所有发生于第一剂给药的时间开始至试验最后一剂给药结束4周后的严重不良事件（SAE）必须被上报"。

该方案进一步规定针对每个SAE，研究者必须在发现受试者发生SAE24小时内通过电话或电子病例报告表（CRF）方式报告给研究合同组织（CRO）。研究者必须将所有严重不良事件（SAE）以及突发事件上报伦理委员会（IRB）。同时，方案9.5.3.1.6不良事件（AE）随访中规定"在出现原因不明，需紧急治疗，具有临床意义的异常实验室检测结果或有临床意义的实验室检测结果显著变化的情况下，应立即重复实验室检测并跟进，直至检测结果恢复至试验方案规定的范围或至该受试者的基线。"

（1）在2008年2月18日采集的受试者389204第8周访视的实验室检测结果，及在2008年2月20日传真到贵试验场所相应实验室报告中受试者的肌酐（CR）测定值为3.2mg/dL。2008年2月20日的病程记录显示，在审阅了第8周的访视实验室报告后，因升高的肌酐（CR）值，决定对受试者终止研究。病程记录进一步指出，受试者将停用研究药物并且终止访视。2008年2月20日以及21日的病程记录显示，贵研究中心给受试者留言，请受试者就异常实验结果与您办公室联系。受试者直到2008年2月26日才联系贵试验场所，而早前所计划的访视终止日期为2008年2月27日。对此严重不良事件（SAE），我们发现了以下几点：

（a）在2008年2月22日至2月26日之间，当受试者联系试验场所时，您并没对受试者的异常实验结果做出随访。受试者最后一剂给药是在2008年2月26日。

（b）您直到2008年2月27日才将急性肾衰竭严重不良事件（SAE）上报CRO。其超出方案中所要求的24小时内汇报要求。此外，给CRO的报告显示，严重不良事件（SAE）发生以及您的研究人员获知的日期为2008年2月26日。这与您的病程记录中所提及贵试验场所在2008年2月20日得知严重不良事件（SAE）不符。

（c）您直到2008年2月27日才将该SAE报告给伦理委员会，而您的进度记录显示您获知该SAE的时间为2008年2月20日。

您指出当时是立即以电话留言与受试者联系，并且最终在6天内取得口头联系。您还指出，您不能在手机

1 （b）（4）涉及商业秘密，根据法规内容不予公开。

上留下有关研究给药的说明，因为这会违反HIPAA法规。为了防止这一问题再次发生，您表示，当收到受试者的关键实验室数值时，将立即电话通知受试者该数值。同时，将指导受试者如何处理研究药物。您还指出，若无法联系到受试者，您会留言，并且每天致电受试者，以及通过（b）（4）向受试者发出邮件通知受试者。

您的回复是不可接受的。我们注意到，贵试验场所于2008年6月19日发送了受试者医疗审阅表给CRO，文中表明“受试者于2008年2月20日接受检测。检测结果未及时发布。受试者进入肾衰竭。”因此，贵试验场所承认这起严重不良事件（SAE）并未得到妥善的处理。此外，您未提供任何有关您将采取的纠正措施的细节，以及如何保证在方案特指时间范围内向申办者以及伦理委员会（IRB）上报严重不良事件（SAEs）。您也未提供如何保证给申办者关于严重不良事件（SAEs）的信息与原始记录的纠正措施一致。

（2）2007年10月9日对受试者389062进行采样，实验结果于2007年10月10日传真至贵试验场所。记录显示，您直到2008年4月22日才记录您的审查化验结果。

您延迟审查受试者的化验结果违反了方案中9.5.3.1.6对不良事件的随访。由于您直到收到检测结果6个月后才进行审查，您没有恰当及时地判定报告中异常的实验结果是否在临床上有显著意义，因而要立即重复检测和随访直到数值恢复至试验方案规定的范围或受试者的基线。这些样本是否反映不良事件或者严重不良事件事实上已无关紧要，因为即使是有，您也无法及时做记录或是妥善跟进处理，这是由于您在收到检测结果的6个月后才进行审查。

您的书面回复指出，您原先在实验结果页签字，划掉错误的日期，并写下“审查了试验结果10/23/2007，写错了日期。”然后，这个批注以您名字缩写的形式签字，并注明日期“4/10/2007。”为了防止这一问题再次发生，您指出，当检测结果以传真形式接收时，它们将被放置在一个篮子里供临床研究者审查并即时签署日期。您还指出，将对装传真的篮子全天定期检查；在周末收到的实验结果，从接收到实验结果和对它们进行审查的最长时间为2天。

您的回复是不可接受的。由于在FDA检查期间提供的检测报告显示，2007年10月9日收集的试验样品报告上只有一个签名，以及2008年4月22日的审核日期；因此无法核实您对试验结果标注日期的书面回复。我们还注意到，您未提供您不在期间所收到的实验报告审查的纠正措施。

b. 试验方案9.3.1，入组标准，试验方案9.4.7，既往和伴随治疗，指出入组试验前30天内使用非甾体抗炎药（NSAID）的受试者，将不能参与试验。FDA对您原始记录的审查显示6位受试者（389058，389069，389080，389090，389143和389218）曾于进入试验的前30天内使用非甾体抗炎药（NSAID），但均入组试验。

此外，在贵试验场所提交给CRO的医疗审查表，（b）（4），以及提交给伦理委员会（IRB）的方案偏差记录中，您声明受试者389040和389111曾于进入试验的前30天使用非甾体抗炎药（NSAID），但入组了试验。

您的书面回复指出，作为涉及两个非处方药物（OTC）的研究，您已经观察到受试者往往没有意识到使用这些药物是违反了方案，尽管您已经告知受试者。您表示未来您会加强管理，让受试者在未通知您的情况下不使用任何非处方药物。您表示，作为一个纠正措施，每次访视，所有受试者将按照指示携带所有伴随用药，并对其做出排除用药审查，临床研究者将在随机化时审查入组/排除标准，并记录符合随机选择的受试者。

您的回复是不可接受的。FDA的审查记录发现贵试验场所对几个受试者曾于进入试验的前30天使用非甾体抗炎药（NSAID）的行为知情，但仍将其纳入试验。您的回复未提及对未来类似情况的处理方式。此外，您所提供的纠正措施的工作表，没有提供任何关于如何验证所有受试者是否符合所有方案入组标准的流程。

c. 试验方案9.4.7，既往和伴随治疗，方案9.3.2，排除标准，第7节，指出所有于进入研究的前14天使用抑酸剂的受试者不能参与试验。FDA对您原始记录的审查显示，4位受试者（389086，389094，389173和389234）曾于进入研究的前14天使用抑酸剂，但均入组试验。此外，在贵试验场所提交给CRO的医疗审查表，以及提交给伦理委员会的方案偏差记录中，和/或是在备忘录中您表示4位随机受试者（389085，389092，389142和389247）曾于进入研究的前14天内使用抑酸剂。

您的书面回复指出，您确认受试者389173，389142，389092，389094和389234曾于进入试验的前14天使用抑酸剂。您指出受试者389086并未告知贵试验场所，她当时服用埃索美拉唑（Nexium）和雷尼替丁

（Zantac），此事实是在收到她的家庭医生所发的医疗记录才被发现。对受试者389085，您表示受试者的家庭医生，在筛查访视后和随机前开了埃索美拉唑（Nexium）以及法莫替丁（Pepcid AC）。此举一直到受试者随机后才被发现。

您提出，作为一个纠正措施，每次访视，所有受试者将按照指示携带所有的伴随用药，并对其做出审查，临床研究员将和其他人员共同审查排除药物清单。

您的回复是不可接受的。您的纠正措施没有提供任何关于如何验证医疗记录（如果可以从家庭医生那里获得），及在受试者入组和或被随机前如何验证伴随用药。此外，您所提供的作为纠正措施的工作表，没有提供任何关于如何检查出受试者的所有伴随用药。您也未提供任何您将使用的纠正措施或流程，以更好地指导受试者避免使用方案规定的排除药物。

d. 试验方案9.5.3.4，临床实验室检验，规定在筛选访视时，对受试者进行现场血液采集，检测血清幽门螺杆菌。试验方案9.3.2，第6节，进一步指出感染血清幽门螺杆菌的受试者不能入组研究。原始记录显示至少两位受试者（389127和389135）在筛选访视时没有证明血清幽门螺杆菌为阴性的记录下，入组研究。

此外，在您试验场所提交给CRO的受试者医疗审查表，以及提交给伦理委员会的方案偏差记录中，您指出除了受试者389129、389137，以及389142，还有其他在筛选访视时没有证明血清幽门螺杆菌为阴性的受试者，也入组研究。

您的书面回复，这个方案违背是个独立的个案。那位因疏忽没有记录检测结果的临床协调员（CRC），已经被“再培训”。您也表示，作为一个纠正措施，任何内部检测都将在原始记录中对批号、有效期限，以及结果做记录。

您的回复是不可接受的。您指出临床协调员（CRC）因疏忽未将结果记录，意味着临床协调员（CRC）实际上进行了检测，只是未将结果记录在原始记录中。根据检查报告，您告诉FDA检查员Smith，在观察这位临床协调员（CRC）的工作时，您发现她并没有使用任何检测血清幽门螺杆菌所需的材料，而是在原始记录中记录她确实做过的那些测试。您的试验场所的文件，也显示涉及的临床协调员（CRC），要么是在筛选访视时没有做过血清幽门螺杆菌检测，要么就是没有使用相关测试所需的材料。您还告知FDA检查员Smith，当您对该研究协调员提出您的质疑时，提议她应该接受培训并且在其他协调员的指导下工作时，她就立即辞职了。因此，FDA不能确认是否如您在您的书面回复所提到的这位受质疑的临床协调员（CRC）有被“再培训”。

e. 除了上述的方案违背，通过书面备忘录文件，提交给CRO的受试者医疗审查表，以及提交给伦理委员会的方案偏差记录中，您的试验场所承认数个方案违背：在筛选访视时对接受抗凝治疗的受试者（例如，389017和389085）包括但不仅限于缺少国际标准化比率（INR）的检测；向受试者分配不正确的试验药物（例如，389013、389041和389091）；研究访视未按照方案进行（例如，389162和389040）；以及未能实施筛查血清妊娠试验（例如，受试者389075和389211）

在您的书面回复，您承认了上述的发现。您的纠正措施包括：①承诺通过更好地了解每个方案以及所有的步骤，并完全遵守方案以减低人为失误。②创建一个原始文件附录，以便第二个协调员能对试验用药（IP）或交互式话音应答系统（IVRS）为特定受试者所分配的试验药物编号进行参照。如此两位协调员才能验证受试者分配正确的试验药物（IP）。③设计“访视计划”表，其中包括预计的日期，以及每次访视的实际日期，包括+/–窗口期。④在每次访视结束时，设计新的原始记录，证明该研究者已经审查所有原始文件的准确性和正确记录。

虽然这些纠正措施看似合适，但因为在这些试验中缺乏这些措施导致以上列出的违规行为，增加了我们对您的措施是否真正能对受试者进行正确保护产生担忧。

2. 您未能保存对研究中使用试验药物或对照组的受试者的所有研究观察结果和其他相关数据的足够及准确的病历记录［21 CFR 312.62（b）］

a. 受试者389137筛选访视原始记录上的签名似乎是属于授权研究者Dr.（b）（4），记录他于2007年10月

11日进行了一次体检。然而，您的记录显示，Dr.（b）（4）确认筛选访视原始记录上的签名不是他的，并且否认执行了检查。

对此，您未提出任何书面回复。

b. 原始记录显示受试者89230于2007年12月18日的筛选访视进行了体检。然而，您直到2008年4月21日才在原始体检报告上签字。

您的书面回复，显示该体检是在筛选访视时进行的，然而，您因疏忽忘记填写原始记录。您的预防纠正措施是，要求所有研究者对所有体检进行实时充分的记录，并签名和注明日期。您的回复是不充分的。您未提供，任何关于保证文件在每次访视时完成，并签名和日期的流程或者培训的信息。

c. 关于受试者（如389198和389168）在第24周的访视超窗的记录是矛盾的。尤其是，在2008年5月20日的贵研究中心的受试者医疗审查表，受试者389168（随机号5168）的第24周访视，早了3周。在这份表格的右上角，有一个手写备注"389198号"。根据入组表，受试者389168的随机号不是5168；这个随机号是受试者389198的。在（b）（4）的IVRS失效表中，您再次申明受试者389168的第24周访视超窗。

本警告信的目的并非是罗列您在试验药物临床研究中存在的所有缺陷。确保遵循法律和FDA相关法规的每一项要求是您的职责，您应当解决所存在的缺陷，并建立规程，以确保任何正在进行或将来进行的研究均符合FDA的法规。

自收到这封信的15个工作日内，您应当书面告知本办公室为预防将来发生类似违规行为而采取的措施。如果不能充分、迅速地解释上述违规问题，可能导致我们在不再通知的情况下采取监管措施。如果您认为您已经遵循了FDA的法规要求，请陈述理由，并提供所有支持资料，以供我们参考。

附：英文原文

Mancha, Vaughn H. Jr. M. D.

WARNING LETTER

FEB 17, 2011

CERTIFIED MAIL
RETURN RECEIPT REQUESTED

Ref: 11-HFD-45-02-03

Vaughn H. Mancha, Jr., M.D.
339 Saint Lukes Drive
Montgomery, AL 36117

Dear Dr. Mancha:

Between September 7 and September 23, 2010, Ms. Patricia Smith, representing the Food and Drug Administration (FDA), conducted an investigation and met with you to review your conduct of a clinical investigation (Protocol **(b)(4)**, entitled **(b)(4)**) of the investigational drug **(b)(4) (b)(4)**, performed for **(b)(4)**.

This inspection is a part of FDA's Bioresearch Monitoring Program, which includes inspections designed to evaluate the conduct of research and to help ensure that the rights, safety, and welfare of the human subjects of those studies have been protected.

From our review of the establishment inspection report, the documents submitted with that report, and your written response dated October 4, 2010, we conclude that you did not adhere to the applicable statutory requirements and FDA regulations governing the conduct of clinical investigations. We are aware that at the conclusion of the inspection, Ms. Smith presented and discussed with you Form FDA 483, Inspectional Observations. We wish to emphasize the following:

1. You failed to ensure that the investigation was conducted according to the investigational plan [21 CFR 312.60].

a. Protocol Section 9.5.3.1.5, Reporting and Documenting Serious Adverse Events, specified that "all Serious Adverse Events (SAEs) that occur beginning with the time of administration of the first dose of study medication and continuing until four weeks after administration of the final dose of study medication must be reported." The protocol further specified that each SAE was to be reported to the Contact Research Organization (CRO) by telephone or via the electronic case report form (CFR) within 24 hours of becoming aware that a subject had experienced an SAE, and that the investigator must report all SAEs and unexpected problems promptly to the IRB. Also, in Section 9.5.3.1.6, Follow-Up of Adverse Events, the protocol stated that "in the event of an unexplained, treatment-emergent, clinically significant abnormal laboratory test results [sic] or clinically significant changes in laboratory test results, the tests should be repeated immediately and followed up until the values have returned to within the reference range or to baseline for that subject."

(1)Subject #389204 had Week 8 laboratory tests collected on February 18, 2008, and the corresponding laboratory report that was faxed to your site on February 20, 2008, showed that the subject's creatinine (CR) level measured 3.2 mg/dL. A progress note dated February 20, 2008, stated that subsequent to the review of the Week 8 visit laboratory report, the decision was made to terminate the subject from the study due to the elevated CR level. The progress note further stated that the subject will hold the study drug and proceed with the end of termination visit. The February 20 and 21, 2008, progress notes indicated that your site left messages for the subject to contact your office regarding the abnormal laboratory results. The subject did not contact your site until February 26, 2008, and the end of termination visit was scheduled for February 27, 2008. With respect to this SAE, we note the following:

(a) In the time period between February 22 and February 26, 2008, when the subject called your site, you had no follow-up with the subject regarding the abnormal laboratory results. The subject's last dose of study drug was on February 26, 2008.

(b) You did not report the SAE of acute renal failure to the CRO until February 27, 2008. This was not within the 24-hour reporting period required by the protocol. In addition, the report to the CRO stated that the onset of the SAE and the date your staff was notified of the SAE was February 26, 2008. This is contradictory to your progress note, which stated that your site became aware of the SAE on February 20, 2008.

(c) Your site did not report the SAE to the IRB until February 27, 2008, even though your progress note indicated that your site was aware of the SAE on February 20, 2008.

You stated that contact was made with the subject immediately by phone message, and that final verbal contact was made within 6 days. You further stated that instructions regarding study medication could not be left on phone message because it would violate HIPAA regulations. To prevent the recurrence of this finding, you indicated that when critical laboratory values are returned for a subject, the subject would be called immediately to report the values, and that the subject would be instructed on what to do regarding the investigational product. You further indicated that if the subject is not reached, you would leave messages and continue to call the subject daily, and also send a letter via **(b)(4)** to the subject's address to notify the subject.

Your response is unacceptable. We note that your site sent a Subject Medical Review Form dated June 19, 2008, to the CRO, stating that the "Subject had labs drawn on 20 Feb 2008. They were not accessed in a timely manner. Subject went into renal failure." Thus, your site acknowledged that this SAE was not handled properly. In addition, you provided no detail regarding corrective actions you will take to ensure that reporting of SAEs to the sponsor and to the IRB are within the protocol-specified timeframes. You also failed to describe corrective actions to ensure that the information provided to the sponsor regarding SAEs would be accurate and consistent with the source records.

(2) Subject 389062 had samples collected on October 9, 2007, and the laboratory results were faxed to your site on October 10, 2007. Records indicate that you did not document your review of the laboratory results until April 22, 2008. Your delayed review of this subject's laboratory results is a violation of Protocol Section 9.5.3.1.6, Follow-up

of Adverse Events. Specifically, since your review did not take place until over six months after you received the test results, you did not adequately determine contemporaneously whether the abnormal laboratory results reported were clinically significant and therefore were required to be repeated immediately and followed up until the values were returned to within the reference range or to the baseline for that subject. The fact that these particular samples may not have, in fact, indicated an adverse or serious adverse event is irrelevant because, if they had, they would not have been documented or followed through properly, since your review did not take place until over six months after you received the test results.

Your written response indicated that you originally signed the laboratory result page, crossed out the wrong date, and wrote "reviewed labs on 10/23/07, wrote wrong date." This notation was then initialed and dated "4/10/07." To prevent the recurrence of this finding, you indicated that as laboratory results are received by fax, they will be placed in a basket for the clinical investigator to review and date immediately. You further stated that the basket of faxes is checked regularly throughout the day, and the longest time between receiving the labs and reviewing them is 2 days, when labs are received during the weekend.

Your response is unacceptable. Your written response regarding the dating of the laboratory result could not be verified, because the laboratory report provided during the FDA inspection showed that for the laboratory specimens collected on October 9, 2007, there was only one signature, with a date of review of April 22, 2008. We further note that you provided no corrective actions concerning the review of laboratory reports received when you would not be available.

b. Protocol Section 9.3.1, Inclusion Criteria, and Protocol Section 9.4.7, Prior and Concomitant Therapy, specified that subjects who had used a nonsteroidal anti-inflammatory drug (NSAID) within the 30 days prior to study entry were ineligible for enrollment into the study. FDA's review of your source records indicated that 6 subjects (389058, 389069, 389080, 389090, 389143, and 389218) had used an NSAID within the 30 days prior to study entry but were enrolled into the study.

Furthermore, in Subject Medical Review Forms submitted by your site to the CRO, **(b)(4)**, and in a protocol deviation list submitted to the IRB, you reported that Subjects 389040 and 389111 had taken an NSAID within the 30 days prior to study entry but were enrolled into the study.

Your written response stated that as the study involved two readily available over-the-counter (OTC) medications, it was your observation that subjects often took these medications not realizing that this was a protocol violation, despite your instructing the subject otherwise. You stated that you would work better in the future by asking the subject not to take any OTC medication without notifying you prior to taking it. You indicated that as a corrective action, all subjects would be instructed to bring all concomitant medications to each visit, where they will be reviewed for exclusionary medications, and that the clinical investigator will review the inclusion/exclusion criteria at randomization and will document that the subject is qualified to be randomized.

Your response is unacceptable. FDA's review of the records found that your site was aware that several subjects had taken NSAIDs within the 30 days prior to study entry, but your site continued to enroll the subjects into the study. Your response does not address how a similar situation would be handled in the future. In addition, the worksheet you provided as your corrective action provided no information as to the procedures you would use to verify that subjects met all protocol eligibility criteria.

c. Protocol Section 9.4.7, Prior and Concomitant Therapy, and Protocol Section 9.3.2, Exclusion Criteria, Subsection 7, specified that subjects who used an acid suppressant agent within 14 days prior to study entry were ineligible for enrollment into the study. FDA's review of your source records indicated that 4 subjects (389086, 389094, 389173, and 389234) had used an acid suppressant agent within 14 days prior to study entry but were enrolled into the study.

Furthermore, in Subject Medical Review Forms submitted by your site to the CRO, in a protocol deviation list submitted to the IRB, and/or in memos to files, you reported that 4 other randomized subjects (389085, 389092, 389142, and 389247) had taken an acid suppressant agent within 14 days prior to study entry.

Your written response stated that you confirmed that Subjects 389173, 389142, 389092, 389094, and 389234 had used an acid suppressant agent within 14 days prior to study entry. For Subject 389086, you stated that the subject did not notify your site that she was taking Nexium and Zantac, and this was discovered when her medical records were received from her primary care provider. For Subject 389085, you stated that the subject was prescribed Nexium and Pepcid AC by the primary care provider after the screening visit and prior to randomization, and this was not discovered until the subject had been randomized. You indicated that the corrective action for this was to have a review of the concomitant medications at every visit, and that the investigator would review the excluded medication list with all staff.

Your response is unacceptable. Your corrective actions provided no information as to how your site will verify medical records, if obtainable and received from the primary care provider, prior to enrolling and/or randomizing subjects into the study to verify the subject's concomitant medications. In addition, you provided no corrective actions regarding procedures you will utilize to elicit from subjects all the medications they are currently taking. You also provided no corrective actions or procedures you would utilize to better instruct subjects against taking protocol-specified, excluded medications.

d. Protocol Section 9.5.3.4, Clinical Laboratory Tests, specified that at the screening visit, blood samples were to be collected from study subjects for on-site testing for serum H. pylori. Protocol Section 9.3.2, Exclusion Criteria, Subsection 6, further specified that subjects with a documented current H. pylori infection were ineligible for enrollment into the study. Source records indicated that at least 2 subjects (389127 and 389135) were enrolled into the study without documentation of a current negative H. pylori test at the screening visit.

Furthermore, in Subject Medical Review Forms submitted by your site to the CRO, in a protocol deviation list submitted to the IRB, and/or in memos to files, you reported that additional subjects, including but not limited to Subjects 389129, 389137, and 389142, were enrolled into the study without documentation of a current negative H. pylori test performed at the screening visit.

Your written response stated that this protocol violation was an isolated issue and that the clinical research coordinator (CRC) who inadvertently did not document the results was "re-educated." You also indicated that, as a corrective action, any in-house test to be performed will have the lot number, expiration date, and results documented in the source documents.

Your response is unacceptable. Specifically, your statement that the CRC inadvertently did not document the result implies that the CRC actually performed the testing, but did not record the results in the source records. According to the establishment inspection report, you informed FDA Investigator Smith that while observing this particular CRC's work, you noticed that she was not using any of the supplies needed for the H. pylori test but was writing on the source records that she had in fact conducted those tests. Documentation found at your site also stated that the CRC in question either did not conduct any H. pylori testing at the screening visit, or that the testing was questionable because the supplies needed for the test were not used. You further informed FDA Investigator Smith that when you questioned the study coordinator about your discovery and suggested that she would have to undergo training and work under the supervision of other coordinators, she abruptly resigned. Therefore, FDA cannot confirm that the CRC in question was "re-educated," as you stated in your written response.

e. In addition to the above protocol violations, in written memos to file, Subject Medical Review Forms submitted to the CRO, and/or protocol deviations sent to the IRB, your site acknowledged numerous protocol deviations, including but not limited to lack of international normalized ratio (INR) testing at the screening visit for subjects on anticoagulant therapy (e.g., 389017 and 389085); dispensing incorrect test articles to subjects (e.g., 389013, 389041, and 389091); study visits not being scheduled according to the protocol (e.g., 389162 and 389040); and failure to conduct screening serum pregnancy tests (e.g., Subjects 389075 and 389211).

In your written response, you confirmed the findings noted above. Your corrective actions included (1) a commitment to reduce human error by having a better understanding of each protocol and all of its procedures, and by total adherence to the protocol; (2) creation of a source document appendix to allow a second coordinator to cross-reference the investigational product (IP) or kit number assigned by the interactive voice recognition system (IVRS) for a particular subject, so that two coordinators can verify that the correct IP is dispensed to the subject; (3) development of a worksheet entitled "Visit Schedule" that includes the projected dates and actual dates of each visit including +/- windows; and (4) development of a new source document to be used at the end of every visit, certifying that the investigator has reviewed the source documents in their entirety for accuracy and correct documentation.

While these corrective actions appear appropriate, it was the absence of such measures during the conduct of these trials that led to the violations listed here, and that increases our concerns over your approach to ensuring appropriate human subject protection.

2. You failed to maintain adequate and accurate case histories that record all observations and other data pertinent to the investigation on each individual administered the investigational drug or employed as a control in the investigation [21 CFR 312.62(b)].

a. The screening visit source record for Subject 389137 had a signature which appeared to be that of sub-investigator, Dr. **(b)(4)**, documenting that he had performed a physical exam on October 11, 2007. Your records indicated, however, that Dr. **(b)(4)** confirmed that the signature on the screening visit source record was not his and denied performing the examination.

You provided no written response to address this finding.

b. Source records indicated that Subject 389230 had a physical exam at the screening visit on December 18, 2007. However, you did not sign the source physical exam record until April 21, 2008.

Your written response indicated that the physical exam was done at the screening visit, but that you inadvertently forgot to fill out the source document. Your corrective action to prevent this finding was to have the investigator thoroughly document, sign, and date all of the physical exams in real time.

Your response is inadequate. You provided no information regarding procedures and/or training that you would require to ensure that documents are completed, signed, and dated at the time of the study visit.

c. Records at your site are discrepant concerning which subject (i.e., 389198 or 389168) had the Week 24 visit out of window. Specifically, your site reported in the Subject Medical Review Form dated May 20, 2008, that Subject 389168 (randomization number 5168) had the Week 24 visit scheduled 3 weeks early. In the upper right-hand corner of this same form, there is a handwritten note stating "#389198." According to the enrollment log, Subject 389168's randomization number was not 5168; this randomization number belonged to Subject 389198. In the **(b)(4)** IVRS Deactivation worksheet, you again stated that Subject 389168's Week 24 visit was out of window.

This letter is not intended to be an all inclusive list of deficiencies with your clinical study of an investigational drug. It is your responsibility to ensure adherence to each requirement of the law and relevant FDA regulations. You should address these deficiencies and establish procedures to ensure that any ongoing or future studies will be in compliance with FDA regulations.

Within fifteen (15) working days of your receipt of this letter, you should notify this office in writing of the actions you have taken to prevent similar violations in the future. Failure to adequately and promptly explain the violations noted above may result in regulatory action without further notice.

If you have any questions, please contact Constance Cullity, M.D., M.P.H., at 301-796-3397; FAX 301-847-8748. Your written response and any pertinent documentation should be addressed to:

Constance Cullity (formerly Lewin), M.D., M.P.H.
Branch Chief
Good Clinical Practice Branch I
Division of Scientific Investigations
Office of Compliance
Center for Drug Evaluation and Research
Food and Drug Administration
Building 51, Room 5354
10903 New Hampshire Avenue
Silver Spring, MD 20993

Sincerely yours,

{See appended electronic signature page}

Leslie K. Ball, M.D.

Director
Division of Scientific Investigations
Office of Compliance
Center for Drug Evaluation and Research
Food and Drug Administration

第104封　给Ratzan, Judith医学博士的警告信

2011年2月16日

参考号：11-HFD-45-02-04

尊敬的Ratzan博士：

2010年7月19日至9月13日，Craig Garmendia先生和Nicole Bell女士代表FDA与您会面，对您所开展的试验药物为（b）（4）[1]，申办者为（b）（4）的以下临床研究进行了审查：试验方案（b）（4），标题为（b）（4）。

本次现场检查是FDA的生物研究监查项目的一部分。该项目通过设定的检查方法，对相关研究的实施情况进行评估，以确认研究数据在科学上是有效和准确的，并帮助确保这些研究中受试者的权益、安全和福利得到了保护。

经对现场检查报告及该报告的附件进行审查，我们认为，您没有遵循适用的法律要求和监管临床研究实施的FDA法规。我们想强调以下几点：

在现场检查结束时，Garmendia先生和Bell女士向您出示了FDA483表，即现场检查发现的问题，并与您进行了讨论。您2010年10月14日对该FDA483表的书面回复已收悉，但我们注意到收到回复的时间已超过检查后15个工作日。因此，尽管我们已经审查了该回复，但是按照2009年8月11日发布的局长执行倡议，本警告信中没有包含对该回复的讨论。我们想强调以下几点。

1. 您未能亲自进行临床研究或对研究进行监督［21 CFR 312.60］

当您为上述临床研究签署研究者声明（FDA 1572表）时，您同意在您的中心担当临床研究者职责。作为一名临床研究者，您的总体职责包括确保临床试验的操作按照您签署的研究者声明、研究计划和适用法规实施；保护您医疗照顾下的受试者的权益、安全和福利；确保研究中的药物的管控［21 CFR 312.60］。通过签署FDA 1572表，您具体地确认您亲自操作的临床试验部分或监督那些您不亲自操作的部分。您可以授权您的一些研究任务给那些有资质来完成任务的个人，但作为一名临床研究者，您不可以授权您的总体职责。我们检查发现，您对于您授权了研究任务的人员的监督不足以确保临床试验的操作按照您签署的研究者声明、研究计划和相关法规实施，也不足以来保护受试者的权益、安全和福利。

具体来说，您没有充分地监督您授权研究任务的研究人员。很多，可能不是所有，在此警告信中列出的其他违背可以追溯到您的在充分监督研究人员和研究操作的失职。例如，发生在3/3例入组的受试者的多次的化疗错误给药，包括一例受试者研究结束后的试验药物的6周期给药。仔细的审阅化疗医嘱可以预防错误给药，或至少让您可以发现您系统中的那些导致重复方案偏离的缺陷。充分的监督也会预防或减少重复的不良事件漏报和重复的未按方案要求程序的操作。您的研究人员向检查员Garmendia报告，本研究的大多数时间您不在试验场所，且一年中有6个月您不住在佛罗里达州。很明显没有相关流程来弥补您不在的情况。

2. 您没有确保按照研究计划进行研究［21 CFR 312.60］

a. 我们检查发现3/3位受试者，化疗药给药的方案没有按照研究计划。我们看到以下情况：

i. 受试者4067803，随机到B组，有多次给药方案的偏离，包括处方剂量、输液速度，或两者都有。

周期/日期/药物	方案剂量	给药剂量	方案的静脉注射速度	实际的静脉注射速度
1 11/19/2008（b）（4）	400 mg/m^2	200 mg/m^2		
2 12/3/2008（b）（4）			60分钟（第2周期）	30分钟
3 12/17/2008（b）（4）	85 mg/m^2	100 mg/m^2		
4 12/31/2008（b）（4）			2小时	快速推注
7 2/11/2009（b）（4）			2小时	8分钟

1 (b)(4)涉及商业秘密，根据法规内容不予公开。

ⅱ. 受试者2564977，随机到B组，有多次给药方案的偏离，包括处方剂量或输液速度方面：

周期/日期/药物	方案剂量	给药剂量	方案的静脉注射速度	实际的静脉注射速度
4 4/27/2009（b）（4）	400 mg/m^2	320 mg/m^2		
5 5/11/2009				
6 5/26/2009				
7 6/8/2009	0mg/kg	5mg/kg		
8 6/22/2009				
9 7/6/2009				
10 7/20/2009（b）（4）				

在2009年4月27日检查受试者2564977第4周期时，我们发现（b）（4）使用剂量是320mg/m^2，而不是方案要求的剂量400mg/m^2。在化疗医嘱上，我们注意到受试者剂量由于腹泻有所调整。然而，在化疗给药记录中，护士的记录报告受试者没有腹泻主诉。而且，即使受试者发生过腹泻，方案中没有关于（b）（4）减量要求。在方案5.5.1部分，化疗剂量调整A组和B组，说明了因毒性反应而减少剂量的要求。方案那部分明确，“（b）（4）剂量保持恒定不用调整。”

另外，在方案5.5.1.1部分的剂量调整表详细说明了对于1级和2级腹泻，研究者维持原剂量；对于3级腹泻,（b）（4）丸剂和注射剂都减低一个剂量标准；对于4级腹泻,（b）（4）丸剂和注射剂都减低一个剂量标准。

在检查受试者2564977第5~10周期时我们发现，重复的错误给药给受试者2564977。您声明您和您的“研究团队没有弄清此案例中申办者关于研究结束的定义和意图。”然而，在看了2009年4月29日（b）（4）关于结束研究的公告后，我们不同意您的声明。我们看到（b）（4）公告清晰地阐明了，“对正在接受试验用（b）（4）合并（b）（4）治疗的患者，（b）（4）须终止……，患者应继续方案规定的标准的术后的系统治疗。”

ⅲ. 受试者4065381，随机到A组［（b）（4）］，有多次给药方案的偏离，包括处方剂量或输液速度，以及错误（b）（4）给药。

周期/日期/药物	方案剂量	给药剂量	方案的静脉注射速度	实际的静脉注射速度
3 12/3/2008（b）（4）	0 mg/kg	5 mg/kg		
4 12/17/2008（b）（4）	85 mg/m^2	100 mg/m^2		
4 12/17/2008（b）（4）			2小时	12 分钟
6 1/14/2009（b）（4）	0mg/kg	5mg/kg	2小时	5 分钟
9 2/25/2009（b）（4）			2 小时	5 分钟

b. 试验方案7.1部分，治疗参数，列明了必需的评估时间点，我们看到3/3入组的受试者没有执行必需的评估。

ⅰ. 受试者4067803没有以下评估：

a）第6、9和12周期尿蛋白/肌酐（UPC）比率；

b）随访9、15和21个月访视的癌胚抗原（CEA）测试；

c）第2、4、8、9和11周期的病史，身体和（b）（4）性能状态；

d）6个月的随访期访视。

ⅱ. 受试者2564977没有以下评估：

a）第1、3和6周期的UPC比率；

b）随访9、12、15和18个月访视的癌胚抗原（CEA）测试；

c）第6和7周期以及15个月随访期访视的病史，身体和（b）（4）性能状态；

d）6个月的随访期访视。

iii. 受试者4065381没有以下评估：

a）第1、2、3和5周期访视的病史，身体和（b）（4）性能状态；

b）6个月的随访期访视；

c）方案5.3部分，不良事件报告要求，讲到“在试验过程中不良事件须按规定的时间点常规报告……”我们看到您在3/3入组受试者的病例报告中没有报告以下不良事件：

i. 受试者4065381　第3周期（2008年11月22日至2008年12月5日）：恶心，呕吐。

ii. 受试者4067803

a）第1周期（2008年11月19日至2008年12月2日）：恶心。

b）第2周期（2008年12月3日至2008年12月16日）：排尿困难，关节痛，直肠瘙痒。

c）第7周期（2009年2月11日至2009年2月24日）：恶心。

d）第9周期（2009年3月11日至2009年3月24日）：血红蛋白（CTCAE Attribution），白细胞。

iii. 受试者2564977

a）第3周期（2009年4月13日至2009年4月26日）：脱水，腹泻，呕吐。

b）第5周期（2009年5月11日至2009年5月25日）：过度流泪。

没有执行研究相关程序和没有按要求执行化疗方案是置受试者安全和健康于风险中，也损害了研究终点的解释和有效性。

3. 您未能保存对研究中使用试验药物或对照组的受试者的所有研究观察结果和其他相关数据的足够及准确的病历［21 CFR 312.62（b）］

a. 在受试者4065381第3周期（2008年11月22日）病例报告表中，记录了指甲改变的不良事件，然而没有相关原始文件作为证据来支持此事件的发生。

b. 所有3例研究受试者的病例报告表中，（b）（4）丸剂和注射剂的剂量值被互换了，（b）（4）注射剂剂量值被错误地记录在（b）（4）丸剂的剂量值的位置，（b）（4）丸剂的剂量值被错误记录在（b）（4）注射剂剂量值的位置。而且，错误记录在注射剂位置的（b）（4）丸剂，单位“mg”被错误转换为“g”。我们还发现（b）（4）的给药，原始文件中和病例报告表中是不一致的，具体如下表。

受试者	周期	剂量互换	错误单位标签（g）	其他
4065381（b）（4）	2~4，6，9~11	是	是	
52282	1	是		
4067803（b）（4）	1，4，7	是	是	
52286	2	是	是	（b）（4）剂量是183，但在CRF是138；（b）（4）剂量是483，但在CRF是274；（b）（4）剂量是860，但在CRF是648
	3	是	是	
2564977（b）（4）	3，4，7~12	是	是	（b）（4）丸剂剂量是374，但在CRF是598；（b）（4）注射剂剂量是1496，但在CRF是1870
	5，6	是	是	

不能保存完整和准确的病历损害了临床研究终点的解释和有效性。

本警告信的目的并非是罗列您在试验药物临床研究中存在的所有缺陷。确保遵循法律和相关FDA法规的每一项要求是您的职责，您应当解决这些缺陷，并建立规程，以确保任何正在进行或将来进行的研究均符合FDA的法规。

自收到这封信的15个工作日内，您应当书面告知本办公室为预防将来发生类似违规情况而采取的措施。如果不能充分、迅速地解释上述违规问题，可能导致我们在不再通知的情况下采取监管措施。如果您确信您于2010年10月14日签署的针对FDA483表的书面回复能充分解释您为避免将来再次发生此类违规而已经采取的措施，请在15个工作日内就此与我们沟通。您需要把2010年10月14日的书面回复作为此沟通的附件。

附：英文原文

Ratzan, Judith M.D.

WARNING LETTER

FEB 16, 2011

CERTIFIED MAIL
RETURN RECEIPT REQUESTED

Ref: 11-HFD-45-02-04

R. Judith Ratzan, M.D.
1475 NW 12th Avenue
Miami, Florida 33136

Dear Dr. Ratzan:

Between July 19 and September 13, 2010, Mr. Craig Garmendia and Ms. Nicole Bell, representing the Food and Drug Administration (FDA), conducted an investigation and met with you to review your conduct of a clinical investigation (Protocol (b)(4), entitled (b)(4)) of the investigational drug (b)(4), performed for (b)(4).

This inspection is a part of FDA's Bioresearch Monitoring Program, which includes inspections designed to evaluate the conduct of research and to help ensure that the rights, safety, and welfare of the human subjects of those studies have been protected.

From our review of the establishment inspection report and the documents submitted with that report, we conclude that you did not adhere to the applicable statutory requirements and FDA regulations governing the conduct of clinical investigations. We are aware that at the conclusion of the inspection, Mr. Garmendia and Ms. Bell presented and discussed with you Form FDA 483, Inspectional Observations. We acknowledge receipt of your response dated October 14, 2010, to Form FDA 483, but note that this response was received past the 15 working days from close of the inspection. Thus, while we have reviewed the response, we have not included a discussion of the response in this letter as per the Commissioner's Enforcement Initiative announced August 11, 2009. We wish to emphasize the following:

1. You failed to personally conduct or supervise the clinical investigation [21 CFR 312.60].

When you signed the Statement of Investigator (Form FDA 1572) for the above referenced clinical trial you agreed to take on the responsibilities of a clinical investigator at your site. Your general responsibilities as a clinical investigator include ensuring that the clinical trial is conducted according the signed investigator statement, the investigational plan, and applicable regulations; protecting the rights, safety, and welfare of subjects under your care; and ensuring control of drugs under investigation [21 CFR 312.60]. By signing Form FDA 1572, you specifically agreed to personally conduct the clinical trial or to supervise those aspects of the trial that you did not personally conduct. While you may delegate certain study tasks to individuals qualified to perform them, as a clinical investigator you may not delegate your general responsibilities. Our investigation indicates that your supervision of personnel to whom you delegated study tasks was not adequate to ensure that the clinical trial was conducted according to the signed investigator statement, the investigational plan, and applicable regulations, and in a manner that protects the rights, safety, and welfare of human subjects.

Specifically, you failed to adequately supervise the study staff to whom you delegated tasks. Many, if not all, of the other violations listed in this letter are traceable to your failure to adequately supervise staff and the conduct of the investigation. For example, multiple episodes of chemotherapy misadministration occurred for 3 of 3 subjects enrolled, including administration of 6 cycles of an investigational drug to a subject after closure of the study. Adequate review of the chemotherapy orders could have prevented misadministrations, or at a minimum allowed you to discover flaws in your systems that led to repeated departures from the investigational protocol. Adequate supervision also could have prevented or minimized repeated failures to report adverse events and to conduct procedures required by the protocol. We note that your staff reported to Investigator Garmendia that you were not present at the clinical site for a majority of the study, and that you live outside of the State of Florida for six months of the year. It is apparent that procedures were not in place to compensate for your absence.

2. You failed to ensure that the investigation was conducted according to the investigational plan [21 CFR 312.60].

a. Our investigation revealed that for 3 out of 3 subjects, the administration schedule of chemotherapeutic agents was not conducted according to the investigational plan. We note the following examples:

i. Subject 4067803, who was randomized to Arm B, had multiple administration schedule deviations of either prescribed dose, infusion rate, or both:

Cycle/Date/Drug	Protocol Dose	Received Dose	Protocol IV Infusion Rate	Received IV Infusion Rate
1 on 11/19/08 (b)(4)	400 mg/m^2	200 mg/m^2		
2 on 12/3/08 (b)(4)			60 minutes for cycle 2	30 minutes
3 on 12/17/08 (b)(4)	85 mg/m^2	100 mg/m^2		
4 on 12/31/08 (b)(4)			2 hours	Boluspush
7 on 2/11/09 (b)(4)			2 hours	8 minutes

ii. Subject 2564977, who was randomized to Arm B, had multiple administration schedule deviations of either prescribed dose or infusion rate:

Cycle/Date/Drug	Protocol Dose	Received Dose	Protocol IV Infusion Rate	Received IV Infusion Rate
4 on 4/27/09 (b)(4)	400 mg/m^2	320 mg/m^2		
5 on 5/11/09				
6 on 5/26/09				
7 on 6/8/09	0mg/kg	5mg/kg		
8 on 6/22/09				
9 on 7/6/09				
10 on 7/20/09 (b)(4)				

Our investigation of Cycle 4 on April 27, 2009, for Subject 2564977 revealed that the **(b)(4)** was dosed at 320 mg/m^2 instead of the protocol required dose of 400 mg/m^2. In the chemotherapy orders, it is noted that the subject's dose was modified due to diarrhea. However, in the chemotherapy administration notes from your clinic, the nurse's notes report that the subject had no complaints of diarrhea. Moreover, even if the subject did experience diarrhea, the protocol did not call for a reduction in **(b)(4)** dosage. Section 5.5.1 of the protocol, Chemotherapy Dose Modifications Arms A and B, outlines the required dose reductions due to toxicity. That section of the protocol states, "Note that **(b)(4)** dose remains constant and without modification." Furthermore, the dose modification table in Section 5.5.1.1. of the protocol specifically instructs the clinical investigator to maintain dose levels for grades 1 and 2 diarrhea; to reduce both bolus **(b)(4)** and infusional **(b)(4)** one dose level for grade 3 diarrhea; and to reduce both bolus and infusional **(b)(4)** and **(b)(4)** by one dose level for grade 4 diarrhea.

Our investigation of Cycles 5~10 for Subject 2564977 identified the repeated misadministration of **(b)(4)** to Subject 2564977. You stated that you and your "study team did not have clarity in this case regarding the definition and intent of the sponsor upon study closure." However, after our review of the **(b)(4)** announcement dated April 29, 2009, closing the trial, we disagree with your statement. We note that the **(b)(4)** announcement clearly stated, "For patients currently being treated with the experimental regimen of **(b)(4)** in combination with **(b)(4)**, the **(b)(4)** must be discontinued.... Patients should continue on standard postoperative systemic therapy **(b)(4)** per protocol."

iii. Subject 4065381, who was randomized to Arm A (**(b)(4)**), had multiple administration schedule deviations of prescribed dose or infusion rate, as well as the wrongful administration of **(b)(4)**

Cycle/Date/Drug	Protocol Dose	Received Dose	Protocol iv Infusion Rate	Received iv Infusion Rate
3 on 12/3/08 (b)(4)	0 mg/kg	5 mg/kg		
4 on 12/17/08 (b)(4)	85 mg/m^2	100 mg/m^2		
4 on 12/17/08 (b)(4)			2 hours	12 minutes
6 on 1/14/09 (b)(4)	0mg/kg	5mg/kg	2 hours	5 minutes
9 on 2/25/09 (b)(4)			2 hours	5 minutes

b. Section 7.1 of the protocol, Therapeutic Parameters, outlines the timing of the required assessments. We note that 3 of 3 subjects enrolled did not have the required assessments performed.

i. Subject 4067803 did not have the following:

a. Urine Protein/Creatinine (UPC) ratio performed for Cycles 6, 9, and 12.

b. Carcinoembryonic Antigen (CEA) test was not performed for followup at the 9, 15, and 21month visits.

c. History, physical, and (b)(4) performance status performed for Cycles 2, 4, 8, 9, and 11.

d. A 6 month followup visit.

ii. Subject 2564977 did not have the following:

a. UPC ratio performed for Cycles 1, 3, and 6.

b. CEA test was not performed for followup at the 9, 12, 15, and 18month visits.

c. History, physical, and (b)(4) performance status performed for Cycles 6 and 7, as well as the 15month follow-up visit.

d. A 6month follow-up visit.

iii. Subject 4065381 did not have the following:

a. History, physical, and (b)(4) performance status performed for Cycles 1, 2, 3, and 5.

b. A 6month followup visit.

c. Section 5.3 of the protocol, Adverse Event Reporting Requirements, states, "Adverse events are reported in a routine manner at scheduled times during a trial...." We note that you failed to report the following adverse events to the sponsor in your CRFs for 3 of 3 subjects enrolled:

i. Subject 4065381: Cycle 3 (11/22/08 12/05/08): Nausea, Vomiting

ii. Subject 4067803:

a. Cycle 1 (11/19/08 12/02/08): Nausea

b. Cycle 2 (12/03/08 12/16/08): Dysuria, Joint Pain, Rectal Itching

c. Cycle 7 (02/11/09 02/24/09): Nausea

d. Cycle 9 (03/11/09 03/24/09): Hemoglobin (CTCAE Attribution), Leukoc

iii. Subject 2564977

a. Cycle 3 (04/13/09 04/26/09): Dehydration, Diarrhea, Vomiting

b. Cycle 5 (05/11/09 05/25/09): Hyperlacrimation

Failure to perform study-related procedures and to administer chemotherapy regimens as required jeopardizes subject safety and welfare, and compromises the interpretation and validity of the investigational endpoints.

3. You failed to maintain adequate and accurate case histories that record all observations and other data pertinent to the investigation on each individual administered the investigational drug or employed as a control in the investigation [21 CFR 312.62(b)].

a. The Cycle 3 (11/22/08) Case Report Form (CFR) for Subject 4065381 documented the adverse event of Nail Change, yet no evidence was available in the source documents to support the event's occurrence.

b. All three study subjects had Case Report Forms (CRFs) in which the doses of **(b)(4)** bolus and **(b)(4)** infusion values were transposed. The value for **(b)(4)** infusion dose was incorrectly recorded in the **(b)(4)** bolus dose box, and the value for **(b)(4)** bolus was incorrectly recorded in the **(b)(4)** infusion. Furthermore, the (b)(4) bolus, which was recorded in the infusion box, was incorrectly converted from milligrams to grams. We also note that the dosing for **(b)(4)**, as noted in the source documents, is inconsistent with what was reported in the CRFs for the subjects and cycles, as noted in the table below.

Subject	Cycles(s)	Dose transposed	Incorrect unit label (gram)	Other
4065381 (b) (4)	2-4,6,9-11	yes	Yes	
52282	1	yes		
4067803 (b) (4)	1,4,7	yes	Yes	
52286	2	yes	Yes	(b)(4) dose was 183, but CFR says 138; (b)(4) dose was 483, but CFR says 274; (b)(4) dose was 860, but CFR says 648
	3	yes	Yes	
2564977 (b)(4)	3,4,7-12	yes	Yes	(b)(4) bolus dose was 374, but CFR says 598; (b)(4) infusion dose was 1496, but CFR says 1870
	5,6	yes	Yes	

Failing to maintain adequate and accurate case histories compromises the interpretation and validity of the clinical investigational endpoints.

This letter is not intended to be an all-inclusive list of deficiencies with your clinical study of an investigational drug. It is your responsibility to ensure adherence to each requirement of the law and relevant FDA regulations. You should address these deficiencies and establish procedures to ensure that any ongoing or future studies will be in compliance with FDA regulations.

Within fifteen (15) working days of your receipt of this letter, you should notify this office in writing of the actions you have taken to prevent similar violations in the future. Failure to adequately and promptly explain the violations noted above may result in regulatory action without further notice. If you believe that your written response to the Form FDA 483 dated October 14, 2010, fully explains the actions you have taken to prevent similar violations in the future, please communicate that to us in writing within fifteen (15) business days. You may reference the written response dated October 14, 2010, in your response to this letter.

If you have any questions, please contact Constance Cullity, M.D., M.P.H., at 301-796-3397; FAX 301-847-8748. Your written response and any pertinent documentation should be addressed to:

Constance Cullity (formerly Lewin), M.D., M.P.H. Branch Chief
Good Clinical Practice Branch I Division of Scientific Investigations Office of Compliance
Center for Drug Evaluation and Research
Food and Drug Administration
Building 51, Room 5354
10903 New Hampshire Avenue
Silver Spring, MD 20993

Sincerely yours,

{See appended electronic signature page}

LeslieK.Ball,M.D.
Director
Division of Scientific Investigations
Office of Compliance
Center for Drug Evaluationand Research
Food and Drug Administration
Reference ID:2903500

第105封 给Lippton, Howard医学博士的警告信

2010年10月20日

参考号：11-HFD-45-10-01

尊敬的Lippton博士：

2010年2月2日至2月4日，Barbara Wright女士和Tiana McKinley女士代表FDA与您会面，对您所开展的试验药物为（b）（4）[1]，申办者为（b）（4）的以下临床试验进行了现场检查：试验方案（b）（4），标题为“（b）（4）”。

本次现场检查是FDA的生物研究监查项目的一部分。该项目通过设定的检查方法，对研究的实施情况进行评估，以确认研究数据在科学上是有效和准确的，并帮助确保这些研究中受试者的权益、安全和福利得到了保护。

在现场检查结束时，Wright和McKinley女士向您出示了FDA483表，即现场检查发现的问题，并与您进行了讨论。您2010年2月5日对该FDA483表的书面回复已收悉。

经对现场检查报告、该报告的附件，以及您2010年2月5日的书面回复进行审查，我们认为，您没有遵循适用的法律要求和监管临床研究实施的FDA法规。我们想强调以下几点：

1. 您未能确保符合21 CFR 56所列要求的IRB对试验方案（b）（4）进行初始审查、跟踪审查和批准［21 CFR 312.66］

FDA法规21 CFR 312.66要求研究者确保伦理委员会符合21CFR 56要求，审查和批准提议的临床研究。FDA法规21 CFR 56.109要求伦理委员会顺应FDA监管审查研究活动。为了让伦理委员会有效地实施审阅，伦理委员会需要有关临床研究的准确信息用以审阅。因此，确保伦理委员会审阅，作为研究者的义务部分，研究者必须提供给伦理委员会准确的信息；如果研究者不能提供给伦理委员会准确的信息，伦理委员会则不能有效地审阅研究活动，研究者也不能确保伦理委员会已审阅过提议的研究。

2009年4月2日您签署并确认的真实和准确的试验场所提交表，并且您递交给（b）（4）伦理委员会以批准试验方案（b）（4）的实施，其信息是不准确的。具体来说，您在那张表上对问题29（d）和29（e）错误地回答了“否”。这些问题问道“自您上次提交（b）（4）或者如果这是您第一次提交（b）（4），对于和这研究中的相关研究者……（d）他/她会被定为或指控为犯罪（轻罪或重罪）吗？……（e）州医学审查委员会是否就他/她的执照有过惩戒措施，或是否有中止的研究？”根据（b）（4）伦理委员会，您在2009年4月2日之前的递交是在2000年10月。2002年2月6日，您涉及了一起犯罪诉讼，被定为医疗诈骗（18 USC 1347），2002年6月19日，您被宣判18个月有期徒刑。2003年6月17日，路易斯安那州审查委员会医学检查官吊销了您在路易斯安那州的行医执照，从您监禁日（2002年7月15日）开始为期2年。因此您在递交表上对问题29（d）和29（e）的回答应该是“是”，并且，根据填表指南，您应该附一份书面解释和所有与您罪行和执照吊销相关文件的复印件。

在获知您2009年4月2日试验场所递交表错误后，（b）（4）伦理委员会撤销了其关于试验方案（b）（4）批件，否决了您关于实施第二个提议临床研究的申请。在一封2009年8月7日给（b）（4）伦理委员会的信中，您陈述是研究协调员填写了2009年4月2日试验场所递交表，并且完成了对问题29（d）和29（e）的回答，您并没有参与。然而，通过签署2009年4月2日试验场所递交表，您确认了您“已审阅了在‘试验场所递交

1 （b）（4）涉及商业秘密，根据法规内容不予公开。

表’中所有回答，并且所有回答都是真实和准确的。”（以原文强调）因此，研究协调员填写此表的事实并不能减轻您在签署时确保其准确性的职责。另外，在您的2009年8月7日给（b）（4）伦理委员会的信中，您承认了您在2009年4月2日的表中对问题29（d）和 29（e）的回答是不准确的，以及您在“确认表格的准确填写方面没有尽职。”

您没有确保在2009年4月2日试验场所递交表中提供准确信息给（b）（4）伦理委员会，从而妨碍了（b）（4）伦理委员会审阅您的实施试验方案（b）（4）的申请，并且做出申请充分的决定。因此您没能确保伦理委员会按照21 CFR 312.66要求审阅试验方案（b）（4）。

2. 您未能保护在您的监护下的受试者的权益、安全和福利［21 CFR 312. 66］

根据21 CFR 312.66，研究者负责保护研究中受试者的权益、安全和福利。遵守21 CFR 312.66，包括21 CFR 56.109规定伦理委员会的审查要求，旨在保护涉及临床研究的受试者的权益、安全和福利（21 CFR 56.101）。为了充分保护受试者的权益、安全和福利，需要关于他们正在审查的提议研究的准确信息，以及将会参与到研究中的个人的准确信息。因此，作为研究者的职责部分，为了保护受试者的权益、安全和福利，研究者必须提供准确的信息给伦理委员会，从而伦理委员会才能充分履行其职责来保护受试者的权益、安全和福利。

如上所述，您2009年4月2日签署并确认正确的试验场所递交表，您给（b）（4）伦理委员会提供了有关您2002年罪行和执照吊销的错误信息。由于您未能确保试验场所递交表提供准确信息给（b）（4）伦理委员会，您也因此未能按21CFR 312.60要求保护您研究中的受试者的权益、安全和福利。

本警告信的目的并非是罗列您在临床研究和遵守相关FDA法规上存在的缺陷。确保遵循法律和相关FDA法规的每一项要求是您的职责，您应当解决这些缺陷，并建立规程，以确保任何正在进行或将来进行的研究均符合FDA的法规。

自收到这封信的15个工作日内，您应当书面告知本办公室为预防将来发生类似违规情况已采取的措施。如果不能充分、迅速地解释上述违规问题，可能导致我们在不预先通知的情况下采取监管措施。

附：英文原文

Lippton, Howard M.D.

WARNING LETTER

OCT 20, 2010

CERTIFIED MAIL
RETURN RECEIPT REQUESTED

Ref: 11-HFD-45-10-01

Howard L. Lippton, M.D.
2326 Line Avenue
Shreveport LA 71104-2131

Dear Dr. Lippton:

Between February 2 and February 4,2010,Ms. Barbara Wright and Ms. Tiana McKinley, representing the Food and Drug Administration (FDA),conducted an investigation and met with you to review your conduct of the following clinical investigation of the investigational drug (b)(4), performed for (b)(4):

• Protocol (b)(4),entitled "(b)(4)"

This inspection is a part of FDA's Bioresearch Monitoring Program, which includes inspections designed to evaluate the conduct of research and to help ensure that the rights, safety, and welfare of the human subjects of those studies have been protected.

At the conclusion of the inspection, Ms. Wright and Ms. McKinley presented and discussed with you the items listed on Form FDA 483, Inspectional Observations. We have reviewed the inspection report, the documents submitted with that report, and your written response to the Form FDA 483 dated February 5, 2010. We conclude that you did not adhere to the applicable statutory requirements and FDA regulations governing the conduct of clinical investigations. We wish to emphasize the following:

1. You failed to assure that an Institutional Review Board (IRB) that complies with the requirements set forth in part 56 was responsible for the initial review and approval of Protocol (b)(4) [21CFR 312.66].

FDA regulations at 21CFR 312.66 require investigators to assure that an IRB that complies with 21CFR part 56 reviews and approves a proposed clinical investigation. FDA regulations at 21CFR 56.109 require that IRBs review research activities subject to FDA oversight. In order for IRBs to conduct suet reviews effectively, IRBs need accurate information regarding the clinical investigations under their review. Therefore, as part of an investigator's obligation to assure IRB review, that investigator must provide the IRB with accurate information; if the investigator does not provide the IRB with accurate information, the IRB cannot effectively review the research activity, and the investigator has not assured that an IRB has reviewed the proposed investigation.

The Research Site Submission Form that you signed and certified as true and accurate on April 2, 2009 and submitted to the (b)(4) Institutional Review Board ((b)(4) IRB) for approval to conduct Protocol (b)(4), was inaccurate. Specifically, you incorrectly answered "no" to questions 29(d) and 29(e) on that form. These questions asked, "Since your last submission to (b)(4) or if this is your first submission to (b)(4), for any investigator associated with this study ... (d) Has he/she been convicted or charged with a crime (misdemeanor or felony)? ... (e) Has a state medical board taken a disciplinary action against his/her license, or is there a current investigation pending?" According to the (b)(4) IRB, your last submission to the (b)(4) IRB before April 2, 2009, was in October 2000. On February 6, 2002, you entered a plea of guilty and were convicted of one count of health care fraud (ll USC 1347), and on June 19, 2002, you were sentenced to be imprisoned for 18 months. On June 17, 2003, the Louisiana State Board of Medical Examiners suspended your license to practice medicine in the state of Louisiana for a period of 2 years, starting from the date of your incarceration (July 15, 2002). Therefore, your responses to questions 29(d) and 29(e) on the April 2, 2009 Research Site Submission Form should have been "yes," and, as instructed by the form, you should have attached a written explanation and copies of all the relevant documentation regarding your conviction and medical license suspension.

After the (b)(4) IRB learned that your April 2, 2009 Research Site Submission Form was inaccurate,it withdrew it sapproval for Protocol (b)(4) and denied your application for approval to conduct a second proposed clinical study. In an August 7, 2009 letter to the (b)(4) IRB[1], you stated that a study coordinator completed the April 2, 2009 Research Site Submission Form, and completed questions 29(d) and 29 (e) without your input. However, by signing the April 2, 2009 Research Site Submission Form, you certified that you "had reviewed all responses provided in this 'Research Site Submission Form' and that all responses are true and accurate." (emphasis in original) Therefore, the fact that a study coordinator completed the form did not relieve you of your responsibility for ensuring its accuracy before you signed it. Moreover, in your August 7, 2009 letter to the (b)(4) IRB, you admitte that the responses to questions 29(d) and 29(e) in the April 2, 2009 form were inaccurate, and that you were "not diligent to the level required to certify complete accuracy of the forms."

Your failure to ensure that the April 2, 2009 Research Site Submission Form provided accurate information to the (b)(4) IRB impeded the IRB's ability to review your application to conduct Protocol (b)(4), and make a determination regarding the adequacy of that application. Therefore, you failed to assure IRB review of Protocol (b)(4) as required

---

1　Your August-7, 2009 leter appealed the (b)(4) IRB's decision to deny your application for approval to conduct the second proposed clinical study.

under 21CFR 312.66.

2. You failed to protect the rights, safety, and welfare of the subjects under your care [21CFR 312.60].

Under 21CFR 312.60, an investigator is responsible for protecting the rights, safety, and welfare of human subjects under the investigator's care. Compliance with 21CFR part 56, including the requirement for IRB review under 21CFR 56.109, is intended to protect the rights, safety, and welfare of human subjects involved in clinical investigations (21CFR 56.101). In order to adequately protect the rights, safety, and welfare of human subjects, IRBs need accurate information about the proposed investigations they are reviewing and the individuals who will be involved in conducting those investigations. Therefore, as part of an investigator's responsibility to protect the rights, safety, and welfare of human subjects, an investigator must provide accurate information to the IRB so that the IRB can fulfill its responsibilities with respect to protecting the rights, safety, and welfare of human subjects.

As explained above, the Research Site Submission Form that you signed and certified as accurate on April 2, 2009, provided false information to the (b)(4) IRB about your 2002 conviction and medical license suspension. By failing to ensure that the Research Site Submission Form provided accurate information to the (b)(4) IRB, you failed to protect the rights, safety, and welfare of the human subjects under your care, as required by 21CFR 312.60.

This letter is not intended to be an all-inclusive list of deficiencies with your clinical study of an investigational drug It is your responsibiligy to ensure adherence to each requirment of law and relevant FDA regulations. You should address these deficiencies and establish procedures to ensure that any ongoing or future studies will be in compliance with FDA regulations.

Within fifteen (15) working days of your receipt of this letter, you should notify this office in writing of the actions you have taken to prevent similar violations in the future. Failure to adequately and promptly explain the violation noted above may result in regulatory action without further notice.

If you have any questions, please contact Constance Cullity, M.D., M.P.H., at 301-796-3397; FAX 301-847-8748. Your written response and any pertinent documentation should be addressed to:

Constance Cullity (for merly Lewin),M.D.,M.P.H.
Branch Chief
Good Clinical Practice Branch I
Division of Scientific Investigations
Office of Compliance
Center for Drug Evaluation and Research
Food and Drug Administration
Building 51, Room 5354
10903 New Hampshire Avenue
Silver Spring, MD20993

Sincerely-yours,

{See appended electronic signature page}

Leslic-K.Ball, M.D. Director
Division of Scientific Investigations
Office of Compliance
Center for Drug Evaluation and Research
Food and Drug Administration

第106封　给David F. Scott医学博士的警告信

2010年10月20日

参考号：11-HFD-45-10-06

尊敬的Scott博士：

2010年3月15日至3月24日，S. Lori Brown博士和Sunitha Rajaram博士代表FDA与您会面，对您所开展的以下临床研究进行了现场检查：

- 试验方案（b）（4）[1]，“（b）（4）”，试验药物为（b）（4），申办者为（b）（4）。
- 试验方案（b）（4），“（b）（4）”，试验药物为（b）（4），申办者为（b）（4）。

本次现场检查是FDA的生物研究监查项目的一部分。该项目通过设定的检查方法，对研究的实施情况进行评估，并帮助确保这些研究中受试者的权益、安全和福利得到了保护。

经对现场检查报告、该报告的附件，以及您2010年4月6日的书面回复进行审查，我们认为您没有遵循适用的法律要求和监管临床研究实施及受试者保护的FDA法规。

在现场检查结束时，S. Lori Brown博士和Sunitha Rajaram博士向您出示了FDA483表，即现场检查发现的问题，并与您进行了讨论。我们想强调以下几点：

1. 您未能确保按照签署的研究者声明和研究计划进行研究［21 CFR 312.60］

a. 试验方案（b）（4）

i. 方案指出，“一旦受试者满足所有的入选标准且不满足任何排除标准，同时已完成膝关节置换手术，研究者或研究者的指派人将通过IVRS系统对受试者进行随机入组。”2008年5月7日，未经申办者批准您的豁免请求，十个受试者（受试者002，003，004，005，006，008，009，010，011和013）在手术前被随机入组，违背了方案。

ii. 方案要求在第10天（结束研究）或在提前终止，早于静脉造影，为每个随机受试者安排一次全面的体格检查，因为当天（第10天，第7次访视）要进行静脉造影。您没有为研究中的任何一个随机入组的受试者安排体格检查。

iii. 方案指出，第五次访视：“仅采集随机入组到（b）（4）研究中的受试者的血液样本进行药代动力学试验。样本应该在服药前，服药后2小时、6小时、12小时进行采集。”药代动力学（PK）的数据是（b）（4）研究的次要研究终点。

13个受试者中的11个（002，003，004，006，010，011，013，014，015，016和017）没有根据要求进行PK试验。（b）（4）试验的实验室文档表明没有收到样本，同时电子病例报告表表明没有采集PK样本。

iv. 申办者专门为每个临床研究设计了入/排标准，以优化研究中疾病进展数据的解释性，并最小化由于合并症和合并用药可能产生的相互作用对参与试验的受试者造成的可预见的危害。

方案的排除标准 #16 指出，“受试者正在服用阿司匹林的量大于162mg/d。”原始文件表明受试者4033017参与研究的同时，正在服用阿司匹林。

- 百服宁含有的阿司匹林剂量为325mg，在病例报告表（CFR）的合并用药中列出，开始日期为2006年，结束日期为(b)(6)。
- 此外，百服宁包含在原始文件(b)(6)中：在目前用药中，病史日期为(b)(6)。

1 (b) (4) 涉及商业秘密，根据法规内容不予公开。

- (b)(6)中还包含了医疗沟通和入院医嘱的文件：需要时口服1~2片阿司匹林（拜耳）[日期：(b)(6)]；且(b)(6)中，医疗沟通和入院医嘱指出：需要时口服1~2片阿司匹林（拜耳），最后服药为：(b)(6)。

ⅴ. 方案要求治疗结束或提前终止时进行双边静脉造影。16个随机受试者中的7位没有进行静脉造影检查。例如：

受试者017，018和019由于时间冲突和/或放射科诊所的技术问题，没有在治疗结束/第10天（第7次访视）时进行静脉造影。

ⅵ. 申办者在2008年6月16日发送给您一封信，指导您暂停筛选新的受试者进入研究中。但是，您在2008年7月23日筛选了受试者4033021进入研究中。

b. 试验方案（b）(4）

ⅰ. 方案要求在第6次访视（结束治疗）时，也就是静脉造影当天，进行体格检查。

受试者72001在2008年8月19日进行第6次访视（结束治疗），但是他/她没有在这次访视中进行体格检查。

ⅱ. 方案要求在第5次访视或出院当日将肝功能（LFT）监测的血液样本送到中心实验室。由于医院的失误，2008年7月25日（第5次访视），受试者72001的LFT血液样本没有被送到中心实验室。取而代之，这些实验室检测于2008年8月8日在当地实验室进行。

ⅲ. 方案要求在第1次访视/筛选访视时收集血液样本进行实验室评估。受试者72004在2008年7月18日进行了第1次访视，但直到2008年8月22日才收集到血液样本。

未能执行相关研究步骤危害了受试者的安全和福利，同时也影响了研究终点的解释性和有效性。

2. 您未能在实施研究的变更之前，获得伦理委员会的批准［21 CFR 312.66］

试验方案（b）(4）要求受试者的随机化在手术完成后进行。所有受试者均在手术前随机。在16个受试者中的10个随机后，申办者批准了您对此方案提出的豁免请求（于2008年5月7日）。但您未能获得IRB对这一变更的批准意见。

未经IRB批准对研究进行变更损害了参加临床研究的受试者的安全和福利。

3. 您未能保存研究中试验药物的受试者或对照组的受试者的所有研究观察结果和其他相关数据的足够准确的病历［21 CFR 312.62（b）］

a. 对于试验方案（b）(4），交互语音应答系统（IVRS）研究中心的用户手册中说明："联系IVRS之前完成电话工作表；再将完成的工作表与每个受试者的原始文件归档。"IVRS的工作表未被保存在受试者的文件中或在研究中心存档。

b. 对于试验方案（b）(4），原始文件中受试者的合格评定表没有填写。根据方案 6.2.1，第1次访视时："筛选阶段（−14到−天），根据入选/排除标准对患者是否合格进行预筛。"例如，受试者72003和72008的原始文件表明排除标准清单中的除了和血小板减少历史相关的排除标准之外的所有项目都已检查，包括肝素诱导的血小板减少，或血小板数量小于100000cell/μL。然而，电子病例报告表表明所有的排除/入选标准都已检查。

未能保存足够和准确的病历，影响了研究终点的解释性和有效性。

本警告信的目的并非是罗列您在试验药物临床研究中存在的所有缺陷。确保遵循法律和相关FDA法规的每一项要求是您的职责，您应当解决这些缺陷，并建立规程，以确保任何正在进行或将来进行的研究均符合FDA的法规。

自收到这封信的15个工作日内，您应当书面告知本办公室为预防将来发生类似违规情况而采取的措施。如果不能充分、迅速地解释上述违规问题，可能导致我们在不再通知的情况下采取监管措施。

附：英文原文

David F. Scott, M.D.

WARNING LETTER

OCT 20, 2010

CERTIFIED MAIL
RETURN RECEIPT REQUESTED

Ref: 11-HFD-45-10-06

David F. Scott, M.D.
785 E Holland Avenue
Spokane, WA 99218-1257

Dear Dr. Scott:

Between March 15 and March 24, 2010, Dr. S. Lori Brown and Dr. Sunitha Rajaram, representing the Food and Drug Administration (FDA), conducted an investigation and met with you to review your conduct of the following clinical investigations:

- Protocol (b)(4),"(b)(4)" of the investigational drug (b)(4), performed for (b)(4).
- Protocol (b)(4),"(b)(4)" of the investigational drug (b)(4), performed for (b)(4).

This inspection is a part of the FDA' s Bioresearch Monitoring Program, which includes inspections designed to evaluate the conduct of research and to help ensure that the rights, safety, and welfare of the human subjects of those studies have been protected.

From our review of the establishment inspection report, the documents submitted with that report, and your written response dated April 6, 2010, we conclude that you did not adhere to the applicable statutory requirements and FDA regulations governing the conduct of clinical investigations and the protection of human subjects. We are aware that at the conclusion of the inspection, Drs. Brown and Rajaram presented and discussed with you Form FDA 483, Inspectional Observations. We wish to emphasize the following:

1. You failed to ensure that the investigations were conducted according to the signed investigator statements and the investigational plans [21 CFR 312.60].

a. Protocol (b)(4):

i. The protocol states, "Once the subject meets all of the inclusion criteria and none of the exclusion criteria, and the knee replacement surgery has been completed, the investigator or the investigator' s designee will contact the IVRS to randomize the subject into the study." Ten subjects (Subjects 002, 003, 004, 005, 006, 008, 009, 010, 011, and 013) were randomized into the study before surgery, contrary to the protocol, prior to sponsor's approval of your request for exemption, dated May 7, 2008.

ii. The protocol required a complete physical examination for each randomized subject at Day 10 (completion of study) or upon early termination, prior to venography, for the day that the venogram was to be performed (Day 10, Visit 7). You failed to perform this physical examination for any of the randomized subjects in this study.

iii. The protocol states, for visit 5: "Collect blood samples for Pharmacokinetic testing for subjects randomized to (b)(4) only. The samples should be collected at pre-dose, 2, 6, and 12 hours post-dose." Pharmacokinetic (PK) data was a secondary endpoint of the (b)(4) study.

PK testing was not performed on 11 of the 13 subjects for whom it was required (002, 003, 004, 006, 010, 011, 013, 014, 015, 016, and 017). The (b)(4) laboratories document indicates that the sample was not received, and the eCRF indicates that PK collection was not performed.

iv. Eligibility criteria are designed specifically for each clinical investigation by the sponsor to optimize the interpretability of the data to the disease process under study and to minimize foreseeable harm to enrolled subjects due to comorbidities and possible interactions with concomitant medications.

Protocol exclusion criterion # 16 states, "The subject is taking aspirin > 162 mg/day." Source documents indicate that subject 4033017 was taking aspirin while participating in the study.

- Bufferin brand aspirin, with a dose of 325 mg, is listed in the case report form (CFR) under Concomitant Medication, with a start date of 2006 and an end date of (b)(6).
- In addition, Bufferin is included in the source documents (b)(6): Medical History dated (b)(6), under Current Medications.
- Documentation is also found in (b)(6), Medication Reconciliation, Admission Medication Orders: Aspirin (Bayer) 1-2 By Mouth As Needed (date: (b)(6)); and (b)(6), Medication Reconciliation, Admission Medication Orders: Aspirin (Bayer) 1-2 By Mouth As Needed, Last Taken: (b)(6).

v. The protocol indicates that a bilateral venography procedure was required at the End of Treatment or at Early Termination. Venography was not performed for 7 of 16 randomized subjects. For example:

Subjects 017, 018, and 019 did not have venography at the End of Treatment/Day 10 (Visit 7) due to scheduling conflicts and/or technical problems at the radiology clinic.

vi. The sponsor sent you a letter dated June 16, 2008, instructing you to suspend screening new subjects into the study. However, you screened Subject 4033021 into the study on July 23, 2008.

b. Protocol (b)(4):

i. The protocol requires a physical examination at Visit 6 (end of treatment) on the day of the venography procedure.

Subject 72001 had Visit 6 (end of treatment) on August 19, 2008. A physical examination was not conducted at this visit.

ii. The protocol requires a blood sample to be sent to the central laboratory for Liver Function Test (LFT) monitoring at Visit 5 or Day of Discharge. A blood sample for LFT was not drawn and sent to the central laboratory for Subject 72001 on July 25, 2008 (Visit 5) due to hospital error. Instead, these laboratory tests were performed in a local laboratory on August 08, 2008.

iii. The protocol requires a blood sample for laboratory evaluations at Visit 1/Screening Visit. Subject 72004 had Visit 1 on July 18, 2008, but blood samples were not collected until August 22, 2008.

Failure to perform study-related procedures jeopardizes subject safety and welfare, and compromises the interpretation and validity of the investigational endpoints.

2. You failed to obtain Institutional Review Board approval for changes in the research prior to implementing the changes [21 CFR 312.66].

Protocol (b)(4) required randomization of subjects after completion of the surgery. All of the subjects were randomized prior to surgery. After the randomization of 10 of the 16 subjects, sponsor approved your request for an exemption from this protocol requirement (dated May 7, 2008). You failed to obtain the IRB approval for this change.

Making changes in the research without IRB approval compromises the safety and welfare subjects enrolled in the clinical investigation.

3. You failed to maintain adequate and accurate case histories that record all observations and other data pertinent to the investigation on each individual administered the investigational drug or employed as a control in the investigation [21 CFR 312.62(b)].

a. For Protocol (b)(4), the Integrated Voice Response System (IVRS) site's user manual states: "Complete call worksheets prior to contacting the IVRS; then file completed worksheets with each subject's source documentation." The IVRS worksheets were not kept in the subjects' files or maintained at the site.

b. For Protocol (b)(4), subject eligibility forms in the source document were not filled out. The protocol states in Section 6.2.1, Visit 1: Screening period (Days -14 to Day -1),"Pre-Screen patient for eligibility by checking inclusion/ exclusion criteria." For example, source documents for Subjects 72003 and 72008 show that all the items in the exclusion criteria checklist are checked except for the exclusion criterion related to the history of thrombocytopenia, including heparin-induced thrombocytopenia, or a platelet count < 100,000 cells/micro liter. However, the eCRFs show that all the exclusion/inclusion criteria are checked.

Failing to maintain adequate and accurate case histories compromises the interpretation and validity of the investigational endpoints.

This letter is not intended to be an all-inclusive list of deficiencies with your clinical study of an investigational drug. It is your responsibility to ensure adherence to each requirement of the law and relevant FDA regulations. You should address these deficiencies and establish procedures to ensure that any ongoing or future studies will be in compliance with FDA regulations.

Within fifteen (15) working days of your receipt of this letter, you should notify this office in writing of the actions you have taken to prevent similar violations in the future. Failure to adequately and promptly explain the violations noted above may result in regulatory action without further notice.

If you have any questions, please contact Constance Cullity, M.D., M.P.H., at 301-796-3397; FAX 301-847-8748. Your written response and any pertinent documentation should be addressed to:

Constance Cullity (formerly Lewin), M.D., M.P.H.
Branch Chief
Good Clinical Practice Branch I
Division of Scientific Investigations
Office of Compliance
Center for Drug Evaluation and Research
Food and Drug Administration
Building 51, Room 5354
10903 New Hampshire Avenue
Silver Spring, MD 20993

Sincerely yours,

{See appended electronic signature page}

Leslie K. Ball, M.D.
Director
Division of Scientific Investigations
Office of Compliance
Center for Drug Evaluation and Research
Food and Drug Administration

第 107 封　给 O' Barr, Thomas Jr. 医学博士的警告信

2010年9月30日

参考号：10-HFD-45-09-05

尊敬的O' Barr博士：

2009年9月16日至9月30日，Stephanie Hubbard女士代表FDA与您会面，对您所开展的试验药物为（b）（4）[1]，申办者为（b）（4）的以下临床研究进行了审查：

试验方案（b）（4），标题为“（b）（4）”；

试验方案（b）（4），标题为“（b）（4）”。

本次现场检查是FDA的生物研究监查项目的一部分。该项目通过设定的检查方法，对研究的实施情况进行评估，以确认研究数据在科学上是有效和准确的，并帮助确保这些研究中受试者的权益、安全和福利得到了保护。

经对现场检查报告、该报告的附件，以及您2009年10月2日的书面回复进行审查，我们认为您没有遵循适用的法律要求和监管临床研究实施的FDA法规。在现场检查结束时，Hubbard女士向您出示了FDA483表，即现场检查发现的问题，并与您进行了讨论。我们想强调以下几点：

1. 您未能确保按照研究计划进行研究［21 CFR 312.60］

试验方案（b）（4）规定了在研究结束时，用于重建或者评定研究报告所需要的所有原始观察和研究活动所产生的原始数据，应在研究中心安全保存，在ICH区域的最终上市批准后至少保存两年，直到在ICH区域不再有任何未决的或预期的上市申请；或在试验药物的临床开发正式终止后至少保存两年。您未按照试验方案要求保存所有研究记录。

a. 特别是现场检查中发现，您未能提供试验方案（b）（4）中筛选的20名受试者或入组的10名受试者的病例报告表。

b. 在FDA的现场检查中，没有发现受试者500010的原始文件。

在您的书面回复中，您提到对受试者的评估中，您会收集受试者的病历，和受试者讨论此研究，并基于受试者的病历确定受试者是否适合参与研究。您提到您依靠研究协调员确保原始数据充分体现和记录了这些信息。此外，您还提到您应该自己查看这些记录，确保其恰当性。

您提到的您依靠研究协调员确保原始数据充分体现和记录了这些信息是不被接受的。作为临床研究者，您是最终的责任人，来确保研究按照研究计划规定的要求进行。

2．您没有保存研究中使用试验药物或对照组的受试者所有研究和观察结果及其他相关数据的足够和准确的病历［21 CFR 312.62（b）］

以下是试验方案（b）（4）中病历不完整和不准确的例子：

a. 以下是关于受试者500006的发现：

i. 有临床意义的实验室异常值的表格上有标注，确认第2周的访视没有发现有临床意义的实验室异常值。但是，第2周访视（2005年6月29日）的实验室报告以及第2周病程记录的手写注释说明，由于156mg/μL的异常高血糖值，您建议该受试者移交给他/她的主治医师。

在您对这一发现的书面回复中，您提到在审查实验室检查报告时，您会签名表明您已审阅。如果发现有

1 (b) (4) 涉及商业秘密，根据法规内容不予公开。

临床意义的实验室检查结果，您会和研究协调员讨论，再和受试者讨论。您提到您相信虽发现异常实验室检查结果，但任何一个都不具有临床意义，除了收到具体指导的需跟进特定值的患者。但您也承认记录没有临床意义的实验室检查结果的文件丢失了。

ii. 该受试者的第2周访视有两个视觉模拟量表。我们未能辨别哪个视觉模拟量表可以作为准确的原始记录。

b. 受试者500008的有临床意义的实验室非正常值的表和第4周访视的实验报告都表明，没有相关信息显示，是否在此次访视中发现了有临床意义的实验室非正常值。但在FDA对此次访视收集样品的实验室检查报告的审查中，却发现报告上的一些实验检测值超出了正常值范围，包括肌酸激酶、钾，以及血单核细胞的检测结果。

在您对这一发现的书面回复中，您提到在审查实验室报告时，您会签名，表明您已审查。如果发现有临床意义的实验室检测结果，您会和研究协调员讨论，再和受试者讨论。您提到，您相信虽发现异常实验室检查结果，但没有一个具有临床意义，除了收到具体指导的需跟进特定值的患者。但您也承认，记录没有临床意义的实验室检查结果的文件丢失了。

3. 您未能保存足够的包括日期、数量和受试者使用情况的药品处置记录［21 CFR 312.62（a）］

以下是试验方案（b）（4）中发现的例子：

a. 根据药品计数表，受试者500006在2005年7月12日被分配了瓶A和瓶B中的各66片药，且这些药片都没有被归还。但是，2005年7月22日的病程记录显示，该受试者归还了瓶A和瓶B中的各48片药。

b. 根据药品计数表，2005年7月9日，受试者500008归还了瓶A和瓶B中的各22片药，同时又被分配了瓶A和瓶B中的各66片新药。但第4周的研究文件显示，受试者500008试验药物的回收和分发发生在2005年7月12日。

c. 根据药品计数表，受试者500013在2005年6月28日被分配了瓶A和瓶B中的各66片药，这些药片均没有被归还。但是，2005年7月21日的病程记录显示，该受试者归还了瓶A中的31片药和瓶B中的29片药。

d. 根据药品计数表，受试者500015在2005年7月5日（基线访视）被分配了瓶A和瓶B中的各66片药；且在2005年7月20日（第2周访视），归还了瓶A和瓶B中的各35片药。但第1周访视（2005年7月12日）的病程记录显示，此次访视中在本研究中心发现了每瓶中都仅剩33片药。

在您的书面回复中，您认可这些发现。您提到您没有亲自审查药品计数表中每个受试者的分发和回收的药品数量，确保它们与临床病程记录数字一致。您也提到此项工作由研究协调员完成，这显然是不符合标准的，是您做出的一个错误判断。

您没有亲自审查药品计数表中每个受试者的分发和回收的药品数量，确保它们与临床病程记录数字一致的回复是不被接受的。作为临床研究者，确保完整保存药品分发记录是您的职责。

本警告信的目的并非是罗列您在试验药物临床研究中存在的所有缺陷。确保遵循法律和相关FDA法规的每一项要求是您的职责，您应当解决这些缺陷，并建立规程，以确保任何正在进行或将来进行的研究均符合FDA的法规。

自收到这封信的15个工作日内，您应当书面告知本办公室为预防将来发生类似违规情况而采取的措施。如果不能充分、迅速地解释上述违规问题，可能导致我们在不再通知的情况下采取监管措施。

附：英文原文

O'Barr, Thomas Jr. M.D.

WARNING LETTER

Sep 30, 2010

CERTIFIED MAIL
RETURN RECEIPT REQUESTED

Ref: 10-HFD-45-09-05

Thomas O'Barr, Jr., M.D.
1431 White Circle NW,
Marietta, GA 30066

Dear Dr. O'Barr:

Between September 16 and 30, 2009, Ms. Stephanie Hubbard, representing the Food and Drug Administration (FDA), conducted an investigation and met with you to review your conduct of the following clinical investigations of the investigational drug (b)(4) performed for (b)(4):

Protocol (b)(4), entitled "(b)(4)"

Protocol (b)(4), entitled "(b)(4)"

This inspection is a part of the FDA' s Bioresearch Monitoring Program, which includes inspections designed to evaluate the conduct of research and to help ensure that the rights, safety, and welfare of the human subjects of those studies have been protected.

From our review of the establishment inspection report, the documents submitted with that report, and your written responses to the Form FDA 483 dated October 2, 2009, we conclude that you did not adhere to the applicable statutory requirements and FDA regulations governing the conduct of clinical investigations. We are aware that at the conclusion of the inspection, Ms. Hubbard presented and discussed with you Form FDA 483, Inspectional Observations. We wish to emphasize the following:

1. You failed to ensure that the investigation was conducted according to the investigational plan [21 CFR 312.60].

Protocol (b)(4) specified that at conclusion of the study, all primary data that are a result of the original observations and activities of the study that are necessary for the reconstruction and evaluation of any study report will be retained in a secure archive at the study site, for a period not less than two years after the last approval of a marketing application in an ICH region, and until there are no pending or contemplated marketing applications in an ICH region; or, at least two years have elapsed since the formal discontinuation of the clinical development of the investigational product. You failed to maintain all study records as required by the study protocol.

a.Specifically, during the inspection you were unable to provide case report forms for Protocol (b)(4) for any of the 20 subjects screened or 10 subjects enrolled into the study.

b.There were no source documents found for Subject 500010 during the FDA inspection.

In your written response, you stated that in your evaluation of a subject, you would take the subject's clinical history, discuss the study with the subject, and make certain that based on the subject's clinical history, the subject was appropriate for the study. You stated that you counted on the study coordinators to make sure that the source data adequately represented and documented this information. You further stated that you clearly should have looked at the records yourself to ensure that they had been done appropriately.

Your statement that you counted on the coordinators to be sure that the source data adequately represented and documented this information is unacceptable. As the clinical investigator, it is your ultimate responsibility to ensure that the study was conducted according to the requirements set forth in the investigational plan.

2. You failed to maintain adequate and accurate case histories that record all observations and other data pertinent to the investigation on each individual administered the investigational drug or employed as a control in the investigation [21 CFR 312.62(b)].

The following are examples of inadequate and inaccurate case histories noted for Protocol (b)(4):

a. The following was noted for Subject 500006:

ⅰ. The Clinically Significant Abnormal Lab Values form had a checkmark in a box that confirmed there were no clinically significant abnormal lab values identified for the Week 2 visit. However, the laboratory report for the Week 2 visit (June 29, 2005) and the Week 2 progress note had handwritten notes stating that you recommended that this subject be referred to his/her primary care physician due to the abnormally high glucose value of 156 mg/dL.

In your written response to this finding, you stated that in your review of the labs, you would sign your name indicating that you had reviewed them. If there were labs of any clinical significance, you would discuss them with the study coordinators and then with the subjects. You stated that you believed while abnormal labs were indicated, none of them are clinically significant, except patients that received specific instructions to follow up for specific values. You, however, concurred that the documentation for the lack of significance in these laboratory values was missing.

ⅱ.There were two Visual Analog Scales for this subject for the Week 2 visit. We were unable to tell from the documents which Visual Analog Scale served as the accurate source record.

b. Subject 500008's Clinically Significant Abnormal Lab Values form and the laboratory report for the Week 4 visit showed no information related to whether clinically significant abnormal labs were identified at this visit. In FDA's review of the lab report for samples collected at this visit, however, there were some test measurements that were noted on the report as being outside the reference range, including the measurements for creatine kinase, potassium, and blood monocytes.

In your written response to this finding, you stated that in your review of the labs, you would sign your name indicating that you had reviewed them. If there were labs of any clinical significance, you would discuss them with the study coordinators and then with the subjects. You stated that you believed while abnormal labs were indicated, none of them are clinically significant, except patients that received specific instructions to follow up for specific values. You, however, concurred that the documentation for the lack of significance in these laboratory values was missing.

3. You failed to maintain adequate records of the disposition of the drug, including the dates, quantity, and use by subject [21 CFR 312.62(a)].

The following are examples noted for Protocol (b)(4):

a. Per the drug accountability log, Subject 500006 was dispensed 66 tablets of medication in Bottle A and 66 tablets in Bottle B on July 12, 2005, and none of these tablets were ever returned. However, the progress note dated July 22, 2005, states that the subject returned 48 tablets in Bottle A and 48 tablets in Bottle B.

b. Per the drug accountability log, on July 9, 2005, Subject 500008 returned 22 tablets of medication in Bottle A and 22 tablets in Bottle B, and was also dispensed 66 new tablets in Bottle A and 66 new tablets in Bottle B. However, a Week 4 study document shows that this exchange of study drug tablets for Subject 500008 occurred on July 12, 2005.

c. Per the drug accountability log, Subject 500013 was dispensed 66 tablets of medication in Bottle A and 66 tablets in Bottle B on June 28, 2005, and none of these tablets were ever returned. However, the progress note dated July 21, 2005, states that the subject returned 31 tablets in Bottle A and 29 tablets in Bottle B.

d. Per the drug accountability log, Subject 500015 was dispensed 66 tablets of medication in Bottle A and 66 tablets in Bottle B on July 5, 2005 (Baseline Visit); and on July 20, 2005 (Week 2 visit), 35 tablets of medication in Bottle A and 35 tablets in Bottle B were returned. The Week 1 visit (July 12, 2005) progress note, however, shows that your site identified only 33 tablets remaining in each bottle at this visit.

In your written response, you acknowledged these findings. You stated that you did not personally review the numbers for each subject in the Drug Accountability Log reports and ensure that they corresponded to the numbers entered in the progress notes in the clinical records. You also stated that counting on the work of the coordinators, which was obviously substandard, was clearly a misjudgment on your part.

Your response that you did not review the numbers for each subject in the Drug Accountability Log reports and ensure that they corresponded to the numbers entered in the progress notes in the clinical records, is unacceptable. As the clinical investigator, it is your responsibility to ensure the maintenance of adequate records of the disposition of the drug.

This letter is not intended to be an all-inclusive list of deficiencies with your clinical study of an investigational drug. It is your responsibility to ensure adherence to each requirement of the law and relevant FDA regulations. You should address these deficiencies and establish procedures to ensure that any ongoing or future studies will be in compliance with FDA regulations.

Within fifteen (15) working days of your receipt of this letter, you should notify this office in writing of the actions you have taken to prevent similar violations in the future. Failure to adequately and promptly explain the violations noted above may result in regulatory action without further notice.

If you have any questions, please contact Constance Cullity, M.D., M.P.H., at 301-796-3397; FAX 301-847-8748. Your written response and any pertinent documentation should be addressed to:

Constance Cullity (formerly Lewin), M.D., M.P.H.
Branch Chief
Good Clinical Practice Branch I
Division of Scientific Investigations
Office of Compliance
Center for Drug Evaluation and Research
Food and Drug Administration
Building 51, Room 5354
10903 New Hampshire Avenue
Silver Spring, MD 20993

Sincerely yours,

{See appended electronic signature page}

Leslie K. Ball, M.D.
Director
Division of Scientific Investigations
Office of Compliance
Center for Drug Evaluation and Research
Food and Drug Administration

第108封 给Snow, Lamar L.医学博士的警告信

2010年9月29日

参考号：10-HFD-45-09-05

尊敬的Snow博士：

2009年4月27日至5月7日，Barbara Wright女士代表FDA与您会面，对您所开展的试验药物为布洛芬（Amelior），申办者为Cumberland制药公司的临床研究进行了审查：试验方案008，A和B部分，标题均为“多中心随机双盲安慰剂对照的布洛芬注射液（IVIb）用于治疗成年患者术后镇痛的研究”。

本次现场检查是FDA的生物研究监查项目的一部分。该项目通过设定的检查方法，对研究的实施情况进行评估，并帮助确保这些研究中受试者的权益、安全和福利得到了保护。

经对现场检查报告、该报告的附件，以及您2009年10月16日的书面回复进行审查，我们认为，您没有遵循适用的法律要求和监管临床研究实施的FDA法规。在现场检查结束时，Wright女士向您出示了FDA483表，即现场检查发现的问题，并与您进行了讨论。

1. 您未能确保按照签署的研究者声明进行研究，您未能亲自参与或监管临床研究［21 CFR 312.60］

当您签署临床研究的研究者声明（FDA1572表）时，您同意承担该试验场所的临床研究者的职责。您的临床研究者的总体职责包括确保临床研究按照签署的研究者声明、临床试验计划及相关适用的法规进行；保护在您的监护下受试者权益、安全和福利并确保用于研究的药物受到控制（21 CFR 312.60）。基于签署的FDA 1572表，明确规定研究者将亲自参与或监管无法参与的部分试验。虽然研究者可以授权部分研究职责给有相关资质的人来执行，但作为临床研究者，您不能授权您的总体职责。检查员发现您对被授权人员的监管，不能充分确保所开展的临床研究遵守了签署的研究者声明、临床试验计划和相关适用的法规，以确保受试者的权益、安全和福利得到了保护。

我们认为，由于您的监管不利，导致该研究中发现了如下重大问题。

2. 您未能保存研究中使用试验药物或对照组的受试者的所有研究观察结果和其他相关数据的足够及准确的病历［21 CFR 312.62（b）］

a. 方案中规定，该研究的首要药效终点为通过监测总吗啡量，来考察患者在术后24小时内吗啡需求量相对安慰剂的降低。通过比较受试者的住院病历和受试者研究文件，检查员无法确定受试者接受吗啡的总剂量。例子包括但不局限于以下：

i. 入组在试验方案008号，A组中的受试者3255，住院病历和病例报告表（CRF）中记录的总吗啡数量不一致。在术后CPI-CL-008疼痛原始记录和CRF中包括，在1小时后持续给药吗啡40分或41分钟时（比如1340，1440，1541，2241等）的记录，并提示受试者在（b）（6）之间接受吗啡的总剂量为37mg。然而，综合医院麻醉后监护病房（PACU）在（b）（6）（完整年份不清晰）打印的报告和医院吗啡患者自控镇痛泵（PCA）报告发现，受试者在（b）（6）期间共接受了18mg吗啡。另外，根据医院麻醉废弃物记录，仅给予受试者15mg的吗啡。CRC备注表中在受试者病例病史页中有提出上述医院记录的不一致处，但未能提供任何解释；此外，也没有解决医院记录与CRF中总吗啡剂量不一致的问题。

ii. 入组在试验方案008，B组中的受试者7060，CRF中记录在（b）（6）期间，给予该受试者吗啡的总剂量为20mg。然而，这与医院记录中吗啡的总量不一致。举例说明，在（b）（6）天的医院PACU报告显示受试者服用了10mg 吗啡；在MAR中记录受试者在（b）（6）期间通过自控镇痛泵共服用了31.75mg的吗啡。综合MAR和PACU报告这两份医院记录表明，受试者总共服用了41.75mg的吗啡，而并非CRF中报告的20mg。

ⅲ. 入组在试验方案008，B组中的受试者6057，CRF中记录在（b）（6）期间术后24小时内，给予受试者总剂量为26mg的吗啡。然而，（b）（6）天的医院PACU报告表明，该受试者接受了 4mg的吗啡；在医院MAR记录显示，该受试者通过PCA共服用了总计39mg的吗啡。综合MAR和PACU报告这两份医院记录表明，受试者共服用了43mg 的吗啡，而并非CRF中报告的 26mg。

ⅳ. 入组在试验方案008，B组中的受试者8058，CRF记录在（b）（6）期间总共给予该受试者48mg的吗啡（40mg 通过PCA，8mg通过PACU给予）。然而，PCA患者术后24小时评价表中显示患者在（b）（6）期间通过PCA给予的吗啡总量为 17mg，而不是CRF中报告的 40mg。

b. 试验方案008，A组中受试者2256文件中，存在给药时间在医院原始记录和其他记录的不一致问题。具体而言，医院MAR记录明确表明预计14:20给予试验用药剂量 2，而实际发生时间为15:30。然而，术后疼痛原始记录CPI-CL-008表明，受试者在 14:20到14:50之间服用剂量 2。

c. 试验方案008，B组中受试者5059文件中，存在联合用药舒马曲坦服用时间在医院记录和其他记录的不一致问题。医院MAR记录明确表明，在（b）（6）天上午8:00给予舒马曲坦。然而，CRF中联合用药页记录的舒马曲坦服用时间为上午9:40。

3. 您未能确保按照进行计划研究［21 CFR 312.60］

a. 试验方案008，A组规定，如果在试验药物服药过程中或服药后出现任何不良反应（AE），研究者应在CRF相应处记录如下信息：AE描述；该AE是否与试验药物相关；发生日期和时间；缓解的日期和时间（或提示该AE正在继续发生的声明）；AE的严重性；AE的严重程度，AE与服用试验药物的关系；采用的治疗方法和AE的结果。治疗结束后的总结记录了受试者1252 48小时发生呕吐，需要输液治疗。然而，在CRF中该呕吐并没有被报告为一次AE。

b. 试验方案008，A组规定该研究为双盲，受试者、研究者和申办者都将对分配的治疗保持盲态，直到所有受试者都已经完成该方案且研究数据都已经被分析以后。方案还规定，受试者分配的治疗只在紧急情况下、有必要知道被分配的治疗时才被揭盲。尽管没有任何迹象表明会有例外，医院的用药记录（MAR）将受试者2251和4251的特别治疗（400mg布洛芬）暴露给研究人员，这违背了方案。

c. 试验方案008，A组规定在筛选期需要进行体格检查（-72小时到0小时）。受试者2251在2006年1月18日进行了方案规定的筛选期体格检查。然而，该患者直至（b）（6）才接受手术及后续的研究药物治疗，这期间的间隔大于72小时。

本警告信的目的并非是罗列您在试验药物临床研究中存在的所有缺陷。确保遵循法律和相关FDA法规的每一项要求是您的职责，您应当解决这些缺陷，并建立规程，以确保任何正在进行或将来进行的研究均符合FDA的法规。

自收到这封信的15个工作日内，您应当书面告知本办公室为预防将来再次发生类似违规情况而采取的措施。如果不能充分、迅速地解释上述违规问题，可能导致我们在不再通知的情况下采取监管措施。

附：英文原文

Snow, Lamar L. M.D.

WARNING LETTER

SEP 29, 2010

CERTIFIED MAIL
RETURN RECEIPT REQUESTED

Ref: 10-HFD-45-09-05

L. Lamar Snow, M.D
(b)(6) (home address)

DearDr.Snow:

Between April 27 and May 7, 2009, Ms. Barbara Wright, representing the Food and Drug Administratiol1 (FDA),conducted an investigation and met with you, to review your conduct of clinical investigations [protocol 008,parts A and B, both entitled "A multi-center randomized, double-blind, placebo-controlled trial of ibuprofen injection (IVIb) for treatment of pain in post-operative adult patients"] of the investigational drug ibuprofen (Amelior), performed for CumberlandPharmaceuticals.

This inspection is a part of the FDA' s Bioresearch Monitoring Program, which includes inspections designed to evaluate the conduct of research and to ensure that the rights, safety, and welfare of the human subjects of those studies have been protected.

From our review of the establishment inspection report, the documents submitted with that report, and your written response dated October 16, 2009, we conclude that you did not adhere to the applicable statutory requirements and FDA regulations governing the conduct of clinical investigations. We are aware that at the conclusion of the inspection, Ms. Wright presented and discussed with you Form FDA 483, Inspectional Observations.

1. You failed to ensure that the investigation was conducted according to the signed investigator statement, in that you failed to personally conduct or supervise the clinical investigation [21 CFR 312.60].

When you signed the Statement of Investigator (Form FDA 1572) for the above referenced clinical trial you agreed to take on the responsibilities of a clinical investigator at your site. Your general responsibilities as a clinical investigator include ensuring that the clinical trial is conducted according to the signed investigator statement, the investigational plan, and applicable regulations; protecting the rights, safety, and welfare of subjects under your care; and ensuring control of drugs under investigation [21 CFR 312.60]. By signing Form FDA 1572, you specifically agreed to personally conduct the clinical trial or to supervise those aspects of the trial that you did not personally conduct. While you may delegate certain study tasks to individuals qualified to perForm them, as a clinical investigator you may not delegate your general responsibilities. Our investigation indicates that your supervision of personnel to whom you delegated study tasks was not adequate to ensure that the clinical trial was conducted according to the signed investigator statement, the investigational plan, and applicable regulations, and in a manner that protects the rights, safety, and welfare of human subjects.

We note that your failure to adequately supervise this study led to significant problems identified below with the conduct of the study.

2. You failed to maintain adequate and accurate case histories that record all observations and other data pertinent to the investigation on each individual administered the investigational drug or employed as a control in the investigation [21 CFR 312.62(b)].

a. The primary efficacy endpoint of the protocol was to measure the reduction in the requirement for morphine use in the 24 hours following surgery measured by total morphine usage compared to placebo. We are unable to determine the total morphine dose administered to subjects as documented in the hospital records, compared to the documents in the subject's files. Examples include, but are not limited to, the following:

i. Regarding Subject 3255, enrolled in protocol 008, partA, there are discrepancies in the total administered dose of morphine, as reflected in hospital records and the Case Report Form (CRF). The CPI-CL-008 Post Operative Pain Source Document and the CRF contain documentation of morphine administered consistently 40 or 41minutes after the hour (e.g.1340, 1440, 1541, 2241, etc.), and indicate that the subject was given a total dose of 37mg of morphine between (b)(6). However, summing up the doses in the hospital Post Anesthesia Care Unit (PACU) report printed on (b)(6) (full year not legible) and the hospital Morphine Patient Control Analgesia (PCA) report reveals that the subject received a total of 18 mg of morphine between (b)(6). In addition, based on the hospital's narcotic waste documentation, only a total of 15 mg of morphine was administered to this subject. , CRC Notes Form in the subject's case history addresses the discrepancy in the hospital records but does not offer any explanation; furthermore, it does not address the discrepancy between the total doses of morphine reflected in these hospital records and the CRF.

ii. Regarding Subject 7060, enrolled in protocol 008, part B, the CRF contains documentation to indicate that the subject was given a total of 20 mg of morphine between (b)(6). However, hospital records indicate that the subject received a different total amount of morphine. For example, the hospital PACU report dated (b)(6), indicates that the subject received a 10 mg dose of morphine; and the hospital Medication Administration Record (MAR) reveals that a total dose of 31.75 mg of morphine was administered to the subject via patient controlled analgesia between (b)(6). Viewed together, these two hospital records (the MAR and PACU reports) indicate that the subject received a total dose of 41.75 mg of morphine, not the 20 mg reported in the CRF.

iii. Regarding Subject 6057, enrolled in protocol 008, partB, the CRF contains documentation to indicate that the subject was given a total of 26 mg of morphine between (b)(6), in the 24 hours following surgery. However, the hospital PACU report dated (b)(6) revealed that the subject received a 4 mg dose of morphine; and the hospital MAR revealed that a total dose of 39 mg of morphine was administered to the subject via PCA between (b)(6). Viewed together, these hospital records indicate that the subject received a total dose of 43 mg of morphine, not the 26 mg reported in the CRF.

iv. Regarding Subject 8058, enrolled in protocol 008, part B, the CRF indicates that the subject was given a total of 48 mg of morphine (40 mg from PCA and 8 mg from PACU) between (b)(6). However, the PCA Patient Assessment 24 Hour Flow sheet indicates that a total dose of 17 mg of morphine was administered to the subject via PCA between (b)(6),not the 40 mg reported in the CRF.

b. Regarding protocol 008, part A, there were discrepancies between the hospital records and other documentation in Subject 2256's file regarding the time of study drug administration. Specifically, the hospital MAR indicates that Dose 2 of the study drug was to be administered at 14:20, but was given at 15:30. However, the CPI-CL-008 Post Operative Pain Source Document indicates that the subject received Dose 2 from 14:20-14:50.

c. Regarding protocol 008, part B, there was a discrepancy between the hospital records and other documentation in subject 5059's file regarding the time of Imitrex administration, a concomitant medication. Specifically, the hospital MAR indicates that Imitrex was given at 8:00 a.m. on (b)(6). However, the concomitant medications page of the CRF indicates that Imitrex was dispensed at 9:40 a.m.

3. You failed to ensure that the investigation was conducted according to the investigational plan [21 CFR 312.60].

a. Protocol 008, part A specified that if any adverse event (AE) occurs during or after dosing with the study drug, the investigator will record the following information on the appropriate pages of the CRF: the AE; whether or not the AE was judged to be study drug related; the date and time of occurrence; date and time of resolution (or a statement to indicate that it is still ongoing); severity of the AE; seriousness of the AE; relationship of the AE to study drug administration; treatment used; and outcome of the AE. The Discharge Summary noted that Subject 1252 had an episode of about 48 hours of vomiting requiring intravenous fluids. However, vomiting was not reported as an adverse event on the CRF.

b. Protocol 008, part A specified that the study will be double-blind and that the subject, investigator, and sponsor will be blinded to the assigned treatment until all subjects have completed the protocol and after the study database has been analyzed. The protocol also specified that a subject's treatment assignment will be revealed only in the case of an emergency, when it would be imperative for the assignment to be known. Despite the absence of any indication that an exception was warranted, the hospital Medication Administration Record (MAR) for Subjects 2251and 4251revealed their particular treatment arm (400 mg of ibuprofen) to study staff, in violation of the protocol.

c. Protocol 008, part A specified that a physical examination was required during the screening/baseline period (Hour -72 to Hour 0). The protocol-required screening/baseline physical examination for Subject 2251was performed on January 18, 2006. However, the surgery and subsequent treatment with study drug did not take place until (b)(6), which is more than 72 hours from the date of the screening physical examination.

This letter is not intended to be an all-inclusive list of deficiencies with your clinical study of an investigational drug. It is your responsibility to ensure adherence to each requirement of the law and relevant FDA regulations. You should address these deficiencies and establish procedures to ensure that any ongoing or future studies will be in compliance with FDA regulations.

Within fifteen (15) working days of your receipt of this letter, you should notify this office in writing of the actions you have taken to prevent similar violations in the future. Failure to adequately and promptly explain the violations noted above may result in regulatory action without further notice. If you have any questions, please contact Constance Cullity,M.D.,M.P.H., at 301-796-3397; FAX 301-847 8748. Your written response and any pertinent documentation should be addressed to:

Constance Cullity (formerly Lewin), M.D., M.P.H.
Branch Chief
Good Clinical Practice Branch
Division of Scientific Investigations
Office of Compliance
Center for Drug Evaluation and Research
Food and Drug Administration
Building 51, Room 5354
10903 New Hampshire Avenue
Silver Spring, MD 20993

Sincerely yours,

{See appended electronic signature page}

Leslie K. Ball, M.D.
Director
Division of Scientific Investigations
Office of Compliance
Center for Drug Evaluation and Research
Food and Drug Administration

第 109 封　给 Picus, Joel 医学博士的警告信

2010年9月20日

参考号：10-HFD-45-09-02

尊敬的Picus博士：

2009年10月14日至10月28日，Katheleen Swat女士代表FDA与您会面，对您所开展的以下临床研究进行了现场检查：

试验方案（b）（4）[1]，标题为（b）（4），试验药物为（b）（4），申办者为（b）（4）。

试验方案（b）（4），标题为（b）（4），试验药物为（b）（4），申办者为（b）（4）。

试验方案（b）（4），标题为（b）（4），试验药物为（b）（4），申办者为（b）（4）。

本次现场检查是FDA的生物研究监查项目的一部分。该项目通过设定的检查方法，对研究的实施情况进行评估，并帮助确保这些研究中受试者的权益、安全和福利得到了保护。

经对现场检查报告及该报告的附件进行审查，我们认为，您没有遵循适用的法律要求和监管临床研究实施及受试者保护的FDA法规。在现场检查结束时，Swat女士向您出示了FDA483表，即现场检查发现的问题，并与您进行了讨论。您于2009年11月11日和2010年1月6日对该FDA483表的书面回复已收悉。我们想强调以下几点：

1. 您未能亲自参与进行临床研究或对研究进行监管［21 CFR 312.60］

当您签署上述临床试验研究者声明（FDA1572表）时，您同意承担该试验场所的临床研究者职责。作为临床研究者，您的总体职责包括确保临床试验按照签署的研究者声明、临床试验计划及适用的法规进行；并保护您监管下的受试者权益、安全和福利［21 CFR 312.60］。基于签署的FDA 1572表，您明确同意将亲自参与临床试验或对您不能亲自实施的部分进行监督。尽管您可以将某些研究任务授权给有相关资质的人来执行，但作为临床研究者，您不能授权您的总体职责。我们的检查发现，您对授权人员的监管不足以确保所开展的临床试验按照签署的研究者声明、临床试验计划和适用的法规进行，并达到了受试者的权益、安全和福利的程度。

由于您的监管不利，导致以下所述的重大问题。

2. 您未能确保按照研究计划进行研究，未能保护在您的监护下的受试者的权益、安全和福利［21 CFR 312.60］

作为临床研究者，您有责任确保研究按照签署的研究者声明、研究计划，以及适用的法规进行，并研究受试者的权益、安全和福利。遵守方案规定的流程损害了人组该研究的受试者的安全和福利。具体而言：

a. 试验方案（b）（4）规定在受试者给药前24小时前需采集血样标本进行血常规和生化检查，并对检查结果进行审查。方案进一步规定肝功能检查（LFT）结果必须进行审查，以确定剂量调整和停止治疗。

我们的检查发现，没有文件证明受试者040-001 的肝功能检查结果按照方案规定的剂量改变或者暂停被您或者您的研究团队审阅，受试者于2009年4月3日给药了。

在（b）（6），受试者040-001因呕吐和发热的症状而进行紧急医疗抢救。受试者040-001在（b）（4）被主治医生宣告死亡。死因为多器官衰竭造成的严重代谢酸中毒导致的心跳骤停。

在病例报告表随访页日期为2009年10月7号，您报告了受试者040-001死于肝衰竭。您报告该死亡不是缘

1 （b）（4）涉及商业秘密，根据法规内容不予公开。

于胃肠道间质瘤（GIST），且死亡和试验药物的关系是“可能”。您同时记录一个方案违背：受试者040-001于2009年4月3日肝功能检查升高，尽管方案规定应当停药，但仍进行了治疗。

b. 试验方案（b）（4）规定试验药物需要由药师或者受过细胞毒性药物安全处理和管理培训的指定人员来配制。

受试者040-001的输液配制表显示，该试验药物于2009年的3月24，27，31和4月3日分别由一个首字母简写为（b）（6）的人员配制。试验记录了该人员为药师或者授权者，且被培训过细胞毒性药物的安全处理和给药。

在您2009年11月11日的回复中，您承认了有些流程并没有得到良好的执行，在给予受试者治疗前异常的实验室结果也没有被研究人员审阅过，且试验药物没有按照方案的规定暂停。另外，您指出您未能保存准确的人员授权表，其中标识出（b）（6）以及授权给他的责任。

我们收到您的回复，您已经实施了一个正式的双重检查流程，需要证明药房在分发试验药物前，一个注册护士（RN）记录他/她对实验室检查结果的审查，而且另一个注册护士进行一次独立和自主的审查。您的回复已收到，如果是按照此回复来执行，那么此回复是可以接受的。此外，您还进一步指出您正在修改人员编制，以便所有与研究有关的事项都由受过培训的研究人员中的限定人员来执行。我们担心此回复不足以预防上述违规情况再次发生。

3. 您未能按 21 CFR 50 的要求获得知情同意［21 CFR 312.60］

除了21 CFR 50.23和21 CFR 50.24规定的之外，不允许研究者让任何人类作为受试者参与到临床试验中，除非该研究者已经获取了受试者或者受试者的合法授权代表的合法有效的知情同意［21 CFR 50.20］。知情同意必须使用IRB批准的知情同意书来进行记录，并由受试者或其合法授权代表在知情时签署姓名及日期［21 CFR 50.27（a）］。

对于试验方案（b）（4），受试者040-001的筛选日期被报告为2009年3月19日。受试者2009年3月24日签署了伦理委员会批准的知情同意书。但是，受试者040-001的原始记录显示和试验相关的检测和流程在该知情日期前就开展了。2009年3月12日采集了一个血样标本用于试验筛选。2009年3月20日开具处方试验药物，2009年3月23日受试者随机入组到试验中。研究资格合格的心电图、眼部检查和一个血样的采集于2009年3月23日完成。

在您2009年11月11日的回复中，您承认了您未能在开展筛选流程前即获取受试者书面知情的事实，但是您在试验记录材料中记录了受试者的口头知情过程。法规中要求受试者在加入到试验前必须由他本人或合法授权代表在知情同意书上签名以及日期［21 CFR 50.20］。未能获取充分的知情同意。不给予受试者一个评估参与研究带来的风险和收益的机会，损害了入组受试者的安全和福利。

我们收到了您的回复。但是，这个回复是不充分的，因为您并没有提供纠正措施以预防上述的违规再次出现。尤其是您的回复并没有表明您正确理解了获取受试者合法有效的知情同意的法规。

4. 您未能保存足够的，包括日期、数量以及受试者的使用情况的药物处置记录［21 CFR 312.62（a）］

对于试验方案（b）（4）的药物计数表是不完整、不准确的。在日期、序列标签号以及药物的鉴认标签码上都有差异。例子包括但不限于以下：

a. 试验药物的主计数表没有记录2009年9月29日接收的所有药物。接收单上有药盒754083，765462以及842798的记录，但是在试验药物的主计数表上没有记录。

b. 2009年10月7日接收的试验药物，箱号为00690997和00696204在试验药物的主计数表记录了两次。

c. 受试者6111-08201的受试者专用试验药物计数表中，缺少受试者Ⅳ包的尺寸、配制的总剂量以及使用的IV包数量的完整记录。

我们注意到，您承认您未能充分、正确记录药物计数记录的事实。我们也收到您在书面回复描述的您已经采取的预防将来药物计数不一致的纠正措施。如果实施恰当的话，我们认为这些纠正措施是充足的。

本警告信的目的并非是罗列您在药物临床研究中存在的所有缺陷。确保遵循法律和相关FDA法规的每一项要求是您的职责，您应当解决这些缺陷，并建立规程，以确保任何正在进行或将来进行的研究均符合FDA的法规。

自收到这封信的15个工作日内，您应当书面告知本办公室为预防将来发生类似违规情况而采取的措施。如果不能充分、迅速地对上述违规问题进行解释，可能导致我们在不再通知的情况下采取监管措施。

附：英文原文

Picus, Dr. Joel

WARNING LETTER

SEP 20, 2010

CERTIFIED MAIL
RETURN RECEIPT REQUESTED

Ref: 10-HFD-45-09-02

Joel Picus, M.D
Washington University of St. Louis
660 South Euclid, Box 8056
St. Louis, MO 63110

Dear Dr. Picus:

Between October 14 and 28, 2009, Ms. kathleen Swat, representing the Food and Drug Administration (FDA), conducted an investigation and met with you, to review your conduct of the following clinical investigations:

Protocol (b)(4), entitled (b)(4) of the investigational drug (b)(4), performed for (b)(4).

Protocol (b)(4), entitled (b)(4) of the investigational drug (b)(4), performed for (b)(4).

Protocol (b)(4), entitled (b)(4) of the investigational drug (b)(4), performed for (b)(4).

This inspection is a part of FDA's Bioresearch Monitoring Program, which includes inspections designed to evaluate the conduct of research and to help ensure that the rights, safety, and welfare of the human subjects of those studies have been protected.

From our review of the establishment inspection report and the documents submitted with that report, we conclude that you did not adhere to the applicable statutory requirements and FDA regulations governing the conduct of clinical investigations and the protection of human subjects. We are aware that at the conclusion of the inspection, Ms. Swat presented and discussed with you Form FDA 483, Inspectional Observations. We acknowledge receipt of your responses dated November 11, 2009, and January 6, 2010, to Form FDA 483. We wish to emphasize the following:

1. You failed to personally conduct or supervise the clinical investigation [21 CFR 312.60].

When you signed the Statement of Investigator (Form FDA 1572) for the above-referenced clinical trials, you agreed to take on the responsibilities of a clinical investigator at your site. Your general responsibilities as a clinical investigator include ensuring that the clinical trial is conducted according to the signed investigator statement, the investigational plan, and applicable regulations; protecting the rights, safety, and welfare of subjects under your care; and ensuring control of drugs under investigation [21 CFR 312.60]. By signing a Form FDA 1572, you specifically agreed to personally conduct the clinical trial or to supervise those aspects of the trial that you did not personally conduct. While you may delegate certain study tasks to individuals qualified to perform them, as a clinical investigator, you may not delegate your general responsibilities. Our investigation indicates that your supervision of personnel to whom you delegated study tasks was not adequate to ensure that the clinical trial was conducted according to the signed investigator statement, the investigational plan, and applicable regulations, and in a manner that protected the rights, safety, and welfare of human subjects. Your failure to adequately supervise led to significant problems with the conduct of the study described below.

2. You failed to ensure that the investigation was conducted according to the investigational plan, and you failed to protect the rights, safety, and welfare of the subjects under your care [21 CFR 312.60].

As the clinical investigator, you are responsible for ensuring that the investigation is conducted according to the signed investigator statement, the investigational plan, and applicable regulations, and for protecting the rights, safety, and welfare of study subjects. Failure to adhere to protocol-specified procedures compromises the safety and welfare of subjects enrolled in the clinical investigation. Specifically:

a. Protocol (b)(4) specified that blood samples for chemistry and hematology should be drawn and the test results should be reviewed within the 24 hours prior to dose administration. The protocol further specified that Liver Function Test (LFT) results must be reviewed for dose modification and withholding of treatment.

Our investigation found no documentation that Subject 040-001's LFT results were reviewed by you or your research staff for the protocol-specified procedures for dose modification and withholding treatment, and the subject was dosed on April 3, 2009.

On (b)(6), Subject 040-001 was taken for emergency medical care with symptoms of vomiting and fever. Subject 040-001 was pronounced dead on (b)(6), by the attending physician, with the cause of death being attributed to cardiac arrest due to severe metabolic acidosis due to multiorgan failure.

In a follow-up case report form dated October 7, 2009, you reported that Subject 040-001 died of liver failure. You reported that the death was not due to a gastrointestinal stromal tumor (GIST), and that the relationship of the death to the study drug was "probable." You also documented the protocol deviation that Subject 040-001 was treated on April 3, 2009, with elevated LFT, although the protocol specified that the dose should have been withheld.

b. Protocol (b)(4) specified that study drugs were to be prepared by the pharmacist or designee who was trained in the safe handling and administration of a cytotoxic agent.

The Infusion Preparation Log for Subject 040-001 documents that study drugs were prepared on March 24, March 27, March 31, and April 3, 2009, by an individual identified only by the initials (b)(6). There was no documentation in the study records that (b)(6) was the pharmacist or designee, or that (b)(6) had been trained in the safe handling and/or administration of a cytotoxic agent.

In your response dated November 11, 2009, you acknowledge that a number of procedures were not appropriately followed, that the abnormal laboratory results were not reviewed by staff prior to treatment, and that the study drug was not withheld as the protocol specified. Further, you indicated that you failed to maintain an accurate Delegation of Authority log that identified (b)(6) and the responsibilities delegated to (b)(6).

We acknowledge your response that you have implemented a formal double check process that requires proof that one registered nurse (RN) documents his/her review of the laboratory values and that a second RN documents a separate and independent review, prior to the Pharmacy dispensing study medications. Your response is acknowledged and is acceptable if implemented as proposed. In addition, you further indicated that you are revising staffing, so that all matters pertaining to studies will be performed by a restricted subset of trained research staff members. We acknowledge your response. However, we are concerned that the response is not adequate to prevent future recurrence of the violation noted above.

3. You failed to obtain informed consent in accordance with the provisions of 21 CFR Part 50 [21 CFR 312.60].

Except as provided in 21 CFR 50.23 and 21 CFR 50.24, no investigator may involve a human being as a subject in research unless the investigator has obtained the legally effective informed consent of the subject or the subject's legally authorized representative [21 CFR 50.20]. Informed consent must be documented by the use of a written consent form approved by the IRB and signed and dated by the subject or the subject's legally authorized representative at the time of consent [21 CFR 50.27(a)].

For Protocol (b)(4), Subject 040-001's screening date was reported as March 19, 2009. The subject signed the IRB-approved informed consent on March 24, 2009. However, source records for Subject 040-001 document that study-related tests and procedures were performed prior to the date of consent. A blood sample was collected for study screening on March 12, 2009; the investigational dose was prescribed on March 20, 2009; and subject randomization occurred on March 23, 2009. Study-qualifying electrocardiograms (ECG), an eye examination, and a blood draw were performed on March 23, 2009.

In your response dated November 11, 2009, you acknowledge that you failed to obtain written consent from the subject prior to conducting all screening procedures, but that you documented the subject's verbal consent process in study records.The regulations require that informed consent be signed and dated by the subject or the subject's legal representative prior to the subject's involvement in the investigation [21 CFR 50.20]. Failing to obtain adequate informed consent jeopardizes the safety and welfare of enrolled subjects by denying them an opportunity to assess the risks and benefits of their participation in the clinical investigation.

We acknowledge your response. However, the response is not adequate, because you did not propose corrective actions to prevent future recurrence of the violation noted above. In particular, your response did not indicate that you properly understand the regulations for obtaining the legally effective informed consent of the subject.

4. You failed to maintain adequate records of the disposition of the drug, including dates, quantity, and use by subjects [21 CFR 312.62(a)].

Drug accountability records are incomplete and inaccurate for Protocol (b)(4). There are discrepancies in dates, lot numbers, and drug identification numbers. Examples include but are not limited to the following:

a. Master Investigational Product Accountability Records do not account for all study drug received on September 29, 2009. Kits 754083, 765462 and 842798 listed on the Proof of Receipt record were not documented in the Master Investigational Product Accountability Record.

b. Investigational drug received on October 07, 2009, boxes 00690997 and 00696204, are documented twice in the Drug Accountability Records.

c. Subject Specific Investigational Product Accountability Records for Subject 6111-08201 lack complete documentation for IV Bag Size, Total Volume Prepared, and Number of IV Bags Used.

We note your acknowledgment that you failed to maintain adequate and accurate drug accountability records. We also acknowledge the corrective actions, described in your written response, that you have taken to prevent drug accountability discrepancies in the future. We find these corrective actions adequate, if implemented as proposed.

This letter is not intended to be an all-inclusive list of deficiencies with your clinical study of an investigational drug. It is your responsibility to ensure adherence to each requirement of the law and relevant FDA regulations. You should address these deficiencies and establish procedures to ensure that any ongoing or future studies will be in compliance with FDA regulations.

Within fifteen (15) working days of your receipt of this letter, you should notify this office in writing of the actions you have taken to prevent similar violations in the future. Failure to adequately and promptly explain the violations noted above may result in regulatory action without further notice.

If you have any questions, please contact Constance Cullity, M.D., M.P.H., at 301-796-3397; FAX 301-847-8748. Your written response and any pertinent documentation should be addressed to:

Constance Cullity (formerly Lewin), M.D., M.P.H.
Branch Chief
Good Clinical Practice Branch I
Division of Scientific Investigations
Office of Compliance
Center for Drug Evaluation and Research
Food and Drug Administration
Building 51, Room 5354
10903 New Hampshire Avenue

Silver Spring, MD 20993

Sincerely yours,

/S/

Leslie K. Ball, M.D.
Director
Division of Scientific Investigations
Office of Compliance
Center for Drug Evaluation and Research

第110封　给Nemechek Do Pa, Patrick的警告信

2010年6月28日

参考号：CBER -10-06

尊敬的Nemechek博士：

这封信特告知您2010年2月22日至3月22日FDA现场检查的结果。一名FDA检查员与您会面，并对您所实施的以下临床研究：试验方案（b）(4）进行了审查。本次检查是FDA的生物研究监查项目的一部分。该项目通过设定的检查方法，对研究的实施情况进行了评估，并确保这些研究中受试者的权益、安全和福利得到了保护。

在现场检查结束时，检查员向您出示并讨论了FDA483表，即现场检查发现问题。经对FDA现场检查报告、该报告附件进行审查，我们认为，您违反了发布在美国联邦法规第21篇312和50部分（21 CFR 312，50，法规详见http://www.gpoaccess.gov/cfr/index.html）、临床研究监管相关的法规。

以下列出的每个违规项均指出了CFR中的相应条款。我们想强调以下几点：

1. 您未能确保按照签署的研究者声明和研究计划来进行研究［21 CFR 312.60］

A. 在这项研究中招募的17名受试者中，有7名受试者不符合方案中规定的合格标准，如下面所述：

受试者编号	知情同意签署日期	疫苗接种日期	内容	入选/排除标准
(b)(6)	2007年5月25日	2007年6月20日	受试者曾被诊断为慢性丙肝病毒感染	入选要求丙肝病毒抗体阴性(anti-HCV)
(b)(6)	2007年5月30日	2007年6月20日	受试者在筛选期的CD4计数为537	如有 CD4细胞 350 t 500/Pl (组2a)将排除
(b)(6)	2007年5月30日	2007年6月20日	受试者在入组和筛查之前经抗病毒治疗（ARV）5个月	入组前经抗病毒治疗（ARV）后病情稳定期大于6个月方可入选
(b)(6)	2007年7月11日	2008年3月13日	受试者在筛选期和访视期重筛期病毒载量均大于400个拷贝	入选要求受试者抗病毒治疗中病毒载量低于400个拷贝
(b)(6)	2008年1月29日	2008年2月20日	受试者在2008年2月20日入选，2007年8月17日病毒载量为640个拷贝，2007年8月17和2007年9月17日病毒载量为640个拷贝	受试者要求保持病毒载量640个拷贝在2007年8月17日至少6个月
(b)(6)	2008年2月19日	2008年4月10日	受试者曾在2007年2月有过心肌梗死的病史	排除标准10：心肌梗死病史
(b)(6)	2008年2月27日	2008年3月19日	受试者筛选时的血糖低于正常值	第2和第6组入选标准：血糖在正常范围内

B. 在第4次随访时受试者（b）(4）未按方案要求进行病毒载量计数。

C. 在第5次随访时受试者（b）(4）未按方案要求进行尿妊娠测试。

D. 本方案第4.2节中，对HIV感染者入选标准，要求在研究之前由（b）(4）记录并确认HIV 1感染者情况。然而，在研究开始之前，您没有记录受试者（b）(4）的感染情况。

2. 您未能按 21 CFR 50 要求获得知情同意［21 CFR 312.60］

A. 从您2007年12月3日审阅伦理委员会有关知情同意书的信中了解到，这封信指导您使用有伦理委员会盖章的更新版知情同意书，重新获取所有正在参加研究及任何新的可能参加研究的受试者的知情同意。知情同意书更新是由于要执行方案修正版# 5。在以下7名受试者的后续访视中，您使用了旧版的知情同意书。

B.

	知情同意书签署日期	知情同意缺陷
(b)(6)	2007年12月13日	未使用2007年11月26日更新的现行版本的知情同意书
(b)(6)	2007年12月13日	未使用2007年11月26日更新的现行版本的知情同意书
(b)(6)	2008年2月19日	未使用2007年11月26日更新的现行版本的知情同意书
(b)(6)	2008年2月26日	未使用2007年11月26日更新的现行版本的知情同意书
(b)(6)	2008年2月27日	未使用2007年11月26日更新的现行版本的知情同意书
(b)(6)	2008年2月27日	未使用2007年11月26日更新的现行版本的知情同意书
(b)(6)	2008年4月24日	未使用2007年11月26日更新的现行版本的知情同意书

C. 受试者（b）(6）使用的知情同意书的版本适用于HIV阳性受试者。然而，这些受试者是以非HIV阳性受试者入组的，在第1组接种或未曾接种过疫苗（b）(4）。这些受试者分别在2008年1月30日和2007年5月25日签署了错误的签署同意书版本。

3. 您未能按要求保留记录，直至研究药物按拟定适应症上市申请获得批准后 2 年，如果没有提交上市申请或药物用于该适应症的上市申请未批准，则在研究终止者后 2 年［21 CFR 312.62（c）］

在您签署的FDA1572表，研究者声明，您同意对于研究按照21 CFR 312.62要求保留完整和准确的记录，并按照21 CFR 312.68要求，这些记录可供现场检查。然而，在现场检查过程中，因为计算机“死机”您不能提供原始文件。您还表示该研究的数据未记入病例报告表。为了保存未来的研究记录，我们要求您解释您的纠正措施计划。

本警告信的目的并非是罗列您在试验药物临床研究中存在的所有缺陷。确保遵循法律和相关FDA法规的每一项要求，并在您的监护下保护受试者的权益、安全和福利是您的职责。

您应当解决这些缺陷，并建立规程，以确保任何正在进行或将来的研究均能符合FDA的法规。

自收到这封信的15个工作日内，您应当书面告知本办公室为纠正违规并防止在当前或将来作为临床研究者的研究中发生类似违规行为已经采取或将要采取的措施。未能对本警告信进行回复并采取适当的纠正措施，可能导致我们在不再通知的情况下采取监管措施。根据21 CFR 312.70的规定，可能包括启动吊销资格的流程。

附：英文原文

Nemechek Do Pa, Patrick

Warning Letter

June 28, 2010

Ref: CBER -10-06

Patrick Nemechek,
D. O., PA 8101
W. 135th Street
Overland Park, Kansas 66223

Dear Dr. Nemechek:

This letter describes the results of a Food and Drug Administration (FDA) inspection that was conducted from February 22 through March 22, 2010. The FDA investigators, met with you to review your conduct of the following clinical study: **(b)(4)** This inspection was conducted as part of the FDA' s Bioresearch Monitoring Program, which includes inspections designed to review the conduct of research involving investigational drugs and to ensure that the rights, safety, and welfare of the human subjects of these studies have been protected.

At the end of the inspection, a Form FDA 483, Inspectional Observations, was issued and discussed with you. From our review of the establishment inspections report, and the documents submitted with the report, we have determined that you violated regulations governing the proper conduct of clinical studies involving investigational drugs, as published in Title 21, **Code of Federal Regulations (CFR)**, Parts 312 and 50 (available at http://www.gpoaccess.gov/cfr/index.html[1]).

The applicable provisions of the CFR are cited for each violation listed below. We wish to emphasize the following:

1. You failed to ensure that the investigation was conducted according to the signed investigator statement and the investigational plan. [21 CFR 312.60].

A. Of the seventeen subjects you enrolled in the study, seven did not meet the enrollment eligibility criteria set forth in the protocol, as described below:

Subject #	Date consent signed	Vaccination Date	Comments	Inclusion/Exclusion Criteria
(b)(6)	5-25-07	6-20-07	Subject had previous diagnosis of chronic hepatitis C virus infection.	Negative antibody to hepatitis C virus (anti-HCV) required for inclusion.
(b)(6)	5-30-07	6-20-07	Subject had a screening CD4 count of 537 during the screening visit.	Exclude if CD4 cells 350 t 500/Pl (Group 2a).
(b)(6)	5-30-07	6-20-07	Subjcct was on antiretroviral therapy (ARV) for 5 months prior to screening and enrollment.	On stable ARV for greater than 6 months prior to enrollment required for inclusion.
(b)(6)	7-11-07	3-13-08	Subject had a detectable viral load greater than 400 copies at both screening and complete rescreening visits.	Viral load less than 400 copies for subjects on ARV therapy required for inclusion.
(b)(6)	1-29-08	2-20-08	Subject was enrolled on 2-20-08 with a viral load of 640 copies on 08-1707 a viral load of 640 copies on 08-17-07 and 9-17-07.	Subjects are required to maintain viral a viral load of 640 copies on 08-17-07 greater than six months.

(Contd.)

Subject #	Date consent signed	Vaccination Date	Comments	Inclusion/Exclusion Criteria
(b)(6)	2-19-08	4-10-08	Subject had a past medical history of myocardial infraction in 02-07.	Exclusion criteria #10: History of Myocardial infarction.
(b)(6)	2-27-08	3-19-08	Subject had a serum glucose result that was below normal limits at screening.	Inclusion Criteria Group 2 # 6: Serum glucose within normal institutional limits.

B. The protocol-required viral load count was not performed for Subject (b)(4) at visit 4.

C. The protocol-required urine pregnancy test was not performed for Subject (b)(4) at visit 5.

D. Section 4.2 of the protocol, inclusion criteria for HIV infected subjects, requires HIV1 infection documented by (b)(4) and confirmed by (b)(4) prior to study entry. However, you failed to document the HIV infection of Subject (b)(4) prior to study entry.

2. You failed to ensure that informed consent was obtained in accordance with 21 CFR Part 50. [21 CFR 312.60].

A. A letter from your reviewing IRB dated 12-3-2007 instructed you to use the updated IRB-stamped consent forms and to reconsent all current and any new prospective subjects. The consent forms were updated to implement protocol amendment #5. You obtained informed consent using an obsolete consent form from the following seven subjects, at the time of their follow-up visits.

B.

	Signature Date of Informed Consent	Informed Consent Deficiency
(b)(6)	12-13-07	Failed to use the current version of the informed consent form dated 11-26-07.
(b)(6)	12-13-07	Failed to use the current version of the informed consent form dated 11-26-07.
(b)(6)	02-19-08	Failed to use the current version of the informed consent form dated 11-26-07.
(b)(6)	2-26-08	Failed to use the current version of the informed consent form dated 11-26-07.
(b)(6)	2-27-08	Failed to use the current version of the informed consent form dated 11-26-07.
(b)(6)	2-27-08	Failed to use the current version of the informed consent form dated 11-26-07.
(b)(6)	4-24-08	Failed to use the current version of the informed consent form dated 11-26-07.

C. You obtained informed consent from Subjects (b)(6) and (b)(6) with the version of the informed consent form intended for HIV positive individuals. However, these subjects were enrolled in the study as non-HIV positive subjects with or without previous (b)(4) vaccination in group 1. The subjects signed the wrong consent form on 1-30-08 and 5-25-07, respectively.

3. You failed to retain records required to be maintained for the period of two years following the date a marketing application is approved for the indication for which the drug is being investigated; or, if no application is filed or if the application is not approved for such indication, until two years after the investigation is discontinued. [21 CFR 312.62(c)].

At the time you signed the Form FDA 1572, Statement of Investigator, for the study, you agreed to maintain adequate and accurate records in accordance with 21 CFR 312.62 and to make these records available for inspection in accordance with 21 CFR 312.68. However, during the inspection, you stated that the source documents were not available because the computer "crashed." You also stated that the study data were not entered into the case report form directly. We request that you explain your corrective action plan for maintaining study records in the future.

This letter is not intended to contain an all-inclusive list of deficiencies in your clinical study of investigational drugs.

It is your responsibility as the clinical investigator to ensure adherence to each requirement of the law and applicable regulations, and to protect the rights, and welfare of subjects under your care.

Within fifteen (15) working days of receiving this letter, please provide written documentation of the actions you have taken or will take to correct these violations and prevent the recurrence of similar violations in current or future studies for which you are the clinical investigator. Failure to respond to this letter and to take appropriate corrective action could result in the FDA taking regulatory action without further notice to you. This could include the initiation of disqualification proceedings in accordance with 21 CFR 312.70.

Please send your written response to:

Solomon Yimam
Division of Inspections and Surveillance (HFM-664)
Office of Compliance and Biologics Quality
Center for Biologics Evaluation and Research
Food and Drug Administration
1401 Rockville Pike, Suite 200N
Rockville, Maryland, 20852-1448
Telephone (301) 827-1948

We also request that you send a copy of your response to the FDA office listed below.

Sincerely,

/S/

Mary A. Malarkey, Director
Office of Compliance and Biologics Quality
Center for Biologics Evaluation and Research
Cc: John Thorsky, Director
Kansas City District Office
Food and Drug Administration
11510 West 80th Street
Lenexa, Kansas 66214-3340

第111封　给Deitz, Robert医学博士的警告信

2010年4月1日

参考号：10-HFD-45-03-03

尊敬的Deitz博士：

2009年5月19日至28日，Aneel K.Sandhu 代表FDA进行了检查，与您会面并对您所实施的一项临床研究试验方案（b）(4)，题为“(b)(4)”，试验药物（b）(4)，申办者为（b）(4)进行了审查。

本次现场检查是FDA的生物研究监查项目的一部分。该项目通过设定的检查方法，对FDA所监管的相关研究的实施情况进行评估，并确保这些研究中受试者的权益、安全和福利得到了保护。

经对现场检查报告和该报告附件进行审查，我们认为，您没有遵循适用的法律要求和监管临床研究实施及受试者保护的FDA法规。我们注意到，现场检查结束时，Aneel K.Sandhu向您出示并讨论了FDA483表，即现场检查发现的问题。我们想强调以下几点：

1. 您未能保存研究中使用试验药物或对照组的受试者的所有研究观察结果和其他相关数据的足够及准确的病历［21 CFR 312.62（b）］

所有入选的临床研究（b）(4)的6个受试者的记录均存在缺陷，导致严重怀疑您实施的临床研究数据的可靠性。

a. 受试者34002，缺陷项如下：

ⅰ. 2005年1月20日，受试者34002入选本研究并服用试验药物。您于2005年5月2日递交伦理委员会的方案偏离/违规报告声明入选的受试者没有签署知情同意书（ICF）。此受试者病历中包含2份知情同意书复印件。一份知情同意书签于2005年5月10日，另一份知情同意书复印件经过修改的签字日期显示为2005年1月10日。FDA 现场检查时您提供给现场检查员担保书声明您认为签字日期为2005年1月10日的为修改的文件。您还阐明您没有修改这份文件，也不知该文件由谁修改。

ⅱ. 电子病例报告表的基线访视期记录这个受试者于 2005年1月20日签署知情同意书（ICF），然而根据基线访视工作记录清单，受试者于 2003年9月18日签署知情同意书（ICF）。受试者病历中无2003年9月18日和2005年1月20日签署知情同意书（ICF）。此外，如1（a）(ⅰ) 所述，此受试者病历中包含2份知情同意书复印件。一份知情同意书文件签于2005年5月10日，另一份知情同意书复印件经过修改显示签字日期为2005年1月10日。因此，显然基线访视期的电子病例报告表和基线访视工作记录清单没有准确记录受试者于 2005年5月20日签署知情同意书（ICF）。

ⅲ. 电子病例报告表中第12 个月访视记录描述2005年1月17日进行支气管舒张试验前肺活量测定，2006年1月17日进行支气管舒张试验后肺活量测定。然而第12个月访视工作记录清单记录显示2006年7月17日进行了这两次肺活量测定。我们注意到，您办公室经理在现场检查阐明这工作记录清单错误用于第24个月访视记录，实际应为第12个月访视记录。

ⅳ. 签字日期为2005年5月10日和2005年1月10日的1～5页知情同意书丢失了。

b. 受试者60060，缺陷项如下：2006年2月9日的30个月工作记录，在“过去6个月患者有以下问题？”的标记框标记“是”，有4个选项：非严重恶性肿瘤、严重恶性肿瘤、严重哮喘恶化，或其他严重不良事件。工作记录同一页指示如对这个问题的答案为“是”，需填写完成每个不良事件的工作记录，但是该受试者的病历中没有完成不良事件记录。

c. 受试者34004，缺陷项如下：

ⅰ. 第6个月访视工作表中不良事件内容矛盾，不能确认该受试者是否有不良事件发生。一页描述患者无非严重恶性肿瘤、严重恶性肿瘤、严重哮喘恶化，或其他严重不良事件。然而另一页答复不良事件是何类型的问题时，标记为非严重恶性肿瘤。

ⅱ. 知情同意书的1~8页丢失。

d. 受试者60667，第12个月访视工作表没有记录受试者在过去6个月内是否发生不良事件。

e. 受试者62694，缺陷项如下：

ⅰ. 第12 个月电子病例报告表中的访视记录描述2007年6月26日进行肺活量测定，然而第12个月访视工作记录清单记录2007年7月26日进行了肺活量测定。

ⅱ.知情同意书的第9页丢失。

2. 您未能按照 21 CFR 50 的要求获得知情同意［21 CFR 312.62（b）］

a. 在没有获取受试者34002法定有效的知情同意书之前，将受试者入选到临床试验，这违反了21 CFR 50.20法规。在1（a）（ⅰ）项中解释，受试者34002于2015年1月20 日入选到临床试验并服用了试验药物。您在2005年5月2日递交伦理委员会方案偏离/违背报告，描述这名受试者没有签署知情同意书。受试者病历中含有2份知情同意书复印件。一份知情同意书签于2015年5月10日，另一份知情同意书复印件签改日期为2015年1月10日。您在递交给FDA 现场检查员的担保书声明签字日期为2015年1月10日的知情同意书为修改文件，您也声明您没有修改此文件，不知是谁修改此文件。因此可见您在2015年5月10日受试者入选这项临床试验几个月后才获得知情同意书。

b. 对于3个受试者，您没有按照21 CFR 50.27 要求记录使用伦理委员会批准的知情同意书文件。具体而言下列受试者签署的知情同意书是未经伦理委员员批准的样本 ICF。

ⅰ. 受试者34002，签于2007年2月7日。

ⅱ. 受试者34004，签于2006年5月29日。

ⅲ. 受试者60060，签于2006年10月12日。

3. 您未能及时向 IRB 报告研究活动中的所有变更［21 CFR 312.66］

您没有递交伦理委员会审核并批准下列临床试验方案修正案。

a. 2007年10月15日A3方案修正案新增了肿瘤专家审查所有恶性肿瘤不良事件。

b. 2008年4月14日A4方案修正案增加了体格检查频率、系统频率、实验室检查结果审查频率和从仅在筛选、基线到每6个月的放射检查的审查。

4. 您未能确保按照签署的研究者声明、研究计划进行研究［21 CFR 312.60］

a. 方案规定临床试验由研究者（您）实施。您签署的研究者声明FDA1572 表证明您是研究者，没有授权研究者，然而下列受试者访视的临床检查是由（b）（4）医学博士实施的。

ⅰ. 受试者62694第12个月的访视。

ⅱ. 受试者34004第18个月的访视。

ⅲ. 受试者34004第30个月的访视。

ⅳ. 受试者60667第18个月的访视。

ⅴ. 受试者60060第12个月的访视。

b. 方案规定电话联系错失访视的受试者。受试者60667错失第6个月的访视，然而没有文件证明您试图联系这名受试者。

c. 方案规定在基线期访视时实施肺活量测定，然而您对下列受试者基线期访视时没有实施肺活量测定。

ⅰ. 受试者 34002：2005年1月20日基线期访视。2003年8月23日肺活量测定。

ⅱ. 受试者 34004：2005年5月12日基线期访视。2005年7月21日肺活量测定。

ⅲ. 受试者60060：2003年8月8日基线期访视。2004年6月24日肺活量测定。

5. 您未能保存足够的包括日期、数量、受试者的使用情况的药物处置记录［21 CFR 312.62（a）］

您没有保存受试者62694和34004的药物处置记录。

6. 您未能按照 21 CFR 312 的要求保存临床研究记录，直至临床研究终止并告知 FDA 后 2 年［21 CFR 312.62（c）］

申办者2008年6月13日信函通知您，终止您参加的试验方案（b）（4）的临床研究，因此您停止您的这项临床研究。申办者同日也书面通知了FDA，您参加的试验方案（b）（4）的临床研究终止了。然而2009年5月19日至28日，在FDA收到这一通知不到2年的时间内，Aneel K. Sandhu代表FDA对您参与实施的试验方案（b）（4）的临床试验进行现场检查。受试者60060、34004和34003 电子病例报告表没有保存。现场文件证明您没有保存受试者60060、34004和34003 电子病例报告表至临床试验终止后和FDA被通知后2年。

本警告信的目的并非是罗列您在试验药物临床研究中存在的所有缺陷。确保遵循法律和相关FDA法规的每一项要求是您的职责。您应当解决这些缺陷，并建立规程，以确保任何正在进行或将来的研究均能符合FDA的法规。

自收到这封信的15个工作日内，您应当书面告知本办公室为预防将来发生类似违规情况已经采取的措施。如果不能充分、迅速地解释上述违规问题，可能导致我们在不再通知的情况下采取监管措施。

附：英文原文

Deitz, Robert, M.D.

WARNING LETTER

APR 1, 2010

CERTIFIED MAIL
RETURN RECEIPT REQUESTED

Ref: 10-HFD-45-03-03

Robert Deitz, M.D.
2001 Union Street
Suite 625
San Francisco, CA 94123

Dear Dr. Deitz:

Between May 19 and 28, 2009, Aneel K. Sandhu, representing the Food and Drug Administration (FDA), conducted an investigation and met with you to review your conduct of a clinical investigation [Protocol (b)(4) entitled "(b)(4)"] of the investigational drug (b)(4), performed for (b)(4).

This inspection is a part of FDA' s Bioresearch Monitoring Program, which includes inspections designed to evaluate the conduct of research and to ensure that the rights, safety, and welfare of the human subjects of the study have been protected.

From our review of the establishment inspection report and the documents submitted with that report, we conclude that you did not adhere to the applicable statutory requirements and FDA regulations governing the conduct of clinical investigations and the protection of human subjects. We are aware that at the conclusion of the inspection, Aneel K. Sandhu presented and discussed with you Form FDA 483, Inspectional Observations. We wish to emphasize the following:

1. You failed to maintain adequate and accurate case histories that record all observations and other data pertinent to the investigation on each individual administered the investigational drug or employed as a control in the investigation [21 CFR 312.62(b)].

Discrepancies in records were found in all six subjects enrolled in Protocol (b)(4), raising significant questions about the reliability of data at your site.

a. For Subject 34002, the following deficiencies were noted:

i. On January 20, 2005, this subject was enrolled in the study and was administered the study drug. You submitted a protocol deviation/violation report to the Institutional Review Board (IRB) on May 2, 2005 stating that this subject was enrolled without having signed an Informed Consent Form (ICF). The subject's records contained two copies of the ICF. One was signed on May 10, 2005, and another copy was an altered version which reflected a signature date of January 10, 2005. You stated in your affidavit obtained by the field investigator during the FDA inspection that you believe that the ICF with a signature date of January 10, 2005 is an altered document. You stated that you did not alter the document and that you do not know who altered it.

ii. The electronic Case Report Form (eCRF) for the Baseline Visit states that the subject signed the ICF on January 20, 2005. However, according to the Baseline Visit worksheet, the ICF was signed on September 18, 2003. The subject's records did not contain an ICF dated September 18, 2003 or January 20, 2005. In addition, as stated above under 1(a)(i), the subject's records contained two copies of the ICF, one copy was signed on May 10, 2005 and the other was altered to indicate it was signed on January 10, 2005. Thus, it appears that the subject signed the ICF on May 10, 2005, which was not accurately recorded in the Baseline Visit eCRF or worksheet.

iii. The eCRF for the 12-Month Visit states that pre-bronchodilator spirometry was conducted on January 17, 2005 and that post-bronchodilator spirometry was conducted on January 17, 2006. However, the 12-Month Visit worksheet states that both of these spirometries were conducted on July 17, 2006. We note that your office manager stated during the inspection that this worksheet was mistakenly documented as the 24-month visit, but was in fact the 12-Month Visit worksheet.

iv. Pages 1 through 5 were missing from the ICFs dated May 10, 2005 and January 10,2005.

b. For Subject 60060, the following deficiency was noted: The February 9, 2006 30-Month Visit worksheet contains a check mark in the box labeled "Yes" for the question, "Has the patient had any of the following during the past 6 months?" These four choices follow the question: non-serious malignancy, serious malignancy, serious asthma exacerbation, and other serious adverse event. The same page of the worksheet indicates that if the answer to this question is "yes," an adverse event (AE) worksheet packet is to be completed for each AE. However, no completed AE worksheet packet was in the subject's records.

c. For Subject 34004, the following deficiencies were noted:

i. The AE section of the 6-Month Visit worksheet contained conflicting information about whether the subject suffered an AE or not. On one page, it states that the patient did not have a non-serious malignancy, serious malignancy, serious asthma exacerbation, or other serious adverse event. However, on another page, in response to the question "What type of adverse event was this?" the "non-serious malignancy" box is checked.

ii. Pages 1 through 8 were missing from the ICF.

d. For Subject 60667, the12-Month Visit worksheet did not document the subject's response regarding whether an adverse event had been experienced in the previous six months.

e. For Subject 62694, the following deficiencies were noted:

i. The eCRF for the 12-Month Visit states that spirometry was conducted on June 26,2007. However, the 12-Month Visit worksheet states that the spirometry was conducted on July 26, 2007.

ii. Page 9 was missing from the ICF.

2. You failed to obtain informed consent in accordance with the provisions of 21 CFR part 50 [21 CFR 312.60].

a. Subject 34002 was enrolled in the study before you obtained the subject's legally effective informed consent, in violation of 21 CFR 50.20. As explained above under 1(a) (i), on January 20, 2005, Subject 34002 was enrolled in the study and was administered the study drug. You submitted a protocol deviation/violation report to the IRB on May 2,

2005 stating that this subject was enrolled without having signed an informed consent form. The subject's records contained two copies of the informed consent form. One was signed on May 10, 2005, and another copy was an altered version which reflected a signature date of January 10, 2005. You stated in your affidavit obtained by the field investigator during the FDA inspection that you believe that the ICF with a signature date of January 10, 2005 is an altered document. You stated that you did not alter the document and that you do not know who altered it. Thus, available documentation indicates that you did not obtain the subject's informed consent until May 10, 2005, months after the subject was enrolled in the study.

b. For three subjects, you failed to document informed consent by the use of a written consent form approved by the IRB, as required by 21 CFR 50.27. Specifically, ICFs, signed by the following subjects on the indicated dates, were sample ICFs, which were not approved by the IRB:

i. Subject 34002, signed on February 7, 2007

ii. Subject 34004, signed on May 29, 2006

iii. Subject 60060, signed on October 12, 2006

3. You failed to promptly report to the IRB all changes in the research activity [21 CFR 312.66].

The following Protocol Amendments were not submitted to the IRB for review and approval:

a. Amendment A3 dated October 15, 2007, which contained additional information regarding expert oncology review of all malignancy adverse events.

b. Amendment A4 dated April 14, 2008, which increased the frequency of physical examination, review of systems, review of laboratory results, and review of radiologic findings from only at screening and baseline to every 6 months.

4. You failed to ensure that the investigation was conducted according to the signed investigator statement and the investigational plan [21 CFR 312.60].

a. The protocol specified that clinical examinations were to be performed by the investigator (you), and you signed the Form FDA 1572, Investigator Statement, indicating that you were the investigator and that there were no sub-investigators. However, the clinical examinations for the following visits were performed by (b)(4), M.D:

i. 12-Month Visit for Subject 62694

ii. 18-Month Visit for Subject 34004

iii. 30-Month Visit for Subject 34004

iv. 18-Month Visit for Subject 60667

v. 12-Month Visit for Subject 60060

b. The protocol specified that subjects who miss any visit were to be contacted by telephone. There is no documentation that you attempted to contact Subject 60667 after the subject missed the 6-Month visit.

c. The protocol specified that spirometry was to be performed at the baseline visit. You did not perform spirometry at the baseline visit for the following subjects:

i. Subject 34002: Baseline visit on January 20, 2005; spirometry on August 23, 2003

ii. Subject 34004: Baseline visit on May 12, 2005; spirometry on July 21, 2005

iii. Subject 60060: Baseline visit on August 8, 2005; spirometry on June 24, 2004

5. You failed to maintain adequate records of the disposition of the drug, including dates, quantity, and use by subjects [21 CFR 312.62(a)].

You did not maintain records of study drug disposition for Subjects 62694 and 34004.

6. You failed to retain records required to be maintained under 21 CFR part 312 until 2 years after the investigation was discontinued and FDA was notified [21 CFR 312.62(c)].

By a letter dated June 13, 2008, the sponsor notified you that your participation in Protocol (b)(4) was terminated, thereby discontinuing your investigation. The sponsor also notified FDA, by a letter dated June 13, 2008, that your participation in Protocol (b) (4) was terminated. Between May 19 and 28, 2009, Aneel K. Sandhu, representing the Food and Drug Administration (FDA), conducted an investigation and met with you to review your conduct of

Protocol (b)(4). At the time of the inspection, which was less than2 years after your investigation was discontinued and FDA was notified, there were no eCRFs in the records for Subjects 60060, 34004, and 34003. Available documentation indicates that you failed to retain eCRFs for Subjects 60060, 34004, and 34003 for therequired period of 2 years after the investigation was discontinued and FDA was notified.

This letter is not intended to be an all-inclusive list of deficiencies with your clinical study of an investigational drug. It is your responsibility to ensure adherence to each requirement of the law and relevant FDA regulations. You should address these deficiencies and establish procedures to ensure that any on-going or future studies will be in compliance with FDA regulations.

Within fifteen (15) working days of your receipt of this letter, you should notify this office in writing of the actions you have taken to prevent similar violations in the future. Failure to adequately and promptly explain the violations noted above may result in regulatory action without further notice.

If you have any questions, please contact Constance Cullity, M.D., M.P.H., at 301-796-3397; FAX 301-847-8748.

Your written response and any pertinent documentation should be addressed to:

Constance Cullity (formerly Lewin), M.D., M.P.H.
Branch Chief, Good Clinical Practice Branch I
Division of Scientific Investigations
Office of Compliance
Center for Drug Evaluation and Research
Food and Drug Administration
Bldg 51, Room 5354
10903 New Hampshire Avenue
Silver Spring, MD 2099

Sincerely yours,

/S/

Leslie K. Ball, M.D.
Director
Division of Scientific Investigations
Office of Compliance
Center for Drug Evaluation and Research

第112封　给Chawla, Sant P. 医学博士的警告信

2010年3月17日

参考号：10-HFD-45-03-02

尊敬的Chawla博士：

2009年8月5日至27日，Diane Van Leeuwen女士代表FDA与您会面并审查了您实施的以下临床研究情况：

- 试验方案（b）(4)，题为"（b）(4)"，试验药物（b）(4)，申办者为（b）(4)。
- 试验方案（b）(4)，题为"（b）(4)"，试验药物（b）(4)，申办者为（b）(4)。

本次现场检查是FDA的生物研究监查项目的一部分。该项目通过设定的检查方法，对研究的实施情况进行评价，并确保这些研究中受试者的权益、安全和福利得到了保护。

经对现场检查报告，该报告的附件，以及您2009年9月14日的书面回复进行审查，我们认为，您没有遵循适用的法律要求和监管临床研究实施的FDA法规。在现场检查结束时，Diane Van Leeuwen女士向您出示并讨论了FDA483表，即现场检查发现的问题。我们想强调以下几点：

关于试验方案（b）(4)：

1. 您未能进行研究，或者确保研究按照研究计划进行［21 CFR 312.60］

a. 试验方案（b）(4)的7.4.1部分（剂量增加与调整）规定，根据分配组来给予试验药物的剂量。受试者008被分配到第4组，规定试验药物剂量为150mg/m^2。2008年9月3日，第4周期、第1天，受试者008身高、体重分别记录为5英尺[1]、132磅[2]。受试者的体表面积记录为1.59m^2，药物剂量被不准确地计算并记录为274.5mg。正确的剂量本应该计算为238.5mg（150mg/m^2×1.59m^2）。受试者的化疗流程表记录：2008年9月3日，受试者接受了274.5mg的试验药物治疗。按错误计算的药量给药，不必要将受试者置于过量用药的境地，有可能增加不良事件的风险。

在2009年9月14日的书面回复中，您表示和研究护士及药师一起对受试者的图表进行审查，药物剂量错误得到了确认。作为纠正措施，您表示对护士和药师进行了再次培训，内容是关于研究剂量要求和计算参数（身高/体重）图表文件，并提醒要确保数据和剂量变化的一致性。此外，您指出您机构已经实施了一项政策，即在进行所有与研究相关的输液前，由一名护士或药师对剂量进行复核。我们收到了您的回复，并且认为您为防止将来再次发生而采取的纠正措施是可以接受的。

b. 试验方案（b）(4)的10.1.1部分（药物代谢动力学）要求，样品抽取应在第1天给药前和试验药物输液开始后15分钟、30分钟、45分钟、1小时、2小时。以下受试者的药物代谢动力学（PK）样品在不正确的时间间隔被抽取。具体来说，样品是在输液完成之后而不是在输液开始之后采集。

试验方案规定的PK抽样时间安排（输液开始后）	按照试验方案PK抽样时间（2400小时）	实际的PK抽样时间（2400小时）
受试者002第1天试验药物输液时间：1330～1405	受试者002第1天试验药物输液时间：1330～1405	受试者002第1天试验药物输液时间：1330～1405
给药之前	给药之前	1325
15分钟（输液开始之后）	1345	1420

1　1英尺＝0.3048米；

2　1磅＝0.4535924千克。

续表

试验方案规定的PK抽样时间安排（输液开始后）	按照试验方案PK抽样时间（2400小时）	实际的PK抽样时间（2400小时）
受试者002第1天试验药物输液时间：1330～1405	受试者002第1天试验药物输液时间：1330～1405	受试者002第1天试验药物输液时间：1330～1405
30分钟（输液开始之后）	1400	1435
45分钟（输液开始之后）	1415	1450
1小时（输液开始之后）	1430	1505
2小时（输液开始之后）	1530	1605

试验方案规定的PK抽样时间安排（输液开始后）	按照试验方案PK抽样时间（2400小时）	实际的PK抽样时间（2400小时）
受试者003第1天试验药物输液时间：1420~1452	受试者003第1天试验药物输液时间：1420~1452	受试者003第1天试验药物输液时间：1420~1452
给药之前	给药之前	1330
15分钟（输液开始之后）	1435	1510
30分钟（输液开始之后）	1450	1525
45分钟（输液开始之后）	1505	1540
1小时（输液开始之后）	1520	1555
2小时（输液开始之后）	1620	1655

试验方案规定的PK抽样时间安排（输液开始后）	按照试验方案PK抽样时间（2400小时）	实际的PK抽样时间（2400小时）
受试者004第1天试验药物输液时间：1440~1514	受试者004第1天试验药物输液时间：1440~1514	受试者004第1天试验药物输液时间：1440~1514
给药之前	给药之前	1330
15分钟（输液开始之后）	1455	1530
30分钟（输液开始之后）	1510	1545
45分钟（输液开始之后）	1525	1600
1小时（输液开始之后）	1540	1615
2小时（输液开始之后）	1640	1716

试验方案规定的PK抽样时间安排（输液开始后）	按照试验方案PK抽样时间（2400小时）	实际的PK抽样时间（2400小时）
受试者005第1天试验药物输液时间：1245~1316	受试者005第1天试验药物输液时间：1245~1316	受试者005第1天试验药物输液时间：1245~1316
给药之前	给药之前	1220
15分钟（输液开始之后）	1300	1335
30分钟（输液开始之后）	1315	1347
45分钟（输液开始之后）	1330	1403
1小时（输液开始之后）	1345	1418
2小时（输液开始之后）	1445	1518

试验方案规定的PK抽样时间安排（输液开始后）	按照试验方案PK抽样时间（2400小时）	实际的PK抽样时间（2400小时）
受试者006第1天试验药物输液时间：1222~1254	受试者006第1天试验药物输液时间：1222~1254	受试者006第1天试验药物输液时间：1222~1254
给药之前	给药之前	1140
15分钟（输液开始之后）	1237	1310
30分钟（输液开始之后）	1252	1325
45分钟（输液开始之后）	1307	1340
1小时（输液开始之后）	1322	1355
2小时（输液开始之后）	1422	1455

试验方案规定的PK抽样时间安排（输液开始后）	按照试验方案PK抽样时间（2400小时）	实际的PK抽样时间（2400小时）
受试者010第1天试验药物输液时间：1330~1402	受试者010第1天试验药物输液时间：1330~1402	受试者010第1天试验药物输液时间：1330~402
给药之前	给药之前	1315
15分钟（输液开始之后）	1345	1417
30分钟（输液开始之后）	1400	1432
45分钟（输液开始之后）	1415	1447
1小时（输液开始之后）	1430	1502
2小时（输液开始之后）	1530	1602

试验方案规定的PK抽样时间安排（输液开始后）	按照试验方案PK抽样时间（2400小时）	实际的PK抽样时间（2400小时）
受试者012第1天试验药物输液时间：1521~1555	受试者012第1天试验药物输液时间：1521~1555	受试者012第1天试验药物输液时间：1521~1555
给药之前	给药之前	1420
15分钟（输液开始之后）	1536	1611
30分钟（输液开始之后）	1551	1632
45分钟（输液开始之后）	1606	1648
1小时（输液开始之后）	1621	1700
2小时（输液开始之后）	1721	1758

在2009年9月14日的书面回复中，您提出贵试验场所误解了PK抽样的时间计划。您表示贵试验场所解读试验方案要求的PK抽样是从试验药物输液时间的终点开始，而不是试验药物输液时间的起点。您表示贵试验场所在以后将特别注意对PK抽样的试验方案要求。我们收到了您的回复，但是，我们关注的是您的答复不足以防止上述违规将来再次发生。尤其，我们关注的是从研究开始您就没有正确地理解试验方案规定的PK抽样时间安排，您没有确保在整个研究过程中PK样品按照试验方案进行采集。您未能按照规定的试验方案采集PK样品，这严重破坏了在贵试验场所获取的数据的可靠性和完整性。

关于试验方案（b）（4）和（b）（4）：

2. 您未能保存研究中使用试验药物或对照组的受试者的所有观察结果和其他数据的足够及准确病历［21 CFR 312.62（b）］

现场检查中发现，有很多不良事件记录在受试者病程记录中，而没有报告在病例报告表（CRF），对于这种不一致的情况没有任何解释。以下是现场检查时发现的、没有在电子CRF中报告的不良事件的一些举例。请注意现场检查是在2009年8月，以下的举例意味着将不良事件由病程记录转录成eCRF，延迟了至少8个月到15个月。

a.（b）（4）受试者071 003：2008年5月7日病程记录记录上肢和下肢无力。

b.（b）（4）受试者071 005：2008年7月2日病程记录记录恶心和呕吐。

c.（b）（4）受试者071 008：2008年8月14日病程记录记录脱发，2008年10月28日指甲发暗。

d.（b）（4）受试者071 012：2008年11月3日病程记录记录吞咽困难，2008年12月31日恶心和呕吐。

e.（b）（4）受试者071 001：2008年9月10日病程记录记录呼吸音减少伴哮鸣，2008年12月8日恶心和呕吐。

f.（b）（4）受试者071 004：2009年1月5日病程记录记录阅读困难。

g.（b）（4）受试者071 005：2009年1月12日体格检查记录左后部头皮小肿物，2009年1月28日病程记录记录脱发。

h.（b）（4）受试者071 006：2008年12月10日病程记录记录由于左大腿疼痛，睡眠困难。

在您2009年9月14日的书面回复中，您表示贵试验场所工作人员会在每次访视时将所有的不良事件和合并用药都记入受试者图表。您指出在研究开始时，贵试验场所工作人员会在申办者的监查访问前将数据（不良事件和合并用药）记入CRF中。但是，您指出贵试验场所工作人员在申办者的监查访问前停止将数据记入CRF，这样他们就能在监查员在场的情况下录入数据，以避免额外的系统查询。作为一项纠正措施，您表示工作人员已经实施了一项政策，要求不管预定的监查访问计划，所有的CRF都在研究访视后的30天内及时完成。

我们收到了您的回复。但是，eCRF中缺乏及时的不良事件信息，可能已经危及受试者的安全，也危害到在贵试验场所CRF中采集的数据的可靠性和完整性。如果按照提出的方案实施，我们认为您为防止将来再次发生而采取的纠正措施是可以接受的。

本警告信的目的并非是罗列您在试验药物临床研究中存在的所有缺陷。确保遵循法律和相关FDA法规的每一项要求是您的职责。您应当解决这些缺陷，并建立规程，以确保任何正在进行或将来的研究均能符合FDA的法规。

自收到这封信的15个工作日内，您应当书面告知本办公室您为预防将来发生类似违规情况已经采取的措施。如果不能充分、迅速地解释上述违规问题，可能导致我们在不再通知的情况下采取监管措施。

附：英文原文

Chawla, Sant P, M.D.

WARNING LETTER

MAR 17, 2010

CERTIFIED MAIL
RETURN RECEIPT REQUESTED

Ref: 10-HFD-45-03-02

Sant P. Chawla, M.D.
Sarcoma Oncology Center
2811 Wilshire Boulevard, Suite 414
Santa Monica, CA90403

Dear Dr. Chawla:

Between August 5 and 27, 2009, Ms. Diane Van Leeuwen, representing the Food and Drug Administration (FDA), conducted an investigation and met with you to review your conduct of the following clinical investigations:

- Protocol (b)(4), entitled "(b)(4)" of the investigational drug (b)(4), performed for (b)(4).; and
- Protocol (b)(4), entitled "(b)(4)," of the investigational drug (b)(4), performed for (b)(4).

This inspection is a part of the FDA's Bioresearch Monitoring Program, which includes inspections designed to evaluate the conduct of research and to ensure that the rights, safety, and welfare of the human subjects of those studies have been protected.

From our review of the establishment inspection report, the documents submitted with that report, and your September 14, 2009 written response, we conclude that you did not adhere to the applicable statutory requirements and FDA regulations governing the conduct of clinical investigations. We are aware that at the conclusion of the inspection, Ms. Van Leeuwen presented and discussed with you Form FDA 483, Inspectional Observations. We wish to emphasize the following:

Regarding Protocol (b)(4):

1. You failed to conduct the studies or ensure they were conducted according to the investigational plans [21 CFR 312.60].

a. Protocol (b)(4), Section 7.4.1 (Dose Escalation and Modification) specified study drug dosages to be administered based on assigned cohort. Subject 008 was assigned to Cohort 4, with a study drug dose specification of 150 mg/m^2. For Cycle 4, Day 1 on September 3, 2008, the subjects height and weight were recorded as 5'0" and 132 lbs., respectively. The subject' s body surface area was documented as 1.59 m^2, and the dose was inaccurately calculated and recorded as 274.5 mg. The correct dosage should have been calculated as 238.5 mg [150 mg/m^2 × 1.59 m^2]. The subject' s chemotherapy flow sheet documents that the subject received 274.5 mg of study drug on Septembe 3, 2008. The administration of this miscalculated dose unnecessarily exposed the subject to an overdose, with the potential for increased adverse events.

In your September 14, 2009, written response, you indicated that the subject' s chart was reviewed with the study nurses and pharmacists, and the dosing error was confirmed. As corrective measures, you indicated that your site' s nurses and pharmacists were retrained on study dosing requirements and chart documentation of calculation parameters (height/weight), with a reminder to ensure consistency of data and dosing changes. Additionally, you noted that your site has implemented a policy whereby a nurse or pharmacist double-checks dosages prior to all study- related infusions. We acknowledge your response and find your corrective measures to prevent future recurrence acceptable.

b. Protocol (b)(4) Section 10.1.1 (Pharmacokinetics) required samples to be drawn on Day 1 at pre dose, and at 15 minutes, 30 minutes, 45 minutes, 1 hour, and 2 hours after study drug infusion was initiated. The following subjects' pharmacokinetic (PK) samples were drawn at the incorrect time intervals. Specifically, the samples were collected after the completion of the infusion rather than after the initiation of the infusion:

Protocol-specified PK sampling schedule (post infusion initiation)	PK sampling time according to protocol (2400 hours)	Actual time of PK sampling (2400 hours)
Subject 002 Day 1 Study Drug Infusion Time: 1330-1405	**Subject 002 Day 1 Study Drug Infusion Time:1330-1405**	**Subject 002 Day 1 Study Drug Infusion Time:1330-1405**
Just prior to dose	Just prior to dose	1325
15 minutes (post infusion initiation)	1345	1420
30 minutes (post infusion initiation)	1400	1435
45 minutes (post infusion initiation)	1415	1450
1 hour (post infusion initiation)	1430	1505
2 hour (post infusion initiation)	1530	1605

Protocol-specified PK sampling schedule (post infusion initiation)	PK sampling time according to protocol (2400 hours)	Actual time of PK sampling (2400 hours)
Subject 003 Day 1 Study Drug Infusion Time: 1420-1452	**Subject 003 Day 1 Study Drug Infusion Time: 1420-1452**	**Subject 003 Day 1 Study Drug Infusion Time: 1420-1452**
Just prior to dose	Just prior to dose	1330
15 minutes (post infusion initiation)	1435	1510
30 minutes (post infusion initiation)	1450	1525
45 minutes (post infusion initiation)	1505	1540
1 hour (post infusion initiation)	1520	1555
2 hour (post infusion initiation)	1620	1655

Protocol-specified PK sampling schedule (post infusion initiation)	PK sampling time according to protocol (2400 hours)	Actual time of PK sampling (2400 hours)
Subject 004 Day 1 Study Drug Infusion Time: 1440-1514	**Subject 004 Day 1 Study Drug Infusion Time: 1440-1514**	**Subject 004 Day 1 Study Drug Infusion Time: 1440-1514**
Just prior to dose	Just prior to dose	1330
15 minutes (post infusion initiation)	1455	1530
30 minutes (post infusion initiation)	1510	1545
45 minutes (post infusion initiation)	1525	1600
1 hour (post infusion initiation)	1540	1615
2 hour (post infusion initiation)	1640	1716

Protocol-specified PK sampling schedule (post infusion initiation)	PK sampling time according to protocol (2400 hours)	Actual time of PK sampling (2400 hours)
Subject 005 Day 1 Study Drug Infusion Time: 1245-1316	**Subject 005 Day 1 Study Drug Infusion Time: 1245-1316**	**Subject 005 Day 1 Study Drug Infusion Time: 1245-1316**
Just prior to dose	Just prior to dose	1220
15 minutes (post infusion initiation)	1300	1335
30 minutes (post infusion initiation)	1315	1347
45 minutes (post infusion initiation)	1330	1403
1 hour (post infusion initiation)	1345	1418
2 hour (post infusion initiation)	1445	1518

Protocol-specified PK sampling schedule (post infusion initiation)	PK sampling time according to protocol (2400 hours)	Actual time of PK sampling (2400 hours)
Subject 006 Day 1 Study Drug Infusion Time: 1222-1254	**Subject 006 Day 1 Study Drug Infusion Time: 1222-1254**	**Subject 006 Day 1 Study Drug Infusion Time: 1222-1254**
Just prior to dose	Just prior to dose	1140
15 minutes (post infusion initiation)	1237	1310
30 minutes (post infusion initiation)	1252	1325
45 minutes (post infusion initiation)	1307	1340
1 hour (post infusion initiation)	1322	1355
2 hour (post infusion initiation)	1422	1455

Protocol-specified PK sampling schedule (post infusion initiation)	PK sampling time according to protocol (2400 hours)	Actual time of PK sampling (2400 hours)
Subject 010 Day 1 Study Drug Infusion Time: 1330-1402	**Subject 010 Day 1 Study Drug Infusion Time: 1330-1402**	**Subject 010 Day 1 Study Drug Infusion Time: 1330-1402**
Just prior to dose	Just prior to dose	1315
15 minutes (post infusion initiation)	1345	1417
30 minutes (post infusion initiation)	1400	1432
45 minutes (post infusion initiation)	1415	1447
1 hour (post infusion initiation)	1430	1502
2 hour (post infusion initiation)	1530	1602

Protocol-specified PK sampling schedule (post infusion initiation)	PK sampling time according to protocol (2400 hours)	Actual time of PK sampling (2400 hours)
Subject 012 Day 1 Study Drug Infusion Time: 1521-1555	**Subject 012 Day 1 Study Drug Infusion Time: 1521-1555**	**Subject 012 Day 1 Study Drug Infusion Time: 1521-1555**
Just prior to dose	Just prior to dose	1420
15 minutes (post infusion initiation)	1536	1611
30 minutes (post infusion initiation)	1551	1632
45 minutes (post infusion initiation)	1606	1648
1 hour (post infusion initiation)	1621	1700
2 hour (post infusion initiation)	1721	1758

In your September 14, 2009, written response, you indicated that your site misunderstood the timing of the PK samples. You noted that your site interpreted the protocol-required PK sampling to begin at the end of the drug infusion time rather than at the start of the drug infusion time. You stated that your site will pay particular attention to the protocol requirement for PK sampling in the future. We acknowledge your response. However, we are concerned that the response is not adequate to prevent future recurrence of the violation noted above. In particular, we are concerned that you did not properly understand the protocol specified PK sampling schedule from the start of the study, and that you did not ensure that the PK samples were collected according to the protocol throughout the study. Your failure to collect PK samples as specified in the protocol significantly undermines the reliability and integrity of the data captured at your site.

Regarding Protocols (b)(4) and (b)(4)

2. You failed to maintain adequate and accurate case histories that record all observations and other data pertinent to the investigation [21 CFR 312.62(b)].

The inspection revealed that there were numerous adverse events recorded in progress notes of subject's records that had not been reported on the case report forms (CRFs), and there was no explanation regarding this discrepancy. The following are examples of adverse events that had not been reported on the electronic CRFs at the time of the inspection. Note that since the inspection occurred in August 2009, the examples below represent delays in transcribing adverse events from progress notes to electronic CRFs that range from at least 8 months to 15 months.

a. Subject (b)(4) 071 003: Progress notes documented weakness of upper and lower extremities on May 7, 2008.

b. Subject (b)(4)071 005: Progress notes documented nausea and vomiting on July 2, 2008.

c. Subject (b)(4)071 008: Progress notes documented alopecia on August 14, 2008, as well as dark nails on October 28, 2008.

d. Subject (b)(4) 071 012: Progress notes documented difficulty swallowing food on November 3, 2008f as well as nausea and vomiting on December 31, 2008.

e. Subject (b)(4) 071 001: Progress notes documented decreased breath sounds with wheezing on September 10, 2008, as well as nausea and vomiting on December 8, 2008.

f. Subject (b)(4) 071 004: Progress notes documented difficulty reading on January 5, 2009.

g. Subject (b)(4) 071 005: Physical examination notes documented a small lump on the left posterior scalp on January 12, 2009; progress notes documented alopecia on January 28, 2009.

h. Subject (b)(4) 071 006: Progress notes documented difficulty sleeping on December 107 2008, due to left thigh pain.

In your September 14, 2009 written response, you stated that your site staff enters all adverse events and concomitant medications in subject' s charts at the time of each visit. You indicated that at the start of the study, your site staff members were entering data (adverse events and concomitant medications) in CRFs prior to the sponsor's monitoring visits. However, you indicated that your site staff stopped entering data in CRFs in advance of the monitoring visits so that they could enter data with the monitors present, to avoid additional system queries. As a corrective measure, you noted that your site staff members have implemented a policy requiring that all CRFs be completed in a timely manner, defined as 30 days following a study visit, regardless of scheduled monitoring visits.

We acknowledge your response. However, the lack of timely adverse event information in the electronic CRFs may have jeopardized subject safety as well as the reliability and integrity of the data captured on the CRFs at your site. We find your corrective measures to prevent future recurrence to be acceptable, if implemented as proposed.

This letter is not intended to be an all-inclusive list of deficiencies with your clinical study of an investigational drug. It is your responsibility to ensure adherence to each requirement of the law and relevant FDA regulations. You should address these deficiencies and establish procedures to ensure tha any ongoing or future studies will be in compliance with FDA regulations.

Within fifteen (15) working days of your receipt of this letter, you should notify this office in writing of the actions you have taken to prevent similar violations in the future. Failure to adequately and promptly explain the violations noted above may result in regulatory action without further notice.

If you have any questions, please contact Constance Cullity (formerly Lewin), M.D.,at 301-7963397; FAX 301-847-8748. Your written response and any pertinent documentation should be addressed to:

Constance Cullity (formerly Lewin), M.D., M.P.H.
Branch Chief, Good Clinical Practice Branch I
Division of Scientific Investigations
Office of Compliance
Center for Drug Evaluation and Research
Food and Drug Administration
Building 51, Room 5354
10903 New Hampshire Avenue
Silver Spring, MD20993

Sincerely yours,

{See appended electronic signature page}

Leslie K. Ball, M.D.
Director
Division of Scientific Investigations
Office of Compliance
Center for Drug Evaluation and Research
Food and Drug Administration

第113封　给Toledo, Charles H. 医学博士的警告信

2010年3月11日

参考号：CBER-10-05

尊敬的Toledo博士：

这封信特告知您2009年8月3日到2009年9月30日FDA进行现场检查的结果。一名FDA检查员与您会面，审查了您实施的以下临床研究的情况：（b）（4）。

本次现场检查是FDA的生物研究监查项目的一部分，该项目通过设定的检查方法，审查试验药物相关研究的实施情况。

在Sylva Pediatric Associates现场检查结束时，FDA检查员与您当面讨论了FDA 483表（即现场检查发现的问题）上的项目。您在2009年10月22日给亚特兰大地区办公室的信函中对该FDA 483表进行了回复。我们对现场检查报告、随报告所附的支持性文件以及您2009年10月22日的回复函进行了审查。

我们认为，您违反了美国联邦法规（CFR）第21篇第312部分关于正确开展新药临床研究相关的监管规定（详见http://www.gpoaccess.gov/cfr/index.html）。

以下列出的每项违规均指明了CFR中的相应条款。

1. 您未能确保按照签署的研究者声明、研究计划、适用法规进行研究，以保护在您的监护下的受试者的权益、安全和福利［21 CFR 312.60］

研究1

A. 方案中8.5部分要求“每次给予研究疫苗后的31天内（Days 0-30）出现的所有AE，不论严重与否以及是否与疫苗相关，都必须记录在受试者eCRF中的AE表上。”但下表中所列的AE未列入受试者的eCRFs中向申办者报告。

受试者	不良反应	日期
(b)(6)	呕吐、腹泻、发热	2/2/2004
(b)(6)	疥疮	11/11/2004
(b)(6)	两侧中耳炎	3/21/2006
(b)(6)	臂部、腿部、躯干部和脸部圆点/皮疹	11/12/2005
(b)(6)	右中耳炎	12/1/2005
(b)(6)	左中耳炎	6/27/2005

B. 方案中8.5部分提到“必须报告所有在活动期和扩展的安全性随访期新发的慢性疾病以及其他医学上具有显著意义的事件”。但下表所列事件在eCRFs中未报告。

受试者	不良反应	日期
(b)(6)	伴发热的癫痫	3/13/2005
(b)(6)	热性癫痫发作	6/8/2005
(b)(6)	昏迷状态下被送到急诊室	12/14/2005

C. 方案中6.9部分要求“所有合并用药，除维生素或营养补充剂外，无论在首次给予研究疫苗后42天内以及随后每次给予研究疫苗后31天内的任何时间发生，均进行记录…”。但下表所列的合并用药并未记录在相应受试者eCRF中向申办者报告。

受试者	合并用药	日期	末次研究疫苗日期
(b)(6)	异丙嗪	2/20/2004	1/6/2004
(b)(6)	氯菊酯乳膏	11/11/2004	11/11/2004
(b)(6)	马来酸美吡拉敏	5/24/2004	4/27/2004
(b)(6)	奥格门汀和环丙沙星地塞米松	3/21/2006	2/20/2006
(b)(6)	头孢地尼	12/1/2005	11/8/2005
(b)(6)	头孢地尼	6/27/2006	5/30/2006

D. 方案中9.2.1部分要求“对于没有返回医院完成计划访视或随访的受试者，研究者将联系他们。”受试者（b）（6）的原始记录表明，其在2005年11月15日第2次访视后已从研究中退出，而直至2008年8月17日给其致电前，均未尝试联系该受试者。相应电话联系记录见该受试者的病历，同时确认该受试者在第2次访视结束后从研究中退出，未返回进行第3、第4或第5次访视。

E. 方案中4.4部分提到该试验的排除标准包括“在每次给予研究疫苗前31天内和给予研究疫苗后31天内接种研究方案中不允许的疫苗”。受试者（b）（6）在2004年10月22日接种了研究疫苗，在2004年11月10日接种了流感疫苗。尽管受试者（b）（6）符合排除标准，但其仍继续参与此项研究。

研究2

“试验药物分发及对账表”以及“研究授权表”显示该研究疫苗由未被授权的人员进行接种。

受试者	日期	初始给药者
(b)(6)	7/18/2007	(b)(6)
(b)(6)	11/13/2007	(b)(6)
(b)(6)	11/13/2007	(b)(6)

您的回复函中称，您未获得查看研究1和研究2记录的权限。

2. 您未能保存与研究相关的记录所有研究观察结果和其他研究相关的数据的足够准确的病历［21 CFR 312.62（b）］

研究1

A. 受试者病历中记录的AEs、新发生的具有显著医学意义的事件以及合并用药均未在受试者eCRF中报告。参见1A、1B和1C。

B. 如第3点所述，原始记录和eCRFs、试验药物分发记录以及试验药物统计和核对记录之间存在不一致之处。

C. 方案中4.4部分提到此试验的排除标准包括“在每次给予研究疫苗前31天内和给予研究疫苗后31天内接种方案中不允许的疫苗”。受试者（b）（6）在2004年10月22日接种了研究疫苗，在2004年11月10日接种了流感疫苗。直至2008年7月22日，该项排除标准未在受试者的eCRF中报告。

研究2

D. 检查发现在研究2中出现下列原始记录与eCRF不一致的情况。

i. 作为方案的一部分，受试者在2007年11月13日接种了（b）（4）疫苗。在2007年11月23日，此受试者被诊断为“（b）（4），疫苗引发”。eCRF向申办者报告了此情形为“（b）（4）”，但并未通知申办者此受试者出现了疫苗引发的（b）（4）。

ii. 受试者SAE报告表提示，某受试者分别在2007年12月21日至2007年12月24日出现了反应性气道病和湿性咳嗽。但胸部X射线报告为肺门区域病毒性肺炎。

您在回复函中称，您无权获得这些试验的记录。

3. 您未能保存足够的试验药物处置记录［21 CFR 312.62（a）］

检查发现，研究1中有以下原始记录和eCRFs、试验药物分发记录以及试验药物统计和核对记录之间存在的不一致之处。

受试者	原始记录和eCRF疫苗接种情况	试验药物分发记录	试验药物统计和核对
(b)(6)	(b)(4)在1/8/2004和 7/21/2004	(b)(4)在1/8/2004 和 7/21/2004	返回4空瓶
(b)(6)	(b)(4)和(b)(4)在3/8/2004	(b)(4)在1/8/2004 和 7/21/2004	返回4空瓶
(b)(6)	(b)(4)在5/4/2004; (b)(4)和(b)(4)在3/22/2004	(b)(4)在5/4/2004; (b)(4) 和(b)(4)在3/22/2004	返回4空瓶
(b)(6)	因协议撤销而无疫苗	未发现记录	返回4空瓶
(b)(6)	因协议撤销而无疫苗	未发现记录	返回4空瓶
(b)(6)	(b)(4)在11/10/2005和5/30/2006	(b)(4)在5/30/2006	10/12/2004: 因过期返回; 未更换

您在回复函中称，您无权获得这些试验的记录。

4. 您未能保存记录，直至试验药物按拟定适应症上市申请获得批准后 2 年；如果没有提交上市申请或药物用于该适应症的上市申请未被批准，则在研究终止后 2 年［21 CFR 312.62（c）］

在您签署试验1和试验2 的FDA1572表，即研究者声明时，您已同意按21 CFR 312.62的规定保存足够、准确的记录，并按21 CFR 312.68规定，在现场检查时可以提供这些记录。在您的回复函中解释称，由于您与Sylva Pediatric Associates（SPA）的隶属关系于（b）（6）结束，因此您无法获得此项研究记录的权限。我们调查发现，在您离开SPA后，您所完成的试验记录由（b）（4）保存。在（b）（4）关闭后，记录被重新保存在SPA，而未在您目前任职的北卡罗来纳州Sylva的Western North Carolina Pediatric and Adolescent Care中处于您的监管之下。

由于您无获取研究记录的权限，因此您在信中对FDA 483表中提出的多个发现项的回复是“在未获得研究记录的情况下，就我所知，此种不一致一定是抄写/人为错误”。但该回复是不充分的，因为作为一名研究者，FDA法规要求您保存这些记录，直至研究的适应症上市批准后两年；或在未进行注册申请或未获FDA批准情况下，保存至研究结束后两年。

本警告信的目的并不是罗列您在试验疫苗开展的临床研究中存在的所有缺陷。确保遵循法律和相关FDA法规的每一项要求是您的职责。

您在信中描述了对未来进行试验的纠正计划，其中包括工作实践指南、流程图以及对研究人员进行额外的培训。我们要求您解释将来对研究记录保存的纠正措施计划。

自收到这封信的15个工作日内，作为临床研究者您应当书面告知本办公室，您为预防将来发生类似违规行为准备采取的措施。未能对本警告信进行回复并采取适当的纠正措施，可能导致FDA在不再通知的情况下采取监管措施。FDA可根据21 CFR 312.70启动吊销您的资格的程序。

附：英文原文

Toledo, Charles H., M.D.

WARNING LETTER

MAR 11, 2010

Ref: CBER-10-05

Dear Dr. Toledo:

This letter describes the results of a Food and Drug Administration (FDA) inspection that was conducted between August 3, 2009, and September 30, 2009. An FDA investigator met with you to review your conduct of the following clinical studies:

(b)(4)

This inspection was conducted as part of the FDA' s Bioresearch Monitoring Program, which includes inspections designed to review the conduct of research involving investigational drugs.

At the end of the inspection conduct at Sylva Pediatric Associates, the FDA investigator contacted you and met with you to discuss the items listed on the Form FDA 483, Inspectional Observations. You responded to the Form FDA 483 in a letter to the Atlanta District Office dated October 22, 2009. We reviewed the inspection report, the supporting documents submitted with that report, and your October 22, 2009 letter.

We have determined that you violated regulations governing the proper conduct of clinical studies involving investigational new drugs, as published in Title 21, Code of Federal Regulations (CFR) Part 312 (available at http://www.gpoaccess.gov/cfr/index.html).

The applicable provisions of the CFR are cited for each violation listed below.

1. You failed to ensure that the investigation was conducted according to the signed investigator statement, the investigational plan, and the applicable regulations in order to protect the rights, safety, and welfare of subjects under your care. [21 CFR § 312.60].

Study 1

A. Section 8.5 of the protocol requires that all adverse events "occurring within 31 days (Days 0-30) following administration of each dose of study vaccine must be recorded on the 'Adverse Event' form in the subject' s eCRF, irrespective of severity or whether or not they are considered related to vaccination." The following adverse events were not reported to the sponsor in the subject' s electronic Case Report Form (eCRF).

Subject	Adverse Event(s)	Date
(b)(6)	Vomiting, diarrhea, fever	02/02/04
(b)(6)	Scabies	11/11/04
(b)(6)	Bilateral otitis media	03/21/06
(b)(6)	Dots/rash on arms, legs, trunk, face	11/12/05
(b)(6)	Right otitis media	12/01/05
(b)(6)	Left otitis media	06/27/05

B. Section 8.5 of the protocol specifies that "All new onset chronic illnesses and other medically significant events occurring during the Active Phase and the Extended Safety Follow-up Phase must also be reported." The following events were not reported in the eCRFs.

Subject	Adverse Event(s)	Date
(b)(6)	Seizure with fever	03/13/05
(b)(6)	Febrile seizure	06/08/05
(b)(6)	Admitted to ER unconscious	12/14/05

C. Protocol Section 6.9 requires that "All concomitant medications, with the exception of vitamins or dietary supplements, administered at ANY time during the period starting with administration of each dose of study vaccine(s) and ending 42 days following the first dose of study vaccine(s) and 31 days following subsequent doses of study vaccine are to be recorded..." The following concomitant medications were not reported to the sponsor in the eCRF for the following subjects:

Subject	Concomitant Medication	Date	Date of Last Study Vaccine
(b)(6)	Phenergan	2/204	1/6/04
(b)(6)	Permethrin cream	11/11/04	11/11/04
(b)(6)	Triaminic	5/24/04	4/27/04
(b)(6)	Augmentin and Ciprodex	3/21/06	2/20/06
(b)(6)	Omnicef	12/1/05	11/8/05
(b)(6)	Omnicef	6/27/06	5/30/06

D. Section 9.2.1 of the protocol requires that "Investigators will make an attempt to contact those subjects who do not return for scheduled visits or follow-up."Source documents for Subject **(b)(6)** show that this subject dropped from the study after Visit 2 on November 15, 2005. An attempt to contact this subject did not occur until a phone call on August 17, 2006. The phone call is documented in the subject' s medical record and confirms that the subject dropped from the study after Visit 2. Subject **(b)(6)** did not return for Visits 3, 4, or 5.

E. Protocol Section 4.4 describes elimination criteria during the study and includes "Administration of a vaccine not foreseen by the study protocol during the study period starting from 31 days before each dose of study vaccine(s) and ending 31 days after". Subject (b)(6) received a study vaccine on October 22, 2004 and an influenza vaccine on November 10, 2004. Although Subject (b)(6) met the elimination criterion this subject was continued in the study.

Study 2

The "Investigational Product Dispensing and Reconciliation Form" and the "Delegation of Authority Log" show that study vaccines were administered by individuals not authorized to dispense the study vaccine.

Subject	Date	Dispenser Initials
(b)(6)	07/18/07	(b)(6)
(b)(6)	11/13/07	(b)(6)
(b)(6)	11/13/07	(b)(6)

In your letter, you explain that you do not have access to the records for Studies 1 and 2.

2. You failed to prepare and maintain adequate and accurate case histories that record all observations and other data pertinent to the investigation. [21 CFR § 312.62(b)].

Study 1

A. Adverse events the onset of new medically significant events, and concomitant medications recorded in subject's medical records were not reported in the subject' s eCRFs. Refer to Item 1 A, B, and C.

B. Discrepancies were observed between source documents and eCRFs, the "Investigational Product(s) Dispensing Record," and the "Investigational Product Accountability and Reconciliation" Records as described in Item 3.

C.Protocol section 4.4 describes elimination criteria during the study and includes "Administration of a vaccine not foreseen by the study protocol during the study period starting from 31 days before each dose of study vaccine(s) and ending 31 days after". Subject (b)(6) received a study vaccine on October 22, 2004 and an influenza vaccine on November 10, 2004. This elimination criterion was not reported in the subject' s eCRF until July 22, 2008.

Study 2

D. The following discrepancies were noted between source documents and eCRFs in Study 2:

i. Subject (b)(6) received a (b)(4) vaccination as part of the study protocol on November 13, 2007. On November 23, 2007 this subject was diagnosed with "(b)(4), vaccine induced". The eCRF reported this occurrence to the sponsor as "(b)(4)" and failed to inform the sponsor that the subject developed vaccine induced (b)(4).

ii. The "Serious Adverse Event Reporting Form" for subject shows a diagnosis of reactive airway disease and wet cough beginning December 21, 2007 and December 24, 2007, respectively. However, the chest x-ray reports perihilar viral pneumonia for this subject.

In your letter, you explain that you do not have access to the records for these studies.

3. You failed to maintain adequate records of the disposition of the investigational drug. [21 CFR § 312.62(a)].

The following discrepancies were observed between source documents and eCRFs, the "Investigational Product(s) Dispensing Record", and the "Investigational Product Accountability and Reconciliation" Records in Study 1:

Subject	Vaccines Administered per Source Document and eCRF	Investigational Product(s) Dispensing Record	Investigational Product Accountability and Reconciliation
(b)(6)	(b)(4) on 1/8/04 and 7/21/04	(b)(4) on 1/8/04 and 7/21/04	4 empty vials returned
(b)(6)	(b)(4) and (b)(4) on 3/8/04	(b)(4) on 1/8/04 and 7/21/04	4 empty vials returned
(b)(6)	(b)(4) on 5/4/04; (b)(4) and(b)(4) on 3/22/04	(b)(4) on 5/4/04; (b)(4) and (b)(4) on 3/22/04	4 empty vials returned
(b)(6)	No vaccinations due to withdrawal of consent	No record found	4 empty vials returned
(b)(6)	No vaccinations due to withdrawal of consent	No record found	4 empty vials returned
(b)(6)	(b)(4) on 11/10/05 and 5/30/06	(b)(4) on 5/30/06	10/12/04: Returned due to expiration; Not replaced

In your letter, you explain that you do not have access to the records for this study.

4. You failed to retain records required to be maintained for a period of two years following the date a marketing application is approved for the indication for which the drug is being investigated; or, if no application is to be filed or if the application is not approved for such indication, until two years after the investigation is discontinued. [21 CFR § 312.62(c)].

At the time you signed the Form FDA 1572, Statement of Investigator, for Studies 1 and 2, you agreed to maintain adequate and accurate records in accordance with 21 CFR 312.62 and to make these records available for inspection in accordance with 21 CFR 312.68. In your letter, you explain that you do not have access to the study record because your affiliation with Sylva Pediatric Associates (SPA) ended in (b)(6). Our investigation revealed that after your departure from Sylva Pediatrics records of your completed studies were stored by (b)(4). After (b)(4) closed, your records were relocated to SPA and did not remain under your supervision at your current position at Western North Carolina Pediatric and Adolescent Care in Sylva, North Carolina.

Because you do not have access to the study records, your response to many of the items cited on the Form FDA 483 in your letter is "To the best of my knowledge without access to the study records this must have been transcription/ human error." This response is not adequate, because FDA' s regulations require you, as an investigator, to retain these records for two years after the date a marketing application is approved for the indication for which the drug is being investigated or for two years after the discontinuation of the study if no marketing application is filed and approved by the FDA.

This letter is not intended to be an all-inclusive list of deficiencies with your clinical studies of investigational vaccines. It is your responsibility to ensure adherence to each requirement of the law and relevant regulations.

In your letter, you described a corrective action plan for future trials that included work practice guides, flow charts, and additional training of study personnel. We request that you explain your corrective action plan for maintaining study records in the future.

Within fifteen (15) business days of receipt of this letter, please provide written documentation of the actions you will take to correct these violations and prevent the recurrence of similar violations in current and future studies for which you are the clinical investigator. Failure to respond to this letter and to take appropriate corrective action could result in FDA taking regulatory action without further notice to you. FDA could initiate disqualification proceedings against you in accordance with 21 CFR 312.70.

Please send your written response to:

Christine Drabick
Division of Inspections and Surveillance (HFM-664)
Office of Compliance and Biologics Quality
Center for Biologics Evaluation and Research
1401 Rockville Pike, Suite 200N
Rockville, Maryland 20852-1488
Telephone: 301-827-6323

We also request that you send a copy of your response to the FDA District Office listed below.

Sincerely,

/S/

Mary A. Malarkey, Director
Office of Compliance and Biologics Quality
Center for Biologics Evaluation and Research

Cc:
John Gridley, District Director
60 Eighth Street NE
Atlanta, Georgia 30309

第114封　给Summers, Timothy医学博士的警告信

2010年2月24日

参考号：10-HFD-45-01-02

尊敬的Summers博士：

2009年3月25日至27日，Barbara Wright女士代表FDA进行了现场检查，与您会面并对您实施的一项临床研究进行了审查：试验方案（b）(4)，题目为"（b）(4)"，试验药物（b）(4)，申办者为（b）(4）股份有限公司。

本次现场检查是FDA的生物研究监查项目的一部分。该项目通过设定的检查方法，对相关研究的实施情况进行评估，以确保这些研究中受试者的权益、安全和福利得到了保护。

经对FDA现场检查报告、该报告附件进行审查，我们认为，您没有遵循适用的法律要求和监管临床研究实施及受试者保护的FDA法规。在现场检查结束时，Wright女士向您出示并讨论了FDA483表，即现场检查发现问题。您还没有提交对FDA483表的书面回复。鉴于您及机构未能对某些方案进行充分解释，健康联盟中心（AHC）2009年4月27日对该FDA483表作出回复。AHC也指出您已经不再在AHC机构进行临床研究。我们想强调以下几点：

1．您未能进行研究或者确保按照签署的研究者声明、研究计划进行研究，未能保护在研究者监管下的受试者的权益、安全和福利［21 CFR 312.60］

a. 方案中的入组标准，是申办者在设计临床研究方案时特意规定的，从而可以确保最好地解读研究疾病进展中的数据，并且把由于伴随用药引起的药物之间的相互作用或者共致病性而对入组受试者造成的可预见的伤害降到最低。在贵研究场所随机的六名受试者中，三名没有符合入组标准，即他们都患有Ⅰ型躁狂症，这样就会使这些受试者因为参与到临床试验而承担伤害的风险。具体而言：

ⅰ. 方案中筛选标准要求，"受试者必须按照SDM-Ⅳ的标准进行初步的Ⅰ型躁狂症的诊断，且诊断需要按照K-SADS的标准核实。"受试者1001筛选和随机的时候，没有按照K-SADS的标准进行全面的Ⅰ型躁狂症的初步评估，而且K-SADS评估中，没有显示受试者是否患有抑郁和躁狂。

ⅱ. 方案的筛选标准要求，受试者在筛选和基线随访时必须进行YMRS评估，评分应大于或等于17分。受试者1009和1010被随机进入本次临床研究中，在基线随访时，YMRS评分都是8。

b. 方案要求在基线访视时，受试者必须经过严格的入组评估，然后服用首次试验药物，之后进行用药后的药代动力学的血样采集。受试者1010在2006年12月11日完成基线随访，而基线访视的前三天，在三天前的2006年12月8日，即接受了第一剂研究药物，这就意味着受试者没有完成筛选评估，并且之后的药代动力学的血样也没有采集。

c. 方案要求在每次随访时，用YMRS、CGAS、CGI进行治疗有效性的评估。受试者1010在第一周的随访中，没有进行CGI的评估。

d. 您没有完全遵循方案中有关弱势群体入组的要求。在递交到伦理委员会的"首次审评表"上的第28项"弱势群体的分类"，您没有声明您要入组受试者1001和1007处于受监护状态，都是弱势群体。所以，伦理委员会就没能按照21 CFR 50.56的规定，合理恰当地评估是否可以入组这两个来自弱势群体的受试者，或者给每一个受试者都指定一个代诉人。

如果入组了没有完全符合方案要求的受试者，并且没有执行方案所求的步骤，就会危害到受试者的安全和福利，而且还会影响到试验结束后对于临床研究数据解读的真实性和有效性。

2．您未能保存研究中使用试验药物或对照组的受试者的所有研究观察结果和其他相关数据的足够及准确的病历［21 CFR 312.62（b）］

在现场检查中，我们发现研究文件（包括研究表格和评估用的工具）中记录的数据不充分，而且缺少管理，比如数据记录在错误的访视表中，同一个访视有多个版本的表。我们还发现，在受试者的资料中出现页码的缺失，多次出现信息更改，但没有必要的解释，彼此信息不一致。在病程记录上，我们发现的问题列举如下：

a. 方案的筛选标准要求，受试者在筛选和基线随访时必须进行YMRS评估，并且评分应大于或等于17。受试者1006的研究文件包含两套原始资料，其中记录了2006年10月31日访视的两个不同的YRMS评分结果，一个YMRS的评分是11，另一个评分是23。对于两者之间的不同，您没有给出必要的解释。

b. KSADS-PL评估是一个多方位的诊断，包括筛选访视时的面试和五次附加的诊断。基于受试者在筛选访视面试时给出的答案，可以提示附加诊断的结果。受试者1001，1004和1006在KSADS-PL的评估中，发生了隔页缺失和/或没有进行附加评估。

c. 受试者1004的病历记录中，受试者编号、研究方案编号和访视日期的记录有如下错误：

i. 受试者编号1002数次出现在原始资料中而不是正确的受试者编号1004。

ii. 用于记录“筛选访视”“第一周访视”“第四周访视”表格的日期，都是2006年10月31日。

iii.“第一周访视”的表格用来记录CDRS-R的评估结果，但是却有两个不同的版本，记录日期分别是2006年10月31日和2006年11月8日。

iv. 您使用了另外一个研究项目中名字为“研究”的表格，来记录受试者参加本次临床研究的检查。

因为没有保存足够、准确的病历，这会影响到本次临床研究中对于终点解读的有效性。

3．您未能按照21 CFR 50的要求获得知情同意［21 CFR 312.60］

除了在21 CFR 50.23和50.24规定的那些例外，在所有涉及人类的临床研究中，研究者必须从受试者或者受试者的法定代表获取合法有效的知情同意书。

除了21 CFR 56.109（C）规定的那些情况，作为一个研究者，您的职责就是按照21 CFR 50的要求，从所有的受试者那里获得经过伦理委员会审批的书面知情同意书，书面知情同意书上必须有受试者或者受试者法定代表在签署知情同意书时的签字，签署知情同意书的人应该存有一份签署的知情同意书［21 CFR 50.27（a）］。

您没有获取受试者1001的合法有效的知情同意书，而您却给这个受试者服用了临床试验用新药（b）（4），特别是在临床试验方案（b）（4）中，受试者1001的知情同意书只有受试者的一位家长签字，而没有来自密西西比州人类服务部代表的签字。在临床研究进展的时候，参与到研究中的受试者受到密西西比州人类服务部的监护，所以只有来自密西西比州的人类服务部可以作为法定代表在知情同意书上签字，决定孩子是否可以参与到临床研究当中。

没有获得足够的知情同意，会危害到入组受试者的安全和福利，因为这没有给他们机会去充分地评估参与到临床研究中的风险和收益。

4．您未能快速地向伦理委员会报告研究活动中的所有变更，而且您在未得到伦理委员会批准的情况下对研究进行了变更［21 CFR 312.66］

FDA法规要求，研究者应确保及时向伦理委员会报告在临床研究中所做出的各种变更，所有非预期的可以使受试者陷于风险的问题，只有得到伦理委员会的批准后才可以作出适当的变更，除非是为了立刻解除受试者的危害［21 CFR 312.66］。

您没有遵从上述法规的要求，在没有得到伦理委员会关于修正知情同意书的批准之前，就给受试者1010服用了临床试验用新药（b）（4）。特别是伦理委员会为试验方案（b）（4）批准的知情同意书，被手工做了一些更改，声称受试者在出院之前，不能在知情同意书上列出的时间点得到报酬。受试者1010在变更的知情同意书上签了字。

没有及时向伦理委员会报告临床研究中的各种变更，以及各种变更没有获得伦理委员会的批准，会危害到入组受试者的安全和福利。

本警告信的目的并非是罗列您在试验药物临床研究中存在的所有缺陷。确保遵循法律和相关FDA法规的每一项要求是您的职责。您应当解决这些缺陷，并建立规程，以确保任何正在进行或将来的研究均能符合FDA的法规。

自收到这封信的15个工作日内，您应当书面告知本办公室为预防将来发生类似违规情况已经采取的措施。如果不能充分、迅速地解释上述违规问题，可能导致我们在不再通知的情况下采取监管措施。

附：英文原文

Summers, Timothy, M.D.

WARNING LETTER

FEB 24, 2010

CERTIFIED MAIL
RETURN RECEIPT REQUESTED

Ref: 10-HFD-45-01-02

Timothy Summers, M.D.
Alliance Health Center
5000 Highway 39 N
Meridian, MS 39301-1021

Dear Dr. Summers:

Between March 25 and 27, 2009, Ms. Barbara Wright, representing the Food and Drug Administration (FDA), conducted an investigation and met with you to review your conduct of a clinical investigation [Protocol (b)(4), entitled "(b)(4)"] of the investigational drug (b)(4) performed for (b)(4) Inc.

This inspection is a part of the FDA's Bioresearch Monitoring Program, which includes inspections designed to evaluate the conduct of research and to ensure that the rights, safety, and welfare of the human subjects of those studies have been protected.

From our review of the establishment inspection report and the documents submitted with that report, we conclude that you did not adhere to the applicable statutory requirements and FDA regulations governing the conduct of clinical investigations and the protection of human subjects. We are aware that at the conclusion of the inspection, Ms. Wright presented and discussed with you Form FDA 483, Inspectional Observations. You have not provided a written response to the Form 483. By letter of April 27, 2009, Alliance Health Center (AHC) responded to the Form 483, recognizing that the facility and you failed to adequately address certain protocols. ACH also indicated that you were no longer conducting clinical research at the AHC facility. We wish to emphasize the following:

1. You failed to conduct the studies or ensure they were conducted according to the signed investigator statement and the investigational plan, and to protect the rights, safety, and welfare of subjects under the investigator's care [21 CFR 312.60].

a. Eligibility criteria are designed specifically for each clinical investigation by the sponsor to optimize the interpretability of the data to the disease process under study and to minimize foreseeable harm of enrolled subjects due to co-morbidities and possible interactions with concomitant medications. Three of the six subjects randomized in this clinical investigation did not meet eligibility criteria of having Bipolar I Disorder and as such were placed at risk of injury from participation in the study. Specifically:

i. The protocol eligibility criteria state that a "subject must have a primary diagnosis of Bipolar I Disorder … as defined by the DSM-IV criteria and confirmed by the [Kiddie-Schedule for Affective Disorders and Schizophrenia (K-SADS)]." Subject 1001 was screened and randomized to the study without a primary diagnosis of Bipolar I disorder confirmed by a fully-completed K-SADS assessment. In particular, the K-SADS assessment for Subject 1001 did not contain the indicated Depressive Disorders and the Mania supplements.

ii. The protocol eligibility criteria state that a subject must have a Young Mania Rating Scale (YMRS) score greater than or equal to 17 at the screening and baseline visits. Subjects 1009 and 1010 were each randomized to the study with a YMRS score of 8 at baseline.

b. The protocol states that the first dose of the study medication is taken at the baseline visit after completion of baseline visit procedures to confirm subject eligibility and to perform post-dosing pharmacokinetic (PK) sampling. Subject 1010 was dosed on December 8, 2006, three days prior to the baseline visit on December 11, 2006 and as such did not have eligibility confirmed and did not have PK sampling performed.

c. The protocol requires that efficacy be assessed using the YMRS, the Children's Global Assessment Scale (CGAS), and Clinical Global Impression (CGI) scale at each visit. The CGI assessment was not performed at the Week 1 study visit for Subject 1010.

d. You failed to follow protocols related to the enrollment of wards of the state. The Institutional Review Board (IRB) "Initial Review Submission Form" Box 28 in this study addressed "vulnerable" subject categories. You failed to indicate that you intended to enroll Subjects 1001 and 1007, both wards of the state and thus vulnerable subjects, to the IRB on the Initial Review Submission Form. In turn, the IRB was prevented from assessing whether it was appropriate to enroll wards of the State in this particular clinical investigation and was prevented from requiring that an advocate be appointed for each child who is a ward pursuant to 21 CFR 50.56.

Enrollment of subjects who do not meet eligibility criteria, and not performing study-related procedures jeopardize subject safety and welfare and compromise interpretation and validity of the investigational endpoints.

2. You failed to maintain adequate and accurate case histories that record all observations and other data pertinent to the investigation on each individual administered the investigational drug or employed as a control in the investigation [21 CFR 312.62(b)].

During the inspection, the study records (including study templates and assessment tools) were observed to be unbound and appeared to lack a system of controls, with entries posted to the wrong visit form and multiple versions completed for the same visit. Subject records contained missing pages, numerous unexplained corrections and conflicting information. Few progress notes were observed Violations included, but were not limited to, the following:

a. The protocol eligibility criteria state that a subject must have a YMRS score greater than or equal to 17 at the screening and baseline visits. Study records for Subject 1006 contained two sets of original records with different scoring for the YMRS assessments reportedly obtained during the October 31, 2006 study visit. One of the copies of the YMRS for Subject 1006 dated October 31, 2006 has a score of 11 and the other copy has a score of 23. You provided no explanation for the discrepancies in these records.

b. The K-SADS-Present and Lifetime Version is a multi-part diagnostic interview instrument that consists of a screening interview and five additional diagnostic supplements. The additional diagnostic supplements may be indicated based upon scores obtained as determined by the answers given by the subject during the screening interview. The KSADS-PL for Subjects 1001, 1004 and 1006 were missing every other page and/or the required supplements.

c. The records for Subject 1004 contained numerous errors in subject number, protocol number, and date or identity of study visit. For example:

i. Numerous records reflect that subject number 1002 was used instead of the correct subject number 1004.

ii. Forms marked "Screening Visit," "Week 1 Visit," and "Week 4 Visit" all are dated October 31, 2006.

ⅲ. There are two forms marked “Week 1 Visit” documenting the Children’s Depression Rating Scale Revised (CDRS-R) evaluation with two different dates, October 31, 2006 and November 8, 2006.
ⅳ. You utilized a form from another study entitled “Study” to document testing completed on this subject for this study.
Failing to maintain adequate and accurate case histories compromises the interpretation of and the validity of the clinical investigational endpoints.

3. You failed to obtain informed consent of each subject in accordance with the provisions of 21 CFR Part 50 [21 CFR 312.60].

Except as provided in 21 CFR 50.23 and 50.24, no investigator may involve a human being as a subject in research unless the investigator has obtained the legally-effective informed consent of the subject or the subject’s legally authorized representative [21 CFR 50.20].

As an investigator, it is your responsibility to obtain informed consent in accordance with 21 CFR Part 50. Except as provided in 21 CFR 56.109(c), informed consent shall be documented by the use of a written consent form approved by the IRB and signed and dated by the subject or the subject’s legally authorized representative at the time of consent. A copy shall be given to the person signing the form [21 CFR 50.27(a)].

You failed to obtain legally-effective informed consent from Subject 1001 to whom you prescribed the investigational new drug, (b)(4). Specifically, the informed consent form for Subject 1001 in Protocol (b)(4) was signed only by a parent and not by a representative of the Mississippi State Department of Human Services. At the time of the clinical investigation, the child was in the legal custody of the Mississippi State Department of Human Services and thus only the Mississippi State Department of Human Services could serve as the child’s legally-authorized representative and grant permission for the child to participate in the clinical investigation.

Failing to obtain adequate informed consent jeopardizes the safety and welfare of enrolled subjects by denying them an opportunity to assess the risks and benefits of their participation in the clinical investigation.

4. You failed to promptly report to the IRB all changes in the research activity and you made changes in the research without IRB approval [21 CFR 312.66].

FDA regulations require that the clinical investigator shall assure that he will promptly report to the IRB all changes in the research activity and all unanticipated problems involving risk to human subjects or others, and that he or she will not make any changes in the research with IRB approval, except where necessary to eliminate apparent immediate hazards to human subjects [21 CFR 312.66].

You violated this requirement by administering the investigational new drug (b)(4), to Subject 1010 without obtaining IRB approval of the modified informed consent document. Specifically, the IRB-approved version of the informed consent document for Protocol (b)(4) was altered by hand to state that the subject would not receive payment for participation in accordance with the schedule listed on the form unless treated as an outpatient, and this altered form was signed by the parent of Subject 1010.

Failure to promptly report changes in the research activity to the IRB and making changes in the research without IRB approval compromises the safety and welfare of subjects enrolled in the clinical investigation.

This letter is not intended to be an all-inclusive list of deficiencies with your clinical study of an investigational drug. It is your responsibility to ensure adherence to each requirement of the law and relevant FDA regulations. You should address these deficiencies and establish procedures to ensure that any on-going or future studies will be in compliance with FDA regulations. Within fifteen (15) working days of your receipt of this letter, you should notify this office in writing of the actions you have taken to prevent similar violations in the future. Failure to adequately and promptly explain the violations noted above may result in regulatory action without further notice.

If you have any questions, please contact Constance Lewin, M.D., M.P.H., at 301-796-3397; FAX 301-847-8748. Your written response and any pertinent documentation should be addressed to:

Constance Lewin, M.D., M.P.H.

Branch Chief, Good Clinical Practice Branch I
Division of Scientific Investigations
Office of Compliance
Center for Drug Evaluation and Research
Food and Drug Administration
Bldg 51, Room 5354
10903 New Hampshire Avenue
Silver Spring, MD 20993

Sincerely yours,

{See appended electronic signature page}

Leslie K. Ball, M.D.
Director
Division of Scientific Investigations
Office of Compliance
Center for Drug Evaluation and Research

第115封　给Punjwani, Sohail S. 医学博士的警告信

2010年2月4日

参考号：10-HFD-45-01-04

尊敬的Punjwani博士：

2009年1月20日至2月18日，Brunilda Torres女士和 Colleen Aspinwall女士代表FDA进行了现场检查，与您会面并对您实施的以下临床研究进行了审查：

试验方案（b）(4)，题为“（b）(4)”，试验药物为（b）(4)，申办者为（b）(4)；

试验方案（b）(4)，题为“（b）(4)”，试验药物为（b）(4)，申办者为（b）(4)；

试验方案（b）(4)，题为“（b）(4)”，试验药物为（b）(4)，申办者为（b）(4)。

本次现场检查是FDA的生物研究监查项目的一部分。该项目通过设定的检查方法，对相关研究的实施情况进行评估，以确保这些研究中受试者的权益、安全和福利得到了保护。

经对FDA现场检查报告、该报告的附件，以及您2009年3月13日的书面回复及附件进行审查，我们认为，您没有遵循适用的法律要求和监管临床研究实施的FDA法规。我们知道，在现场检查结束时，Brunilda Torres女士和 Colleen Aspinwall女士向您出示并讨论了FDA483表，即现场检查发现的问题，我们想强调以下几点：

1. 您未能进行研究或者确保按照研究计划进行研究，未能保护受试者的权益、安全和福利［21 CFR 312.60］

a. 试验方案（b）(4)第三部分详细说明，对于体重低于45kg的受试者，试验药物的目标剂量是60～80mg/d；对于体重等于或高于45kg的受试者，试验药物的目标剂量是120~160mg/d。方案同时详细说明，不应在第8天前达到160mg/d的剂量。您并没有一直遵照这些给药限定。

所提供的试验药物及相对应的安慰剂的剂量分别为20mg、40mg、60mg和80mg的胶囊，不同剂量药物的包装外观和大小稍有不同。药物按照“早上”和“晚上”的服用时间分别放于吸塑卡中，药量为7天加上额外3天的服用量。吸塑卡上用不同颜色及字母A、B、C、D来标记四栏，用于区分不同剂量。每一栏包含一个剂量（20mg、40mg、60mg和80mg），这样在一个吸塑卡上就包含四种不同剂量的胶囊。根据方案，护士和家长或监护人将取出1粒胶囊早上服用，1粒胶囊下午服用，其余的留在吸塑卡中。整个研究过程中，当需要调整剂量时，受试者将得到明确详细的说明，然后在早上和晚上从药物吸塑卡中取出相应剂量的胶囊。当有必要改变起初的用药量方案时，建议进行计划外访视，以便研究者观察受试者并向受试者和家长或监护人充分解释用药量方案调整。

关于试验方案（b）(4)，7名入组受试者中，6名患者的服药剂量超出了方案规定的给药限定。

i. 受试者1001，入组时年龄13岁，2006年5月9日随机，2006年6月5日完成试验，停止服药。受试者1001，记录的体重为46.8kg，参加研究（b）(4)期间，连续20天过量用药。

具体而言，2006年5月16日和17日（治疗第8天和第9天），该受试者的给药剂量是180mg/d；2006年5月18日和19日（治疗第10天和第11天），该受试者的给药剂量是240mg/d；2006年5月20日和21日（治疗第12天和第13天），给药剂量是320mg/d；2006年5月22日（治疗第14天），给药剂量是400mg/d，从5月23日直至2006年6月4日（治疗第15天和第27天），这名受试者的给药剂量是180mg/d。研究过程中，该受试者曾出现嗜睡和眩晕。

ii. 受试者1003，入组时15岁，2006年6月1日随机，2006年6月27日完成试验停止服药。受试者1003，记

录的体重为65kg，参加研究（b）（4）期间，连续21天过量给药。

具体而言，2006年6月7日（治疗第7天），该受试者给药剂量为180mg/d，而方案规定第8天前最大给药剂量是160mg/d。2006年6月8日和9日（治疗第8天和第9天），该受试者给药剂量是240mg/d。从6月10日至26日（治疗第10天和第26天），该受试者的给药剂量是400mg/d。在2006年6月27日（治疗第27天），该受试者的给药剂量是280mg/d。

ⅲ. 受试者1004，入组时16岁，2006年6月1日随机，因缺乏疗效和嗜睡，未完成试验，于2006年6月14日结束。受试者在参加研究（b）（4）期间，连续3天超出最大目标剂量（160mg/d）给药。具体而言，2006年6月9日（治疗第9天），该受试者给药剂量是320mg/d。2006年6月10日和11日（治疗第10天和第11天），该受试者的给药剂量是240mg/d。该受试者在研究过程中出现嗜睡状态。

ⅳ. 受试者1005，入组时15岁，2006年6月14日随机，因受试者依从性差，未完成试验，于2006年7月18日结束。受试者在参加研究（b）（4）期间，连续16天超出最大目标剂量（160mg/d）给药。具体而言，2006年6月21日和22日（治疗第8天和第9天），该受试者给药剂量是180mg/d。2006年6月23日至27日（治疗第10天和第14天），该受试者的给药剂量是240mg/d。2006年6月28日至7月3日，7月5日至7月6日（治疗第15天至第20天，第22天至第23天），该受试者的给药剂量是400mg/d。2006年7月4日（治疗第21天），该受试者的给药剂量是200mg/d。

ⅴ. 受试者1006，入组时13岁，2006年6月26日随机，2006年7月25日完成试验停止服药。受试者1005，记录的体重低于45kg，受试者在参加研究（b）（4）期间，总共连续7天超剂量给药。具体而言，2006年7月11日至17日（治疗第16天至第22天），该受试者的给药剂量是400mg/d。

ⅵ. 受试者1007，入组时10岁，2006年6月27日随机，2006年7月25日完成试验停止服药。受试者1007，记录的体重为39.5kg，受试者在参加研究（b）（4）期间，连续13天超剂量给药。具体而言，2006年7月12日至24日（治疗第16天至第28天），该受试者的给药剂量是120mg/d。

关于试验方案（**b**）（**4**），纳入一名受试者，该受试者的给药剂量超出了方案的限定。

ⅶ. 受试者1001为青少年，2006年5月1日随机，2006年5月23日因幻听加重并导致其刮伤手腕而在试验完成前停止给药。受试者1001，记录的体重为66.5kg，受试者在参加研究（b）（4）期间，连续17天超剂量给药。具体而言，2006年5月5日（治疗第5天），该受试者给药320mg/d。2006年5月6日至21日（治疗第6天至第21天），该受试者给药400mg/d。

在您2009年3月13日的回复中，您表示2006年7月26日您第一次从数据管理人员处获知研究开展过程中出现了给药错误，您推测这是由于您误认为吸塑卡中胶囊的剂量均为20mg。您说明，在获知这一问题之后，您立即电话告知了每一位受试者的家长或监护人，并向那些回答说没有不良事件的家长，询问了任何可能存在的安全性事件。您声明，在电话中，您通知家长和监护人停止按照之前的给药剂量服药，开始正确的服药剂量。2006年8月4日，您给家长和监护人发了跟踪函。您还声明，在2006年7月26日，（b）（4）研究的监查员、您的研究人员和您一起针对正确的给药剂量和药物发放进行了核实。此外，2006年7月31日，您的研究人员参加了由方案组（b）（4）组织的（b）（4）招募问题解答会，包括针对上述您参加的所有的（b）（4）临床研究中心研究的有关给药剂量和发药的培训。

作为您纠正措施计划的一部分，您正式地修改了您的标准操作规程。具体而言，您指出修订“研究药物剂量和发放标准操作规程”更具体地说明了住院患者和门诊患者的剂量流程，特别要求在整个研究期间，研究者或指定人员应记录给药剂量（mg）及给药片数，以及清楚的药量计算和后续的剂量滴定。您还说明，对“研究启动标准操作规程”进行了修改：①强调研究者会议上收到并审阅的文件；②增加审阅伦理委员会给研究者的操作手册；③增加模拟对一名受试者从筛选到完成的给药剂量和流程的记录。此外，您说还修订了“质量保证/质量控制标准操作规程”，确保对2名受试者，或10%的随机受试者进行监查，内容包括持续进行的给药和发药情况监查，方案依从性、既往/合并用药和禁忌用药情况的监查。

我们认可您的回复。但是，我们担心您的回复还不足以预防将来再次发生上述违规事件。尤其是从研究一开始，您没有充分了解药物的包装，在整个研究期间，也没能给予参加本次临床试验的受试者以正确的给药剂量。我们了解到，在申办者发现研究者未能正确给药之后，改变了试验药物的包装。尽管是包装的问题，但作为研究者，您负有确保遵循方案的职责，包括确保每位受试者的给药是正确的。

b. 试验方案（b）（4）和（b）（4）第5.3.3节规定，对于两周内如何将受试者每日的用药剂量，从起始剂量20mg（基线访视时）增加至目标剂量，您应有一个大致的滴注计划。在制订该计划时，您应考虑受试者的精神疾病史、目前精神疾病状态，以及体重。方案允许您根据受试者的临床反应和耐受性调整滴定计划。您或您的研究人员应向受试者解释滴定计划，并向受试者清楚地解释，在滴定计划的最初7天里，如何从“上午”和“下午”的吸塑卡中取出胶囊。而且，试验方案（b）（4）和（b）（4）5.3.4还规定了您应在第一周及之后的访视中评估受试者服药的依从性。此外，受试者每次归还的试验药物，您应计数清点，核对分发给受试者的药物与受试者汇报的服药情况的一致性。没有证据证明您根据方案要求，为纳入的受试者制订了剂量滴定计划，或评估了受试者服药依从性，并对用药的一致性进行了必要的核对。

在您2009年3月13日的回复中，您承认您未能完整记录详细的给药指示和滴定计划。您说您认识到为了确保准确的给药剂量，详细的记录是必要的。作为纠正措施，您说您将修改“研究药物剂量和发放标准操作规程”，针对有关如何、为什么，以及何时调整剂量的详细记录予以详细说明。我们认可您保证将会采取这些纠正措施。然而，我们注意到，您的回复中没有包括您将要实施的具体流程或程序的要点，以预防将来再次发生上述违规情况，尤其是，我们担心您在制订剂量滴定计划、评估受试者的依从性以及核对药物数量一致性时，不能做到遵循方案，这会造成严重的超剂量给药，导致在您纳入的儿童受试者身上再次出现上述不良事件。如您在您的回复中所说，2006年7月26日您第一次从（b）（4）数据管理人员处获知在您开展儿科研究过程中出现了给药错误。可能的情况是，您未能遵循方案导致了在您未能意识到出现了超剂量给药，直至被申办者的数据管理人员发现才引起您的注意。尽管可能存在试验药物包装方面的问题，说到底，还是由于您未能采取必要的安全措施，以至于儿童受试者被暴露于不必要的严重过量给药中，危害了受试者的权益、安全和福利。

c. 试验方案（b）（4）6.2要求在基线完成血清妊娠和尿液药物筛查检测。没有对下列受试者进行上述检测：

i. 受试者1002的基线血清妊娠和尿液药物筛查检测；

ii. 受试者1003的基线血清妊娠和尿液药物筛查检测；

iii. 受试者1004的基线尿液药物筛查检测；

iv. 受试者1007的基线尿液药物筛查检测。

在您2009年3月13日的回复中，您说受试者1002、1003、1004和1007在基线时是住院患者。考虑到筛选时他们的妊娠试验和尿液药物筛查是阴性，您指出您的研究人员推测这些受试者的检测结果不可能会有改变，因此没有在基线时重复检测。您写道，贵研究场所创建了访视清单，以确保实施每次访视所要求的全部研究相关流程，而完成这份清单是贵研究场所的标准工作常规。我们认可您的回复。然而，无论筛选检查结果如何，都应按方案规定在基线时应进行血清妊娠和尿液药物筛查检测。制定的访视清单作为贵研究场所的标准常规，避免将来发生类似问题的做法，可以被接受。

2. 您未能快速地向伦理委员会报告研究实施过程中的所有变更［21 CFR 312.66］

2006年8月2日，在确认了试验药物剂量错误时，申办者要求您停止贵研究场所的受试者入组。2007年2月7日，因为出现给药错误以及持续性地不及时回复疑问和完成数据澄清表等违背GCP的问题，申办者通知您终止在贵研究场所开展的（b）（4）儿科研究，包括试验方案（b）（4）。您未能将申办者的这些决定告知伦理委员会。贵研究场所的文件记录显示，您报告伦理委员会的仅限于有关受试者给药错误的方案违背事件，您没有在跟踪审查报告和结题报告中将申办者的决定报告伦理委员会。

在您2009年3月13日的回复中，您说您承担未能及时报告伦理委员会的全部责任。为了确保能继续遵循伦理委员会的准则，您说贵研究场所于2007年3月17日进行了关于伦理委员会的正式培训，并分发了西部伦理委员会的研究者指南（第1.5和1.6版）供独立审阅。我们认可您的回复并认为您的纠正计划是可被接受的。

本警告信的目的并非是罗列您在试验药物临床研究中存在的所有缺陷。确保遵循法律和相关FDA法规的每一项要求是您的职责。您应当解决这些缺陷，并建立规程，以确保任何正在进行或将来的研究均能符合FDA的法规。

自收到这封信的15个工作日内，您应当书面告知本办公室为预防将来发生类似违规情况已经采取的措施。如果不能充分、迅速地解释上述违规问题，可能导致我们在不再通知的情况下采取监管措施。

附：英文原文

Punjwani, Sohail S. M.D.

WARNING LETTER

FEB 04, 2010

CERTIFIED MAIL
RETURN RECEIPT REQUESTED

Ref:10-HFD-45-01-04

Sohail Punjwani, M.D.
Professional Clinical Research
1065 NE 125th Street, Suite 221
North Miami, Florida 33161

Dear Dr. Punjwani:

Between January 20 and February 18, 2009, Ms. Brunilda Torres and Ms. Colleen Aspinwall, representing the Food and Drug Administration (FDA), conducted an investigation and met with you, to review your conduct of the following clinical investigations:

Protocol (b)(4), entitled "(b)(4)," of the investigational drug (b)(4) performed for (b)(4).;

Protocol (b)(4), entitled, "(b)(4)" of the investigational drug (b)(4) performed for (b)(4).; and

Protocol (b)(4), entitled "(b)(4)" of the investigational drug (b)(4) performed for (b)(4)

This inspection is a part of the FDA' s Bioresearch Monitoring Program, which includes inspections designed to evaluate the conduct of research and to ensure that the rights, safety, and welfare of the human subjects of those studies have been protected. From our review of the establishment inspection report, the documents submitted with that report, and your March 13, 2009 written response and its attachments, we conclude that you did not adhere to the applicable statutory requirements and FDA regulations governing the conduct of clinical investigations. We are aware that at the conclusion of the inspection, Ms. Brunilda Torres and Ms. Colleen Aspinwall presented and discussed with you Form FDA 483, Inspectional Observations. We wish to emphasize the following:

1. You failed to conduct the studies or ensure they were conducted according to the investigational plans, and to protect the rights, safety and welfare of subjects [21 CFR 312.60].

a. Section 3 of Protocols (b)(4) specified that for subjects with a body weight less than 45 kg, the target dose of study drug was 60-80 mg/day; and for subjects with a body weight greater than or equal to 45 kg, the target dose of study drug was 120-160 mg/day. These protocols also specified that the dose level of 160 mg/day was not to be achieved before Day 8 of treatment. These study drug administration limits were not always followed.

The study drug and matching placebo were supplied as 20-, 40-, 60-, and 80-mg capsules, with the appearance and size slightly different among the dosage strengths. All medications were packaged in AM (morning dosing) and PM (evening dosing) blister cards that supplied medication for seven days plus three extra days. Each blister card was marked with four different-colored columns labeled with the letters A, B, C, and D to distinguish the different potencies. Each column contained one potency (20-, 40-, 60-, and 80-mg), such that four capsule strengths were available for each dose. Per protocol, the nursing staff and subject' s parent(s) or guardian(s) were to select one capsule for the morning administration and one capsule for the afternoon administration, and leave the remaining capsules in the blister pack. Throughout the study and when dosing modifications were necessary, subjects were to receive clear specifications regarding which capsule was to be taken from the morning and afternoon blister cards. When changes to the original dosage plan were necessary, unscheduled visits were recommended so that subjects could be observed and so that changes to the dosage plan could be fully explained to the subjects and to his or her parent(s) or guardian(s).

Regarding Protocol (b)(4): Six of the seven randomized subjects received dosages in excess of protocol-specified limits:

i. Subject 1001, age 13 at the time of enrollment, was randomized on May 9, 2006, and discontinued on June 5, 2006, upon completion of the study. Subject 1001, with a documented weight of 46.8 kg, was overdosed on study medication for 20 consecutive days while participating in study (b)(4).

Specifically, on May 16 and 17, 2006 (Treatment Days 8 and 9), this subject received 180 mg/day; on May 18 and 19, 2006 (Treatment Days 10 and 11), this subject received 240 mg/day; on May 20 and 21, 2006 (Treatment Days 12 and 13), this subject received 320 mg/day; on May 22, 2006 (Treatment Day 14), this subject received 400 mg/day; and from May 23 through June 4, 2006 (Treatment Days 15 through 27), this subject received 180 mg/day. This subject experienced sedation and dizziness during the study.

ii. Subject 1003, age 15 at the time of enrollment, was randomized on June 1, 2006, and discontinued on June 27, 2006, upon completion of the study. Subject 1003, with a documented weight of 65 kg, was overdosed on study medication for 21 consecutive days while participating in study (b)(4) Specifically, on June 7, 2006 (Treatment Day 7), this subject received 180 mg/day, in excess of the protocol-specified maximum dose of 160 mg/day prior to Day 8 of treatment. On June 8 and 9, 2006 (Treatment Days 8 and 9), this subject received 240 mg/day. From June 10 through 26, 2006 (Treatment Days 10 through 26), this subject received 400 mg/day. On June 27, 2006 (Treatment Day 27), this subject received 280 mg/day.

iii. Subject 1004, age 16 at the time of enrollment, was randomized on June 1, 2006, and discontinued on June 14, 2006, prior to study completion, due to lack of efficacy and sedation. Subject 1004 received doses in excess of the maximum target dose (160 mg/day) for 3 consecutive days while participating in Study (b)(4). Specifically, on June 9, 2006 (Treatment Day 9), this subject received 320 mg/day. On June 10 and 11, 2006 (Treatment Days 10 and 11), this subject received 240 mg/day. This subject experienced sedation during the study.

iv. Subject 1005, age 15 at the time of enrollment, was randomized on June 14, 2006, and discontinued on July 18, 2006, prior to study completion, due to noncompliance. Subject 1005 received doses in excess of the maximum target dose (160 mg/day) for 16 consecutive days while participating in study (b)(4). Specifically, on June 21 and 22, 2006 (Treatment Days 8 and 9), this subject received 180 mg/day. From June 23 through 27, 2006 (Treatment Days 10 through 14), this subject received 240 mg/day. From June 28 through July 3, and July 5 through July 6, 2006 (Treatment Days 15 through 20 and Days 22 through 23), this subject received 400 mg/day. On July 4, 2006 (Treatment Day 21), this subject received 200 mg/day.

v. Subject 1006, age 13 at the time of enrollment, was randomized on June 26, 2006, and discontinued on July 25, 2006, upon study completion. Subject 1006, with a documented weight less than 45 kg, was overdosed on study medication for a total of 7 consecutive days while participating in study (b)(4). Specifically, from July 11 through 17, 2006 (Treatment Days 16 through 22), this subject received 400 mg/day.

vi. Subject 1007, age 10 at the time of enrollment, was randomized on June 27, 2006, and discontinued on July 25, 2006, upon study completion. Subject 1007, with a documented weight of 39.5 kg, was overdosed on study medication for 13 consecutive days while participating in study (b)(4) Specifically, from July 12 through 24, 2006 (Treatment Days 16 through 28), this subject received 120 mg/day.

Regarding Protocol (b)(4): The only subject randomized in this study received dosages in excess of protocol-specified limits:

ⅶ.Subject 1001, an adolescent, was randomized on May 1, 2006, and discontinued on May 23, 2006, prior to study completion, due to worsening auditory hallucinations that apparently caused the subject to lacerate her wrists. Subject 1001, with a documented weight of 66.5 kg, was overdosed on study medication for 17 consecutive days while participating in study (b)(4). Specifically, on May 5, 2006 (Treatment Day 5), this subject received 320 mg/day. From May 6 through 21, 2006 (Treatment Days 6 through 21), this subject received 400 mg/day.

In your March 13, 2009 response, you stated that you were first notified on July 26, 2006 by (b)(4) data management personnel that there were dosing errors in the conduct of the studies, stemming from your mistaken assumption that all capsules contained in the study drug blister pack were of the same 20 mg strength. Immediately upon becoming aware of this issue, you stated that you telephoned each subject's parent or guardian to inform him or her of this error, and inquired about any possible safety concerns or issues, of which there were none. You stated that during these calls, you instructed the parents and guardians to stop dispensing the currently prescribed dosage and begin the corrected dosage amount. A follow-up letter was also sent to the parents and guardians on August 4, 2006. You noted that the (b)(4) study monitor conducted a targeted review with you and your research staff on the correct dosing and dispensing of study medication on July 26, 2006. Additionally, on July 31, 2006, your research staff attended the (b)(4)-hosted Question and Answer (b)(4) Recruitment meeting that included training on the dosing and dispensing for all (b)(4) research sites conducting the above-referenced studies in which you were involved.

As part of your corrective action plan, you made formal revisions to your Standard Operating Procedures (SOPs). Specifically, you indicated that the Dosing and Dispensing of Investigational Product SOP was revised to add a more detailed inpatient and outpatient dosing process and to further specify how the clinical investigator, or designee, should document dosing instructions in both milligrams and tablets/capsules, as well as clearly document original dosing schematics and any titration throughout the study. You also noted that the Study Launch Procedures SOPs were revised to: (1) emphasize the materials reviewed and received at the investigator meetings, (2) include the review of the applicable Institutional Review Board (IRB) manuals for investigators, and (3) include internal documentation of the dosing and procedures to be performed on a mock subject from screening through study completion. Additionally, you stated that the Quality Assurance/Quality Control (QA/QC) Program SOP was also revised to ensure the oversight of two subjects, or 10% of the population randomized, with ongoing review of dosing and dispensing, protocol compliance, prior/concomitant medications, and prohibited medications.

We acknowledge your response. However, we are concerned that the response is not adequate to prevent future recurrence of the violation noted above. In particular, we are concerned that you did not properly understand the study drug packaging from the start of the study and you did not ensure that the appropriate dose was administered throughout the study. We are aware that the sponsor subsequently changed the packaging for the investigational product following observations that clinical investigators were not properly dosing subjects. Notwithstanding the packaging concerns, as clinical investigator, you retain responsibility for ensuring that the protocol is followed, including ensuring that the proper dose is administered to subjects.

b. Section 5.3.3 of Protocols (b)(4) and (b)(4) specified that you were to have developed a titration plan to increase the subject' s total daily dose of study medication from a 20 mg starting dose (at the baseline visit) to a target dose achieved over 2 weeks, in general. In developing the titration plan, you were to have considered the subject's psychiatric history, current psychiatric status, and weight. The Protocol also permitted you to modify the plan at any time based on a subject's clinical response and toleration. You or a staff member were to have explained the titration plans to subjects, and to have clearly specified which capsules the subjects were to have taken from each AM and PM column for the first seven days of the titration plan. Furthermore, Section 5.3.4 of Protocols (b)(4) and (b)(4) specified that you were to have assessed subject' s compliance with study medication administration at Week 1 and at each subsequent visit. Additionally, you were to have counted medication returned by subjects to reconcile medication dispensed with subject' s reported usage. There is no evidence that you developed dosing titration plans for the subjects enrolled in these studies, or that you assessed subject' s compliance and performed the requisite drug reconciliation as specified in the protocols.

In your March 13, 2009 response, you acknowledged your failure to fully document specific dosing instructions and titration plans. You stated that you recognized that this specific documentation was necessary in order to ensure accurate dosing. As a corrective measure, you stated that your Dosing and Dispensing of Investigational Product SOP will be revised to include more specific information on how, why, and when dosing changes are documented. We acknowledge your assurance that corrective actions will be taken. However, we note that your response did not contain a detailed outline of procedures or processes that would be implemented to prevent future recurrence of the violation noted above. Specifically, we are concerned that your lack of adherence to the protocol in developing dosing titration plans, assessing subject's compliance, and performing drug reconciliation led to the significant overdoses and resultant adverse events experienced by the pediatric subjects enrolled at your site as described above. As you noted in your response, you were first notified on July 26, 2006 by (b)(4) data management personnel that there were dosing errors in your conduct of these pediatric studies. It is likely that your lack of adherence to the protocols led to your failure to recognize the overdosing at your site, until it was discovered and brought to your attention by the sponsor's data management unit. While there may have been concerns with the packaging of the study drug, your failure to conduct the requisite safety measures contributed to the unnecessary exposure of pediatric subjects to significant overdoses, which jeopardized the subject' s rights, safety, and welfare.

c. Section 6.2 of Protocol (b)(4) required serum pregnancy and urine drug screening tests to be performed at baseline. These tests were not performed for the following subjects:

i. Subject 1002' s serum pregnancy and urine drug-screening tests were not performed at baseline.

ii.Subject 1003' s serum pregnancy and urine drug-screening tests were not performed at baseline.

iii.Subject 1004' s urine drug-screening tests were not performed at baseline.

iv.Subject 1007' s urine drug-screening tests were not performed at baseline.

In your March 13, 2009 response, you stated that Subjects 1002, 1003, 1004, and 1007 were inpatients at baseline. Given that the pregnancy and urine drug screen tests were negative for these subjects at the time of screening, you indicated that your research staff did not repeat the tests at baseline as they assumed there was no opportunity for the results to change. You noted that a Visit Checklist was created to ensure that all study-related procedures are being conducted for each visit, and that completion of this checklist is now standard work practice at your site. We acknowledge your response. However, regardless of the results obtained at screening, the serum pregnancy and urine drug tests should also have been performed at baseline as specified in the protocol. The Visit Checklist you have instituted as standard practice at your site to prevent any similar future occurrences is acceptable.

2. You failed to promptly report to the Institutional Review Board (IRB) all changes in the research activity [21 CFR 312.66].

On August 2, 2006, upon confirming study drug dosing errors, the sponsor instructed you to cease subject enrollment at your site. On February 7, 2007, the sponsor notified you of its decision to terminate your investigational site's participation in the (b)(4) pediatric studies, including Protocols (b)(4) due to good clinical practice (GCP) noncompliance related to dosing errors and continued delays in resolution of queries and data-clarification forms. You failed to notify the IRB of these decisions made by the sponsor. Documentation available at your site indicates that notification of the IRB was limited to the submission of protocol deviation reports concerning subject's overdosing errors. Furthermore, you failed to notify the IRB of the sponsor' s decisions in the continuing review reports and study close-out letters.

In your March 13, 2009 response, you stated that you assume full responsibility for the lack of notification to the IRB. To ensure continued compliance with IRB guidelines, you noted that formal training concerning IRBs was conducted at your site on March 17, 2007, and the Western Institutional Review Board Guide for Researchers Versions 1.5 and 1.6 was distributed at your site for independent review. We acknowledge your response and find your corrective actions acceptable.

This letter is not intended to be an all-inclusive list of deficiencies with your clinical study of an investigational drug. It is your responsibility to ensure adherence to each requirement of the law and relevant FDA regulations. You should address these deficiencies and establish procedures to ensure that any on-going or future studies will be in compliance with FDA regulations.

Within fifteen (15) working days of your receipt of this letter, you should notify this office in writing of the actions

you have taken to prevent similar violations in the future. Failure to adequately and promptly explain the violations noted above may result in regulatory action without further notice.

If you have any questions, please contact Constance Cullity (formerly Lewin), M.D., M.P.H., at 301-796-3397; FAX 301-847-8748. Your written response and any pertinent documentation should be addressed to:

Constance Cullity (formerly Lewin), M.D., M.P.H.
Branch Chief, Good Clinical Practice Branch I
Division of Scientific Investigations
Office of Compliance
Center for Drug Evaluation and Research
Food and Drug Administration
Building 51, Room 5354
10903 New Hampshire Avenue
Silver Spring, MD 20993

Sincerely yours,

/S/

Leslie K. Ball, M.D.
Director
Division of Scientific Investigations
Office of Compliance
Center for Drug Evaluation and Research

第116封　给Nasr, Samya医学博士的警告信

2010年1月28日

参考号：10-HFD-45-01-03

尊敬的Nasr博士：

2009年7月20日至8月25日，Barbara Rusin 和 L'Oreal Fowlkes女士代表FDA进行了现场检查，与您会面并对您所实施的以下临床研究进行了审查：

试验方案CP-AI-005，题目为“一项双盲、多中心、随机、安慰剂对照赖氨酸氨曲南吸入治疗肺部假单胞菌感染并需要持续使用抗生素的囊性纤维化患者的Ⅲ期试验（AIR-CF2）”，其中试验药物是赖氨酸氨曲南，申办者为Corus制药。

试验方案CP-AI-007，题目为“评价肺部假单胞菌感染的囊性纤维化患者赖氨酸氨曲南吸入治疗的双盲、多中心、多国家、随机、安慰剂对照的Ⅲ期试验（AIR-CF1）”，试验药物赖氨酸氨曲南，申办者为Corus制药。

试验方案08-108，题目为“评价地纽福索四钠盐吸入溶液治疗轻度囊性纤维化肺疾病患者的多中心、双盲、安慰剂对照、随机有效性和安全性研究（INS37217）”，试验药物地纽福索四钠盐，申办者为Inspire制药。

试验方案08-110，题目为“一项评价地纽福索四钠盐吸入溶液治疗预期FEV1≥75%但≤110%的囊性纤维化肺部疾病患者的Ⅲ期、国际多中心、随机、双盲、安慰剂对照、平行组的有效性和安全性研究”，试验药物地纽福索四钠盐，申办者为Inspire制药。

试验方案0000726，题目为“一项评价ALTU-135治疗囊性纤维化相关的胰腺外分泌功能不全患者有效性和安全性的Ⅲ期、随机、双盲、安慰剂对照的临床研究”，试验药物ALTU-135，申办者为Altus制药。

试验方案0000767，题目为“一项评价ALTU-135治疗囊性纤维化相关的胰腺外分泌功能不全患者长期安全性的开放临床研究”，试验药物ALTU-135，申办者为Alnara制药。

本次现场检查是FDA的生物研究监查项目的一部分，该项目通过设定的检查方法，评估相关研究的实施情况，以确认这些研究中受试者的权益、安全和福利得到了保护。

经对FDA现场检查报告、该报告的附件，以及您2009年9月16日和11月24日的书面回复进行审查，我们认为，您没有遵循适用的法律要求和监管临床研究实施的FDA法规。我们获知，在现场检查结束时，检查员向您出示并讨论了FDA483表，即现场检查发现的问题。我们想强调以下几点：

1. 您未能按21 CFR 50的要求来获得知情同意［21 CFR 312.60］

FDA法规21 CFR 50.20声明除21 CFR 50.23和21 CFR 50.24规定的情况外，除非研究者获取了受试者或受试者法定代表人法律上有效的知情同意，否则研究者不能把患者入组为在法规指导下的研究的受试者。法规特别说明研究者获取知情同意应该提供给可能的受试者或者受试者代理人充分的机会考虑是否参加，并且最小化受胁迫或者受不当影响的可能性。

FDA法规的50.27部分进一步声明，除非如21 CFR 56.109（c）情况下，知情同意都应该使用一个书面知情文件进行记录，并且这一文件要由受试者或者受试者代理人在做知情时进行签署。

a. 试验方案CP-AI-005的目的是为了评价对有肺部假单胞菌感染的囊性纤维化患者在给予28天托普霉素溶液吸入治疗后用赖氨酸氨曲南吸入（Cayston™）治疗28天的安全性和有效性以及其维持或者改善临床状况的能力。IRB在2005年4月7日批准了原版知情同意书，但是，研究的目的被错误地写为观察一种研究用吸入性抗生素，赖氨酸氨曲南吸入剂是否“可以阻止PA［假单胞菌］重回患者的肺部”。

在2005年6月28日的一封邮件中（b）（4）告知您，申办者需要对已经批准的知情同意书做几项修改，包

括："（目的）：第2句到最后一句，请把'新药'改为'研究或试验药物'。请修改这部分的最后一句以便能正确地反映此研究的目的——来观察是否AL［赖氨酸氨曲南］在有肺部感染的CF患者中是安全和有效的，而不是看AL［赖氨酸氨曲南］是如何很好地阻止PA［假单胞菌］重回患者［原文如此］的肺部"。您的研究中心重新提交了一份修改的知情同意书（第2版）给IRB，并且在2005年8月25日获得了批准。

但在2005年9月12日的一封邮件中，申办者告知您关于修改后的知情同意书还是存在问题。申办者强调知情同意书中2.1部分的声明，宣称赖氨酸氨曲南可以阻止假单胞菌重回肺部可以看作是无依据的，因为赖氨酸氨曲南还仍然是试验药物。根据这封邮件，您要求申办者同意运送试验药物和容许受试者用现在IRB批准版本的知情同意书入组患者。申办者批准了向您的研究中心运送试验药物，条件是您提交一份能把所有问题都解决的修改版知情同意书给IRB，并且对所有入组患者重做知情。申办者还批准了您可以使用现在IRB批准版本的知情同意书，如果您能在ICF上记录：①潜在生育女性患者要被告知在随访1做血清妊娠检查；②用现在版本已经做过知情的所有患者要被告知在稍晚日期需要用修改后的知情同意书重做知情；③所有用现在版本已经做过知情的患者要被告知赖氨酸氨曲南没有被证明能如2.1部分说明的那样阻止假单胞菌重回肺部，并且此研究的目的实际上是观察是否赖氨酸氨曲南能成功治疗CF患者假单胞菌的肺部感染。在2005年9月14日的邮件中，您又一次被提醒要把更新的、正确的知情同意书发给IRB。IRB在2006年3月9日批准了3.1版的知情同意书。

FDA的现场检查发现对所有已经入组研究的6位受试者，其知情同意书或者是同意书上没有任何记录表明您已按照申办者的要求就此次研究的真正目的告知了这些受试者。除此之外，记录申办者关于血清妊娠检测和对受试者重做知情的要求的手写记录或是：①没有记录在知情同意书上和/或同意书上；或是②与所有知情同意书和/或同意书副本上的不一致。而且，受试者004、005和006直到2006年7月才用3.1版修改后的知情同意书重做知情，这大约比IRB批准3.1版 ICF晚了3个月。

在您的书面回复中，您承认没有意识到在知情同意书2版中和在方案中对研究目的的解释存在实质上的不同。您也承认当申办者在2005年7月第一次让这个问题引起您的注意时，您没有及时修正。您进一步声明手写的声明在受试者知情前已经添加到同意书中，您现在可以意识到并理解这些声明在任何时候都不应该被加进到知情中。对这一缺陷，您的纠正措施包括制定了新的SOP，其中包括要求"完成电子研究申请"来保证研究团队中一位成员审阅了方案、研究者手册、知情文件和电子研究提交中的信息一致性。"对监查报告的回复"要求对任何的发现要做出快速反应，并且向IRB提交正式报告，以做进一步考虑；"获取知情同意"将会禁止知情同意书上手写声明。

您的回复是不充分的。在审阅题目为"电子研究提交标准操作规程"的SOP中，在您承诺的纠正措施中，没有流程详细说明您中心使用何种方法来证明在知情同意书、方案、研究者手册和电子研究提交中所有要素的一致性。您关于在给受试者做知情前，手写声明已被添加的主张也不能被证实。很多情况下，在您研究记录中保留的知情同意书副本与医疗记录中发现的副本是不同的。

b. 受试者385-003和385-007的知情同意书和/或同意书未找到，他们是为08-108方案筛选的。但是，这两位受试者与研究相关的筛选流程已经完成。（分别在2007年2月22日和2007年9月5日）

在您的书面回复中，您承认了这一缺陷。您强调包括"获取知情同意""文件管理和保存""患者完成研究/提前结束/筛选失败"在内的新的SOP的生成；和对研究团队就这些SOP进行培训等纠正措施是为了防止这一错误的再次发生。这些纠正措施看起来是很充分的。

c. 对于08-110方案，注意到了如下问题：

i. 受试者385-101和385-102的知情同意文件没有在方框上做选择来体现受试者是否愿意参加或者不参加P2Y2基因分型测试唾液的收集。但是，您却收集这两位受试者的唾液标本并把它们送到中心实验室进行检测。

ii. 由受试者385-104签署的日期为2009年1月9日原版知情同意书在受试者是否选择参加或者放弃参加P2Y2基因分型检测的唾液收集的方框内没有做选择。但您收集了此受试者的唾液标本并把它送到中心实验室进行检测。表明受试者选择参加基因分型测试的唾液收集的选项标记是在随后的2009年2月13日完成的，但这已经是在唾液标本被收集之后了。

在您的书面回复中，您承认了这一缺陷并声明您的研究中心已经发现了从受试者那里取得标本做“任何的基因分析之前”没有取得充分知情的错误。您的纠正措施包括修改知情同意文件的最后一页可选择性检查的选项框的策略。您声称如果IRB同意这种新方法，就会将它包括在关于“获取知情同意”而新制定的SOP中。

您的回复是不充分的。我们发现，没有证据表明研究中心在取得标本进行基因分析前发现了这一错误。更有甚者，在FDA现场检查中似乎还发现了在取标本进行检测之前缺少知情同意的情况。而且，在现场检查过程中，您提供的文件表明，在2009年7月23日的邮件中当申办者被告知385-101和受试者385-102缺少做基因检测的知情时，申办者声明这些样本将要被销毁。申办者的邮件没有提到这些样本没有进行过任何基因检测。另外，您没有提供表明这个错误在检测发生之前已经被发现的证据。我们也注意到，即使没做基因分析检测，也不能否认在没有取得他们知情同意时已经从受试者那里收取样本的这个事实。

d. 对于试验方案0000726，受试者009-001和009-002签署的知情同意文件中没有包括测定维生素K水平而进行血样检测的参考说明。但是，您却对这两位受试者血样进行了维生素K检测。

在您的书面回复中，您承认了这一缺陷并声称已经制定了一个“研究材料和供应管理”的SOP以此作为纠正措施来防止这一错误的再次发生。

您的回答是不充分的。您没有提供纠正措施计划来保证给研究受试者做那些只包括在知情同意书中的检查。而且，在对“研究材料和供应管理”的SOP审阅时，流程声称您的人员将会通过检查“研究试剂盒的内容来验证只有经过IRB批准的检测收集试管包括在试剂盒中，此后它们再被运送到研究采血团队”。然而没有明确的流程来表明您中心如何证明试剂盒中的检测项目与当试剂盒运达时，已生效的当前已批准的方案或方案修证案中的检测项目是一致的。

2. 您未能确保按照研究计划进行研究［21 CFR 312.60］

a. 试验方案08-110声明在访视1胸部X射线检查必须完成，除非是访视1之前12个月之内受试者做过的胸部X射线，高分辨率计算机断层扫描（HRCT），胸部CT扫描或者肺部磁共振检查。受试者385-101在2008年9月10日入组本研究并在2008年9月17日访视2时收到试验药物，但是，这名受试者在访视1时，没做X射线检查，也没有显示在访视1之前的12个月内有做过胸部X射线、高分辨率计算机断层扫描（HRCT）、胸部CT扫描或者是肺部磁共振检查的文件记录。原始文件确认此受试者的胸X射线检查是在2008年9月17日完成的，大概在受试者接受首剂的试验药物一个小时之后。

在您的书面回复中，您承认了这一缺陷并声称已经制定了关于“方案偏离和研究修正”以及“文件管理和保存”的SOP，以此作为纠正措施防止这一错误的再次发生。我们承认在您的信中，您说明已经采取了纠正措施来防止这一错误的再次发生。尽管这些纠正措施看上去恰当，但正是由于在做试验的过程中缺乏相应措施才导致了以上所列违规情况的发生，也引起我们对研究中心受试者受保护的充分性的担忧。

b. 试验方案0000726定义，不良事件是指在患者或者临床研究患者身上发生的任何的不良的医学事件，不管其是否与试验药物有关。按照方案，从研究开始第一天所有的不良事件都要收集，一直持续到为期2周的追踪随访。而且，方案声称所有的研究人员都要负责确保足够的安全性信息都要记录在CRF上。FDA现场检查发现在进展报告中注明的几个AE没有记录在CRF上。例如：

受试者	不良事件	原始记录上记录的AE日期
009-001	胃肠胀气	10/22/2007、10/29/2007、11/05/2007
009-001	右肺啰音和呼吸减弱	10/24/2007、10/29/2007
009-002	双肺基底部啰音	12/03/2007
009-002	暗色痰	12/03/2007
009-002	双侧肺上下叶显著干啰音	12/06/2007

续表

受试者	不良事件	原始记录上记录的AE日期
009-005	中等程度干啰音	03/03/2008
009-005	鼻甲肿胀	03/05/2008 ~ 03/07/2008

在您的书面回复中，声称有些例外，包括以上用（*）注明的条款，您承认了这一缺陷。您声称将会提供文件说明这些例外已经被记录。您进一步声明，在制定方案时，您将“非预期医疗事件”理解为患者身上发生的新的或者不同的事件，防止这一缺陷的纠正措施就是对不清晰的语言要更仔细分析解释方案。而且，您制定了“不良事件”的SOP来确保类似的偏移和误解避免在将来的研究中再次发生。

以上用（*）注明的条款，在您书面回复中提供的信息中没有发现支持性文件来证明这些不良事件已经记录在CRF中，但是，我们认可在您的回复函中您说明已经采取了纠正措施来防止这一事件在将来再次发生。尽管这些纠正措施看起来是合适的，但正是在试验操作过程中缺少相应措施才导致了以上违规情况的发生。

c. 试验方案08-108特别说明患者在访视1（筛选访视）之前28天到跟踪随访期间所有的药物都要记录在CRF上。每种药物的通用名、剂量、给药途径、治疗时间（包括起止日期）、频率和适应症都要记录。

i. 对于受试者385-002，其服用的Lacinex口嚼片，被记录在了2007年11月1日的病程记录上，但并没有列在治疗前用药、合并用药和疗法记录上。

ii. 对于受试者385-004，其服用的Benadryl，被记录在了2007年5月23日的病程记录上，但并没有列在治疗前用药、合并用药和疗法记录上。

在您的书面回复中您承认这一缺陷。但是，您没有提供纠正措施来防止这一错误的再次发生。

3. 您未能快速地向伦理委员会报告研究活动中所有变更，而且您在未得到伦理委员会的批准的情况下对研究进行了变更［21 CFR 312.66］

FDA21 CFR 312.66法规声称研究者没有IRB同意不能对研究做任何改动，除非是必须要消除对受试者造成的明显的即刻的危害。试验方案CP-AI-005是由IRB在2005年4月7日批准的。但在日期为2006年2月26日、5月9日、7月18日和9月1日的监查信中，您被问到是否就已经发给受试者的大手提袋、患者日记卡和受试者日历申请IRB的批准。直到研究结束告知IRB（2007年4月12日）之前的一个月，即2007年3月22日，您才通知IRB进行这项研究时分发这些物资所做的变化。

在您的书面回复中，您承认了这些缺陷并声明IRD最终批准了使用患者日记卡，但那时，入组已经结束。您的纠正措施是制定了关于“方案偏离和研究修正”的新SOP来保证遵循合适的流程以避免未经授权的偏离和此类事件一旦发生时，确保遵循正确的流程快速地报告和纠正错误。您也声称将会就关于“IRB申请和修正过程”和所有给予试验受试者的资料和服务必须要事先得到IRB批准等问题对研究团队委员再进行指导和培训。这些纠正措施看来是恰当的。

本警告信的目的并非是罗列您在试验药物研究中存在的所有缺陷。确保遵循法律和相关FDA法规的每一项要求是您的职责。您应当解决这些缺陷，并建立规程，以确保任何正在进行或将来的研究均能符合FDA的法规。

自收到这封信的15个工作日内，您应当书面告知本办公室为预防将来发生类似违规情况已经采取的措施。如果不能充分、迅速地解释上述违规问题，可能导致我们在不再通知的情况下采取监管措施。

附：英文原文

Nasr, Samya, M.D.

WARNING LETTER

JAN 28, 2010

CERTIFIED MAIL
RETURN RECEIPT REQUESTED

Ref: 10-HFD-45-01-03

Samya Nasr, M.D.
1500 East Medical Center Drive
L2221 Women's Hospital, SPC 5212
Ann Arbor, MI 48109-5212

Dear Dr. Nasr:

Between July 20 and August 25, 2009, Ms. Barbara Rusin and Ms. L'Oreal Fowlkes, representing the Food and Drug Administration (FDA), conducted an investigation and met with you to review your conduct of the following clinical investigations:

Protocol CP-AI-005, entitled "A Phase 3, Double-Blind, Multicenter, Randomized, Placebo-Controlled Trial with Aztreonam Lysinate for Inhalation in Cystic Fibrosis Patients with Pulmonary P. *aeruginosa* Requiring Frequent Antibiotics (AIR-CF2)." of the investigational drug Aztreonam Lysinate, performed for Corus Pharma.

Protocol CP-AI-007, entitled "A Phase 3, Double-Blind, Multicenter, Multinational, Randomized, Placebo-Controlled Trial Evaluating Aztreonam Lysinate for Inhalation in Cystic Fibrosis Patients with Pulmonary P. *aeruginosa* (AIR-CF1)," of the investigational drug Aztreonam Lysinate, performed for Corus Pharma.

Protocol 08-108, entitled "A Multi-Center, Double-Blind, Placebo-Controlled Randomized, Efficacy and Safety Study of Denufosol Tetrasodium (INS37217) Inhalation Solution in Patients With Mild Cystic Fibrosis Lung Disease," of the investigational drug Denufosol Tetrasodium, performed for Inspire Pharmaceuticals.

Protocol 08-110, entitled "A Phase 3, International, Multi-Center, Randomized, Double-Blind, Placebo-Controlled, Parallel-Group, Efficacy and Safety Study of Denufosol Tetrasodium Inhalation Solution in Patients With Cystic Fibrosis Lung Disease and FEV1 ≥ 75% but ≤ 110% Predicted," of the investigational drug Denufosol Tetrasodium, performed for Inspire Pharmaceuticals.

Protocol 0000726, entitled "A Phase Ⅲ, Randomized, Double-Blind, Placebo-Controlled Clinical Study Evaluating the Efficacy and Safety of ALTU-135 Treatment in Patients with Cystic Fibrosis-Related Exocrine Pancreatic Insufficiency," of the investigational drug ALTU-135, performed for Altus Pharmaceuticals.

Protocol 0000767, entitled "An Open-Label Clinical Study Evaluating the Long-Term Safety of ALTU-135 for the Treatment of Patients with Cystic Fibrosis-Related Exocrine Pancreatic Insufficiency (ALTUS-767)," of the investigational drug ALTU-135, performed for Alnara Pharmaceuticals.

This inspection is a part of the FDA's Bioresearch Monitoring Program, which includes inspections designed to evaluate the conduct of research and to ensure that the rights, safety, and welfare of the human subjects of those studies have been protected. From our review of the establishment inspection report, the documents submitted with that report, and your written responses dated September 16, 2009, and November 24, 2009, we conclude that you did not adhere to the applicable statutory requirements and FDA regulations governing the conduct of clinical investigations. We are aware that at the conclusion of the inspection, FDA investigators presented and discussed with you Form FDA 483, Inspectional Observations. We wish to emphasize the following:

1. You failed to obtain the informed consent of each human subject, in accordance with 21 CFR part 50 [21 CFR 312.60].

FDA' s regulations at 21 CFR 50.20 state that except as provided in 21 CFR 50.23 and 21 CFR 50.24, no investigator may involve a human being as a subject in research covered by the regulations unless the investigator has obtained the legally effective informed consent of the subject or the subject's legally authorized representative. The regulation specifies that an investigator shall seek such informed consent only under circumstances that provide the prospective subject or the subject's representative sufficient opportunity to consider whether or not to participate and that minimize the possibility of coercion or undue influence.

Section 50.27 of FDA's regulations further states that except as provided in 21 CFR 56.109(c), informed consent shall be documented by the use of a written consent document, which is to be signed by the subject or the subject's representative at the time of consent.

a. The objective of Protocol CP-AI-005 was to assess the safety and efficacy of a 28-day treatment with Aztreonam Lysinate for Inhalation (Cayston™) and the ability of this treatment to maintain or improve clinical status following a 28-day course of Tobramycin Solution for Inhalation therapy in cystic fibrosis (CF) patients with pulmonary *Pseudomonas aeruginosa*. The original informed consent form approved by the IRB on April 7, 2005, however, incorrectly stated that the purpose of the study was to see if an investigational inhaled antibiotic, Aztreonam Lysinate for Inhalation, "can stop Pa [*Pseudomonas aeruginosa*] from coming back into your lungs."

You were notified by (b)(4) in an e-mail dated June 28, 2005, that the sponsor required a number of revisions to be made to the approved informed consent form, including these: "(Purpose): 2nd to last sentence, please change 'new drug' to 'investigational or experimental drug'. Please change the last sentence in this section to correctly reflect the purpose of this study - to see if Al [Aztreonam Lysinate] is safe and effective in CF patients with lung infections, not to see how well Al [Aztreonam Lysinate] can stop PA [*Pseudomonas aeruginosa*]from coming back into patients [sic] lungs." Your site resubmitted a revised informed consent form (version 2) to the IRB; that form was approved on August 25, 2005.

In an e-mail dated September 12, 2005, however, the sponsor informed you that there were still problems with the revised informed consent form. The sponsor noted that the statement in section 2.1 of the informed consent form stating that Aztreonam Lysinate can stop *Pseudomonas aeruginosa* from coming back to your lungs could be considered coercive because Aztreonam Lysinate was still an investigational drug. According to the e-mail, you had requested that the sponsor approve shipment of the study drug and allow patients to be enrolled with the current IRB-approved version of the informed consent form. The sponsor approved the shipment of study drug to your site with the conditions that you submit a revised informed consent form addressing all outstanding issues to the IRB and that you reconsent all patients enrolled in the study. The sponsor further approved your use of the current IRB-approved version of the informed consent form, provided that on the informed consent form you document that (1) female patients of childbearing potential were notified of the serum pregnancy test at Visit 1; (2) all patients consented with the current version were notified that they would be required at a later date to reconsent, using a revised consent form; and (3) all patients consented with the current IRB-approved version of the informed consent form were notified that Aztreonam Lysinate has not been proven to stop *Pseudomonas aeruginosa* from coming back into the lungs, as is implied in section 2.1, and that the purpose of the study was actually to see if Aztreonam Lysinate is successful in treating Pseudomonas aeruginosa lung infections in CF patients. In an e-mail dated September 14, 2005, you were again reminded to send the updated, corrected informed consent form to the IRB. The IRB approved version 3.1 of the informed consent form on March 9, 2006.

FDA' s investigation found that for all six subjects enrolled into the study, there was no documentation on either the informed consent form or the assent forms that you told the subjects about the true purpose of the study, as required by the sponsor. In addition, handwritten notes documenting the sponsor's requirements regarding the serum pregnancy test and the reconsenting of subjects were either (1) not documented on the informed consent form and/or the assent form, and/or (2) not consistently documented on all copies of the informed consent form and/or the assent form. Furthermore, Subjects 004, 005 and 006 were not reconsented with revised informed consent form version 3.1 until July 2006, approximately three months after the IRB had approved version 3.1.

In your written responses, you acknowledged that you failed to recognize any substantive difference between articulations of the study purpose as stated in informed consent form version 2 versus that in the protocol. You also acknowledged that you failed to correct this oversight in a timely manner when the sponsor first brought it to your attention in July 2005. You further stated that while handwritten statements were added to the consent forms prior to the subject's/parent's consent, you now recognized and understand that these statements should not have been added to the consents at any time. Your corrective actions to this finding included the development of new standard operating procedures (SOPs) including: "Completing the eResearch Application" to ensure that a member of the study team reviewed the consistency of the information in the protocol, investigator's brochure, consent document and the eResearch submission; "Responding to Monitoring Reports" which required prompt response to any observations and a formal report to the IRB for further consideration; and "Obtaining Informed Consent" which will prohibit handwritten statements on the informed consent form.

Your response is inadequate. In review of the SOP entitled "Standard Operating Procedure for eResearch Submissions", there were no procedures detailing the methods used by your site to verify consistency of all elements between the informed consent form, protocol, investigator's brochure and eResearch submission as noted in your promised corrective action. Your assertion that handwritten statements were added prior to consents being given to the subjects could also not be verified. In many cases the copy of the informed consent form in your research record was different from the copy found in the medical record.

b. No informed consent form and/or assent form could be found for Subjects 385-003 and 385-007, who were screened for Protocol 08-108. However, study-related screening procedures were performed on these subjects (on February 22, 2007, and September 5, 2007, respectively).

In your written responses, you acknowledged this finding. You noted that your corrective action to prevent the recurrence of this finding included the development of new SOPs including "Obtaining Informed Consent", "Document Management and Storage", and "Patient Completion/Early Termination/Screen Failure" and the education of your study team on these SOPs. These corrective actions appear adequate.

c. The following was noted for Protocol 08-110:

i. The informed consent documents for Subjects 385-101 and 385-102 did not have check marked responses to show whether consent was given either to participate in or to abstain from having saliva collected for P2Y2 genotyping. However, you collected these subjects' saliva samples and sent them to the central laboratory for testing.

ii. The original informed consent document signed by Subject 385-104 and dated January 9, 2009, did not have a checkmark in the box noting whether the subject elected to participate in or to abstain from having saliva collected for P2Y2 genotyping. However, you collected a saliva sample from this subject and sent it to the central laboratory for testing. A checkmark showing that the subject elected to participate in the collection of saliva for genotyping was subsequently made on February 13, 2009, which was after the time of saliva sample collection.

In your written responses, you acknowledged this finding and stated that your site detected the error in failing to get appropriate consent "before any genetic analysis" was performed on the samples from these subjects. Your corrective action included a policy for changing the check box for the optional tests to the last page of the informed consent document. You stated that if the IRB endorsed this new approach, it would be included in the newly created SOP on "Obtaining Informed Consent".

Your response is inadequate. We found no evidence that your site detected this error before genetic analysis was performed on these samples. Rather, it appears that the lack of consent of subjects to having samples taken for testing was identified during the FDA inspection. Furthermore, documents provided by you during the inspection showed that when the sponsor was informed of the lack of consent of Subjects 385-101 and 385-102 to the testing in an email dated July 23, 2009, the sponsor stated that the samples were to be destroyed. The sponsor's email made no mention that the samples had not undergone any genetic testing. In addition you provided no evidence to show that the error was detected before testing occurred. We also note that even if genetic analysis was not performed, this does not negate the fact that samples should not have been drawn from subjects without their consent.

d. The informed consent documents signed by Subjects 009-001 and 009-002 for Protocol 0000726 did not include a reference to testing of blood samples for Vitamin K levels. However, you tested these subjects' blood samples for Vitamin K.

In your written responses, you acknowledged this finding and stated that you had developed an SOP for "Managing Investigational Materials and Supplies" which would serve as corrective actions to prevent the recurrence of this finding.

Your response is inadequate. You provided no corrective action plan to ensure that only those tests included in the informed consent document would be performed on study subjects. In addition, in review of the SOP for "Managing Investigational Materials and Supplies", your procedure stated that your staff would examine the "contents of study kits to validate that only collection tubes for IRB-approved tests are included in the kit before it is delivered to the research phlebotomy team." There were no clear procedures for how your site would verify that the test or tests in the kit are in line with the currently approved protocol or protocol amendment that is in effect at the time of arrival of the kit.

2. You failed to ensure that the investigations were conducted according to the investigational plans [21 CFR 312.60].

a. Protocol 08-110 stated that either a chest X-ray must be performed at Visit 1, or there must be a chest X-ray, high resolution computed tomography (HRCT), chest CT scan, or MRI of the lung performed 12 months before Visit 1. Subject 385-101 was enrolled into the study on September 10, 2008, and received study drug on September 17, 2008 at Visit 2. However, no chest X-ray was performed for this subject at Visit 1, and there is no documentation indicating that either a chest X-ray, high resolution computed tomography (HRCT), chest CT scan, or MRI of the lung had been performed 12 months before Visit 1. Source documents confirm that the chest X-ray for this subject was taken on September 17, 2008, approximately an hour after the subject had received the first dose of investigational drug.

In your written responses, you acknowledged this finding and stated that you had developed SOPs for "Protocol Deviations and Study Amendments" and "Document Management and Storage" which would serve as corrective actions to prevent the recurrence of this finding.

We acknowledge that in your letters, you describe the corrective actions you have taken to prevent the recurrence of this finding. While these corrective actions appear appropriate, it was the absence of such measures during the conduct of these trials that led to the violations listed here, raising concerns regarding the adequacy of human subject protections at your site.

b. Protocol 0000726 defined an Adverse Event (AE) as any untoward medical occurrence in a patient or clinical investigation patient, regardless of its causal relationship to study drug. According to the protocol, all AEs were to be collected beginning on Study Day B1, and would continue inclusive of the 2-week follow-up visit. In addition, the protocol stated that all study staff were responsible for ensuring that complete safety information was recorded on the case report form (CRF). FDA's investigation found that several AEs noted in the progress reports were not recorded onto the CRF. Examples include the following:

Subject	AE	Date(s) AE noted in the source records
009-001	Flatulence	10/22/07 10/29/07 11/05/07
009-001	Crackles and Diminished Breath in Right Lung	10/24/07 10/29/07
009-002	Bilateral Crackles in Bases of Lungs	12/03/07
009-002	Darkened Sputum	12/03/07
009-002	Bilateral rhonchi noted in the upper and lower lobes of the lungs	12/06/07
009-005	Mild Rhonchi	03/03/08
009-005	Boggy, swollen turbinates with cloudy discharge	03/05/08 - 3/07/08

In your written responses, you stated that with some exceptions, including the items noted with an asterisk (*) above, you acknowledged this finding. You stated that you would provide documentation that those exceptions were reported. You further stated that as you were conducting the protocol, you interpreted "untoward medical occurrence" to mean something new or different in a patient, and your corrective action to prevent this finding is to more carefully analyze the protocol for unclear language. In addition, you developed an SOP for "Adverse Events" to ensure that similar deviations and misunderstandings were avoided in future studies.

For the items noted with an asterisk (*) above, there was no supporting documentation found in the information you provided in your written responses to verify that these AEs were reported in the CRF. However, we acknowledge that in your response letters you describe the corrective actions you have taken to prevent this from happening in the future. While these corrective actions appear appropriate, it was the absence of such measures during the conduct of these trials that led to the violations listed here.

c. Protocol 08-108 specified that all medications that the patient has taken from 28 days prior to Visit 1 (screening visit) through the follow-up visit were to be recorded in the CRF. The generic name of the drug, dose, route of administration, duration of treatment (including start and stop dates), frequency, and indication were also to be recorded for each medication.

i. For Subject 385-002, Lacinex chewable tablets, taken by the subject and identified in the progress note dated November 1, 2007, were not listed on the prior and concurrent medication and therapies log.

ii. For Subject 385-004, Benadryl, taken by the subject and identified in the progress note dated May 23, 2007, was not listed on the prior and concurrent medication and therapies log.

In you written responses you acknowledged this finding. You, however, provided no corrective action to prevent the recurrence of this finding.

3. You failed to promptly report to the IRB all changes in research activities and made changes in the research without IRB approval [21 CFR 312.66].

FDA' s regulations at 21 CFR 312.66 state that an investigator shall not make any changes to the research without IRB approval, except where necessary to eliminate apparent immediate hazards to human subjects. Protocol CP-AI-005 was approved by the IRB on April 7, 2005. In monitoring letters dated February 26, May 9, July 18, and September 1, 2006, you were asked whether you had requested approval from the IRB for tote bags, diary cards, and subject calendars that were given to subjects participating in the study. You failed to inform the IRB of the changes you had implemented to the research by distributing these items. The IRB was not made aware of these changes until March 22, 2007, which was one month before the study was terminated with the IRB (on April 12, 2007).

In your written response, you acknowledged these findings and stated that while the IRB eventually approved the use of the subject diary cards, by that time, enrollment had ended. Your corrective action was the development of a new SOP for "Protocol Deviations and Study Amendments" to assure appropriate procedures are followed to avoid unauthorized deviations, and in the event they occur, proper procedures were followed for promptly reporting and correcting them. You also state that study team members will be re-educated about "the IRB application and amendment processes" and to the fact that all items and services given to study subjects must be approved by the IRB in advance. These corrective actions appear appropriate.

This letter is not intended to be an all-inclusive list of deficiencies with your clinical study of an investigational drug. It is your responsibility to ensure adherence to each requirement of the law and relevant FDA regulations. You should address these deficiencies and establish procedures to ensure that any ongoing or future studies will be in compliance with FDA regulations.

Within fifteen (15) working days of your receipt of this letter, you should notify this office in writing of the actions you have taken to prevent similar violations in the future. Failure to adequately and promptly explain the violations noted above may result in regulatory action without further notice.

If you have any questions, please contact Constance Lewin, M.D., M.P.H., at 301-796-3397; FAX 301-847-8748. Your written response and any pertinent documentation should be addressed to:

Constance Lewin, M.D., M.P.H.
Branch Chief, Good Clinical Practice Branch I
Division of Scientific Investigations
Office of Compliance
Center for Drug Evaluation and Research

Food and Drug Administration
Building 51, Room 5354
10903 New Hampshire Avenue
Silver Spring, MD 20993

Sincerely yours,

{See appended electronic signature page}

Leslie K. Ball, M.D.
Director
Division of Scientific Investigations
Office of Compliance
Center for Drug Evaluation and Research
Food and Drug Administration

第 117 封　给 Ward, John A. 医学博士的警告信

2009年12月3日

参考号：10-HFD-45-12-01

尊敬的Ward博士：

2009年5月12日至5月20日，Patricia Smith女士代表FDA进行了现场检查，与您会面并对您所实施的以下临床研究：试验方案（b）(4)，题目为（b）(4)，试验药物（b）(4)，申办者为（b）(4）进行了审查。

本次现场检查是FDA的生物研究监查项目的一部分。该项目通过设定的检查方法，评估相关研究的实施情况，以确保这些研究中受试者的权益、安全和福利得到了保护。

经对现场检查报告、该报告的附件，以及您2009年7月17日对FDA483表的书面回复进行审查，我们认为，您没有遵循适用的法律要求和监管临床研究实施及受试者保护的FDA法规。在现场检查结束时，Smith女士向您出示并讨论了FDA483表，即现场检查发现的问题。我们想强调以下几点：

1. 您未能确保按照研究计划进行研究［21 CFR 312.60］

方案要求应在手术前一天，即第0天筛选后随机化。但是贵中心的受试者是在手术后而不是手术前随机化，违背了方案的要求。2007年5月30日的方案违背报告中，贵中心通知伦理委员会受试者5001至5139均于手术后被随机。

另外，受试者的病程记录显示2007年5月30日后，您仍然授权在受试者手术后随机化。示例包括但不局限于这些受试者：5205，5209，5212，5215，5223 和 5229。

您2009年7月17日对FDA483表，即现场检查发现的问题回复中，您声明收到申办者于2007年5月11日发出的说明后，贵中心在受试者手术前随机化，大部分受试者随机化和手术在同一天，但是都在术前。您提出在新的研究中，贵中心会按照方案要求随机受试者，并通过和申办者更紧密的合作来纠正任何可能引起歧义的问题。我们认为您关于这方面的解释是不能接受的。我们注意到您未能提供任何文件支持贵中心关于2007年5月11日后在手术后随机受试者的声明。

2. 您未能确保符合 21 CFR 56 所列要求的 IRB 负责对临床研究进行初始审查、跟踪审查和批准［21 CFR 312.66］

您在伦理委员会批准失效后仍然继续进行临床试验。伦理委员会于2006年5月31日初始审查并批准试验方案（b）(4)，批准有效期为12个月，即2007年5月31日起失效。2007年6月18日，您向伦理委员会递交了研究者年度报告；但是，伦理委员会直到2007年7月2日才给予批准。伦理委员会批准失效的2007年5月31日至7月2日期间，以下47例受试者参加了临床研究的相关活动，包括但不限于筛选、给药和研究程序：受试者5109，5126，5127，5128，5129，5130，5131，5132，5133，5135，5136，5137，5138，5139，5140，5141，5142，5143，5144，5145，5146，5147，5148，5149，5151，5152，5154，5155，5156，5157，5158，5159，5160，5161，5162，5163，5164，5165，5166，5167，5168，5169，5170，5171，5172，5173和5174。

您2009年7月17日对FDA483表，即现场检查发现的问题的回复中，您声明了伦理委员会批件失效是由于委员会人员的失误，而且该问题是自查时发现并已确认。我们认可您采取纠正措施以预防类似问题在将来的研究中重复发生。

本警告信的目的并非是罗列您在试验药物临床研究中存在的所有缺陷。确保遵循法律和相关FDA法规的每一项要求是您的职责。您应当解决这些缺陷，并建立规程，以确保任何正在进行或将来的研究均能符合FDA的法规。

自收到这封信的15个工作日内，您应当书面告知本办公室为预防将来发生类似违规情况已经采取的措施。如果不能充分、迅速地解释上述违规问题，可能导致我们在不再通知的情况下采取监管措施。

附：英文原文

Ward, John A., M.D.

WARNING LETTER

Dec 03, 2009

CERTIFIED MAIL
RETURN RECEIPT REQUESTED

Ref:10-HFD-45-12-01

John A. Ward, M.D.
Capstone Clinical Trials, Inc.
2018 Brookwood Medical Center Drive, Suite 314
Birmingham, AL 35209-6870

Dear Dr. Ward:

Between May 12 and May 20, 2009, Ms. Patricia Smith, representing the Food and Drug Administration (FDA), conducted an investigation and met with you to review your conduct of a clinical investigation [Protocol (b)(4) entitled (b)(4)of the investigational drug (b)(4)performed for (b)(4).

This inspection is a part of the FDA' s Bioresearch Monitoring Program, which includes inspections designed to evaluate the conduct of research and to ensure that the rights, safety and welfare of the human subjects of those studies have been protected.

From our review of the establishment inspection report, the documents submitted with that report, and your July 17, 2009, written response to the Form FDA 483, Inspectional Observations, we conclude that you did not adhere to the applicable statutory requirements and FDA regulations governing the conduct of clinical investigations and the protection of human subjects. We are aware that at the conclusion of the inspection, Ms. Smith presented and discussed with you Form FDA 483, Inspectional Observations.We wish to emphasize the following:

1. You failed to ensure that the investigation was conducted according to the investigational plan [21 CFR 312.60].

The protocol required that randomization take place following screening on Day 0, one day prior to surgery. However, subjects at your site were randomized postoperatively, as opposed to preoperatively, in violation of the protocol. In a Protocol Deviations report dated May 30, 2007, your site notified the Institutional Review Board (IRB) that subjects 5001 through 5139 were randomized post-surgery.

In addition, subject' s progress notes revealed that after May 30, 2007, you continued to authorize randomization of subjects post-surgery. Examples include, but are not limited to, Subjects 5205, 5209, 5212, 5215, 5223, and 5229.

In your July 17, 2009, response to the Form FDA 483, Inspectional Observations, you stated that after receiving clarification from the sponsor on May 11, 2007, your site randomized subjects pre-surgery, many on the same day as surgery , but preoperatively. You proposed that during future studies, yoursite would randomize subjects as required by the protocol, and would work more closely with the sponsor to correct any perceived ambiguities. We do not find your response to be acceptable in addressing this manner. We note that you have not provided any documentation to support your statement that the subjects were randomized preoperatively after May 11, 2007.

2. You failed to ensure that an Institutional Review Board (IRB) that complies with the requirements set forth in 21 CFR Part 56, was responsible for the initial and continuing review and approval of the clinical study [21 CFR 312.66].

You continued to perform research activities during periods of time when IRB approval had expired. Initial IRB approval for Protocol (b)(4) was granted on May 31, 2006, and continued for twelve consecutive months, with an expiration date of May 31, 2007. On June 18, 2007, you submitted the Investigator's Annual Report Review to the IRB; however , IRB approval was not granted until July 2, 2007. The following 47 subjects participated in research study activities including, but not limited to, screening , dosing, and study procedures between May 31, 2007, and July 02, 2007, when IRB approval had lapsed: Subjects 5109, 5126, 5127, 5128, 5129, 5130, 5131, 5132, 5133, 5135, 5136, 5137, 5138, 5139, 5140, 5141, 5142, 5143, 5144, 5145, 5146, 5147, 5148, 5149, 5151, 5152, 5154, 5155, 5156, 5157, 5158, 5159, 5160, 5161, 5162, 5163, 5164, 5165, 5166, 5167, 5168, 5169, 5170, 5171, 5172, 5173, and 5174.

In your July 17, 2009, response to the Form FDA 483, Inspectional Observations, you stated that the lapse in IRB approval was the error of a staff member and that it was self-identified and self acknowledged. We acknowledge your assurance that corrective actions have been taken to prevent this observation during future studies.

This letter is not intended to be an all-inclusive list of deficiencies with your clinical study of an investigational drug. It is your responsibility to ensure adherence to each requirement of the law andrelevant FDA regulations. You should address these deficiencies and establish procedures to ensure that any ongoing or future studies will be in compliance with FDA regulations.

Within fifteen (15) working days of your receipt of this letter, you should notify this office in writing of the actions you have taken to prevent similar violations in the future. Failure to adequately and promptly explain the violations noted above may result in regulatory action without further notice.

If you have any questions, please contact Constance Lewin, M.D., M.P.H., at 301-796-3397; FAX 301- 847-8748. Your written response and any pertinent documentation should be addressed to:

Constance Lewin, M.D., M.P.H.
Branch Chief, Good Clinical Practice Branch 1
Division of Scientific Investigations
Office of Compliance
Center for Drug Evaluation and Research
Food and Drug Administration
Building 51, Room 5354
10903 New Hampshire Avenue
SiIver Spring, MD 20993

Sincerely yours,

{See appended electronic signature page}

Leslie K. Ball, M.D.
Director
Division of Scientific Investigations
Office of Compliance
Center for Drug Evaluation and Research

第 118 封　给 Buettner, Craig M. 医学博士的警告信

2009年11月24日

参考号：10-HFD-45-11-03

尊敬的Buettner博士：

2009年5月4日至6日，Patricia Smith女士代表FDA进行了现场检查，与您会面并对您所实施的一项临床研究进行了审查：试验方案（b）（4），题目为"（b）（4）"，试验药物（b）（4），申办者为（b）（4）。

本次现场检查是FDA的生物研究监查项目的一部分。该项目通过设定的检查方法，评估相关研究的实施情况，以确保这些研究中受试者的权益、安全和福利得到了保护。

经对FDA现场检查报告、该报告的附件进行审查，我们认为，您没有遵循适用的法律要求和监管临床研究的FDA法规。在现场检查结束时，Smith女士向您出示并讨论了FDA483表，即现场检查发现的问题。我们想强调以下几点：

您未能确保按照研究计划进行研究［21 CFR 312.60］

受试者是在手术后，而不是手术前随机化，违背了方案的要求。按照方案第4.6.4.1章节，应在手术前一天即第0天筛选后随机化。在一封2009年4月8日的备注文件中记录，您的试验人员告知伦理委员会，有44名受试者在手术后随机化，违背了方案要求。以下是在手术后随机化的受试者的举例：受试者001，002，003，004，005，006，010，011，030，031，040，058，061和064。

在您2009年6月3日的书面回复中，您声明该方案违背源于对方案的错误理解；您希望在确认所有入选和排除标准符合之后才对受试者进行随机化。您理解方案要求受试者已经经历（b）（4），您错误地在受试者手术后进行随机化，以核实他们确实已经经历了方案要求的特别步骤。但是，在2007年5月11日，贵的研究中心收到了监查员重申受试者应在手术前随机化的邮件。尽管如此，您继续在受试者手术后随机化，直至2007年10月。此外在您的书面回复中，您提到您将此方案违背告知了伦理委员会。我们注意到按照方案第5.2章节，任何方案违背应被尽快告知伦理委员会。但是，您直到2009年4月8日才告知伦理委员会，距离2008年4月24日结束该项目研究已经将近一年，距离监查员通知您受试者应在手术前随机化已经将近两年。在您的回复中，作为纠正措施，您承诺将来按照方案要求对受试者进行随机化，并且对方案特定要求的不确定之处向申办者寻求进一步澄清。

我们确认收到了您的回复。但是，我们担忧该回复不足以预防将来上述违规情况再次发生，因为它没有提供特定或详细的计划或步骤来预防将来类似违规的再次发生。在此，您不仅从试验开始时没有正确理解方案随机化步骤，从而没有确保随机化步骤按照方案进行；而且在您收到方案要求澄清后的四个多月内没有对问题进行纠正。

本警告信的目的并非是罗列您在试验药物临床研究中存在的所有缺陷。确保遵循法律和相关FDA法规的每一项要求是您的职责。您应当解决这些缺陷，并建立规程，以确保任何正在进行或将来的研究均能符合FDA的法规。

自收到这封信的15个工作日内，您应当书面告知本办公室为预防将来发生类似违规情况已经采取的措施。如果不能充分、迅速地解释上述违规问题，可能导致我们在不再通知的情况下采取监管措施。

附：英文原文

Buettner, Craig M., M.D.

WARNING LETTER

Nov 24, 2009

CERTIFIED MAIL
RETURN RECEIPT REQUESTED

Ref: 10-HFD-45-11-03

Craig M. Buettner, M.D.
100 Rice Mine Road Loop Suite 104
Tuscaloosa, AL 35406-2421

Dear Dr. Buettner:

Between May 4 and 6, 2009, Ms. Patricia Smith, representing the Food and Drug Administration (FDA), conducted an investigation and met with you to review your conduct of a clinical investigation [protocol(b)(4) entitled (b)(4) of the investigational drug (b)(4) performed for (b)(4)

This inspection is a part of the FDA' s Bioresearch Monitoring Program, which includes inspections designed to evaluate the conduct of research and to ensure that the rights, safety, and welfare of the human subjects of those studies have been protected.

From our review of the establishment inspection report and the documents submitted with that report, we conclude that you did not adhere to the applicable statutory requirements and FDA regulations governing the conduct of clinical investigations. We are aware that at the conclusion of the inspection, Ms. Smith presented and discussed with you Form FDA 483, Inspectional Observations. We wish to emphasize the following:

1. You failed to ensure that the investigation was conducted according to the investigational plan [21 CFR 312.60].

Subjects were randomized postoperatively, as opposed to preoperatively, in violation of the protocol. Per Section 4.6.4.1 of the protocol, randomization was to take place following screening on Day 0, a day prior to surgery. In a Note to File dated April 8, 2009, your site staff notified the Institutional Review Board (IRB) that 44 subjects were randomized post-surgery, in violation of the protocol. The following are examples of subjects that were randomized postoperatively: Subjects 001, 002, 003, 004, 005, 006, 010, Oil, 030, 031, 040, 058, 061, and 064.

In your June 3, 2009 written response, you stated that this violation occurred due to a misunderstanding of the protocol. You noted that you intended to randomize subjects only after verifying that all inclusion and exclusion criteria were met. You indicated that you understood that the protocol required subjects to have had a (b)(4) and as such, you mistakenly randomized subjects postoperatively to verify that they had indeed undergone the protocol-specified procedure. However, on May 11, 2007, your site was forwarded a monitor' s email reiterating that subjects were to be randomized before surgery. Nonetheless, you continued to randomize subjects postoperatively until October 2007. Additionally, in your written response, you indicated that you notified the IRB of this protocol deviation. We note that under section 5.2 of the protocol, any protocol deviations were to be submitted to the IRB as soon as possible. However, you did not notify the IRB until April 8, 2009, almost a year following notification of your site's closure of the study on April 24, 2008, and almost two years after you were notified by the monitor that randomization was to occur prior to surgery. In your response, as corrective measures, you promised to randomize subjects as required by the protocol in the future, and to seek further clarification from the sponsor for any future ambiguities in protocol specifications.

We acknowledge your response. However, we are concerned that the response is not adequate to prevent future recurrence of the violation noted above because it provides no specific or detailed plans or procedures to prevent future recurrence of this or similar violations. In this case, not only did you fail to properly understand the protocol randomization procedure from the start of the study, and therefore did not ensure that the randomization procedure was carried out according to the protocol from the outset, but also you did not remedy the problem for more than four months after having received clarification of the protocol.

This letter is not intended to be an all-inclusive list of deficiencies with your clinical study of an investigational drug. It is your responsibility to ensure adherence to each requirement of the law and relevant FDA regulations. You should address these deficiencies and establish procedures to ensure that any on-going or future studies will be in compliance with FDA regulations.

Within fifteen (15) working days of your receipt of this letter, you should notify this office in writing of the actions you have taken to prevent similar violations in the future. Failure to adequately and promptly explain the violations noted above may result in regulatory action without further notice.

If you have any questions, please contact Constance Lewin, M.D., M.P.H., at 301-796-3397; FAX 301- 847-8748. Your written response and any pertinent documentation should be addressed to:

Constance Lewin, M.D., M.P.H.
Branch Chief, Good Clinical Practice Branch I
Division of Scientific Investigations
Office of Compliance
Center for Drug Evaluation and Research
Food and Drug Administration
Building 51, Room 5354
10903 New Hampshire Avenue
Silver Spring, MD 20993

Sincerely yours,

{See appended electronic signature page}

Leslie K. Ball, M.D.
Director
Division of Scientific Investigations
Office of Compliance
Center for Drug Evaluation and Research

第119封　给Gazda, Thomas医学博士的警告信

2009年11月24日

参考号：10-HFD-45-11-02

尊敬的Gazda博士：

2009年1月20日至2月6日，Tonia Sawyer女士代表FDA进行了现场检查，与当前的Meadowbrook研究股份有限公司的临床人员Dr.（b）(6)、公司总裁及CEO Pamela Larson女士会面，并对您所实施的临床研究进行了审查：试验方案（b）(4)，试验药物（b）(4)，申办者（b）(4)。

本次现场检查是FDA的生物研究监查项目的一部分。该项目通过设定的检查方法，评估相关研究的实施情况，以确保这些研究中受试者的权益、安全和福利得到了保护。

经对现场检查报告和该报告的附件进行审查，我们认为，您没有遵循适用的法律要求和监管临床研究实施的FDA法规。在现场检查结束时，由于您已不再是Meadowbrook研究股份有限公司的雇员，Tonia Sawyer女士向助理研究者Dr.（b）(6)出示并讨论了FDA483表，即现场检查发现的问题。我们注意到Tonia Sawyer女士于2009年6月6日向您现雇主的地址：7275 E. Earll Drive，Scottsdale，Arizona 85251邮寄了一份FDA483表的复印件。

我们确认收到了Meadowbrook研究股份有限公司CEO Pamela Larson女士和助理研究者Dr.（b）(6)日期为2009年2月17日和2009年2月26日的两封对FDA483表的书面回复，即现场检查发现的问题。这些回复函描述了Meadowbrook研究股份有限公司已经采取或即将采取的措施，以预防由Meadowbrook研究股份有限公司未来实施的研究发生类似的违规情况。然而，截至2009年11月20日，FDA没有收到您对于FDA483表的书面回复。作为主要研究者的您本人，而不是Meadowbrook研究股份有限公司，需要对临床研究负责。

您书面回复说明，您将如何确保类似的违规在未来您所实施的研究中不再发生。

我们希望强调如下几点：

1．您未能确保按照研究计划进行研究［21 CFR 312.60］

具体而言，大量的方案偏离导致对数据可靠性的严重怀疑。

a. 方案规定获得知情同意的人员必须对于医学事件有充分的培训，以确保提出的问题能够获得充分地解决。方案明确要求这个人需要有博士或RN（注册护士）学位；如果这个人未能有如上学位，此人必须由（b）(4)批准才可获得知情同意。入组本研究的所有受试者（受试者1001～1008和1010～1013），知情同意文件及年龄在10～17的儿童同意表，均未按照方案要求由博士或RN学位的人员获得，且您亦未获得（b）(4)对于这些人获得知情同意或儿童同意书的批准。

b. 方案入组标准明确规定受试者需要按照（b）(4)定义获得关于（b）(4)的主诊断。而根据（b）(4)确认受试者1008、1010、1012和1013因为错误使用诊断仪器而未能按照方案要求在筛选阶段确认诊断。

c. 方案要求（b）(4)必须由主要研究者或是（b）(4)或者与（b）(4)等价的博士学位的授权研究者执行。

ⅰ受试者1001～1007，（b）(4)未由方案要求的主要研究者或助理研究者执行，而使用不符方案标准的研究协调员执行。

ⅱ. 没有文件记录主要研究者和助理研究者按照方案要求参与（b）(4)或（b）(4)等价模式的培训。

d. 方案要求自基线访视后研究开始第2周，研究者或指定人员需要每天通过电话或者亲临与受试者和受试者的父母或监护人联系，以确保受试者在合适的时候服用合适的胶囊，并观察给药方案的耐受性和有效性。

对于11个入组受试者中的10名，未有文件记录您或者您指定的人员按照方案要求每天通过电话或者亲临与受试者和受试者父母或监护人联系。

e. 方案明确规定，当受试者体重低于45kg时，目标剂量是60～80kg/d。2006年10月5日，受试者1010的体重记录为40.1kg，依据方案受试者的起始用药剂量为每次20mg，每天两次，每天总剂量为40mg。2006年10月12日受试者的用药剂量提高至每次40mg，每天两次，达到研究对于此受试者的最大耐受量。然而，2006年10月15日，这名受试者用药剂量再次提高到每次60mg，每天两次，以至一日总剂量为120mg，超出受试者的最大耐受量。这名受试者在参加研究期间连续5天接受了120mg/d的研究药物。

f. 方案要求筛选访视检测一次ECG并在基线访视时连续检测3次ECG。基线访视需要在筛选访视之后1～10天进行。受试者1010未在2006年9月29日的筛选访视时检测ECG。替代筛选访视ECG检测，在2006年10月5日的基线访视时完成3次基线ECG检测。

g. 方案要求所有受试者应在首次用药（第一天）20mg之后获得两份PK血样，第一份血样在首剂用药后0.5～1.5小时采集，第二份血样在首剂用药后1.5～3小时采集。相关血样未能经常按照方案规定时限采集。如：

ⅰ. 受试者1010在2006年10月5日17:30首剂用药。然而，受试者原始记录显示第一次PK血样仅在首剂用药后5分钟17:35采集，第一份血样应该在首剂之后于2006年10月5日18:00～19:00采集。

ⅱ. 受试者1011在2006年10月31日16:15首剂用药。然而，受试者原始记录显示第一次PK血样仅在首剂用药后15分钟16:30采集，第一份血样应该在首剂之后于2006年10月31日16:45～17:45采集。

h. 方案明确规定在基线访视受试者应首次用药（第一天）20mg。之后获得两份PK血样，第一份血样在首剂用药后0.5～1.5小时采集，第二份血样在首剂用药后1.5～3小时采集。方案要求在4周访视时，受试者晨起用药后，将检测ECG，之后在用药后0.75～3.0小时采集PK血样。在用药后5～7小时，受试者将回访诊所，当生命体征检测稳定后，检测另一次ECG，此后10分钟，采集另一份PK血样。同时，方案要求在4周前终止研究的受试者应按照4周访视流程采集PK血样、检测ECG和血压和脉搏（生命体征）检测。11名入组受试者有9名未能按照方案规定流程实施。如下表，按照受试者列明未能按照方案规定流程实施的情况。

受试者	日期	访视	PK血样缺失	ECG缺失	生命体征缺失
1002	7/08/2006	4周	5～7小时	5～7小时	5～7小时
1003	8/23/2006	4周	5～7小时	不适用	5～7小时
1004	8/16/2006	第一天	1. 5～3小时	不适用	不适用
1004	9/14/2006	终止治疗	5～7小时	5～7小时	5～7小时
1005	8/31/2006	终止治疗	5～7小时	5～7小时	5～7小时
1007	9/28/2006	终止治疗	5～7小时		
1008	10/11/2006	4周	5～7小时	5～7小时	5～7小时
1010	10/20/2006	终止治疗	5～7小时	5～7小时	5～7小时
1012	3/01/2007	第一天	0. 5～1.5小时	不适用	不适用
1012	3/01/2007	第一天	1. 5～3小时	不适用	不适用
1013	3/02/2007	第一天	0. 5～1.5小时	不适用	不适用
1012	3/02/2007	第一天	1. 5～3小时	不适用	不适用

2．您未能保存研究中使用试验药物或对照组的受试者的所有研究观察结果和其他相关数据的足够及准确的病历［21 CFR 312.62（b）］

具体而言，在11名入组研究的受试者中的10名的记录中，存在大量不准确的记录。引起对数据可靠性的重大质疑。

a. 如受试者1001的不准确病历，包括但不限于以下：

i. 于2006年6月2日筛选访视的原始记录中记录脉搏为98；而在相应的CRF中记录脉搏为82。筛选访视的原始记录关于家族疾病史的记录在“同胞”一栏中NA（4）处记录X，而在相应的CRF同意栏目中Yes（1）处记录X。

ii. 于2006年6月23日的2周访视原始记录记录脉搏为100，而相应的CRF中记录脉搏为88。

iii. 关于（b）（4）时间的不良事件原始表格记录结束日期为2006年7月5日；而相应CRF在AE的结果日期记录解决日期为2006年7月11日。

b. 如受试者1002不准确的病历，包括但不限于以下：

i. 于2006年6月2日筛选访视的初步诊断的原始记录，记录上初步诊断的时间（月）为0及之前的主诊断数量为0，而相应的CRF上主诊断的时间（月）为1及之前的主诊断数量为2。

ii. 于2006年6月6日的第一天（基线）访视的原始记录，记录血压为179/99，而相应的2006年6月9日的CRF记录血压为119/99。

iii. 于2006年7月5日的4周访视的原始记录，记录体温为37.1℃，而相应的CRF记录体温为31.7℃。

c. 如受试者1003的不准确病历，包括但不限于以下：

i 于2006年7月21日筛选访视的主诊断原始记录，记录上主诊断的时间（月）为0及之前的主诊断数量为0，而相应的CRF上主诊断的时间（月）为4及之前的主诊断数量为1。

ii. 于2006年8月23日的4周访视的原始记录，记录卧位血压为114/72及脉搏为76，标准血压为111/70及脉搏为90（用药前）而相应的CRF记录血压为卧位血压为108/78及脉搏为78，标准血压为100/64及脉搏为80（用药前）。

d. 如受试者1004不准确的病历，包括但不限于以下：

i. 于2006年8月1日的筛选访视原始记录，在病史问题的第5部分家族史（b）（4），第一个问题，（b）（4），在uncle/aunt处记录Yes，而在CRF上的同一问题，此处记录No。

ii. 于2006年8月16日的第一天（基线）访视的原始记录，第2题，附属（b）（4）记录为“（2）”，第3题，附属（b）（4）记录为“（1）（b）（4）”。相应地电子CFR录入第2题，记录“（1）（b）（4）”及第3天记录为“（0）（b）（4）”。

e. 如受试者1005的不准确病历，包括但不限于以下信息：

i. 于2006年8月1日筛选访视的主诊断的原始记录，记录上主诊断的时间（月）为0及之前的主诊断数量为0，而相应的CRF上主诊断的时间（月）为2。

ii.于2006年8月17日的1周访视原始记录，记录第9题的回复为（b）（4），而相应的电子CRF第9题回复留空（无任何记录）。

f. 如受试者1007不准确的病历，包括但不限于以下：

于2006年8月31日筛选访视的主诊断的原始记录，记录主诊断数量为1，而相应的CRF上主诊断数量为2。

g. 如受试者1008的不准确病历，包括但不限于以下：

i. 于2006年9月8日筛选访视的主诊断的原始记录，记录上主诊断的时间（月）为0及之前的主诊断数量为3，而相应的CRF上主诊断的时间（月）为1及之前的主诊断数量为0。

ii.于2006年9月8日筛选访视中关于合并用药的原始记录，百忧解（prozac）的记录但由R.M.于2006年11月9日删除，而相应的CRF将百忧解（prozac）列于‘既往精神药物治疗’表中。

h. 如受试者1010不准确的病历，包括但不限于以下：

i. 于2006年9月29日筛选访视的主诊断的原始记录，记录上主诊断的时间（月）为0，而相应的CRF现主诊断的时间（月）为2。

ii. 于2005年9月29日的筛选访视原始记录，记录腰围为“26.5=67.3cm”，而相应的电子CRF记录腰围为26.5。

iii. 于2006年10月20日的早期终止访视原始记录，记录身高为60.5英寸，而相应的电子CRF记录身高为

152.9cm，取代准确的身高153.7cm。

i. 如受试者1011不准确的病历，包括但不限于：

于2006年10月20日筛选访视的主诊断的原始记录，记录之前的主诊断数量为3，而相应的CRF上主诊断的时间（月）为0。

j. 如受试者1012不准确的病历，包括但不限于以下：

于2007年2月21日筛选访视的主诊断的原始记录，记录之前的主诊断的时间（月）为0而相应的CRF上主诊断的时间（月）为2。

本警告信的目的并非是罗列您在试验药物临床研究中存在的所有缺陷。确保遵循法律和相关FDA法规的每一项要求是您的职责。您应当解决这些缺陷，并建立规程，以确保任何正在进行的研究或将来的研究均能符合FDA的法规。

自收到这封信的15个工作日内，您应当书面告知本办公室为预防将来发生类似违规情况已经采取的措施。如果不能充分、迅速地解释上述违规问题，可能导致我们在不再通知的情况下采取监管措施。

附：英文原文

Gazda, Thomas M.D.

WARNING LETTER

Nov 24, 2009

CERTIFIED MAIL
RETURN RECEIPT REQUESTED

Ref: 10-HFD-45-11-02

Thomas Gazda, M.D.
4383 N. 75th Street
Scottsdale, Arizona 85251

Dear Dr. Gazda:

Between January 20 and February 6, 2009, Ms. Tonia Sawyer, representing the Food and Drug Administration (FDA), conducted an investigation and met with Dr. (b)(6), current Meadowbrook Research, Inc. clinical staff member; and Ms. Pamela Larson, President and CEO of Meadowbrook Research, Inc., to review your conduct of a clinical investigation (b)(4) of the investigational drug (b)(4) performed for (b)(4).

This inspection is a part of the FDA's Bioresearch Monitoring Program, which includes inspections designed to evaluate the conduct of research and to ensure that the rights, safety, and welfare of the human subjects of those studies have been protected.

From our review of the establishment inspection report and the documents submitted with that report, we conclude that you did not adhere to the applicable statutory requirements and FDA regulations governing the conduct of clinical investigations. We are aware that at the conclusion of the inspection, as you were no longer an employee of Meadowbrook Research, Inc., Ms. Tonia Sawyer presented and discussed with the sub-investigator, Dr. (b)(6), Form FDA 483, Inspectional Observations. We note that on June 6, 2009, Ms. Tonia Sawyer delivered a copy of the Form FDA 483 to you at your current employer's address: 7575 E. Earll Drive, Scottsdale, Arizona 85251.

We acknowledge receipt of two letters, dated February 17, 2009, and February 26, 2009, from Meadowbrook Research, Inc' s CEO, Ms. Pamela Larson, and the sub-investigator, Dr. (b)(6), that were intended to respond to the Form FDA 483, Inspectional Observations. The response letters describe the actions that have been taken or that will be taken by Meadowbrook Research, Inc. to prevent similar violations in future studies conducted at Meadowbrook Research, Inc. However, as of November 20, 2009, FDA has not received a written response from you to the Form FDA 483, Inspectional Observations. As the principal clinical investigator, you are personally responsible for the conduct of the study, not Meadowbrook Research, Inc.

You should respond in writing explaining how you will ensure that such violations do not occur in any future clinical studies you conduct.

We wish to emphasize the following:

1. You failed to ensure that the investigation was conducted according to the investigational plan [21 CFR 312.60].

Specifically, there were numerous violations of the protocol that raise significant questions regarding the reliability of the data.

a. The protocol specified that the person obtaining informed consent must be sufficiently trained on medical issues, so that questions could be adequately addressed. The protocol specifically required that this person have an M.D., Ph.D., or RN degree; if the person did not have one of these degrees, then this person must have been approved by (b)(4) to obtain informed consent. For all subjects enrolled into this study (Subjects 1001-1008 and 1010-1013), the informed consent document and the assent form for children 10-17 years of age were not obtained by an M.D., Ph.D., or RN, as required by the protocol. In addition, you did not obtain (b)(4) approval for these persons to obtain informed consent and assent of the study subjects.

b. The protocol inclusion criteria specified that the subject must have a primary diagnosis of (b)(4) as defined by (b)(4) criteria and confirmed by the (b)(4) For Subjects 1008, 1010, 1011, 1012, and 1013, (b)(4) for (b)(4) diagnostic instrument was used in error to confirm diagnosis at screening, instead of the (b)(4) instrument as required by the protocol.

c. The protocol required that the (b)(4) be administered by the principal investigator or a sub-investigator who was a (b)(4) or a Ph.D.-level (b)(4), and who had participated in the (b)(4) rater-qualification program.

ⅰ. For Subjects 1001-1007, (b)(4) was not administered by the principal investigator or a sub-investigator, as required by the protocol. Instead, the (b)(4) was administered by a study coordinator, contrary to the criteria specified in the protocol.

ⅱ. There was no documentation of (b)(4) training for the principal investigator or sub-investigators participating in the (b)(4) rater-qualification program, as required by the protocol.

d. The protocol required that after the baseline visit and through Study Week 2, the investigator or designated staff contact the subject and the subject's parent(s) and/or guardian(s) on a daily basis, either by telephone or in person, to ensure that the subject was taking the proper capsules at the proper time, and to monitor the tolerability and efficacy of the titration plan.

For 10 of the 11 enrolled subjects, there is no documentation that you or your designated staff contacted the subject and the subject's parent(s) and/or guardian(s) on a daily basis, either by telephone or in person, as required by the protocol.

e. The protocol specified that for subjects with a body weight $<$ 45 kg, the target dose was 60-80 kg/day. On 10/5/06, Subject 1010's body weight was documented as 40.1 kg, and per protocol, the subject's initial study medication dose was 20 mg twice a day for a total of 40 mg/day. On 10/12/06, the subject's study medication dose was increased to 40 mg twice a day, which was the maximum allowable limit for this subject on study. However, on 10/15/06, this subject's study medication dose was increased again to 60 mg twice a day for a total of 120 mg per day, thus exceeding the maximum allowable study medication limit for this subject. This subject received 120 mg/day of study medication for five consecutive days while participating in this study.

f. The protocol required that one ECG be done at the screening visit and that three consecutive ECGs be done at the baseline visit. The baseline visit was to occur 1-10 days after the screening visit. Subject 1010 did not have an ECG performed at the screening visit on 9/29/06. Instead the screening ECG was completed on the same date that the three baseline ECGs were completed, at the baseline visit on 10/05/06.

g. The protocol required that all subjects have two pharmacokinetic samples drawn after taking the first dose of study medication (Day 1), 20 mg; the first sample was to be collected at 0.5-1.5 hours post first dose, and the second sample was to be collected 1.5-3 hours post first dose. These samples were not always collected within the protocol-required time periods. For example:

i. Subject 1010 took the first dose of study medication on 10/5/06 at 1730 hours; however, the source record for this subject showed that the first pharmacokinetic sample was collected at 1735 hours, only 5 minutes after taking the first dose. The pharmacokinetic post first dose draw time for this subject should have been between the hours of 1800-1900 on 10/5/06.

ii. Subject 1011 took the first dose of study medication on 10/31/06 at 1615 hours; however, the source record for this subject showed that the first pharmacokinetic sample was collected at 1630 hours, only 15 minutes after taking the first dose. The pharmacokinetic post first dose draw time for this subject should have been between the hours of 1645-1745 on 10/31/06.

h. The protocol specified that at the baseline visit, Day 1, subjects take their first dose of study medication, 20 mg. Following this first study medication dose, the subject was to have a pharmacokinetic sample drawn 0.5-1.5 hours post dose, and a second pharmacokinetic sample drawn at 1.5-3 hours post the first study medication dose. The protocol required that at the Week 4 visit, subjects take their morning dose of study medication. An ECG was to be administered, followed by a pharmacokinetic sample at 0.75-3.0 hours post study medication dose. Subjects were then to present at the clinic between 5-7 hours post study medication dose, when blood pressure and pulse (vitals) were to be measured, followed by another ECG. Ten minutes after the ECG administration, another pharmacokinetic sample was to be drawn. Finally, the protocol required that subjects who terminated from the study prior to Week 4 (Early Termination: ET) were to have pharmacokinetic samples taken and ECG and vital signs measured, as per the Week 4 visit procedures. These protocol-specified procedures were not always followed for 9 of 11 enrolled subjects. The table below lists, by subject, protocol-specified procedures that were not conducted at your site.

Subject	Date	Protocol Visit	PK Sample Missed	ECG Missed	Vital Signs Missed
1002	7/08/06	Week 4	5 hrs to 7 hrs	5 hrs to 7 hrs	5 hrs to 7 hrs
1003	8/23/06	Week 4	5 hrs to 7 hrs	N/A	5 hrs to 7 hrs
1004	8/16/06	Day 1	1 hrs 30 min to 3 hrs	N/A	N/A
1004	9/14/06	ET	5 hrs to 7 hrs	5 hrs to 7 hrs	5 hrs to 7 hrs
1005	8/31/06	ET	5 hrs to 7 hrs	5 hrs to 7 hrs	5 hrs to 7 hrs
1007	9/28/06	ET	5 hrs to 7 hrs		
1008	10/11/06	Week 4	5 hrs to 7 hrs	5 hrs to 7 hrs	5 hrs to 7 hrs
1010	10/20/06	ET	5 hrs to 7 hrs	5 hrs to 7 hrs	5 hrs to 7 hrs
1012	3/01/07	Day 1	30 min to 1 hrs 30 min	N/A	N/A
1012	3/01/07	Day 1	1 hrs 30 min to 3 hrs	N/A	N/A
1013	3/2/07	Day 1	30 min to 1 hrs 30 min	N/A	N/A
1013	3/2/07	Day 1	1 hrs 30 min to 3 hrs	N/A	N/A

ET Early Termination
Day 1 Baseline Date per Protocol
hrs Hours
min Minutes
N/A Not Applicable (not cited as a violation)

2. You failed to prepare and maintain adequate and accurate case histories that record all observations and other data pertinent to the investigation on each individual administered the investigational drug or employed as a control in the investigation [21 CFR 312.62(b)].

Specifically, there were numerous inaccuracies in recordkeeping noted in records for 10 of 11 subjects enrolled into the study, which raises significant questions regarding the reliability of the data.

a. Examples of inaccurate case histories for Subject 1001 include, but were not limited to the following:

i. The screening visit source record, dated 6/2/06, documented the standing pulse as 98; however, the corresponding electronic CRF (eCRF) documented the standing pulse as 82. The screening visit source record entry for Family History of Disease documented (b)(4) under the "Biological Siblings" heading with "NA (4)" marked with an X; however, the corresponding eCRF had the same heading with "yes (1)" marked with an X.

ii. The Week 2 visit source record, dated 6/23/06, documented the standing pulse as 100; however, the corresponding eCRF documented the standing pulse as 88.

iii. The Adverse Event Log source record for an (b)(4) event recorded the stop date as 7/5/06; however, the eCRF documented the "Outcome of AE to Date" as "Date resolved 7/11/06."

b. Examples of inaccurate case histories for Subject 1002 include, but were not limited to the following:

i. The screening visit Primary Diagnosis source record entry, dated 6/2/06, documented the duration of current Primary Diagnosis episode (months) as zero (0) and number of prior Primary Diagnosis episodes as 0 (zero). However, the corresponding eCRF recorded the duration of current Primary Diagnosis episode (months) as 1 and the number of prior Primary Diagnosis episodes as 2.

ii. The Day 1 (Baseline) visit source record, dated 6/6/06, documented the standing blood pressure as 179/99; however, the corresponding eCRF, dated 6/9/06, documented the standing blood pressure as 119/99.

iii. The Week 4 visit source record, dated 7/05/06, documented the temperature as 37.1°C. However, the corresponding eCRF documented the temperature as 31.7°C.

c. Examples of inaccurate case histories for Subject 1003 include, but were not limited to the following:

i. The screening visit Primary Diagnosis source record, dated 7/21/06, documented the duration of current Primary Diagnosis episode (months) as zero (0) and number of prior Primary Diagnosis episodes as 0 (zero). However, the corresponding eCRF recorded the duration of current Primary Diagnosis episode (months) as 4 and the number of prior Primary Diagnosis episodes as 1.

ii. The Week 4 visit source record, dated 8/23/06, documented the supine blood pressure as 114/72 and pulse as 76, and the standing blood pressure as 111/70 and pulse as 90 (Predose). The corresponding eCRF recorded the supine blood pressure as 108/78 and pulse as78, and the standing blood pressure as 100/64 and pulse as 80 (Pre-dose).

d. Examples of inaccurate case histories for Subject 1004 include, but were not limited to the following:

i. The screening visit source record, dated 8/1/06, titled (b)(4) History Questions," in Section 5: Family History of (b)(4), Question 1 reads, (b)(4)?" The response box is marked "yes, uncle/aunt"; however, for the same question on the eCRF, the box was marked "no."

ii. The Day 1 (Baseline) visit source record, dated 8/16/06, for the (b)(4), Question 2, pertaining to (b)(4) was marked "(2)." The (b)(4) Question 3, pertaining to (b)(4), was marked "(1) (b)(4)." The corresponding eCRF (b)(4) entry for Question 2, (b)(4) was marked "(1) (b)(4)," and Question 3, (b)(4), was marked "(0) (b)(4)."

e. Examples of inaccurate case histories for Subject 1005 include, but were not limited to the following:

i. The screening visit Primary Diagnosis source record, dated 8/1/06, documented the duration of current Primary Diagnosis episode (months) as 0 (zero) and number of prior Primary Diagnosis episodes as 0 (zero). However, the corresponding eCRF recorded the duration of current Primary Diagnosis episode (months) as 2 (two).

ii. The Week 1 visit source record, dated 8/17/06, for (b)(4) Question 9, pertaining to (b)(4), documented the response as (b)(4). However, the corresponding eCRF (b)(4) Question 9 response was blank (i.e., nothing was marked).

f. Examples of inaccurate case histories for Subject 1007 include, but were not limited to the following:

The screening visit Primary Diagnosis source record, dated 8/31/06, documented the number of prior Primary Diagnosis episodes as 1 (one). However, the corresponding eCRF recorded the number of prior Primary Diagnosis episodes as 2 (two).

g. Examples of inaccurate case histories for Subject 1008 include, but were not limited to the following:

i. The screening visit Primary Diagnosis source record, dated 9/8/06, documented the duration of current Primary Diagnosis episode (months) as 0 (zero) and the number of prior Primary Diagnosis episodes as 3 (three). However, the corresponding eCRF recorded the duration of current Primary Diagnosis episode (months) as 1 (one) and the number of prior Primary Diagnosis episodes as 0 (zero).

ii. The screening visit Log Concomitant Drug Treatment source record, dated 9/8/06, had Prozac listed but then crossed out by R.M. on 11/9/06; however, the corresponding eCRF has Prozac listed on the "Previous Psychotropic Drug Treatment" form.

h. Examples of inaccurate case histories for Subject 1010 include, but were not limited to the following:

i. The screening visit Primary Diagnosis source record, dated 9/29/06, documented the duration of current Primary Diagnosis episode (months) as 0 (zero). However, the corresponding eCRF recorded the duration of current Primary Diagnosis episode (months) as 2 (two).

ii. The screening visit source record, dated 9/29/06, documented waist circumference as "26.5 = 67.3 cm." However, the corresponding eCRF recorded the waist circumference (cm) as 26.5.

iii. The early termination visit source record, dated 10/20/06, documented height as 60.5. However, the corresponding eCRF recorded the height as 152.9 (cm) instead of the correct height in cm of 153.7.

i. Examples of inaccurate case histories for Subject 1011 include, but were not limited to the following:

The screening visit Primary Diagnosis source record, dated 10/20/06, documented the duration of the number of prior Primary Diagnosis episodes as 3 (three). However, the corresponding eCRF recorded the duration of the number of prior Primary Diagnosis episodes as 0 (zero).

j. Examples of inaccurate case histories for Subject 1012 include but were not limited to the following:

The screening visit Primary Diagnosis source record, dated 2/21/07, documented the duration of current Primary Diagnosis episode (months) as 0 (zero). However, the corresponding eCRF recorded the duration of current Primary Diagnosis episode (months) as 2 (two).

This letter is not intended to be an all-inclusive list of deficiencies with your clinical study of an investigational drug. It is your responsibility to ensure adherence to each requirement of the law and relevant FDA regulations. You should address these deficiencies and establish procedures to ensure that any ongoing or future studies will be in compliance with FDA regulations.

Within fifteen (15) working days of your receipt of this letter, you should notify this office in writing of the actions you have taken to prevent similar violations in the future. Failure to adequately and promptly explain the violations noted above may result in regulatory action without further notice.

If you have any questions, please contact Tejashri Purohit-Sheth, M.D., at 301-796-3402; FAX 301-847-8750. Your written response and any pertinent documentation should be addressed to:

Tejashri Purohit-Sheth, M.D.
Branch Chief
Good Clinical Practice Branch Ⅱ
Division of Scientific Investigations
Office of Compliance
Center for Drug Evaluation and Research
Food and Drug Administration
Building 51, Room 5358
10903 New Hampshire Avenue
Silver Spring, MD 20993

Sincerely yours,

{See appended electronic signature page}

Leslie K. Ball, M.D.
Director
Division of Scientific Investigations
Office of Compliance
Center for Drug Evaluation and Research

This is a representation of an electronic record that was signed electronically and this page is the manifestation of the electronic
signature.

/S/

LESLIE K BALL
11/24/2009

第120封　给Dallas Jr, Anthony V. 医学博士的警告信

2009年11月9日

参考号：10-HFD-45-11-01

尊敬的Dallas博士：

2009年3月16日至4月8日，Donna Gallien女士代表FDA进行了现场检查，与您会面并对您所实施的以下临床研究进行了审查：

试验方案（b）(4)，题为“（b）(4)”，试验药物（b）(4)，申办者为（b）(4)；

试验方案（b）(4)，题为“（b）(4)”，试验药物（b）(4)，申办者为（b）(4)。

本次现场检查是FDA的生物研究监查项目的一部分。该项目通过设定的检查方法，评估临床研究的实施情况，并确保此研究中受试者的权益、安全和福利得到了保护。

经对现场检查报告、该报告的附件和您2009年5月7日的书面回复进行审查，我们认为，您未遵循适用的法律要求和监管临床研究实施的FDA法规。我们注意到现场检查结束时，Gallien女士向您出示并与您讨论了FDA 483表，即现场检查发现的问题。我们想强调以下几点：

1．您未能亲自进行临床研究或对研究进行监督［21 CFR 312.60］

您在签署上述临床研究的研究者声明（FDA 1572表）时，您同意承担贵临床研究机构的临床研究者职责。您的总体职责（21 CFR 312.60）包括确保临床研究按照签署的研究者声明、研究计划和适用的法规进行，保护在您的监护下的受试者的权益、安全和福利，确保对试验药物进行管控。您明确同意将亲自进行临床研究或监管不是由您亲自进行的临床研究。虽然作为研究者，您可以授权有资质的人员进行某些研究任务，但您不能授权您的总体职责。我们的调查表明，您对被授权了研究任务的全体人员的监督不足，未能确保临床研究按照签署的研究者声明、研究计划和适用的法规进行，并在某种程度上保护受试者的权益、安全和福利。

特别是您签署了临床研究试验方案（b）(4)的受试者0011，008 和003的多个空白原始工作记录表，但原始文件应在填写数据和审查后签字确认。您签署的文件表明，您已审核了此文件。

我们还注意到，在您的书面回复中确认，您依赖临床研究协调员跟踪研究计划和通信信息，此通信方式无适当的发送流程。我们确认您已描述纠正措施，如所有研究通信信息直接发送给您，以预防上述缺陷的再发生。然而，此纠正措施未阐明确保您以后亲自参加临床研究或监管临床研究以及确保其他临床协调员参与的临床研究的研究程序正确。

2. 您未能进行研究或确保按照签署的研究者声明、研究计划进行研究［21 CFR 312.60］

a. 试验方案（b）(4)声明，绝经后口服激素替代疗法的受试者应从临床研究中排除。试验方案附件I禁止的合并用药列出口服激素替代疗法和雌激素、孕激素。受试者0011在2005年8月16日随机入组，尽管2006年8月6日和2007年1月24日受试者门诊病历记载使用了禁止的合并药物，Prempro和一个口服激素替代疗法，但是此受试者被允许参与这项临床研究。

b. 试验方案（b）(4)声明，新诊断的受试者或未治疗的4周以上受试者可合并第1、2次访视。试验方案（b）(4)也声明，受试者使用（b）(4)药物必须经历洗脱期和必须进入第2次访视前至少停用一周以前服用的药物。

i. 受试者0001的2006年10月12日门诊病历记录此人当前服用药物，然而他进入第2次访视，但未遵循方案经历洗脱期。

ii. 受试者0001在2006年10 月13日合并第1次访视和第2次访视接受试验方案（b）(4)的治疗，然而根据试验方案（b）(4)新诊断的受试者或未治疗4周以上的受试者可合并第1次和第2次访视。无证据表明受试者

0001符合这条标准，因此这名受试者不能合并第1、2次访视。

我们注意到，您承认未按照签署的临床研究声明和研究计划实施临床研究。我们也确认在您的书面回复中已提供充分的纠正措施，以预防未来再次发生上述事件。

3. 您未能准备和维护研究中使用试验药物或对照组的受试者的所有研究观察结果和其他相关数据的足够及准确的病历［21 CFR 312.62（b）］

多个参与临床试验的受试者的病历的准确性存在缺陷：

a. 受试者0008　2004年11月22日门诊病历准确记载了基底细胞瘤，然而2005年6月8日筛选期第2次访视的病例报告表未将此疾病作为疾病史记录，无文件解释这项不一致性。

b. 受试者0003

ⅰ. 早期终止临床试验的受试者003的记录和受试者签署的声明相矛盾。如在2006年10月18日第7次访视原始文件中，研究协调员记录该受试者不在本市并拒绝安排最后一次访视。2007年7月19日的第8.1次访视原始文件中，研究协调员声明，该受试者不再服用临床试验药物，因为受试者撤回知情同意书不继续参加临床研究；然而受试者声明描述和上述原始文件所述的受试者因撤回知情同意书而不继续参加临床研究相矛盾。受试者声明记载，受试者003第3次访视后就未见过临床研究协调员。受试者声明记载，受试者未拒绝最后1次访视，未撤回知情同意书，这名受试者试图继续参加临床研究，但这一电话信息未得到回复。

ⅱ.病例报告表记录此受试者多项合并用药的起始日期和停止日期相矛盾。无文件解释此不一致性。

c. 受试者0011

ⅰ. 在（2006年9月7日）第6次访视后的（2007年2月20日）第7次访视的原始文件未记载任何不良事件，然而CRF列出了大量不良事件。

ⅱ. 2007年9月19日进行了第8次访视，这次访视的原始文件记录不一致。一些文件记录受试者用药发生了变化并接收了（b）（6）鼻窦炎手术，但其他文件记录药物和健康无变化。

ⅲ. 病例报告表未记录第6.1次访视，所附文件也未解释这一记录缺失。

无文件记录解释受试者0011记录的不一致性。

参加试验方案（b）（4）临床研究的多名受试者的病历准确性存在缺陷。

d. 受试者003

ⅰ. 不良事件日志未记载2007年1月23日到6月13日的门诊病历记录的不良事件。

ⅱ. 2006年12月5日的第1次访视筛选期的病例报告表中的吸烟变更为不吸烟，然而2007年6月27日门诊记录受试者约一月前停止吸烟。无文件解释受试者停止吸烟时间的不一致事件。

e. 受试者005　不良事件日志未记载2006年10月31日第2次访视到2007年1月3日第6次访视的门诊病历记录的大量不良事件。

f. 受试者001　病例报告表试验药物（b）（4）未记录在第1次访视（2006年10月12日）前6个月内使用（b）（4），然而同一时间的门诊病历记载了使用试验药物（b）（4）并声明这次访视的目的是为了继续获得服用（b）（4）。

g. 受试者004　2006年10月23日第1次访视用右臂测量的平均坐位收缩压被错误计算为150mmHg 和84mmHg，正确的舒张压和收缩压应为147mmHg 和86mmHg。

h. 受试者0006　试验方案7.5.2阐明，研究者在第11次访视实施全面的体格检查。临床试验机构的原始文件必须记录体格检查的信息，然而您临床试验机构的原始文件未记录第11次访视体格检查的信息。

我们注意到，您承认您未保存足够和准确的记录。我们也承认在您的书面回复中描述的将来采取的改进记录保存管理的纠正措施。

4. 您未能保存足够的包括日期、数量和受试者的使用情况的药物处置记录［21 CFR 312.62（a）］

a. 对于入组试验方案（b）（4）的受试者0011

ⅰ. 第4次访视：2005年11月14日第4次访视的原始文件工作表药物使用部分记载分发药物，第4次访视的用药依从性检查记录编号5097765的药物发放日期在2005年11月15日。药瓶标签也记录药物发放日期为2005年11月15日。无文件解释此差异。

ii. 第7次访视：第7次访视的病例报告表药物章节记录2007年2月20日返还200片药物。第7次访视的药物依从性检查记录返还38片药物。

b. 入组（b）（4）临床研究的受试者00002：第5次访视的病例报告表药物标签表记录2006年11月21日分发编号513548药物，然而药物清点表未记载这一药物编号。

c. 入组（b）（4）临床研究的受试者00004，2007年3月5日的第8次访视。

i. 药物再供应电话工作表记录编号515201，519282，519101的药物在2007年3月5日发放。但是2007年3月18日临床再供应确认表未记录编号515201药物的发放。无文件解释此差异。

ii. 药物清点表记载编号519282和519101的药物于2007年3月19日发放。2008年4月29日药物汇总记录记载未发放编号519101的药物。此外，药物标签表也未记录编号519101标签和使用编号519282的受试者号。

我们注意到，您承认您未保存足够和准确的药物登记管理记录。我们也承认在您的书面回复中描述了已采取充分的措施，以预防将来的药物管理缺陷。

本警告信的目的并非是罗列您在试验药物临床研究中存在的所有缺陷。确保遵循法律和相关FDA法规的每一项要求是您的职责。您应当解决这些缺陷，并建立规程，以确保任何正在进行或将来的研究均能符合FDA的法规。

自收到这封信的15个工作日内，您应当书面告知本办公室为预防将来发生类似违规情况已经采取的措施。如未能正确地、快速地解释上述违规问题，可能导致我们在不再通知的情况下采取监管措施。

附：英文原文

Dallas Jr, Anthony V. M.D.

WARNING LETTER

Nov 9, 2009

CERTIFIED MAIL
RETURN RECEIPT REQUESTED

Ref: 10-HFD-45-11-01

Anthony Dallas, M.D.
Family Health Care of Hendersonville
353 New ShackleIsland Road, Suite141C
Hendersonville, TN37075

Dear Dr. Dallas:

Between March 16 and April 8,2009,Ms. Donna Gallien, representing the Food and Drug Administration (FDA),conducted an investigation and met with you to review your conduct of the following clinical investigations:

- Protocol (b)(4) entitled (b)(4) of the investigational drug (b)(4) performed for (b)(4),and
- Protocol (b)(4) entitled (b)(4) of the investigational drug (b)(4) performed for (b)(4)

This inspection is a part of the FDA' s Bioresearch Monitoring Program, which includes inspections designed to evaluate the conduct of research and to ensure that the rights, safety, and welfare of the human subjects of those studies have been protected.

From our review of the establishment inspection report, the documents submitted with that report, and your written response dated May 7, 2009, we conclude that you did not adhere to the applicable statutory requirements and FDA regulations governing the conduct of clinical investigations. We are aware that at the conclusion of the inspection, Ms. Gallien presented and discussed with you Form FDA 483, Inspectional Observations. We wish to emphasize the following:

1. You failed to personally conduct or supervise the clinical investigations referenced above [21 CFR 312.60].

When you signed the investigator statements (Form FDA 1572) for the above referenced clinical investigations, you agreed to take on the responsibilities of a clinical investigator at your site. Your general responsibilities (21 CFR 312.60) include ensuring that the investigation is conducted according to the signed investigator statement, the investigational plan, and applicable regulations; protecting the rights, safety and welfare of subjects under your care; and ensuring control of drugs under investigation. You specifically agreed to personally conduct the clinical studies or to supervise those aspects of the studies that you did not personally conduct. While you may delegate certain study tasks to individuals qualified to perform them, as clinical investigator, you may not delegate your general responsibilities. Our investigation indicates that your supervision of personnel to whom you delegated study tasks was not adequate to ensure that clinical trials were conducted according to the signed investigator statement, the investigational plan, and applicable regulations, and in a manner that protected the rights, safety, and welfare of human subjects.

Specifically, multiple blank source document worksheets for Protocol (b)(4) were signed by you for subjects #0011, #008, and #003. Your signature on a document indicates that you have reviewed the data within; thus, source documents should not be signed until relevant data has been added and reviewed.

We note your acknowledgment in your written response that you relied on the study coordinator to follow the investigational plan as well as that the correspondence regarding the various studies was sent to the study coordinator without an appropriate flow of information. We also acknowledge that you have described corrective actions such as having all study correspondence sent directly to you to prevent recurrence of the findings noted above in the future. However, these corrective procedures do not address how you will assure that you personally conduct or supervise investigational studies in the future as well as ensure the integrity of the investigational procedures in the other clinical investigations in which the study coordinator may have been involved.

2. You failed to conduct the studies or ensure they were conducted according to the signed investigator statement and the investigational plan [21 CFR 312.60].

a. Protocol **(b)(4)** specifically stated that subjects with current use of postmenopausal oral hormone replacement therapy were to be excluded from the clinical investigation. Furthermore, Appendix I of the protocol, Disallowed Concomitant Medications, lists "oral hormone replacement therapy" and specifies "estrogens and progestins". Subject #0011 was randomized on 8/16/05 and allowed to continue in the clinical investigation despite clinic records dated 8/8/06 and 1/24/07 documenting the use of the disallowed concomitant medication, Prempro, an oral hormone replacement therapy.

b. Protocol **(b)(4)** states that newly diagnosed **(b)(4)** subjects or subjects currently untreated for greater than 4 weeks may combine visits 1and 2. The protocol also states that subjects on current (b] (4) medication must undergo a washout period and must be completely off their previous **(b)(4)** medication for at least one week before entering visit 2.

i. The clinic chart dated 10/12/06 documents subject #0001 as currently taking the medication, yet he did not undergo a washout period prior to visit 2, as required in the protocol.

ii. Visits 1 and 2, which occurred on 10/13/06, were combined for subject #0001, who was currently treated with **(b)(4)** against protocol guidelines that state combined visits 1 and 2 are only for subjects who are newly diagnosed as **(b)(4)** or are currently untreated for at least 4 weeks. There is no evidence that subject #0001 met these criteria, and therefore he should not have combined visits 1and 2.

We note your acknowledgment that the investigation was not conducted in accordance with the signed statement and investigational plan. We also acknowledge that you have described adequate corrective actions in your written response to prevent recurrence of the findings noted above in the future.

3. You failed to prepare and maintain adequate and accurate case histories that record all observations and other data pertinent to the investigation on each individual administered the investigational drug or employed as a control in the investigation [21 CFR 312.62(b)].

Deficiencies were noted in the accuracy of the case histories of multiple subjects participating in Protocol (b)(4):

a. Subject #0008: Clinic chart on 11/22/04 documented excision of basal cell carcinoma yet screen visit 2 Case Report Form (CRF) on 6/8/05 fails to document this as past medical history. There is nc written documentation to explain this inconsistency.

b. Subject #0003:

i. The documentation in the records for the early termination of subject #003 contradicts an affidavit signed by subject #003. For example, the source document for visit 7 dated 10/18/06 written by the study coordinator states that the subject was out of town and declined to schedule the final study visit. Additionally, source document for visit 8.1 dated 7/19/07 written by the study coordinator states that subject #003 was no longer taking the study medication due to discontinuation from the study because the subject withdrew consent. However, the affidavit of subject #003 contradicts the above mentioned source documents regarding the subject' s discontinuation from the study due to withdrawal of consent. The affidavit of subject #003 states that the subject never saw the study coordinator after the third visit. Furthermore, the affidavit states that the subject did not decline the final study visit, did not withdraw consent, and that the subject had attempted to continue participation in the study but that the telephone messages were not returned.

ii. Multiple concomitant therapy case report forms documenting medications used by subject #0003 contain conflicting information with respect to start and stop dates. There is no written documentation to explain these inconsistencies.

c. Subject #0011:

i. For Visit 7 (2/20/07), the source document fails to document any adverse events after Visit 6 (9/7/06), yet the CRF documents numerous adverse events.

ii. Visit 8 was conducted on 9/19/07. Source documents from that visit are inconsistent in that some records document that the subject underwent medication changes and sinus surgery on (b) (6), but other records state there were no changes in medication or health.

iii. CRF fails to include documentation of visit 6.1 and the accompanying memo-to-file does not explain this lack of documentation.

There is no written documentation to explain these inconsistencies for Subject #0011.

Deficiencies were noted in the accuracy of the case histories of multiple subjects participating in Protocol (b)(4):

d. Subject #003:

i. The adverse event log fails to document adverse events listed in the clinic chart between 1/23/07 through 6/13/07.

ii Visit 1 screening form CRF was changed from smoker to non-smoker on 12/5/06, yet clinic records dated 6/27/07 document that subject stated she stopped smoking "about 1 month ago". There is no explanation for the different dates recorded in the subject's records.

e. Subject #005: Adverse event log fails to document numerous adverse events listed in the clinic chart between visit 2 (10/31/06) and visit 6 (1/3/07).

f. Subject #001: failure to document use of (b)(4) in the six months prior to visit 1 (10/12/06) on Prior (b)(4) Medication case report form, yet clinic notes from same date list the use of (b)(4) and state that the purpose of the subject's visit was for a (b)(4) refill.

g. Subject #004: The Mean Sitting Systolic Blood Pressure using the right arm was miscalculated as 150 mmHg and MSDBP as 84 mmHg for Visit 1 on 10/23/06 instead of the correct values of 147 and 86, respectively.

h. Subject #0006: Section 7.5.2 of the protocol states that a complete physical examination be performed by the investigator at Visit 11. Furthermore, information about the physical examination must be present in the source documentation at the study site. The Visit 11 complete physical examination was not documented in source documents at your site.

We note your acknowledgment that you failed to maintain adequate and accurate records. We also acknowledge the corrective actions, described in your written response, that you have taken to improve record keeping in the future.

4. You failed to maintain adequate records of the disposition of the drug, including dates, quantity and use by subjects [21 CFR 312.62(a)].

a. For subject #0011enrolled in Protocol (b)(4)

i. Visit 4: The study medication section of the source document worksheet documents medication dispensed for visit 4 on 11/14/05, yet the study medication compliance check for visit 4 documents kit number 5097765 was dispensed on 11/15/05. The medication bottle label for kit number 5097765 also documents that it was dispensed on 11/15/05. There is no written documentation to explain this discrepancy.

ii. Visit 7: The study medication case report form for visit 7 documents 200 tablets returned on 2/20/07, yet the study medication compliance check for visit 7 documents 38 tablets returned on 2/20/07.

b. For subject #00002 enrolled in Protocol (b)(4): Visit 5 CRF Drug Labels form documents that kit number 513548 was dispensed on 11/21/06, yet the Drug Accountability Log fails to document this kit.

c. For subject #00004 enrolled in Protocol (b)(4), Visit 8 on 3/5/07:

i. Medication Re-Supply Call Worksheet dated 3/5/07 documents kit numbers 515201, 519282, and 519101as being dispensed but ClinPhone Re-Supply Confirmation form dated 3/18/07 does not list kit number 515201as being dispensed. There is no written documentation to explain this discrepancy.

ii. Drug Accountability Log documents kit numbers 519282 and 519101 as being dispensed 3/19/07 but the Drug Summary Log dated 4/29/08 documents kit number 519101 as not dispensed. Additionally, Drug Labels forms fail to document the label for kit number 519101 and the study subject number for kit number 519282.

We note your acknowledgment that you failed to maintain adequate and accurate drug accountability records. We also acknowledge the adequate corrective actions, described in your written response, that you have taken to prevent drug accountability discrepancies in the future.

This letter is not intended to be an all-inclusive list of deficiencies with your clinical study of an investigational drug. It is your responsibility to ensure adherence to each requirement of the law and relevant FDA regulations. You should address these deficiencies and establish procedures to ensure that any on-going or future studies will be in compliance with FDA regulations.

Within fifteen (15) working days of your receipt of this letter, you should notify this office in writing of the actions you have taken to prevent similar violations in the future. Failure to adequately and promptly explain the violations noted above may result in regulatory action without further notice.

If you have any questions, please contact Constance Lewin, M.D., M.P.H., at 301-796-3397; FAX 301-847-8748. Your written response and any pertinent documentation should be addressed to:

Constance Lewin, M.D., M.P.H.
Branch Chief, Good Clinical Practice Branch I
Division of Scientific Investigations
Office of Compliance
Center for Drug Evaluation and Research
Food and Drug Administration
Bldg 51, Room 5354
10903 New Hampshire Avenue
Silver Spring, MD 20993

Sincerely yours,

{See appended electronic signature page}

Leslie K. Ball.M.D.
Director
Division of Scientific Investigations
Office of Compliance
Center for Drug Evaluation and Research

第121封 给McKay, Charles医学博士的警告信

2009年10月23日

参考号：10-HFD-45-10-03

尊敬的McKay博士：

2009年2月24日至3月6日，Diane Van Leeuwen女士和Trushani Shah女士代表FDA进行了现场检查，与您会面并对您实施的一项临床研究（b）(4)，申办者为（b）(4）进行了审查。

本次现场检查是FDA的生物研究监查项目的一部分。该项目通过设定的检查方法，评估相关研究的实施情况，并确保这些研究中受试者的权益、安全和福利得到了保护。

经对现场检查报告、该报告的附件进行审查，我们认为，您没有遵循适用的法律要求和监管临床研究实施的FDA法规。我们知道，在现场检查结束时，Van Leeuwen女士和Shah女士向您出示并讨论了FDA483表，即现场检查发现的问题。我们想强调以下几点：

1. 您未能亲自进行研究或对临床研究进行监督［21 CFR 312.60］

您在签署上述临床研究的研究者声明（FDA1572表）时，您同意承担作为本研究场所的临床研究者的职责。您的总体职责包括确保临床研究按照签署的研究者声明、研究计划以及相关法规要求进行，保护您监管下的受试者的权益、安全和福利，确保对试验药物进行管控（21 CFR 312.60)。在签署的研究者声明中，您明确同意将亲自进行研究或者将对不是您亲自进行的研究工作予以监督和管理。虽然作为研究者您可以授权有资质的人员进行某些研究任务，但您不能授权总体职责。我们的调查显示，您对授权进行研究任务的全体人员的监督不足以确保临床试验是按照签署的研究者声明、研究计划和适用的法规进行，并在某种程度上保护受试者的权益、安全和福利。

在审查现场检查报告以及随该报告提交的其他文件时，我们发现您未能充分参与或者监督研究的进行，以确保数据的可靠性并保护参与本研究的受试者的权益、安全和福利，如下条目2～4所述。

在FDA现场检查期间，您签署的书面宣誓书上，您指出，您认为监查员提供给您和研究协调员的培训是充分的，而且在有问题的时候监查员会让您知道。您进一步声称，您不知道您需要监督研究的进行并确保研究协调员正确地进行诸如完成原始记录和病例报告表（CRF)、填写不良事件和住院病历并且及时通知伦理委员会和申办者等工作。您同时指出，直至2008年秋天您才知道发生在贵研究中心的问题，并参与到试图识别可用数据的工作中，以及雇佣有经验的人员帮助实施改进。

我们想再次强调，作为研究者，确保研究按照FDA的要求正确地执行并保护研究中受试者的权益、安全和福利是您最基本的职责。

2. 您未能及时向IRB报告研究活动中的所有变更［21 CFR 312.66］

在受试者入组到研究中的时间范围内，贵研究中心已被申办者告知几次方案变更。例如，在日期为2007年7月20日的一封信中，申办者告知您方案修正案#2。在另一封日期为2008年8月5日的信中，申办者提醒您告知伦理委员会关于方案修正案#2和#3。此外，在日期为2008年2月21日的信中，申办者告知您方案修正案#4。最后，在日期为2008年8月5日的信中，申办者告知您关于方案修正案#5。然而，伦理委员会的记录显示，您未能及时报告这些变更。在几封日期为2009年1月6日的信中，伦理委员会指出其直到2008年12月才收到方案修正案#2到#5。而且，在2008年12月份伦理委员会承认收到这些方案修正案的时候，由一封申办者在2008年10月22日发出的信函证实该研究已经在贵研究中心结束了。

在一份书面的承诺书中，您阐明了依据方案修正案#4和#5，您已经知道了方案修正案中指出的使用（b）

（4）和其他药物的危害，以及外科手术的风险。因此，您已经审查了受试者的病历记录并与受试者讨论了这些风险以确定他们没有风险。在承诺书中您指出了您相信这些方案修正案已经被递交给伦理委员会。

FDA的检查员未能发现证据证实本研究在贵研究场所结束之前向伦理委员会递交了方案修正案#2到#5，并获批准。未能立即递交这些方案修正案给伦理委员会是对FDA法规的重大违背。

3. 您未能进行研究或者确保按照签署的研究者声明或研究计划进行研究［21 CFR 312.60］

a. 方案规定了严重不良事件（SAE）为任何导致死亡，危及生命，导致永久或严重地残疾/能力丧失，需住院治疗或延长住院时间，导致先天畸形/出生缺陷，或因其他原因被视作严重地反映了重大风险的不良事件。方案进一步阐明了所有的AE，严重或者不严重，需要足够地记录在适当的CRF中，严重不良事件需要填写严重不良事件报告表汇报给申办者，并且记录尽可能详细的因果关系判断。当收到后续增补信息后，所有SAE表上剩余的部分需要填写完整或者更新。所有严重的或者重大的AE，无论是否认为与试验药物相关，无论是否服用过试验药物，需要马上通过电话/传真等方式汇报给申办者。您未能遵循方案的要求，例子包括但不仅限于如下：

i. 受试者001

（1）受试者因充血性心力衰竭导致了住院（b）（6）。根据FDA检查员对这名受试者原始资料的审核发现，这个事件并未记录在SAE报告表中，没有进行因果关系判断并且直至7月13日（没有记录年份）才报告申办者，并于2008年11月12日再次报告。

（2）在2007年8月7日，贵研究中心被告知这个受试者发生心脏停搏已经住院，并且情况不佳。在FDA检查人员审查这名受试者的原始资料时，没有证据显示您已经向申办者报告了该SAE。受试者住院后随即死亡。原始记录显示在2007年9月贵研究中心已经知晓了这名受试者死亡的信息。但是这个新增的SAE也未在SAE报告表中记录并对因果关系进行评价，直至2008年11月12日才向申办者报告了该SAE。

ii. 受试者007在研究（b）（4）期间曾几次住院，FDA检查人员未能发现任何记录显示这些事件已经报告了申办者。

b. 方案明确规定，在受试者筛选访视的时候应采集和评估用于安全分析的实验室样品。FDA指出有记录显示，在您审查的七名受试者中，有四名受试者的记录审查是严重滞后的。在您完成方案要求的、筛选相关记录的审查时，该四名受试者不是已进入随机研究就是已经完成了研究。例如，

i. 文件显示直至2007年8月15日，您才审查了受试者002在2007年6月4日筛选访视时采集样本的实验室报告。在您审查原始记录时，这名受试者已经被发放了试验药物（发药时间2007年6月11日）。

ii. 文件显示直至2007年11月9日，您才审查了受试者007在2007年11月1日筛选访视时采集样本的实验室报告。在您审查原始记录时，这名受试者已经被随机到研究中并被发放了试验药物（发药时间2007年11月8日）。

c. 方案明确规定，在筛选访视时（例如访视1），关键的基线特征需要进行记录，包括人口统计学信息，既往病史，体格检查和生命体征。

i. 对受试者002，筛选访视中没有进行体格检查的记录，并且在既往病史中仅有有限的信息。

ii. 受试者007直至随机进入到研究后才进行体格检查。这名受试者的体格检查是在2007年12月6日进行的，晚于筛选访视（2007年10月29日）和受试者随机进入研究和发放试验药物的时间（2007年11月8日）。

d. 方案明确规定，在研究过程中，受试者需要按方案中的流程图所规定的时间回到诊所完成定期随访计划（在随机后的第1，3，6，9和12个月），之后的试验过程中为每四个月一次，以评估试验药物的依从性和数量，进行伴随治疗或干预，以及进行疗效和安全相关的评估。此外，方案还要求所有随机的患者应按照随机时制订的计划执行直至终末访视，无论治疗状态是什么（例如永久的或者暂时的中止）。以下受试者没有充分地遵循每一个方案：

i. 受试者002，记录显示在访视6之后（2007年12月6日），贵研究中心的研究人员没有在随机后的第9、第12和第16个月见到该受试者。您的研究人员没有对该受试者进行任何方案要求的访视，直至这名受试者在2008年11月21日终止研究。

ⅱ. 受试者004，记录显示在2007年10月16日第3个月的随机访视后，贵研究中心的研究人员没有在随机后的第6、第9、第12个月的访视见到该受试者。直至2008年10月16日您才再次见到该受试者。

ⅲ. 受试者005，随机后第12个月的访视发生时间比方案要求的晚了两个月。

ⅳ. 受试者007，在2008年2月的随机后3个月访视，贵研究人员没有在随机后6个和9个月访视见到该受试者。直至2008年10月10日您才再次见到该受试者。

鉴于受试者到贵研究中心访视的间隔时间，我们不确定您如何充分保护入组本研究的受试者的权益、安全以及福利。

e. 方案要求实验室样本采集品应包括每四周检测一次国际标准化比率（INR），每月检测肝功能相关指标。对如下受试者，实验室检查没有按照方案要求进行检测。

ⅰ. 受试者002，记录显示在2008年3月20日之后，没有进行月度INR检测。此外，没有记录显示在访视6（2007年12月6日）和受试者2008年11月21日终止研究期间对该受试者进行过月度肝功能检测。

ⅱ. 受试者004，在2007年10月16日后至受试者在2008年10月24日这段时间没有发现受试者进行过月度肝功能检测的任何证据。

ⅲ. 受试者007，在2008年2月3日后至受试者在2008年10月24日这段时间没有发现受试者进行过月度肝功能检测的任何证据。

4. 您未能保存足够的包括日期、数量和受试者的使用情况的药物分发记录［21 CFR 312.62（a）］

FDA调查发现，您未能足够地保存随机在此研究中的五名受试者的药物发放记录。

a. 受试者001，在2007年3月23日进行了药物发放。记录未包含此受试者使用的试验药物数量的任何信息。

b. 受试者002，关于受试者发放研究药物的日期和数量的记录存在不一致。根据发放/回收登记表，受试者在2007年6月11日、2007年8月10日和2007年12月6日进行了发放研究药物，但这几次发药均没有返还。根据试验药物发放报告，受试者在2007年6月11日、2007年9月7日和2007年12月6日进行了发药。此外，根据发放/回收登记，受试者在2007年6月11日仅发放了一瓶药物，然而试验药物发放报告中显示受试者被发放了3瓶药物，每一瓶分别来自不同的记录批号。

c. 受试者004，记录中未包含受试者在随访后3个月访视中使用药物的数量信息，同时也没有任何关于在2007年7月13日、2007年10月16日和2007年12月12日发放药物返还给研究中心的日期信息。此外，在2007年12月12日发放试验药物的信息是“估算的”，并且这个信息是直至受试者终止研究（2008年10月24日）之后的2008年12月11日才进行填写的。

d. 受试者005，记录未包含在2007年8月3日（随机访视）和2007年12月3日（随机后3个月访视）发药后试验药物使用数量的信息。此外，在2007年12月之后的某个未知日期发放的6瓶试验药物在2008年10月10日空瓶返还给贵研究中心。没有详细记录何时发放了这几瓶药物以及受试者使用药物的数量。

e. 受试者007，记录未包含试验药物在2007年11月8日（随机访视）和2008年2月15日（随机后3个月访视）发放后的使用数量信息。

f. 原始记录显示2瓶（b）（4）和6瓶（b）（4）在贵研究中心的总药物库存中丢失。

您未能保存足够和准确的药物发放记录，这令我们担心随机药物是否适当地发放给受试者，并对采集数据的可靠性产生了怀疑。

本警告信的目的并非是罗列您在试验药物临床研究中存在的所有缺陷。确保遵循法律和相关FDA法规的每一项要求是您的职责。您应当解决这些缺陷，并建立规程，以确保任何正在进行或将来的研究均能符合FDA的法规。

自收到这封信的15个工作日内，您应当书面告知本办公室为预防将来发生类似违规情况已经采取的措施。如果不能充分、迅速地解释上述违规问题，可能导致我们在不再通知的情况下采取监管措施。

附：英文原文

McKay, Charles M.D.

WARNING LETTER

OCT 23, 2009

CERTIFIED MAIL
RETURN RECEIPT REQUESTED

Ref: 10-HFD-45-10-03

Charles McKay, M.D.
1124 West Carson Street, RB2
Torrance, CA 90502

Dear Dr. McKay:

Between February 24 and March 6, 2009, Ms. Diane Van Leeuwen and Ms. Trushani Shah, representing the Food and Drug Administration (FDA), conducted an investigation and met with you to review your conduct of a clinical investigation (b)(4) performed for (b)(4)

This inspection is a part of the FDA' s Bioresearch Monitoring Program, which includes inspections designed to evaluate the conduct of research and to ensure that the right, safety, and welfare of the human subjects of those studies have been protected. From our review of the establishment inspection report and the document submitted with that report, we conclude that you did not adhere to the applicable statutory requirement and FDA regulations governing the conduct of clinical investigations. We are aware that at the conclusion of the inspection, Ms. Van Leeuwen and Ms. Shah presented and discussed with you Form FDA 483, Inspectional Observations. We wish to emphasize the following:

1. You failed to personally conduct or supervise the clinical investigation [21 CFR 312.60].

When you signed the investigator statements (Form FDA 1572) for the above referenced clinical investigations,you agreed to take on the responsibilities of a clinical investigator at your site. Your general responsibilities include ensuring that the investigation is conducted according to the signed investigator statement, the investigational plan, and applicable regulations; protecting the rights, safety, and welfare of subject under your care; and ensuring control of drugs under investigation (21 CFR 312.60). In the signed investigator agreement, you specifically agreed to personally conduct the clinical studies or to supervise those aspects of the studies that you did not personally conduct. While you may delegate certain study tasks to individuals qualified to perform them, as clinical investigator, you may not delegate your general responsibilities. Our investigation indicates that your supervision of personnel to whom you delegated study tasks was not adequate to ensure that clinical trials were conducted according to the signed investigator statement, the investigational plan, and applicable regulations, and in a manner that protected the right, safety, and welfare of human subjects.

In our review of the inspection report and the documents submitted with that report, we find that you failed to have adequate involvement in and oversight of the study to ensure data integrity and to protect the rights, safety, and welfare of subjects enrolled in the study, as noted in Items 2 through 4 below.

In a written affidavit signed by you during the FDA inspection, you noted that you thought the training provided by the monitors to you and your study coordinators was sufficient, and that if there were problems, the monitors would let you know. You further asserted that you did not know that you had to supervise the study and ensure that the study coordinators were correctly doing such things as completing source records and case report forms (CRFs), filling out adverse event and hospitalization forms, and notifying the IRB and sponsor on time. You also noted that it was not until the fall of 2008 that you became aware of the problems at your site, got involved in trying to identify usable data, and hired experienced people to help make improvements.

We wish to emphasize again that as the clinical investigator, it was your ultimate responsibility to ensure that the studies were conducted properly and in compliance with FDA regulations in order to protect the rights, safety, and welfare of study subjects.

2. You failed to promptly report to the IRB all changes in research activity [21 CFR 312.66].

Your site had been notified by the sponsor of several changes in the protocol during the time period when subjects were enrolled in the study. For example, the sponsor notified you of Protocol Amendment #2 in a letter dated July 20, 2007. In another letter, dated January 21, 2008, the sponsor reminded you to notify the IRB about Protocol Amendments #2 and #3. In addition, in a letter dated February 21, 2008, the sponsor notified you of Protocol Amendment #4. Finally, in a letter dated August 5, 2008, the sponsor notified you of Protocol Amendment #5. However, IRB records indicate that you failed to promptly report these changes. In several letters dated January 6 2009, the IRB noted that it had not received notice of Protocol Amendment #2 through #5 until December 2008. Furthermore, by the time the IRB acknowledged receipt of these Protocol Amendments from you in December 2008, the study had already been closed at your site, as evidenced by a letter from the sponsor dated October 22, 2008.

In a written affidavit, you stated that with regard to Protocol Amendments #4 and # 5, you were aware of the hazards of the use of (b)(4) and other drugs, as well as the risk of surgeries, as note in the amendments. Thus, you had reviewed the subject's charts and discussed these risks with the subject to determine that they were not at risk. Per the affidavit, you noted that you did believe that the Protocol Amendment had been submitted to the IRB.

FDA' s investigators were unable to find evidence that prior to the study being closed at your site, Protocol Amendments #2 through #5 were submitted to and approved by the IRB. Failure to submit these Protocol Amendments promptly to the IRB is a significant violation of FDA' s regulations.

3. You failed to conduct the studies or ensure they were conducted according to the signed investigator statement and investigational plan [21 CFR 312.60].

a. The protocol defined a serious adverse event (SAE) as any adverse event (AE) that resulted in death, was immediately life-threatening, resulted in persistent or significant disability/incapacity required or prolonged patient hospitalization,was a congenital anomaly/birth defect, or was deemed to be serious for any other reason representing a significant hazard. The protocol further stated that all AEs, serious and nonserious, were to be fully documented on the appropriate CRFs; and SAEs were to be reported to the sponsor using the Serious Adverse Event Report Form, with a documented causal relationship assessment and in as much detail as possible. Upon receipt of follow-up information, all remaining fields on the SAE form were to be completed or updated. Any serious or significant AE, whether or not it was thought to be related to the investigational product, and whether or not the investigational product had been administered, was to be reported immediately by telephone/fax to the sponsor. You failed to follow the protocol requirements.

Examples include but were not limited to the following:

ⅰ. For Subject #001:

1. The subject had congestive heart failure that resulted in a hospitalization on (b)(6) Based on the FDA investigator's review of your source documents for this subject, it appears that this event was not documented on a Serious Adverse Event Report Form with a documented causal relationship assessment and was not reported to the sponsor until July 13 (no year documented) and again on November 12, 2008.

2. On August 7, 2007, your site was informed that this subject had suffered cardiac arrest, has been hospitalized, and was not doing well. In the FDA investigator's review of your source documents for this subject, there was no evidence that you informed the sponsor of this SAE.

Subsequent to the subject's hospitalization, the subject died. Source records indicate that in September 2007 your site was aware of the subject's death. However, this additional SAE was not documented on the Serious Adverse Event Report Form with a documented causal relationship assessment, and was not reported to the sponsor until November 12, 2008.

ⅱ. Subject #007 was hospitalized several times during the course of the study on (b)(4) FDA's investigators were unable to find documentation that these events were reported to the sponsor.

b. The protocol specified that laboratory samples for safety analysis were to be collected and evaluated at the screening visit. FDA notes that the documentation reveals a significant delay in your review of four of seven subject records, such that subjects were either randomized into the study or had completed the study by the time you reviewed the protocol-required, screening-related documents. For example:

i. Documentation shows that you did not review the laboratory reports of samples taken at the screening visit on June 4, 2007, for Subject #002 until August 15, 2007. By the time you reviewed the source records, the subject had already been dispensed study drug (on June 11, 2007).

ii. Documentation shows that you did not review the laboratory reports of samples taken at the screening visit on November 1, 2007, for Subject #007 until November 9, 2007. By the time you reviewed the lab report, the subject had been randomized into the study and had been dispensed study medication (on November 8, 2007).

c. The protocol specified that at the screening visit (i.e., Visit 1), key baseline characteristics were to be recorded, including demographics, medical history, physical exam, and vital signs.

i. For Subject #002, there was no documentation that a physical examination was performed at the screening visit, and only limited information is documented in the subject's medical history.

ii. Subject #007's physical examination was not conducted until after the subject was randomized into the study. The subject's physical examination was performed on December 6, 2007, which was after the screening visit (on October 29, 2007) and after the subject had been randomized into the study and dispensed study drug (on November 8, 2007).

d. The protocol specified that during the study, the patients were to return to the clinic for regularly scheduled follow-up visits (at 1, 3, 6, 9, and 12 months from randomization) and then every 4 months for the duration of the trial, as specified in the protocol flow chart, to assess study medication compliance and accountability, concomitant therapy or intervention, and conduct of efficacy and safety-related assessments. Furthermore, the protocol required that all randomized patients be followed through to the final follow-up visit in accordance with the schedule established at the time of randomization, regardless of treatment status (i.e., permanent or temporary discontinuation). The following subjects were not adequately followed per the protocol:

i. For Subject #002, records indicate that after Visit 6 (on December 6, 2007), your site staff did not see the subject for the 9-, 12-, and 16-month post randomization visits. Your site staff did no conduct any protocol-required visits for this subject again until the subject was terminated from the study on November 21, 2008.

ii. For Subject #004, records indicate that after the 3-month post-randomization visit on October 16, 2007, your site staff did not see the subject for the 6-, 9-, and 12-month post-randomization visits. You did not see this subject again until October 16, 2008.

iii. For Subject #005, the 12-month post-randomization visit occurred two months later than prescribed by the protocol.

iv. For Subject #007, after the 3-month post-randomization visit in February 2008, your site staff did not see the subject for the 6- and 9-month post randomization visits. You did not see this subject again until October 10, 2008.

Given the length of time between clinic visits, we are unsure how you adequately protected the rights, safety, and welfare of the subjects enrolled into the study.

e. The protocol required that laboratory sampling to include International Normalized Ratio (INR) testing be done at least every four weeks, and that hepatic tests be done monthly. For the following subjects, laboratory testing was not performed as specified in the protocol:

i. For Subject #002, records indicate that after March 20, 2008, there were no monthly INR tests conducted on this subject. In addition, no documentation was found that monthly hepatic tests were performed on this subject between Visit 6 (on December 6, 2007) and the time the subject terminated from the study on November 21, 2008.

ii. For Subject #004, no evidence was found that monthly hepatic function tests were performed after October 16, 2007, to the time the subject terminated from the study on October 24, 2008.

iii. For Subject #007, no evidence was found that monthly hepatic function tests were performed after February 3, 2008, to the time the subject terminated from the study on October 24, 2008.

4. You failed to maintain adequate records of the disposition of the drug, including dates, quantity, and use by subjects [21 CFR 312.62(a)].

FDA's investigation found that you failed to maintain adequate records of the disposition of the drug for all five subjects randomized in the study.

a. Subject #001 was dispensed study medication on March 23, 2007. Records contained no imformation concerning the quantity of study drug used by this subject.

b. For Subject #002, records were discrepant concerning the dates on which the subject was dispensed study medication, and the quantities dispensed. Per the dispensing/returning log, the subject was dispensed study drug on June 11, 2007; August 10, 2007; and December 6, 2007, none of which were returned. Per the study medication dispensation report, the subject was dispensed study drug on June 11, 2007; September 7, 2007; and December 6, 2007. In addition, per the dispensing/returning log, the subject was dispensed only of drug on June 11, 2007; however, the study medication dispensation report shows that the subject was dispensed 3bottles of study drug, each from a different record kit number.

c. For Subject #004, records contained no information related to the quantity of drug used by the subject at the 3-month follow-up visit. There was also no information concerning the dates on which the investigational drugs that had been dispensed on July 13, 2007; October 16, 2007; and December 12, 2007, were returned to the site. In addition, the information related to the dispensation of study drugs on December 12, 2007, was "estimated" and was not filled out until December 11, 2008, after the subject was terminated from the study (on October 24, 2008).

d. For Subject #005, records contained no information related to the quantity of study drug used by the subject after dispensation of the study drug on August 3, 2007 (randomization visit) and 0 December 3, 2007 (3-month post randomization visit). In addition, 6 bottles of drug were dispensed on some unknown date after December 2007 and were returned to your site empty on October 10, 2008. Records did not specify when the bottles were dispensed or the quantity of study drug used by the subject.

e. For Subject #007, records contained no information related to the quantity of study drug used by the subject after dispensation of the study drug on November 8, 2007 (randomization visit) and on February 15, 2008 (3-month post-randomization visit).

f. Source records indicate that 2 bottles of (b)(4) and 6 bottles of (b)(4) were missing from the total drug inventory at your site.

Your failure to maintain adequate and accurate drug disposition records raises concerns regarding adequate disposition of randomized drug to subjects, and calls into question the integrity of the data collected.

This letter is not intended to be an all-inclusive list of deficiencies with your clinical study of an investigational drug. It is your responsibility to ensure adherence to each requirement of the law and relevant FDA regulations. You should address these deficiencies and establish procedures to ensure that any ongoing or future studies will be in compliance with FDA regulations.

Within fifteen (15) working days of your receipt of this letter, you should notify this office in writing of the actions you have taken to prevent similar violations in the future. Failure to adequately and promptly explain the violations noted above may result in regulatory action without further notice.

If you have any questions, please contact Constance Lewin, M.D., M.P.H., at 301-796-3397; FAX 301-847-8748. Your written response and any pertinent documentation should be addressed to:

Constance Lewin, M.D., M.P.H.
Branch Chief, Good Clinical Practice Branch I
Division of Scientific Investigations
Office of Compliance
Center for Drug Evaluation and Research
Food and Drug Administration
Building 51, Room 5354
10903 New Hampshire Avenue
Silver Spring, MD 20993

Sincerely yours,

{See appended electronic signature page}

Leslie K. Ball, M.D.
Director
Division of Scientific Investigations
Office of Compliance
Center for Drug Evaluation and Research

第 122 封　给 Kirkwood, John M. 医学博士的警告信

2009年9月15日

参考号：CBER-09-08

尊敬的Kirkwood博士：

这封信特告知您2009年3月18日至4月24日FDA进行现场检查的结果。一位FDA检查员与您会面并对您所实施的以下临床研究的情况进行了审查：

- （b）（4）的Ⅰ期临床评价［研究（b）（4）以下简称“研究1”］，在该研究中您是临床研究者；
- （b）（4）的随机Ⅱ期临床评价［研究（b）（4）以下简称“研究2”］，在该研究中您是申办者和临床研究者。

本次现场检查是FDA的生物研究监查项目的一部分。该项目通过设定的检查方法，审查与试验药物相关的临床研究的实施情况。在现场检查结束时，检查员向您和您机构的工作人员发出并讨论了FDA 483表，即现场检查发现的问题。我们审阅了FDA 483表、您2009年5月1日对FDA483表的书面回复以及现场检查报告。

我们认为您违背了对试验新药相关的临床研究的正确实施进行监管的法规，美国联邦法规（CFR）第21篇第312部分（参见http://www.access.gpo.gov/nara/cfr/index.html）。

针对每项违规而援引的CFR适用性规定列举如下：

1. 您未能确保按照签署的研究者声明、研究计划和适用法规来进行研究，以保护在您的监护下的受试者的权益、安全和福利［21 CFR 312.60］

A. 您没有遵循研究1和研究2的研究方案。研究1研究方案5.1 ~ 5.4部分，研究2研究方案第4.1、4.2、4.3和6.0部分介绍了必需的筛选、治疗和随访程序。下表列出了您没有执行方案要求的程序情况：

受试者# 临床研究#	方案要求，而实际未执行的程序
（b）（6） 研究1	筛选：尿常规，磷酸肌酸激酶（CPK），血清无机磷和镁 疗程1: 第 2，5，6，和 7周: 体格检查 (PE) 和体力状况评分(PS) 第 10:用抗核抗体（ANA），癌症干细胞（CSC），分类，血小板，血生化，凝血酶原时间/部分凝血活酶时间（PT/PTT），迟发型过敏反应（DTH） 疗程 3:第1 和 2周随访PE和PS 疗程 4:第 1，2 和 4周 随访的PE和PS
（b）（6） 研究1	筛选：血清乳酸脱氢酶 疗程1:第2和3周 PE和PS
（b）（6） 研究1	筛选：CPK和尿常规 疗程1:第2，3和4周，PE和PS
（b）（6） 研究1	研究1 疗程1：第 2 和 3周 随访PS
（b）（6） 研究1	研究1筛选：LDH，γ-谷氨酰转肽酶(GGT),CPK，血清无机磷和镁
（b）（6） 研究2	筛选：尿常规和CPK 周期 1: 疫苗 1，2，3，4 血糖, CPK, 血清无机磷、镁和钙 第5周：PE和所有实验室检验 第6周：PE和血糖, CPK, 血清无机磷、镁和钙 周期2: 疫苗1, 2, 3, 4 血糖, CPK, 血清无机磷、镁和钙

续表

受试者# 临床研究#	方案要求，而实际未执行的程序
（b）（6） 研究2	筛选：CPK, 血清无机磷、镁和尿常规 周期1: 疫苗1 CPK, LDH, 血清无机磷和镁 疫苗2 PE, CPK, 血清无机磷和镁 疫苗3和4 CPK, LDH, 血清无机磷、镁 周期2: 疫苗1, 2, 3和 4 LDH, CPK, 血清无机磷、镁 第5和6周随访CPK, LDH, 血清无机磷、镁 第8周随访PE和实验室检验 周期3: 疫苗1和4 CPK, 血清无机磷、镁疫苗2 CPK 疫苗3 血清无机磷、镁

在2009年5月1日的来信中，您表示两项试验方案都已经进行了修订，原因是您认为部分检验项目是医疗上不需要的，或者不适合用于筛选或持续评估受试者的资格。您还说明您开发了新的试验方案专用的表格，以确保适当的检验得到执行。但是，只有研究的申办者可以对研究方案进行修订删减检验项目，同时，申办者有责任按照21 CFR 312.30（b）的要求，将修订后的试验方案提交给FDA和伦理委员会（IRB）进行审查。您不是研究1的申办者，因此您无权对研究方案进行修订删减检验项目。此外，既然您是研究2的申办者，您需要按照21 CFR 312.30（b）的要求，将修订后的试验方案提交给FDA和伦理委员会（IRB）进行审查。我们还要提醒您的是，任何这种关于研究程序的修订都要反映在知情同意书中，并获得IRB的批准。

B. 您未按照研究1试验方案的要求，随访并收集不良事件信息。试验方案3.2部分，“风险管理规程”中要求您监督受试者并审查研究数据和受试者安全性问题；试验方案5.4部分要求，（每疗程）疫苗接种后的第一、二、四周，然后每月一次、持续6个月对受试者进行观察，查找意外反应的证据，这是以发现潜在疾病为目的对受试者常规随访的一部分内容。

试验方案还要求您按照专门的研究计划与受试者保持联系并进行随访，直至受试者死亡。至少有5名受试者您没有按照要求进行随访，而他们还被当成是研究中的积极参与者。

- 受试者(b)(6)于2006年10月10日开始治疗，并死于(b)(6)。只有在现场检查期间，您的研究人员才报告这例受试者于2006年11月因为疾病进展从研究中剔除。
- 受试者(b)(6)于2007年1月29日入组，并于2007年1月30日至2007年3月9日接受了研究疫苗疗程1，2的治疗。现场检查期间，在一份日期为2009年4月15日的备忘录上，您报告说这例受试者因疾病进展于2007年3月28日从研究中剔除。该受试者病历中没有记录您按照试验方案要求对受试者进行过随访。
- 受试者(b)(6) 于2007年7月17日开始接受研究疫苗治疗。一份日期为2009年4月20日的记录显示该受试者取消了所有访视。您递交给FDA检查员的一份日期为2009年4月15日的文件承认：没有被取消的研究访视的记录，受试者死于(b)(6)。
- 受试者(b)(6)于2007年9月24日开始治疗。您日期为2009年4月15日的文件表明，该受试者于2007年11月13日从该研究中剔除，该受试者死于(b)(6)。该受试者病历中没有记录您按照试验方案要求对受试者进行过随访。
- 受试者(b)(6)于2008年2月12日开始治疗。您日期为2009年4月15日的文件表明该受试者于2008年3月14日从该研究中剔除，该受试者死于(b)(6)。该受试者病历中没有记录您按照试验方案要求对受试者进行过随访。

我们建议您来信所附的范例“治疗随访表”也记录与受试者们的所有联系，以清楚地确定是否或者何时受试者们已经退出研究或从研究中剔除。

C. 您未按试验方案要求，及时向数据安全监查委员会（DSMC）报告发生在研究1中3名受试者的严重不良事件（SAE）。试验方案6.2部分要求研究者和研究人员每周会面来审查研究数据和受试者的安全性问题，并按照已确立的IRB指导原则，每年向IRB提交一份研究中发生的所有不良事件的情况汇总。直到这次现场检查时，您才报告以下严重不良事件：

ⅰ. 2006年11月6日，受试者（b）（6）发生黑色素瘤病灶感染，并导致2006年11月27日手术切除。这些严重不良事件直到2年后的2009年4月14日才报告给DSMC。

ⅱ. 受试者（b）（6）于2008年3月发生胸腔积液、左侧胸痛及后来手术的严重不良事件。这些严重不良事件直到2009年4月1日才报告给DSMC。

ⅲ. 受试者（b）（6）于2008年12月19日发生小腿蜂窝组织感染，并导致入院治疗的严重不良事件。这一严重不良事件直到2009年4月1日才报告给DSMC。

在您5月1日的来信中，您承认在遵照试验方案要求向DSMC报告严重不良事件方面存在失误，并且提出了要实施的纠正措施计划，包括研究者、护理人员、临床研究协调员和助理们之间的定期会议。我们建议所有会议应包括了解日常研究活动的研究人员，建议您对会议进行记录，记下与研究受试者安全性相关的任何讨论内容。

D. 研究2中，在疫苗和DTH抗原被发现受污染后，您未进行试验方案要求的血培养。试验方案3.7.3 部分介绍了在疫苗接种后，当遇到无菌试验结果为阳性时应采取的措施。受试者（b）（6），2008年9月9日周期1，疫苗1和2008年10月28日的DTH都已发现被痤疮丙酸杆菌污染以后，您未进行血培养。

E. 研究1试验方案的5.4部分要求，基线评估应在按试验方案的治疗开始前1周内进行，而且在受试者病情出现恶化的情况下，应当在下一疗程的治疗开始前48小时内再次进行实验室评估。对于下列受试者，您未遵守试验方案的要求。

ⅰ. 受试者（b）（6）于2006年10月10日给予研究药物治疗，但基线评估于2006年8月30日治疗开始前近6周进行。

ⅱ. 受试者（b）（6）于2007年7月17日给予研究药物治疗，但现场检查期间在该受试者病历档案中未查见基线评估记录，仅查见一份未注明日期、未经确认的合格清单。

2. 您未能保存研究中使用试验药物或对照组的受试者的所有观察结果和其他数据的足够及准确的病历［21 CFR 312.62（b）］

A. 研究1试验方案3.1部分要求备选受试者ECOG体力状况评分在0～1之间方可入选进入研究。下列受试者，ECOG体力状况评分要么未记录，要么不同文件间不一致。

ⅰ. 受试者（b）（6），2006年8月30日病程记录中ECOG体力状况评分为3。但是一份未注明日期、未签名的合格清单上记录的评分为1。

ⅱ. 受试者（b）（6），尽管受试者于2007年9月25日进行了疫苗1疗程1的药物治疗，2007年9月13日的病程记录中未查见ECOG体力状况评分。但是一份未注明日期、未签名的合格清单上记录的评分为1。

ⅲ. 受试者（b）（6），2009年1月14日病程记录中ECOG体力状况评分为3。2009年3月4日的治疗随访表没有记录ECOG体力状况评分，但现场检查中这份表格被修改了，显示ECOG体力状况评分为1。

B. 研究1试验方案3.1部分要求治疗前实验室检验，包括AST、ALT、GGT、LDH和血清碱性磷酸酶，到小于或等于正常上限值的2.5倍。没有对受试者（b）（6）筛选LDH值的记录。

C. 研究2试验方案4.4部分介绍了对完成第一疗程疫苗接种的受试者进行再次治疗的要求。按照试验方案要求，再次治疗以前，受试者们应当在免疫治疗后第1、2、4周接受评估，病情稳定的受试者方可进行其余周期的疫苗治疗。受试者（b）（6）从2005年12月6日开始进行周期2，疫苗1～4的治疗。

但是，没有文件表明该受试者为再次治疗接受了评估。

D. 在研究2中，您给两位受试者分配了相同的研究识别代码（b）（6）。

3. 您未能及时地向 IRB 报告研究活动中的所有变更［21 CFR 312.66］

在2009年5月1日信中，您表示您修订了研究1和研究2的试验方案，原因是您认为部分检验项目是医疗上不需要的，或者不适合用于筛选或持续评估受试者的资格。但是您没有按照要求，将研究活动的变更向IRB报告。

4. 您未能取得在研究项目进行过程中协助研究者授权研究者的名单［21 CFR 312.53（c）（1）（ⅷ）］

您未能证明（b）（4）是研究2中的授权研究者。（b）（4）分别于2005年10月19日和2005年12月28日对受试者（b）（6）进行了（b）（4）疫苗注射。

5. 您未能对 IND 下属开展的临床研究的进展情况进行监查［21 CFR 312.56（a）和 312.50］

作为研究2的申办者，您未像上述1.中介绍的那样，按照IND中包含的总体研究计划和方案的要求，监查研究的过程。

我们注意到您正在参与的临床研究至少有37项。您有责任监督研究人员，并确保研究正常开展。我们建议您建立并保存日志或其他记录，前瞻性地确定每位研究人员的角色和职责，每人参与研究的开始和结束日期，以及他们的签名和缩写。我们还建议您在研究过程中对研究工作人员进行适当的培训，对培训进行记录并按需要进行更新。

本警告信的目的并非是罗列您在开展的临床研究中存在的所有缺陷。确保遵循法律和所有适用法规的每一项要求是您的职责。

在收到这封警告信15个工作日内，请提供以下书面文件：您为纠正上述违规行为并防止在目前和将来您作为临床研究者的研究中再次发生类似违规情况，已经采取的或将要采取的措施。未能对警告信进行回复并采取适当的纠正性措施，可能导致FDA在不再通知的情况下采取监管措施。FDA可根据21 CFR 312.70对您启动取消资格程序。

附：英文原文

Kirkwood, John M., M.D.

By Certified Mail - Return Receipt Requested
And By Facsimile Transmission

CERTIFIED MAIL
RETURN RECEIPT REQUESTED

CBER - 09-08

Warning Letter

SEP 15, 2009

John M. Kirkwood, M.D.
University of Pittsburgh Cancer Institute
Hillman Cancer Research Pavilion Suite 1.32c
5115 Centre Avenue
Pittsburgh, Pennsylvania 15213-2584

Dear Dr. Kirkwood:

This letter describes the results of a Food and Drug Administration (FDA) inspection that was conducted from March 18 through April 24, 2009. An FDA investigator met with you to review your conduct of the following clinical studies:

- Phase I Evaluation of (b)(4) (Study (b)(4) hereinafter "Study 1"), in which you were the clinical investigator; and,
- Randomized Phase Ⅱ Evaluation of (b)(4) (Study (b)(4) hereinafter "Study 2"), in which you were the sponsor and clinical investigator.

FDA conducted this inspection under the agency's Bioresearch Monitoring Program, which includes inspections designed to review the conduct of clinical research involving investigational drugs.

At the end of the inspection, a Form FDA 483, Inspectional Observations, was issued to and discussed with you and the staff from your institution. We reviewed the Form FDA 483, your letter dated May 1, 2009, responding to the Form FDA 483, and the inspection report.

We have determined that you violated regulations governing the proper conduct of clinical studies involving investigational new drugs, as published in Title 21, Code of Federal Regulations (CFR), Part 312 (available at http://www.access.gpo.gov/nara/cfr/index.html).

The applicable provisions of the CRF are cited for each violation listed below.

1. You failed to ensure that the investigation was conducted according to the signed investigator statement, the investigational plan, and the applicable regulations in order to protect the rights, safety, and welfare of subjects under your care. [21 CFR § 312.60].

A. You failed to follow the protocols for Studies 1 and 2. The required screening, treatment, and follow-up procedures are described in Study 1 protocol sections 5.1 to 5.4, and in Study 2 protocol sections 4.1, 4.2, and 4.3, and 6.0. You failed to perform the protocol-required procedures as illustrated in the following table.

Subject # Study #	Missing protocol procedures
(b)(6) Study1	Screening: urinalysis, CPK, phosphorous and magnesium Course #1: Weeks # 2, #5, #6, and #7: physical examination (PE) and performance status (PS) Week #10: ANA, CSC, differential, platelet, chemistry, PT/PTT, DTH Course #3: Weeks #1 and #2 follow-up PE and PS Course #4: Weeks #1, #2, and #4 follow-up PE and PS
(b)(6) Study1	Screening: LDH Course #1: Weeks #2 and #3 PE and PS
(b)(6) Study1	Screening: CPK and urinalysis Course #1: Weeks #2, #3, and #4 PE and PS
(b)(6) Study1	Study 1 Course #1: Weeks #2 and #3 follow-up PS
(b)(6) Study1	Study 1 Screening: LDH, GGT, CPK, phosphorous and magnesium
(b)(6) Study2	Screening: urinalysis and CPK Cycle #1: Vaccine #1, #2, #3, and #4 glucose, CPK, phosphorous, magnesium, and calcium Week #5 PE and all laboratory tests Week #6 PE and glucose, CPK, phosphorous, magnesium, and calcium Cycle #2: Vaccine #1, #2, #3, and #4 glucose, CPK, phosphorous, magnesium, and calcium
(b)(6) Study2	Screening: CPK, phosphorous, magnesium, and urinalysis Cycle #1: Vaccine #1 CPK, LDH, phosphorous, and magnesium Vaccine #2 PE, CPK, phosphorous, and magnesium Vaccine #3 and #4 CPK, LDH, phosphorous, and magnesium Cycle #2: Vaccine #1, #2, #3, and #4 LDH, CPK, phosphorous, and magnesium Weeks #5 and #6 follow-up CPK, LDH, phosphorous, and magnesium Week #8 follow-up PE and laboratory tests Cycle #3: Vaccine #1 and #4 CPK, phosphorous, and magnesium Vaccine #2 CPK Vaccine #3 phosphorous and magnesium

In your letter of May 1, 2009, you state that the protocols have been amended because you determined that some tests were not medically required or appropriate for the screening or ongoing assessment of the eligibility of subjects. You also described that you have developed new protocol-specific forms to ensure that the appropriate tests are performed. However, only a sponsor of a study may amend a study protocol requiring omission of tests and that the sponsor is responsible for submitting such amended protocols to the FDA and the Institutional Review Board (IRB) for review as required by 21 CFR 312.30 (b). You are not the sponsor of Study 1 and therefore are not authorized to amend a study protocol requiring omission of tests. Furthermore, while you are the sponsor of Study 2, you are required to submit the amended protocol to FDA and the IRB for review under 21 CFR 312.30(b). We further remind you that any such revisions made to the protocol regarding study procedures be reflected on the consent form and approved by the IRB.

B. You failed to follow-up and collect adverse event information as required by the Study 1 protocol. Section 3.2 of the protocol, "Risk management procedures", requires you to monitor the subjects and review the study data and subject safety issues, and section 5.4 requires that "subjects will be observed one, two, and four weeks after a course of vaccination, and then monthly for 6 months for evidence of untoward responses as part of routine follow-up of subjects for underlying disease." The protocol further requires you to contact and follow-up with subjects until their deaths and according to a specific study schedule. You failed to follow-up with at least five subjects as required while they were still considered to be active participants in the study.

- Subject #(b)(6) was initiated therapy on 10/10/06 and died on (b)(6) Only during the inspection did your study staff report that the subject was removed from the study in November 2006 due to progressive disease.
- Subject #(b)(6) was enrolled in the study on 1/29/07 and received course #1 and #2 of the study vaccines between 1/30/07 and 3/9/07. During the inspection, in a memo dated 4/15/09, you report that the subject was removed from the study on 3/28/07 due to progressive disease. The case history for this subject does not document that you followed up with this subject as required by the protocol.
- Subject #(b)(6) received the study vaccine starting on 7/17/07. A note dated 4/20/09 indicated that the subject cancelled all visits. A document dated 4/15/09 that you sent to the FDA investigator acknowledged that there was no documentation of the cancelled study visits and that the subject died on (b)(6)
- Subject #(b)(6) was initiated therapy on 9/24/07. Your document dated 4/15/09 states that the subject was removed from the study on 11/13/07 and that the subject died on (b)(6). The case history for this subject does not document that you followed up with this subject as required by the protocol.
- Subject #(b)(6) was initiated therapy on 2/12/08. Your document dated 4/15/09 indicates that the subject was removed from the study on 3/14/08 and the subject died on (b)(6). The case history for this subject does not document that you followed up with this subject as required by the protocol.

We recommend that the sample Treatment Visit Follow-up Form attached to your letter also document all contacts made to subjects in order to clearly identify if or when subjects have withdrawn or are removed from a study.

C. You failed to report serious adverse events (SAEs) experienced by three subjects enrolled in Study 1 in a timely manner to the Data Safety Monitoring Committee (DSMC) as required by the protocol. Protocol section 6.2 requires the investigator and study staff to meet weekly to review the study data and subject safety issues, and to submit a cumulative summary of all adverse events occurring during the study to the IRB according to the established IRB guidelines on an annual basis. You failed to report the following SAEs until this inspection:

i. On 11/6/06, subject #(b)(6) experienced infected melanoma lesions which resulted in amputation on 11/27/06. These SAEs were not reported to the DSMC until 4/14109, more than 2 years later.

ii. Subject #(b)(6) experienced the SAEs of pleural effusion, left sided chest pain, and subsequent surgery in March 2008. These SAEs were not reported to the DSMC until 4/1/09.

iii. Subject #(b)(6) experienced the SAE of a lower leg cellulitis infection which resulted in hospitalization on 12/19/08. This SAE was not reported to the DSMC until 4/1/09.

In your May 1 letter you acknowledged the lapses in your reporting of the SAEs to the DSMC as required by the protocol and describe corrective action plans to be implemented, including regular meetings between the investigators, nursing staff, clinical research coordinators, and associates. We recommend that all meetings include the study staff with knowledge of the day-to-day study activities and that you document your meetings, describing any discussion relating to the safety of study subjects.

D. You failed to perform the protocol-required blood cultures in Study 2 after the vaccine and the DTH antigen were found to be contaminated. Protocol section 3.7.3 describes the actions to be taken when positive sterility tests are encountered after a vaccine has been administered. For subject #(b)(6), you did not perform blood cultures after tests for both cycle #1, vaccine #1 on 9/9/08 and the DTH on 10/28/08 were found to be contaminated with Propionibacterium acnes.

E. Section 5.4 of the Study 1 protocol requires that baseline evaluations be conducted within 1 week prior to the start of protocol therapy, and that in the event a subject's condition is deteriorating, laboratory evaluations should be repeated within 48 hours prior to the initiation of the next course of therapy. You did not follow this protocol requirement for the subjects listed below.

i. Subject (b)(6) was administered the study drug on 10/10/06, but baseline evaluations were conducted on 8/30/06, nearly 6 weeks prior to the start of the therapy.

ii. Subject (b)(6) was administered the study drug on 7/17/07, but no baseline evaluation was found in the case file during the inspection except an undated and unidentified eligibility checklist.

2. You failed to prepare and maintain adequate and accurate case histories that record all observations and other data pertinent to the investigation. [21 CFR § 312.62(b)].

A. Section 3.1 of the protocol for Study 1 requires that prospective subjects have an ECOG performance status of 0 or 1 to be included in the study. For the following subjects the ECOG status was either not documented or was discrepant between documents.

i. For subject #(b)(6) the progress note on 8/30/06 indicates an ECOG status of 3. However, an undated and unsigned eligibility checklist indicates an ECOG status of 1.

ii. For subject (b)(6) the progress note dated 9/13/07 does not include an ECOG status even though the subject received the vaccine #1 for course #1 on 9/25/07. However, an undated and unsigned eligibility checklist indicates an ECOG status of 1.

iii. For subject (b)(6), the progress note dated 1/14/09 denotes an ECOG status of 3. The Treatment Visit Follow-up form dated 3/4/09 did not document the ECOG status, but during the inspection this form was changed to indicate an ECOG status of 1.

B. Study 1 protocol section 3.1 requires pretreatment laboratory tests, including AST, ALT, GGT, LDH, and Alkaline Phosphatase, to be less than or equal to 2.5 times the upper limit of normal. There is no documentation of screening LDH values for subjects (b)(6):

C. Study 2 protocol section 4.4 describes the re-treatment requirements for subjects who finished the first course of vaccination. According to the protocol, before re-treatment, subjects should be evaluated at 1, 2, and 4 weeks post-immunization, and subjects with stable disease may be retreated with additional cycles of the vaccine. Subject (b)(6) was administered the Cycle #2 vaccines #1 through #4 starting 12/6/05.

However, there is no documentation to indicate that the subject was evaluated for re-treatment.

D. You assigned duplicate study identification (b)(6) for two subjects in Study 2.

3. You failed to promptly report all changes in the research activity to the IRB. [21 CFR § 312.66].

In your May 1 letter you state that you amended the research protocols for Study 1 and Study 2 because you determined that some tests were not medically required or appropriate for the screening or ongoing assessment of the eligibility of subjects. However, you did not report these changes in the research activity to the IRB as required.

4. You failed to obtain a list of the names of the sub-investigators who will be assisting the investigator in the conduct of the investigation. [21 CFR § 312.53(c)(1) (viii)].

You failed to identify (b)(4) as sub-investigators for Study 2. (b)(4) performed (b)(4) vaccine injections for subject (b)(6) on 10/19/2005 and 12/28/2005, respectively.

5. You failed to monitor the progress of the clinical investigation conducted under your IND. [21 CFR § 312.56(a) and 312.50].

As a sponsor for Study 2, you failed to monitor the progress of the investigation as required by the general investigational plan and protocols contained in the IND, as described in item 1, above.

We note that you are currently participating in at least 37 clinical studies. You are responsible for supervising study staff and ensuring proper study conduct. We recommend that you develop and maintain logs or other records that prospectively identify each study staff member's roles and responsibilities, the beginning and end dates of each person's involvement, and their signatures and initials. We further recommend that the study personnel be provided appropriate training in study procedures and that the training be documented and updated as needed.

This letter is not intended to contain an all-inclusive list of violations that may exist with your conduct of clinical studies. It is your responsibility to ensure compliance with the Act and all applicable regulations.

Within fifteen (15) business days of receiving this letter, please provide written documentation of the actions you have taken or will take to correct these violations and prevent the recurrence of similar violations in current and future studies for which you prevent the recurrence of similar violations in current and future studies for which you are the clinical investigator. Failure to respond to this letter and to take appropriate corrective action could result in FDA taking regulatory action without further notice to you. FDA could initiate disqualification proceedings against you in accordance with 21 CFR 312.70.

Please send your written response to:

Ms. Bhanu Kannan
Division of Inspections and Surveillance (HFM-664)
Office of Compliance and Biologics Quality
Center for Biologics Evaluation and Research
Food and Drug Administration
1401 ockville Pike, Suite 200N
Rockville, Maryland, 20852-1448
Telephone: (301) 827-6221

We also request that you send a copy of your response to the FDA District Office listed below.

Sincerely,

/S/

Mary A. Malarkey, Director
Director
Office of Compliance and Biologics Quality
Center for Biologics Evaluation and Research
cc: Karyn Campbell
Acting District Director, HFR-CE100
Food and Drug Administration
900 US Customhouse
200 Chestnut Street Philadelphia, Pennsylvania 19106

第123封　给Harris, Barbara A.的警告信

2009年7月27日

参考号：09-HFD-45-07-0

尊敬的Harris博士：

2009年1月13日至16日，Mark C. Saale先生和Michelle Chuen博士，2009年3月25日，Cheryl D. McCall女士代表FDA进行了现场检查，与您会面并对您实施的一项临床研究进行了审查：试验方案（b）(4)，题目为“（b）(4)”，试验药物（b）(4)，申办者为（b）(4)。

本次现场检查是FDA的生物研究监查项目的一部分，该项目通过设定的检查方法，评估相关研究的实施情况，以确认这些研究中受试者的权益、安全和福利得到了保护。

经对FDA现场检查报告和该报告的附件进行审查，我们认为，您没有遵循适用的法律要求和监管临床研究开展及受试者保护的FDA法规。我们获知，在现场检查结束时，Mark C. Saale先生和Michelle Chuen博士向您出示并讨论了FDA 483表，即现场检查发现的问题。我们想强调以下几点：

1. 您未能准备和保存研究中使用试验药物或对照组的受试者的所有研究相关观察结果和其他数据的足够及准确的病历［21 CFR 312.62（b）］

a. 根据研究方案，受试者服用试验药物后约1.5小时要进行一次脑电图。但病历有多处不符，许多试验药物的给药时间由间隔1.5小时以上改为1.5小时以内，也没有支持性文件解释这些修改。另外，病例报告表（以下简称CRF或CRFs）记录时间和病程记录登记时间竟然不一致。

i. 受试者002，2007年6月20日脑电图扫描时间为13:18，病程记录的给药时间为11:40，由研究协调员（b）(6）签名加注日期。此处时间后被修改为11:50，并由BH首字母签名加注日期。然而，CRF记录时间仍为11:40。

ii. 受试者002，2007年6月27日脑电图扫描时间为11:37，记录在实验室申请单的试验药物给药时间，由研究协调员（b）(6）签名加注日期为9:30。这一时间在病程记录和实验室申请单上被改为10:00，并由BH首字母签名加注日期。病程记录中，由（b）(6）签名加注日期的记录如下：“由于患者及其护理人员晚到脑电图室，导致超窗32分钟”。此记录与病程和实验室申请单修改的10:00不符。

iii. 受试者002，2007年7月25日脑电图扫描时间为13:40，记录在实验室申请单的试验药物给药时间，由研究协调员（b）(6）签名加注日期的是12:00。这一时间被改为12:10，并由BH首字母签名加注日期2007年1月25日（此日期早于访视日期6个月）。

iv. 受试者008，2011年11月2日脑电图扫描时间为10:24。记录在实验室申请单的试验药物给药时间为8:00，该时间被改为9:00。然而，CRF记录时间仍为8:00。

b. 受试者002病历中，第一次访视时CRF第12页出现两份不同副本。一份为粉色副本，由Barbara Harris签名加注日期表明于2007年5月10日完成。另一份为影印副本，同样由Barbara Harris签名加注日期2007年5月10日。但第二份副本内容显然由不同人填写（笔迹不同），且填写信息与第一份副本不同。病史无相关解释为何受试者002有两份不同版本原始记录。一位给定受试者的单个CRF页却有两份版本，这影响了病历的准确性。

c. 受试者008，2007年11月2日，实验室心电图申请单上最初记录的时间是8:22，后被修改为10:22。尽管如此，在心电图和CRF上记录的时间仍为8:22，并无支持性文件说明实验室申请单ECG时间的修改。

d. 受试者002（2007年5月30日）第二次访视，脑电图报告丢失。

e. 受试者014，根据2007年12月4日心电图扫描记录显示，P-R间期为175毫秒，QRS间期为108毫秒，Q-T间期为456毫秒，Q-Tc间期为438毫秒。在相应的CRF上，P-R间期，QRS间期，Q-T间期的首次记录与脑电

图扫描记录一致，但分别被修改为174毫秒、104毫秒和470毫秒。Q-Tc间期的首次记录与脑电图扫描记录一致，但是于2008年3月21日及2008年6月10日被分别修改成444毫秒和452毫秒。以上修改由（b）（6）首字母签名，但没有相关支持文件解释CRF上ECG结果的修改。

f. 受试者002，CRF第54页，错误地将受试者编号标识为001。

g. 受试者007，CRF第84页（访视7，第12周）未记录CIBC-plus的起止时间，尽管CRF要求记录。

2. 您未能确保按照研究计划进行研究［21 CFR 312.60］

研究方案要求：关于患者发生不良事件的所有发现，无论疑似缘由，都应在病例报告表的不良事件（即AE）页进行报告。受试者2007年6月13日病程记录中记录受试者主诉在家服药2小时后有轻度头痛，但未被记录在病例报告表的不良事件页。我们注意到您在现场检查时解释是，医生认为该患者的轻度头痛极有可能是酒精引起。然而，没有该观点的记录。方案要求在CRF/AE页中报告患者发生的关于不良事件的所有发现，无论怀疑的缘由如何。

3. 您未能保存足够的包括日期、数量和受试者使用情况的药物处置记录［21 CFR 312.62（a）］

a. 研究计量日志上表明2007年11月2日，受试者008获得分发药物84片；然而，该天的CRF显示受试者获得分发药物为42片。正确数量不明，且记录中未解释这一差异。

b. 受试者002病历中，第七次访视CRF第77页有两份不同副本。一份记录了2007年8月22日受试者获得药物168片，然而另一份记录上在2007年10月10日168片被划掉，手写为140片。但没有文件支持这一修改。

本警告信的目的并非是罗列您在试验药物临床研究中存在的所有缺陷。确保遵循法律和相关FDA法规的每一项要求是您的职责。您应当解决这些缺陷，并建立规程，以确保任何正在进行或将来的研究均能符合FDA的法规。

自收到这封信的15个工作日内，您应当书面告知本办公室为预防将来发生类似违规情况已经或将要采取的措施。如果不能充分、迅速地解释上述违规问题，可能导致我们在不再通知的情况下采取监管措施。

附：英文原文

Harris, Barbara A. Ph.D

WARNING LETTER

JUL 27, 2009

CERTIFIED MAIL
RETURN RECEIPT REQUESTED

Ref: 09-HFD-45-07-0

Barbara A. Harris, Ph.D.
Psypharma Clinical Research, Inc.
4045 E. Union Hills, # 122
Phoenix, AZ 85050

Dear Dr. Harris:

Between January 13 and 16, 2009, Mr. Mark C. Saale and Dr. Michelle Chuen and, on March 25, 2009,Ms. Cheryl D. McCall, representing the Food and Drug Administration (FDA), conducted an investigator and met with you to review your conduct of a clinical investigation (Protocol Number (b)(4) entitled“(b)(4)”) of the investigational drug (b)(4), performed for (b)(4).

This inspection is a part of FDA's Bioresearch Monitoring Program, which includes inspections designed to evaluate the conduct of research and to ensure that the rights, safety, and welfare of the human subjects of the study have been protected. From our review of the establishment inspection report and the documents submitted with that report, we conclude that you did not adhere to the applicable statutory requirements and FDA regulations governing the conduct of clinical investigations and the protection of human subjects. We are aware that at the conclusion of the inspection, Mr. Mark C. Saale and Dr. Michelle Chuen presented and discussed with you Form FDA 483, Inspectional Observations. We wish to emphasize the following:

1. You failed to prepare and maintain adequate and accurate case histories that record all observations and other data pertinent to the Investigation on each Individual administered the Investigational drug or employed as a control in the investigation [21 CFR 312.62(b)].

a. According to the protocol, an electroencephalogram (EEG) was to be performed on subjects approximately 1.5 hours after study drug administration. The case histories demonstrated multiple inconsistencies in instances where the study drug administration time was changed from a time outside of the 1.5 hours interval to a time within the interval. There was no supporting documentation that explains these study drug administration time changes. In addition, the times recorded on the Case Report Forms (CRFs) were not necessarily consistent with the times recorded on the progress notes.

i. For Subject #002, on 6/20/07, the time of EEG recording was 13:18, and the study drug administration time documented in the progress notes, signed and dated by the study coordinator, (b)(6) was 11:40. This time was changed to 11:50, and initialed and dated by BH. However, the time recorded on the CRF was 11:40.

ii. For Subject #002, on 6/27/07, the time of EEG recording was 11:37, and the study drug administration time documented on the laboratory request sheet and in the progress notes, signed and dated by (b)(6), was 09:30. This time was changed to 10:00 on the laboratory request sheet and in the progress notes, and was initialed and dated by BH. The following is documented in the progress notes signed and dated by (b)(6): "pt & caregiver arrived to EEG lal late pt out of window by 32 min." The amended time of 10:00 is inconsistent with this note.

iii. For Subject #002, on 7/25/07, the time of EEG recording was 13:40, and the study drug administration time documented on the laboratory request sheet, signed and dated by (b)(6), was 12:00. This time was changed to 12:10, initialed and dated 1/25/07 (i.e., 6 months before the visit date) by BH.

iv. For Subject #008, on 11/2/07, the time of EEG recording was 10:24, and the study drug administration time documented on the laboratory request sheet was 8:00. This time was changed to 9:00. However, the time recorded on the CRF was 8:00.

b. The case history for Subject #002 had two different copies of CRF page 12 from Visit 1. One copy was a pink duplicate copy of CRF page 12, signed and dated as having been completed by BarbaraHarris on May 10, 2007. The second copy was a photocopy of CRF page 12, also signed and dated as having been completed by Barbara Harris on May 10, 2007, but apparently filled out by a different person (as evidenced by different handwriting) and contains different information from the first copy. There was no explanation in the case history for the existence of two different versions of the same source record for Subject #002. Having 2 versions of a single CRF page for a given subject compromises case history accuracy.

c. For Subject #008, on 11/2/07, the time of electrocardiogram (ECG) originally documented on the laboratory request sheet was 8:22. This time was changed to 10:22. However, the time recorded on the ECG and on the CRF was 8:22. There was no supporting documentation for the ECG time change on the laboratory request sheet.

d. For Subject #002, the EEG report was missing for Visit 2 (5/30/07).

e. For Subject #014, according to the ECG tracing obtained on 12/4/07, the P-R interval was 175 msecs, the QRS interval was 108 msecs, the QT interval was 456 msecs, and the QTc interval was 438 msecs. On the corresponding CRF, the P-R interval, QRS interval, and QT interval were initially documented in accordance with the ECG tracing, but were changed to 174 msecs, 104 msecs, and 470 msecs, respectively. The QTc interval on this CRF was initially documented in accordance with the ECG tracing, but was changed to 444 msecs on 3/21/08 and to 452 msecs on 6/10/08. These changes appear to be initialed by (b)(6). There was no supporting documentation to explain these changes to the ECG results on the CRF.

f. CRF page 54 for Subject #002 incorrectly identifies the subject number as #001.

g. There was no start or finish time documented for the CIBC-plus on page 84 of the CRF (Visit 7, Week 12) for Subject #007, despite the fact that the CRF indicated that this information should be entered.

2. You failed to ensure the investigation was conducted according to the investigational plan [21 CFR 312.60].

The protocol required that all findings regarding adverse events experienced by a patient, irrespective of the suspected causality, be reported on the Adverse Events (AE) page in the CRF. Progress notes dated 6/13/07 for Subject #002 document that the patient complained of light headedness 2 hours after dosing at home. This was not reported on the AE page in the CRF. We note your statement during the inspection interview that it was the opinion of the doctor that the light headedness was most probably due to alcohol. However, there is no documentation of this opinion. The protocol required that all findings regarding adverse events experienced by a patient, irrespective of the suspected causality, be reported on the AE page in the CRF.

3. You failed to maintain adequate records of the disposition of the drug, including dates, quantity, and use by subjects [21 CFR 312.62(a)].

a. The investigational accountability log on 11/2/07 for Subject #008 indicates that 84 tablets were dispensed; however, the CRF for that date indicates that the amount dispensed was 42. It is unclear which number is correct, and there is no explanation in the record for this discrepancy.

b. The case history for Subject #002 had two different copies of CRF page 77 from Visit 7. One copy indicated that 168 tablets were dispensed on 8/22/07, while the other copy had 168 crossed out and 140 written instead on 10/10/07, with no documentation to support this change.

This letter is not intended to be an all-inclusive list of deficiencies with your clinical study of an investigational drug. It is your responsibility to ensure adherence to each requirement of the law and relevant FDA regulations. You should address these deficiencies and establish procedures to ensure that any on-going or future studies will be in compliance with FDA regulations.

Within fifteen (15) working days of your receipt of this letter, you should notify this office in writing of the actions you have taken or will be taking to prevent similar violations in the future. Failure to adequately and promptly explain the violations noted above may result in regulatory action without further notice.

If you have any questions, please contact Constance Lewin, M.D., M.P.H., at 301-796-3397; FAX 301- 847-8748. Your written response and any pertinent documentation should be addressed to:

Constance Lewin, M.D., M.P.H.
Branch Chief, Good Clinical Practice Branch I
Division of Scientific Investigations
Office of Compliance
Center for Drug Evaluation and Research
Food and Drug Administration
Bldg 51, Room 5354
10903 New Hampshire Avenue
Silver Spring, MD 20993

Sincerely yours,

{See appended electronic signature page}

Leslie K. Ball, M.D.
Director
Division of Scientific Investigations
Office of Compliance
Center for Drug Evaluation and Research

第 124 封　给 Mark F. Gordon 医学博士的警告信

2009年6月26日

参考号：09-HFD-46-04-03

尊敬的Gordon博士：

2009年1月12日至29日，Robert C. Steyert先生代表FDA进行了现场检查，与您当前的工作人员会面，并对您实施的一项临床研究进行了审查：试验方案（b）(4)，题目为（b）(4)，关于试验药物（b）(4)，申办者为（b）(4)。

本次现场检查是FDA的生物研究监查项目的一部分。该项目通过设定的检查方法，评估相关研究的实施情况，并确保这些研究中受试者的权益、安全和福利得到了保护。

经对FDA现场检查报告、该报告的附件，以及您2009年2月26日对FDA 483表的书面回复进行审查，我们认为，您没有遵循适用的法律要求和监管临床研究实施的FDA法规。我们获悉，在现场检查结束时，Steyert先生向您出示并讨论了FDA483表，即现场检查发现的问题。我们想强调以下几点：

1. 您未能保存与研究相关的所有观察结果和其他数据的记录，例如病例报告表、医生的病程记录和护士的护理记录，直至试验药物按拟定适应症上市申请获得批准后 2 年［21 CFR 312.62（c）］

您没有保存病例报告表（CRF）和原始文件（即您用来填写病例报告表的记录），这些文件对于试验药物上市申请中数据完整性和研究活动对联邦法规的依从性的确证是必要的。您必须保存这些研究相关的记录，直至用于研究受试者的适应症的试验药物上市申请批准，或直到研究被停止且FDA被告知后两年。您的研究在2000年终止，但由于（b）(4）用于适应症（b）(4）的上市申请尚未批准或未被批准，并且FDA没有得到该研究停止通知，您必须保存您的研究记录。

我们收到您对FDA 483表的回复，您认同影印病例报告表（CRF）无法找到。您表示您的员工能够找到受试者的医疗记录，然而，这些医疗记录不足以替代按照312部分第62条（c）您需要保存的CRF和其他原始文件。

我们同样也认可您在回复中提交了将来用于在您以前的机构对记录归档时使用的“归档研究数据和记录的登记册”的草案的复印件，然而您没有说明您本人如何确保未来在FDA监管的临床研究实施中类似违规不再发生。

2. 您未能按照 21 CFR 50 的要求获得知情同意［21 CFR 312.60］

入组的16个受试者中有10个（P02，P08，P09，P10，P11，P12，401，402，403和404）签署了过期版本的知情同意文件，而不是在他们签署的日期之前已经被IRB批准的修订版本。由于这些受试者没有机会签署包含了研究程序的新信息的修订版知情同意文件，他们没有足够的机会，按照21 CFR 50.20去考虑是否继续参与研究，在您对FDA 483表的回复中您认同这个发现。我们注意到在您书面回复中，您有解释您以前的机构将如何确保类似违规不再发生。然而您没有解释本人如何确保未来在FDA监管的临床研究实施中类似违规不再发生。

本警告信的目的并非是罗列您在试验药物临床研究中存在的所有缺陷。确保遵循法律和相关FDA法规的每一项要求是您的职责。您应当解决这些缺陷，并建立规程，以确保任何正在进行或将来的研究均能符合FDA的法规。

自收到这封信的15个工作日内，您应当书面告知本办公室为预防将来发生类似违规情况已经或将要采取的措施。如果不能充分、迅速地解释上述违规问题，可能导致我们在不再通知的情况下采取监管措施。

尊敬的Gordon博士：

2009年6月1日的信中，FDA药品评价和研究中心通过认证邮件发布的警告信至您以前的地址，900 Ridgebury Road，Ridgefied，CT 06877-0368。

根据您的要求，我们正重新发布警告信至您目前的地址。除了地址的变化，这种警告信与2009年4月20号警告信是一样的。

附件为警告信的副本。

附：英文原文

Mark F. Gordon, M.D.

WARNING LETTER

JUN 26, 2009

CERTIFIED MAIL
RETURN RECEIPT REQUESTED

Ref: 09-HFD-46-04-03

Mark F. Gordon, M.D.
C/o Office of Research Compliance
350 Commumity Drive
Manhasset, NY 11030

Dear Dr. Gordon:

Between January 12 and 29, 2009, Mr. Robert C. Steyert, representing the Food and Drug Administration (FDA), conducted an investigation and met with the current staff, to review your conduct of a clinical investigation (Protocol (b)(4)), entitled (b)(4) of the investigational drug (b)(4), performed for (b)(4).

This inspection is a part of FDA's Bioresearch Monitoring Program, which includes inspections designed to evaluate the conduct of research and to ensure that the rights, safety, and welfare of the human subjects of those studies have been protected.

From our review of the establishment inspection report, the documents submitted with that report, and your February 26, 2009, written response to the Form FDA 483, Inspectional Observations, we conclude that you did not adhere to the applicable statutory requirements and FDA regulations governing the conduct of clinical investigations. We are aware that at the conclusion of the inspection, Mr. Steyert presented and discussed with you Form FDA 483, Inspectional Observations. We wish to emphasize the following:

1. You failed to retain records that record all observations and other data pertinent to the investigation, such as case report forms, progress notes of the physician, and nurses'notes, for a period of 2 years following the date a marketing application is approved for the drug for the indication for which it is being investigated [21 CFR 312.62(c)].

You failed to retain case report forms (CRFs) and source documents (i.e. the notes you used to fill out case report forms) that are necessary for the verification of data integrity and compliance of study activities with federal regulations for the marketing application of the investigational drug. You are required to keep these study-related records for two years following the approval of a marketing application for the study drug for the indication that was the subject of your investigation, or until the study was discontinued and FDA was notified. Your study terminated in

2000, but because a marketing application has not yet been approved or not approved for (b)(4) for the indication of (b)(4), and because FDA has not been notified that the study was discontinued, you were required to retain your study records.

We acknowledge your response to the FDA Form 483 in which you agreed that the photocopied case report forms (CRFs) could not be found. You stated that your staff was able to find the subjects'medical records. However, these medical records are not an adequate substitute for the CRFs and other source documents, which you were required to retain per 312.62(C).

We also acknowledge that with your response you submitted a draft copy of "Register of Archived Research Data & Record" for future use when archiving records at your former institution.However, you have not addressed how you, personally, will ensure that a similar violation does not recur in your conduct of FDA regulated clinical research in the future.

2. You failed to obtain informed consent in accordance with the provisions of 21 CFR Part 50 [21 CFR 312.60].

Ten of sixteen subjects enrolled (P02, P08, P09, P10, P11, P12, 401, 402, 403, and 404) signed an outdated version of the informed consent documents, as opposed to a revised version which the IRB had approved prior to the date of signing. Because these subjects were not given the opportunity to sign the revised informed consent documents, which contained new information about study procedures, they did not have sufficient opportunity to consider whether or not to continue their participation in the study, per 21 CFR 50.20. You agreed with this observation in your response to the FDA Form 483. We note that in your written response, you have explained how your former institution will ensure that a similar violation does not recur. However, you have not addressed how you, personally, will ensure that a similar violation does not recur in your conduct of FDA regulated clinical research in the future.

This letter is not intended to be an all-inclusive list of deficiencies with your clinical study of an investigational drug. It is your responsibility to ensure adherence to each requirement of the law and relevant FDA regulations. You should address these deficiencies and establish procedures to ensure that any ongoing or future studies will be in compliance with FDA regulations.

Within fifteen (15) working days of your receipt of this letter, you should notify this office in writing of the actions you have taken or will be taking to prevent similar violations in the future. Failure to adequately and promptly explain the violations noted above may result in regulatory action without further notice.

If you have any questions, please contact Constance Lewin, M.D., M.P.H., at 301-796-3397; FAX 301-847-8748. Your written response and any pertinent documentation should be addressed to:

Constance Lewin, M.D., M.P.H.
Branch Chief, Good Clinical Practice Branch I
Division of Scientific Investigations
Office of Compliance
Center for Drug Evaluation and Research
Food and Drug Administration
Building 51, Room 5354
10903 New Hampshire Avenue
Silver Spring, MD 20993

Sincerely yours,

Leslie K. Ball, M.D.

Director
Division of Scientific Investigations
Office of Compliance
Center for Drug Evaluation and Research

JUN 26 2009
Mark F. Gordon, M.D.
C/o Office of Research Compliance
350 Commumity Drive
Manhasset, NY 11030

Dear Dr. Gordon:By letter dated June 1, 2009, the Food and Drug Administration (FDA), Center for Drug Evaluation and Research, issued a Warning Letter sent by certified mail to you at your former address of 900 Ridgebury Road, Ridgefied, CT 06877-0368.

Per your request, we are re-issuing the Warning Letter to you at your current address. Except for the change of address, this Warning Letter is identical to the one dated April 20, 2009.

Enclosed you will find a copy of the Warning Letter.

Sincerely yours,

Leslie K. Ball, M.D.
Director
Division of Scientific Investigations
Office of Compliance
Center for Drug Evaluation and Research

第 125 封　给 Zosa, Noli R. 医学博士的警告信

2009年6月16日

参考号：09-HFD-45-06-02

尊敬的Zosa博士：

2008年10月2日至2008年10月7日，Sonya Karsik女士和Brian Putz先生代表FDA进行了现场检查，并对您为实施的申办者为Bausch & Lomb股份有限公司，试验药物为盐酸贝西沙星混悬型滴眼剂（ISV-403）的临床研究（试验方案编号433，试验名称为“一项评估0.6% ISV-403相比空白辅料治疗细菌性结膜炎的临床和微生物有效性研究”）进行了审查。

本次现场检查是FDA的生物研究监查项目的一部分，该项目通过设定的检查方法，评估研究的实施情况，以确保这些研究中受试者的权益、安全和福利得到了保护。

经对FDA现场检查报告、该报告的附件进行审查，我们认为，您没有遵循适用的法律要求和监管临床研究实施的FDA法规。我们知道，在现场检查结束时，Karsik女士和Putz先生向您出示并讨论了FDA 483表，即现场检查发现的问题。我们想强调以下几点：

1. 您未能进行研究或确保按照签署的研究者声明、研究计划开展研究［21 CFR 312.60］

具体而言，您入组的4位受试者中有3位不符合入组标准。

a. 方案入组标准中要求受试者“具有急性细菌性结膜炎的临床诊断，并表现为结膜有化脓性分泌物（眼睑有硬壳或发黏），至少一只眼发红。分泌物等级至少为1分，球结膜充血等级至少1分”。

FDA检查发现，尽管受试者0154和0155电子病例报告表（eCRF）中临床评估部分，双眼的眼分泌物等级均记录为“0=没有”，但他们仍入组了研究并接受了首剂试验药物。具体而言：

ⅰ）对于受试者0154，eCRF访视1——第1天部分记录，受试者被诊断为“鼻部翼状胬肉”。没有记录显示该受试者患有方案中规定的细菌性结膜炎。

ⅱ）对于受试者 0155，根据eCRF第36页记录，该受试者不符合入组标准，而且2008年2月11日产生的审计追踪报告指出，该受试者被诊断患有“巩膜外层炎,”属于方案的排除标准之一。

b. 方案排除标准排除“疑似病毒性或过敏性结膜炎的受试者（即重度发痒或急性滤泡性结膜炎），或患有任何其他可能干扰试验药物有效性和安全性评估的疾病病症的受试者。”我们的检查发现，两名受试者0154 和 0155在eCRF“排除标准部分”，上述排除标准均标记为“是”。

检查期间您就此给出的解释不可接受。您辩称，您的“筛选潜在研究受试者的系统是与受试者初步会面，进行部分筛选，给予首剂试验药物，发放供受试者回家使用的试验药物，然后在1天内或在第一天访视的时候将受试者送给眼科医师看，进而完成筛选过程。”我们注意到，方案第12和15页特别指出，“首次第1天的试验药物应在初次眼部检查和结膜培养后，在办公室给予。”

c. 方案要求受试者至少年满1岁。根据eCRF记录，受试者0156 入组时仅10个月大。我们的检查发现，尽管受试者0156不符合年龄要求，但仍被入组了研究。

当您签署研究者声明，FDA1572表时，您同意承担一名临床研究者的职责，这些责任包括确保研究按照研究计划和签署的研究者声明实施，以保护受试者的安全、权益或福利，并履行临床研究者的所有义务和21 CFR 312中所有其他的相关要求。我们提醒您，作为一名临床研究者，您担负着实施研究的责任。

2. 您未能准备和保存记录了服用试验药物的每个人与试验有关的所有研究观察结果和其他相关数据的足够准确的病历［21 CFR 312.62（b）］

试验方案433指出如下事项：

临床数据将被输入到电子病例报告表（eCRF）中。eCRF上的数据必须与保存在研究中心的原始文件对应一致并获得后者的支持，除非中心直接输入没有保存其他最初或原始文件的数据。这种情况下，中心应记录哪些eCRF是属于直接输入数据产生的，并应设置程序，以获取并保留通过直接输入数据所提交信息的副本。

FDA调查发现，贵研究中心没有原始文件可证实输入到所有入组受试者eCRF中的数据，我们也没有查见记录哪些eCRF是属于直接输入数据产生的相关文件，或者为获取并保留通过直接输入数据所提交信息的副本而设置的程序。举例来说，在受试者档案中未查见下列项目：眼科医师的评估报告，视力评估报告，实验室报告，受试者的病历，所有采集的培养物样本的细菌和病毒培养实验室报告，以及记录每日服用试验药物情况的受试者日记卡。因此，我们无法核实提交给申办者的数据的准确性。

3. 您未能按照21 CFR 50的要求保存知情同意的记录［21 CFR 50.27（a）］

具体而言，21 CFR 50.27（a）规定，除去21 CFR 56.109（c）中规定的例外情况，知情同意应采用一份经IRB批准并经受试者或受试者合法授权代理人在表示同意时签字并签署日期的书面同意书来证明。

FDA检查发现，对于所有入组的4名受试者，您均未采用一份经IRB批准并经受试者或受试者合法授权代理人在表示同意时签字并签署日期的书面同意书来证明其已知情同意。贵研究中心现有可证明其已知情同意的唯一证据是所有4名受试者eCRF知情同意部分记录的日期。检查期间，您辩称因您的办公室搬迁而不能找到这些记录。

本警告信的目的并非是罗列您在试验药物临床研究中存在的所有缺陷。确保遵循法律和相关FDA法规的每一项要求是您的职责。您应当解决这些缺陷，并建立规程，以确保任何正在进行或将来的研究均能符合FDA的法规。

自收到这封信的15个工作日内，您应当书面告知本办公室为预防将来发生类似违规情况已经或将要采取的措施。如果不能充分、迅速地解释上述违规问题，可能导致我们在不再通知的情况下采取监管措施。

附：英文原文

Zosa, Noli R., M.D.

WARNING LETTER

Jun 16, 2009

CERTIFIED MAIL
RETURN RECEIPT REQUESTED

Ref: 09-HFD-45-06-02

Noli R. Zosa, M.D.
12444 East Washington Boulevard
Whittier, California 90602

Dear Dr. Zosa:

Between October 2, 2008 and October 7, 2008, Ms. Sonya Karsik and Mr. Brian Putz, representing the Food and Drug Administration (FDA), conducted an investigation and met with you to review your conduct of a clinical investigation (Protocol #433 entitled“A Study to Evaluate the Clinical and Microbial Efficacy of 0.6% ISV-

403 Compared toVehicle in the Treatment of Bacterial Conjunctivitis") of the investigational drug besifloxacin hydrochloride ophthalmic suspension (ISV-403), performed for Bausch & Lomb Incorporated.

This inspection is a part of the FDA's Bioresearch Monitoring Program, which includes inspections designed to evaluate the conduct of research and to ensure that the rights,safety, and welfare of the human subjects of those studies have been protected.

From our review of the establishment inspection report and the documents submitted with that report, we conclude that you did not adhere to the applicable statutory requirements and FDA regulations governing the conduct of clinical investigations. We are aware that at the conclusion of the inspection, Ms. Karsik and Mr. Putz presented and discussed with you Form FDA 483, Inspectional Observations. We wish to emphasize the following:

1. You failed to conduct the study or ensure the study was conducted according to the signed investigator statement and investigational plan [21 CFR 312.60]

Specifically, 3 of 4 subjects you enrolled failed to meet enrollment criteria.

a. The protocol inclusion criteria required subjects to "have a clinical diagnosis of acute bacterial conjunctivitis and exhibit purulent conjunctival discharge (crusty or sticky eyelids) and redness in at least one eye. A minimum score of 1 should be present for discharge and a minimum score of 1 for bulbar conjunctival injection".

FDA's investigation found that Subjects 0154 and 0155 were enrolled and received the initial dose of investigational drug despite having the ocular discharge rating of "0 = Absent" for both eyes as documented for both subjects in the Clinical Assessment portion of the electronic case report form (eCRF).

Specifically,

i) For Subject 0154, the Visit 1-Day 1 portion of the eCRF, documented that the subject was diagnosed with "Pterygium nasal". There is no documentation that this subject had bacterial conjunctivitis as specified by the protocol.

ii) For Subject 0155, the eCRF, pg 36 documented that the subject did not meet enrollment criteria and the Audit Trail Report generated on February 11,2008, documented that the subject was diagnosed with "Episcleritis," one of the exclusion criteria in the protocol.

b. The protocol exclusion criteria excluded "subjects with suspected viral or allergic conjunctivitis (i.e, severe itching or acute follicular conjunctivitis), or any other disease conditions that could interfere with the efficacy and safety evaluations of the study medication." Our investigation found that both Subjects 0154 and 0155 had the above exclusion criteria marked as "Yes" on the "Exclusion Criteria section of the eCRF.

Your explanation provided during the inspection is unacceptable. You stated that your "system for screening potential study subjects was to see the subject initially, conduct partial screening, administer the initial dose of study drug, dispense study medication for home use to the subject, and then send the subject to be seen by the ophthalmologist within a day or so of the Day 1 Visit to complete the screening process." We note that pages 12 and 15 of the protocol specifically state, "The first Day 1 dose of study medication will be administered in the office after the initial eye exam and conjunctival culture."

c. The protocol required subjects to be at least one year of age. The eCRF documented that Subject 0156 was only 10 months of age at the time of enrollment. Our investigation found that Subject 0156 was enrolled despite not meeting the age requirement.

When you signed the Statement of Investigator, Form FDA 1572, you agreed to the responsibilities of a clinical investigator that included ensuring that the study is conducted according to the investigational plan and the signed Investigator Statement, to protect the safety, rights or welfare of the subjects and to comply with all the obligations of a clinical investigator and all other pertinent requirements in 21 CFR 312. We remind you that as a clinical investigator, you retain responsibility for the conduct of the study.

2. You failed to prepare and maintain adequate and accurate case histories that record all observations and other data pertinent to the investigation on each individual administered the investigational drug [21 CFR 312.62(b)].

Protocol #433 stated the following:

Clinical data will be entered into electronic Case Report Forms (eCRFs). Data on eCRFs must correspond to and be supported by source documentation maintained at the investigational site, unless the site makes direct data entry for which no other original or source documentation is maintained. In such cases, the site should document which eCRFs are subject to direct data entry and should have in place procedures to obtain and retain copies of the information submitted by direct data entry.

FDA's investigation found that there was no source documentation at your site to corroborate data entered into the eCRF for any of the enrolled subjects, nor did we find documentation regarding which eCRFs were subject to direct data entry, or which procedures were in place to obtain and retain copies of information submitted by direct data entry. The following items, for example, were not found in subjects' files: ophthalmologist assessment reports, visual acuity assessment reports, laboratory reports, subjects' medical charts, bacterial and viral culture laboratory reports for all culture samples collected, and subject's worksheets documenting daily administration of study drug. Therefore, we are unable to verify the accuracy of the data submitted to the sponsor.

3. You failed to maintain documentation of informed consent in accordance with21 CFR 50 [21 CFR 50.27(a)]

Specifically, 21 CFR 50.27(a) states that except as provided in 21 CFR 56.109(c), informed consent shall be documented by the use of a written consent form approved by the IRB and signed and dated by the subject or the subjects' legally authorized representative at the time of consent.

FDA's investigation found that for all four subjects enrolled, you did not document informed consent by the use of a written consent form approved by the IRB and signed and dated by the subject or the subject's legally authorized representative at the time of consent. The only documentation available at the site to document informed consent was the date recorded in the Informed Consent Section of the eCRFs for all four subjects. During the inspection, you stated that you were unable to locate these records due to the relocation of your office.

This letter is not intended to be an all-inclusive list of deficiencies with your clinical study of an investigational drug. It is your responsibility to ensure adherence to each requirement of the law and relevant FDA regulations. You should address these deficiencies and establish procedures to ensure that any on-going or future studies will be in compliance with FDA regulations.

Within fifteen (15) working days of your receipt of this letter, you should notify this office in writing of the actions you have taken or will be taking to prevent similar violations in the future. Failure to adequately and promptly explain the violations noted above may result in regulatory action without further notice.

If you have any questions, please contact Tejashri Purohit-Sheth, M.D., at 301-796-3402;FAX 301-847-8748. Your written response and any pertinent documentation should be addressed to:

Tejashri Purohit-Sheth, M.D.
Branch Chief
Good Clinical Practice Branch Ⅱ
Division of Scientific Investigations
Office of Compliance
Center for Drug Evaluation and Research
Food and Drug Administration
Bldg 51, Room 5358
10903 New Hampshire Avenue
Silver Spring, MD 20993

Sincerely yours,

{See appended electronic signature page}

Leslie K. Ball, M.D.
Director
Division of Scientific Investigations
Office of Compliance
Center for Drug Evaluation and Research

第126封　给Linzer, Dov医学博士的警告信

2009年6月12日

参考号：09-HFD-45-06-01

尊敬的Linzer博士：

2008年12月3日至15日，CDR Ileana Barreto-Pettit女士，代表FDA进行了现场检查，与您会面并对您所实施的一项临床研究［试验方案（b）（4）[1]，试验名称为（b）（4），试验药物（b）（4），申办者为（b）（4）］，进行了审查。

本次现场检查是FDA的生物研究监查项目的一部分，该项目通过设定的检查方法，评估研究的实施情况，以确保这些研究中受试者的权益、安全和福利得到了保护。

经对FDA现场检查报告、该报告的附件，以及您2008年12月29日的书面回复进行审查，我们认为，您没有遵循适用的法律要求和监管临床研究实施的FDA法规。我们获知，在现场检查结束时，CDR Barreto-Pettit女士向您出示并讨论了FDA 483表，即现场检查发现的问题。我们想强调以下几点：

1. 您未能亲自进行临床研究或对研究进行监督［21 CFR 312.60］

当您为上述临床试验签署研究者声明（FDA 1572表）时，您同意将在您的临床研究场所承担临床研究者的职责。您的总体职责（21 CFR 312.60）包括确保按签署的研究者声明、研究计划和适用的法规实施试验；保护您在您的监护下的受试者的权益、安全和福利；以及确保试验药物受控。您还特别同意将亲自实施该项临床研究或监督那些您未亲自实施的研究事项。尽管您可以将特定的研究任务授权给有资质的人员实施，但作为临床研究者，您不能转移您的总体职责。我们的检查显示，您未能对接受研究任务授权的人员实施充分的监督，以确保该项临床试验按照签署的研究者声明、研究计划和适用法规进行，并以保护受试者权益、安全和福利的方式进行。而且，FDA的检查还发现您几乎未参与这项研究。

根据试验方案（b）（4）的试验人员清单，您的临床研究协调员，（b）（4）和（b）（4），被授权了以下职责（包括但不限于），确定入排标准以及评估不良事件（AEs），严重不良事件（SAEs）和研究终点。您告知FDA检查员，您缺乏实施临床试验的经验，因此您主要依靠您的临床研究协调员来实施研究并完成研究的相关书面工作。（b）（4）先生和（b）（4）女士根据FDA对他们是受试者入组和参与试验其间的主要研究协调员简历的检查，这些人员似乎没有资格认证，或者明显接受过医学培训并具有执照可独立作出与受试者入组该项研究的资格确认相关的判断和/或对不良事件是否与使用试验药物相关做出判断。

另外，监查报告证明，当这项研究在贵研究场所关闭且（b）（4）先生和（b）（4）女士停止研究工作后，您的中心试图就监查员在监查访视中发现的大量问题进行改正。我们注意到新的研究协调员被指派去依据原始记录改正病例报告表（CRFs）和填写不良事件和严重不良事件病例报告表。原始记录显示，在改正这些信息时，您的新研究协调员也对受试者在研究期间发生的AEs和SAEs是否与使用试验药物相关进行了判断。FDA指出，鉴于您的新研究协调员并未参与最初的研究，因此不清楚他们何以能充分改正您中心受试者的病历并就受试者在研究期间发生的AEs和SAEs是否与使用试验药物相关进行判断。

正由于您对研究过程缺乏监督，导致了下述的重大问题，并且显著增加了我们关于数据可靠性以及您如何保护入组该项研究的受试者权益、安全和福利等问题的担忧。

---

1 （b）（4）代表涉及商业秘密根据法规不予披露内容的标注。

2. 您未能按 21 CFR 50 的要求，获得每位接受药物治疗的受试者的知情同意［21 CFR 312.60］

FDA 的法规在21 CFR 50.20中规定，除外 21 CFR 50.23和21 CFR 50.24中所列特例，除非研究者在受试者或受试者的合法授权代理人处获得了合法有效的知情同意，研究者不得入选人类作为法规监管范围内的研究的受试者。法规明确了研究者只有在给予潜在的受试者或受试者代理人充分的机会来思考是否要参与，并且应当在最大程度地减少强迫或不当影响的可能性的情况下，才能寻求这种知情同意。FDA法规50.27进一步说明知情同意应当使用书面的同意文件进行记录，并且该文件应该在受试者或受试者代理人被给予充分的机会进行阅读后再由其签署。

在日期为2005年12月14日的信函中，伦理委员会通知贵研究场所他们已经批准了版本为2005年10月19日的试验方案和知情同意书。在日期为2006年5月26日的信函中，伦理委员会通知贵研究场所他们又批准了修订的知情同意书（版本为2006年5月23日），其中包括了与研究背景和目的、研究治疗访视，以及妊娠风险相关的新信息，并要求贵研究场所"所有现已入组的受试者在下次计划访视时签署该修订版同意书，并且所有新的入组受试者都使用新版知情同意书。"

A. 您未使用修订后的2006年5月23日版知情同意书再次获得7名受试者（020，022，025，033，042，044和045）的同意。

B. 您没有按照 IRB的要求，及时在下次计划访视时再次获得11名受试者（001，007，013，024，036，041，043，048，049，053和056）的同意。具体而言，方案规定，受试者被随机分配入研究后，应对受试者每月进行一次肝功能检查；因此，要求贵研究场所与受试者至少每月会面一次。在FDA对文件审查过程中，我们注意到贵研究场所使用修订版知情同意书再次获得这些受试者的同意时，已过去数月之久。修订版知情同意书，版本为2006年5月23日，含有可能影响受试者继续参与研究意愿的信息，因为其中警告他们参与研究具有的额外风险，并提供了关于研究的新信息。因此，您拖延使用修订版知情同意书再次获得这些受试者的同意，导致我们对于您是否对研究进行了充分监督，以确保入组该项研究受试者的权益、安全和福利等得到保护的问题产生了严重担忧。

C. 受试者060 于2006年8月17日签署了知情同意书并入组该项研究。贵研究场所采用失效的2005年10月19日版知情同意书获得了该受试者参与研究的同意。而您本应采用在该受试者入组该项研究时已经生效的2006年5月23日版知情同意书。

根据您2008年12月29日的书面回复，您承诺，未来将使用各修订版知情同意书获得所有受试者的同意。此外，您还提供了一个标准操作规程（SOP），详细说明贵研究场所将如何处理知情同意文件和过程。FDA已收到您的保证，即您已采取纠正措施，防止任何将来研究中发生类似问题。虽然这些纠正措施似乎妥当，但正是在这些试验实施过程中缺乏这样的措施，从而造成了上述违规行为，并增加了我们对于您确保受试者获得适当保护的方法的关注。

3. 您未能进行研究或者确保按照研究计划进行研究［21 CFR 312.60］

A. 方案规定，受试者必须具有如下（b）（4）记录才可被纳入该项研究：

（1）筛选或随机日具有记录了（b）（4）的心电图（ECG）。

（2）根据12-导联ECG记录，患者在随机化之前6个月之内曾有有症状的阵发性或持续性（b）（4）发作；

（3）有记录证明患者在2个单独的、至少间隔1天的场合中，且其中一次在随机化之前6个月之内，发生有症状或无症状的阵发性或持续性（b）（4）发作。

原始文件显示，受试者003 和 015 不符合这项入组标准，但被随机进入研究且被分配了试验药物。

B. 方案规定，重度肾损伤（经评估肌酐清除率＜ 30mL/min）的受试者应被排除。实验室检查结果证实，受试者003筛选时的肌酐清除率为 21mL/min，故符合这项排除标准。然而我们注意到，贵研究场所对该受试者进行了随机，并将其分配进入了研究。

C. 方案指出，活动性肝病受试者，包括但不限于：（a）持续性的 ALT，AST，碱性磷酸酶＞2倍正常上限（ULN）；（b）已知活动性丙型肝炎；（c）活动性乙型肝炎；（d）活动性甲型肝炎，应被排除。方案进一步指出，已知具有乙型肝炎或丙型肝炎病史的患者，必须在入组研究前接受乙型和丙型肝炎血清学检查。

（1）记录显示，2006年5月4日受试者047采集了筛选访视实验室样本，用于肝炎检查，2006年6月13日传真到贵研究场所的筛选实验室检查结果显示，该受试者丙型肝炎阳性。但是，我们注意到，在收到这项肝炎筛选结果之前，贵研究场所已对该受试者进行了随机，并将其分配进入了研究，并于2006年5月17日开始使用试验药物进行治疗。

（2）贵研究场所未在对受试者进行随机分配入组前，对受试者033、042和056进行肝炎筛查，以确保这些受试者不符合这条排除标准。

D. 方案指出，对于（b）（4）治疗具有禁忌症的受试者应被排除。记录表明，受试者062入组之前，于（b）（6）因（b）（6）的（b）（4）毒性而住院，因此符合这条排除标准。但贵研究场所于2006年9月7日对该受试者进行了随机，并将其分配进入了研究。

E. 方案指出，除了被记录的（b）（4），受试者必须至少具有一个方案规定的额外的（b）（4）风险因素，才可被纳入这项研究。原始记录显示，受试者009不符合入组研究所需要的任何方案规定的额外的（b）（4）风险因素。但是，贵研究场所对该受试者进行了随机，并将其分配进入了研究。

F. 方案规定，肝功能检查是入组受试者应进行的安全性检查之一。具体而言，方案要求在治疗的前12个月期间每月一次，此后每4个月一次对肝功能（ALT，AST，碱性磷酸酶，胆红素）进行评估。基于对这些检查结果的审查，可能需要实施额外的流程，以确保受试者安全。在贵研究场所检查原始文件时，FDA不能核实贵研究场所每月进行了肝功能检查。

示例包括，但不限于以下：

受试者 #	缺失肝功能检查的月份
003	2006年4月
011	2006年4月
018	2006年10月、11月、12月
024	2006年8月、9月、11月和12月
033	2006年5月和6月
049	2006年9月和10月
056	2006年8月和10月
062	2006年10月

G. 方案规定，不论患者何时终止参与研究（提前或根据方案），均应进行一次末次访视（访视98）。这次访视时，① 不良事件、出血事件、有效性事件，以及上次访视以来合并用药的变化等信息应予以记录② 实施例如体格检查、生命体征检查、标准安全性实验室检查和12-导联ECG检查等研究流程；③ 回收试验药物，计算依从性；④ 采集安全性实验室检查样本，如有说明，完成INR测量。记录显示，当受试者009和042在贵研究场所接受末次访视时，未对这些受试者实施所有的末次访视研究流程。

H. 方案规定，研究基线时，每年一次以及在末次访视或彻底停用试验药物时，所有受试者均进行 12-导联 ECG检查。在FDA审查受试者024原始文件时，未查见基线ECG结果，也未查见有进行了基线ECG检查的相关信息。

I. 方案规定，对于该项临床研究期间（即从签署知情同意书开始直到观察期［治疗后期］结束）发生的所有AE，研究者均需根据研究中心文件中“不良事件报告”章节中详细规定的特定定义和说明进行采集、记录，并报告申办者。此外，方案还指出，对于所有AE，不论是严重还是非严重事件，均需在适当的CRF上进行完整记录。方案进一步指出，发生任何严重或重要AE时，不论是否被认为与试验药物有关，也不论是否给予过试验药物，都必须通过电话/传真形式立即报告申办者。FDA检查发现，贵研究场所未遵循方案的AE报告要求。示例包括但不限于以下：

（1）医疗记录表明，贵研究场所于2006年6月29日会见了受试者033，并发现该受试者存在偶见前方闪光，心率稍慢，以及有点晕头转向。医学记录还表明，在2006年8月17日，贵研究场所也会见了该受试者，发现该受试者存在疲劳，偶有咳痰和黏液问题，还因其使用的（b）（4）药物而胀气。FDA在检查中未发现这些AE被报告给申办者的记录。

（2）原始记录显示，在受试者059 于（b）（6）被随机分配到（b）（4）后，该受试者因（b）（6）的（b）（6）毒性而住院。我们注意到，贵研究场所于（b）（6）填写了关于该受试者住院的SAE报告。FDA在检查中未发现这份SAE报告已提交至申办者的记录。

根据您2008年12月29日的书面回复，您指出，您和您的临床研究协调员加入了2009年（b）（4）项目，而且贵研究场所也自2008年1月以来建立了标准操作规程（SOP）。关于检查发现的问题，您指出，判定受试者临床试验入选资格所需的最终的入组和排除标准，以及仔细审查和评估所有的资格评估原始文件和安全性检查结果都是研究者应单独承担的责任。此外，您还指出其他纠正措施包括：① 对临床研究协调员（CRCs）进行培训，并执行将来的方案；② 研究者按研究方案要求，在规定时间内审查评估所有安全性检查的书面承诺；③ 对于所有筛选的排除性结果均进行复查、比较和核实，而且如检测值不在正常范围内，立即将受试者退出研究，并给予临床治疗的书面承诺；④ 对于所有早期终止的受试者实施所有早期终止访视流程的书面承诺。

FDA注意到，接受培训是一个有助于您和贵研究场所理解相关法规中开展临床研究相关的监管要求的积极步骤。但是FDA注意到，在我们对贵研究场所SOPs的审查过程中发现与您所承诺的纠正措施存在差异。具体而言，在审查标题为“研究团队职责标准操作规程”的SOP时，研究者的个人职责中没有包括确保并核实受试者入组研究的资格。根据这份SOP显示，确定入组资格的责任由研究护士、协调者和/或数据管理员承担。这与您书面承诺的纠正措施中确定入组资格为临床研究者单独承担的责任的表述迥然不同。

此外，在审查标题为“研究期间受试者管理标准操作规程”的SOP A和B部分时，FDA不能确定您将询问和记录受试者的病史，进行完整或规定的体检，确定受试者的基线体征和症状，开列方案要求的检查/操作，评估受试者任何并发性疾病的体征和症状，妥善记录不良事件，以及如受试者的状况需要，给予其适当的治疗等责任，授权给了谁。具体而言，FDA不能确定这些责任是否共同授权给了研究者和研究护士、协调员，或者研究者或研究护士、协调员是否可在他人未获知或监督的情况下独立处理这些职责。FDA注意到，后者，即允许研究护士、协调员独立开展这些活动，是不适当的，并与您的书面承诺纠正措施直接抵触。请在回复中给予说明。

4. 您未能保存研究中使用试验药物或对照受试者的所有观察结果和其他数据的足够及准确的病历［21 CFR 312.62（b）］

A. 贵研究场所选用了申办者的标准化表格作为原始文件来记录并证明与受试者研究访视有关的信息。根据标准化表格，贵研究场所需“填写入组/排除标准工作表，以评估研究资格”。FDA检查员在贵研究场所审查65名受试者中的16名受试者的记录时，未查见这些受试者中任何一人的入组/排除标准工作表。

B. FDA检查员审查的贵研究场所所有这16名受试者的病历均有严重问题。示例包括但不限于以下：

（1）受试者003

i. 未填写完成访视4原始记录表格。

ii. 该受试者记录中没有任何受试者访视的病例报告表（CRFs）。

（2）受试者015，筛选访视（2006年3月15日）血红蛋白计数为 10.7g/dL，2006年4月3日采集的实验室血样显示血红蛋白计数为7.8g/dL。因此，该受试者的血红蛋白计数下降 2.9g/dL，根据方案，这应被视为一次重大出血事件。但贵研究场所错误地在CRF中，将该事件报告为一次轻微出血事件。

（3）受试者024

i. 受试者记录中，访视6的CRF缺失第20，22和62页。

ii. 贵研究场所于2008年5月对受试者024的数份CRFs进行了改动，彼时距离该受试者末次研究访视

（2007年1月9日）已逾1年。FDA检查员不能根据原始记录确认，在贵研究场所对CRFs进行改动后，已将那些变动后的CRFs提交给了申办者。

（4）受试者033

ⅰ. 在筛选访视的原始文件中，贵研究场所对于“过去6个月内该患者的心室功能做过评估吗？”的问题，勾选了“否”。但是，贵研究场所随后又提供了2005年12月12日进行的一次评估的相关信息，该次评估中确认其“LV射血分数”为40%。FDA对该受试者记录的核查，未发现其记录中有任何支持性的文件可证实在2005年12月12日进行过任何心室功能评估。

ⅱ. 在访视2的原始记录中，存在大量的日期矛盾。具体而言，根据发放/返还日志，访视日期和向受试者发放试验药物的日期为2006年4月27日。

然而，2006年4月26日被列为是向交互式语音应答系统（IVRS）致电，以对受试者进行随机化的日期，受试者首次服用试验药物的日期，以及贵研究场所记录为您填写访视2原始记录的日期。根据这些原始记录显示，受试者在向其发放试验药物之前已服用了首剂药物。

在审查您的标题为“法规档案和受试者记录标准操作规程”和“数据管理标准操作规程”SOP时，我们注意到：① 收集临床研究数据的责任主要由研究护士、协调员承担；② 将数据转录到CRF中的责任授权给了研究护士、协调员和/或辅助员工；③ 质量保证以确保仅第一组完成CRF的受试者病历完整、准确的责任授权给了研究管理员和/或研究护士/协调员。我们注意到，这些SOP不要求研究者审查这些文件，以确保原始记录中信息的准确和完整。此外，根据SOP，贵研究场所为确保病史完整、准确而进行的唯一的质量保证程序仅限于第1组完成的CRF。我们进一步注意到，鉴于研究护士/协调员也被授权了收集研究数据的责任，这可能导致出现这样的情形，即采集并记录研究数据的个人也稽查其自己的原始记录。您的回复未充分解决这些疑虑。

5. 您未能及时向 IRB 报告给受试者或其他人带来风险的所有非预期事件［21 CFR 312.66］

A. 原始记录表明，受试者015于2006年3月15日入组该研究，2006年3月24日被随机分配，并于2006年3月30日接受了首剂试验药物。在一个2006年4月6日的归档备忘录中，您的授权研究者（b）（6）医生，指出在2006年4月2日，该患者致电贵研究场所并报告过去2天他发生了直肠出血，且当他次日到达贵研究场所办公室，贵研究场所发现该受试者的血红蛋白水平为7.8 g/dL，血细胞比容（HCT）水平为 24.8。然后该患者被转至初级保健医师，在门诊接受了输血治疗，并接受了一次检查以排除胃肠道（GI）出血。在一份日期也是2006年4月6日的跟进书面备忘录中，（b）（6）医生指出GI检查显示该受试者患有结肠癌。

FDA注意到，贵研究场所在该受试者停止参与研究前已意识到其有胃肠道出血（不同原始记录中停止的日期不同：在2份不同的原始文件中记录为2006年3月31日，另一份原始文件中为2006年4月2日，还有一份原始文件中为2006年4月3日），并且在贵研究场所获悉受试者患有结肠癌后，应及时向IRB报告这一未预期的问题。FDA的核查未能查见证明这一事件已报知IRB的文件。

B. 原始记录显示受试者059于2006年8月10日入组该研究，2006年8月17日被随机分配到（b）（4）。一份2006年9月6日产生，以提供2006年9月5日所采集样本相关信息的实验室报告，显示该受试者：①（b）（4）值异常增高；② 红细胞计数、血红蛋白和血细胞比容值异常降低。原始记录进一步表明，该受试者于（b）（4）因（b）（6）诊断而住院。贵研究场所于2008年6月17日准备了一份关于此次住院的严重不良事件报告。FDA的核查未能查见证明这一不良事件已报知IRB的文件。

根据您2008年12月29日的书面回复，您承诺将在要求的时间限度内向申办者和IRB报告及记录发生的严重和非严重AE，并且贵研究场所已创建了将来研究中使用的关于SAE报告指南和报告结构要求的SOP，并对所有研究团队委员作了相应培训。您在信中进一步指出，研究者将对研究受试者密切跟进，如研究期间作出癌症诊断，将立即采取所有的安全措施，并且研究者将确定和评估其与试验药物的联系。试验相关各方将共同作出是否早期终止访视的决定，受试者的安全始终将优先予以考虑。

您的标题为“与伦理委员会沟通标准操作规程”的SOP指出，所有关于研究进程中发生的AE和SAE的沟通均由研究护士、协调员和/或辅助员工与IRB进行。基于对您SOP的审查，FDA不能确定这份SOP中授权的这些责任是研究护士、协调员和/或辅助员工的共享责任，还是每个人均可以在没有其他人监督或获悉的情况下独立承担的责任。请在您的回复中对此予以说明。FDA进一步注意到，这份SOP未要求研究者审查AE和SAE和/或核实提交给IRB的报告中包含了准确和足够的信息，包括事件是否与使用试验药物有关的信息。

此外，在标题为“不良事件报告标准操作规程”的SOP中，将研究受试者相比基线或治疗前状况发生任何不良变化时进行随访的责任授权给了主要研究者、授权研究者和/或研究护士、协调员。跟进确认，以确保在进行中研究的批准阶段，贵研究场所发生的所有严重或危急事件已通知了IRB的责任被授权给了主要研究者、研究护士、协调员和/或辅助员工。但是根据这份SOP，不能确定这些责任是共享责任，还是每个人均可以在没有其他人监督或获悉的情况下独立承担的责任。如是后者，那么研究者未能承担充分监督向IRB报告非预期问题的责任。请在您的回复中对此予以说明。

6. 您未能及时向申办者报告有理由判断与药物有关或者可能有关的不良反应［21 CFR 312.64（b）］

A. 原始记录表明，2006年9月，贵研究场所被告知受试者033因胃部不适停用了试验药物，包括有胃痛，胀气和腹泻症状。贵研究场所填写了一份CRF，指出这些AE与使用试验药物有关。FDA检查员Barreto-Pettit未查见可证明已向申办者报告这些AE的文件。

B. 原始记录显示，在受试者024参与研究期间，其于2006年6月30日发生腹痛，2006年8月28日发生恶心和呕吐。贵研究场所直到2007年12月12日才填写不良事件CRF，这距该受试者终止参与研究已有很长时间（即终止参与研究日期为2007年1月9日）。此外，FDA检查员未查见可证明已向申办者提交这些不良事件的文件。

根据您2008年12月29日的书面回复，您承诺，所有可被合理关联为因，或可能因试验药物引起的严重和非严重AE均将在要求的时间限度内报知申办者并记录在案。您还进一步指出，对所有研究团队委员均进行了贵研究场所创建的SOP的培训，这些SOP讨论了SAE报告指南和报告结构要求。

在FDA对于您的SOP的审查中，我们注意到根据标题为“不良事件报告标准操作规程”的SOP章节A“管理不良事件”中要求，向申办者报告严重和/或非预期AE，在原始记录中记载AE详情，以及填写完成CRF的责任由主要研究者和/或研究护士、协调员承担。FDA不能确定这些责任是由研究者和研究护士/协调员共享，还是一方可在没有其他方的情况下独立处理的责任。FDA指出，允许研究护士/协调员在没有研究者监督的情况下独立处理SAE记录和报告的作法是不可接受的。请在您的回复中对此予以说明。

此外，FDA还注意到，在标题为“中心-申办者/CRO沟通标准操作规程”的SOP，章节C“研究进行中的沟通”中，似乎研究护士、协调员负责立即向申办者/CRO通报发生的SAE。然而我们注意到，在该章节中，研究者没有对试验药物与AE或SAE关系作出任何评估的责任。此外，关于研究者在审查SAE报告以确保报告信息准确方面的作用亦无相关信息。关于主要研究者在不良事件记录，报告和不良事件判断方面的监督作用，您的回复尚不充分。

7. 您未能及时向 IRB 报告研究活动中所有的变更［21 CFR 312.66］

原始记录显示，贵研究场所开始要求受试者签署一份备忘录，表明贵研究场所不再参与这项研究，并要求受试者选择或者在另一个中心继续参与该项研究，或者撤出他们的参与/同意并完成一次最终的检查。在许多受试者签署该表时，您尚未收到IRB关于研究活动这一变更的批准。

根据您2008年12月29日的书面回复，您承诺在分发和/或向研究受试者出示任何物品之前将首先获得IRB的批准。

在贵研究场所标题为“与伦理委员会沟通标准操作规程”的SOP中，研究进行中与IRB的所有沟通均委托给研究护士、协调员和/或辅助员工。未发现临床研究者参与研究过程中与IRB的任何通讯往来，或对任何通讯往来进行审查的相关信息。临床研究者应参与与IRB的交流，以确保向IRB提供信息的准确性。此外，FDA不能确定临床研究者如何确保研究团队妥善地遵循方案修订，因为SOP未提供研究者如何持续了解已获得IRB批准的方案修订中的新要求。您的回复尚不充分，因为主要研究者在与IRB沟通交流方面的充分监督未明确得到解决。

本警告信的目的并非是罗列您在试验药物临床研究中存在的所有缺陷。确保遵循法律和相关FDA法规的每一项要求是您的职责。您应当解决这些缺陷，并建立规程，以确保任何正在进行或将来的研究均能符合FDA的法规。

自收到这封信的15个工作日内，您应当书面告知本办公室为预防将来发生类似违规情况已经或将要采取的措施。如果不能充分、迅速地解释上述违规问题，可能导致我们在不再通知的情况下采取监管措施。

附：英文原文

Linzer, Dov M.D.

WARNING LETTER

Jun 12, 2009

CERTIFIED MAIL
RETURN RECEIPT REQUESTED

Ref: 09-HFD-45-06-01

Dov Linzer, M.D.
302 NW 179th Avenue, Suite 102
HealthwoRx
Pembroke Pines, FL 33029

Dear Dr. Linzer:

Between December 3 and 15, 2008, CDR Ileana Barreto-Pettit, representing the Food and Drug Administration (FDA), conducted an investigation and met with you, to review your conduct of a clinical investigation (Protocol (b) (4) entitled (b) (4) of the investigational drug (b) (4) performed for (b) (4).

This inspection is a part of the FDA's Bioresearch Monitoring Program, which includes inspections designed to evaluate the conduct of research and to ensure that the rights, safety, and welfare of the human subjects of those studies have been protected.

From our review of the establishment inspection report, the documents submitted with that report, and your written response dated December 29, 2008, we conclude that you did not adhere to the applicable statutory requirements and FDA regulations governing the conduct of clinical investigations. We are aware that at the conclusion of the inspection, CDR Barreto-Pettit presented and discussed with you Form FDA 483, Inspectional Observations. We wish to emphasize the following:

1. You failed to personally conduct or supervise the clinical investigation [21 CFR 312.60].

When you signed the investigator statement (Form FDA 1572) for the above referenced clinical investigation, you agreed to take on the responsibilities of a clinical investigator at your site. Your general responsibilities (21 CFR 312.60) include ensuring that the investigation is conducted according to the signed investigator statement, the investigational plan, and applicable regulations; protecting the rights, safety and welfare of subjects under your care;and ensuring control of drugs under investigation. You specifically agreed to personally conduct the clinical studies or to supervise those aspects of the studies that you did not personally conduct. While you may delegate certain study tasks to individuals qualified to perform them, as clinical investigator, you may not delegate your general responsibilities. Our investigation indicates that your supervision of personnel to whom you delegated study tasks was not adequate to ensure that the clinical trial was conducted according to the signed investigator statement, the investigational plan, and applicable regulations, and in a manner that protected the rights, safety, and welfare of human subjects. Furthermore, FDA's investigation found that you had little involvement in this study.

According to the trial staff list for Protocol (b) (4), your clinical research coordinators, (b) (4) and (b) (4), were delegated responsibilities, including but not limited to, affirmation of inclusion and exclusion criteria and assessment of adverse events (AEs), serious adverse events (SAEs), and study endpoints. You had informed the FDA investigator that as you were inexperienced in conducting clinical trials, you mainly relied on your clinical research coordinators to conduct the study and complete the study's paperwork. In FDA's review of the resumes of Mr. (b) (4) and Ms. (b) (4), who were the primary study coordinators during the time of enrollment and participation of the subjects in the study, these individuals did not appear to be qualified, certified, or significantly medically trained and licensed to be independently making judgments related to determination of eligibility of subjects for enrollment into the study and/ or making the determination as to whether or not adverse events were related to the use of the investigational drug.

In addition, monitoring reports identified that, subsequent to the closure of this study at your site and the termination of both Mr. (b) (4) and Ms. (b) (4), your site attempted to rectify the numerous deficiencies that were identified by the monitors during the monitoring visits. We note that new study coordinators were assigned the tasks of rectifying the case report forms (CRFs) with the source documentation and filling out AE and SAE Case Report Forms. In rectifying this information, source documents show that your new study coordinators were also making determinations as to whether AEs and SAEs experienced by subjects during the course of the study were related to the use of the investigational drug. FDA notes that it is unclear how your new study coordinators could adequately rectify the case histories at your site and also make the determinations that AEs and SAEs experienced by the subjects during the course of the study were related or not related to the use of the investigational drug, as they were not part of the original study.

Your lack of supervision over the study resulted in the significant findings as detailed below, and raises significant concerns with respect to data integrity and how you protected the rights, safety, and welfare of subjects who were enrolled into this study.

2. You failed to obtain the informed consent of each human subject in accordance with 21 CFR part 50 [21 CFR 312.60].

FDA's regulations at 21 CFR 50.20 state that, except as provided in 21 CFR 50.23 and 21 CFR 50.24, no investigator may involve a human being as a subject in research covered by the regulations unless the investigator has obtained the legally effective informed consent of the subject or the subject's legally authorized representative. The regulation specifies that an investigator shall seek such consent only under circumstances that provide the prospective subject or the subject's representative sufficient opportunity to consider whether or not to participate and that minimize the possibility of coercion or undue influence. Section 50.27 of FDA's regulations further provides that informed consent shall be documented by the use of a written consent document, which is to be signed by the subject or subject's representative only after the subject or the subject's representative is given adequate opportunity to read the document.

In a letter dated December 14, 2005, the IRB informed your site that they had approved the protocol and the informed consent document version 10/19/05. In a letter dated May 26, 2006, the IRB informed your site that they had approved the revised informed consent document (version 5/23/06), which included new information related to the background and purpose of the study, study treatment visits, and pregnancy risks, and requested that your site "have all currently enrolled subjects sign the revised consent at their next scheduled visit and use it for all new enrolles."

A. You failed to re-consent 7 subjects (#020, 022, 025, 033, 042, 044, and 045) with revised informed consent document version 5/23/06.

B. You failed to re-consent 11 subjects (#001, 007, 013, 024, 036, 041, 043, 048, 049, 053, and 056) in a timely manner at their next scheduled visit per the IRB's requirement. Specifically, the protocol specified that subsequent to the randomization of subjects into the study, subjects were to have monthly hepatic function tests performed; thus, your site was required to see the subjects at least monthly. In FDA's review of the documents, we note that several months had elapsed prior to your site re-consenting these subjects with the revised consent form. The revised informed consent document, version 5/23/06, provided information that may have affected the subjects' willingness to stay in the study, because it warned them of additional risks of participating in the study and also provided new information about the study. Thus, your delay in re-consenting these subjects with the revised consent document leads to significant concerns about the adequacy of your oversight over the study to ensure the protection of the rights, safety and welfare of the subjects enrolled in this study.

C. Subject #060 signed the informed consent document to be enrolled into the study on August 17, 2006. Your site consented this subject into the study utilizing the outdated informed consent version 10/19/05.You should have utilized informed consent document version 5/23/06, which was in effect at the time the subject enrolled into the study.

Per your December 29, 2008 written response, you promised that in the future all subjects will be consented with all of the revised versions of the informed consent forms. In addition, you provided a standard operating procedure (SOP) detailing how your site will handle the informed consent documentation and process. FDA acknowledges your assurances that corrective actions have been taken to prevent similar findings from occurring in any future studies. While these corrective actions appear appropriate, it was the absence of such measures during the conduct of these trials that led to the violations listed above, and which raises our concern for your approach to assuring appropriate human subject protection.

3. You failed to conduct the studies or ensure they were conducted according to the investigational plan [21 CFR 312.60].

A. The protocol specified that to be included in the study, the subject was to have documentation of (b) (4) as follows:

1. There is electrocardiogram (ECG) documented (b) (4) on the day of screening or randomization;
2. The patient has had a symptomatic episode of paroxysmal or persistent (b) (4) documented by 12 lead ECG within six months prior to randomization; or
3. There is documentation of symptomatic or asymptomatic paroxysmal or persistent (b) (4) on two separate occasions, at least one day apart, one of which is within six months prior to randomization.

Source documents showed that Subjects #003 and #015 did not meet this inclusion criterion, but were randomized into the study and dispensed study drug.

B. The protocol specified that subjects with severe renal impairment (estimated creatinine clearance $<$ 30 mL/min) were to be excluded from the study. Lab results identified that Subject #003's screening creatinine clearance was 21 mL/min and thus met this exclusionary criterion. We note, however, that your site randomized this subject into the study.

C. The protocol stated that subjects with active liver disease, including but not limited to (a) Persistent ALT, AST, Alkaline Phosphatase $>$ 2 X Upper Limit of Normal (ULN); (b) known active Hepatitis C; (c) active Hepatitis B; and (d) active Hepatitis A were to be excluded from the study. The protocol further noted that patients with a known history of Hepatitis B or C must undergo hepatitis serology for Hepatitis B and C prior to inclusion in the study.

1. Records indicate that Subject #047 had screening visit lab samples taken for hepatitis testing on May 4, 2006 and the results of the screening labs faxed to your site on June 13, 2006 showed that the subject was positive for Hepatitis C. We note, however, that prior to receiving the results of the hepatitis screening, your site had already randomized the subject into the study and initiated treatment with the investigational drug on May 17, 2006.
2. Your site failed to perform hepatitis screening tests on Subjects #033, #042, and #056 to ensure that these subjects did not meet this exclusion criterion prior to randomization of the subjects into the study.

D. The protocol stated that subjects with contraindications to (b) (4) treatment were to be excluded from the study. Records indicate that Subject #062 had been hospitalized for (b) (4) toxicity with (b) (6) on (b) (6), prior to enrollment into the study, and thus met this exclusion criterion. Your site, however, randomized this subject into the study on September 7, 2006.

E. The protocol stated that in addition to documented (b) (4), the subject must have at least one protocol specified additional risk factor for (b) (4) in order to be included into the study. Source records indicate that Subject #009 did not meet any of the protocol specified additional risk factors for (b) (4) required for inclusion into the study. However, your site randomized this subject into the study.

F. The protocol specified that one of the safety tests to be conducted on subjects enrolled into the study was hepatic function testing. Specifically, the protocol required that hepatic function (ALT, AST, Alkaline Phosphatase, Bilirubin) testing was to be evaluated every month during the first 12 months of treatment and every four months thereafter. Based on the review of the results from these tests, additional procedures may be performed to ensure the safety of the subjects. In the review of the source documents at your site, FDA could not verify that your site performed hepatic function tests at monthly intervals.

Examples include, but were not limited to the following:

Subject #	Month(s) of missing hepatic function tests
003	April 2006
011	April 2006
018	October, November & December 2006
024	August, September, November and December 2006
033	May and June 2006
049	September and October 2006
056	August and October 2006
062	October 2006

G. The protocol specified that whenever a patient terminated from the study, either prematurely or according to the protocol, a final follow-up visit (visit 98) was to be performed. At this visit, (1) information such as adverse events, bleeding events, efficacy events, and changes in concomitant medication since last visit were to be recorded, (2) study procedures such as a physical exam, vital signs, standard safety lab, and 12-lead ECG were to be performed, (3) study medication was to be collected and compliance calculated; and (4) laboratory sampling was to be done for safety and, if indicated, INR measurements were to be done. Records indicate that when Subjects #009 and #042 had their final follow up visit with your site, not all final follow up study procedures were performed on these subjects.

H. The protocol specified that all subjects were to have a 12-lead ECG done at baseline, annually, and at the final follow-up visit or upon permanent discontinuation of study medication. In FDA's review of the source documents for Subject #024, no baseline ECG could be found and no information could be found that a baseline ECG was performed.

I. The protocol specified that all AEs occurring during the course of the clinical study (i.e. from signing the informed consent onwards through the observational phase [post-treatment]) were to be collected, documented and reported to the Sponsor by the investigator according to the specific definitions and instructions detailed in the 'Adverse Event Reporting' section of the Investigator Site File. In addition, the protocol stated that all AEs, serious and non-serious, were to be fully documented on the appropriate CRFs. The protocol further stated that any serious or significant AE, whether or not considered related to the investigational product, and whether or not the investigational product had been administered, must be reported immediately by telephone/fax to the Sponsor. FDA's investigation found that your site failed to follow the protocol requirements for reporting of AEs. Examples include, but are not limited to, the following:

1. Medical records indicate that your site saw Subject #033 on June 29, 2006 and identified that the subject was experiencing occasional flashing lights in front of her, that her heart rate was a little bit slow, and that she felt a little bit disoriented. Medical records further indicate that on August 17, 2006, your site also saw this subject and identified that the subject had fatigue, occasional problems with phlegm and mucous, and also had gas from the (b)(4) medication the subject was taking. FDA's investigation found no documentation that these AEs were reported to the sponsor.

2. Source records showed that after randomization of Subject #059 to (b)(4) on (b)(6), the subject was hospitalized due to (b)(6) with (b)(6) toxicity. We note that your site filled out the SAE report concerning this subject's hospitalization on (b)(6). FDA's investigation found no documentation that this SAE report had been submitted to the sponsor.

Per your December 29, 2008 written response, you noted that you and your clinical research coordinators have enrolled in the (b)(4) program for 2009, and that your site also created standard operating procedures (SOP) since January 2008. With respect to the findings, you noted that the final inclusion and exclusion criteria and the careful review and assessment of all the qualifying source documents and safety tests needed to qualify a subject for a clinical trial would be the sole responsibility of the investigator. In addition, you noted other corrective actions to include: (1) Implementation of training and execution of future protocols to the clinical research coordinators (CRCs); (2) A written promise that all safety tests are to be reviewed and assessed by the investigator during the required time frame as per the study protocol; (3) A written promise that all screening exclusionary results are to be repeated, compared and verified, and if values are not within the normal ranges, the subject is to be withdrawn from the study immediately and treated clinically; and (4) A written promise that all early termination visit procedures will be conducted for all early termination subjects.

The FDA notes that obtaining education serves as a positive step in helping you and your site understand the regulatory requirements related to conducting clinical research covered by the regulations. FDA notes, however, that there were discrepancies identified in our review of your SOPs with your noted promised corrective actions. Specifically, in review of the SOP entitled "Standard Operating Procedure for Responsibilities of the Research Team," the investigator's individual responsibility does not include ensuring and verifying eligibility of the subject into the study. From this SOP, it appears that the responsibility for determination of eligibility is left to the research nurse/coordinator and/or the data manager. This would be in direct contrast to your written promised corrective action that eligibility determination is to be the sole responsibility of the clinical investigator.

In addition, in review of Sections A and B of the SOP entitled "Standard Operating Procedure for Subject Management While on Study," FDA could not determine to whom you delegated the responsibilities for eliciting and documenting the subject's medical history, performing a complete or directed physical examination, establishing a subject's baseline signs and symptoms, ordering the tests/procedures that were directed by the protocol, assessing the subject for signs and symptoms of any intercurrent illness, documenting adverse events appropriately, and instituting appropriate therapy if required by the subject's condition. Specifically, FDA was unsure if the responsibility was jointly delegated to the investigator and research nurse/coordinator, or if the investigator or the research nurse/coordinator could independently handle these responsibilities without the knowledge or oversight by the other. FDA notes that the latter, which would allow the research nurse/coordinator to perform these activities alone, is inadequate and is in direct contrast to your written promised corrective actions. Please clarify this in your response.

4. You failed to maintain adequate and accurate case histories that record all observations and other data pertinent to the investigation on each individual administered the investigational drug or employed as a control in the investigation [21 CFR 312.62(b)].

A. Your site chose to use the sponsor's standardized forms as source documents to record and document information related to the subjects' study visits. Per the standardized form, your site was to "Complete the Inclusion/Exclusion Criteria Worksheet to evaluate for study eligibility." In the FDA investigator's review of 16 of 65 subject records at your site, there was no Inclusion/Exclusion Criteria Worksheet found for any of these subjects.

B. There were significant problems with the case histories at your site for all 16 subject records reviewed by the FDA investigator. Examples include, but were not limited to, the following:

1. For Subject #003:
   i. The source document worksheets for Visit 4 were not completed.
   ii. There were no case report forms (CRFs) in the subject's records for any of the subject's visits.
2. For Subject #015, the screening visit (March 15, 2006) hemoglobin count was 10.7 g/dL and the labs taken on April 3, 2006 showed the hemoglobin count as 7.8 g/dL. Thus, the subject's hemoglobin count decreased 2.9 g/dL, which, per the protocol, was considered a major bleeding event. Your site, however, inaccurately reported in the CRF that this event was a minor bleeding event.
3. For Subject #024:
   i. Pages 20, 22, and 62 of the CRF for Visit 6 were missing from the subject's records.
   ii. Your site made changes to several CRFs for Subject #024 in May 2008, which was over one year after the

Subject's last study visit (January 9, 2007.) FDA's investigation was unable to confirm from the source records that after your site made the changes to the CRFs, that your site submitted those changed CRFs to the sponsor.

4. For Subject #033:

i. Your site checkmarked "No" to the question in the source documents for the Screening Visit that asked "Has the patient's ventricular function been assessed in the past 6 months?" However, your site then provided information related to an assessment that was made on December 12, 2005 that identified an "LV Ejection Fraction" of 40%. FDA's audit of this subject's record found no supporting documentation in this subject's records to verify any ventricular function assessment that was made on December 12, 2005.

ii. There were numerous date discrepancies in the source records for Visit 2. Specifically, the visit date and the date the subject was dispensed study medication per the dispensing/returning log was April 27, 2006.

However, April 26, 2006 was listed as the date the interactive voice response system (IVRS) was called to randomize the subject, the date the subject took the first dose of study medication, and the date your site documented that you filled out the source record for Visit 2. From the source records it appears that the subject took the first dose of study drug prior to it being dispensed to them.

In review of your SOPs entitled "Standard Operating Procedure for Regulatory Files and Subject Records" and "Standard Operating Procedure for Data Management," we note that the responsibilities of (1) the collection of the clinical research data reside mainly with the research nurse/coordinator; (2) the transcription of the data to the CRFs is delegated to the research nurse/coordinator and/or support staff; and (3) the quality assurance to ensure adequate and accurate case histories of only the first sets of completed CRFs is delegated to either the research manager and/or the research nurse/coordinator. We note that these SOPs provide no requirement for the investigator to review the documents to ensure the accuracy and adequacy of the information in the source records. In addition, per the SOP, the only quality assurance performed at your site to ensure adequate and accurate case histories is limited to only the first sets of completed CRFs. We further note that given that the research nurse/coordinator is also delegated to collect the study data, this could lead to the situation whereby the individual who is collecting and recording the study data is also auditing their own source records. Your response does not adequately address these concerns.

5. You failed to promptly report to the IRB all unanticipated problems involving risk to human subjects or others [21 CFR 312.66].

A. Source records indicate that Subject #015 was enrolled into the study on March 15, 2006, was randomized on March 24, 2006, and took the first dose of study medication on March 30, 2006. In a memo to file dated April 6, 2006, your subinvestigator, Dr. (b)(6), noted that on April 2, 2006, the patient called your site and reported that he had experienced rectal bleeding for the past 2 days and when he came to the office the following day, your site identified that the subject's hemogloblin level was 7.8g/dL and the hematocrit (HCT) level was 24.8. The patient was then referred to the primary care physician, treated with transfusions in an outpatient setting, and underwent a workup to rule out a GI bleed. In a follow up written memo that was also dated April 6, 2006, Dr. (b)(6) noted that the GI workup revealed that the subject had colon cancer.

FDA notes that as your site was aware of the gastrointestinal bleed prior to the subject being discontinued from the study (dates of discontinuation were discrepant between source records: March 31, 2006 on two different source documents, April 2, 2006 on another source, April 3, 2006 on another source), and promptly after your site became aware the subject had colon cancer, your site should have reported this unanticipated problem to the IRB. FDA's investigation was unable to find documentation that this event had been reported to the IRB.

B. Source records show that Subject #059 was enrolled into the study on August 10, 2006 and was randomized to (b)(4) on August 17, 2006. The laboratory report generated on September 6, 2006, which provided information related to the samples that were collected on September 5, 2006, showed that the subject had (1) abnormally high values for the (b)(4) and (2) abnormally low values for the red blood cell count, hemoglobin and hematocrit. Source records further indicated that the subject was hospitalized on (b)(4) with a diagnosis of (b)(6). A Serious Adverse Event report concerning the hospitalization was prepared by your site and dated June 17, 2008. FDA's investigation was unable to find documentation that this adverse event was reported to the IRB.

Per your December 29, 2008 written response, you promised that serious and nonserious AEs will be reported and documented in the required timeframe to both the sponsor and the IRB, and that your site has created and trained all members of the research team on the SOP that discussed the SAE reporting guidelines and reporting structure requirements for future studies. Your letter further noted that the study subjects will be carefully followed by the investigator, and if the diagnosis of cancer is made during the study, all of the safety measures are to take place immediately, and the association to the investigational product will be determined and evaluated by the investigator. The decision for an early termination visit will be determined by all parties involved, and the subject's safety will always be the priority.

Your SOP entitled "Standard Operating Procedure for Interactions with the Institutional Review Board" states that all communications about AEs and SAEs that occur during the course of the study are to be communicated to the IRB by either the research nurse/coordinator and/or support staff. Based upon the review of your SOP, FDA is unsure whether the responsibilities delegated in this SOP are shared responsibilities between the research nurse/coordinator and/or support staff or whether each could individually take on the responsibility without oversight or knowledge by the other. Please clarify this in your response. FDA further notes that this SOP does not provide a role for the investigator to review the AEs and SAEs and/or verify that the reports submitted to the IRB have accurate and adequate information, which would include information about whether or not the event was associated with the use of the investigational drug.

In addition, in the SOP entitled "Standard Operating Procedure for Adverse Event Reporting," the responsibility for follow up when the research subject experiences any adverse change from baseline or pretreatment condition is delegated to the principal investigator, subinvestigator, and/or research nurse/coordinator. Follow up for ensuring that the IRB is notified of all serious or alarming events occurring at the site during the approval period for the ongoing study is delegated to the principal investigator, research nurse/coordinator, and/or support staff. From the SOP, however, it cannot be determined if these responsibilities are shared responsibilities or whether one individual can take on the responsibility without oversight or knowledge by the others. If it is the latter, then the investigator does not have adequate oversight over the responsibility for reporting to the IRB unanticipated problems. Please clarify this in your response.

6. You failed to report promptly to the sponsor adverse effects that may reasonably be regarded as caused by, or probably caused by, the drug [21 CFR 312.64(b)].

A. Source records indicate that in September 2006, your site was informed that Subject #033 had stopped taking study medication due to stomach discomfort, which included symptoms of stomach pain, bloating and diarrhea. Your site filled out a CRF that noted that these AEs were related to the use of the study drug. FDA investigator Barreto-Pettit was unable to find documentation that these AEs were reported to the sponsor.

B. Source records indicate that during Subject #024's enrollment in the study, the subject experienced abdominal pain on June 30, 2006 and nausea and vomiting on August 28, 2006. Your site did not fill out the Adverse Event CRF until December 12, 2007, which was a significant amount of time after the subject was terminated from the study (i.e. date of termination from the study was January 9, 2007). In addition, the FDA investigator was unable to find documentation that these adverse events were submitted to the sponsor.

Per your December 29, 2008 written response, you promised that all serious and nonserious AEs that may be reasonably be regarded as caused by, or probably caused by, an investigational product will be reported and documented in the required timeframe to the sponsor. You further noted that all members of the research team had been trained and received education on the SOP created by your site, which discussed SAE reporting guidelines and reporting structure requirements.

In FDA's review of your SOPs, we note that per Section A entitled "Managing Adverse Events" in the SOP entitled "Standard Operating Procedure for Adverse Event Reporting," the responsibilities of informing the sponsor about serious and/or unexpected AEs, recording the details of AEs in the source documentation, and completion of the CRFs is given to the principal investigator and/or the research nurse/coordinator. FDA could not determine if these responsibilities are to be shared between the investigator and research nurse/coordinator or if one or the other could handle the responsibility without the other party. FDA notes that allowing the research nurse/coordinator to independently handle the SAE recording and reporting without oversight by the investigator is unacceptable. Please clarify this in your response.

In addition, FDA notes that in Section C, entitled "Communications while the study is ongoing," of the SOP entitled "Standard Operating Procedure for Site-Sponsor/CRO Communications," it appears that the research nurse/coordinator is responsible for informing the sponsor/CRO about SAE(s) immediately. We note, however, that in this section the investigator does not have responsibility for making any assessments as to the relationship of the investigational drug to the AE or SAE. In addition, there is no information related to the investigator's role in reviewing the SAE reports to ensure the accuracy of the information within that report. Your response is inadequate to address the principal investigator's oversight over adverse event recording, reporting, and adjudication of adverse events.

7. You failed to promptly report to the IRB all changes in research activity [21 CFR 312.66].

Source records indicate that your site began having subjects sign a memorandum of notification indicating that your site was no longer participating in the study and requesting that the subject choose the option of either continuing to participate in the study at another site or withdrawing their participation/consent from the study and completing a final exam. At the time that many of the subject's signed this form, you had not yet received IRB approval for this change in research activity.

Per your December 29, 2008 written response, you promised that you will obtain IRB approval prior to distributing and/or presenting anything to the study subjects.

In your site's SOP entitled "Standard Operating Procedure for Interactions with the Institutional Review Board," all communication with the IRB while the study is ongoing is delegated to the research nurse/coordinator and/or support staff. There appears to be no information related to the involvement of the clinical investigator in any correspondence, or review of any correspondence, to or from the IRB while the study is ongoing. The clinical investigator should be involved in IRB correspondence, in order to ensure the accuracy of the information that is being provided to the IRB. In addition, FDA cannot determine how the clinical investigator will ensure that the study team is adequately following protocol amendments, as the SOP does not provide information as to how the investigator will maintain knowledge about new requirements noted in the protocol amendments that have been approved by the IRB. Your response is inadequate, as adequate oversight by the principal investigator over IRB communications is not clearly addressed.

This letter is not intended to be an all-inclusive list of deficiencies with your clinical study of an investigational drug. It is your responsibility to ensure adherence to each requirement of the law and relevant FDA regulations. You should address these deficiencies and establish procedures to ensure that any on-going or future studies will be in compliance with FDA regulations.

Within fifteen (15) working days of your receipt of this letter, you should notify this office in writing of the actions you have taken or will be taking to prevent similar violations in the future. Failure to adequately and promptly explain the violations noted above may result in regulatory action without further notice.

If you have any questions, please contact Tejashri Purohit-Sheth, M.D., at 301-796-3402; FAX 301-847-8748. Your written response and any pertinent documentation should be addressed to:

Tejashri Purohit-Sheth, M.D.
Branch Chief
Good Clinical Practice Branch Ⅱ
Division of Scientific Investigations
Office of Compliance
Center for Drug Evaluation and Research
Food and Drug Administration
Bldg 51, Room 5358
10903 New Hampshire Avenue
Silver Spring, MD 20993

Sincerely yours,

{See appended electronic signature page}

Leslie K. Ball, M.D.
Director
Division of Scientific Investigations
Office of Compliance
Center for Drug Evaluation and Research

第127封　给Hijazi, Saad医学博士的警告信

2009年5月19日

参考号：09-HFD-45-05-01

尊敬的Hijazi博士：

2008年10月27日至12月2日，Thomas Gordon先生代表美国FDA，对您所实施的以下临床研究：试验方案（b）（4）题为（b）（4），申办者（b）（4）进行了审查。

本次现场检查是FDA的生物研究监查项目的一部分。该项目通过设定的检查方法，评估研究的实施情况，以确保这些研究中受试者的权益、安全和福利得到了保护。

经对现场检查报告及该报告提交的附件进行审查，我们认为，您没有遵循适用的法律要求和监管临床研究实施的FDA法规。在检查结束后，Gordon先生向您出示并与您讨论了FDA 483表，即现场检查发现的问题。我们希望强调以下几点：

1. 您未能保存对研究中每个受试者的所有研究观察结果和其他相关数据的足够准确的病历［21 CFR 312.62（b）］

FDA对现场检查过程中被稽查的记录的原始文件进行了审查，发现数起如下情况：①病例报告表（CRF）中录入的信息与原始文件中的信息不匹配；②原始文件中的信息在受试者完成研究后被修改，最长直至研究完成两年后，我们无法判定这些被修改的数据的来源。例证包括但不限于以下内容：

A. 受试者0001：

访视日期	与受试者接触方式	临床症状	慢性支气管炎急性加重(AECB)相关的体征和症状的评估日志	病例报告表(CRF)
2006年1月25日	电话	呼吸困难 痰液产生 痰液产生	更重 一样 大部分是清痰[1]	一样 更重 黄色，绿色的浑浊脓痰
2006年1月26日	电话	咳嗽 呼吸困难 痰液产生	更重[2] 更重[2] 一样	更重 一样 更重
2006年2月13日	诊室	咳嗽 喘息 啰音	不存在 轻度[1] 轻度[1]	轻度 轻度 轻度

1. 日志条目于2006年3月15日被修改；
2. 没有日期显示日志上的信息何时被修改。

我们注意到，以上以脚注1或2标示的项目，原始记录中的信息在受试者已经完成研究之后（研究于2006年2月13日完成）被修改。FDA在审查这位受试者的原始记录后，不能确定贵研究场所从何处获得相关信息，以证实贵研究场所对原始记录所做的修改（即慢性支气管炎急性加重相关体征和症状的评估日志）。

B. 受试者0002：

访视日期	与受试者接触方式	临床症状	慢性支气管炎急性加重(AECB)相关的体征和症状评估日志	病例报告表(CRF)
2006年1月29日	电话	咳嗽 呼吸困难 痰液产生	改善[1] 改善[1] 改善[1]	改善 改善 改善
2006年1月31日	诊室访视	痰液产生 脓痰 喘息 啰音 喘鸣音 呼吸音减低	轻度[1] 黄色，绿色的浑浊脓痰 轻度[1] 轻度[1] 不存在[1] 不存在[1]	轻度 没有列出 轻度 轻度 不存在 不存在

注：1. 日志条目于2006年3月16日被修改。

以上以脚注1标示的项目，原始记录中的信息在受试者已经完成研究之后（研究于2006年2月14日完成）被修改。FDA在审查这位受试者的原始记录后，不能确定贵研究场所从何处获得相关信息，以证实贵研究场所对原始记录所做的修改（即慢性支气管炎急性加重相关体征和症状的评估日志）。

C. 受试者0003：

访视日期	与受试者接触方式	临床症状	慢性支气管炎急性加重(AECB)相关的体征和症状的评估日志	病例报告表(CRF)
2006年2月6日	电话	咳嗽 呼吸困难 痰液产生 脓痰	没有列出 没有列出 没有列出 没有列出	改善 改善 改善 大部分是清痰

根据递交伦理委员会（IRB）的试验方案违背报告显示，贵研究场所于2006年2月6日对受试者0003进行电话访视时，未能收集到慢性支气管炎急性加重相关的体征和症状。鉴于贵研究场所未能收集到慢性支气管炎急性加重相关的症状和体征，我们无法确定您如何将信息填入病例报告表（CRF）中。

D. 受试者0004：

访视日期	与受试者接触方式	临床症状	慢性支气管炎急性加重(AECB)相关的体征和症状的评估日志	病例报告表(CRF)
2006年2月10日	电话	脓痰	大部分是清痰[1]	大部分是清痰
2006年2月11日	电话	咳嗽 呼吸困难 痰液产生 脓痰	改善[2] 改善[2] 改善[2] 大部分是清痰[1]	改善 改善 改善 大部分是清痰

注：1 日志条目于2008年6月24日被修改；2 日志条目于2006年11月被修改。

我们注意到，以上以脚注1或2标示的项目，原始记录中的信息在受试者已经完成研究之后（研究于2006年3月7日完成）被修改。关于2008年6月24日所做的修改，记录显示该数据修改是由研究协调员（b）（6）完成的，然而根据递交给中心的报告，他并未参与原始研究。此外，FDA在审查这位受试者的原始记录后，不能确定贵研究场所从何处获得相关信息，以证实贵研究场所对原始记录所做的修改（即慢性支气管炎急性加重相关体征和症状的评估日志）。

E. 受试者0010，2006年4月13日基线诊室访视

加重前的体征和症状	（b）（4）原始文件	病例报告表(CRF)
咳嗽	不存在*	轻度
痰液产生	不存在*	轻度
脓痰	不存在*	中度（又名黏液脓痰）

以上以*号标示的项目，原始文件于2008年6月24日，即研究完成两年后，由研究协调员（b）（6）修改，然而根据递交给中心的报告，他并未参与最初的研究。

F. 受试者0012，2006年6月27日治疗访视检查

临床症状	慢性支气管炎急性加重(AECB)相关的体征和症状的评估日志	病例报告表(CRF)
痰液产生	黏痰*	不存在

以上以*标示的项目，原始文件于2008年7月2日，即研究完成两年后，由研究协调员（b）（6）修改，然而根据递交给研究场所的报告，他并未参与原始研究。FDA在审查这位受试者的原始记录后，不能确定贵研究场所从何处获得相关信息，以证实贵研究场所对原始记录所做的修改（即慢性支气管炎急性加重相关症状和体征的评估日志）。

G. 受试者0015，2006年7月14日诊室访视期间

临床症状	慢性支气管炎急性发作相关的体征和症状评估日志	病例报告表
咳嗽	一样	重度
呼吸困难	改善	中度
痰液产生	改善	中度
脓痰	浑浊/脓痰 黏痰未作为反应勾选	黏痰

目前还不清楚在受试者完成研究后，贵研究场所如何或为何更改原始文件。鉴于贵研究场所被稽查的原始文件和病例报告表（CRF）中出现的多处信息不准确，FDA无法认定贵研究场所收集的数据具有可靠性。

2. 您未能按 21 CFR 50 的要求获得每位受试者的知情同意［21 CFR 312.60］

21 CFR 312.60规定，研究者必须按照21 CFR第50部分征得每一位受试者的知情同意。FDA法规21 CFR 50.20规定，除符合21 CFR 50.23和21 CFR 50.24规定的情况下，研究者必须在征得由受试者或其合法授权代表签署的具有法律效力的知情同意书后，方可将受试者入组研究。法规明确指出，研究者只有在给潜在受试者或其代表充分考虑是否参加研究的机会，且最小化强迫或施加影响的可能的情况下，才能征求知情同意。FDA法规50.27进一步规定，知情同意书须使用由伦理委员会（IRB）批准的书面同意文件的格式，由受试者或其代表在充分阅读后签署。

受试者0004在2006年2月7日签署了最初的书面知情同意书，并入组该研究。伦理委员会（IRB）于2006年3月1日致信贵研究场所，告知其已批准了2006年2月17日版的知情同意书，该版本中对风险部分做出了修

改。伦理委员会（IRB）在信中进一步提出，现有和新的受试者均须签署更新的知情同意书。FDA在检查过程中没有找到记录表明贵研究场所让当时仍入组试验的受试者0004重新签署了更新的知情同意书，以告知其受试者可能承受的额外风险。

3. 您未能进行研究或者确保按照研究计划进行研究［21 CFR 312.60］

A. 试验方案修订2和3指出，接受包括但不仅限于HMG-CoA还原酶抑制剂（如辛伐他汀、洛伐他汀或阿托伐他汀）联合治疗药物的受试者将被排除在研究之外。此外，两个试验方案均指出，在研究的过程中，应避免HMG-CoA还原酶抑制剂与泰利霉素的联合用药。在审查的10位受试者记录中，5位受试者（受试者0001，0005，0010，0015和0017）的原始记录表明，虽然他们在入组研究前正接受HMG-CoA还原酶抑制剂联合疗法，或在入组研究后开始使用上述疗法，他们依然被入组了该研究。

关于受试者0001，一份原始文件中指出，您的研究协调员于2006年2月7日通过电话联系研究申办者，就该受试者已开始使用试验药物，但直至试验的第2天才停止使用HMG-CoA抑制剂的情况，询问是否应该让其退出研究。在一封日期为2006年2月7日的电子邮件中，申办者就您的研究协调员提出的问题回复，该受试者无需退出研究。但是，FDA在审查记录后发现，您的研究协调员向申办者提出问题的时候，受试者0001已经使用了所有试验药物（2006年1月28日），完成治疗访视检查（2006年2月2日），仅剩随访还未进行。此外，记录显示HMG-CoA抑制剂并未向申报者报告的那样在研究的第2天停止使用。

B. 试验方案修订3指出，入组研究的受试者需有气流阻塞的证据（当前加重前一年内，或当前加重过程中以及恢复后再次被确诊），其定义为：

1秒钟用力呼气容积（FEV1）占预计值%＞35。

1秒钟用力呼气容积（FEV1）与用力肺活量（FVC）之间的比值＜0.70。

原始记录表明，受试者0017的FEV1/FVC比值为0.72，因此不符合入组标准，且未得到申办者给予的可允许其参加研究的豁免，但是贵研究场所仍将该受试者随机入组到研究中。

C. 试验方案修订3指出，试验药物必须存储在限制出入的区域或上锁的柜子中，适宜的环境条件为≤25°C（77°F）。我们检查发现，2006年4月6日后，没有记录可以证实试验药物根据试验方案的要求妥善储存。因此，FDA无法确认2006年4月6日之后发放给受试者的试验药物的完整性。

D. 受试者0021于申办者“暂停”研究期间签署知情同意书并入组研究。（b）（4）在2006年12月22日的一份传真中告知贵研究场所，FDA咨询委员会开会讨论了泰利霉素的使用后，（b）（4）和（b）（4）决定从试验方案中去除泰利霉素，不再将其作为活性对照药物。信中特别指出：“对您最直接的就是截至写下本信时，暂停对现有试验方案的受试者入组。此次暂停并非监管机构要求。互动语音应答系统（IVRS）将暂时‘关闭’，您将无法对受试者进行随机分组。现已参与研究的所有受试者应完成所有计划访视。”在贵研究场所找到的记录显示（b）（4）直至2007年2月27日才取消了暂停入组。

原始文件显示，贵研究场所于2007年1月5日，即申办者要求暂停期间，将受试者0021招募入组，并对其执行了与研究相关的程序，包括但不限于记录生命体征，记录病史、进行肺功能测试，拍胸部X射线片，收集痰液和实验室样本，审查受试者是否有资格入组研究。检查中找到的病程记录显示，直至贵研究场所人员试图使用IVRS系统将受试者随机分组进入研究时，才发现由于（b）（4）已暂停使用IVRS系统对受试者进行随机分组，因此无法完成上述工作。根据在贵研究场所获得的记录显示，贵研究场所于2006年12月22日，即该受试者入组之前，已得知申办者已经暂停试验方案的受试者招募，贵研究场所不应将受试者0021入组研究。

4. 您未能确保符合适用法规要求的IRB负责对临床研究进行跟踪审查和批准［21 CFR 312 66］

根据伦理委员会（IRB）发送给贵研究场所的最初批准函IRB已经通知贵研究场所，研究于2007年1月3日到期。我们注意到，您的研究场所在日期为2007年1月31日的信中获知IRB已批准对研究的跟踪审查。因此，在2007年1月3日和2007年1月31日之间，贵研究场所并未被告知研究的跟踪审查被再次批准，故在这段时间内，贵研究场所不应再入组任何新的受试者。而如上所述，贵研究场所于2007年1月5日入组了受试者0021。

本警告信的目的并非是罗列您对试验药物临床研究中存在的所有缺陷。确保遵循法律和相关FDA法规的每一项要求是您的职责。您应当解决这些缺陷，并建立规程，以确保任何正在进行或将来的研究均能符合FDA的法规。

自收到这封信的15个工作日内，您应当书面告知本办公室为预防将来发生类似违规情况已经采取或将会采取的措施。如果不能充分地、及时地解释上述违规问题，可能导致我们在不再通知的情况下采取监管措施。

附：英文原文

Hijazi, Saad, M.D.

WARNING LETTER

May 19, 2009

CERTIFIED MAIL
RETURN RECEIPT REQUESTED

Ref.: 09-HFD-45-05-01

Saad Hijazi, M.D.
1151 Hospital Way
Building D, Suite 100
Pocatello, ID 83201-5091

Dear Dr. Hijazi:

Between October 27 and December 2, 2008, Mr. Thomas Gordon, representing the Food and Drug Administration (FDA), conducted an investigation to review your conduct of a clinical investigation (Protocol **(b)(4)** entitled **(b)(4)** performed for **(b)(4)**).

This inspection is a part of the FDA's Bioresearch Monitoring Program, which includes inspections designed to evaluate the conduct of research and to ensure that the rights, safety, and welfare of the human subjects of those studies have been protected.

From our review of the establishment inspection report and the documents submitted with that report, we conclude that you did not adhere to the applicable statutory requirements and FDA regulations governing the conduct of clinical investigations. We are aware that at the conclusion of the inspection, Mr. Gordon provided and discussed with you Form FDA 483, Inspectional Observations. We wish to emphasize the following:

1. You failed to maintain adequate and accurate case histories that record all observations and other data pertinent to the investigation on each individual [21 CFR 312.62(b)].

In FDA's review of the source documents for the records audited during the inspection, there were numerous instances where either (a) information entered into the case report forms (CRFs) did not match the information in the source documents or (b) information in the source documents was changed after the subject had completed the study, up to two years post-completion, and it could not be determined where the information related to the change was derived. Examples include but were not limited to the following:

A. For Subject #0001:

Date of visit	Type of contact with subject	Clinical symptom	AECB related signs and symptoms assessment log	CRF
January 25, 2006	Telephone contact	Dyspnea	Worse	Same
		Sputum Production	Same	Worse
		Sputum Purulence	Mostly clear[1]	yellow, green, cloudy and thick
January 26, 2006	Telephone contact	Cough	Worse[2]	Worse
		Dyspnea	Worse[2]	Same
		Sputum Production	Same	Worse
February 13, 2006	Clinic visit	Cough	Absent	Mild
		Wheezing	Mild[1]	Mild
		Rales	Mild[1]	Mild

1 Log entry changed on March 15, 2006

2 No date to show when the information was changed on the Log

For those items noted with the footnotes [1] or [2] above, we note that the information in the source record was changed after the subject had already completed the study (study completion February 13, 2006). FDA's review of the source records for this subject could not determine where your site obtained the information to corroborate the noted changes your site made to the original source record (i.e. the AECB related signs and symptoms assessment log).

B. For Subject #0002:

Date of visit	Type of contact with subject	Clinical symptom	AECB related signs and symptoms assessment log	CRF
January 29, 2006	Telephone	Cough	Improved[1]	Improved
		Dyspnea	Improved[1]	Improved
		Sputum Production	Improved[1]	Improved
January 31, 2006	Clinic visit	Sputum Production	Mild[1]	Mild
		Sputum Purulence	Yellow, green, cloudy and thick	Nothing Listed
		Wheezing	Mild[1]	Mild
		Rales	Mild[1]	Mild
		Ronchi	Absent[1]	Absent
		Decreased Breath Sounds	Absent[1]	Absent

1 Log entry changed on March 16, 2006

For those items noted with the footnote [1], the information in the source record was changed after the subject had already completed the study (study completion February 14, 2006). FDA's review of the source records for this subject could not determine where your site obtained the information to corroborate the noted changes your site made to the original source record (i.e. the AECB related signs and symptoms assessment log).

C. For Subject #0003:

Date of visit	Type of contact with subject	Clinical symptom	AECB related signs and symptoms assessment log	CRF
February 6, 2006	Telephone	Cough	Nothing listed	Improved
		Dyspnea	Nothing listed	Improved
		Sputum Production	Nothing listed	Improved
		Sputum Purulence	Nothing listed	Mostly Clear

Per the protocol deviation form sent to the IRB, you noted that for the telephone contact your site made to Subject #0003 on February 6, 2006, you did not capture the AECB signs and symptoms of disease. As your site did not capture the AECB signs and symptoms of disease, it could not be determined how you could have reported information to the CFR.

D. For Subject #0004:

Date of visit	Type of contact with subject	Clinical symptom	AECB related signs and symptoms assessment log	CRF
February 10, 2006	Telephone	Sputum Purulence	Mostly Clear[1]	Mostly Clear
February 11, 2006	Telephone	Cough	Improved[2]	Improved
		Dyspnea	Improved[2]	Improved
		Sputum Production	Improved[2]	Improved
		Sputum Purulence	Mostly Clear[1]	Mostly clear

1 Log entry changed on June 24, 2008

2 Log entry changed in November 2006

For those items noted with the footnotes [1] or [2] above, we note that the information in the source record was changed after the subject had already completed the study (study completion March 7, 2006). With respect to the changes made on June 24, 2008, records indicate the changes were made by study coordinator **(b)(6)**, who per the report to the Center, was not a part of the original study. In addition, FDA' s review of the source records for this subject could not determine where your site obtained the information to corroborate the noted changes your site made to the original source record (i.e. the AECB related signs and symptoms assessment log).

E. For Subject #0010, for the baseline office clinic visit on April 13, 2006:

Pre-Exacerbation signs and symptoms	(b)(4) Source Document	CRF
Cough	Absent*	Mild
Sputum Production	Absent*	Mild
Sputum Purulence	Absent*	Moderate (aka mucopurulent)

For those items noted with an * above, the changes to the source document were made on June 24, 2008, two years after the completion of the study, by study coordinator **(b)(6)**, who per the report to the Center, was not a part of the original study.

F. For Subject #0012 for the Test of Cure Visit on June 27, 2006:

Clinical symptom	AECB related signs and symptoms assessment log	CRF
Sputum Purulence	Mucoid*	Absent

For the item noted with an * above, the change to the source document was made on July 2, 2008, two years after the completion of the study, by study coordinator **(b)(6)**, who per the report to the Center, was not a part of the original study. FDA' s review of the source records for this subject could not determine where your site obtained the information to corroborate the noted changes your site made to the original source record (i.e. the AECB related signs and symptoms assessment log).

G. For Subject #0015, for the during study clinic visit on July 14, 2006:

Clinical symptom	AECB related signs and symptoms assessment log	CRF
Cough	Same	Severe
Dyspnea	Improved	Moderate
Sputum Production	Improved	Moderate
Sputum Purulence	Cloudy/thick Mucoid not circled as a response.	Mucoid

It is unclear how or why changes to source documents were made at your site following subject completion from the study. Given the numerous inaccuracies noted in the source documents and CRFs audited at your site, FDA is unable verify the integrity of data collected at your site.

2. You failed to obtain the informed consent of each human subject in accordance with 21 CFR part 50 [21 CFR 312.60].

Under 21 CFR 312.60, an investigator is required to obtain the informed consent of each human subject in accordance with 21 CFR part 50. FDA's regulations at 21 CFR 50.20 state that except as provided in 21 CFR 50.23 and 21 CFR 50.24, no investigator may involve a human being as a subject in research covered by the regulations unless the investigator has obtained the legally effective informed consent of the subject or the subject's legally authorized representative. The regulation specifies that an investigator shall seek such consent only under circumstances that provide the prospective subject or the subject's representative sufficient opportunity to consider whether or not to participate and that minimize the possibility of coercion or undue influence. Section 50.27 of FDA' s regulations further provide that informed consent shall be documented by the use of a written consent document approved by the IRB, which is to be signed by the subject or subject's representative only after the subject or the subject's representative is given adequate opportunity to read the document.

Subject #0004 signed the original informed consent form to be enrolled into the study on February 7, 2006. In a letter dated March 1, 2006, the IRB informed your site that they had approved informed consent form version 021706 which included modifications that were made to the risks section. The IRB's letter further stated that current and new subjects were to sign the revised informed consent form. There was no documentation found during the FDA inspection to show that your site re-consented Subject #0004, who was still enrolled into the study at the time, with the revised informed consent form to inform them of the possible additional risks the subject may experience.

3. You failed to conduct the studies or ensure they were conducted according to the investigational plan [21 CFR 312.60].

A. Protocol Amendment #2 and #3 stated that subjects receiving concomitant therapy with medications including but not limited to HMG-CoA reductase inhibitors (e.g. simvastatin, lovastatin, or atorvastatin) were to be excluded from the study. In addition, both protocols noted that during the study, concomitant administration of HMG-CoA reductase inhibitors with telithromycin should be avoided. For five of ten subject records reviewed (Subject #0001, #0005, #0010, #0015, and #0017), source records indicate that these subjects were enrolled into the study even though they were either receiving concomitant therapy with HMG-CoA reductase inhibitors prior to enrollment into the study or began their use after your site had enrolled them into the study.

With respect to Subject #0001, a source document noted that your study coordinator contacted via telephone, the study sponsor, on February 7, 2006 requesting information as to whether this subject who had started study medication but did not discontinue the use of a HMG-CoA inhibitor until Day 2 should be withdrawn from the study. In an email dated February 7, 2006, the sponsor noted that subsequent to the question posed by your study coordinator, this subject should not be discontinued from the study. In review of the records, however, FDA notes that by the time the question was posed by your study coordinator to the sponsor, Subject #0001 had completed taking all study drug (January 28, 2006), completed the test of cure visit (February 2, 2006) and only had the follow up visit remaining. In addition, records indicate that the HMG-CoA inhibitor was not withdrawn on Day 2 of the study as was reported to the sponsor.

B. Protocol Amendment #3 stated that to be included into the study, the subject was to have evidence of airflow obstruction (within the year prior to the current exacerbation or during the current exacerbation and then reconfirmed after recovery), defined as:

- Forced expiratory volume in one second (FEV1) % predicted $>$ 35 and
- Ratio of FEV1 to forced vital capacity (FVC) $<$ 0.70

Source records indicate that Subject #0017 had an FEV1/FVC ratio of 0.72 and thus did not meet this inclusion criterion and further was also not granted a waiver by the sponsor for enrollment into the study, but your site continued to randomize the subject into the study.

C. Protocol Amendment #3 stated that the study drug was to be stored in a limited access area or in a locked cabinet under appropriate environmental conditions at or below 25°C (77°F). Our inspection found that there were no records after the date of April 6, 2006 to confirm that the study medication was stored appropriately per the protocol requirements. Therefore, FDA is unable to confirm the integrity of the investigational product that was dispensed to the subjects following April 6, 2006.

D. Subject #0021 was consented and enrolled into the study during a time when the study was placed on "hold" by the sponsor. In a fax dated December 22, 2006 to your site, (b)(4) informed you that due to an FDA advisory committee meeting that discussed the use of telithromycin, (b)(4) and (b)(4) made the decision to remove telithromycin as the active comparator drug from the protocol. The letter specifically stated "What this means most immediately to you is that enrollment in the current protocol will be temporarily stopped as of the writing of this letter. This is not a regulatory "hold" in that no regulatory agency has requested this action. The Interactive Voice Response System (IVRS) will be temporarily "shut off" and you will be unable to randomize any further subjects. Any subjects currently active in the study should complete all scheduled visits". Documentation found at your site showed that this hold on enrollment was not removed by (b)(4) until February 27, 2007.

Source documents show that your site enrolled Subject #0021 into the study on January 5, 2007 during the time of the sponsor's hold and further that your site performed study related procedures including but not limited to taking vitals, performing a medical history, spirometry test and chest x-ray, collecting sputum and laboratory samples, and reviewing the subject's eligibility into the study. Per the progress note found during the inspection, it was only after someone at your site contacted the IVRS to try to randomize this subject were you were unable to do so as (b)(4) had temporarily stopped randomization of subjects into the study using the IVRS. As records obtained at your site showed that your site had been informed on December 22, 2006, prior to this subject's enrollment, that the sponsor had temporarily stopped enrollment of subjects into the protocol, your site should not have enrolled Subject #0021 into the study.

4. You failed to assure that an Institutional Review Board (IRB) complying with applicable regulatory requirements was responsible for the continuing review and approval of a clinical study [21 CFR 312.66].

Per the original IRB approval letter sent to your site, the IRB had informed your site that the study expired on January 3, 2007. We note that your site was informed of the IRB's approval of the continuing review of the study in a letter dated January 31, 2007. Thus, between January 3, 2007 and January 31, 2007, your site had not been informed that the study was re-approved for continuing review and thus during this time your site should not have enrolled any new subjects into the study. As noted above, your site enrolled Subject #0021 into the study on January 5, 2007.

This letter is not intended to be an all-inclusive list of deficiencies with your clinical study of an investigational drug. It is your responsibility to ensure adherence to each requirement of the law and relevant FDA regulations. You should address these deficiencies and establish procedures to ensure that any on-going or future studies will be in compliance with FDA regulations.

Within fifteen (15) working days of your receipt of this letter, you should notify this office in writing of the actions you have taken or will be taking to prevent similar violations in the future. Failure to adequately and promptly explain the violations noted above may result in regulatory action without further notice.

If you have any questions, please contact Tejashri Purohit-Sheth, M.D., at 301-796-3402; FAX 301-847-8748. Your written response and any pertinent documentation should be addressed to:

Tejashri Purohit-Sheth, M.D.
Branch Chief
Good Clinical Practice Branch Ⅱ
Division of Scientific Investigations
Office of Compliance
Center for Drug Evaluation and Research
Food and Drug Administration
Bldg 51, Room 5358
10903 New Hampshire Avenue

Silver Spring, MD 20993

Sincerely yours,

/S/

Leslie K. Ball, M.D.
Director
Division of Scientific Investigations
Office of Compliance
Center for Drug Evaluation and Research

第 128 封　给 Hernandez, Francisco 医学博士的警告信

2009年4月20日

参考号：09-HFD-45-04-02

尊敬的Hernandez博士：

2008年2月19日至2008年3月13日，Dianiris Ayala女士代表FDA进行了现场检查，并对您实施的试验药物为赖谷胰岛素（艾倍得）、申办者为美国赛诺菲-安万特的下列临床研究进行了审查。

- 试验方案［（b）（4）］：每日注射一次、两次、三次速效胰岛素注射液艾倍得（赖谷胰岛素）联合来得时及口服增敏剂基础疗法治疗2型糖尿病：一项多中心、随机、平行和开放的临床研究。
- 试验方案［（b）（4）］：将来得时（甘精胰岛素）作为基础胰岛素治疗2型糖尿病的成年患者的餐前和餐后艾倍得（赖谷胰岛素）治疗比较：一项多中心、随机、平行和开放的临床研究。

本次现场检查是FDA的生物研究监查项目的一部分。该项目通过设定的检查方法，评估研究的实施情况，以确保这些研究中受试者的权益、安全和福利得到了保护。

经对FDA现场检查报告、该报告的附件，以及您2008年4月16日对FDA 483表的书面回复，您2008年6月14日和2008年10月6日的书面回复进行审查，我们认为，您没有遵循适用的法律要求和监管临床研究实施及受试者保护的FDA法规。我们获知，在现场检查结束时，Ayala女士向您出示并讨论了FDA 483表，即现场检查发现的问题。我们想强调以下几点：

1. 您未能确保按照签署的研究者声明和研究计划进行研究［21 CFR 312.60］

关于试验方案［（b）（4）］：

a. 试验方案［（b）（4）］中随机的15名受试者中，有12名违背方案的入组/排除标准而入组，详细描述如下：

i. 试验方案排除上一年度使用胰岛素的受试者，以下这些受试者在他们第一次到达临床中心时报告使用胰岛素，但是全部违背试验方案的入组/排除标准而入组：

（1）受试者3511-001虽然于2006年6月5日接受6单位的优泌乐皮下注射，但是在2006年8月7日签署知情同意并被筛选。

（2）受试者3511-005于2006年8月14日接受5单位的诺和锐皮下注射，同一天签署知情同意并被筛选。

（3）受试者3511-011于2006年10月17日接受诺和锐皮下注射，同一天签署知情同意并被筛选。

（4）受试者3511-012于2006年10月18日接受5单位的优泌乐皮下注射，同一天签署知情同意并被筛选。

（5）受试者3511-013于2006年11月2日接受5单位的胰岛素皮下注射，同一天签署知情同意并被筛选。

（6）受试者3511-015于2006年11月22日接受8单位的诺和锐皮下注射，同一天签署知情同意并被筛选。

（7）受试者3511-016虽然于2006年11月15日接受7单位的优泌乐皮下注射，但是在2006年12月15日签署知情同意并被筛选。

（8）受试者3511-019于2007年1月22日接受4单位的胰岛素，同一天签署知情同意并被筛选。

在贵研究场所2009年4月16日的回复函中，您提到标准办公室规程要求当受试者有明确水平的高血糖时需要单次注射胰岛素。此外，您声称这些入组的受试者均是普通的门诊患者，这样做也是为了为了避免入组的“专业的临床受试者”。该回复也已收悉。但在入组前这一年内使用胰岛素违背方案的排除标准，且对试验结果有潜在的影响。在回复函中，贵研究场所提出了针对如何避免今后违背入组和排除标准的纠正措施。

您具体罗列了计划明确入组和排除标准，详细审查过往病历，并就处于临界值的受试者的入组决定与工作人员和申办者进行了详细讨论。此外，中心提出了区分标准操作规程和临床实践的一些纠正措施。若能如实落实，上述整改计划是可接受的。

ⅱ.方案中要求受试者参加入组筛选前口服至少3个月稳定剂量的2或3个下面药物：磺酰脲类药物、双胍类药物、噻唑烷二酮类药物。

下列受试者是违背标准而入组的：

（1）受试者3511-007一直到签署知情同意和筛选之前，没有按照方案要求口服稳定剂量的上述种类的口服药物，却口服了Glyset米格列醇，这是研究中不被允许的口服药物。

Glyset（米格列醇）是一种α-葡萄苷酶抑制剂，而不是磺酰脲类，双胍类或噻唑烷二酮类药，在贵研究场所2008年4月16日的回复函中指出Glyset（米格列醇）在方案中没有被列入排除药物，但即使如此仍然违背了研究方案。也就是说，受试者并没有口服2～3个稳定剂量的下列种类的药物：磺酰脲类药物、双胍类药物、噻唑烷二酮类药物。若能切实执行，贵研究场所的关于避免未来就纳入和排除标准的违规行为的纠正措施是可以接受的。

（2）受试者3511-012，同样没有按照方案要求口服稳定剂量的上述种类的口服药物，却口服了米格列醇，这是在获得知情和筛选前不被批准的口服药物。

如上文1. a. ⅱ（1）所述，贵研究场所关于米格列醇不被列入排除药物的声明与是否违反方案并不相干，即受试者没有口服2～3个稳定剂量的方案要求的下列种类的药物（磺酰脲类药物、双胍类药物、噻唑烷二酮类药物），另外，贵研究场所为避免以后在入组和排除标准方面的违规行为采取的纠正措施的计划业已收悉。

b. 研究过程中发现的疾病、伴发疾病的恶化及伴随用药没有按照方案规定报告。

具体而言：

ⅰ. 受试者3511-008由于病毒性感染并发症（肺炎）于2006年12月入院，直到2007年7月13日，这一严重不良事件才报给申办者。根据方案，导致住院治疗或延长已有住院治疗的不良事件均被认为是严重不良事件（SAE）。同样，方案要求SAE必须记录在“严重不良事件或临床试验快速报告”表中，24小时内传真给申办者的药物警戒性部门，并抄送给研究监查员。严重不良事件或临床试验快速报告表记录受试者肺炎不良事件始于［（b）（6）］，止于［（b）（6）］。但是，此表日期为2007年7月13日，大约在不良事件之后的6个半月时间。

在2008年4月16日的回复函中指出，您提到与医院访视相关的细节和相关诊断具有不确定性，且获得这方面的核实花费了超预期的时间，您同时也声称研究协调员不清楚不良事件一经发现就需要立即报告，即使只能提供一般性描述。然而，作为临床研究者，您有责任按照批准的方案执行相关研究。该SAE并未按照方案的要求进行报告。在您的回复函中提供了一个纠正措施，避免以后此类事件的发生，即有任何不利事件立即报告，不管重要性如何或与试验药物相关与否均需立即报告，并更新后续信息。如果能够落实，此纠正措施是可接受的。

ⅱ. 受试者3511-019的病例报告表（CRF）中缺少使用欣百达的报告信息和相应地使用此药物的临床情况。根据方案，除试验药物外，受试者进入研究或研究期间的任何时间的治疗，都应该视作伴随治疗，记录在CRF相关页码中。

在您2008年4月16日的回复函中，您提出研究后期发现了一些慢性疾病药物（包括精神药物，即抗抑郁药），这些药物用在了非精神病原因的地方，如神经性疼痛。该回复已经收悉。但是，受试者3511-019使用了欣百达，不论何时使用此药物或适应症为何，都没有按照方案要求记录在CRF中。您提供了计划，以理顺工作人员对记录的管理，并提供了政策确保随访结束后作出修订并将材料正确放回受试者记录。此外，您还提供了记录针对质疑进行修改和提交的次数的措施，您的纠正措施收悉并可以接受。

关于试验方案［（b）（4）］：

c. 试验方案［（b）（4）］中随机抽查了7个受试者，有3个入组受试者违背方案的入组和排除标准，以下为这些受试者的细节描述。

该试验方案需要排除在入组前3个月内服用磺酰脲类、噻唑烷二酮类，或其他任何口服治疗糖尿病药物的受试者，服用胰岛素类似物伴随或不伴随使用二甲双胍的受试者不包含在内。以下受试者违背了本试验方案的排除标准，他们服用了这些被排除的口服抗糖尿病药物，却被筛选和入组这项研究中。

（1）受试者3503-0005服用文迪雅（马来酸罗格列酮，一种噻唑烷二酮类药物）直到2006年4月10日，随后在2006年6月5日签署知情同意并通过筛选进入研究。

（2）受试者3503-0007服用梵蒂美锭（马来酸罗格列酮，一种噻唑烷二酮类药物和盐酸二甲双胍）直到2006年5月22日，随后在2006年6月8日签署知情同意并通过筛选进入研究。

（3）受试者3503-0009服用文迪雅（马来酸罗格列酮，一种噻唑烷二酮类药物）直到2006年6月12日，在同一天他签署知情同意并被筛选。

贵研究场所在2008年4月16日的回复函中表示：根据贵研究场所的审查，受试者可能未使用这些被排除药物并达3个月以上，但日期却没有明确的记录。该回复已收悉。然而，上述研究记录中的日期表明：上述3位受试者使用被排除的药物是在进入试验前的3个月内。如上所示，在回复函中提出了对于未来研究中可以避免违反有关入组和排除标准的修正措施。具体而言，贵研究场所提出计划列明入组和排除标准，彻底审查过往病史，在入组决策之前与工作人员和申办者详细讨论临界候选人。如切实执行，这些纠正措施可以被接受。

d. 在研究过程中所发现的疾病，以及伴发疾病在研究期间的恶化，伴随药物都没有按照试验方案的要求被记录在案。具体而言：

受试者3503-0010由于起搏器部位感染所导致心力衰竭的严重不良事件，并没有按照方案的要求在24小时内报告给申办者。按照方案，“严重不良事件/临床试验快速报告”表格应该是在24小时内完成并传真至申办者的药物安全监察部门，并将传真副本抄送至研究监查员。在临床试验中心完成的表格说明该不良反应事件是威胁受试者生命的，符合方案规定的严重不良事件的定义。不良事件开始日期的记录如［（b）（6）］所示，然而，该表格的填写日期却是2007年7月2日，大约是不良事件发生后的两个月。

在贵研究场所2008年4月16日的回复函中指出，医院记录和详细资料有时需要花费几个月时间才能获得，尽管贵研究场所已努力去争取最快，该回答已收悉。尽管如此，不论医院的记录和详细资料是否可以获得，这个严重不良反事件的一般性报告并没有在方案规定的24小时的时间段内开展和实施。在贵研究场所的回复函中提出了一个补救措施，以避免未来发生类似的事件。具体而言，贵研究场所描述了一个计划，利用现有的信息立即报告任何不良事件，无论是否意义重大或与试验药物是否相关的均立即上报，并随时更新，如切实实施，这些纠正措施可以被接受。

2. 您未能保存对研究中每个受试者的所有研究观察结果和其他相关数据的足够及准确的病历［21 CFR 312.62（b）］

a. 原始记录中审查和签署的日期和研究行为实际发生的日期存在差异，例如：

关于试验方案［（b）（4）］：

i. 受试者3511-018来到临床试验中心做6# 随访的时间是2007年4月23日，然而临床研究者登记原始记录的日期为2007年4月11日。

在贵研究场所2008年4月16日的回复函中指出，临床研究者偶尔在研究活动进行过程中会出现手写日期和签字，但是在其他日期打印表格，且没有以草签对差异作出任何解释。贵研究场所承认应该遵守和执行规范的记录形式。这一回答已收悉。然而，这并不能解释为什么受试者3511-018的6# 随访是发生在签署随访的原始记录之后。作为临床研究者，贵研究场所有责任保证原始记录的足够和准确。如前所述，贵研究场所提供了计划以理顺工作人员对记录的管理，制定政策确保随访结束后作出修改并将材料正确放回受试者记录。此外，贵研究场所还提供了纠正措施记录所有修改和回答质疑的次数，贵研究场所的纠正措施收悉并可以接受。

ⅱ. 受试者3511-002访视1#体检原始记录的日期为2006年8月8日，六个月之后即2007年2月8日修改增加关于存在心脏收缩期射出杂音的信息。该杂音是在2006年11月21日第5次随访的体检原始记录中被注意到。一份日期为2007年11月11日的备忘录文件中提到，主要研究者在该受试者1随访的体检原始记录因疏忽而未记录心脏异常情况，在第5次随访期间意识到错误时这份记录才发生了改变。然而，对1# 随访体检原始记录的日期进行修改的日期为2007年2月8日，与2007年11月11日的备忘录中说明改变开始发生的日期2006年11月21日并不一致。

在贵研究场所2008年4月16的回复函中承认，开始观察到杂音出现是在首次体检中，但是那次检查原始记录出现缺失，而随后的说明很难去评估发现杂音的具体时间。这一回答已经收悉，但FDA再一次重申，贵研究场所的责任是保存完整和准确的记录。如上2. a. ⅰ. 所述，如果切实执行，贵公司关于预防将来记录差异的纠正措施和计划是可以接受的。

关于试验方案［（b）（4）］：

ⅲ. 受试者3503-0001访视1# 体检是在2006年4月26日进行的。体检的原始记录在2006年5月10日被修改，加入了甲状腺可被触及的信息。然而没有相关的原始记录解释在体检实际发生后再做出修改的原因。我们注意到在您的回复函中并没有对这一项问题作出具体说明。

ⅳ. 受试者3503-0001发生甲状腺囊肿的不良事件被记录在患者报告中的日期为2006年9月21日，然而CRF里记录这个不良事件的开始日期是2007年8月22日。

在贵研究场所2008年4月16日的回复函中您指出，会对受试者随访正在进行过程中的病情，如甲状腺疾病，其确诊有时是在对于现有疾病的检查中完成的。贵研究场所指出，这些情况在试验地点被发现的时候应该记录下来，但是医院的记录和详细资料有时候需要数月才可获得，尽管贵方已努力争取更快。该回答已经收悉。然而，这并不能解释上述文件中所存在的矛盾。特别说明的是，它不足以解释为什么患者报告中记录甲状腺囊肿的日期是2006年9月21日，而CRF里记录的开始日期是2007年8月22日，几乎晚了一年之久。

b. 受试者3511-007的电子日志信息没有及时取回，因此在FDA检查期间，没有相关信息供审查，2007年3月1日的文件说明：从2006年11月1日到2006年12月4日期间所丢失的数据不可用是因为研究协调员从网站上打印阅读日志的失误，从而导致后来出现无法访问的情况。尽管如此，作为临床研究者，贵研究场所有责任确保记录的完整和准确。我们注意到在贵研究场所的回复函中没有对这一问题进行专门解决。

3. 您未能及时向伦理委员会报告给受试者或他人带来风险的所有非预期事件［21 CFR 312.66］

IRB要求严重不良事件需在贵研究场所发现此不良事件的三个工作日之内报告。贵研究场所并没有将下列严重不良事件要求的在三个工作日期限内上报伦理委员会：

关于试验方案［（b）（4）］：

a. 受试者3511-018于2006年12月因病毒感染（肺炎）住院。此严重不良事件没有报告给IRB。

关于试验方案［（b）（4）］：

b. 受试者3503-0010在［（b）（4）］因植入心脏起搏器住院，并在［（b）（4）］发生了继发性的植入部位感染。这些严重不良事件直到2007年7月31日才报告给IRB，大约是第一个可报告的严重不良事件3个月后。

在2008年4月16日的回复函中，您声称，尽管已经努力去获得有关医院访视和相关文档的详细内容，但还是很困难，且通常这个过程会花费比预期更长的时间。虽然我们承认这个很困难，但及时向IRB报告严重不良事件依旧是您作为研究者的责任，您提出的“通过理顺现场人员对记录的处理来预防未来的违规行为”之纠正措施已收悉。贵方表示，这些措施包括在随访结束后作出修改并确保材料正确放回到受试者记录中的政策。另外，贵方提出的“记录任何修改和回复质疑的次数，确保IRB等第三方以适时的方式接受数据”的措施，是可以接受的。

我们收到您2008年4月16日、6月14日、10月6日的回复函，以及您对可能导致上述违规事件的解释。特别是，我们收到您的声明，称您的临床研究协调员有个人问题，并且和临时临床研究协调员也有问题。此外，我们注意到在本次回复中，八个月的时间里贵研究场所共有六个不同的监查员。我们也收到了您已采取的或正在采取的纠正措施，特别是，我们承认在这些纠正措施中，一旦意识到有违规，您就停止了新的试验来解决违规，并从方案关联的工作中调离协调研究员，委派新的人员去完成待解决的问题，并使被授权研究者了解在研究实施过程中发现的监管漏洞。此外，我们还注意到您已经制订了将研究流程与临床实际操作分开的计划，以及对研究人员实施正式的培训。除了以上特别提到的外，是可以接受的。

本警告信的目的并非是罗列您在试验药物临床研究中存在的所有缺陷。确保遵循法律和相关FDA法规的每一项要求是您的职责。您应当解决这些缺陷，并建立规程，以确保任何正在进行或将来的研究均能符合FDA的法规。

自收到这封信的15个工作日内，您应当书面告知本办公室为预防将来发生类似违规情况已经或将要采取的措施。如果不能充分、迅速地解释上述违规问题，可能导致我们在不再通知的情况下采取监管措施。

附：英文原文

Hernandez, Francisco M.D.

WARNING LETTER

April 20, 2009

CERTIFIED MAIL
RETURN RECEIPT REQUESTED

Ref: 09-HFD-45-04-02

Francisco Hernandez, M.D.
777 E. 25th Street, Suite 118
Hialeah, FL 33013-3850

Dear Dr. Hernandez:

Between February 19, 2008 and March 13, 2008, Ms. Dianiris Ayala, representing the Food and Drug Administration (FDA), conducted an investigation and met with you, to review your conduct of the following clinical investigations of the investigational drug insulin glulisine (Apidra), performed for Sanofi-Aventis U.S.:

- Protocol [(b)(4)]: One versus two versus three daily rapid-acting insulin injections of Apidra® (insulin glulisine) as add-on to Lantus® and oral sensitizer basal therapy in type 2 diabetes: a multi-center, randomized, parallel, open-label clinical study; and
- Protocol [(b)(4)]: Apidra® (insulin glulisine administered premeal versus postmeal in adult subjects with type 2 diabetes mellitus receiving Lantus® (insulin glargine) as basal insulin: a multi-center, randomized, parallel, open-label clinical study.

This inspection is a part of the FDA's Bioresearch Monitoring Program, which includes inspections designed to evaluate the conduct of research and to ensure that the rights, safety, and welfare of the human subjects participating in those studies have been protected.

From our review of the establishment inspection report and the documents submitted with that report, your April 16, 2008 written response to Form FDA 483, your June 14, 2008 written response, and your October 6, 2008 written response, we conclude that you did not adhere to the applicable statutory requirements and FDA regulations governing the conduct of clinical investigations and the protection of human subjects. We are aware that at the conclusion of the inspection, Ms. Ayala presented and discussed with you Form FDA 483, Inspectional Observations.

We wish to emphasize the following:

1. You failed to ensure that the investigations were conducted according to the signed investigator statement and investigational plans [21 CFR 312.60].

Regarding Protocol [(b)(4)]:

a. Of fifteen subjects randomized in Protocol [(b)(4)], twelve subjects were enrolled in violation of protocol inclusion and exclusion criteria. The details for these subjects are described below.

ⅰ. The protocol excluded subjects that had received insulin within the prior year. The following subjects reportedly received insulin at their first visit to the clinical site, but were enrolled in the study in violation of protocol exclusion criteria:

(1)Subject # 3511-001 was consented and screened on August 7, 2006, even though he received 6 units of Humalog® subcutaneously on June 5, 2006.

(2)Subject # 3511-005 received 5 units of Novolog® subcutaneously on August 14, 2006, the same day she was consented and screened in the study.

(3)Subject # 3511-011 received Novolog® subcutaneously on October 17, 2006, the same day she was consented and screened in the study.

(4)Subject # 3511-012 received 5 units of Humalog® subcutaneously on October 18, 2006, the same day he was consented and screened in the study.

(5)Subject # 3511-013 received 5 units of insulin subcutaneously on November 2, 2006, the same day he was consented and screened in the study.

(6)Subject # 3511-015 received 8 units of Novolog® subcutaneously on November 22, 2006, the same day he was consented and screened in the study.

(7)Subject # 3511-016 was consented and screened on December 15, 2006, even though he received 7 units of Humalog® subcutaneously on November 15, 2006.

(8)Subject # 3511-019 received 4 units of insulin on January 22, 2007, the same day he was consented and screened in the study.

In your April 16, 2008 response letter, you noted that standard office procedures dictated that subjects receive an isolated dose of insulin when they presented with a defined level of hyperglycemia. Additionally, you stated that subjects were regular clinic patients who enrolled in research as subjects, and that this was an attempt to avoid the enrollment of "professional patients". Your responses are acknowledged. Nonetheless, the administration of insulin within the year prior to enrollment remains a violation of protocol exclusion criteria, and had the potential to influence study results. In your response letter, you proposed corrective measures to avoid future violations pertaining to inclusion and exclusion criteria. Specifically, you outlined plans to present inclusion and exclusion criteria, thoroughly review past medical histories, and discuss borderline candidates in detail with your staff and the sponsor prior to enrollment decision-making. Additionally, you proposed measures to provide a clear separation of study procedures and clinical practice visits. These corrective measures are acceptable if implemented as proposed.

ⅱ. The protocol required subjects to be on a stable dose of two or three of the following oral agents for at least three months before the screening visit: Sulfonylureas, Biguanides, or Thiazolidinediones. The following subjects were enrolled in the study in violation of this criterion:

(1) Subject # 3511-007 was not on a stable dose of the protocol-required classes of oral agents, but was reportedly using Glyset® (miglitol), an oral agent that was not approved for the study, up to the time of consent and screening.

In your April 16, 2008 response letter, you noted that Glyset® (miglitol) was not listed as an exclusionary medication in the protocol. While this is true, it is irrelevant to the protocol violation noted above, namely that the subject was not on a stable dose of two or three of the following classes of oral agents: sulfonylureas, biguanides, and thiazolidinediones. Glyset® is an alpha glucosidase inhibitor, and is not a sulfonylurea, biguanide, or thiazolidinedione. As noted in 1. a. i. above, your plan for corrective measures regarding violations pertaining to inclusion and exclusion criteria is acceptable if implemented as proposed.

(2) Subject #3511-012 was similarly not on a stable dose of the protocol-required classes of oral agents, but was

reportedly using Glyset® (miglitol), an oral agent that was not approved for the study, up to the time of consent and screening.

As noted in 1. a. ii. (1) above, your statement that Glyset® was not listed as an exclusionary medication is irrelevant to the protocol violation of the subject not having been on a stable dose of two or three of the protocol-required classes of oral agents (sulfonylureas, biguanides, and thiazolidinediones). Again, your plan for corrective measures to avoid future violations pertaining to inclusion and exclusion criteria is acknowledged.

b. Illnesses detected during the study, concomitant illnesses that worsened during the study, and concomitant medications were not reported as required by the protocol.

Specifically:

i. Subject # 3511-008 was hospitalized in December 2006 due to complications of a viral infection (pneumonia), but this serious adverse event was not reported to the sponsor until July 13, 2007. Per the protocol, an adverse event that required in-subject hospitalization or prolongation of existing hospitalization was considered a serious adverse event (SAE). As such, the protocol required this SAE to be recorded on the "Serious Adverse Event/ Expedited Report from a Clinical Trial" form, and faxed to the sponsor's Pharmacovigilance department within 24 hours, with a copy faxed to the study monitor. The "Serious Adverse Event/Expedited Report from a Clinical Trial" form documents that the subject's adverse event of pneumonia started on [(b)(6)], and ended on [(b)(6)]. However, the form is dated July 13, 2007, approximately six and a half months following the onset of the adverse event.

In your April 16, 2008 response letter, you noted that elucidating details pertaining to hospital visits and associated diagnoses were erratic, and obtaining verification took longer than expected. You also stated that it was not clear to your clinical research coordinator that there was a need to report these events immediately upon discovery even if only a general statement could be made. However, as clinical investigator, it was your responsibility to ensure the investigation was conducted according to the approved protocol. This SAE was not reported as required by the protocol. In your response letter, you proposed a corrective measure to avoid future occurrences of this nature, namely to use available information to immediately report any adverse event, regardless of significance or relation to the study drug, with updates to follow. This corrective measure is acceptable if implemented as proposed.

ii. Subject # 3511-019' s case report form (CRF) lacks information on the reported use of Cymbalta® and the clinical condition corresponding to the use of this medication. Per the protocol, all treatments taken by subjects on entry to the study, or at any time during the study, in addition to the investigational product, are regarded as concomitant treatments and must be documented on the appropriate pages of the CRF.

In your April 16, 2008 response letter, you indicated that some chronic medications were discovered late in the course of the study (including psychiatric medications, i.e., antidepressants), and that they had been in use for non-psychiatric reasons such as neuropathic pain. Your response is acknowledged. However, Subject #3511-019's use of Cymbalta® was not documented on the CRF as required by the protocol, regardless of when its use was discovered and its specific indication in this case. You have proposed a plan to clarify your staff member's handling of records, as well as a policy to make revisions and ensure that materials are returned properly to subject's charts at the conclusion of monitoring visits. Additionally, you proposed measures to record times of any revisions and submissions to queries. Your corrective measures are acknowledged and acceptable.

Regarding Protocol [(b)(4)]:

c. Of seven subjects randomized in Protocol [(b)(4)], three subjects were enrolled in violation of protocol inclusion and exclusion criteria. The details for these subjects are described below.

i. The protocol excluded subjects who were treated with sulfonylureas, thiazolidinediones, or any other oral antidiabetic drugs, except for insulin analogues with or without metformin, within the three months before study entry. The following subjects reportedly were treated with exclusionary oral antidiabetic agents and were screened and enrolled in the study, in violation of this exclusion criterion:

(1) Subject # 3503-0005 was treated with Avandia® (rosiglitazone maleate, a thiazolidinedione) until April 10, 2006, and was later consented and screened for the study on June 5, 2006.

(2) Subject # 3503-0007 was treated with Avandamet® (rosiglitazone maleate, a thiazolidinedione, and metformin hydrochloride) until May 22, 2006, and was later consented and screened on June 8, 2006.

(3) Subject # 3503-0009 was treated with Avandia (rosiglitazone maleate, a thiazolidinedione) until June 12, 2006, the same day he was consented and screened.

In your April 16, 2008 response letter, you indicated that based on your review, subjects were probably off treatment with these exclusionary medications for over three months, but that the dates were not clearly documented. Your response is acknowledged. However, the dates of use noted above were documented in study records, and indicate that these three subject' s use of the exclusionary medications was within three months prior to study entry, in violation of the protocol. As noted above, you proposed corrective measures to avoid future violations pertaining to inclusion and exclusion criteria in your response letter. Namely, you outlined plans to present inclusion and exclusion criteria, thoroughly review past medical histories, and discuss borderline candidates in detail with your staff and the sponsor prior to enrollment decision-making. These corrective measures are acceptable if implemented as proposed.

d. Illnesses detected during the study, concomitant illnesses that worsened during the study, and concomitant medications were not reported as required by the protocol. Specifically:

i. Subject # 3503-0010' s SAE of heart failure related to a pacemaker site infection was not reported to the sponsor in the 24-hour timeframe required by the protocol. Per the protocol, the "Serious Adverse Event/Expedited Report from a Clinical Trial" form was to be completed and faxed to the sponsor' s Pharmacovigilance department within 24 hours, with a copy faxed to the study monitor. The form completed at the clinical site documents that the adverse event was life-threatening, and therefore, met the protocol-specified definition of an SAE. The start date of the adverse event is documented as [(b)(6)]; however, the form is dated July 2, 2007, approximately two months after the onset of the adverse event.

In your April 16, 2008 response letter, you noted that hospital records and details sometimes took months to obtain despite efforts to secure them promptly. Your response is acknowledged. Nonetheless, general reporting of this SAE was not carried out within the protocol-specified 24-hour timeframe, regardless of whether hospital records and details were available. In your response letter, you proposed a corrective measure to avoid any such future occurrences. Specifically, you outlined a plan to use available information to immediately report any adverse event, regardless of significance or relation to the study drug, with updates to follow. This corrective measure is acceptable if implemented as proposed.

2. You failed to maintain adequate and accurate case histories that record all observations and other data pertinent to the investigation on each individual [21 CFR 312.62(b)].

a. There are discrepancies in the dates the source records were reviewed and signed and the dates when the study activities actually occurred. For example:

Regarding Protocol [(b)(4)]:

i. Subject # 3511-018 came to the clinical site on April 23, 2007 for visit # 6; however the source document was signed by the study coordinator on April 11, 2007.

In your April 16, 2008 response letter, you noted that it appeared that the clinical research coordinator occasionally dated and signed forms at the time study activities occurred, but printed forms on other dates, and that no initialing was done to explain any discrepancies. You acknowledged that proper record keeping should have been carried out. Your response is acknowledged. However, it does not explain how Subject #3511-018's visit #6 occurred after the source document for that visit was signed. As clinical investigator, it is your responsibility to ensure that adequate and accurate records are maintained. As stated earlier, you proposed a plan to clarify your staff member's handling of records, as well as a policy to make revisions and ensure that materials are returned properly to subject's charts at the conclusion of monitoring visits. Additionally, you proposed measures to record times of any revisions and submissions to queries. Your corrective measures are acknowledged and acceptable.

ii. Subject # 3511-002' s visit # 1 physical exam source documents dated August 8, 2006 were amended six months later, on February 8, 2007, to add information regarding the presence of a systolic ejection murmur. The murmur was noted on the November 21, 2006 physical exam source documents for visit # 5. A memo-to-file dated October 11, 2007 notes that the principal investigator inadvertently forgot to add the abnormal heart condition to the subject' s visit # 1 physical exam source documents, and that the records were changed during visit # 5 when the error was realized. However, given that the amendment to the visit #1 physical exam source document is dated February 8, 2007, the amendment does not comport with the October, 11, 2007 memo stating that the change was made on November 21, 2006.

In your April 16, 2008 response letter, you acknowledged this observation, stating that the murmur was observed during the original physical examination, but that the exam records failed to document it, and a later explanation was documented in such a way that it was difficult to assess the specific time of findings. Your response is acknowledged, and your responsibility to maintain adequate and accurate records is reiterated. As stated in 2. a. i. above, your plan for corrective actions to prevent future record keeping discrepancies is acceptable if implemented as proposed.

Regarding Protocol [(b)(4)]:

iii. Subject # 3503-0001' s visit # 1 physical exam was conducted on April 26, 2006. The physical exam source document was amended on May 10, 2006 to include information that the thyroid was palpable. However, no source documentation was included to explain the reason for the change after the actual evaluation was conducted. We note that you did not specifically address this observation in your response letters.

iv. Subject # 3503-0001' s adverse event of a thyroid cyst was documented in a patient note dated September 21, 2006. However, the CRF records the start date of this adverse event as August 22, 2007.

In your April 16, 2008 response letter, you indicated that subjects were followed for conditions that were in the process of being worked up, such as thyroid conditions, and that diagnoses were sometimes made during the course of the study for pre-existing conditions. You noted that these conditions should have been reported at the time your site was aware of them, but that hospital records and details sometimes took months to obtain despite efforts to secure them promptly. Your response is acknowledged. However, it does not explain the discrepancy in the documentation noted above. Specifically, it does not adequately explain how the thyroid cyst was documented in a patient note on September 21, 2006, but that the CRF recorded the start date as August 22, 2007, almost one year later.

b. The electronic diary information for Subject #3511-007 was not retrieved in a timely manner, such that the information was not available for review during the FDA inspection. A Note to File, dated March 1, 2007, indicates that missing data from November 1, 2006 to December 4, 2006 was not available due to the failure of the study coordinator to print the diary readings from the website, which was later rendered inaccessible. Nonetheless, as clinical investigator, you are required to maintain adequate and accurate study records. We note that you did not specifically address this observation in your response letters.

3. You failed to report promptly to the Institutional Review Board (IRB) all unanticipated problems involving risk to human subjects or others. [21 CFR 312.66].

The IRB required serious adverse events to be reported within three business days of your site becoming aware of the event. Your site failed to report the following SAEs to the IRB within the requisite three-day period:

Regarding Protocol [(b)(4)]:

a. Subject # 3511-018 was hospitalized in December 2006 due to a viral infection (pneumonia). This SAE was not reported to the IRB.

Regarding Protocol [(b)(4)]:

b. Subject # 3503-0010 was hospitalized for implantation of a pacemaker on [(b)(4)] and suffered a subsequent infection of the implant pocket on [(b)(6)]. These SAEs were not reported to the IRB until July 31, 2007, approximately three months after the start of the first reportable serious adverse event.

In your April 16, 2008 response letter, you indicated that your site had difficulty in obtaining details pertaining to hospital visits and associated documentation despite conscious efforts to obtain them, and that this process often took longer than expected. While we acknowledge this, it remains your responsibility as clinical investigator to report SAEs to the IRB in a timely manner. Your proposed corrective actions to prevent future violations through the clarification of site personnel' s record handling are acknowledged. You indicated that these measures include a policy to make revisions and ensure that materials are returned properly to subject' s charts at the conclusion of monitoring visits. Additionally, you proposed measures to record times of any revisions and submissions to queries such that third parties, such as the IRB, receive data in a timely manner. Your corrective measures are acceptable.

We acknowledge your April 16, June 14, and October 6, 2008 responses, and your explanations of the events that may have led to the violations noted herein. Specifically, we acknowledge your statement that your clinical research coordinator had personal problems, and that there were also problems with an interim clinical research coordinator. Additionally, we note your response that your site had six different monitors in a period of eight months. We also acknowledge corrective actions you have undertaken or are in the process of undertaking. Specifically, we acknowledge that among these actions, you halted new trials to address violations once you became aware, removed a clinical research coordinator from working with protocols, assigned new personnel to complete pending tasks, and made a sub-investigator aware of supervising flaws found in the course of study conduct. Additionally, we also note that you have instituted plans for the separation of study procedures and clinical practice visits as well as the implemention of formal training of study personnel. These corrective measures, in addition to those addressed specifically above, are acceptable.

This letter is not intended to be an all-inclusive list of deficiencies with your clinical study of an investigational drug. It is your responsibility to ensure adherence to each requirement of the law and relevant FDA regulations. You should address these deficiencies and establish procedures to ensure that any on-going or future studies will be in compliance with FDA regulations.

Within fifteen (15) working days of your receipt of this letter, you should notify this office in writing of the actions you have taken or will be taking to prevent similar violations in the future. Failure to adequately and promptly explain the violations noted above may result in regulatory action without further notice.

If you have any questions, please contact Constance Lewin, M.D., M.P.H., at 301-796-3397; FAX 301-847-8748. Your written response and any pertinent documentation should be addressed to:

Constance Lewin, M.D., M.P.H .
Branch Chief, Good Clinical Practice Branch I
Division of Scientific Investigations
Office of Compliance
Center for Drug Evaluation and Research
Food and Drug Administration
Bldg 51, Room 5354
10903 New Hampshire Avenue
Silver Spring, MD 20993

Sincerely yours,

{See appended electronic signature page}

Leslie K. Ball, M.D.
Director
Division of Scientific Investigations
Office of Compliance
Center for Drug Evaluation and Research

第129封 给Branitz, Bruce医学博士的警告信

2009年4月9日

参考号：09-HFD-45-03-03

尊敬的Branitz博士：

2007年9月14日至11月6日，Stephanie Hubbard女士代表FDA实施了调查，与您会面并审查了您实施的以下临床研究的情况：

试验方案［（b）（4）］，名称为“一项Ⅱ期、随机、多中心、安慰剂对照、双盲、剂量范围临床试验，旨在评估［（b）（4）］对治疗［（b）（4）］的有效性和安全性，试验药物为［（b）（4）］，申办者为［（b）（4）］，以及试验方案［（b）（4）］，名称为［（b）（4）］。

本次现场检查是FDA的生物研究监查项目的一部分。该项目通过设定的检查方法，评估研究的实施情况，以确保这些研究中受试者的权益、安全和福利得到了保护。

经对FDA现场检查报告、该报告的附件，以及您2007年11月23日的书面回复进行审查，我们认为，您没有遵循适用的法律要求和监管临床研究并保护受试者的FDA法规。在现场检查结束时，Hubbard女士向您出示并讨论了FDA 483表，即现场检查发现的问题。我们想强调以下几点：

1. 您未能按照研究计划进行研究［21 CFR 312.60］

试验方案［（b）（4）］

a. 下列受试者的入组是不合适的，因为按照方案他们的病情或实验室检查结果是应该被排除的：

i. 受试者8201的病例报告表筛选页中注明有右下叶肺癌，且LDH水平为242u/L。

ii. 2006年6月21日的实验室报告显示，2006年6月15日收集的受试者8202的筛选样本BUN和肌酐值分别为41mg/dL和1.8mg/dL。

iii. 2006年6月20日的实验室报告显示，2006年6月15日收集的受试者8204的筛选样本BUN值为36mg/dL。

iv. 受试者8205在入组研究时已有肺癌。

v. 2006年6月24日的实验室报告显示，2006年6月15日收集的受试者8208的筛选样本BUN和肌酐值分别为33mg/dL和1.6mg/dL。

vi. 2006年6月30日的实验室报告显示，2006年6月20日收集的受试者8209的筛选样本肌酐值为1.8mg/dL。

b. 方案要求按合格患者加入研究的顺序进行随机化。研究受试者没有按顺序进行随机化。例如，受试者8201，是第一个入组本研究的受试者，被分配的随机化号码10007并不是第一个随机数字。大部分剩余受试者也同样没有按顺序进行随机化。

上述方案违背的例子并非是对试验方案［（b）（4）］中受试者符合的所有排除标准的全部列表。类似违背情况在试验方案［（b）（4）］实施中也有被发现。例如，下列受试者的入组违背了方案：

c. 受试者0003和0014的病历中记载受试者有［（b）（4）］腺癌。但方案要求排除有（b）（4）癌症病史的受试者。

d. 受试者0002不符合入组标准，即在访视3前的5天研究日志中，每24小时平均8个或更多的［（b）（4）］，但在2006年7月24日访视3时被随机给予治疗并分发药品。

e. 受试者0002和0013，访视3日志记录他们不满足入组标准，即每天平均8个或更多的［（b）（4）］。

f. 基于受试者0005在访问3即受试者入组研究时的心电图，您记录该受试者有一个异常心电图，其重要性需要参考心脏病医生的意见。方案排除那些“有重大医学问题”的人员，包括心脏问题。该受试者入组该

研究时，没有对受试者异常心电图严重性的评估文件。

g．受试者0010的病程记录表明，受试者有［（b）（4）］腺癌、体外放射治疗［（b）（4）］和放射疗法植入物的病史。排除标准规定有［（b）（4）］癌或［（b）（4）］辐射治疗史的受试者不能参加研究。

h．受试者0010和0012的病程记录表明，受试者以前接受过达非那新治疗；因此这些受试者不满足入组标准，即受试者未使用过达非那新。

i．受试者0013，2007年6月27日采集的血样中的血糖浓度为219mg/dL。方案规定葡萄糖水平大于200 mg/dL具有临床意义，要进行随访以解决。转诊时传真给研究者的化验报告表明有“提示有未受控制的糖尿病的程度”。没有对该受试者进行糖尿病情随访的记录，违背了方案。

2. 您未能保存研究中每个受试者的所有研究观察结果和其他数据的完整和准确的病历［21 CFR 312. 62（b）］

试验方案［（b）（4）］

a. 关于受试者［（b）（4）］

i. 没有对访视1心电图的解释记录。访视6的心电图申请和心电图图谱是存在的；然而，申请中心脏病史部分没有完成，也没有对访视6心电图图谱进行审阅的记录。

ii. 日期为2006年6月7日的原始病历显示为正常心血管系统；但是，这个记录于2006年11月6日被修订为两例心脏搭桥手术。日期为2006年8月24日的方案偏差表显示存在一个下壁梗塞和可能的侧壁缺血。

iii. 有两份日志都记录了2006年6月14日到6月21日间的［（b）（4）］数量和严重性。目前还不清楚为什么受试者在这段时间完成了两份日志，此外，两份日志记录［（b）（4）］的数量和严重性是不一致的。完成了两份CRF来报告这些［（b）（4）］。这两份CRF记录的数据也不一致，并且有一份CRF不符合任何一份日志所报告的数据。另外，在受试者记录中查见一份手写的［（b）（4）］日志在数量和严重程度上不同于任何一份CRF记录的（b）（4）日志。这些多重的不一致，使我们无法确定这个受试者经历［（b）（4）］实际数量/严重性。

b. 受试者8202、8203、8205，在知情同意书中受试者签名旁的日期由初始的2006年6月8日改为2006年6月15日，受试者8202的日期又改回到2006年6月8日，这些受试者筛查访视的原始文件的大多数页面更改了日期，并没有提供文档来解释这些更改。

c. 对于受试者8203、8204、8205、8207和8208，研究协调员在多次研究访视的多次时间修改了Karnofsky评分数值，且没有提供文档解释这些更改。

d. 受试者8205的“病史”日期为2006年6月8日（后来修正为2006年6月15日）原始文档，显示为正常心血管和呼吸系统，然而，这个受试者的病史中包括原始文件提示有冠状动脉疾病、慢性阻塞性肺疾病（COPD）和肺癌。

e. 受试者8206的CRF筛选页最初显示正常呼吸、心血管、胃肠道、内分泌系统。2006年6月15日进行筛选访视。2007年5月10日CRF页被筛选修正为提示受试者有肺气肿、冠状动脉疾病、胃食管反流疾病、憩室炎、糖尿病。

f. 受试者8208的CRF病史筛选页记录呼吸系统的“咳嗽、鼻窦引流”和心血管系统的“阻塞”，所有其他系统都显示正常。受试者有高血压、冠状动脉疾病、成人型糖尿病、肺气肿、肾结石、异常心电图和实验室检测数据，这些情况没有在CRF病史筛选页中记录。2006年6月15日收集筛选的血液样本有众多临床实验室指标被记录为有临床意义；然而，CRF实验室评估筛选页中显示没有有临床意义上的实验检测值。这个受试者入组该研究中并接受治疗。

g. 受试者8209，2006年6月20日CRF病史筛选页中，最初提示所有的身体系统是正常的。2007年6月20日，CRF被修订为提示有慢性阻塞性肺病、尿道支架、肾结石、勃起功能障碍、膀胱过动症、膀胱癌、骨退化。没有文件表明已经对这些医疗问题进行评估，以确定受试者参与研究的资格。此外，2006年6月20日收集筛选的血液样本有众多临床实验室指标被记录为有临床意义；然而，实验室评估筛选CRF中显示没有有临床意义的实验室检测值。这个受试者在入组该研究并接受治疗。

h. 受试者8210，访视5的原始记录被划掉并注明“没有进行”，但是，您的2006年9月6日的病程记录中显示受试者参加了访视5，进行了研究相关的程序并且受试者返还了访视5日志。

试验方案［（b）（4）］

i. 受试者0003的CRF病史页指出，除了在寒冷的天气下需鼻窦引流，所有的身体系统，包括泌尿系统正常，然而，受试者病史包括有前列腺癌（包括经尿道前列腺切除术）、高血压、哮喘、肾结石和关节炎。

j. 受试者0010的CRF病史页指出所有的身体系统正常，然而，从另外一个提供者得到的受试者病史包括有前列腺癌、类风湿关节炎、高血压、胃炎和高胆固醇。

k. 受试者0011的日期为2007年5月16日的［（b）（4）］登记确认表和［（b）（4）］参考表提示，受试者上一次膀胱过动症（OAB）治疗包括使用奥西布丁缓释制剂；然而，日期为2007年10月15日的登记确认表提示受试者的上一次治疗OAB 药物是Detrol LA。

l. 受试者0012，患者既往治疗评估问卷调查表明，Detrol是最后使用的OAB药物，然而，［（b）（4）］参考表和［（b）（4）］登记确认表都表明，受试者最后使用的是奥西布丁缓释制剂。

受试者0012的病史提示，由于脊髓受到过枪伤，存在神经性膀胱功能障碍。排除标准第六条明确排除患有影响膀胱功能的神经疾病（包括脊髓损伤）的受试者。该受试者入组研究且接受了治疗。您在检查时表示受试者没有神经性膀胱功能障碍。然而，受试者的研究记录中没有相关文档。

受试者0012的访视1的实验室报告完成于2007年5月17日。然而，您在2007年5月15日草签了姓名和日期，代表已经审阅过这些记录。

m. 受试者0013的CFR病史页提示所有的身体系统是正常的，但受试者自诉报告有糖尿病、青光眼、心脏病、静脉疾病、肾脏疾病、心脏搭桥手术病史。

n. FDA检查员审查的诺华研究的电子CRF（eCRFs）显示存在不符情况。当FDA检查员要求提供eCRF的硬盘备份时，您无法提供eCRF副本。您的协调研究员告知我们的检查员，eCRFs由另一家公司保留，您不能访问eCRF数据库。因此，您不能证明您准备和保存了完整和准确的病历。

3. 您未能按 21 CFR 54 的要求获得知情同意［21 CFR 312.60 和 21 CFR 50］

受试者821于2006年6月12日被随机分配至试验方案［（b）（4）］。您直到2006年6月26日才获得这个受试者的知情同意。

4. 您未能保存足够的药物处置记录，包括日期、数量和受试者的使用情况［21 CFR 312.62（a）］

试验方案［（b）（4）］

a. 您没有保存足够的药物处置记录。例如，药物分发的总日志（MDDL）中不含任何受试者在访视5及以后的药物的计数文件。

b. 受试者8202，按照原始工作表和药物分发的日志（MDDL），其随机号为10002。在运单上标明发给随机号10002的瓶或盒号为248752，343193和218605，号码为24875，343193，218605的瓶标签也附在受试者8202的CRF标签页，表明这几个号码的药物瓶已经发给该受试者。运送单上标明瓶号899686的药物发给随机号10003的受试者，试验药物回收表格表明899686的药物没有返还，根据同一张表格，瓶号为343193也没有返还，患者编号“UNK”。瓶号248752的标签上的患者的标号和首字母被黑色涂抹。尽管如此，CRF记录受试者8202的依从性为100%。这些药物分发和记录不一致的结果是无法保证受试者［（b）（6）］的药物是按指定分发的，也无法保证受试者用药是符合药物给药方案的。

c. 受试者8204，其随机号为10001，在运送单上标明发给随机号为10001的瓶盒号分别为864628，104632和591691，前两个号码的标签被放置在CFR标签页上，但瓶号591691的标签没有放置在CRF标签页上；然而，研究药物回收表表明这个瓶子被使用过，因为14片被返还。

d. 受试者8208，CRF药品标签页提示该受试者被分发的瓶号是168130；然而，研究药物回收表表明患者编号是“UNK”，瓶子没有返还。

试验方案［（b）（4）］

e. 根据当前的研究协调员向FDA检查员的陈述，由她入组的那些受试者的药品计数日志是她在研究访视前按照计划访视日期和计划剩余药物数量提前准备好的，这些预先填写的表格然后根据需要进行修改，以反映实际访视日期和返还药物的数量。

不充分的药物处置记录，包括日期、数量和受试者的使用情况，不限于上面所列的例子。两个方案的药物记录都不足以证明试验药物的计数情况。

本警告信的目的并非是罗列您在试验药物临床研究中存在的所有缺陷。确保遵循法律和相关FDA法规的每一项要求是您的职责。您应当解决这些缺陷，并建立规程，以确保任何正在进行或将来进行的研究均能符合FDA的法规。

自收到这封信的15个工作日内，您应当书面告知本办公室为预防将来发生类似违规情况已经或将要采取的措施。如果不能充分、迅速地解释上述违规问题，可能导致我们在不再通知的情况下采取监管措施。

附：英文原文

Branitz, Bruce, M.D.

WARNING LETTER

APR 9, 2009

CERTIFIED MAIL
RETURN RECEIPT REQUESTED

Ref: 09-HFD-45-03-03

Bruce Branitz, M.D.
2121 Fountain Drive, Suite D
Snellville, GA 30078

Dear Dr. Branitz:

Between September 14 and November 6, 2007, Ms. Stephanie Hubbard, representing the Food and Drug Administration (FDA), conducted an investigation and met with you, to review your conduct of the following clinical investigations:

Protocol [(b)(4)], entitled "A Phase 2, Randomized, Multicenter, Placebo-Controlled, Double-Blind, Dose-Ranging Clinical Trial To Study The Efficacy And Safety of [(b)(4)] For The Treatment of [(b)(4)] of the investigational drug [(b)(4)] sponsored by [(b)(4)]., and Protocol [(b)(4)], entitled "A [(b)(4)].

This inspection is a part of the FDA's Bioresearch Monitoring Program, which includes inspections designed to evaluate the conduct of research and to ensure that the rights, safety, and welfare of the human subjects of those studies have been protected.

From our review of the establishment inspection report, the documents submitted with that report, and your November 23, 2007, written response, we conclude that you did not adhere to the applicable statutory requirements and FDA regulations governing the conduct of clinical investigations and the protection of human subjects. We are aware that at the conclusion of the inspection, Ms. Hubbard presented and discussed with you Form FDA 483, Inspectional Observations. We wish to emphasize the following:

1. You failed to conduct the studies in accordance with the investigational plan [21 CFR 312.60].

Protocol [(b)(4)]

a. The following subjects were enrolled inappropriately as they had conditions or laboratory values which were exclusionary according to the protocol:

i. A Screening Case Report Form (CRF) for subject 8201 noted the presence of right lower lobe lung cancer and an LDH level of 242 U/L.

ii. The laboratory report dated June 21, 2006, for the screening sample collected on June 15, 2006, for subject 8202 indicated values for BUN and creatinine of 41 mg/dL and 1.8 mg/dL, respectively.

iii.The laboratory report dated June 20, 2006, for the screening sample collected on June 15, 2006, for subject 8204 indicated a value for BUN of 36 mg/dL.

iv. Subject 8205 had lung cancer on the date of enrollment in the study.

v. The laboratory report dated June 24, 2006, for the screening sample collected on June 15, 2006, for subject 8208 indicates values for BUN and creatinine of 33 mg/dL and 1.6 mg/dL, respectively.

vi. The laboratory report dated June 30, 2006, for the screening sample collected on June 20, 2006, for subject 8209 indicates a value for creatinine of 1.8 mg/dL.

b. The protocol required that randomization be done in sequential order as the patients qualified for entry into the study. Study subjects were not randomized sequentially; for example, subject 8201, the first subject enrolled in the study, was assigned randomization number 10007 which was not the first randomization number. The majority of the remaining subjects were also randomized out of sequence.

The above examples of protocol violations are not intended to he a comprehensive listing of all exclusionary criteria met by subjects in protocol [(b)(4)]. Similar violations were found in the conduct of protocol [(b)(4)]. For example, the following subjects were enrolled in violation of the protocol:

c. The medical histories for subjects 0003 and 0014 note that the subjects had [(b)(4)] adenocarcinoma. The protocol excluded subjects with any history of carcinoma of the [(b)(4)].

d. Subject 0002 did not meet the inclusion criterion of eight or more [(b)(4)] on average every 24 hours for the five day study diary period leading up to Visit 3 but was randomized to treatment and dispensed medication at Visit 3 on July 24, 2006.

e. For subjects 0002 and 0013, Visit 3 diaries documented that they did not meet the inclusion criterion of an average of eight or more [(b)(4)] per day.

f. For subject 0005, based upon an EKG performed during visit 3, the visit during which subjects were enrolled in the study, you noted that the subject had an abnormal EKG and that its significance would require referral to a cardiologist. The protocol excluded those individuals with "significant medical problems" including cardiac problems. This subject was enrolled in the study without documentation of an assessment of the significance of the subject's abnormal EKG findings.

g. For subject 0010 the progress notes indicated that the subject had a history of [(b)(4)] adenocarcinoma, external beam radiation therapy for [(b)(4)], and brachytherapy implants. Exclusion criteria specified that subjects with any history of carcinoma of the [(b)(4)] or [(b)(4)] radiation would not be allowed in the study.

h. For subjects 0010 and 0012 progress notes indicated that the subjects had been treated previously with darifenacin; therefore, these subjects did not meet the inclusion criterion which stated that subjects must be naive to darifenacin treatment.

i. For subject 0013, a blood sample taken on June 27, 2007, revealed a blood glucose level of 219 mg/dL. The protocol defined glucose levels greater than 200 mg/dL as clinically significant and to be followed to resolution. A laboratory report faxed to the Investigator at the time of referral noted a "degree of uncontrolled diabetes indicated". In violation of the protocol, there is no documentation that the diabetic condition of this subject was followed up.

2. You failed to maintain adequate and accurate case histories that record all observations and other data pertinent to the investigation on each individual [21 CFR 312.62(b)].

Protocol [(b)(4)]

a. Regarding Subject [(b)(4)]:

i. There was no documentation of the interpretation of the Visit 1 EKG. The requisition and EKG tracing for Visit 6 were available; however, the Cardiac History portion of the requisition was not completed nor was there any documentation of the review of the Visit 6 EKG tracing.

ii. The Medical History source document dated June 7, 2006, indicated a normal cardiovascular system; however, this notation was revised on November 6, 2006 to indicate two instances of cardiac bypass surgery. A Protocol Deviation form dated August 24, 2006, noted an inferior infarct and possible lateral ischemia.

iii. Two diaries were present which recorded the number and severity of [(b)(4)] between the periods of June 14 and June 21, 2006. It is unclear why the subject completed two diaries for this period of time. Furthermore, these two diaries are not in agreement with each other in terms of number and severity of [(b)(4)]. Two CRFs were completed to report these [(b)(4)]. These CRFs were not in agreement with each other, and one of the CRFs did not agree with the data reported in either diary. In addition, a handwritten log of [(b)(4)] that did not agree with either CRF in number or severity was observed in the subject' s records. These multiple discrepancies make it impossible to determine the actual number/severity of [(b)(4)] experienced by this subject.

b. For subjects 8202, 8203, and 8205, the dates next to the subject's signatures on the consent forms were initially dated 6/8/06 and then changed to 6/15/06. For subject 8202, the date was then revised back to 6/8/06 and multiple date changes were made to most of the pages in the Screening Visit Source Documents for these subjects. No documentation was provided to explain these changes.

c. For subject 8203, 8204, 8205, 8207 and 8208, Karnofsky performance scores were revised by the study coordinator at various times for various study visits without documentation explaining the changes.

d. The "Medical History" source document dated June 8, 2006 (later revised to June 15, 2006), for subject 8205 indicated normal cardiovascular and respiratory systems; however, the subject's medical history included source documents indicating the presence of coronary artery disease, chronic obstructive pulmonary disease (COPD), and lung cancer.

e. The Medical History Screening CRF for subject 8206 originally indicated normal respiratory, cardiovascular, gastrointestinal, and endocrine systems. The screening visit occurred on June 15, 2006. On May 10, 2007, the screening CRF was revised to indicate that the subject had emphysema, coronary artery disease, gastroesophageal reflux disease, diverticulitis, and diabetes.

f. The Medical History Screening CRF for subject 8208 noted "cough, sinus drainage" for the respiratory system and "congested w/ cough" for the cardiovascular system. All other systems were indicated to be normal. The subject had a history of hypertension, coronary artery disease, adult onset diabetes, emphysema, kidney stones and abnormal EKG and laboratory results. These conditions were not noted on the Medical History Screening CRF. Numerous clinical laboratory parameters were noted as being clinically significant for the blood sample collected at screening on June 15, 2006; however, the Lab Assessments Screening CRF indicated that there were no clinically significant laboratory values. This subject was enrolled and treated in the study.

g. The Medical History Screening CRF of June 20, 2006, for subject 8209 originally indicated all body systems to be normal. On June 20, 2007, the CRF was revised to indicate the presence of COPD, urinary stents, kidney stones, erectile dysfunction, overactive bladder, bladder cancer, and osseous degeneration. There is no documentation that these medical problems were assessed to determine the subject' s eligibility for study participation. In addition, numerous clinical laboratory parameters were noted as being clinically significant for the blood sample collected at screening on June 20, 2006; however, the Lab Assessments Screening CRF indicated that there were no clinically significant laboratory values. This subject was enrolled and treated in the study.

h. For subject 8210, the Visit 5 Source Worksheets were lined through and noted as "Not Done"; however, a progress note in your clinical chart dated September 6, 2006, indicates that the subject was present for Visit 5, that study-related procedures were performed, and that the subject returned his Visit 5 diary.

Protocol [(b)(4)]

i. The Medical History CRF for subject 0003 noted all body systems, including the urologic system, to be normal except for sinus drainage during cold weather; however, the subject's history included prostate cancer (including a trans-urethral resection of the prostate), hypertension, asthma, kidney stones, and arthritis.

j. The Medical History CRF for subject 0010 noted all body systems to be normal despite the subject's medical history from another provider which indicated that the subject had prostatic adenocarcinoma, rheumatoid arthritis, hypertension, gastritis, and high cholesterol.

k. For subject 0011 the [(b)(4)] Registration Confirmation form dated May 16, 2007, and the [(b)(4)] Reference Sheet indicated that the subject' s last overactive bladder (OAB) treatment consisted of oxybutynin extended release; however, a note dated October 15, 2007, on the Registration Confirmation form indicated that the subject's last treatment for OAB was Detrol LA.

l. For subject 0012 the Patient' s Previous Treatment Assessment questionnaire indicated that Detrol was the last OAB drug taken; however, both the [(b)(4)] Reference Sheet and the [(b)(4)] Registration Confirmation form indicated that the subject was last treated with oxybutynin extended release.

The medical history for subject 0012 indicated the presence of a neurogenic bladder as the result of a gunshot wound to the spinal cord. Exclusion criteria number 6 specifically excluded those subjects with neurological diseases affecting urinary bladder function (including spinal cord injury). This subject was enrolled and treated in the study. You stated during the inspection that the subject did not have a neurogenic bladder; however, there was no documentation in the subject' s study records to that effect.

The laboratory reports for subject 0012 for Visit 1 were completed on May 17, 2007; however, you initialed and dated these records as having reviewed them on May 15, 2007.

m. The Medical History CRF for subject 0013 indicated all body systems to be normal despite the subject's self-reported history of diabetes, glaucoma, heart trouble, vein trouble, kidney disease, and bypass surgery.

n. The FDA investigator' s review of the electronic CRFs (eCRFs) for the Novartis study revealed discrepancies. When the FDA investigator requested hard copies of the eCRFs, you were unable to provide copies of the eCRFs. Your study coordinator informed our investigator that the eCRFs were maintained by another firm and that you had no access to that eCRF database. Accordingly, you could not show that you prepared and maintained adequate and accurate case histories.

3. You failed to obtain informed consent in accordance with the provisions of 21 CFR Part 50 [21 CFR 312.60 and 21 CFR 50].

Subject 8210 was randomized to protocol [(b)(4)] on June 12, 2006. You did not obtain informed consent from this subject until June 26, 2006.

4. You failed to maintain adequate records of the disposition of the drug including dates, quantity, and use by subjects [21 CFR 312.62(a)].

Protocol [(b)(4)]

a. You did not maintain adequate records of the disposition of the drug. For example, the Master Drug Dispensation Log (MDDL) contained no drug accountability documentation for any subject in the study at Visit 5 or later.

b. For subject 8202, the randomization number was 10002 according to the source worksheet and the MDDL. The bottle/kit numbers identified on the shipment form for randomization number 10002 were 248752, 343193, and 218605. Bottle labels with numbers 248752, 343193, and 899686 were attached to the Label CRF for subject 8202 indicating that those bottles had been dispensed to the subject. The shipment form identified 899686 as a bottle number for the subject with randomization number 10003 and the Investigational Product Return Form indicated that reference number 899686 was not returned. According to the same form, bottle number 343193 was also not returned and the Patient No. was "UNK" . The patient number and initials on the label of 248752 were obliterated in black. Nonetheless, the CRF documented 100% compliance for Subject 8202. The result of these discrepancies in drug dispensation and documentation is that there is no assurance that subject [(b)(6)] was dispensed the study drug as allocated nor is there any assurance that the subject was compliant with the drug regimen.

c. For subject 8204, the randomization number was 10001. The bottle/kit numbers identified on the shipment form for randomization number 10001 were 864628, 104632, and 591691. Labels for the first two numbers were placed on the label CRF but not the label for bottle 591691; however, the Product Return Form indicates that this bottle was used since 14 tablets were returned.

d. For subject 8208, the Drug Label CRF indicates that this subject was dispensed bottle number 168130; however, the Product Return Form indicates that Patient No. was "UNK" and that the bottle was not returned.

Protocol [(b)(4)]

e. According to statements made by the current study coordinator to the FDA investigator, drug accountability logs for those subjects she enrolled were prepared in advance of study visits with projected visit dates and projected amounts of remaining drug, and that these pre-filled forms were then revised as necessary to reflect actual visit dates and amounts of drug returned.

Inadequate records of the disposition of the drug including dates, quantity, and use by subjects, are not limited to the examples listed above. The drug records for both protocols are inadequate to document study drug accountability.

This letter is not intended to be an all-inclusive list of deficiencies with your clinical study of an investigational drug. It is your responsibility to ensure adherence to each requirement of the law and relevant FDA regulations. You should address these deficiencies and establish procedures to ensure that any on-going or future studies will be in compliance with FDA regulations.

Within fifteen (15) working days of your receipt of this letter, you should notify this office in writing of the actions you have taken or will be taking to prevent similar violations in the future. Failure to adequately and promptly explain the violations noted above may result in regulatory action without further notice.

If you have any questions, please contact Constance Lewin, M.D., M.P.H., at (301) 796-3397; FAX (301) 847-8748. Your written response and any pertinent documentation should be addressed to:

Constance Lewin, M.D., M.P.H.
Branch Chief
Good Clinical Practice Branch I
Division of Scientific Investigations
Office of Compliance
Center for Drug Evaluation and Research
Food and Drug Administration
Building 51, Room 5354
10903 New Hampshire Avenue
Silver Spring, MD 20993

Sincerely yours,

{See appended electronic signature page}

Leslie K. Ball, M.D.
Director
Division of Scientific Investigations
Office of Compliance
Center for Drug Evaluation and Research

第130封　给Bukowski, Ronald M. 医学博士的警告信

2009年3月30日

参考号：09-HFD-45-03-02

尊敬的Bukowski博士：

2008年8月4日至9月15日，Benjamin Dastoli先生代表FDA进行了现场检查，对您所实施的以下临床研究进行了审查：试验方案（b）（4）名称为“一项二期、多中心、随机、双盲临床研究，评估（b）（4）合并（b）（4）与（b）（4）单独使用对治疗（b）（4）肉瘤的有效性和安全性”，试验药物为（b）（4），申办者为（b）（4）。

本次现场检查是FDA的生物研究监查项目的一部分，该项目通过设定的检查方法，对研究的实施情况进行评估，并确保这些研究中受试者的权益、安全和福利得到了保护。

FDA注意到，从2004年4月6日伦理委员会（IRB）批准，到2007年1月31日IRB批准关闭本研究期间，您是本项目的研究者，（b）（6）医生是授权研究者。因为您于2008年1月退休，所以本次检查由（b）（6）医生配合完成。

经对现场检查报告、该报告的附件进行审查，我们认为，您没有遵循适用的法律要求和监管临床研究实施的FDA法规。在现场检查结束时，Benjamin Dastoli先生向（b）（6）医生出示了FDA483表，即现场检查发现的问题，并与他进行了讨论。

我们注意到在现场检查结束时，一份FDA483表的复印件被邮寄给您，我们想强调以下几点：

1. 您未能按照21 CFR 50的要求取得每个受试者的知情同意［21 CFR 312.60］

FDA法规在21 CFR 50.20中规定，只有在准受试者或其代表有充分的时机考虑是否参与临床研究，以及把胁迫或不当影响的可能性降到最低的情况下，研究者才可以征求知情同意。50.25（a）阐述在寻求知情同意时，应提供给每个受试者任何可合理预见的风险和不适的资料［21 CFR 50.25（a）（2）］。

a. 根据日期为2004年7月14日从您的试验场所到IRB的信件，您提供了下列信息：使用（b）（4）与“严重昏迷”的风险有关，这一点已经从23位其他个体中发现；并且基于这个可能的严重不良事件,知情同意文件正在被修订。我们注意到在2004年7月27日的信中，在IRB批准了修订的知情同意书的通知以后，您的研究场所未能对修订的知情同意书批准之日前入组而且仍继续参与研究的6位受试者［即受试者（b）（6）］重新进行知情同意。结果，这些受试者没有被提供参加该研究的可合理预见的风险的充分描述。

b. 根据日期为2004年8月24日的信件，您的研究场所向IRB提供信息，正在对知情同意书进行修订，以包括除了其他项目外的血栓栓塞事件的风险。在日期为2004年9月20日的信件中，IRB通知您修订的知情同意书已被批准，并且您必须对以前入组的受试者签署修订的知情同意书，以允许其继续参与试验。我们注意到在IRB批准了修订的知情同意书的通知以后，您的研究场所未能使用批准的修订过的知情同意书对已经入组的9位受试者［即受试者（b）（6）］重新进行知情同意。结果，这些受试者没有被提供参加该研究的可合理预见的风险的充分描述。

c. 根据方案修正案# 4的摘要页，该修正案的主要目的是在有里程碑意义的分析之后修改研究的治疗方法，该分析表明，（b）（4）添加到（b）（4）导致与单独使用（b）（4）取得的效果类似的无进展期和响应率。为该修正案所修订的知情同意书中包括与有里程碑意义的分析有关的信息，还包括对选择继续留在（b）（4）

的受试者额外风险有关的信息，这些额外风险包括致命的肺损伤，血液细胞紊乱和某些食物与（b）（4）相互作用。在日期为2006年2月3日的信件中，IRB通知您修订的知情同意已被批准，并且您必须对以前入组的受试者签署修订的知情同意书以允许其继续参与试验。我们注意到在IRB批准修订的知情同意书之日以后，您的研究场所未能使用批准的修订过的知情同意书对受试者（b）（6）重新进行知情同意。结果，该受试者没有被提供参加该研究的可合理预见的风险的充分的描述。

2. 您未能进行研究或者确保研究按照研究计划进行［21 CFR 312.60］

a. 方案修正案#1是在受试者（b）（6）入组该试验期间生效，其规定要加入本研究，受试者要有组织学证实（b）（4）的（b）（4）癌。根据2001年4月17日手术病理报告，该受试者已经被诊断为有（b）（4）细胞的特征（b）（4）癌，因此该受试者不符合入组该研究的入选标准。然而，该受试者入组了该研究，并在您的研究场所向申办者请求并得到允许该受试者可以入组研究之前就给予了研究药物治疗。

b. 原方案和方案修正案都规定，作为一个研究的安全计划的一部分，入组的受试者在整个治疗阶段都要被仔细监控，而且在整个研究的规定访视时，要进行包括医学访谈、不良事件记录、体格检查、血压和实验室检测的安全评估。对体格检查，方案规定在筛选和末次访视，受试者要进行全面的体格检查；在治疗阶段，受试者每两周进行有限的体格检查，直到52周，此后每4周进行。

该方案还规定，在筛选访视、研究期间每6周和治疗末次访视时要进行尿分析和尿蛋白/肌酐比值检测。基于尿分析和尿蛋白/肌酐比值结果,方案进一步规定受试者的剂量要进行修改和/或受试者要进行额外的检测或在末次访视后进行足够的随访。方案进一步规定，如果筛选的尿分析结果显示尿液中蛋白质达到规定的水平，该受试者将被排除。

在FDA审查的12个受试者记录中全部都发现, 在数次研究访视中，您的研究场所的记录没有显示您的研究场所进行了方案规定的体格检查，并且在或者筛选访视，研究治疗期间访视和/或末次访视，未能得到尿分析和/或进行尿蛋白/肌酐比值检测。此外，经审查您的研究场所的记录，CRF中已做过体格检查的注释却找不到文件来证实。例子包括但不限于以下：

受试者编号	没有进行过或者没有证据表明进行过的研究流程	流程没有进行过，或者没有证据表明流程进行过的研究访视
23240	体格检查 尿分析 尿蛋白/肌酐比值	周: 0, 2, 14, 18* 周: 12, 18 筛查, 周: 6, 12, 18
23241	体格检查 尿分析 尿蛋白/肌酐比值	周: 0, 2, 10, 14 筛查, 周18 筛查周: 6, 18
23242	体格检查 尿分析 尿蛋白/肌酐比值	第2*，6*，10*周 第18，42周 筛选，第12，18，42周
23243	体格检查 尿分析 尿蛋白/肌酐比值	第2*，18*，22*周 第18周 筛选，第6，12，18周
23244	体格检查 尿分析 尿蛋白/肌酐比值	第6*，10，26*，42*周 第18周，末次访视 第12，18，24周，末次访视
23245	体格检查 尿分析 尿蛋白/肌酐比值	第0，6*，14*，34*周 第18，36，42周 筛选，第18，36，42周

续表

受试者编号	没有进行过或者没有证据表明进行过的研究流程	流程没有进行过，或者没有证据表明流程进行过的研究访视
23246	体格检查 尿分析 尿蛋白/肌酐比值	第30*周 第24周 筛选，第6，18，24周，末次访视
23247	体格检查 尿分析 尿蛋白/肌酐比值	第0，6*，30*，38*周 第18，60周 第18，24，36，60周
23248	体格检查 尿分析 尿蛋白/肌酐比值	第0，2，22*周 第18，60周 第6，12，18周，末次访视
23249	体格检查 尿分析 尿蛋白/肌酐比值	第2，6周 末次访视 筛选，末次访视
23250	体格检查 尿分析 尿蛋白/肌酐比值	第2，6*周 末次访视 末次访视
23251	体格检查 尿蛋白/肌酐比值	第6*，10*，50*周 筛选

* 对于上述标星号的条目，CRF中记录方案规定的体格检查已经进行，而原始记录中没有发现有文件来证实。

c. 方案修正案# 3规定研究者必须在观察到或者得知48小时内向申办者报告所有严重不良事件（SAE）。此外，对于最初的SAE，研究者还要将所有能收集到的48小时内的情况的细节记录到CRF的SAE页中。方案修正案# 3进一步规定研究者必须让IRB知晓任何重要的不良事件。

一份日期为2005年12月7日的正式访视记录显示，受试者（b）（6）患有4级肾病综合征。我们发现您没有按照方案要求在48小时内向申办者报告这个严重不良事件（SAE），该报告在日期为2006年5月11日的SAE表中提交给申办者。此外，该SAE直到2006年5月3日才报告给IRB。

d. 方案修正案# 2规定该研究给予的（b）（4）剂量为10mg/kg，每2周一次。记录显示2004年9月27日，受试者（b）（6）接受了（b）（4），而不是（b）（4）。

本警告信的目的并未是罗列您在试验药物临床研究中存在的所有缺陷。确保遵循法律和相关FDA法规的每一项要求是您的职责。您应当解决这些缺陷，并建立规程，以确保任何正在进行或将来的研究均能符合FDA的法规。

自收到这封信的15个工作日内，您应当书面告知本办公室为预防将来发生类似违规情况已经或将要采取的措施。如果不能充分地、快速地对上述违规问题作出解释，可能导致我们在不再通知的情况下采取监管措施。

附：英文原文

Bukowski, Ronald M., M.D.

WARNING LETTER

MAR 30, 2009

CERTIFIED MAIL
RETURN RECEIPT REQUESTED

Ref: 09-HFD-45-03-02

Ronald Bukowski, M.D.
28099 Gates Mills Blvd.
Pepper Pike, OH 44124

Dear Dr. Bukowski:

Between August 4 and September 15, 2008, Mr. Benjamin Dastoli, representing the Food and Drug Administration (FDA), conducted an investigation to review your conduct of a clinical investigation (Protocol **(b)(4)** entitled "A Phase Ⅱ, Multicenter, Randomized, Double-Blind Clinical Trial to Evaluate the Efficacy and Safety of **(b)(4)**) in Combination with **(b)(4)** Versus **(b)(4)**. Alone for Treatment of **(b)(4)** Carcinoma) of the investigational drugs **(b)(4)** performed for **(b)(4)**.

This inspection is a part of the FDA' s Bioresearch Monitoring Program, which includes inspections designed to evaluate the conduct of research and to ensure that the rights, safety, and welfare of the human subjects of those studies have been protected.

The FDA notes that during the time period between the IRB's approval of the study on April 6, 2004 am closure of the study with the IRB on January 31, 2007, you served as the clinical investigator of this study and that Dr. **(b)(6)** served as the sub-investigator. As you had retired from your position in January 2008, we note that the FDA inspection of this study was thus facilitated by Dr. **(b)(6)**

From our review of the establishment inspection report and the documents submitted with that report, we conclude that you did not adhere to the applicable statutory requirements and FDA regulations governing the conduct of clinical investigations. We are aware that at the conclusion of the inspection, Mr. Benjamin Dastoli presented and discussed with your Dr. **(b)(6)** a Form FDA 483, Inspectional Observations.

We note that a copy of the Form FDA 483 was mailed to you at the conclusion of the inspection. We wish to emphasize the following:

1. You failed to obtain the informed consent of each human subject in accordance with 21 CFR part 50 [21 CFR 312.60].

FDA' s regulations at 21 CFR 50.20 specify that an investigator shall seek informed consent only under circumstances that provide the prospective subject or the subject's representative sufficient opportunit to consider whether or not to participate and that minimize the possibility of coercion or undue influence. Section 50.25(a) states that in seeking informed consent, certain information shall be provided to each subject, including a description of any reasonably foreseeable risks or discomforts to the subject. [21 CFR 50.25(a)(2)]

a. Per the letter dated July 14, 2004, sent by your site to the IRB, you provided information that the use of **(b)(4)** was associated with the risk of "serious confusion" that had been identified in 23 other individuals, and that based on this possible serious adverse event, the informed consent document was being revised. We note that following notification of the IRB's approval of this revised consent form in July 27, 2004 letter, your site failed to re-consent the 6 subjects (i.e. Subject #**(b)(6)**) who were enrolled prior to the date of the approval of the revised informed consent document and who were still participating in the study. As a result of this failure, those subjects were not provided with an adequate description of the reasonably foreseeable risks of participating in the study.

b. Per the letter dated August 20, 2004, your site provided information to the IRB that the consent form was being revised to include, among other items, the risk of thromboembolic events. In a letter dated September 20, 2004, the IRB informed you that the revised consent form was approved and that you were required to have previously enrolled subjects sign and date the revised consent form in order to allow their continued participation in the study. We note that following notification of the IRB's approva of this revised consent form, your site failed to re-consent the 9 subjects who were already enrolled (i.e. Subject #**(b)(6)**) using the approved revised consent form. As a result of this failure, those subjects were not provided with an adequate description of the reasonably foreseeable risks of participating in the study.

c. Per Protocol Amendment #4's summary page, the primary purpose of this amendment was to modify the study treatment after the landmark analysis, which suggested that the addition of **(b)(4)** to **(b)(4)** resulted in progression-free survival and response rates similar to those achieved with **(b)(4)** alone. The revised informed consent form for this amendment, which included information related to the landmark analysis, also included information related to additional risks to the subjects who opted to remain on **(b)(4)** , including fatal lung injury, disorders of blood cells, and interaction of certain food with **(b)(4)**. In a letter dated February 3, 2006f the IRB informed you that the revised consent form was approved and that you were required to have previously enrolled subjects sign and date the revised consent form in order to allow their continued participation in the study. We note that subsequent to the date of the IRB's approval of this revised consent form, your site failed to re-consen Subject **(b)(6)** using the approved revised consent form. As a result of this failure, that subject was not provided with an adequate description of the reasonably foreseeable risks of participating in the study.

2. You failed to conduct the study or ensure it was conducted according to the investigational plan [21 CFR 312.60].

a. Protocol Amendment #1 which was in effect during the time of Subject **(b)(6)** enrollment into the study, specified that to be included in the study, the subject was to have histologically confirmed **(b) (4)** carcinoma of **(b)(4)**. Per the surgical pathology report dated April 17, 2001, the subject had been diagnosed with **(b)(4)** carcinoma with both **(b) (4)** cell features, and thus the subject did not meet the inclusion criterion for enrollment into the study. However, the subject was enrolled into the study and was administered study medication prior to your site requesting and receiving a waiver from the sponsor that allowed the subject's enrollment in the study.

b. The original protocol and protocol amendments all specified that as a part of the safety plan of the study, enrolled subjects were to be carefully monitored during the entire treatment phase and that safety evaluations which consisted of medical interviews, recording of adverse events, physical examinations, and blood pressure and laboratory measurements, were to be performed on subjects at specified visits throughout the study. With respect to the physical exams, the protocol specified that at the screening and termination visits, the subjects were to have a complete physical exam, and during the treatment phase the subjects were to have limited physical exams every two weeks until 52 weeks into the study and then every 4 weeks thereafter.

The protocols also specified that a urinalysis and urine protein/creatinine ratio were to be performed at the screening visit, every 6 weeks during the study, and at the treatment termination visit. Based on the results of the urinalysis and urine protein/creatinine results, the protocols further specified that the subject's dose was to be modified and/or the subject was to have additional testing or adequate follow up subsequent to the termination visit. The protocols further specified that the results from the screening urinalysis would exclude subjects if a specific level of protein in the urine was reached.

In FDA' s review of 12 of 12 subject records, there were numerous study visits where your site's records do not indicate that your site conducted the protocol specified physical exams and at either the screening visit, during study treatment visits, and/or termination visits, failed to obtain a urinalysis and/or perform a urine protein/creatinine ratio. In addition, in review of your site's records, documentation could not be found to verify comments made in the CFR that a physical exam was done .Examples include but were not limited to the following:

Subject #	Study procedure not conducted or no evidence found to show it was conducted	Study visit the procedure was not conducted or no evidence found to show it was conducted
(b) (6)	Physical Exam Urinalysis Urine Protein/Creatinine Ratio	Weeks: 0, 2, 14, 18* Weeks: 12, 18 Screening, Weeks: 6, 12, 18
(b) (6)	Physical Exam Urinalysis Urine Protein/Creatinine Ratio	Weeks: 0, 2, 10, 14* Screen, Week: 18 Screening, Weeks: 6, 18
(b) (6)	Physical Exam Urinalysis Urine Protein/Creatinine Ratio	Weeks: 2*, 6*, 10* Weeks: 18, 42 Screening, Weeks: 12, 18,42
(b) (6)	Physical Exam Urinalysis Urine Protein/Creatinine Ratio	Weeks: 2*, 18*, 22* Week: 18 Screening, 6, 12, 18
(b) (6)	Physical Exam Urinalysis Urine Protein/Creatinine Ratio	Weeks: 6*, 10, 26*, 42* Week: 18, Termination Weeks: 12, 18, 24, Termination
(b) (6)	Physical Exam Urinalysis Urine Protein/Creatinine Ratio	Weeks: 0, 6*, 14*, 34* Weeks: 18, 36, 42 Screening, Weeks: 18, 36,42
(b) (6)	Physical Exam Urinalysis Urine Protein/Creatinine Ratio	Week: 30* Week: 24 Screening, Weeks: 6, 18, 24, Termination
(b) (6)	Physical Exam Urinalysis Urine Protein/Creatinine Ratio	Weeks: 0, 6*, 30*, 38* Weeks: 18, 60 Weeks: 18, 24, 36, 60
(b) (6)	Physical Exam Urinalysis Urine Protein/Creatinine Ratio	Weeks: 0, 2, 22* Week: 18 Weeks: 6, 12, 18, Termination
(b) (6)	Physical Exam Urinalysis Urine Protein/Creatinine Ratio	Weeks: 2, 6 Termination Screening, Termination
(b) (6)	Physical Exam Urinalysis Urine Protein/Creatinine Ratio	Weeks: 2, 6* Termination Termination
(b) (6)	Physical Exam Urine Protein/Creatinine Ratio	Weeks: 6*, 10*, 50* Screening

* For items noted with an asterisk above, there was no documentation found in the source records to corroborate that a protocol specified physical exam was performed as noted in the CRF.

c. Protocol Amendment #3 specified that the investigator must report all Serious Adverse Events (SAE) to the sponsor within 48 hours of observing or learning of the event. In addition, for the initial SAE, the investigator was to also record all case details that can be gathered within the 48 hours on the SAE page of the CRF. Protocol Amendment #3 further specified that investigators were required to keep the IRB informed of any significant AEs.

An office visit note dated December 7, 2005, stated that Subject, #**(b)(6)** experienced grade 4 nephrotic syndrome. We note that you failed to report this SAE to the sponsor within 48 hours as required by the protocol. The report was submitted to the sponsor on an SAE form dated May 11, 2006. In addition, the SAE was not reported to the IRB until May 3, 2006.

d. Protocol Amendment #2 specified that the dose **(b)(4)** of administered in this study was 10 mg/kg once every 2 weeks. Records indicate that on September 27, 2004, Subject **(b)(6)** received **(b)(4)** instead of **(b)(4)**

This letter is not intended to be an all-inclusive list of deficiencies with your clinical study of an investigational drug. It is your responsibility to ensure adherence to each requirement of the law and relevant FDA regulations. You should address these deficiencies and establish procedures to ensure that any on-going or future studies will be in

compliance with FDA regulations.

Within fifteen (15) working days of your receipt of this letter, you should notify this office in writing of the actions you have taken or will be taking to prevent similar violations in the future. Failure to adequately and promptly explain the violations noted above may result in regulatory action without further notice.

If you have any questions, please contact Tejashri Purohit-Sheth, M.D., at 301-796-3402; FAX 301-847 8748. Your written response and any pertinent documentation should be addressed to:

Tejashri Purohit-Sheth, M.D.
Branch Chief
Good Clinical Practice Branch Ⅱ
Division of Scientific Investigations
Office of Compliance
Center for Drug Evaluation and Research
Food and Drug Administration
Bldg 51, Room 5358
10903 New Hampshire Avenue
Silver Spring, MD 20993

Sincerely yours,

{See appended electronic signature page}

Leslie K. Ball, M.D. Director
Division of Scientific Investigations
Office of Compliance
Center for Drug Evaluation and Research

第131封　给Paulson, Daniel M.医学博士的警告信

2009年3月11日

参考号：09-HFD-45-03-01

尊敬的Paulson博士：

2008年4月21日至2008年5月29日，以及2008年12月4日，Dianne Milazzo女士和Emmanuel Dimanno Jr.先生代表FDA，对您所实施的以下临床研究："试验方案（b）（4），标题为在（b）（4）设定下慢性阻塞性肺病患者每日服用一次18mg规格噻托溴铵胶囊的治疗过程中，一个随机双盲、安慰剂对照、平行组试验评估，慢性阻塞性肺病加重的比例和因一次加重住院治疗超过6个月的患者比例的临床试验"进行了现场检查。试验药物为思力华（噻托溴铵粉吸入剂），申办者为勃林格殷格翰制药有限公司。

本次现场检查是FDA的生物研究监查项目的一部分。该项目通过设定的检查方法，评估研究的实施情况，以确保这些研究中受试者的权益、安全和福利得到了保护。

经对现场检查报告（EIR）及该报告的附件进行审查，我们认为您没有遵循适用的法律要求和监管临床研究实施并受试者保护的FDA法规。在检查结束时，检查员们向您的前任授权研究者（b）（6）医生出示并讨论了FDA483表，即现场检查发现的问题。我们注意到，您通过电话出席的方式参与了FDA483表的讨论。此外，我们还注意到，FDA483表的复印件于2008年5月29日以信函寄给您。关于检查中发现的问题，我们想强调以下几点：

1. 您未能进行研究或确保按照试验计划进行研究［21 CFR 312.60］

A. 试验方案规定，在筛选访视时，所有受试者都要进行心电图（ECG）检查，检查结果由研究者或具有医学资质的指定人员在随机分组前进行确认。此外，试验方案明确规定，"基线心电图检查的目的是获得关于患者的基线情况，以确定是否有资格参与这项临床试验。"试验方案还规定，如果受试者有任何不稳定的身体状况（如神经系统、心脏等方面的问题），致使研究者认为会妨碍其有效参与临床研究，或将其预期寿命降低到小于6个月，则受试者将被排除。

FDA对58名受试者筛选心电图进行了稽查，发现其中38份筛选心电图的审查存在较长延迟现象，如：①受试者在审查以前已经随机分组并领到试验药物；②受试者已经完成研究。鉴于随机分组访视前，心电图的检查结果并未标注为已审查，因此FDA无法评估您是如何判断受试者是否符合试验方案规定的入组条件。有关事例包括但不限于以下内容：

受试者编号	心电图检查日期	受试者领到试验药物日期	受试者完成研究的日期	心电图上标注的结果审查日期	心电图上注意到的异常结果
(b)(6)	5/6/2002	5/29/2002	12/4/2002	9/13/2002	非特异性T波异常；心电图异常
(b)(6)	10/15/2001	10/21/2001	4/8/2002	5/9/2002	窦性心动过缓，电轴不确定；下部心肌梗死，年龄不确定；异常心电图
(b)(6)	9/24/2001	10/17/2001	4/15/2002	6/17/2002	1°房室传导阻滞的窦性心律伴前；室间隔梗死，年龄未定；心电图异常
(b)(6)	1/15/2002	1/23/2002	2/24/2002（受试者死亡）（b）（6）	8/15/2002	心电图左束支传导阻滞，受试者死亡；心电图异常

您对受试者入组临床研究之前对心电图结果的审查的延迟，忽视了在研究过程中受试者的安全性，我们对此深表担忧。

B. 试验方案规定了本临床研究的入组和排除标准。您未能排除根据上述标准不应入组试验的数位受试者，包括：

i. 临床诊断为哮喘的受试者应被排除在本项临床研究之外。受试者（b）（6）的原始文件显示，受试者被诊断为哮喘。

ii. 在过去的一年里因为心脏衰竭而住院治疗的受试者应被排除在本项临床研究之外。受试者（b）（6）于2001年12月10日入组本项临床研究。原始文件表明，在之前一年里该受试者两次［即（b）（6）和（b）（6）］因为充血性心脏衰竭而住院治疗两次。

iii. 试验方案规定，入组本项临床研究的受试者要求被诊断为慢性阻塞性肺病并有中度至重度气道阻塞，1秒钟最大呼气量（FEV 1）≤ 预计正常量的60%，1秒钟用力呼气容积（FEV1）≤最大肺活量（FEVC）的70%。试验方案还规定，在第2，3和4次访视时进行肺功能测试，时间通常为受试者上午服用呼吸系统药物之前约1小时，选取任意3次呼气时获取的最高1秒钟最大呼气量（FEV 1）和最大肺活量（FVC）作为最佳值（根据试验方案允许最多5次呼气）。原始记录表明受试者（b）（6）不符合1秒钟最大呼气量（FEV 1）≤预计正常量60%的入选标准。具体而言，在第2次访视时（2001年10月3日），受试者（b）（6）肺功能测试显示，5次测试中1秒钟用力呼气容积（FEV1）最高值为1.16L。然而，第2次访视的肺功能记录表和其他原始文件错误地将最高值记录为1.12L。FDA指出，若准确录入1秒钟用力呼气容积（FEV1）为1.16L，该受试者应没有资格入组本项临床研究。

C. 试验方案规定，任何严重不良事件（SAE），无论是否与试验用药有关，无论试验药物是否已被使用，必须立即通过电话/传真报告给申办者。试验方案还规定，若发生严重不良事件（SAE），研究者必须填写严重不良事件（SAE）表（病例报告表中的部分），并将表立即传真至研究负责人和申办者。

根据现场检查报告（EIR），FDA检查员在其审查的58位受试者［即受试者（b）（6）和（b）（6）］的记录中，未能找到其中11位受试者的严重不良反应（SAE）表提交至申办者的传真日期。我们注意到，从贵研究场所得知严重不良事件发生，到您签署申办者严重不良事件报告之间的时间间隔从11天到超过51周之间不等。具体例证包括但不限于以下内容：

受试者编号	严重不良事件（SAE）	开始日期	中心得知严重不良事件(SAE)的日期	中心签署严重不良事件(SAE))报告日期
(b)(6)	脑卒中	12/25/2001和1/2002	4/15/2002	4/11/2003
(b)(6)	机动车事故	10/25/2001	11/7/2001	11/18/2001
(b)(6)	充血性心力衰竭恶化	1/8/2002	1/18/2002	1/30/2002
(b)(6)	复发的恶性淋巴瘤	4/1/2002	4/1/2002	4/11/2003

D. 试验方案规定，治疗期间禁用某些药物，包括：（a）单方或复方的吸入式抗胆碱能药物（如爱全乐、氧托溴铵、可必特、能倍乐、Duovent）和（b）鼻内抗胆碱能制剂，如爱全乐异丙托溴铵气雾剂。FDA的检查显示受试者接受过被禁用的联合用药。举例如下：

i. 受试者（b）（6）在2001年11月28日至2001年12月2日，出现了慢性阻塞性肺病急性加重，并使用了可必特。该严重不良事件（SAE）发生于第3次访视，即2002年1月9日之前，但第3次访视的病例报告表（CRF）错误地记录受试者未使用可必特。

ii. 受试者（b）（6）于2002年3月8日出现不稳定型心绞痛，并于（b）（6）住院。记录表明，根据您2002年3月20日签署的严重不良事件（SAE）报告，您对上述严重不良事件知情。原始记录表明，受试者在住院期间使用了可必特。但贵研究场所未能更新严重不良事件（SAE）报告，并通知申办者受试者在住院期间使用了可必特联合用药治疗。

2. 您未能保存足够的包括日期、数量和受试者的使用情况的药物处置记录［21 CFR 312.62（a）］

根据试验方案，受试者在随机分组（即第2次访视）时，领取1个药粉吸入器和110粒编盲的胶囊（每包10粒，共11包），在第3次访视时再领取110粒胶囊（每包10粒，共11包）。试验方案进一步指出，在第3次、第4次访视开始时，所有的研究药物胶囊（使用和未使用的）均需回收。在审查的59位受试者记录中，13位受试者［即受试者（b）（6）］的记录中显示分发的试验药物数量和受试者归还的试验药物数量不一致。例证包括但不限于以下内容：

受试者编号	访视次数	分发的药物胶囊数量	访视次数	归还总量（包括使用和没有使用的药物）	药物胶囊数量差
(b)(6)	3	110	4	91	19
(b)(6)	3	110	4	12	88
(b)(6)	3	110	4	116	16
(b)(6)	2	110	3	99	11
(b)(6)	2	110	3	105	5

本警告信的目的并非是罗列您在试验药物临床研究中存在的所有缺陷。确保遵循法律和相关FDA法规的每一项要求是您的职责。您应当解决这些缺陷，并建立规程，以确保任何正在进行或将来的研究均能符合FDA的法规。

自收到这封信的15个工作日内，您应当书面告知本办公室为预防将来发生类似违规情况已经或即将采取的措施。如果不能充分、迅速地解释上述违规问题，可能导致我们在不再通知的情况下采取监管措施。

附：英文原文

Paulson, Daniel M., MD

Warning Letters

MAR 11, 2009

CERTIFIED MAIL
RETURN RECEIPT REQUESTED

Ref: 09-HFD-45-03-01

Daniel M. Paulson, M.D
3565 Freeland Avenue
Philadelphia, PA 19128

Dear Dr. Paulson:

Between April 21, 2008 and May 29, 2008 and on December 4, 2008, Ms. Dianne Milazzo and Mr. Emmanuel Dimanno Jr., representing the Food and Drug Administration (FDA), conducted an investigation to review your conduct of a clinical investigation (Protocol (b)(4) entitled "A Randomized Double Blind, Placebo-Controlled, Parallel Group Trial Assessing the Proportion of Patients Experiencing an Exacerbation and Proportion of Patients

Hospitalized for an Exacerbation Over 6 months During Treatment with Tiotropium 18 mcg Capsule Once Daily in Patients with COPD in a (b)(4) Setting") of the investigational drug SPIRIVA® Handihaler (tiotropium bromide), performed for Boehringer Ingelheim Pharmaceuticals.

This inspection is a part of the FDA's Bioresearch Monitoring Program, which includes inspections designed to evaluate the conduct of research and to ensure that the rights, safety, and welfare of the human subjects of those studies have been protected.

From our review of the establishment inspection report (EIR) and the documents submitted with that report, we conclude that you did not adhere to the applicable statutory requirements and FDA regulations governing the conduct of clinical investigations and the protection of human subjects. We are aware that at the conclusion of the inspection, our investigators presented and discussed with your previous sub-investigator, Dr. (b) (6), a Form FDA 483, Inspectional Observations. We note that you were present via telephone during the discussion of the Form FDA 483. In addition, we note that a copy of the Form FDA 483 was sent to you in a letter dated May 29, 2008. In reference to the findings noted during the inspection, we wish to emphasize the following:

1. You failed to conduct the studies or ensure they were conducted according to the investigational plan [21 CFR 312.60].

A. The protocol specified that at the screening visit, all subjects were to have an Electrocardiogram(ECG) performed, and this ECG was to be interpreted by the investigator or medically qualified designee prior to randomization. In addition, the protocol specifically stated that "the purpose of the baseline ECG is to obtain information about the patient's baseline condition that may determine eligibility for participation in this trial." The protocol further specified that subjects were to be excluded from the study if they had any unstable medical condition (e.g. neurologic, cardiac, etc.,) which the investigator feels would preclude effective participation in the study, or which would be expected to reduce life expectancy to less than six months.

In FDA's audit of 58 subjects' screening ECGs, there was a significant delay in the documentation of your review of 38 screening ECGs such that the subjects had either (1) already been randomized into the study and received investigational drug by the time of your review and/or (2) subjects had already completed the study. The FDA is unable to assess how you could have adequately made the determination that the subjects met the protocol required condition for eligibility into the study given that the ECGs were not documented as having been reviewed prior to the randomization visit. Example include but were not limited to the following:

Subject Number	Date ECG Performed	Date Subject Received Investigational Drug	Date Subject Completed Study	Date Documented on ECG as Reviewed	Abnormal result(s) noted on ECG
(b)(6)	5/6/2002	5/29/02	12/4/02	9/13/2002	Nonspecific T wave abnormality; Abnormal ECG
(b)(6)	10/15/2001	10/21/01	4/8/02	5/9/2002	Sinus bradycardia; Indeterminate axis; Inferior infarct, age undetermined; Abnormal ECG
(b)(6)	9/24/2001	10/17/01	4/15/02	6/17/2002	Sinus rhythm with 1" degree AV block; Septal infarct, age undetermined; Abnormal ECG
(b)(6)	1/15/2002	1/23/02	2/24/02 Subject Died (b)(6)	8/15/2002	Left bundle branch subject Died block; Abnormal ECG

Your delayed review of ECGs prior to enrollment of the subjects into the study leads to significant concerns regarding your oversight over subjects' safety during the course of the study.

B. The protocol specified inclusionary and exclusionary criteria for enrollment in this study. You failed to identify multiple subjects who should have been excluded based on these criteria. This included:

1. Subjects with a clinical diagnosis of asthma were to be excluded from the study. Source documents for Subjects (b)(6) indicated that these subjects had been diagnosed with asthma.

2. Subjects who had been hospitalized for cardiac failure during the past year were to be excluded from the study. Subject (b) (6)was enrolled into the study on December 10, 2001. Source documents identified that this subject was hospitalized twice in the previous year (i.e. (b)(6) and (b)(6) for congestive heart failure.

3. The protocol specified that inclusion in the study required that subjects have a diagnosis of Chronic Obstructive Pulmonary Disease and have moderate to severe airway obstruction with an FEV 1 < 60% of predicted normal and an FEVI < 70% of FVC. The protocol further specified that pulmonary function testing was to be performed at Visits 2, 3 and 4, approximately 1 hr prior to the time the subjects usually took their morning dose of respiratory medication, with the best of 3 efforts being defined as the highest FEV 1 and the highest FVC each obtained on any of the three blows (maximum 5 attempts, was allowed per the protocol). Source records showed that Subject (b) (6) did not meet the inclusion criteria of having an FEV1 < 60% of predicted normal. Specifically, at Visit #2 (October 3, 2001), Subject (b) (6) spirometry showed that the highest FEVI value for 5 tests was 1.16 L. However, the Visit 2 spirometry worksheet and other source documents inaccurately reported the highest value of 1.12 L. FDA notes that had the FEVI value of 1.16 L been accurately transcribed, this subject would have been ineligible for the study.

C. The protocol specified that any serious adverse event (SAE), whether or not considered related to the investigational product, and whether or not the investigational product has been administered, must be reported immediately by telephone/fax to the sponsor. The protocol also stated that in the event of an SAE, the investigator must complete the SAE form (part of the case report form) and send it immediately by fax to the study chairman and to the sponsor.

Per the EIR, FDA investigators could not find a fax date to indicate that the SAE form was submitted to the sponsor for 11 of 58 subjects' records (i.e. Subject (b)(6) and (b)(6) reviewed. We note that the time period between your site becoming aware of an SAE and you signing the sponsor' s SAE report varied between 11 days to greater than 51 weeks. Examples include but were not limited to the following:

Subject Number	SAE	Date of Onset	Date Your Site Become Aware of SAE	Date SAE report signed by your site
(b)(6)	Stroke	12/25/2001 & 1/2002	4/15/2002	4/11/2003
(b)(6)	Motor vehicle accident	10/25/2001	11/7/2001	11/18/2001
(b)(6)	CHF Exacerbation	1/8/2002	1/18/2002	1/30/2002
(b)(6)	Recurrent Malignant lymphoma	4/1/2002	4/1/2002	4/11/2003

D. The protocol specified that certain medications were not allowed during the treatment period including (a) inhaled anticholinergic medications formulated alone or in combination with other medications (e.g. Atrovent, Oxitropium, Combivent, Berodual, Duovent) and (b) Intranasal anticholinergic formulations such as Atrovent Nasal spray. FDA's inspection documented that subjects received prohibited concomitant medications. Specifically,

i. Subject (b) (6) experienced a COPD exacerbation between the dates of November 28, 2001 and December 2, 2001 and was given Combivent. While this SAE occurred prior to Visit 3 on January 9, 2002, the Visit 3 CRF inaccurately noted that the subject did not receive Combivent.

ii. Subject (b) (6) experienced unstable angina on March 8, 2002 and was admitted to the hospital on (b) (6). Records indicate that you were aware of this SAE per the signed SAE report which you dated on March 20, 2002. Source records indicate that the subject received Combivent while hospitalized. Your site, however, failed to update the SAE report to notify the sponsor that Combivent was taken as concomitant therapy during the hospitalization.

2. You failed to maintain adequate records of the disposition of the drug, including dates, quantity, and use by subjects [21 CFR 312.62(a)].

Per the protocol, the subjects were to be provided a handihaler and a supply of 110 blinded capsules (11 packages of 10 capsules) at randomization (i.e. Visit 2), and a new supply of 110 capsules (11 packages of 10 capsules) was to be dispensed at Visit 3. The protocol further stated that at the beginning of Visits 3 and 4, all study medication capsules (used and unused) were to be collected. For 13 of 59 subject records reviewed, however (i.e. Subject (b)(6), there was no documentation of reconciliation between quantities of study drug dispensed and quantities of study drug returned by subject. Examples include but were not limited to the following:

Subject Number	Visit#	Amount of drug capsules dispensed	Visit#	Total amount (used and unused drug) returned	Unreconciled number of drug capsules
(b)(6)	3	110	4	91	19
(b)(6)	3	110	4	12	88
(b)(6)	3	110	4	116	16
(b)(6)	2	110	3	99	11
(b)(6)	2	110	3	105	5

This letter is not intended to be an all-inclusive list of deficiencies with your clinical study of an investigational drug. It is your responsibility to ensure adherence to each requirement of the law and relevant FDA regulations. You should address these deficiencies and establish procedures to ensure that any on-going or future studies will be in compliance with FDA regulations.

Within fifteen (15) working days of your receipt of this letter, you should notify this office in writing of the actions you have taken or will be taking to prevent similar violations in the future. Failure to adequately and promptly explain the violations noted above may result in regulatory action without further notice.

If you have any questions, please contact Tejashri Purohit-Sheth, M.D., at 301-796-3402; FAX 301-847-8748 Your written response and any pertinent documentation should be addressed to:

Tejashri Purohit-Sheth, M.D.
Branch Chief
Good Clinical Practice Branch Ⅱ
Division of Scientific Investigations
Office of Compliance
Center for Drug Evaluation and Research
Food and Drug Administration
Bldg 51, Room 5358
10903 New Hampshire Avenue
Silver Spring, MD 20993

Sincerely yours,

{See appended electronic signature page}

Leslie K. Ball, M.D.
Director
Division of Scientific Investigations
Office of Compliance
Center for Drug Evaluation and Research

第 132 封　给 Quinones, Manue J. 的警告信

2009年3月3日

参考号：09-HFD-45-02-05

尊敬的Quinones博士：

2008年7月21日至8月5日，Diane C. Van Leeuwen女士和Richard W. Tubb先生代表FDA进行了现场检查，与您会面并对您实施的关于罗格列酮药物（Avandia）的临床研究进行审查［试验方案（b）(4)，标题为“一项随机、双盲研究，比较在近期诊断为2型糖尿病无用药史的患者中罗格列酮单一疗法与二甲双胍或优降糖/格列本脲相比降低血糖并保留胰腺β细胞功能的持久性］，该试验由史克必成（SmithKline Beecham）葛兰素史克（GlaxoSmithKline）申办。

本次现场检查是FDA的生物研究监查项目的一部分。该项目通过设定的检查方法，评估研究的实施情况，以确保这些研究中受试者的权益、安全和福利得到了保护。

经对现场检查报告、该报告的附件进行审查，我们认为，您没有遵循适用的法律要求和监管临床研究实施及保护受试者的FDA法规。我们知道在现场检查结束时，Van Leeuwen女士和Tubb先生向您出示并和您讨论了FDA483表，即现场检查发现的问题。我们想强调以下几点：

1. 您未能确保 IRB 符合 21 CFR 56 要求而负责对拟开展的临床研究进行初始审查、跟踪审查和批准［21 CFR 312.66］

具体地说，在研究过程中IRB的审批多次失效，而当时仍有受试者在接受治疗或随访观察。现场检查发现，研究在2000年4月27日启动，在约2006年结束。部分试验受试者参加并被监查了约4年。我们注意到您未能在2001年4月27日到2001年5月28日，2004年4月8日到2004年9月8日，以及2005年9月9日到2005年11月27日期间得到IRB批准。

2. 您未能保存与研究相关的所有观察结果和其他相关数据的足够准确的病历记录［21 CFR 312. 62（b）］

a. 受试者（b）(6）最初签署了英文版的知情同意书，而之后作为一个不同的受试者（b）(6）重新签署了西班牙语版。这一受试者的两个原始图表在生日［（b）(6）和（b）(6）］、2型糖尿病确诊日期（1999年10月和2000年8月）以及吸烟史（1支/天30年和无）等内容上都有冲突。

b. 以下受试者的方案要求的胸部X射线检查缺失：

i. 受试者［（b）(6）］在2000年12月22日进行的检查。

ii. 受试者［（b）(6）］在2001年2月15日进行的检查。

iii. 受试者［（b）(6）］在2001年2月2日进行的检查。

iv. 受试者［（b）(6）］在2001年1月25日进行的检查。

c. 受试者［（b）(6）］2001年7月13日的胸部X射线报告缺失。

3. 您未能确保按照研究计划进行研究［21 CFR 312.60］

方案要求使用药物接收表记录所有已递送的药物的批号、运送数量和接收日期。第一次药物运送在2000年6月28日接收，最后一次运送在2006年1月31日接收。但是，在2003年11月21日之前的要求的记录没有保留。

本警告信的目的并非是罗列您在试验药物临床研究中存在的所有缺陷。确保遵循法律和相关FDA法规的每一项要求是您的职责。您应当解决这些缺陷，并建立规程，以确保任何正在进行或将来的研究均能符合FDA的法规。

自收到这封信的15个工作日内，您应当书面告知本办公室为预防将来发生类似违规情况已经采取或即将采取的措施。如果不能充分、迅速地解释上述违规问题，可能导致我们在不再通知的情况下采取监管措施。

附：英文原文

Quinones, Manue J., M.D.

WARNING LETTER

Mar 3, 2009

CERTIFIED MAIL
RETURN RECEIPT REQUESTED

Ref: 09-HFD-45-02-05

Manuel J. Quinones, M.D.
800 Pacific Coast Highway, #181
Redondo Beach, CA 90277

Dear Dr. Quinones:

Between July 21 and August 5, 2008, Ms. Diane C. Van Leeuwen and Mr. Richard W. Tubb, representing the Food and Drug Administration (FDA), conducted an investigation and met with you to review your conduct of a clinical investigation [Protocol Number (b)(4) entitled "A Randomized, Double-Study to compare the Durability of Glucose Lowering and Preservation of Pancreatic Beta-cell Function of Rosiglitazone Monotherapy Compared to Metformin or Glyburide/Glibenclamide in Patients with Drug-Naïve recently Diagnosed Type 2 Diabetes Mellitus"] of the investigational drug rosiglitazone (Avandia), performed for SmithKline Beecham/GlaxoSmithKline (GSK).

This inspection is a part of FDA's Bioresearch Monitoring Program, which includes inspections designed to evaluate the conduct of research and to ensure that the rights, safety, and welfare of the human subjects of the study have been protected.

From our review of the establishment inspection report and the documents submitted with that report, we conclude that you did not adhere to the applicable statutory requirements and FDA regulations governing the conduct of clinical investigations and the protection of human subjects. We are aware that at the conclusion of the inspection, Ms. Van Leeuwen and Mr. Tubb presented and discussed with you Form FDA 483, Inspectional Observations. We wish to emphasize the following:

1. You failed to assure that an IRB that complies with the requirements set forth in 21 CFR part 56 was responsible for the initial and continuing review and approval of the proposed clinical study (21 CFR 312. 66).

Specifically, IRB approval lapsed on several occasions during the ongoing study where subjects were being treated or seen for follow-up visits. Inspection found that the study was initiated on 4/27/00 and was closed in approximately 2006. Some trial subjects participated and were monitored for up to four years. We note that you failed to have IRB approval from 4/27/01 to 5/28/01, 4/8/04 to 9/8/04, and 9/9/05 to 11/27/05.

2. You failed to maintain adequate and accurate case histories that record all observations and data pertinent to the investigation [21 CFR 312. 62(b)].

a. Subject #(b)(6) was initially consented with an English version of the informed consent form, and later reconsented with a Spanish version, under a different subject number (b)(6). The two source charts for this subject had conflicting dates of birth(b)(6) vs. (b)(6), dates of type Ⅱ diabetes mellitus diagnosis (10/99 vs. 8/00), and smoking history (30 yrs 1 cigar a day vs. none).

b. Protocol-required chest x-rays were missing for the following subjects:

ⅰ (b)(6) reported taken on 12/22/00

ⅱ (b)(6) reported taken on 2/15/01

ⅲ (b)(6) reported taken on 2/2/01

ⅳ (b)(6) reported taken on 1/25/01

c. Chest x-ray report for subject (b)(6) was missing for x-rays dated 7/13/01.

3. You failed to ensure the investigation was conducted according to the investigational plan (21 CFR 312. 60).

The protocol required a Drug Receipt From to be used to record all delivered medication lot numbers, quantity shipped and date of receipt. The first drug shipment was received 6/28/00; the last shipment was received 1/31/06. However, the required records were not kept for the period prior to 11/21/03.

This letter is not intended to be an all-inclusive list of deficiencies with your clinical study of an investigational drug. It is your responsibility to ensure adherence to each requirement of the law and relevant FDA regulations. You should address these deficiencies and establish procedures to ensure that any on-going or future studies will be in compliance with FDA regulations.

Within fifteen (15) working days of your receipt of this letter, you should notify this office in writing of the actions you have taken or will be taking to prevent similar violations in the future. Failure to adequately and promptly explain the violations noted above may result in regulatory action without further notice.

If you have any questions, please contact Constance Lewin, M.D., M.P.H.,at 301-796-3397; FAX 301-847-8748.

Your written response and any pertinent documentation should be addressed to:

Constance Lewin, M. D., M.P.H.
Branch Chief, Good Clinical Practice Branch I
Division of Scientific Investigations
Office of Compliance
Center for Drug Evaluation and Research
Food and Drug Administration
Bldg 51, Room 5354
10903 New Hampshire Avenue
Silver Spring, MD 20993

Sincerely yours,

{See appended electronic signature page}

Leslie K. Ball, M.D.
Director
Division of Scientific Investigations
Office of Compliance
Center for Drug Evaluation and Research

第133封　给Coté, Charles J.医学博士的警告信

2009年3月2日

参考号：09-HFD-45-02-04

尊敬的Cot é 博士：

2008年4月14日至30日，M. Patricia Murphy女士和Michelle M. Noe女士代表FDA进行了现场检查，与您会面，并对您所实施的申办者为Organon、试验药物为Zemuron®（罗库溴铵）的以下临床研究进行了审查：

- 试验方案(b)(4)，标题为："一项开放、随机、ⅢB期、多中心临床试验，在儿童和青少年受试者中，气管插管给药、推注和静脉维持剂量罗库溴铵注射液的药效学参数评价"；
- 试验方案(b)(4)，标题为："一项随机、评估者盲，剂量范围，ⅢB期，多中心临床试验，在全身麻醉下的儿童和青少年受试者中，比较罗库溴铵注射液三种不同的插管剂量（0.45mg/kg，0.6mg/kg和1.0mg/kg）的插管状况和阻滞的时间进程"。

本次现场检查是FDA的生物研究监查项目的一部分。该项目通过设定的检查方法，评估研究的实施情况，以确保这些研究中受试者的权益、安全和福利得到了保护。

经对FDA现场检查报告、该报告的附件，以及您2008年5月22日对FDA483表（现场检查发现的问题）的书面回复进行审查，我们认为，您没有遵循适用的法律要求和监管临床研究实施的FDA法规。我们知道在现场检查结束时，Murphy女士与Noe女士向您出示并讨论了FDA483表，即现场检查发现的问题。我们想强调以下几点：

1. 您未能按照签署的研究者声明进行研究［21 CFR 312.60］

当您签署了上述临床研究的研究者声明（FDA 1572表），即表明您同意承担临床研究者的职责。您明确同意亲自开展研究，或监督研究中某些您未亲自参与的部分，并确保告知所有协助进行试验的助理、同事和员工他们应承担的义务。

a. 您没有对您所授权参与这项研究工作的人员进行充分监督。FDA的检查显示，您没有对被授权这项研究任务的人员进行充分的监督，以确保这项临床试验按照签署的研究者声明和适用的法规来进行。由于您未能进行充分的监督，导致在下面第2条和第3条列举的知情同意等记录不完整和记录不准确的问题。在您2008年5月22日对FDA 483表的回复中提到，虽然您亲自参与了研究，但您未能确保参与人员有充分的培训，也没有对他们在病例报告表中的记录进行核实。我们已收到您的承诺，即已采取纠正措施，以确保记录更加严谨。

b. 关于试验方案［（b）（4）］，您没有按照研究者声明（FDA 1572表）的要求，列出所有参与这项研究的授权研究者们的名字。FDA的规定明确要求，如果一项研究是由一个团队进行的，研究者是该团队的负责人，团队中的任何其他人为授权研究者［21 CFR 312.3（b）］。检查时，您告诉FDA检查员，临床研究方案要求由住院医生在外科手术当天在手术室进行盲法评估。因为住院医生要进行这一重要的研究活动，因此住院医生应作为授权研究者在FDA1572表中列出。我们已收到您的承诺，即将来所有参与临床研究评估的相关人员都将列入FDA 1572表。

2. 您未能获得合法有效的知情同意［21 CFR 50和21 CFR 312.60］

除了21 CFR 50.23和21 CFR 50.24规定的情形外，获得受试者或受试者法定监护人的合法有效同意后，研究者才能把受试者纳入临床研究。知情同意书的内容应该采用受试者或受试者监护人能理解的语言［21

CFR 50.20］。应对知情同意进行记录，采用IRB批准的知情同意书，并经受试者或受试者的法定监护人签名同意并注明日期［21 CFR 50.27（a）］。您还未按IRB的要求取得知情同意［21 CFR 50.55］。

a. 发现在［（b）（4）］试验方案的［（b）（6）］受试者和［（b）（4）］试验方案［（b）（6）］受试者的知情同意书中，伪造受试者法定监护人的签名。我们注意到，您在内部稽查时发现了伪造签名，您分别于2007年9月10日、2007年12月11日写信给受试者［（b）（6）］的父母、受试者［（b）（6）］监护人，要求重新签署知情同意文件。此外，您及时把有关发现报告给伦理委员会。您2008年5月22日回复FDA483表的信中提到，根据机构的规定，您已要求研究协调员确保最初的已签署的知情同意书的复印件放置在受试者的医疗记录中，但您未证实该要求是否得以落实。您还提到该情况发生后，您希望能够找回最初的知情同意书复印件。您还说，估计是您以前的研究护士（研究协调员）遗失了签过名的知情同意书原件，后面伪造了知情同意书的签名。您还表示，您将这些情况已报告给护士注册委员会。作为研究者，您应该负责监督授权研究人员的研究活动。

在您的书面回复中，您还指出，您立即与那些知情同意书签名有明显伪造的家庭联系。您说能联系到2/3的家庭，而且他们已签署确认声明，在研究之前就已经允许他们的孩子参加该项研究。因1/3的家庭已经迁址，您无法与他们取得联系。您提到CRO的文件证实受试者在参加这项临床研究之前，确实在有效的知情同意书上征得了所有受试者家长的同意。因为没有提供足够的书面文件来支持您的上述陈述，我们认为您对本问题的回复尚不充分。

b. 在［（b）（4）］试验中，知情同意书第5页的问题“您同意让您的孩子抽取血液样本吗？”随后是空格让受试者或受试者的法定监护人确认“YES”或“NO”并用其首字母表示。然而，受试者的药代动力学测试样本并没有获得取血样的知情同意，如包括但不限于［（b）（6）］受试者。我们注意到，您于2007年12月11日将这些受试者不同意抽血的情况报告给伦理委员会。在2008年5月22日您对FDA483表的答复中说到，您将会确保在知情同意书正文部分包括所有的选择条款。然而，您没有说明如何保证得到正确的知情同意。

c. 在［（b）（4）］试验中，伦理委员会要求7～13岁的受试者，须签署知情同意书。受试者［（b）（6）］在知情同意的时候7岁，但在入组研究前没有签署知情同意书。我们注意到，您于2007年12月11日致信给该受试者的法定监护人，要求受试者在知情同意书上签署名字和日期。因此，您未按伦理委员会的规定取得知情同意［21 CFR 50.55］。

d. 根据研究记录，受试者［（b）（6）］的监护人不会讲英语。该监护人签署了英文的知情同意书，而非其可以理解的语言的书面知情同意书。您没有给受试者的监护人提供翻译后的知情同意文件或“简化”翻译后的知情同意书。我们注意到，在签署的知情同意书上注明了翻译员的名字。在您对FDA483表的书面回复中，您承认您没有给这些受试者提供翻译后的知情同意书，但您会按照该要求培训您的员工，确保在将来不会发生这种事。已收到您将采取的纠正措施，以确保在将来的任何研究中不会再次发生这些情况。

e. 知情同意书是由研究人员，而不是由入组［（b）（4）］临床试验的［（b）（4）］受试者的法定监护人和入组［（b）（4）］临床试验的［（b）（4）］受试者来签署日期。在您于2008年5月22日对FDA483表的书面回复中承认，这是您们的日常惯例，在父母签名之前先自己填上日期，以简化过程。您称现在已知道受试者和其父母必须自己签署知情同意的日期。已收到您将采取的纠正措施，以确保在将来的任何研究中不会再次发生这些问题。

3. 您未能保存研究中每个使用试验药物或对照组的受试者的所有研究观察结果和其他数据的足够及准确的病历［21 CFR 312.62（b）］

示例包括，但不限于以下内容：

a.［（b）（4）］试验方案中主要疗效参数，是计算最后一次罗库溴铵®插管维持剂量，或罗库溴铵®输液停止后从插管剂量到T3再现时的总剂量。以下受试者用于计算总剂量（mg）的给药持续时间，与TOF监测原始记录中的给药时间间隔不吻合：

受试者编号	四联刺激监测（mcg/kg/min）	四联刺激监测原始记录 时间（h:mm:ss）/持续时间(mm:ss)	用于计算的持续时间
[（b）（6）]	调节到14	10:15:49 ~ 10:23:28/7:39（459秒）	499秒
	调节到12	10:23:28 ~ 10:28:18/4:50（290秒）	429秒
	调节到8	10:31:57 ~ 10:44:58/13:01（781秒）	790秒
[（b）（6）]	从10开始	13:36:52 ~ 13:39:09/2:17（137秒）	177秒
	调节到12	13:39:09 ~ 13:42:01/2:52（172秒）	212秒
	调节到10	13:42:01 ~ 13:44:25/2:24（144秒）	165秒
	调节到8	13:44:25 ~ 13:47:52/3:27（207秒）	186秒
	调节到6	13:47:52 ~ 13:51:02/3:10（190秒）	230秒
	调节到4	13:51:02 ~ 13:54:38/3:36（216秒）	226秒
	调节到2	13:54:38 ~ 14:03:33/8:55（535秒）	565秒
	调节到5	14:03:33 ~ 14:15:01/11:28（688秒）	128秒
	调节到4	14:23:24 ~ 14:46:14/22:50（1370秒）	1402秒
	调节到6	14:46:14 ~ 15:15:39/29:25（1765秒）	1773秒
[（b）（6）]	从10开始	14:42:40 ~ 14:48:07/5:27（327秒）	361秒
[（b）（6）]	调节到8	9:01:32 ~ 9:06:10/4:38（278秒）	318秒
	调节到5	9:26:45 ~ 9:37:25/10:40（640秒）	680秒
	调节到5	9:55:54 ~ 10:07:15/11:21（681秒）	721秒
[（b）（6）]	从10开始	12:56:21 ~ 13:04:20/7:59（479秒）	519秒
	调节到8	13:09:52 ~ 15:25:32/2:15:40（8140秒）	8732秒
[（b）（6）]	调节到8	12:34:59 ~ 12:38:29/3:30（210秒）	220秒
	调节到2	12:41:52 ~ 13:00:45/18:53（1133秒）	1128秒
[（b）（6）]	调节到5	11:43:04 ~ 12:00:49/17:45（1065秒）	1125秒

b.［（b）（4）］临床试验中，随机接受输注维持剂量的10例受试者没有按照方案记录“输液速度（mL/min）”。在您2008年5月22日对FDA483表的答复中，您承认您记录的剂量是从生成四联刺激监测的电脑上获取的以mg/（kg·min）为单位的剂量，而没有进行适当计算而获得以mL/min为单位的输液速度。

c. 研究记录表明，在［（b）（4）］临床试验中入组的［（b）（6）］受试者，于2006年6月2日获得知情同意，在［（b）（4）］临床试验中入组的［（b）（6）］受试者，于2006年11月30日获得知情同意。在上述知情同意书的“获取知情的研究医生或人员”声明上面，都有一个类似您的签名。在检查中，您告知这些文件上的签名不是您的。在您于2008年5月22日对FDA483表的回复中称上述文件上的签名是伪造的。

d. 在［（b）（4）］临床试验中，［（b）（6）］受试者输液量的维持剂量的原始记录上“罗库溴铵®输液浓度（mg/mL）”显示为“1：1”或“0.5：1”。根据这些记录，实际的药物浓度是不确定的。此外，原始记录中的浓度与［（b）（6）］受试者CRF上的浓度不一致。在您对FDA 483表的回复中称这些剂量由研究护理记录。您还称，您将确保以后授权记录具体信息（如稀释过程等）的人员得到充分的训练。

我们获知您保证已经采取纠正措施，以确保在将来的任何研究中不会重复出现项目3中的问题。

本警告信的目的并非是罗列您在试验药物临床研究中存在的所有缺陷。确保遵循法律和相关FDA法规的每一项要求是您的职责。您应当解决这些缺陷，并建立规程，以确保任何正在进行或将来进行的研究均能符合FDA的法规。

自收到这封信的15个工作日内，您应当书面告知本办公室为预防将来发生类似违规情况已经采取或将要采取的措施。如果不能充分、迅速地解释上述违规问题，可能导致我们在不再通知的情况下采取监管措施。

附：英文原文

Coté, Charles J., M.D.

WARNING LETTER

Mar 2, 2009

CERTIFIED MAIL
RETURN RECEIPT REQUESTED

Ref: 09-HFD-45-02-04

Charles J. Coté, M.D.
Massachusetts General Hospital
Department of Anesthesia and Critical Care
55 Fruit Street
Boston, MA 02114

Dear Dr. Coté:

Between April 14 and 30, 2008, Ms. M. Patricia Murphy and Ms. Michelle M. Noe, representing the Food and Drug Administration (FDA), conducted an investigation and met with you to review your conduct of the following clinical investigations of the investigational drug Zemuron® (rocuronium bromide), performed for Organon:

- Protocol [(b)(4)] entitled, "An open-label, randomized, phase ⅢB, multicenter trial to evaluate the pharmacodynamic parameters of intubation bolus, and bolus and infusion maintenance doses of Zemuron® in pediatric and adolescent subjects" and
- Protocol [(b)(4)] entitled, "A randomized, assessor-blind, dose-ranging, phaseⅢB, multicenter trial comparing the intubating conditions and time course of block of three different intubating doses (0.45 mg/kg, 0.6 mg/kg and 1.0 mg/kg) of Zemuron® in pediatric and adolescent subjects under general anesthesia."

This inspection is a part of the FDA's Bioresearch Monitoring Program, which includes inspections designed to evaluate the conduct of research and to ensure that the rights, safety, and welfare of the human subjects of those studies have been protected.

From our review of the establishment inspection report, the documents submitted with that report, and your May 22, 2008 written response to the Form FDA 483, Inspectional Observations, we conclude that you did not adhere to the applicable statutory requirements and FDA regulations governing the conduct of clinical investigations and the protection of human subjects. We are aware that at the conclusion of the inspection, Ms. Murphy and Ms. Noe presented and discussed with you Form FDA 483, Inspectional Observations. We wish to emphasize the following:

1. You failed to conduct the studies according to the signed investigator statement [21 CFR 312.60].

When you signed the investigator statements (Form FDA 1572) for the above-referenced clinical investigations, you agreed to take on the responsibilities of a clinical investigator. You specifically agreed to personally conduct, or supervise those aspects of the study you did not personally conduct, and to ensure that all associates, colleagues, and employees assisting in the conduct of the study were informed about their obligations.

a. You failed to adequately supervise individuals to whom you delegated study tasks. The FDA inspection revealed that your supervision of personnel to whom you delegated study tasks was not adequate to ensure that the clinical trials were conducted according to the signed investigator statement and applicable regulations. Your failure to provide adequate oversight resulted in inadequate informed consent documentation and inadequate and inaccurate records as outlined in items 2 and 3 below. In your May 22, 2008 response to the Form FDA 483, you stated that although you were personally involved in the study, you did not ensure that the delegated staff were fully trained, and you did not verify their performance as documented in the case report forms (CRFs). We acknowledge your assurance that corrective actions have been taken to assure more rigorous documentation.

b. Regarding protocol [(b)(4)], you did not list the names of all subinvestigators who would be assisting in the conduct of the investigation, as required by the Statement of Investigator, Form FDA 1572. The FDA regulations specified that in the event an investigation is conducted by a team of individuals, the investigator is the responsible leader of the team. "Subinvestigator" includes any other individual member of that team [21 CFR 312.3(b)]. During the inspection, you told the FDA investigator that the protocol-required blinded assessments were done by residents present in the operating room on the day of surgery. By performing these significant study activities, the residents should have been listed on the Form FDA 1572 as subinvestigators. We acknowledge your assurance that in the future, the individuals who are involved in research-related assessments will be included on a Form FDA 1572.

2. You failed to obtain legally effective informed consent [21 CFR part 50 and 21 CFR 312.60].

Except as provided in 21 CFR 50.23 and 21 CFR 50.24, no investigator may involve a human being as a subject in research unless the investigator has obtained the legally effective informed consent of the subject or the subject's legally authorized representative. The information that is given to the subject or the representative shall be in language understandable to the subject or the representative [21 CFR 50.20]. Informed consent must be documented by the use of a written consent form approved by the institutional review board (IRB) and signed and dated by the subject or the subject's legally authorized representative at the time of consent [21 CFR 50.27(a)]. You also failed to obtain proper assent as determined to be appropriate by the IRB [21 CFR § 50.55].

a. Fabricated signatures of the subject's legally authorized representative were found on the consent forms for subjects [(b)(6)], who were enrolled in protocol [(b)(4)], and subject [(b)(6)], who was enrolled in protocol [(b)(4)]. We note that you discovered the fabricated signatures through your own internal audit, and that you sent letters dated September 10, 2007 to the parents of subjects [(b)(6)], and a letter dated December 11, 2007 to the representatives of subject [(b)(6)], requesting that the informed consent documents be signed again. In addition, you promptly reported the findings to the IRB. In your May 22, 2008 response to the Form FDA 483, you stated that you asked the study coordinator to ensure that copies of the original, signed consent forms were placed in the subjects' medical records, according to institutional policy, but you did not confirm this action. You stated that had this occurred, you would have been able to retrieve a copy of the original consent forms. You stated that it is presumed that your former research nurse (study coordinator) apparently falsified the signatures after she lost the original, signed consent forms. You also stated that you reported these findings to the Board of Registration in Nursing. As the clinical investigator, you are responsible for oversight of study activities delegated to study staff.

In your written response you also stated that you took immediate action to contact the families that had consent forms with apparently false signatures. You stated that you was able to reach two out of three and they sent confirmatory signed statement that they had allowed their child to participate in a research project prior to study procedure. You stated that the third family had vacated their apartment and you were not able to contact them. You stated that documentation by the CRO exists to confirm that you did in fact obtain consent from all subject parents prior to participation in the study on a valid consent form. We do not find your response to this observation adequate as it does not include documentation to support your statements.

b. Regarding protocol [(b)(4)], page 5 of the informed consent document asks "Do you agree to allow your child to have blood samples taken?" followed by a space for the subject or subject's legally authorized representative to respond by checking "YES" or "NO" and initial. However, pharmacokinetic samples were collected from subjects without obtaining informed consent for blood sampling. Example: include, but are not limited to, subjects [(b)(6)]. We note that you sent a letter dated December 11, 2007 to the IRB informing the IRB that these subjects did not consent to blood draw. In your May 22, 2008 response to the Form FDA 483, you stated that you will ensure that you are aware of any options sections included in the body of the consent form. However, you did not state how you will ensure that proper consent is obtained.

c. Regarding protocol [(b)(4)], the IRB requires that subjects who are 7-13 years old sign a Research Assent form. Subject [(b)(6)] was seven years old at the time of consent, but did not sign a Research Assent form prior to being enrolled in the study. We note that you sent the subject's representative a letter dated December 11, 2007 requesting that the subject sign and date a Research Assent form. Therefore, you failed to obtain proper assent as determined to be appropriate by the IRB [21 CFR § 50.55].

d. According to the study records, representatives for subjects [(b)(6)] were non-English speaking. The subjects' representatives signed informed consent documents written in English rather than a language understandable to the representatives. The subjects' representatives were not provided with either a translated consent document or a "short form" translated consent document. We note that the names of the translators were written on the signed consent documents. In your response to the Form FDA 483, you acknowledged that you failed to provide translated consent documents to these subjects, but stated that you would train your staff on this requirement so it would not happen in the future. We acknowledge your assurance that corrective actions will be taken to ensure that this finding is not repeated in any future studies.

e. Informed consent documents were dated by study personnel rather than the legally authorized representative for subjects [(b)(4)] enrolled in protocol [(b)(4)], and subject [(b)(4)] enrolled in protocol [(b)(4)]. In your May 22, 2008 response to the Form FDA 483, you acknowledged that it was your routine practice to insert the date yourself, prior to the parents' signatures, in order to simplify the process. You stated that you now know that subjects and parents must date the consent forms themselves. We acknowledge your assurance that corrective actions have been taken to ensure that this finding is not repeated in any future studies.

3. You failed to maintain adequate and accurate case histories that record all observations and other data pertinent to the investigation on each individual administered the investigational drug or employed as a control in the investigation [21 CFR 312.62(b)].

Examples include, but are not limited to, the following:

a. Regarding protocol [(b)(4)] the primary efficacy parameter was the total dose from administration of intubating dose to reappearance of T3 after the last maintenance bolus dose of Zemuron®, or discontinuation of Zemuron® infusion. The duration of drug administrations used to calculate the total dose (mg) does not correspond to the time interval of drug administration recorded on the Train-of Four Watch (TOF-Watch) source document for the following subjects:

Subject No.	TOF-Watch（mcg/kg/min）	TOF-Watch Source Document Time (h:mm:ss) / Duration (mm:ss)	Duration Used in Calculation
[(b)(4)]	adjust to14	10:15:49-10:23:28/7:39（459sec）	499sec
	adjust to12	10:23:28-10:28:18/4:50（290sec）	429sec
	adjust to8	10:31:57-10:44:58/13:01（781sec）	790sec
[(b)(4)]	start at 10	13:36:52-13:39:09/2:17（137sec）	177sec
	adjust to12	13:39:09-13:42:01/2:52（172sec）	212sec
	adjust to10	13:42:01-13:44:25/2:24（144sec）	165sec
	adjust to8	13:44:25-13:47:52/3:27（207sec）	186sec
	adjust to6	13:47:52-13:51:02/3:10（190sec）	230sec
	adjust to4	13:51:02-13:54:38/3:36（216sec）	226sec
	adjust to2	13:54:38-14:03:33/8:55（535sec）	565sec
	adjust to5	14:03:33-14:15:01/11:28（688sec）	128sec
	adjust to4	14:23:24-14:46:14/22:50（1370sec）	1402sec
	adjust to6	14:46:14-15:15:39/29:25（1765sec）	1773sec
[(b)(4)]	start at 10	14:42:40-14:48:07/5:27（327sec）	361sec
[(b)(4)]	adjust to8	9:01:32-9:06:10/4:38（278sec）	318sec
	adjust to5	9:26:45-9:37:25/10:40（640sec）	680sec
	adjust to5	9:55:54-10:07:15/11:21（681sec）	721sec
[(b)(4)]	start at 10	12:56:21-13:04:20/7:59（479sec）	519sec
	adjust to8	13:09:52-15:25:32/2:15:40（8140sec）	8732sec
[(b)(4)]	adjust to8	12:34:59-12:38:29/3:30（210sec）	220sec
	adjust to2	12:41:52-13:00:45/18:53（1133sec）	1128sec
[(b)(4)]	adjust to5	11:43:04-12:00:49/17:45（1065sec）	1125sec

b. Regarding protocol [(b)(4)], the "Infusion Rate (mL/min)" was not recorded for the 10 subjects who were randomized and received the infusion maintenance dose for protocol [(b)(4)]. In your May 22, 2008 response to the Form FDA 483, you acknowledged you recorded the dose in mcg/kg/min that was obtained from the computer generated TOF-Watch and did not appropriately calculate the infusion rate in ml/min.

c. The study records indicate that informed consent for subject [(b)(6)] enrolled in protocol [(b)(4)] was obtained on June 2, 2006, and informed consent for subject [(b)(6)] enrolled in protocol [(b)(4)] was obtained on November 30, 2006. Each of these informed consent documents contains a signature similar to yours entered on the line above the statement "Study Doctor or Person Obtaining Consent." During the inspection, you stated that the signatures on these documents were not yours. In your May 22, 2008 response to the Form FDA 483, you stated that the signatures on these documents were fabricated.

d. Regarding protocol [(b)(4)] the "Concentration of Zemuron® Infusion (mg/mL)" on the source document for the administration of (infusion) maintenance dose was recorded as "1:1" or "0.5:1" for subjects [(b)(6)]. Based on this documentation, the actual drug concentration is uncertain. In addition the concentration on the source document does not match the concentration reported on the CRF for subject [(b)(6)]. In your response to the FDA Form 483, you stated that your research nurse recorded these doses. You also stated that, in the future, you will ensure that staff delegated to document specific information, such as dilutions, are adequately trained on how to do so.

We acknowledge your assurance that corrective actions have been taken to ensure that the findings in item 3 are not repeated in any future studies.

This letter is not intended to be an all-inclusive list of deficiencies with your clinical study of an investigational drug. It is your responsibility to ensure adherence to each requirement of the law and relevant FDA regulations. You should address these deficiencies and establish procedures to ensure that any on-going or future studies will be in compliance with FDA regulations.

Within fifteen (15) working days of your receipt of this letter, you should notify this office in writing of the actions you have taken or will be taking to prevent similar violations in the future. Failure to adequately and promptly explain the violations noted above may result in regulatory action without further notice.

If you have any questions, please contact Constance Lewin, M.D., M.P.H., at 301-796-3397; FAX 301- 847-8748. Your written response and any pertinent documentation should be addressed to:

Constance Lewin, M.D., M.P.H.
Branch Chief, Good Clinical Practice Branch I
Division of Scientific Investigations
Office of Compliance
Center for Drug Evaluation and Research
Food and Drug Administration
Bldg 51, Room 5354
10903 New Hampshire Avenue
Silver Spring, MD 20993

Sincerely yours,

{See appended electronic signature page}

Leslie K. Ball, M.D.
Director
Division of Scientific Investigations
Office of Compliance
Center for Drug Evaluation and Research

This is a representation of an electronic record that was signed electronically and this page is the manifestation of the electronic signature.

/S/

Leslie Ball
3/2/2009 06:17:05 PM
Warning Letter Response
Coté, Charles J., M.D. Response Letter 1
Page Last Updated: 12/08/2009
Note: If you need help accessing information in different file formats, see Instructions for Downloading Viewers and Players.
Accessibility Contact FDA Careers FDA Basics FOIA No FEAR Act Site Map Transparency Website Policies
U.S. Food and Drug Administration 10903 New Hampshire Avenue Silver Spring, MD 20993 Ph. 1-888-INFO-FDA (1-888-463-6332)
Contact FDA
LSA.gov
For Government For Press
Combination Products Advisory Committees Science & Research Regulatory Information Safety Emergency Preparedness International Programs News & Events Training and Continuing Education Inspections/Compliance State & Local Officials Consumers Industry Health Professionals FDA Archive
U.S. Department of Health & Human Services
Links on this page:
1. /ICECI/EnforcementActions/WarningLetters/ucm 171367.htm

第 134 封　给 Desai, Virendra M. 医学博士的警告信

2009年3月2日

参考号：09-HFD-45-02-03

尊敬的Desai博士：

2008年3月17日至2008年4月17日，Yvette LaCour-Davis小姐和Yvonne LaCour女士代表FDA进行了现场检查，与您见面并对您进行的由（b）（4）申办，试验方案（b）（4）标题为“一项Ⅲ期，（b）（4）与（b）（4）在试验药物（b）（4）治疗复杂的（b）（4）的随机双盲研究”的临床研究进行了审查。

本次现场检查是FDA的生物研究监查项目的一部分。该项目通过设定的检查方法，评估研究的实施情况，以确保这些研究中受试者的权益、安全和福利得到保护。

经对现场检查报告、该报告的附件、FDA483表（即现场检查发现的问题），以及您2008年6月9日对FDA483表的书面回复进行审查，我们认为，您没有遵循适用的法律要求和监管临床研究实施的FDA法规。我们知道在现场检查结束时，FDA检查员出示并和您讨论了FDA483表，即现场检查发现的问题。我们想强调以下几点：

1. 您未能按照研究计划进行研究［21 CFR 312.60］

a. 我们检查发现，在您研究场所审查和评估受试者基线实验室结果之前，所有18个随机进入研究的受试者接受了研究药物，这样做潜在损害了受试者的安全性。具体而言，［（b）（4）］研究的实验室结果在试验受试者被静脉注射研究药物3天后被您接收和审查，而在某些情况下，［（b）（4）］研究的结果在受试者被静脉注射研究药物20天后也没有被您接收和审查。总结如下表：

知情同意书签署日期	预筛试验的日期/时间	随机进入研究的日期/时间	受试者接受第一个剂量的研究药物的日期/时间	由中心实验室[(b) (4)]得到的基线实验日期	由地方实验室[(b) (4)]报告的基线实验日期	[(b) (4)]研究的基线实验结果P. I. 签署日期
[(b)(6)]7/27/2006	27/07/2006@13:10	27/07/2006@ 13:17	07/27/2006@ 16:55	08/04/2006（由传真）	08/03/2006	[(b)(4)]=8/4/2006 [(b)(4)]=7/28/2006
[(b)(6)]7/27/2006	27/07/2006@15:38	27/07/2006@ 14:56	07/27/2006@ 17:04	09/08/2006 重印/传真	08/03/2006	[(b)(4)]=8/9/2006 [(b)(4)]=8/7/2006
[(b)(6)]8/1/2006	1/08/2006@14:50	1/08/2006@ 15:08	08/01/2006@ 17:05	08/03/2006（由传真）	08/25/2006	[(b)(4)]=8/3/2006 [(b)(4)]=8/25/2006
[(b)(6)]8/1/2006	01/08/2006@15:10	01/08/2006@ 15:09	8/1/2006@ 17:10	08/03/2006（由传真）	08/25/2006	[(b)(4)]=8/3/2006 [(b)(4)]=8/25/2006
[(b)(6)]8/2/2006	02/08/2006@11:30	02/08/2006@ 14:10	8/2/2006@ 16:22	08/09/2006 重印/传真	08/07/2006	[(b)(4)]=8/9/2006 [(b)(4)]=8/3/2006
[(b)(6)]8/3/2006	03/08/2006@11:00	03/08/2006@ 11:14	8/3/2006@ 16:55	08/04/2006（由传真）	08/09/2006	[(b)(4)]=8/4/2006 [(b)(4)]=8/10/2006
[(b)(6)]8/7/2006	07/08/2006@16:30	07/08/2006 (存档未发现传真)	8/7/2006@ 16:45	08/09/2006（由传真）	08/16/2006 仅有	[(b)(4)]=8/9/2006 [(b)(4)]=8/16/2006
[(b)(6)]8/8/2006	08/08/2006@14:02	08/08/2006 (存档未发现传真)	8/8/2006@ 16:38	08/11/2006（由传真）	08/25/2006	[(b)(4)]=8/11/2006 [(b)(4)]=8/25/2006
[(b)(6)]8/9/2006	09/08/2006@13:23	09/08/2006@ 12:41	8/9/2006@ 16:44	08/11/2006（由传真）	08/16/2006	[(b)(4)]=8/10/2006 [(b)(4)]=8/18/2006
[(b)(6)]8/10/2006	10/08/2006@11:23	10/08/2006@ 11:28	8/10/2006@ 16:56	08/15/2006（由传真）	08/17/2006	[(b)(4)]=8/15/2006 [(b)(4)]=8/18/2006

续表

知情同意书签署日期	预筛试验的日期/时间	随机进入研究的日期/时间	受试者接受第一个剂量的研究药物的日期/时间	由中心实验室[(b)(4)]得到的基线实验日期	由地方实验室[(b)(4)]报告的基线实验日期	[(b)(4)]研究的基线实验结果P.I.签署日期
[(b)(6)]8/14/2006	14/08/2006@14:10	14/08/2006@13:46	8/14/2006@16:47	08/17/2006（由传真）	08/30/2006	[(b)(4)]=8/17/2006 [(b)(4)]=8/30/2006
[(b)(6)]8/14/2006	14/08/2006@14:26	14/08/2006@13:48	8/14/2006@16:52	08/16/2006（由传真）	08/30/2006	[(b)(4)]=18/16/2006 [(b)(4)]=8/30/2006
[(b)(6)]8/16/2006	16/08/2006@12:45	16/08/2006@12:18	8/16/2006@16:44	08/20/2006（由传真）	08/28/2006	[(b)(4)]=8/20/2006 [(b)(4)]=8/28/2006
[(b)(6)]8/16/2006	16/08/2006@15:00	16/08/2006@13:52	8/16/2006@16:50	08/18/2006（由传真）	08/25/2006	[(b)(4)]=8/18/2006 [(b)(4)]=8/25/2006
[(b)(6)]8/18/2006	18/08/2006@14:10	18/08/2006@13:13	8/18/2006@16:55	08/21/2006	08/28/2006	[(b)(4)]=8/22/2006 [(b)(4)]=8/28/2006
[(b)(6)]8/18/2006	18/08/2006@15:35	18/08/2006@14:09	8/18/2006@16:58	08/20/2006（由传真）	08/30/2006	[(b)(4)]=8/20/2006 [(b)(4)]=8/30/2006
[(b)(6)]8/21/2006	21/08/2006@11:10	21/08/2006@11:00	8/21/2006@16:44	08/23/2006（由传真）	08/21/2006	[(b)(4)]=8/23/2006 [(b)(4)]=8/30/2006
[(b)(6)]8/21/2006	21/08/2006@12:50	21/08/2006@13:35	8/21/2006@16:50	08/23/2006（由传真）	08/30/2006	[(b)(4)]=8/23/2006 [(b)(4)]=8/30/2006

您对FDA483表的书面回复提供的解释是不被接受的。您在回复中声明，“方案的5.2.2仅表明中心实验室检测需要被获得。另外，方案的5.1.7.4仅提到妊娠试验在试验第一次给药前需要被审查。”若这些声明是真实的，试验方案58页清楚地写着“所有筛选/给药前评估将被认为是基线并且在随机和第一天的给药前应进行实施和审查……”当您签署FDA1572表，即研究者声明的时候，您同意临床研究者的责任包括确保研究按照研究方案和签署的研究者声明实施，以保护受试者安全和权益及福利，并遵循临床研究者的所有义务和21 CFR 312其他相关要求。我们提醒您，作为一个临床研究者，您对研究的实施负有责任。

b. 方案要求已知或可能有肝功能缺陷的受试者（总胆红素≥2×正常范围的上限［ULN］，或丙氨酸氨基转移酶［ALT］≥3 × ULN，或天冬氨酸氨基转移酶［AST］≥3× ULN）应被排除在研究行列之外。

我们的检查发现，尽管［（b）（4）］报告中的受试者［（b）（6）］基线AST110U/L（大于3倍的ULN），仍在2006年8月16日入组的研究中。另外，［（b）（4）］，您当地的实验室，报告受试者基线ALT为120U/L，这也高于了3倍的ULN。您在检查期间声明，受试者并没有已知或疑似肝功能缺陷，也不知道肝功能检查结果升高。但是，在您2008年6月9日的书面回复中，您承认“如果实验结果在2007年8月16日随机前已经获得并审查，受试者将不会满足入选/排除标准”。另外，日期为2006年8月17日@15:00护理的记录说明，“由于有肝功能检查升高，受试者退出研究。受试者有酗酒历史。”根据受试者用药记录（“MAR”），受试者在2006年8月17日退出研究之前，从2006年8月16日16:50到2006年8月17日10:21被输注了5个剂量的试验药物。该受试者入组研究是一个明显研究方案违背。

c. 方案要求所有育龄女性在试验药物第一次给药前有一个基线值的阴性的妊娠试验。但是，受试者［（b）（6）］在没有完成妊娠试验的情况下被随机分配并获得试验药物。在您的FDA483表的回复中，您承认该受试者应该在接受试验药物之前完成妊娠试验。

d. 方案要求在第8天随访时进行“体格检查”“创面评估”和“自基线以来的总体临床评估”。这些受试者［（b）（6）］都没有进行。在您的FDA483回复中，您承认第8天信息没有获得。

2. 您未能保存研究中使用试验药物或对照组的受试者的所有研究观察结果和其他相关数据的足够及准确的病历［21 CFR 312.62（b）］

a. 我们的检查发现，受试者141068的筛选实验室报告记录了［（b）（4）］于2006年8月10日接收样本，实验室于2006年8月11日报告。在报告顶端，出现日期“2006年8月12日”，时间为12:28am的一个章印及

“[（b）（4）]”和“页数4/5”这些显示是报告传真给您的日期。您的签名在2006年8月10日，比报告发给您还早了2天。

b. 我们的检查发现，对于入组研究的18名受试者中的5名，有大量的例子显示，受试者在MAR和/或“护理记录”中的资料被更改，但是没有签日期或没有更改人的首字母签名。这显示这些“覆盖修改”是为了与CRF的时间匹配。照此，很难精确地确定药物什么时候开始被注射。例如，对于受试者[（b）（6）]，以下“注射开始时间的更改”和“停止注射时间”都是被“覆盖修改”的。

注射日期及时长	注射开始时间的修改	停止注射时间
7/28/2006 -2小时注射	17:03	19:06
7/29/2006 -2小时注射	17:10	19:16
7/30/2006 -2小时注射	17:20	19:22
7/31/2006 -2小时注射	17:22	19:27
7/31/2006 -1小时注射	22:38	23:20
8/1/2006 -2小时注射	17:25	19:25
8/2/2006 -2小时注射	17:00	19:03
8/2/2006 -2小时注射	22:30	23:33

c. 我们检查发现，受试者的[（b）（6）]结束治疗随访（EOT）病例报告表（CRFs）记录了TOC评估已经实施，并且“自基线以来的总体临床评估”被记录“已改善”；但是，受试者在最小7天治疗期仅接受了33组试验药物而不是方案中要求的35组。

我们注意到方案中说明如果在“疗效”（TOC）评估中，临床结果被认为“治愈”，则已接受了至少5天治疗的受试者不需要更多的[（b）（4）]治疗。这相当于至少25组试验药物给药。

在您的FDA483表回复中，您说明“在受试者临床条件的审查中，我发现受试者病情已经好转很多，不需要另外的介入治疗。这与方案中提供的‘治愈’的定义是一致的”。但是，您未能充分记录这些评估。我们接受您的解释并提醒您充分精确的案例记录的重要性。

3. 您未能保存足够准确的药物处置记录［21 CFR 312.62（a）］

a. 我们检查发现，未设盲的药房保存的[（b）（4）]给药#/盒#/瓶#/发放记录与药物计数表中记录的有很多不一致，包括7名随机进入[（b）（4）]治疗组中的5名受试者和11名随机进入安慰剂治疗组中的4名受试者。

具体而言，根据记录来自相同药盒的相同发放瓶，在[（b）（4）]表中被发放给一个受试者，在药物计数表中被发放给另一个受试者。另外，药物计数表中若干个受试者的药物发放信息缺失。举例见下表：

同一发放盒发放给不同受试者的例子：

[(b) (4)] 给药# 药物名称，盒#和瓶# 受试者 发放日期	“药物计数表” 药物名称，盒# 和瓶# 受试者 发放日期
给药# 2 盒# 21148-8 发放给受试者[(b)(6)] 01/08/06 (受试者[(b)(6)] 随机分配于 01 /08/2006)	盒# 21148-8 发放给受试者[(b)(6)] 30 /07/ 06 (受试者[(b)(6)] 随机分配于27 /07/ 2006)

续表

[(b) (4)] 给药# 药物名称，盒#和瓶# 受试者 发放日期	"药物计数表" 药物名称, 盒# 和瓶# 受试者 发放日期
给药# 4 盒# 21148-1 发放给受试者[(b)(6)] 01/08/2006	盒# 21148-1 发放给受试者[(b)(6)] 02/08/2006 (记录为"未使用")
给药# 7 盒# 26609-2 发放给受试者[(b)(6)] 2 /08/2006	盒# 26609-2 发放给受试者[(b)(6)] 27 /07/2006
给药# 9 [(b)(4)]- 盒# 22609-1 发放给受试者141059(MPP) 02/08/2006	[(b)(4)]- 盒# 22609-1 发放给受试者141052 (G-D) 27 /07/2006
给药# 12 [(b)(4)]- 盒# 22609-4 发放给受试者[(b)(6)] 03/08/2006	[(b)(4)]- 盒# 22609-4 发放给受试者[(b)(6)] 08/08/2006
给药# 14 [(b)(4)]- 盒# 22609-3 发放给受试者[(b)(6)] 03/08/2006	[(b)(4)]- 盒# 22609-3 发放给受试者[(b)(6)] 09/08/2006 (受试者[(b)(6)] 随机分配于 03/08/ 2006)

不一致或缺失的信息举例：

[(b) (4)] 给药# 药物名称，盒#及瓶# 受试者 发放日期	"药物计数表" 药物名称, 盒# 及瓶# 受试者 发放日期
给药# 17 [(b)(4)]-盒# 23666-13 发放给受试者[(b)(6)] 04/08/2006	[(b)(4)]- 盒# 23666-13 发放给受试者[(b)(6)] 05/08/2006
给药# 11&给药# 15 [(b)(4)]- 盒# 60936-13 (记录了发放2次) 受试者[(b)(6)] 29 /07/2006 (受试者[(b)(6)] 随机分配于27/07/2006)	[(b)(4)]- 盒# 60936-13 发放给受试者[(b)(6)] 29/07/2006
无[(b)(4)]记录, 盒# 60936-12 在 [(b)(4)]表中发放	[(b)(4)]- 盒# 60936-12 发放给受试者[(b)(6)] 29/07/2006

续表

[(b) (4)] 给药# 药物名称，盒#及瓶# 受试者 发放日期	"药物计数表" 药物名称, 盒# 及瓶# 受试者 发放日期
给药# 18 &给药# 20 [(b)(4)]– 盒# 60936–20 (记录了发放2次) 受试者[(b)(6)] 30 /07/2006	[(b)(4)]– 盒# 60936–20 发放给受试者[(b)(6)] 30/07/2006
给药# 33 [(b)(4)]– 盒# 23110–4 发放给受试者[(b)(6)] 14 /08/2006	未记录[(b)(4)] 盒# 23110–4 发放
给药# 26 [(b)(4)]– 盒# 23110–13 发放给受试者[(b)(6)] 15 /08/2006	未记录[(b)(4)] 盒# 23110–13 发放
给药# 28 [(b)(4)]– 盒# 23110–14 发放给受试者[(b)(6)] 15 /08/2006	未记录[(b)(4)] 盒# 24107–12 发放
给药# 30 [(b)(4)]– 盒# 23110–6 发放给受试者[(b)(6)] 15/08/2006	未记录[(b)(4)] 盒# 23110–6 发放
给药# 31 [(b)(4)]– 盒# 24107–13 发放给受试者[(b)(6)] 16/08/2006	未记录[(b)(4)] 盒# 24107–13 发放
给药# 33 [(b)(4)]– 盒# 24107–12 发放给受试者[(b)(6)] 16 /08/2006	未记录[(b)(4)] 盒# 24107–12 发放

b. 我们的检查发现，在"护理记录"和相对应的关于试验药物剂量的MAR记录之间存在大量的差异。部分剂量记录为给药不止一次，部分剂量没有记录在"护理记录"中。例如：

i. 受试者［（b）（6）］的"护理记录"中记录受试者剂量#17、#18和#31给药两次，但是没有剂量#12、#13和#33的给药记录。

ii. 受试者［（b）（6）］的"护理记录"中记录受试者剂量#16和#17给药两次，但是没有剂量#11的给药记录。

本警告信的目的并非是罗列您在试验药物临床研究中存在的所有缺陷。确保遵循法律和相关FDA法规的每一项要求是您的职责。您应当解决这些缺陷，并建立规程，以确保任何正在进行或将来的研究均能符合FDA的法规。

自收到这封信的15个工作日内，您应当书面告知本办公室为预防将来发生类似违规情况已经采取和即将采取的措施。如果不能充分、迅速地解释上述违规问题，可能导致我们在不再通知的情况下采取监管措施。

附：英文原文

Desai, Virendra M., M.D.

WARNING LETTER

March 2, 2009

CERTIFIED MAIL
RETURN RECEIPT REQUESTED

Ref: 09-HFD-45-02-03

Virendra Desai, M.D.
Physician Alliance Research Center
21520 S. Pioneer Blvd.,Suite 203
Hawaiian Gardens, California 90716

Dear Dr. Desai:

Between March 17, 2008 and April 17, 2008, Mrs. Yvette LaCour-Davis and Ms. Yvonne LaCour, representing the Food and Drug Administration (FDA), conducted an investigation and met with you to review your conduct of a clinical investigation (protocol [(b)(4)] entitled " A Phase III, Randomized, Double-Blind Study of [(b)(4)] versus [(b)(4)] in the Treatment of Complicated [(b)(4)] of the investigational drug [(b)(4)], performed for [(b)(4)]

This inspection is a part of the FDA's Bioresearch Monitoring Program, which includes inspections designed to evaluate the conduct of research and to ensure that the rights, safety, and welfare of the human subjects of those studies have been protected.

From our review of the establishment inspection report, the documents submitted with that report, the Form FDA 483, Inspection Observations, and your written response to the Form FDA 483 dated June 9, 2008, we conclude that you did not adhere to the applicable statutory requirements and FDA regulation governing the conduct of clinical investigations. We are aware that at the conclusion of the inspection, FDA personnel presented and discussed with you From FDA 483, Inspectional Observations. We wish to emphasize the following:

1. You failed to conduct the study according to the investigational plan [21 CFR 312. 60].

a. Our investigation found that all 18 subjects randomized into the study received study drug prior to your review and assessment of their baseline laboratory results, thereby potentially compromising the safety of subjects in the study. Specifically, the laboratory results from [(b)(4)] were received and reviewed by you up to 3 days after the study subjects were infused intravenously with study drug and in some instances, results from [(b)(4)] were not received and reviewed by you up to 20 days after the study subjects were infused intravenously with study drug, as summarized in the following table.

Informed consent Document (ICD) Signed	Date/Time Pre-Screen Labs drawn	Date/Time Randomized into study	Date/Time 1st dose of study drug received by subject	Date Baseline labs rec'd from central lab[(b)(4)]	Date Baseline labs reported by local lab[(b)(4)]	Date P.I. signed off on baseline lab results from [(b)(4)]
[(b)(6)]7/27/06	27 Jul 2006@13:10	27 Jul 2006@ 13:17	07/27/06@ 16:55	08/04/06 (by fax)	08/03/06	[(b)(4)]=8/4/06 [(b)(4)]=7/28/06
[(b)(6)]7/27/06	27 Jul 2006@15:38	27 Jul 2006@ 14:56	07/27/06@ 17:04	09/Aug/06 reprint/fax	08/03/06	[(b)(4)]=8/9/06 [(b)(4)]=8/7/06
[(b)(6)]8/1/06	1 Aug 2006@14:50	1 Aug 2006@ 15:08	08/01/06@ 17:05	08/03/06 (by fax)	08/25/06	[(b)(4)]=8/3/06 [(b)(4)]=8/25/06
[(b)(6)]8/1/06	1 Aug 2006@15:10	1 Aug 2006@ 15:09	8/1/06@ 17:10	08/03/06 (by fax)	08/25/06	[(b)(4)]=8/3/06 [(b)(4)]=8/25/06

(Contd.)

Informed consent Document (ICD) Signed	Date/Time Pre-Screen Labs drawn	Date/Time Randomized into study	Date/Time 1st dose of study drug received by subject	Date Baseline labs rec'd from central lab[(b)(4)]	Date Baseline labs reported by local lab[(b)(4)]	Date P.I. signed off on baseline lab results from [(b)(4)]
[(b)(6)]8/2/06	2 Aug 2006@11:30	2 Aug 2006@ 14:10	8/2/06@ 16:22	08/09/06 reprint/fax	08/07/06	[(b)(4)]=8/9/06 [(b)(4)]=8/3/06
[(b)(6)]8/3/06	3 Aug 2006@11:00	3 Aug 2006@ 11:14	8/3/06@ 16:55	08/04/06 (by fax)	08/09/06	[(b)(4)]=8/4/06 [(b)(4)]=8/10/06
[(b)(6)]8/7/06	7 Aug 2006@16:30	7 Aug 2006 (no fax conf found on file)	8/7/06@ 16:45	08/09/06 (by fax)	08/16/06 C&S only	[(b)(4)]=8/9/06 [(b)(4)]=8/16/06
[(b)(6)]8/8/06	8 Aug 2006@14:02	8 Aug 2006 (no fax conf found on file)	8/8/06@ 16:38	08/11/06 (by fax)	08/25/06	[(b)(4)]=8/11/06 [(b)(4)]=8/25/06
[(b)(6)]8/9/06	9 Aug 2006@13:23	9 Aug 2006@ 12:41	8/9/06@ 16:44	08/11/06 (by fax)	08/16/06	[(b)(4)]=8/10/06 [(b)(4)]=8/18/06
[(b)(6)]8/10/06	10 Aug 2006@11:23	10 Aug 2006@ 11:28	8/10/06@ 16:56	08/15/06 (by fax)	08/17/06	[(b)(4)]=8/15/06 [(b)(4)]=8/18/06
[(b)(6)]8/14/06	14 Aug 2006@14:10	14 Aug 2006@ 13:46	8/14/06@ 16:47	08/17/06 (by fax)	08/30/06	[(b)(4)]=8/17/06 [(b)(4)]=8/30/06
[(b)(6)]8/14/06	14 Aug 2006@14:26	14 Aug 2006@ 13:48	8/14/06@ 16:52	08/16/06 (by fax)	08/30/06	[(b)(4)]=18/16/06 [(b)(4)]=8/30/06
[(b)(6)]8/16/06	16 Aug 2006@12:45	16 Aug 2006@ 12:18	8/16/06@ 16:44	08/20/06 (by fax)	08/28/06	[(b)(4)]=8/20/06 [(b)(4)]=8/28/06
[(b)(6)]8/16/06	16 Aug 2006@15:00	16 Aug 2006@ 13:52	8/16/06@ 16:50	08/18/06 (by fax)	08/25/06	[(b)(4)]=8/18/06 [(b)(4)]=8/25/06
[(b)(6)]8/18/06	18 Aug 2006@ 14:10	18 Aug 2006@ 13:13	8/18/06@ 16:55	08/21/06	08/28/06	[(b)(4)]=8/22/06 [(b)(4)]=8/28/06
[(b)(6)]8/18/06	18 Aug 2006@15:35	18 Aug 2006@ 14:09	8/18/06@ 16:58	08/20/06 (by fax)	08/30/06	[(b)(4)]=8/20/06 [(b)(4)]=8/30/06
[(b)(6)]8/21/06	21 Aug 2006@11:10	21 Aug 2006@ 11:00	8/21/06@ 16:44	08/23/06 (by fax)	08/21/06	[(b)(4)]=8/23/06 [(b)(4)]=8/30/06
[(b)(6)]8/21/06	21 Aug 2006@12:50	21 Aug 2006@ 13:35	8/21/06@ 16:50	08/23/06 (by fax)	08/30/06	[(b)(4)]=8/23/06 [(b)(4)]=8/30/06

Your explanation provided in your written response to the Form FDA 483 is unacceptable. You stated in your response that, "section 5.2.2 of the protocol only indicates that central laboratory testing needs to be obtained. In addition, section 5.1.7.4 of the protocol only mentions that the pregnancy tests need to be reviewed prior to first dosing of study medication." While these statements are true, page 58 of the protocol clearly states that "all screening/predose assessments will be considered as baseline and must be performed and reviewed before randomization and dosing on Day 1..." When you signed the Statement of Investigator, Form FDA 1572, you agreed to the responsibilities of a clinical investigator that included ensuring that the study is conducted according to the investigational plan and the signed Investigator Statement, to protect the safety, rights or welfare of the subjects and to comply with all the obligations of a clinical investigator and all other pertinent requirements in 21 CFR 312. We remind you that as a clinical investigator, you retain responsibility for the conduct of the study.

b. The protocol required that subjects with known or suspected hepatic dysfunction (total bilirubin >= 2×upper limit of the normal range [ULN], or alanine aminotransferase [ALT] >= 3×ULN, or aspartate aminotransferase [AST] >= 3×ULN) be excluded from study enrollment.

Our investigation found that Subject [(b)(6)] was enrolled into the study on 8/16/06 despite having a baseline AST of 110 U/L (which was greater than 3×ULN) as reported by [(b)(4)]. In addition, [(b)(4)], your local laboratory, reported the subject's baseline ALT as 120 U/L, which was also greater than 3×ULN. You stated during our inspection that the subject did not have known or suspected hepatic dysfunction and was not known to have elevated liver tests. However, in your written response dated 6/9/08, you admitted that "if the laboratory results had been obtained and reviewed prior to the randomization on August 16, 2007, that this subject would not have meet the inclusion/exclusion criteria."In addition, the Nurse's Notes dated 8/17/06 @ 15:00 state that, "subject discontinued from participation in the study due to elevated liver function test. Subject with history of alcohol abuse." According to the subject's Medication Administration Record ("MAR"), the subject was infused with five (5) doses of study medication from 08/16/06 @16:50 hours through 08/17/06 @ 10:21 hours prior to being withdrawn from the study on 8/17/06. The inclusion of this subject into the study was a clear violation of study protocol.

c. The protocol required that all women of childbearing potential have a negative pregnancy test performed at baseline prior to receiving the first dose of study medication. However, Subject [(b)(6)] was randomized and received study medication without having the pregnancy test completed. In your response to the Form FDA 483, you acknowledged that this subject should have completed a pregnancy test before she received the study drug.

d. The protocol required "physical exam,""wound assessment," and "overall clinical assessment since baseline" at the Day 8 Visit. These were not conducted for Subject [(b)(6)]. In your response to the Form FDA 483, you acknowledged that the Day 8 information was not obtained.

2. You failed to maintain adequate and accurate case histories that record all observations and other data pertinent to the investigation on each individual administered the investigational drug or employed as a control in the investigation [21 CFR 312. 62(b)].

a. Our investigation found that the Screening Laboratory Report for Subject 141068 documented that the sample was received by [(b)(4)] on 8/10/06, and reported by the laboratory on 8/11/06. At the top of the report, there is the date of 8/12/06 with a time stamp of 12:28 am and the words, [(b)(4)] and "PAGE 4 of 5" which appears to be the date the report was faxed to you. Your signature is dated 8/10/06, two days prior to when the report was sent to you.

b. Our investigation found that for 5 of 18 subjects enrolled in the study, there were numerous instances where subject data on the MAR and/or "Nurse's Notes" were changed without dates or the initials of the person making the change. It appears that these "write-overs" were done to match the times on the CRFs. As such, it is difficult to accurately determine when the drug was administered. For example, for Subject [(b)(6)], the following times for the "Change of Start Time of Infusion" and "Stop Time of Infusion were all "write-overs."

Date & length of infusion	Change of Start Time of Infusion	Stop Time of Infusion
7/28/06 -2 hour infusion	1703 hours	1906 hours
7/29/06 -2 hour infusion	1710 hours	1916 hours
7/30/06 -2 hour infusion	1720 hours	1922 hours
7/31/06 -2 hour infusion	1722 hours	1927 hours
7/31/06 -1 hour infusion	2238 hours	2320 hours
8/1/06 -2 hour infusion	1725 hours	1925 hours
8/2/06 -2 hour infusion	1700 hours	1903 hours
8/2/06 1 hour infusion	2230 hours	2333 hours

c. Our investigation found that subjects' [(b)(6)] End-of-Therapy Visit (EOT) case report forms (CRFs) documented that TOC assessment was conducted and the "overall clinical assessment since baseline" was documented as "improved"; however, the subjects only received 33 doses of study medication instead of the protocol required 35 doses of study medication for the minimum 7 day treatment period.

We note that the protocol states that if at the "test of cure" (TOC) assessment, the clinical outcome was deemed "cured", than no further [(b)(4)] therapy was necessary in subjects who had received at least 5 days of treatment. This would equate to at least 25 doses of study medication.

In your response to the Form FDA 483, you stated that "in reviewing the subjects' clinical condition I felt that the subject had improved sufficiently and did not require additional interventional therapy. This is in line with the definition of "cure" provided in the protocol". However, you failed to adequately document this assessment. We acknowledge your explanation and remind you of the importance of adequate and accurate documentation of events.

3. You failed to maintain adequate and accurate records for disposition of drug [21 CFR 312. 62(a)].

a. Our investigation found numerous discrepancies between the [(b)(4)] dose#/kit #/vial # dispensing records kept by the unblinded pharmacy and what was recorded on the Drug Accountability Forms for five (5) of seven (7) subjects randomized into the [(b)(4)] treatment arm and for four (4) of the eleven (11) subjects randomized into the [(b)(4)]/ Placebo treatment arm.

Specifically, the same dispensing vials form the same kits were documented as being dispensed to one subject on the [(b)(4)]s Form and to a different subject on the drug accountability form. In addition, drug dispensing information was missing for several subjects on the Drug Accountability Forms. See the following table for examples.

Examples of the same kit dispensed to different subjects:

[(b)(4)] **Dose#** **Name of drug, Kit# & Vial#** **Subject#** **Date dispensed**	"Drug Accountability Form" Name of drug, Kit# & Vial# Subject# Date dispensed
Dose# 2 Kit# 21148-8 Dispensed to Subject#[(b)(6)] 01Aug06 (Subject#[(b)(6)] randomized on 01 Aug 06)	Kit# 21148-8 Dispensed to Subject#[(b)(6)] 30 Jul 06 (Subject#[(b)(6)] randomized on 27 Jul 06)
Dose# 4 Kit# 21148-1 Dispensed to Subject#[(b)(6)] 01Aug06	Kit# 21148-1 Dispensed to Subject#[(b)(6)] 02Aug06 (documented as "unused")
Dose# 7 Kit# 26609-2 Dispensed to Subject#[(b)(6)] 02 Aug 06	Kit# 26609-2 Dispensed to Subject#[(b)(6)] 27 Jul 06
Dose# 9 [(b)(4)]-Kit# 22609-1 Dispensed to Subject#141059(MPP) 02Aug06	[(b)(4)]-Kit# 22609-1 Dispensed to Subject#141052 (G-D) 27 Jul 06
Dose# 12 [(b)(4)]-Kit# 22609-4 Dispensed to Subject#[(b)(6)] 03Aug06	[(b)(4)]-Kit# 22609-4 Dispensed to Subject#[(b)(6)] 08Aug06
Dose# 14 [(b)(4)]-Kit# 22609-3 Dispensed to Subject#[(b)(6)] 03Aug06	[(b)(4)]-Kit# 22609-3 Dispensed to Subject#[(b)(6)] 09Aug06 (Subject#[(b)(6)] randomized on 03 Aug 06)

Examples of discrepant or missing information:

[(b)(4)] **Dose#** **Name of drug, Kit# & Vial#** **Subject#** **Date dispensed**	"Drug Accountability Form" Name of drug, Kit# & Vial# Subject# Date dispensed
Dose# 17 [(b)(4)]-Kit# 23666-13 Dispensed to Subject#[(b)(6)] 04Aug06	[(b)(4)]-Kit# 23666-13 Dispensed to Subject#[(b)(6)] 05Aug06
Dose# 11& Dose# 15 [(b)(4)]-Kit# 60936-13 (documented as being dispensed twice) Subject#[(b)(6)] 29 Jul 06 (Subject#[(b)(6)] randomized on 27 Jul 06)	[(b)(4)]-Kit# 60936-13 Dispensed to Subject#[(b)(6)] 29 Jul 06

(Contd.)

[(b)(4)] Dose# Name of drug, Kit# & Vial# Subject# Date dispensed	"Drug Accountability Form" Name of drug, Kit# & Vial# Subject# Date dispensed
No record of [(b)(4)], Kit# 60936-12 Being dispensed on the [(b)(4)] Form	[(b)(4)]-Kit# 60936-12 Dispensed to Subject#[(b)(6)] 29 Jul 06
Dose# 18 & Dose# 20 [(b)(4)]-Kit# 60936-20 (documented as being dispensed twice) Subject#[(b)(6)] 30 Jul 06	[(b)(4)]-Kit# 60936-20 Dispensed to Subject#[(b)(6)] 30 Jul 06
Dose# 33 [(b)(4)]-Kit# 23110-4 Dispensed to Subject#[(b)(6)] 14 Aug06	No record of [(b)(4)] Kit# 23110-4 as being dispensed
Dose# 26 [(b)(4)]-Kit# 23110-13 Dispensed to Subject#[(b)(6)] 15 Aug06	No record of [(b)(4)] Kit# 23110-13 as being dispensed
Dose# 28 [(b)(4)]-Kit# 23110-14 Dispensed to Subject#[(b)(6)] 15 Aug06	No record of [(b)(4)] Kit# #23110-14 as being dispensed
Dose# 30 [(b)(4)]-Kit# 23110-6 Dispensed to Subject#[(b)(6)] 15 Aug06	No record of [(b)(4)] Kit# 23110-6 as being dispensed
Dose# 31 [(b)(4)]-Kit# 24107-13 Dispensed to Subject#[(b)(6)] 16 Aug06	No record of [(b)(4)] Kit# 24107-13 as being dispensed
Dose# 33 [(b)(4)]-Kit# 24107-12 Dispensed to Subject#[(b)(6)] 16 Aug 06	No record of [(b)(4)] Kit# 24107-12 as being dispensed

b. Our investigation found numerous discrepancies between the "Nurses Notes" and what was recorded on the corresponding MAR regarding doses of study medication. Some of the doses are documented as being administered more than once, and some doses were not recorded in the "Nurses Notes." For example,

i. The "nurse's notes" for Subject #[(b)(6)] documented that the subject was administered dose #17, #18, &#31 twice, and there is no documentation that doses #12, #13, &#33 were administered.

ii. The "nurse's notes" for Subject #[(b)(6)] documented that the subject was administered dose #16and#17 twice. There is no documentation in the nurses notes that dose 11 was administered.

This letter is not intended to be an all-inclusive list of deficiencies with your clinical study of an investigational drug. It is your responsibility to ensure adherence to each requirement of the law and relevant FDA regulations. You should address these deficiencies and establish procedures to ensure that any on-going or future studies will be in compliance with FDA regulations.

Within fifteen (15) working days of your receipt of this letter, you should notify this office in writing of the actions you have taken or will be taking to prevent similar violations in the future. Failure to adequately and promptly explain the violations noted above may result in regulatory action without further notice.

If you have any questions, please contact Tejashri Purohit-Sheth,M.D., at 301-796-3402; FAX 301-847-8748. Your written response and any pertinent documentation should be addressed to:

Tejashri Purohit-Sheth, M.D.
Branch Chief

Good Clinical Practice Branch Ⅱ
Division of ScientificInvestigations
Office of Compliance
Center for Drug Evaluation and Research
Food and Drug Administration
Bldg 51, Room 5358
10903 New Hampshire Avenue
Silver Spring, M.D 20993

Sincerely yours,

{See appended electronic signature page}

Leslie K. Ball, M.D.
Director
Division of Scientific Investigations
Office of Compliance
Center for Drug Evaluation and Research

第135封　给Wright, Richard A.医学博士的警告信

2009年2月18日

参考号：09-HFD-45-02-01

尊敬的Wright博士：

2008年4月29日至5月28日，Lauren Collins女士代表FDA对您进行了现场检查，与您会面并审查了您实施的一项临床研究的情况，该临床试验方案（b）(4)，题为“一项Ⅲ期临床试验，旨在评估（b）(4)和一个阳性对照药，兰索拉唑（30mg每日一次）对糜烂性食管炎愈合的有效性和安全性”，针对试验药物（b）(4)，申办者为（b）(4)。

本次现场检查是FDA的生物研究监查项目的一部分。该项目通过设定的检查方法，评估研究的实施情况，并确保这些研究中受试者的权益、安全和福利得到了保护。

经对FDA现场检查报告、该报告的附件，以及您2008年6月2日对FDA 483表（现场检查发现的问题）的书面回复，我们认为，您没有遵循适用的法律要求和监管临床研究实施的FDA法规。我们知道在这次检查结束时，Collins女士出示并与您讨论了FDA483表，即现场检查发现的问题。我们想强调以下几点：

1. 您未能进行研究，或者确保按照研究计划进行研究［21 CFR 312.60］

a. 该研究16名入组的受试者中有10名在内镜筛选过程中进行了活检，这一点违背了方案。2006年4月10日伦理委员会（IRB）批准了日期为2006年2月16日的#1行政管理变更信。信中指出，“只有当研究场所中有康复研究维持的情况下，受试者才能进行胃活检”。但是，您的研究场所中没有康复研究维持。因此，以下受试者在2006年4月10日后进行活检，违背了研究方案：

i. 受试者（b）(6)：2006年4月13日进行活检；

ii. 受试者（b）(6)：2006年4月14日进行活检；

iii. 受试者（b）(6)：2006年4月14日进行活检；

iv. 受试者（b）(6)：2006年4月26日进行活检；

v. 受试者（b）(6)：2006年5月8日进行活检；

vi. 受试者（b）(6)：2006年5月10日进行活检；

vii. 受试者（b）(6)：2006年5月8日进行活检；

viii. 受试者（b）(6)：2006年5月18日进行活检；

ix.受试者（b）(6)：2006年5月31日进行活检；

x. 受试者（b）(6)：2006年6月15日进行活检。

b. 该研究16名入组的受试者中，有7名做了CLO检查（空肠弯曲菌样生物检查），该检查需要在筛选内镜检查时进行活检，同样违背了方案。2006年4月10日伦理委员会（IRB）批准了日期为2006年2月16日的#1行政管理变更信。信中指出，“一个确定的CLO检查将只对某些受试者进行——筛查时通过手指血或血清学检查幽门螺杆菌结果为阳性，并且患有糜烂性食管炎（EE）”。以下受试者通过手指血或血清学检查幽门螺杆菌结果为阴性，但是在2006年4月10日以后进行了CLO检查，违背了方案：

i. 受试者（b）(6)：2006年4月13日进行了CLO检查；

ii. 受试者（b）(6)：2006年4月26日进行了CLO检查；

iii. 受试者（b）(6)：2006年5月10日进行了CLO检查；

iv. 受试者（b）(6)：2006年5月8日进行了CLO检查；

ⅴ. 受试者（b）（6）：2006年5月19日进行了CLO检查；

ⅵ. 受试者（b）（6）：2006年5月31日进行了CLO检查；

ⅶ. 受试者（b）（6）：2006年5月31日进行了CLO检查。

c. 方案规定，实验室检查值异常的受试者将被排除在研究外。16名入组的受试者中有5名，您直到受试者已经入组研究的治疗阶段时，才审查了他们的筛选实验室检查结果。因为实验室检查值异常的受试者将被排除在研究外，所以方案要求您在受试者入组研究的治疗阶段之前，审查受试者的实验室检查结果。关于这些受试者的详细资料如下：

ⅰ. 受试者（b）（6）的筛选实验室检查在2006年4月27日，第1天访视在2006年5月10日，实验室筛查结果直到2006年5月12日、受试者入组到研究的治疗阶段以后，才进行了审查。

ⅱ. 受试者（b）（6）的筛选实验室检查在2006年5月1日，第1天访视在2006年5月11日，实验室筛查结果直到2006年6月5日、受试者入组到研究的治疗阶段以后，才进行了审查。

ⅲ. 受试者（b）（6）的筛选实验室检查在2006年5月1日，第1天访视在2006年5月9日，实验室筛查结果直到2006年6月5日、受试者入组到研究的治疗阶段以后，才进行了审查。

ⅳ. 受试者（b）（6）的筛选实验室检查在2006年5月9日，第1天访视在2006年5月19日，实验室筛查结果直到2006年6月5日、受试者入组到研究的治疗阶段以后，才进行了审查。

ⅴ. 受试者（b）（6）的筛选实验室检查在2006年5月15日，第1天访视在2006年6月2日，实验室筛查结果直到2006年6月5日、受试者入组到研究的治疗阶段以后，才进行了审查。

d. 方案规定，在4周访视时要进行全面的体格检查。但是，16名入组受试者中有14名，4周访视检查表中只记录了简要的体格检查结果。4周访视简要的检查结果被用于受试者（b）（6）的记录。

在您2008年6月2日对FDA483表的回复中，您声称您已经采用了一个“合规性检查表”来避免这些错误。我们获知您保证纠正措施已经实施，以防止类似的错误在将来的研究中再次出现。

e. 方案的入选标准规定，受试者必须“同意持续使用双重避孕的措施”。但是对于受试者（b）（6），她们都是育龄期女性受试者，双重避孕措施没有被记录。

2. 您未能及时向 IRB 报告研究活动的所有变更［21 CFR 312.66］

您未能按照法规和方案的要求，及时向伦理委员会报告研究活动中的所有变更。具体来说，2006年6月26日，在您的研究场所中所有筛选工作都被停止、直到不合规问题得到纠正。但是，直到2006年11月递交跟踪审查报告时，您才告知伦理委员会本研究被停止入组。

在您2008年6月2日对FDA483文件的回复中，您声称您已经采用了一个“合规性检查表”来避免这些错误。我们获知您保证纠正措施已经实施，以防止类似的错误在将来的研究中再次出现。

3. 您未能通过使用由伦理委员会批准的书面知情同意书来正确地记录知情同意［21 CFR 50.27（a）］

该研究16名入组受试者中，7名签署了过期的筛选知情同意书。2006年4月25日，伦理委员会批准了一份新版本（2006年4月14日）的知情同意书。但是，在2006年5月和6月间，在您的研究场所的受试者还是使用了过期的知情同意书（该知情同意书2006年3月24日进行了草拟，于2006年4月5日被伦理委员会批准），具体来说：

a. 受试者（b）（6）于2006年5月5日签署了版本为2006年3月24日的知情同意书。

b. 受试者（b）（6）于2006年5月9日签署了版本为2006年3月24日的知情同意书。

c. 受试者（b）（6）于2006年5月9日签署了版本为2006年3月24日的知情同意书。

d. 受试者（b）（6）于2006年5月15日签署了版本为2006年3月24日的知情同意书。

e. 受试者（b）（6）的法定授权代表于2006年5月15日签署了版本为2006年3月24日的知情同意书。

f. 受试者（b）（6）于2006年5月19日签署了版本为2006年3月24日的知情同意书。

g. 受试者（b）（6）于2006年6月6日签署了版本为2006年3月24日的知情同意书。

在您2008年6月2日对FDA483表的回复中，您声称您已经采用了一个“合规性检查表”来避免这些错误。我们获知您保证纠正措施已经实施，以防止类似的错误在将来的研究中再次出现。

4. 您未能确保按照签署的研究者声明（FDA1572 表）进行研究［21 CFR 312.60］

具体来说，研究过程由没有列入FDA1572表（研究者声明）的人员进行。当您签署了上述研究的研究者声明，您就同意在您的研究机构承担临床研究者的职责。临床研究者的职责，包括只允许在FDA1572表中列出的人执行研究过程。由于您将以下这些研究过程交给授权研究者进行，而授权研究者还未被列入FDA1572表中，所以您未能遵循21 CFR 312.60中规定的研究者的总体职责。例如下列研究过程由医师或医师助理完成，而在进行这些研究过程时他们还未被列入FDA1572表中：

a. 2006年5月18日对受试者（b）（6）进行了两次筛选内窥镜检查，而直到2006年8月1日，研究者才被加入到FDA1572表中。

b. 2006年3月29日至5月19日对受试者（b）（6）进行了9次体格检查，而直到2006年6月20日，这些研究者才被加入到FDA1572表中。

c. 2006年4月14日至6月12日对受试者（b）（6）进行了12次第1天访视体格检查，而直到2006年6月20日，这些研究者才被加入到FDA1572表中。

d．2006年5月1日对受试者（b）（6）进行了筛选期GERD症状评估，直到2006年6月20日，研究者才被加入到FDA1572表中。

e. 2006年5月22日至7月3日对受试者（b）（6）进行了3次四周访视内镜检查，直到2006年8月1日，研究者才被列入FDA1572表中。

f. 2006年5月11日至7月3日对受试者（b）（6）进行了8次四周访视体格检查，直到2006年6月20日，这些研究者才被加入到FDA1572表中。

在您2008年6月2日对FDA483表的回复中，您声称您已经采用了一个“合规性检查表”来避免这些错误。我们获知您的保证纠正措施已经实施，以防止类似的错误在将来的研究中再次出现。

本警告信的目的并非是罗列您在试验药物临床研究中存在的所有缺陷。确保遵循法律和相关FDA法规的每一项要求是您的职责。您应当解决这些缺陷，并建立规程，以确保任何正在进行或将来进行的研究均能符合FDA的法规。

自收到这封信的15个工作日内，您应当书面告知本办公室为预防将来发生类似违规情况已经采取或将要采取的措施。如果不能充分、迅速地解释上述违规问题，可能导致我们在不再通知的情况下采取监管措施。

附：英文原文

Wright, Richard A., M.D.

WARNING LETTER

Feb 18, 2009

CERTIFIED MAIL
RETURN RECEIPT REQUESTED
Ref: 09-HFD-45-02-01
Richard A. Wright. M.D.
550 S. Jackson Street
3rd Floor ACB
Louisville, KY 402021622

Dear Dr. Wright:

Between April 29 and May 28, 2008, Ms. Lauren Collins, representing the Food and Drug Administration (FDA), conducted an investigation and met with you to review your conduct of a clinical investigation [protocol (b)(4) entitled "A Phase 3 Study to Evaluate the Efficacy and Safety of (b)(4) and an Active Comparator, Lansoprazole (30 mg QD) on Healing of Erosive Esophagitis"] of the investigational drug (b)(4), performed for (b)(4).

This inspection is a part of the FDA's Bioresearch Monitoring Program, which includes inspections designed to evaluate the conduct of research and to ensure that the rights, safety, and welfare of the human subjects of those studies have been protected.

From our review of the establishment inspection report, the documents submitted with that report, and your June 2, 2008 letter written in response to the Form FDA 483, Inspectional Observations, we conclude that you did not adhere to the applicable statutory requirements and FDA regulations governing the conduct of clinical investigations and the protection of human subjects. We are aware that at the conclusion of the inspection, Ms. Collins presented and discussed with you Form FDA 483, Inspectional Observations. We wish to emphasize the following:

1. You failed to conduct the studies, or ensure they were conducted, according to the investigational plan [21 CFR 312.60].

a. Of sixteen subjects enrolled in the study, ten subjects had biopsies taken during the screening endoscopy in contravention of the protocol. Administrative change letter #1, dated February 16, 2006, was approved by the Institutional Review Board (IRB) on April 10, 2006. The letter states that "gastric biopsies will only be taken if the subject has a maintenance of healing study available at the site."

However, your study site did not have a maintenance of healing study. Therefore, the following subjects had biopsies taken after April 10, 2006, in violation of the protocol:

i. Subject (b)(6): biopsy performed on April 13, 2006
ii. Subject (b)(6): biopsy performed on April 14, 2006
iii. Subject (b)(6): biopsy performed on April 14, 2006
iv. Subject (b)(6): biopsy performed on April 26, 2006
v. Subject (b)(6): biopsy performed on May 8, 2006
vi. Subject (b)(6): biopsy performed on May 10, 2006
vii. Subject (b)(6): biopsy performed on May 8, 2006
viii. Subject (b)(6): biopsy performed on May 18, 2006
ix. Subject (b)(6): biopsy performed on May 31, 2006

x. Subject (b)(6): biopsy performed on June 15, 2006

b. Of sixteen subjects enrolled in the study, seven subjects had a CLO test (Campylobacter-Like Organism test), which involved a biopsy, performed during screening endoscopy, in violation of the protocol. Administrative change letter #1, dated February 16, 2006, was approved by the IRB on April 10, 2006. The letter states that "a definitive CLO test will only be performed for those subjects who tes positive for H. pylori by finger stick or serology at screening and have erosive esophagitis (EE)." CLO tests were performed for the following subjects who had a negative serology or finger stick test for H. pylori after April 10, 2006, in violation of the protocol:

i. Subject (b)(6): CLO test performed on April 13, 2006

ii. Subject (b)(6): CLO test performed on April 26, 2006

iii. Subject (b)(6): CLO test performed on May 10, 2006

iv. Subject (b)(6): CLO test performed on May 8, 2006

v. Subject (b)(6): CLO test performed on May 19, 2006

vi. Subject (b)(6): CLO test performed on May 31, 2006

vii. Subject (b)(6): CLO test performed on May 31, 2006

c. As specified in the protocol, subjects with abnormal laboratory values were to be excluded from the study. For five of sixteen enrolled subjects, you did not review the screening laboratory results until after the subjects were enrolled in the treatment phase of the study. Because subjects with abnormal laboratory values were to be excluded, the protocol required you to review subject's lab results prior to their enrollment in the treatment phase. The details for these subjects are provided below.

i. Subject (b)(6) screening labs were collected on April 27, 2006; the Day 1 visit was conducted on May 10, 2006. The screening labs were not reviewed until May 12, 2006, after the subject was enrolled in the treatment phase of the study.

ii. Subject (b)(6) screening labs were collected on May 1, 2006; the Day 1 visit was conducted on May 11, 2006. The screening labs were not reviewed until June 5, 2006, after the subject was enrolled in the treatment phase of the study.

iii. Subject (b)(6) screening labs were collected on May 1, 2006; the Day 1 visit was conducted mn May 9, 2006. The screening labs were not reviewed until June 5, 2006, after the subject was enrolled in the treatment phase of the study.

iv. Subject (b)(6) screening labs were collected on May 9, 2006; the Day 1 visit was conducted on May 19, 2006. The screening labs were not reviewed until June 5, 2006, after the subject was enrolled in the treatment phase of the study.

v. Subject (b)(6) screening labs were collected on May 15, 2006; the Day 1 visit was conducted on June 2, 2006. The screening labs were not reviewed until June 5, 2006, after the subject was enrolled in the treatment phase of the study.

d. The protocol states that a complete physical exam will be performed at the Week 4 visit. For fourteen of sixteen enrolled subjects, however, the Week 4 exam worksheets document only brief physical exam results. Brief exam results at Week 4 were documented for Subjects (b)(6).

In your June 2, 2008 response to the Form FDA 483 you stated that you have implemented a "Compliance Checklist" to avoid these errors. We acknowledge your assurance that corrective actions have been taken prevent similar findings from occurring in any future studies.

e. The inclusion criteria of the protocol states that subjects must "agree to continued use of a double barrier method of birth control." However, a double barrier method of birth control was not documented for Subjects (b)(6) who were all female subjects of childbearing potential.

2. You failed to promptly report all changes in research activity to the IRB [21 CFR 312.66].

You did not promptly report all changes in research activity to the IRB, as required by the regulations and the protocol. Specifically, on June 26, 2006, all screening activity at your site was stopped until noncompliance issues were corrected. However, you did not notify the IRB that the study was closed to enrollment until you submitted a continuing review report in November 2006.

In your June 2, 2008 response to the Form FDA 483 you stated that you have implemented a "Compliance Checklist" to avoid these errors. We acknowledge your assurance that corrective actions have been taken prevent similar findings from occurring in any future studies.

3. You failed to properly document informed consent by the use of a written informed consent form approved by the IRB [21 CFR 50.27(a)].

Of sixteen subjects enrolled in the study, seven subjects signed an outdated screening informed consent form (ICF). On April 25, 2006, the IRB approved a new (April 14, 2006) version of your ICF.

However, in May and June of 2006, subjects in your study were given an outdated version of the ICF (which was drafted on March 24, 2006 and approved by the IRB on April 5, 2006). Specifically:

a. Subject (b)(6) signed the March 24, 2006 version of the ICF on May 5, 2006.

b. Subject (b)(6) signed the March 24, 2006 version of the ICF on May 9, 2006.

c. Subject (b)(6) signed the March 24, 2006 version of the ICF on May 9, 2006.

d. Subject (b)(6) signed the March 24, 2006 version of the ICF on May 15, 2006.

e. Subject (b)(6) legally authorized representative signed the March 24, 2006 version of the IFC on May 15, 2006.

f. Subject (b)(6) signed the March 24, 2006 version of the ICF on May 19, 2006.

g. Subject (b)(6) signed the March 24, 2006 version of the ICF on June 6, 2006.

In your June 2, 2008 response to the Form FDA 483 you stated that you have implemented a "Compliance Checklist" to avoid these errors. We acknowledge your assurance that corrective actions have been taken prevent similar findings from occurring in any future studies.

4. You failed to ensure that the investigation was conducted according to the signed investigator statement (Form FDA-1572) [21 CFR 312.60].

Specifically, study procedures were conducted by personnel not yet listed on the Form FDA-1572, Statement of Investigator. When you signed the investigator statement for the above referenced clinical investigation, you agreed to take on the responsibilities of a clinical investigator at your site.

The responsibilities of a clinical investigator include allowing only personnel listed on the 1572 to perform study procedures. By allowing the following procedures to be performed by subinvestigators who were not yet listed on the Form FDA-1572, you failed to comply with the general responsibilities of a clinical investigator as stated in 21 CFR 312.60. For example, the following procedures were performed by a physician or physician assistant (PA) not listed on the Form FDA-1572 at the time the procedures were performed.

a. Two screening endoscopies for Subjects (b)(6) were performed on May 18, 2006. The investigator was not added to the Form FDA-1572 until August 1, 2006.

b. Nine screening physical exams for Subject (b)(6) and were performed between March 29, 2006 and May 19, 2006. The investigators were not added to the Form FDA1572 until June 20, 2006.

c. Twelve Day 1 physical exams for Subject, (b)(6) were performed between April 14, 2006 and June 12, 2006. The investigators were not added to the Form FDA-1572 until June 20, 2006.

d. One GERD Symptom Assessment at screening for Subject (b)(6) was performed on May 1, 2006.

The investigator was not added to the Form FDA-1572 until June 20, 2006.

e. Three Week 4 endoscopies for Subjects (b)(6) were performed between May 22, 2006 and July 3, 2006. The investigator was not added to the Form FDA-1572 until August 1, 2006.

f. Eight Week 4 physical exams for Subjects (b)(6) were performed between May 11, 2006 and July 3, 2006. The investigators were not added to the Form FDA-1572 until June 20, 2006.

In your June 2, 2008 response to the Form FDA 483 you stated that you have implemented a "Compliance Checklist" to avoid these errors. We acknowledge your assurance that corrective actions have been taken prevent similar findings from occurring in any future studies.

This letter is not intended to be an all-inclusive list of deficiencies with your clinical study of an investigational drug. It is your responsibility to ensure adherence to each requirement of the law and relevant FDA regulations. You should address these deficiencies and establish procedures to ensure that any on-going or future studies will be in

compliance with FDA regulations.

Within fifteen (15) working days of your receipt of this letter, you should notify this office in writing of the actions you have taken or will be taking to prevent similar violations in the future. Failure to adequately and promptly explain the violations noted above may result in regulatory action without further notice.

If you have any questions, please contact Constance Lewin, M.D., M.P.H., at 301-796-3397; FAX 301-847-8748. Your written response and any pertinent documentation should be addressed to:

Constance Lewin, M.D., M.P.H.
Branch Chief, Good Clinical Practice Branch I
Division of Scientific Investigations
Office of Compliance
Center for Drug Evaluation and Research
Food and Drug Administration
Bldg 51, Room 5354
10903 New Hampshire Avenue
Silver Spring, MD 20993

Sincerely yours,

{See appended electronic signature page}

Leslie K. Ball, M.D.
Director
Division of Scientific Investigations
Office of Compliance
Center for Drug Evaluation and Research

This is a representation of an electronic record that was signed electronically and this page is the manifestation of the electronic signature.

/S/

LESLIE K BALL
02/18/2009

Page Last Updated: 05/08/2009

Note: If you need help accessing information in different file formats, see Instructions for Downloading Viewers and Players.

第 136 封　给 Chappel, Christopher 医学博士的警告信

2009年2月2日

参考号：09-HFD-45-01-02

尊敬的Chappel博士：

2007年10月22日至2007年11月21日，Brunilda Torres女士代表 FDA 实施了现场检查，与您会面并对您实施下列临床研究的情况进行了审查：

试验方案［（b）（4）］，题为“双盲，随机，平行组，剂量范围，多中心研究，评估试验药物［（b）（4）］在轻度到中度高血压患者中的有效性和安全性”，试验药物［（b）（4）］，申办者为［（b）（4）］；

试验方案［（b）（4）］，题为“试验药物［（b）（4）］和阿托伐他汀钙片治疗高胆固醇受试者的合并效应Ⅱ期临床研究”，试验药物［（b）（4）］，申办者为［（b）（4）］；

试验方案［（b）（4）］，题为“一项随机、双盲、双模拟，安慰剂对照的［（b）（4）］临床研究，评估在Ⅰ期和Ⅱ期高血压患者［（b）（4）］和［（b）（4）］联合用药8周，并有［（b）（4）］子研究”，试验药物［（b）（4）］，申办者为［（b）（4）］。

本次现场检查是FDA的生物研究监查项目的一部分。该项目通过设定的检查方法，评估研究的实施情况，并确保这些研究中受试者的权益、安全和福利得到了保护。

我们审查了FDA483表、现场检查报告（EIR）、该报告的附件，对FDA483表的两封书面回复（2007年10月30日和给佛罗里达地区主任Emma Singleton的更新信函）。根据审查，我们认为，您没有遵循适用法律的要求和监管临床研究实施及受试者保护的FDA法规。我们知道在现场检查结束时，Torres女士向您出示并讨论了FDA483表，即现场检查发现的问题。我们想强调以下几点：

1. 您未能亲自进行临床研究或对研究进行监督［21 CFR 312.60］

当您签署上述临床研究的研究者声明（FDA1572表）时，您已同意承担研究场所临床研究者的责任。您的总体责任包括确保该临床研究依照签署的研究者声明、研究计划、适用的法规进行；在职责内保护受试者的权益、安全和福利；并管理好试验中使用的药物（21 CFR 312.60）。尤其是您本应亲自进行这几项临床研究，或对您未亲自实施的临床研究部分进行监督。作为研究者，尽管您可以授权具备相应资质的其他人承担一些研究任务，但您不能将总体责任授权给他人承担。

我们在检查中发现，您允许某些并未授权的人员承担试验任务，且您对这些人员的监管不足以确保研究依照签署的研究者声明、研究计划、适用的法规进行，并且保障受试者的权益、安全和福利。

A. 以下是发现的对试验方案［（b）（4）］的方案违背

（1）我们发现根据“职责分配和授权人员签字表”，您和/或您的授权研究者是您在研究场所指定的仅有的两位有权作出研究相关的医疗决定并执行试验相关关键步骤的人员。然而，您告诉FDA检查员Torres您授权试验协调员［（b）（6）］女士判断受试者是否具备入组资格；她作出这样的决定的情况可以在医疗、研究记录中查到。判断受试者入组资格是研究相关的医学决定，也是研究相关的关键步骤。照此而言，该研究任务不能授权给［（b）（6）］女士。允许［（b）（6）］女士进行她并未得到授权的研究任务证明您未能依照研究计划和相应规范进行试验。

（2）如后文（3、4、6部分）详述的那样，您未能亲自进行试验的某些环节并/或对研究人员进行足够的监管，导致研究出现了严重问题，包括：不合格受试者入组，许多次偏离方案，未能保存足够的病历，未能向伦理委员会报告给受试者带来风险的非预期问题。

另外，您已注意到［（b）（6）］女士进行了她未被授权进行的研究任务（根据“职责分配和授权人员签字表”）。此外，她未能尽职履行她授权范围内的职责。我们注意到申办者［（b）（4）］的监查员给您的信函中发现并记录了这个问题：

ⅰ. 在2006年5月18日、10月13日和2007年2月27日的信函中，监查员记录了［（b）（4）］女士进行了不适当的试验入组评估，未能遵照方案中排除标准，未进行恰当的原始数据的记录。

ⅱ. 在2007年1月19日的信函中，监查员记录了类似的问题，且您的办公室未将这些事件通知伦理委员会。

B. 以下是发现的对试验方案［（b）（4）］的方案违背

（1）与1.A.2部分提到的事件类似，该试验中出现的问题本质和严重性（在以下2，3，4，5部分详述），证明您未亲自实施或有效监督该临床研究。

我们还从您收到的该研究申办者监查员的通知中发现，关于［（b）（4）］女士行为的一些严重问题，如2006年8月8日的信函中，监查员发现：① 受试者研究表中的原始表和全部受试者访视的数据缺失；② 该试验相关文件分几堆散落在研究协调员办公室的地面和/或桌面上，与其他临床研究的文件混杂在一起；③ 受试者访视的原始文件很少，主要包括一张勾选了每次访视需要检查项目的表格；④ 病史、不良事件和合并用药不是没有合理评估就是没有完整记录；⑤ 药物责任日志不完整，研究协调员并不知道该日志的存在。我们发现，在这次监查访视过程中，有21位受试者参加了该试验的筛选。信函中以下内容总结了对您的研究场所的监查员评价：“总而言之，该中心忽视了此项临床研究。受试者安全保障存在问题。大量研究表格缺失之前访视的原始记录文件，而研究协调员需要在当前受试者访视中回顾这些记录，心电图和实验室检测值超限未对其是否有临床意义进行判断，也未对这些受试者进行随访”。

（2）一份2006年9月24日的信函中显示，在对2006年9月19日至21日监查访视的跟踪访视中，监查员注意到，总体上看，研究场所有很大进步。然而，监查发现，在那个时间点，所有受试者都完成了该试验，由于病历记录不定，您的团队在回溯解决关于病史缺漏的来源确认问题方面仍有困难。在我们审阅FDA检查报告和附件时，我们发现就本研究审查的记录来说，原始文件依然存在问题，文件中包括一些之后加入的文件，且难以确认文件的来源。

我们发现［（b）（4）］女士是以上两个试验的主要研究协调员，且［（b）（4）］女士与研究现场的雇佣关系于2006年12月4日终止。我们要强调的是，临床研究者的首要职责是保证试验依照FDA的法规进行，以保护受试者的权益、安全和福利。我们注意到两个不同试验的监查员们都多次告知您［（b）（4）］女士未能依照方案开展试验和/或未能正确完成某些研究相关的工作。在监查员发现的未能正确完成的任务中，一些是她未被授权开展的工作。尽管申办者多次告知您以上情况，但您仍允许她继续担任研究协调员工作，这说明您未能依照研究计划进行试验且未尽到监督的职责。监查员尤其是2006年秋天和2007年初派出的几位监查员都质疑您在10月30日信函中声称的“您努力帮助［（b）（4）］女士纠正她工作中偏差。”我们发现您未能有效参与并监督临床研究，以保证试验依照FDA法规进行。

2. 您未能按照21 CFR 50的要求获得每位受试者的知情同意［21 CFR 312.60］

FDA法规21 CFR 50.20规定，除21 CFR 50.23和21 CFR 50.24提供的情况外，研究者要在受试者或受试者法定代表人签署法律上生效的知情同意书后，才能接受受试者参加临床试验。法规规定，只有潜在受试者或受试者代表有足够机会考虑是否参加试验，并且将产生强迫和不适当的影响的可能性降到最低的情况下，研究者才可以循求这些知情。FDA法规的50.27部分进一步规定知情同意要通过知情同意书这种书面记录的形式进行，并让受试者或受试者代表有足够的机会阅读知情同意书。

A. 对于试验方案［（b）（4）］，我们从研究现场的记录中未能确定知情同意是否在受试者参加试验前进行，另外，也不能确定受试者是否有足够机会考虑是否参加该临床试验。我们特别注意到，研究现场通常使用签到表记录受试者到达的日期、时间。

根据已记录的预约时间、签到时间和方案流程开始时间，下表中的受试者无法依照21 CFR 50.20和50.27的要求进行合法有效的知情同意。其原因是：① 所记录的研究相关的步骤时间早于计划的预约时间或/和受试者的签到时间。② 根据研究记录，预约时间、受试者签到时间和/或方案流程开始时间过于紧凑，在签署知情同意书之前，未能给受试者提供足够的机会阅读知情同意文件，并考虑是否参加该试验。例如，受试者［（b）（6）］于2006年3月25日入组。签到表显示受试者［（b）（6）］在早上9:00到达研究场所。但是原始文件显示，研究相关步骤记录时间早于受试者到达时间（即一份血样于早上8:50抽取）。另外，细节如下：

受试者	知情同意日期	签到日期	签到时间	预约时间	血压测量时间	抽血时间	ECG时间
[(b)(6)]	记录不清	3/23/2006	9:38a.m.	9:30a.m.	9:20 a.m.	9:40a.m.	9:35 a.m.
[(b)(6)]	3/23/2006	3/23/2006	9:38a.m.	9:30a.m.	9:00 a.m.	9:20a.m.	9:15 a.m.
[(b)(6)]	7/20/2006	7/20/2006	9:48a.m.	10:00a.m.	8:30 a.m.	9:30a.m.	8:44 a.m.
[(b)(6)]	8/8/2006	8/8/2006	9:11 a.m.	9:30a.m.	9:05 a.m.	9:45a.m.	8:20 a.m.
[(b)(6)]	8/16/2006	8/16/2006	没有时间记录 根据其他受试者当天签到时间，最可能是在9:00 a.m.和9:30 a.m之间	没有时间记录	8:38 a.m.	8:53a.m.	8:50 a.m.

B. 以下是发现的对试验方案［（b）（4）］的方案违背

（1）与上面2.A.（1）类似，根据已记录的预约时间、签到、知情同意和方案流程开始时间，对下列受试者您无法依照21 CFR 50.20和50.27的要求进行合法有效的知情同意。其原因是：① 所记录的研究相关的步骤时间早于计划的预约时间或/和受试者的签到时间；② 预约时间、受试者签到时间和/或方案流程开始时间过于紧凑，在签署知情同意前未能给受试者提供足够的机会阅读知情同意文件，并考虑是否参加该研究。细节如下：

受试者	知情同意日期	知情同意时间	第1次访视日期	第1次访视签到时间	第1次访视预约时间	受试者坐下测血压时间	ECG时间
[(b)(6)]	6/19/2006	10:15 a. m.	6/19/2006	10:30 a.m.	10:30 a.m.	10:25 a.m.	10:45 a.m.
[(b)(6)]	7/19/2006	8:35 a. m.	7/19/2006	8:50 a.m.	8:30 a.m.	8:37 a.m.	*
[(b)(6)]	8/3/2006	8:25 a. m.	8/3/2006	9:30 a.m.	9:00 a.m.	8:30 a.m.	8:50 a.m.
[(b)(6)]	10/31/2006	9:25 a. m.	10/31/2006	9:50 a.m.	9:00 a.m.	9:30 a.m.	9:50 a.m.
[(b)(6)]	11/1/2006	9:15 a. m.	11/1/2006	9:50 a.m.	10:00 a.m.	9:20 a.m.	9:40 a.m.

（*-ECG检测时间对于违背的发现并非决定性。）

（2）另外，研究场所执行受试者［（b）（6）］试验相关步骤的时间早于该受试者知情同意的时间。原始记录显示受试者收到的方案要求早上8:30测血压并记录读数，但知情同意记录时间为早上8:45。

C. 以下是发现的对试验方案［（b）（4）］的方案违背

您好像没有获得受试者［（b）（6）］知情同意之前就进行了研究相关的步骤。2006年2月10日的签到表显示，受试者［（b）（6）］于下午12:20签到，但试验相关步骤在下午12:15进行。

关于这3个试验中发现的问题，在您未标明日期的信中，您认为每个受试者的到达时间和/或受试者被带离等候室的时间通常不是即时记录，所以导致了似乎受试者到达时间、进行知情同意的时间、研究相关步骤的开始时间存在矛盾，似乎受试者进行知情同意时的时间间隔过短。但是，您陈述到，所有的受试者有足够的时间阅读知情同意书且所有知情同意的过程都是在任何一项研究相关的步骤开始前进行的。

由于以上提到的这些试验方案中的时间记录不一致，我们不能确认您的说法是否准确。但是，如上讨论，我们认为，根据我们已审查的记录，您不可能依照21 CFR 50.20和 50.27的要求得到合法有效的知情同意书。

我们认可您未标明日期的信函中提到的为防止同样缺陷发生采取的纠正措施。虽然这些纠正措施好像是适当的，但在当时进行临床试验时，这些措施的缺失导致了上述违反法律法规的情况，也让我们对您确保对受试者适当保护的措施引起关注。

3. 您未能进行研究或者确保按照研究计划进行研究［21 CFR 312.60］

A. 以下是发现的对试验方案［（b）（4）］的方案违背

（1）研究方案中的入选标准规定：在安慰剂导入期的第一次确定资格的访视（P2访视），受试者有至少3次血压测试结果平均值，坐位收缩压大于140mmHg，小于180mmHg；坐位舒张压大于90mmHg，小于110mmHg。研究方案中的入选标准进一步规定：在安慰剂后导入期的第二次确定资格的访视（P3访视），受试者要有至少3次血压测试结果平均值，坐位收缩压大于140mmHg，小于180mmHg；坐位舒张压大于90mmHg，小于110mmHg。如果受试者在P3访视中不能达到相应的血压标准，方案规定要进行第三次资格确认访视（P4访视）。如果受试者在P4访视中不能达到入选标准，他或她不具有参加随机的资格。

ⅰ. 受试者［（b）（6）］未能符合入选标准，在P2访视时，坐位舒张压为85mmHg；P3访视时，坐位舒张压为87mmHg；但依然入组参加试验。

我们还发现两份原始文件签署时间都为2006年8月28日，都为同一受试者在P3访视中签署。如上所述，根据其中一份原始记录，该受试者［（b）（6）］平均舒张压为87mmHg，不符合要求。病例报告表显示，在血压不符合要求（即舒张压为87mmHg）的情况下参加了随机。另一份原始记录显示，该受试者坐位舒张压平均值为90mmHg，符合入选标准。

ⅱ. 受试者［（b）（6）］未能达到方案规定的血压入选标准：P2访视，坐位收缩压129mmHg，坐位舒张压65mmHg；P3访视，坐位舒张压原记为86mmHg，2007年被划掉改为85mmHg；P4访视，坐位舒张压为85mmHg，但该受试者依然随机入组。申办者最终允许该受试者留在试验中，但这未能改变最初的方案违背。

（2）研究方案规定如果两次确认资格的访视中坐位舒张压平均值相差超过7mmHg，受试者不能入组参加临床研究。

在2006年12月27日进行的P2访视中，受试者［（b）（6）］坐位舒张压平均值为93mmHg；在2007年1月10日进行的P3访视，出现了2份原始记录，受试者坐位舒张压平均值分别为105、106mmHg。我们发现，使用P3访视中的任何一个坐位舒张压平均值，差值都超过了7mmHg。因此，该受试者符合排除标准，且不应入组参加此临床研究。另外，2007年2月7日一份文件的注释中，您承认该受试者在两次访视坐位舒张压平均差值超过7mmHg的情况下依然入组参加临床研究。

（3）试验方案规定育龄期的女性受试者的定义是：非绝经后或未手术绝育的女性患者，血清妊娠试验呈阳性的或不同意使用可接受的避孕手段的女性不能参加临床试验。试验方案还规定妊娠试验需要在P1访视和T1访视时进行。受试者［（b）（6）］和［（b）（6）］在其中一次和/或两次访视中未进行试验方案规定的妊娠试验。

（4）方案规定在T1访视中，研究者需要通过［（b）（4）］得到需要分发的药盒编号，并依据编号将药盒分发给受试者。相关［（b）（4）］记录显示，受试者［（b）（6）］应发给100210药盒，但研究场所把100201药盒发给了他。

（5）研究方案规定在每次计划访视中，研究人员应测量受试者给药前（低谷期）血压和心率。试验方案还规定了测量血压和心率的规定步骤，包括但不限于以下步骤：① 受试者测量血压和心率前应静坐至少5分钟；② 研究人员应在3分钟后测量站姿的心率/血压。我们注意到该研究中数位受试者在数次访视中都未执行上述步骤。例子包括却不限于以下受试者：

受试者	研究访视	坐下的时间	坐式血压/心率测量时间	站起时间	站式血压/心率测量时间
[(b)(6)]	P1	8:55 a.m.*	9:00 a.m.*	9:05 a.m.	9:10 a.m.
[(b)(6)]	V2	9:00 a.m.	9:00 a.m.	9:10 a.m.	9:15 a.m.
[(b)(6)]	V3	9:05 a.m.*	9:10 a.m.	9:19 a.m.	无时间
[(b)(6)]	V4	8:00 a.m.	8:00 a.m.	8:09 a.m.	无时间
[(b)(6)]	V6	9:10 a.m.	9:18 a.m.	9:23 a.m.	无时间
[(b)(6)]	P1	无时间	8:40 a.m.	无时间	8:49 a.m.
[(b)(6)]	V2	7:40 a.m.	7:44 a.m.	7:52 a.m.	无时间
[(b)(6)]	V3	7:33 a.m.	7:33 a.m.	7:40 a.m.	无时间
[(b)(6)]	记录上的T2和T3	7:00 a.m.*	7:05 a.m.*	7:10 a.m.	7:15 a.m.
[(b)(6)]	记录上的T5、T7和T9	7:30 a.m.	7:32 a.m.	无时间	7:38 a.m.
[(b)(6)]	记录上的T5、T7和T9	6:55 a.m.	6:57 a.m.	无时间	7:02 a.m.

*注：为了确保完整性，这些条目列入表格中；但是并不都代表违反相关法律法规。

（6）试验方案要求研究人员对T3访视中采集的血样进行额外的血生化检测。受试者［（b）（4）］未按试验方案要求在T3访视进行抽血。

B. 以下是发现的对试验方案［（b）（4）］的方案违背

（1）试验方案要求研究人员在每位受试者基线访视时查问足够的病史并进行体检。我们不能判断受试者［（b）（6）］在基线访视时是查问了足够的病史或进行了体检。这次访视的原始记录仅限于一些勾选项，几乎没有方案中所规定的受试者体检和病史的相关信息。

（2）试验方案规定受试者发生指定的不良反应事件（DAE）#5，包括：丙氨酸转氨酶（ALT）水平高于正常值上限（ULN）1.5倍，但低于3倍，则需要每周进行跟踪测试，直到ALT降低至ULN1.5倍以下或满足另一标准［DAE#2，3或4］。我们发现受试者［（b）（6）］ALT水平升高，但没有按方案规定的每周进行ALT检测。

（3）试验方案要求在得到心电图（ECG）数据并经过有资质的医生初步阅片后，ECG要送往外包的中心实验室处进行分析。一旦“通读过的”ECG（如方案中所述）从中心实验室返回，研究者或其有资质的代表需负责决定对该患者的治疗方案是否需要改变，并且对他/她的此次审查进行记录并签署名字和日期，以确保受试者的安全。受试者（b）（6）的下列ECG异常中您没有审查并进行临床评估。2016年1月27日发生，直到/并至2006年8月5日；2006年3月30日发生，直到2006年4月12日；2006年5月1日发生，直到2006年8月9日；受试者［（b）（6）］2006年4月17日发生，直到2006年8月5日才审查和评估。因为您对ECG的审查显著滞后于您拿到“被读过的”的ECG的时间，您不可能按照方案要求在研究过程中对受试者的治疗方案进行必要的调整。

（4）试验方案规定在第一次访视时，受试者应被指导按NECP的TLC（国家胆固醇教育计划的治疗性生活方式改变）要求进行饮食。原始文件并不能证明受试者［（b）（6）］被指导进行饮食。

在您未标明日期的信函中，您提出以上缺陷不仅发生在［（b）（6）］女士进行的两项临床研究中。您还提出，在过去研究场所的临床试验步骤依赖于研究协调员100%清楚方案的入排标准。为了纠正这些缺陷，您认为虽然您仍需要研究协调员十分了解试验方案，现在您还委托负责人草拟一份入排标准清单，将此用于临床研究入组开始时，所有适用的前期访视，包括随机化访视。只有在申办者提供类似清单的情况下除外。

您的回复我们认为还不够。首先，如上所述，您没有授权［（b）（4）］女士进行方案中这些步骤。其次，尽管［（b）（6）］女士是两个方案的主要研究协调员，您作为临床试验研究者有责任保证临床试验依照研究方案开展。另外，我们发现上述所有方案违背并非都是由［（b）（6）］女士导致的。

4. 您未能保存研究中每个受试者与研究相关的所有研究观察结果和其他相关数据的足够及准确的病历［21 CFR 312.62（b）］

A. 以下是发现的对试验方案［（b）（4）］的方案违背

（1）我们找到了受试者［（b）（6）］P3访视的两份原始记录，签名时期为2006年8月28日。一份原始记录显示，该受试者坐式舒张压平均值为87mmHg，不符合入选标准。另一份原始记录显示，该受试者坐式舒张压平均值为90mmHg，符合入选标准。病例报告表显示，该受试者在血压不符合要求（即舒张压为87mmHg）的情况下参加了随机化。

在您未标明日期的来信中，您认为文件出现问题是因为旧的流程中在同一访视中使用了多种表格，您在日常工作中没有讨论并强调文件记录问题。现在，在会议中，您将文件记录问题作为常规项进行讨论，并建立和实施了专门的文件管理指导规范。您的回复中还不足够。这不能解释为何一份原始记录显示该受试者不能参加临床试验，而另一份记录显示同一受试者符合入组条件。

（2）我们不能确定受试者［（b）（6）］哪天签署了知情同意书并入组参加临床试验。该受试者和［（b）（6）］女士在2006年3月22日的知情同意文件上签署了日期，且入组日志也显示，该受试者在这天入组参加临床试验。但是，我们发现2006年3月22日的签到表中并未记录该受试者在这天曾来过您的研究场所。然而，筛选原始记录和您研究场所的签到表显示，受试者［（b）（6）］于2006年3月23日来到您研究场所，并进行了入组筛选。

（3）受试者［（b）（6）］于2006年2月1日签署知情同意文件。但是，2006年2月1日的签到表中并未记录该受试者在这天曾来过您的研究场所。

（4）［（b）（6）］女士于2006年11月21日签署的一份记录显示，受试者［（b）（6）］在“2006年11月21日6:45，药盒#203841给药”，且该受试者的下一次访视应该在2007年2月13日的6:00。但是，该试验方案新的研究协调员于2006年12月7日在病程记录中写到，该受试者告诉研究协调员，他/她“退出知情同意”，不再参加该临床研究，并已经向［（b）（6）］女士退还了试验用药。病程记录还提到您新的研究协调员随后在水槽下找到了未打开的药盒。因此，该受试者并未像前一份原始记录显示的那样于2006年11月21日服用试验药物。

在您未标明日期的来信中，您承认［（b）（6）］女士错误记录了这次给药，而实际上将未开封的药盒分发给受试者。您还提到，您现在的规程要求专门记录药物是否发放或使用，且上述的事件在新雇佣的研究协调员培训班上讨论了这一问题，所有新雇佣的研究协调员均出席培训。

您的回复不够充分。具体来说，我们尤其注意到［（b）（6）］女士对按期到研究场所来进行访视的据标是给过试验药物的受试者使用了“给药”这个词。事实上，如您在信中提到的，“给药”这个可以推定为仅把未开启的药盒分发给受试者，而您没有确认受试者是否按试验方案要求在接受访视时实际服用了试验药物。我们不能确认受试者在何种程度上拿到并服用了试验药物。

B. 以下是发现的对试验方案［（b）（4）］的方案违背

（1）受试者的原始记录中很多项目是记录生成很久后再添加的，包括不良反应事件结果、合并用药、吸烟饮酒习惯和/或试验药物给药的信息。但是，没有关于这些信息获取来源和时间的书面记录。例如：

ⅰ. 受试者［（b）（6）］原始记录于2006年9月1日记录该受试者V3访视（2/13/06），V4访视（3/6/06），V5访视（3/13/06）和V6访视（3/27/06）中无不良事件和新的合并用药。该受试者原始记录于2006年7月31日记录该受试者V8访视（4/24/06）和V9访视（5/9/06）中无不良事件和新的合并用药。

ⅱ. 受试者［（b）（6）］于2006年3月30日从临床研究中退出。但是，2006年1月17日访视的原始记录于2006年8月12日加上一条新的内容，即该受试者不吸烟和/或不饮酒。

ⅲ. 受试者［（b）（6）］于2006年5月25日进行了V8访视。一份2006年10月25日的记录显示，该受试者2016年5月25日访视的给药发生于2006年10月23、24、25日。

（2）受试者［（b）（6）］数次访视的合并用药评估并未按试验方案要求进行记录。

5. 您未能保存关于受试者使用情况的试验药物处置记录［21 CFR 312.62（a）］

在试验方案［（b）（4）］中，受试者［（b）（6）］的药物数量登记表未能找到。

我们认可您未标明日期的信中提到的，过去您不使用药物数量登记表，除非申办者提供表格。您还提到，为了纠正这一问题，您已经建立并开始使用药物数量登记表记录药物的分发情况和具体数量。另外，创建了主药物数量登记表，对于负责特定临床试验的协调者，可以逐次更新试验药物的接受和分发情况。您还指出，现有的规程要求协调员需要在发药前请另一名协调者对药盒的编号和［（b）（4）］指定的编号进行交叉复核。虽然这些纠正措施好像是合理的，但正是由于这些管理措施的缺失导致了上述违反相关规定的情况。

6. 您未能及时向IRB报告给受试者或他人带来风险的所有非预期事件［21 CFR 312.66］

在试验方案［（b）（4）］中，贵研究场所于2006年12月12日获知受试者［（b）（6）］因两侧肺栓塞在［（b）（4）］入院治疗，并且在重症监护病房住了一周。按伦理委员会的要求，严重不良事件应在3个工作日内通知伦理委员会，您未能及时通知。您在2007年2月12日将该事作为方案偏离向伦理委员会报告，并未作为不良事件报告。

在您未标明日期的信中，您在回复中提到［（b）（6）］女士是该试验方案的主要研究协调员。您的回复我们认为是不足够的，因为贵研究场所获知该不良事件是在［（b）（6）］女士与您中心的雇佣关系结束后。另外，根据2006年12月12日与受试者的交谈获知，“［（b）（6）］”并非［（b）（6）］女士是实际记录人。

本警告信的目的并非是罗列您在试验药物临床研究中存在的所有缺陷。确保遵循法律和相关FDA法规的每一项要求是您的职责。您应当解决这些缺陷，并建立规程，以确保任何正在进行或将来进行的研究均能符合FDA的法规。

对于上述回复不够充分的情况，自收到这封信的15个工作日内，您应当书面告知本办公室为预防将来发生类似违规情况已经或将要采取的措施。如果不能充分、迅速地解释上述违规问题，可能导致我们在不再通知的情况下采取监管措施。

附：英文原文

Chappel, Christopher, M.D.

WARNING LETTER

Feb 02, 2009

CERTIFIED MAIL
RETURN RECEIPT REQUESTED

Ref: 09-HFD-45-01-02

Christopher Chappel, M.D.
445 West Oak Street
Family Practice Associates
Kissimmee, FL 34741

Dear Dr. Chappel:

Between October 22, 2007 and November 21, 2007, Ms. Brunilda Torres, representing the U.S. Food and Drug Administration (FDA), conducted an investigation and met with you to review your conduct of the following clinical investigations:

Protocol [(b)(4)] ("Protocol [(b)(4)]"), entitled "Double-blind, randomized, parallel-group, dose ranging, multi-center study to evaluate the efficacy and safety of [(b)(4)] in patients with mild to moderate hypertension" of the investigational drug [(b)(4)], performed for [(b)(4)].

Protocol [(b)(4)] ("Protocol [(b)(4)])" entitled "A Phase 2 Study of the Combinatorial Effect of [(b)(4)] and Atorvastatin in Subjects with Hypercholesterolemia" of the investigational drug [(b)(4)]performed for [(b)(4)].

Protocol [(b)(4)] ("Protocol [(b)(4)]"), entitled "A randomized, double-blind. double-dummy, placebo-controlled, [(b)(4)] trial to evaluate [(b)(4)] in combination with [(b)(4)] after eight weeks of treatment in patients with Stage I or II hypertension, with an [(b)(4)] sub-study" of the investigational drugs [(b)(4)], performed for [(b)(4)].

This inspection is a part of the FDA's Bioresearch Monitoring Program, which includes inspections designed to evaluate the conduct of research and to ensure that the rights, safety, and welfare of the human subjects of those studies have been protected.

We have reviewed the Form FDA 483, the establishment inspection report and the documents submitted with that report, and the two letters you wrote in response to the Form FDA 483 [the October 30, 2007 letter (October 30 Letter) and the undated letter to Florida District Director, Emma Singleton (Undated Letter)]. Upon review, we conclude that you did not adhere to the applicable statutory requirements and FDA regulations governing the conduct of clinical investigations and the protection of human subjects. We are aware that at the conclusion of the inspection, Ms. Torres presented and discussed with you Form FDA 483, Inspectional Observations. We wish to emphasize the following:

1. You failed to personally conduct or to supervise the clinical investigation [21 CFR 312.60].

When you signed the investigator statements (Form FDA 1572) for the above-referenced clinical investigations, you agreed to take on the responsibilities of a clinical investigator at your site. Your general responsibilities include ensuring that the investigation is conducted according to the signed investigator statement, the investigational plan, and applicable regulations; protecting the rights, safety, and welfare of subjects under your care; and ensuring control of drugs under investigation (21 CFR 312.60). You specifically agreed to personally conduct the clinical studies or to supervise those aspects of the studies that you did not personally conduct. While you may delegate certain study tasks to individuals qualified to perform them, as clinical investigator, you may not delegate your general responsibilities.

Our investigation indicates that you permitted individuals to conduct study tasks which they had not been delegated the authority to execute, and that your supervision of personnel to whom you delegated study tasks was not adequate to ensure that the clinical trials were conducted according to the signed investigator statement, the investigational plan, and applicable regulations, and in a manner that protected the rights, safety, and welfare of human subjects.

A The following violations were noted for Protocol [(b)(4)]

1. We note that per the "Delegation of Duties & Authorized Signatures Form," you and/or your sub-investigator were the only individuals at your site designated by you to make trial-related medical decisions and to perform critical trial-related procedures. You informed FDA Investigator Torres, however, that you gave to your study coordinator Ms. [(b)(6)] the responsibility to determine subject eligibility into the study; the fact that she made such determinations is also evident in the medical and study records. Determination of subject eligibility is a trial-related medical decision, as well as a critical trial-related procedure. As such, this study task was not delegated to Ms. [(b)(6)] Permitting Ms. [(b)(6)] to conduct study tasks for which she did not have authorization demonstrates your failure to conduct the study in accordance with the study plan and applicable regulations.

2. As discussed in more detail in Sections 3, 4, and 6 below, your failure to personally conduct certain aspects of the study and/or to supervise study personnel adequately resulted in serious problems with the study, including: the enrollment of ineligible subjects, the failure to follow numerous trial protocols, the failure to maintain adequate case histories, and the failure to report to the Institutional Review Board (IRB) unanticipated problems involving risk to human subjects.

Moreover, you had notice that Ms. [(b)(6)] was performing duties for which she did not have authorization, per the Delegation of Duties & Authorized Signatures Form, and that she was not performing adequately duties which she did have authority to perform. Specifically, we note that monitors from [(b)(4)], the sponsor of this study, identified and documented such problems in correspondence to you:

i. In letters of May 18 and October 13, 2006, and February 27, 2007, the monitor documented Ms. [(b)(6)] improperly conducting a study eligibility assessment, failing to follow the protocol in evaluating exclusion criteria, and failing to ensure proper source documentation.

ii. In a January 19, 2007 letter, the monitor documented similar findings, as well as your office's failure to notify the Institutional Review Board of certain events.

B. The following violations were noted for Protocol [(b)(4)]:

1. Similar to the events noted in Paragraph 1.A.2 above, the nature and severity of the problems relating to this study, as detailed in Sections 2, 3, 4, and 5 below, indicate that you failed to personally conduct and/or adequately supervise the clinical investigation.

We note again that you received notice from the study sponsor's monitors that there were significant problems at your site related to Ms. [(b)(6)] activities. For example, in a letter dated August 8, 2006, the monitor found that: (1) source worksheets and data for entire subject visits were missing from subject's research charts; (2) several piles of study-related documents were scattered on the study coordinator's floor and/or desk intermixed with documents from other clinical trials; (3) source documentation for subject visits was minimal and mainly consisted of one sheet of check marks for items required at each visit; (4) medical histories, adverse events, and concomitant medications either were not assessed or were not documented appropriately; and (5) drug accountability logs were not completed, as the study coordinator was not aware of the log. We note that at the time of this monitoring visit, 21 subjects had been screened for this study. The letter summarized the monitor's assessment of your site: "Overall, this study has been neglected at this site. Subject safety has been in question since so many research charts were missing previous visit source documents that the Study Coordinator would need to reflect on for her current Subject visits, and ECG [electrocardiogram] and lab alerts were not assessed for clinical significance or followed up with the Subjects."

2. In a letter dated September 24, 2006, in follow-up to a monitoring visit that occurred between September 19 and 21, 2006, the monitors noted that, overall, your site had shown much improvement. However, it was noted that your staff continued having difficulty going backwards with resolving the source verification problems in terms of scant medical history as all subjects had completed the study at that point. In our review of the FDA inspectional report and the documents submitted with that report, we note that there were still problems with source documentation with respect to records reviewed for this study and that late entries noted within the source documentation could not be verified as to where the information was derived.

We note that Ms. [(b)(6)] served as the primary study coordinator for both of the above-discussed studies and that Ms. [(b)(6)] employment was terminated from your site as of December 4, 2006. We wish to emphasize, however, that as the clinical investigator, it was your ultimate responsibility to ensure that the studies were conducted properly and in compliance with FDA regulations to protect the rights, safety, and welfare of study subjects. We note that the monitors from two different studies notified you on multiple occasions that Ms. [(b)(6)] was failing to follow the protocols and/or incorrectly completing certain study-related tasks. Among the tasks identified by the monitors were those for which she had not been delegated authority. The fact that you permitted her to continue as study coordinator despite these repeated notices indicates your failure to conduct the study in accordance with the investigational plans and the lack of adequate supervision on your part. These letters from the monitors, especially those sent in fall 2006 and early 2007, also call into question your assertion in your October 30 Letter that you "worked diligently to help Ms. [(b)(6)] correct the discrepancies." We find that you failed to have adequate involvement and oversight over the studies to ensure that they were properly conducted in compliance with FDA regulations.

2. You failed to obtain the informed consent of each human subject in accordance with 21 CFR part 50 [21 CFR 312.60].

FDA's regulations at 21 CFR 50.20 state that except as provided in 21 CFR 50.23 and 21 CFR 50.24, no investigator may involve a human being as a subject in research covered by the regulations unless the investigator has obtained the legally effective informed consent of the subject or the subject's legally authorized representative. The regulation specifies that an investigator shall seek such consent only under circumstances that provide the prospective subject or the subject's representative sufficient opportunity to consider whether or not to participate and that minimize the possibility of coercion or undue influence. Section 50.27 of FDA's regulations further provides that informed consent shall be documented by the use of a written consent document, which is to be signed by the subject or subject's representative only after the subject or the subject's representative is given adequate opportunity to read the document.

A. For Protocol [(b)(4)], we were unable to determine from your site records if subjects gave informed consent prior to participation in the study and/or if subjects were given sufficient opportunity to consider whether or not to participate in the study. Specifically, we note that your site routinely used sign-in sheets to document the date and time of arrival of subjects.

Based on the times recorded for appointment time, sign-in, and the commencement of protocol procedures, it does not appear possible that you obtained legally effective informed consent from the subjects in the chart below, in compliance with 21 CFR 50.20 and 50.27. This is because either 1) study-related procedures are listed as having taken place prior to the scheduled appointment time and/or prior to the time the subject signed in, or 2) based on the study records, the time between the appointment time, the time the subject signed in and/or the commencement of the procedure(s) did not provide adequate opportunity for the subjects to read the informed consent document, and to consider whether or not to participate in the study, before signing the informed consent form. For example, Subject [(b)(6)] was enrolled into the study on March 25, 2006. The sign in sheet notes that Subject [(b)(6)] arrived at your site at 9:00 a.m. However, source documents showed that study related procedures were performed prior to the subject's arrival (i.e., a blood sample was drawn at 8:50 a.m. In addition, as detailed below

Subject	Date Informed Consent Obtained	Sign-In Date	Sign-in Time	Appointment Time	Blood Pressure Measured	Blood Samples Taken	ECG Conducted
[(b)(6)]	Unclear from records	3/23/06	9:38 a.m.	9:30 a.m.	9:20 a.m.	9:40 a.m.	9:35 a.m.
[(b)(6)]	3/23/06	3/23/06	9:38 a.m.	9:30 a.m.	9:00 a.m.	9:20 a.m.	9:15 a.m.
[(b)(6)]	7/20/06	7/20/06	9:48 a.m.	10:00 a.m.	8:30 a.m.	9:30 a.m.	8:44 a.m.
[(b)(6)]	8/8/06	8/8/06	9:11 a.m.	9:30 a.m.	9:05 a.m.	9:45 a.m.	8:20 a.m.
[(b)(6)]	8/16/06	8/16/06	No time indicated; most likely between 9:00 a.m. and 9:30 a.m. based on other patients' recorded sign-in times that day	No time indicated	8:38 a.m.	8:53 a.m.	8:50 a.m.

B. The following violations were noted for Protocol [(b)(4)]:

1. Similar to Paragraph 2.A.1. above, it does not appear possible, based on the times recorded for appointment time, sign-in, informed consent, and the commencement of protocol procedures, that you obtained legally effective informed consent from the subjects listed below in compliance with 21 CFR 50.20 and 50.27. This is because 1) study-related procedures are listed as having taken place prior to the scheduled appointment time and/or prior to the time the subject signed in, or 2) because the time between the appointment time, the time the subject signed in, and/or the commencement of the procedure(s) did not provide adequate opportunity for the subjects to read the informed consent document, and to consider whether or not to participate in the study, before signing the informed consent form. As detailed below:

Subject	Consent Date	Consent Time	Visit 1 Date	Visit 1 Sign-In Time	Visit 1 Appointment Time	Patient Seated for Blood Pressure Measurement	ECG Conducted
[(b)(6)]	6/19/06	10:15 a.m.	6/19/06	10:30 a.m.	10:30 a.m.	10:25 a.m.	10:45 a.m.
[(b)(6)]	7/19/06	8:35 a.m.	7/19/06	8:50 a.m.	8:30 a.m.	8:37 a.m.	*
[(b)(6)]	8/3/06	8:25 a.m.	8/3/06	9:30 a.m.	9:00 a.m.	8:30 a.m.	8:50 a.m.
[(b)(6)]	10/31/06	9:25 a.m.	10/31/06	9:50 a.m.	9:00 a.m.	9:30 a.m.	9:50 a.m.
[(b)(6)]	11/1/06	9:15 a.m.	11/1/06	9:50 a.m.	10:00 a.m.	9:20 a.m.	9:40 a.m.

(* - Time ECG Conducted is not dispositive to finding of violation)

2. In addition, your site performed a study related procedure on Subject [(b)(6)] prior to obtaining the subject's informed consent. Specifically, the source records showed that the subject received the protocol specified blood pressure readings at 8:30 am, while informed consent was not documented until 8:45 am.

C. The following violation was noted for Protocol [(b)(4)]:

1. It does not appear that you obtained informed consent from Subject [(b)(6)] prior to conducting study-related procedures. The sign-in sheet for February 10, 2006 indicates that Subject [(b)(6)] signed in at 12:20 p.m., but that study-related procedures were conducted at 12:15 p.m.

With respect to the findings noted above for these three studies, in your Undated Letter, you noted that documentation of arrival time for each subject was not routinely recorded immediately upon arrival and/or before the subject was taken from the waiting room, which you stated resulted in the appearance of contradictory times between arrival, the informed consent process, and the beginning of study-related procedures, as well as the appearance of inadequate time intervals for the informed consent process itself. You stated, however, that all subjects had adequate time to read the informed consent form and that the informed consent process was always completed prior to the start of any other study-related procedures.

We cannot verify the accuracy of your assertion in light of the time discrepancies reflected in the records for these protocols, and as noted above. Therefore, as discussed above, we conclude, based on the records reviewed, that it was not possible for you to obtain legally effective informed consent as specified in 21 CFR 50.20 and 50.27.

We acknowledge that in your Undated Letter you describe the corrective actions you have taken to prevent the recurrence of this finding. While these corrective actions appear appropriate, it was the absence of such measures during the conduct of these trials that led to the violations listed here, and which raises our concern for your approach to assuring appropriate human subject protection.

3. You failed to conduct the studies or to ensure they were conducted according to the investigational plans [21 CFR 312.60].

A. The following protocol violations were noted for Protocol [(b)(4)].

1. The protocol inclusion criteria specified that at the first qualifying visit during the placebo lead-in phase (Visit P2), the subject was to have a mean of at least three readings for seated systolic blood pressure (SeSBP) of > 140 mm Hg and < 180 mm Hg and for seated diastolic blood pressure (SeDBP) of > 90mm Hg and < 110 mm Hg. The protocol inclusion criteria further specified that at the second qualifying visit during the placebo lead-in phase (Visit P3), the subject was to have a mean of at least three readings for the SeSBP to be > 140 mm Hg and < 180 mm Hg, and for SeDBP > 90mm Hg and < 110 mm Hg. If the subject did not meet the qualifying blood pressure criterion at Visit P3, the protocol specified that a third qualifying visit (Visit P4) was to be performed. If the patient did not meet the inclusion criteria at Visit P4, he or she would not be qualified for randomization.

i. Subject [(b)(6)] did not meet the inclusion criterion at either Visit P2, when the SeDBP was 85, or Visit P3, when the SeDBP was 87, but nevertheless was enrolled into the study.

We note further that there were two source documents signed and dated August 28, 2006, found for this subject for the P3 visit. As referenced above, according to one of these source documents, Subject [(b)(6)] had a non-qualifying mean SeDBP of 87. The case report forms (CRF) showed that the subject was initially randomized based on this non-qualifying BP (i.e., SeDBP of87). The second source document listed a qualifying mean SeDBP of 90.

ii. Subject [(b)(6)] did not meet the protocol-specified blood pressure inclusion criterion at either Visit P2 (SeSBP of 129, and SeDBP of 65), Visit P3 (SeDBP of 86 originally, then crossed out in 2007 to read 85), or Visit P4 (SeDBP of 85), but was randomized into the study. That the sponsor ultimately permitted this subject to remain in the trial does not mitigate this initial failure to follow the protocol.

2. The protocol specified that if the variability between the mean blood pressure measurements on two qualifying visits was more than 7 mm Hg for SeDBP, then the subject was to be excluded from the study.

At Visit P2 on December 27, 2006, Subject [(b)(6)] had a mean SeDBP of 93 and at Visit P3 on January 10, 2007, there were two separate source documents listing the mean SeDBP as either 105 or 106, respectively. We note that using either of the mean SeDBPs for Visit P3, the variability was greater than 7 mm Hg, and therefore the subject still met the exclusion criterion and should not have been enrolled into this study. Moreover, in a note to file dated February 7, 2007, you acknowledge that this subject was enrolled into the study despite having variability greater than 7 mm mean SeDBP over two visits.

3. The protocol specified that women of child bearing potential, defined as female patients who were not postmenopausal or surgically sterile, who had a positive serum pregnancy test or who did not agree to use an accepted method of contraception, were to be excluded from the study. The protocol further specified that pregnancy tests were to be taken at the Visits P1 and T1. Protocol-specified pregnancy tests were not performed for Subjects [(b)(6)] and [(b)(6)] on one and/or both of these visits.

4. The protocol specified that at Visit T1, the investigator should call the [(b)(4)] to receive the medication kit number that was to be allocated to the patient and then allocate that kit accordingly. As reflected on the relevant [(b)(4)] record, Subject [(b)(6)] should have been dispensed Kit #100210, but your site dispensed Kit #100201 instead.

5. The protocol specified that at each scheduled study visit, study personnel should measure the pre-dose (trough) blood pressure (BP) and heart rate (HR). The protocol further set forth that certain procedures should be used to measure the BP and HR, including but were not limited to: (1) the patient first should be required to be seated for a minimum of five minutes prior to BP and HR data collection; and (2) study personnel then should take one HR/BP measurement after three minutes in the standing position. We note that this did not occur for several subjects at several visits throughout the course of their participation in the study. Examples include but were not limited to the following:

Subject	Study Visit	Time Seated	Sitting BP/HR Taken	Time Stood	Standing BP/HR Taken
[(b)(6)]	P1	8:55 a.m.*	9:00 a.m.*	9:05 a.m.	9:10 a.m.
[(b)(6)]	V2	9:00 a.m.	9:00 a.m.	9:10 a.m.	9:15 a.m.
[(b)(6)]	V3	9:05 a.m.*	9:10 a.m.	9:19 a.m.	No time indicated
[(b)(6)]	V4	8:00 a.m.	8:00 a.m.	8:09 a.m.	No time indicated
[(b)(6)]	V6	9:10 a.m.	9:18 a.m.	9:23 a.m.	No time indicated
[(b)(6)]	P1	No time indicated	8:40 a.m.	No time indicated	8:49 a.m.
[(b)(6)]	V2	7:40 a.m.	7:44 a.m.	7:52 a.m.	No time indicated
[(b)(6)]	V3	7:33 a.m.	7:33 a.m.	7:40 a.m.	No time indicated
[(b)(6)]	T2 and T3 indicated on record	7:00 a.m.*	7:05 a.m.*	7:10 a.m.	7:15 a.m.
[(b)(6)]	T5, T7, and T9 indicated on record	7:30 a.m.	7:32 a.m.	No time indicated	7:38 a.m.
[(b)(6)]	T5, T7, and T9 indicated on record	6:55 a.m.	6:57 a.m.	No time indicated	7:02 a.m.

(* - Note: for completeness, these items are listed in the table; however, they specifically do not represent a violation)

6. The protocol required study personnel to obtain additional checks for biochemistry from blood samples at Visit T3. Subjects #[(b)(6)] did not have the protocol-specified blood samples drawn at this visit.

B. The following protocol violations were noted for Protocol [(b)(4)]:

1. The protocol specified that study personnel should perform a complete medical history and physical examination at the baseline visit for each subject. We were unable to determine whether Subjects [(b)(6)] had either a complete medical history or a physical examination performed at the baseline visit. The source documents for this visit were limited to checkmarks that provide little to no information concerning the subject's physical examination or past medical history rather than actual documentation of the medical history or physical examination that should have been performed.

2. The protocol specified that subjects who experienced a designated adverse event (DAE) #5 consisting of an elevation in their alanine aminotransferase (ALT) level > 1.5 but < 3 Upper Limits of Normal (ULN) were to have repeat tests done weekly until the ALT dropped to < 1.5 × ULN or met another criterion [DAE# 2, 3, or 4]. We note

that Subjects [(b)(6)] did not have the weekly protocol-specified ALT tests repeated despite elevated ALTs.

3. The protocol specified that subsequent to the collection of an ECG and initial interpretation by a qualified physician, the ECGs were to be sent for analysis to a centralized ECG vendor. Once this "overread" ECG (as described by the protocol) was returned from the centralized ECG vendor, the investigator or qualified designee was responsible for determining if any change to the medical management of the subject was needed, and for documenting his/her review by signing and dating the ECG, to ensure subject safety. You did not review and clinically evaluate the ECG Alerts for Subject [(b)(6)] dated January 27, 2006 until August 5, 2006, March 30, 2006 until April 12, 2006, and May 1, 2006 until August 9, 2006; and an ECG Alert for Subject [(b)(6)] dated April 17, 2006 until August 5, 2006. Because your review took place significantly after you received the "overread" ECG readings, you could not have made the necessary adjustments to subject medical management as required by the protocol over the course of the study.

4. The protocol specified that at Visit 1, subjects should be instructed on being on the NCEP TLC diet. Source documents did not verify that Subjects [(b)(6)] were instructed on the diet.

In your Undated Letter, you noted that the above findings were only found within the two studies conducted by Ms. [(b)(6)]. You further stated that in the past, the procedures at your site were reliant on the study coordinator having 100% knowledge of the protocol inclusion/exclusion criteria. To correct these findings you indicated that while you still require study coordinators have such knowledge of the protocol, you now mandate that the Director of Clinical Operations draft an inclusion/exclusion checklist to be used at all appropriate visits leading up to and including the randomization visit prior to beginning enrollment for a study. The only exception to use of this list is when the sponsor provides such a checklist itself.

This response is inadequate. First, as noted above, you did not delegate to Ms. [(b)(6)] the authority to conduct these procedures in Protocol [(b)(4)]. Second, while Ms. [(b)(6)] was the primary study coordinator for both protocols, it was your responsibility as the clinical investigator to ensure the studies were conducted according to the investigational plans. Further, we note that not all protocol violations delineated above resulted from Ms. [(b)(6)] conduct.

4. You failed to maintain adequate and accurate case histories that record all observations and other data pertinent to the investigation on each individual [21 CFR 312.62(b)].

A. The following violations were noted for Protocol [(b)(4)]:

1. We found two source documents signed and dated August 28, 2006, for Subject [(b)(6)] for Visit P3. One of the source documents listed a non-qualifying mean SeDBP of 87. The other source document listed a qualifying mean SeDBP of 90. The case report forms (CRFs) showed that the subject was initially randomized based on the non-qualifying SeDBP of 87.

In your Undated Letter you noted that the documentation issues arising from multiple worksheets for the same visit resulted from past processes in which you did not routinely discuss or stress documentation, that currently documentation is discussed routinely at staff meetings, and that specific guidelines have been developed and implemented in the arena of documentation. This response is inadequate. It does not explain why one source document shows the subject was ineligible for the study while the other shows the subject was eligible.

2. We cannot determine on what date Subject [(b)(6)] signed the informed consent form and was enrolled into the study. The subject and Ms. [(b)(6)] dated the informed consent document on March 22, 2006, and per the enrollment log the subject was enrolled into the study on this day. We note, however, that the March 22, 2006 sign-in sheet does not document that the subject was present at your site on this date. Rather, screening source documents and your site's sign-in sheet show that Subject [(b)(6)] arrived at your site on March 23, 2006 and was screened for enrollment into the study on this date.

3. Subject [(b)(6)] signed the informed consent document February 1, 2006. However, the February 1, 2006 sign-in sheet does not show that this subject was at your site on this date.

4. Ms. [(b)(6)] signed a November 21, 2006 record stating that Subject [(b)(6)] was "dosed from kit #203841 on 11/21/06 @ 0645" and that the next visit for this subject was going to be February 13, 2007 at 0600. However, the new study coordinator for this protocol recorded in a progress note dated December 7, 2006, that the subject had

notified her that he/she was "withdrawing consent" from participation in the study and already had returned the drug to Ms. [(b)(6)]. The progress note further mentioned that your new study coordinator later had found the medication box unopened under the sink. Thus the subject was never dosed with the study medication on November 21, 2006 as indicated in the initial source record.

In your Undated Letter, you conceded that Ms. [(b)(6)] erroneously recorded that the medication had been administered to the subject when in fact she had dispensed an unopened container. You further stated that your current procedures require specific documentation of whether the drug is dispensed or administered, and that this issue is discussed in the new hire coordinator class that all newly-hired coordinators attend.

This response is inadequate. Specifically, we note that Ms. [(b)(6)] used the word "dosed" for all subjects to whom she purportedly administered investigational drug on days on which the subjects were seen at your site for study-related visits. If in fact as you noted in your letter the word "dosed" could imply the subject only was dispensed an unopened container, and you did not verify that the subjects actually took the study drug during the office study visits as specified in the protocol, we cannot be assured to any degree that subjects enrolled into the study received and/or took the investigational drug.

B. The following violations were noted for Protocol [(b)(4)]:

1. There were entries made on subject source documents long after those documents were created that provided information concerning the results of adverse events, concomitant medication assessments, alcohol and smoking habits, and/or study drug dosing. However, there is no documentation concerning from where or when this information was obtained. For example:

i. An entry dated September 1, 2006 was written on the source documents for Subject [(b)(6)] noting no adverse events and no changes in concomitant medications for Visits V3 (2/13/06), V4 (3/6/06), V5 (3/13/06), and V6 (3/27/06). An entry dated July 31, 2006 was written on the source documents for this subject noting no adverse events and no changes in concomitant medications for Visits V8 (4/24/06) and V9 (5/9/06).

ii. Subject [(b)(6)] withdrew from the study on March 30, 2006. However, an entry dated August 12, 2006 was made on the source record for the January 17, 2006 visit indicating that the subject did not smoke and/or consume alcohol.

iii. Subject [(b)(6)] had his/her Visit V8 on May 25, 2006. An entry dated October 25, 2006 indicated that the subject's dosing for the May 25, 2006 visit occurred on October 23, 24, and 25, 2006.

2. Concomitant medication assessments were not documented in the source records at several visits for Subjects [(b)(6)] as required by the protocol.

5. You failed to maintain investigational drug disposition records with respect to use by subjects [21 CFR 312.62(a)].

In Protocol [(b)(4)], the drug accountability logs for Subjects [(b)(6)] could not be found.

We acknowledge that in your Undated Letter you stated that you maintained drug accountability logs in the past only if the sponsor had provided one. You stated further that to correct this problem you have developed and implemented a drug accountability log to track and document drug dispensing and accountability. drug accountability log that you created that the In addition, there now is a master coordinator responsible for a specific trial will update every time the investigational product is received and dispensed. You also indicated that current procedures require the coordinators to have the medication number and [(b)(4)] assigned number cross checked by another coordinator prior to it being give to the subject. While these corrective actions appear appropriate, it was the absence of such measures that led to the violations listed here.

6. You failed to promptly report to the IRB all unanticipated problems involving risk to human subjects or others [21 CFR 312.66].

In Protocol [(b)(4)], your site was informed on December 12, 2006 that Subject [(b)(6)] had been admitted to the hospital for a bilateral pulmonary embolism on [(b)(4)], and had remained in the intensive care unit for one week. You failed to notify the IRB per IRB requirements within three business days of becoming aware of this serious adverse event, and you reported this event to the IRB on February 12, 2007 as a protocol deviation rather than an adverse event.

In your Undated Letter, you noted in response that Ms. [(b)(6)] was the primary study coordinator for this protocol. This response is inadequate, because your site became aware of this event after Ms. [(b)(6)] employment termination from your site. In addition, "[(b)(6)]," rather than Ms. [(b)(6)], made this notation after speaking to the subject on December 12, 2006.

This letter is not intended to be an all-inclusive list of deficiencies with your clinical study of an investigational drug. It is your responsibility to ensure adherence to each requirement of the law and relevant FDA regulations. You must address these deficiencies and establish procedures to ensure that any on-going or future studies will be in compliance with FDA regulations.

For those responses noted above that were found inadequate you must notify this office in writing within fifteen (15) working days of your receipt of this letter and of the actions you have taken or will be taking to prevent similar violations in the future. Failure to adequately and promptly explain the violations noted above may result in regulatory action without further notice.

If you have any questions, please contact Tejashri Purohit-Sheth, M.D. at 301-796-3402; FAX 301-847-8748. Your written response and any pertinent documentation should be addressed to:

Tejashri Purohit-Sheth, M.D.
Branch Chief
Good Clinical Practice Branch Ⅱ
Division of Scientific Investigations, Bldg 51, Room 5358
Office of Compliance
Center for Drug Evaluation and Research
Food and Drug Administration
10903 New Hampshire Avenue
Silver Spring, MD 20993

Sincerely yours,

{See appended electronic signature page}

Leslie K. Ball, M.D.
Director
Division of Scientific Investigations
Office of Compliance
Center for Drug Evaluation and Research

This is a representation of an electronic record that was signed electronically and this page is the manifestation of the electronic signature.

/S/

LESLIE KBALL
02/02/2009

第137封　给Stewart, Lynette D. 医学博士的警告信

2009年1月21日

参考号：09-HFD-45-01-01

尊敬的Stewart博士：

2007年4月26日至5月18日Myla Chapman女士代表FDA进行了现场检查，与您会面并对您为（b）（4）实施的下列试验药物（b）（4）的临床研究进行了审查。

试验方案（b）（4）：一项在（b）（4）阳性受试者中评价两个（b）（4）剂量组与安慰剂相比的有效性和安全性的为期12个月的随机双盲Ⅲ期临床试验。

试验方案（b）（4）：一项在（b）（4）阳性受试者中评价（b）（4）安全性的为期12个月的Ⅲ期扩展临床试验。

本次现场检查是FDA的生物研究监查项目的一部分。该项目通过设定的检查方法，由FDA监管的相关研究的实施情况，并确保这些研究中受试者的权益、安全和福利得到了保护。

对FDA现场检查报告、该报告的附件，我们认为您未遵守适用的法律要求和监管临床研究实施及受试者保护的FDA法规。在现场检查结束时，Myla Chapman女士向您出示并讨论了FDA483表，即现场检查发现的问题。我们想强调如下几点：

1. 您未能保护在您的监护下的受试者的权益、安全和福利［21 CFR 312.60］

为了评价（b）（4）制剂潜在的临床疗效，方案要求受试者给药后进行（b）（4）和（b）（4）活体组织检查，以确认受试制剂是否具有增生作用。另外，方案要求进行安全性和后续的评估并排除符合一定标准的受试者。遗漏了安全性评价，推迟了随后的评估，让符合排除标准的受试者继续进行试验，您让受试者处于危险处境，具体来说：

a. 受试者（b）（6）在2003年12月2日进行了（b）（4）活检，这是试验方案（b）（4）第12个月访视和试验方案（b）（4）第1天访视所要求的。活检没有得到足够的组织用于检测分析。两个方案均要求在一个月内重复取样。重复活检未进行。

随后，根据试验方案（b）（4）受试者（b）（6）在2004年6月16日第6个月访视时进行了活检，获取了足够的组织用于检测分析。结果检测出（b）（4），根据方案受试者不能继续参加研究，并应作为不良事件记录。然而，您让受试者继续参加研究，并且未记录为不良事件，继续提供随机药物，这可能导致受试者受到伤害。

b. 受试者（b）（6）在2004年4月20日进行（b）（4），这是试验方案（b）（4）第12个月访视和试验方案（b）（4）第1天访视的一部分。（b）（4）耳的结果报告符合排除标准。这些记录显示您审查（b）（4）结果的时间是2004年6月4日。方案允许受试者在等待（b）（4）结果，即（b）（4）肿瘤阴性期间继续参加研究。根据文件记录显示，受试者直到2004年7月30日才按要求进行（b）（4）测试。

此外，方案指定的实验室直到2004年9月3日才收到组织。没有文件对该延时情况做解释。尽管存在这些可能被排除的结果，受试者仍继续参与研究，直到2005年1月失访为止。

2. 您未能进行研究或者确保按照试验计划进行研究［21 CFR 312.60］

除了以上情况，我们发现以下几点：

a. 方案入排标准要求（b）（4）具有一定的（b）（4）水平。以下受试者在试验方案（b）（4）未达到（b）（4）水平却被入组了。

ⅰ）受试者（b）（6）2004年5月4日第1天访视时（b）（4）值为1.7。

该受试者入组该研究，没有文件记录显示您曾经请求豁免。

ⅱ）受试者（b）（6）2004年6月28日第1天访视时（b）（4）值为0.7。

该受试者被入组研究，您在2004年9月30日才请求豁免。申办者允许该受试者在第3个月访视结果出来前继续参加研究。2004年9月24日第3个月访视的（b）（4）值报告为1.0，在2004年10月11日作为排除进行了报告。一个2004年10月26日采集的样本（b）（4）的值为0.08，报告符合排除标准。您直到2004年11月9日才审查第3个月访视结果，并将排除结果归类为无临床意义。受试者最终在2004年12月退出。

b. 您在2004年3月2日第3个月访视时对试验方案（b）（4）的受试者（b）（4）进行了（b）（4）测试。方案在这次访视中没有要求这个操作，在临床记录中没有提及为什么会进行该（b）（4）操作。此外，该研究场所未给该受试者打第二个月的访视电话。

c. 受试者（b）（6）在2004年11月19日第6个月访视时进行试验方案（b）（4）规定的活检组织，没有取得足够的组织量用于检验分析。活检应该在一个月内重复取样，但是没有取。没有关于重复活检的文件记录。

d. 受试者（b）（6）未按照试验方案（b）（4）要求进行原定在2005年3月14日的治疗后随访。记录显示直到2005年5月研究者才为这项失访尝试联系受试者。

e. 2003年12月2日第12个月访视时受试者（b）（6）未按照试验方案（b）（4）完成生活质量调查和（b）（4）功能指数。

f. 在扩展研究期间受试者（b）（6）第5个月电话随访没有完成。

3. 您未能准备和保存研究中的每个受试者的所有研究观察结果和其他相关数据的足够准确的病历记录［21 CFR 312.62（b）］

a. 原始文件显示受试者（b）（6）根据试验方案（b）（4）在第7个月（2005年1月17日）和第8个月（2005年2月17日）有电话随访。基于受试者在2004年12月提前终止了研究，该信息应该报告为治疗后第1个月和第2个月的电话随访。

b. 入组试验方案（b）（4）的受试者（b）（6）第6个月随访记录存在矛盾。第6个月随访，受试者明显在不同的两天（2003年10月6日和7日）访问了办公室。2004年6月8日的一个文件注释声明，原始文件第2页2003年10月7日随访的记录丢失了，而且由于您不在办公室，所以未进行体检。这个注释还声明在2004年12月15日和23日第8个月访视中进行了简单的体检。矛盾的是，2003年10月6日另一研究协调员的记录中声明，由于医生不在办公室，没有进行活检，其他所有相应的操作均已完成。

c. 有2个缩写代号为（b）（6）的受试者根据试验方案（b）（4）进行了入组筛选，两个均筛选失败。这两个受试者的记录在不同的文件夹中混杂在一起，由于这种记录标识方式，很难区分哪些文件是属于哪个受试者的。

本警告信的目的并非是罗列您在试验药物临床研究中存在的所有缺陷。确保遵循法律和FDA相关法规的每一项要求是您的职责。您应当解决这些缺陷，并建立规程，以确保任何正在进行或将来进行的研究均能符合FDA的法规。

自收到这封信的15个工作日内，您应当书面告知本办公室为预防将来发生类似违规情况已经和将要采取的措施。如果不能充分、迅速地解释上述违规问题，可能导致我们在不再通知的情况下采取监管措施。

附：英文原文

Stewart, Lynette D. M.D.

WARNING LETTER

Jan 21, 2009

CERTIFIED MAIL
RETURN RECEIPT REQUESTED

Dr. Lynette Stewart
Georgia Center for Female Health
4775 Jimmy Carter Blvd., Suite 101
Norcross, GA 30093 USA
Ref: 09-HFD-45-01-01

Dear Dr. Stewart:

Between April 26 and May 18, 2007, Ms. Myla Chapman, representing the Food and Drug Administration (FDA), conducted an investigation and met with you, to review your conduct of the following clinical investigation of the investigational drug (b)(4), performed for (b)(4)

- Protocol No. (b)(4): A Phase 3, 12-Month, Randomized, Double-Blind Study to Evaluate the Efficacy and Safety of Two Doses of (b)(4) Versus Placebo in Subjects with (b)(4)
- Protocol No. (b)(4): A Phase 3, 12-Month, Extension Study to Evaluate the Safety of (b)(4) in Subjects with (b)(4)

This inspection is a part of the FDA's Bioresearch Monitoring Program, which includes inspections designed to evaluate the conduct of research and to ensure that the rights, safety, and welfare of the human subjects of those studies have been protected.

From our review of the establishment inspection report and the documents submitted with that report, we conclude that you did not adhere to the applicable statutory requirements and FDA regulations governing the conduct of clinical investigations and the protection of human subjects. We are aware that at the conclusion of the inspection, Ms. Chapman presented and discussed with you Form FDA 483, Inspectional Observations.

We wish to emphasize the following:

1. You failed to protect the rights, safety and welfare of subjects under your care [21 CFR 312.60].

As required in this protocol evaluating a potentially therapeutic (b)(4) agent, subjects were to have (b)(4) and (b)(4) biopsies performed to evaluate for potential proliferative effects of the test agent. In addition, the protocol required conducting safety and follow up evaluations and excluding subjects who met certain criteria. By omitting these safety evaluations, delaying follow up evaluations or continuing subjects in the study despite the presence of exclusion criteria, you placed the study subjects at risk. Specifically,

a. i) Subject (b)(6) had an (b)(4) biopsy on 12/2/03 which was required for the Month 12 visit for protocol # (b)(4) and the Day -1 visit for protocol # (b)(4). The biopsy yielded inadequate tissue for analysis. Both protocols required a repeat of the procedure within one month. The repeat biopsy was not performed.

a. ii) Subsequently, subject (b)(6) had a biopsy at the Month 6 visit for protocol # (b)(4) on 6/16/04 which yielded adequate tissue for analysis. The result indicated a (b)(4), which according to the protocol should have resulted in discontinuation of the subject from the study and should have been recorded as an adverse event. However, you allowed the subject to remain in the study, did not record this an adverse event, and continued to provide randomized medication that may have placed the subject at risk for injury.

b. i) Subject (b)(6) had a (b)(4) on 4/20/04 that was part of the Month 12 visit for protocol (b)(4) and the Day -1 visit for protocol (b)(4). The results of the (b)(4) ear were reported as exclusionary. The records indicate that you reviewed the (b)(4) test results on 6/4/04. The protocol allows for the subject to continue in the study pending a (b)(4) result that is negative for (b)(4)/cancer. Based on the documents in the file, it does not appear as if the subject had the required (b)(4) test until 7/30/04.

b. ii) In addition, it appears that the protocol specified laboratory did not receive the tissue for this test until 9/3/04. There is no explanation in the files for these delays. Despite these potential exclusionary results, the subject remained in the study until January 2005 when she was lost to follow up.

2. You failed to conduct the studies or ensure they were conducted according to the investigational plan [21 CFR 312.60]. In addition to items la.-b. above, we note the following:

a. The protocol inclusion criteria required an (b)(4) level of (b)(4). The following subjects were enrolled in protocol (b)(4) with exclusionary (b)(4) levels:

i) Subject (b)(6) had a Day -1 5/4/04 (b)(4) level of 1.7.

This subject was allowed to enroll in the study and there is no documentation indicating that you ever requested a wavier.

ii) Subject (b)(6) had a Day -1 6/28/04 (b)(4) level of 0.7.

This subject was allowed to enroll in the study. You did not request a waiver for this enrollment until 9/30/04; the sponsor allowed for the subject to stay on the study pending the Month 3 results. An (b)(4) result of 1.0 was reported for the labs drawn at the Month 3 visit on 9/24/04 and reported on 10/11/04 as exclusionary. An (b)(4) sample collected on 10/26/04 was also reported as exclusionary at .08. Your review of the Month 3 results did not occur until 11/9/04 and categorized the exclusionary result as not clinically significant. The subject was ultimately withdrawn December 2004.

b. You performed a (b)(4) on Subject (b)(6) on 3/2/04 at the Month 3 visit for protocol # (b)(4). This procedure was not required by the protocol for that visit and there is no mention in the clinic notes as to why this (b)(4) was done. In addition, thc site did not make the Month 2 phone call to this subject.

c. Subject (b)(6) had a biopsy for the Month 6 treatment visit for protocol # (b)(4) on 11/19/04 that did not yield enough tissue for an analysis. The biopsy should have been repeated within one month, but it was not. There is no documentation regarding performance of a repeat biopsy.

d. Subject (b)(6) missed her scheduled post-treatment follow-up for protocol # (b)(4) on March 14, 2005. The records do not indicate that the site tried to contact the subject until May 2005 regarding the missed visit.

e. The Quality of Life Questionnaire and the (b)(4) Function index were not completed by Subject (b)(6) at the Month 12 visit for protocol # (b)(4) 12/2/03.

f. The Month 5 phone call was not made to Subject (b)(6) during the extension study.

3. You failed to prepare and maintain adequate and accurate case histories that record all subject's observations and other data pertinent to the investigation on each individual [21 CFR 312.62(b)].

a. Source documents show phone calls for Month 7 (dated 1/17/05) and Month 8 (dated 2/17/05) for Subject (b)(6) for # (b)(4). Based on the subject's early termination date in 12/04, the information should have been reported as Month 1 and Month 2 post treatment follow-up phone calls.

b. Month 6 records conflict for Subject (b)(6) enrolled in protocol # (b)(4). For the Month 6 visit, the subject apparently visited the office on two different days, 10/6/03 and 10/7/03. A note to file dated 6/8/04 states that page 2 of the source document for the visit done on 10/7/03 is missing and indicates that the physical exam was not done because you were not at the office. The note also states that a brief physical exam was conducted at the Month 8 visit which took place 12/15/04 and 12/23/04. By contrast, a note written on 10/6/03 by a different study coordinator states that all appropriate procedures were done except for a biopsy because the physician had to leave the office.

c. There were two subjects screened for #(b)(4) with the initials (b)(6) both were screen fails. The records for these two subjects were mixed in the different folders and because of the way that the records are identified, it is difficult to discern which documents belong to which subject.

This letter is not intended to be an all-inclusive list of deficiencies with your clinical study of an investigational drug. It is your responsibility to ensure adherence to each requirement of the law and relevant FDA regulations. You should address these deficiencies and establish procedures to ensure that any on-going or future studies will be in compliance with FDA regulations.

Within fifteen (15) working days of your receipt of this letter, you should notify this office in writing of the actions you have taken or will be taking to prevent similar violations in the future. Failure to adequately and promptly explain the violations noted above may result in regulatory action without further notice.

If you have any questions, please contact Constance Lewin, M.D., M.P.H., at 301-796-3397; FAX 301-847-8748. Your written response and any pertinent documentation should be addressed to:

Constance Lewin, M.D., M.P.H.
Branch Chief, Good Clinical Practice Branch I
Division of Scientific Investigations
Office of Compliance
Center for Drug Evaluation and Research
Food and Drug Administration
Bldg 51, Room 5354
10903 New Hampshire Avenue
Silver Spring, MD 20993

Sincerely yours,

{See appended electronic signature page}

Leslie K. Ball, M.D.
Director
Division of Scientific Investigations
Office of Compliance
Center for Drug Evaluation and Research

第 138 封　给 Spirtos, Nick M. 医学博士的警告信

2009年1月3日

参考号：09-HFD-45-12-01

尊敬的Spirtos博士：

2007年11月12日至12月1日，Anthony Keller陆军上尉，代表FDA进行了现场检查，与您进行了会面，并对您所实施的一项临床研究进行了审查：试验方案［（b）（4）］，名称为"评估［（b）（4）］和［（b）（4）］联合用药作为一线药物治疗［（b）（4）］患者的Ⅱ期临床预试验"，试验药物为［（b）（4）］，申办者为［（b）（4）］。

本次现场检查是FDA的生物研究监查项目的一部分。该项目通过设定的检查方法，对研究的实施情况进行评估，并确保这些研究中受试者的权益、安全和福利得到了保护。

经对FDA现场检查报告（EIR）、随该报告的附件、检查结束时交给检查员Keller的更新信函进行审查，我们认为，您没有遵循适用的法律要求和监管临床研究实施的FDA法规。我们知道在现场检查结束时，检查员Keller向您出示并讨论了FDA483表，即现场检查发现的问题。我们想强调以下几点：

1. 您未能确保按照签署的研究者声明、研究计划进行研究［21 CFR 312.60］

A. 试验方案最初版和修正案#1都规定，研究中试验药物给药都要遵照以下的浓度和时间表：

［（b）（4）］静脉注射30~90分钟，随后［（b）（4）］静脉注射1小时，之后立即静脉注射［（b）（4）］2个小时。

另外，最初的试验方案和试验方案的修正案#1都规定所有试验药物都要在每周期（每周期21天）的第一天注射，注射6个周期或直到疾病进展；6个周期后［（b）（4）］作为单一药物继续注射，每3周一次，至治疗开始后的12个月。试验方案还规定［（b）（4）］的剂量需要根据受试者个人的耐受情况进行调整，［（b）（4）］则需要一直保持在建议剂量的100%。另外，试验方案还规定如果受试者在试验中体重与筛选时相比变化大于10%，则试验药物的剂量需要重新计算。方案违背的例子包括但不限于以下受试者：

ⅰ. 如第2周期，受试者［（b）（6）］按照下列错误的指令接受了试验药物：［（b）（4）］。

ⅱ. 对于受试者［（b）（6）］。

（1）从第1周期到第5周期，您研究场所按照受试者驾照上的信息（即分别是190磅，5英尺3英寸）报告了化疗指令表上受试者的身高、体重测量值。但我们注意到，原始记录显示受试者的在这些周期的体重要比驾照上登记的要轻。

周期	访视工作表上的体重	换算体重（1lbs=453.59g）
1	67.3 kg	148.1 lbs
2	67 kg	147.41bs
3	61.4 kg	135.1 lbs
4	61.4 kg	135.1 lbs
5	58 kg	127.6 lbs

当试验药房按照来自您研究场所的化疗指令表上的体重和身高值准备试验药物时，受试者［（b）（6）］在这些访视期间的试验药物剂量明显过量。

（2）在基线访视（即2006年6月19日）和第5周期第1天访视期间，受试者体重下降超过10%。但是，根据化疗指令表，您没有修正受试者体重值，导致未能重新计算给药剂量。

ⅲ. 受试者［（b）（6）］的第1周期至第6周期，研究场所按照受试者驾照上的信息（即分别是120磅，4英尺10英寸）报告了化疗顺序表上受试者的身高、体重测量值。但我们注意到，原始记录显示受试者在这些访视期量的体重比驾照上登记的要轻。

周期	访视工作表上的体重	换算体重
1	45 kg	99 lbs
2	45 kg	99 lbs
3	45 kg	99 lbs
4	45 kg 根据病程记录 49 kg 根据（b）（4）访视工作表	99 lbs 107.8 lbs
5	45 kg 根据病程记录 48 kg 根据（b）（4）访视工作表	99 lbs 105.6 lbs
6	44.5 kg	97.9 lbs

当试验药房按照来自研究场所的化疗指令表上的体重和身高值准备试验药物时，受试者［（b）（6）］在这些访视期间的试验药物剂量明显过量。

B. 最初的试验方案和试验方案的修正案#1都规定，对所有受试者都要仔细监测试验药物的毒性，［（b）（4）］给药剂量要根据受试者个人耐受情况进行调整。另外，试验方案要求，新周期第1天的推荐剂量调整要根据前一周期观察到的最严重的毒性反应和/或新周期例行实验室检查结果进行。关于［（b）（4）］，试验方案明确而详细地规定，在新周期第1天的给药剂量调整要根据前一周期观察到的最严重的毒性反应类型进行。尤其是当受试者有4级中性粒细胞减少时，需要延迟给药，并且当受试者恢复到中性粒细胞计数（ANC）大于1200时给药剂量下降一个等级。

原始记录显示，受试者［（b）（6）］于第3周期第8天（2006年6月8日）的访视中被研究场所判断为4级中性粒细胞减少。2006年6月13日，ANC上升至0.6 $\times 10^3/\mu L$。实验室检测结果显示2006年6月17日该受试者的ANC升高超过1200限度（即1.2$\times 10^3/\mu L$）。原始记录显示，受试者［（b）（6）］于2006年6月19日进行了第4周期第1天的访视，并于6月20日接受了标准剂量的试验药物给药，并未按试验方案规定，降低给药剂量水平。我们发现，显示该4级中性粒细胞减少已经恢复的实验室检测没有在方案规定的24小时窗口内进行，血常规应该在每个周期的第1天进行（即2006年6月20日）。2006年6月17日，第4周期第1天访视的血常规结果没有依照方案要求进行。

C. 最初的试验方案和试验方案的修正案#1都规定，在严重不良事件出现后的一个工作日内，研究者要填写并提交严重不良事件报告表。表上的信息应包括对严重不良事件与试验药物是否相关的评估，且需要签署姓名和日期。根据［（b）（6）］先生2006年7月27日的书面咨询报告，您的授权研究员知道受试者［（b）（6）］因胸部疼痛入院治疗。住院期间，受试者先后进行了左心插管，两侧选择性的冠状动脉造影和血管搭桥术。您直到2006年12月5日才向申办者提交了SAE的初次报告（由您签署姓名和日期）。

D. 初始的试验方案和试验方案的修正案#1规定，虽然知情同意可以在试验药物给药前14天之前进行，基线研究步骤（包括但不限于［（b）（4）］一般状态评估、体检、感觉神经评估和ECG）需要在研究治疗14天内进行。以下是方案违背的例子：

ⅰ. 受试者［（b）（6）］的原始记录显示，基线研究步骤（包括但不限于［（b）（4）］一般状态评估、体检、感觉神经评估）在2006年3月23日进行。受试者直到2006年4月15日或4月17日才进行第一次给药，超过了方案中规定的14天。

ⅱ. 受试者［（b）（6）］的原始文件显示，基线研究步骤（体检、感觉神经评估、生命体征和［（b）（4）］一般状态评估）在2006年6月16日进行，ECG在2006年6月22日进行。受试者直到2006年7月21日才进行第一次给药，超过了方案中规定的14天。

E. 初始的试验方案和试验方案的修正案#1规定，在基线访视时，需要进行尿检和尿蛋白/肌酸酐（UPC）率检测。原始记录显示，受试者［（b）（6）］在基线访视时未进行这些检测。

F. 初始的试验方案和试验方案的修正案#1规定，所有试验药物都要在每周期（每周期21天）的第一天注射，注射6个周期或直到疾病进展。此后，［（b）（4）］作为单一药物继续注射，每3周一次，至治疗开始后的第12个月。关于第1天访视需要进行的研究步骤，初始的试验方案规定每周期第1天，特定的研究步骤（包括但不限于体检，生命体征和感觉神经评估，［（b）（4）］测试和外周神经毒性量表）要在试验药物给药前进行。试验方案的修正案#1仅修改为：［（b）（4）］测试需要每隔一个周期进行。方案违背包括但不限于：

ⅰ. 对于受试者［（b）（6）］

（1）第1周期第1天的访视没有进行感觉神经评估。

（2）第1周期第1天外周神经毒性量表在2006年4月11日进行，比受试者试验药物给药时间（即2006年4月17日）早了6天。

ⅱ. 对于受试者［（b）（6）］

（1）有很多周期中，研究步骤（包括但不限于体检和感觉神经评估）在周期的第1天进行，但试验药物没有依照方案、在周期的第1天给药：

周期	访视工作表和/或CRF上的周期第一天日期	该周期的试验药物给药日期
1	2006年6月19日	2006年6月26日
2	2006年7月12日	2006年7月17日
3	2006年8月2日	2006年8月7日
4	2006年8月23日	2006年8月28日
5	2006年9月11日	2006年9月18日
6	2006年10月4日	2006年10月9日

（2）每个周期的第1天，当按照方案要求受试者要接受试验药物治疗时，未进行外周神经毒性量表检查。尤其是，原始记录显示第1周期第1天访视未进行该量表检查。另外，第2、5周期的第1天访视，量表检查分别在受试者试验药物给药前的5天和7天进行。

ⅲ. 关于受试者，我们注意到：

（1）很多周期中，研究步骤（包括但不限于体检和感觉神经评估）在周期的第1天进行，但试验药物没有依照方案在周期的第1天给药。

例如：

周期	访视工作表和/或CRF上的周期第一天日期	该周期的试验药物给药日期
2	2006年8月1日	2006年8月11日
3	2006年8月29日	2006年9月1日
4	2006年9月19日	2006年9月22日
6	2006年10月31日	2006年11月3日

（2）每个周期的第1天，当按照方案要求受试者要接受试验药物治疗时，未进行外周神经毒性量表检查。尤其是，第6周期第1天访视未进行该量表检查。另外，第2周期的第1天访视，量表检查在受试者试验药物给

药前的10天进行。

G. 初始的试验方案规定，在进行细胞毒化疗和［（b）（4）］治疗期间，第1天和第8天给药之前，要进行规定的实验室检查：包括血常规（每周期第1天之前的24小时时间窗内；除了第1周期第1天前可在72小时时间窗内），血生化（每周期第1天之前的72小时时间窗内），凝血（每周期第1天之前的72小时时间窗内），尿检和尿蛋白/肌酸酐（UPC）检测（每周期第1天之前的72小时时间窗内）和［（b）（4）］检测（每周期第1天）。试验方案的修正案#1修订了细胞毒化疗和［（b）（4）］给药期间实验室检查的部分要求：血常规（72小时时间窗；需在每周期第1天和第8天进行），血生化（72小时时间窗；第8天不要求），凝血（72小时时间窗；第8天不要求），尿检和尿蛋白/肌酸酐（UPC）检测（72小时时间窗；基线，第1天，以及化疗前每周期；第8天不要求）和［（b）（4）］检测（每周期第1天）对比研究场所病历和每次访视时有效的试验方案，我们发现了存在方案违背。例子包括却不限于：

i. 对于受试者［（b）（4）］

（1）尽管采集了样本进行检测，包括血常规、血生化、凝血和/或［（b）（4）］检测，但第1、2、3、4、5和/或6周期第1天访视时，样本未在方案规定的、受试者给药前的时限内进行检测。

（2）第1周期第8天访视或第6周期第8天的访视，未进行血生化检测。

（3）第1周期的第8天、第2周期的第1天、第3周期的第8天和第5周期的第1天访视，未进行尿检和UPC测定。

（4）第2周期的第8天、第3周期的第1天、第3周期的第8天、第4周期的第1天和第6周期的第1天访视，未进行部分凝血激活酶时间（PTT）测定。

ii. 关于受试者［（b）（6）］，我们注意到：

（1）第4周期第1天的访视没有进行UPC测定。

（2）第2周期第8天的访视没有检查血常规。

H. 初始的试验方案和试验方案的修正案#1都规定，［（b）（4）］瓶应在［（b）（4）］条件下冻存，直到使用前。我们检查发现，2007年1月前没有找到任何记录能证明试验药物按方案规定适合的条件进行保存。

I. 方案规定，［（b）（4）］应储存在［（b）（4）］到［（b）（4）］之间的温度下，经允许后到［（b）（4）］的短途运输中需保持在［（b）（4）］。我们检查发现，2007年4月前没有找到任何记录能证明试验药物按方案规定适合的条件进行保存。

J. 初始的试验方案和试验方案的修正案#1都规定，研究者要确保遵从访视计划和方案规定的步骤，且根据提供的说明来准确、清晰地提交病例报告表（CRF）需要的所有信息，并保证让申办者的代表能直接接触原始文件。两个方案还规定，研究者有责任完整、准确地保持申办者设计的CRF，以记录与临床研究相关的所有观察和其他相关的数据。所有CRF都需要完整的填写，并且保证整洁、清晰，以便准确的分析数据。方案还规定，如果需要进行修改，原数值不能被覆盖，更正后的数值由经过授权的人员誊写在原数值旁，并签署姓名和日期；任何情况下不能使用白色修正液或修改液。

根据FDA检查员Keller的观察，FDA现场检查期间审查的原始材料中，有多处使用修正液和覆盖原数值修改。另外，这些修改未注明原因。例子包括却不限于：

i. CRF中受试者［（b）（6）］试验药物［（b）（4）］的给药剂量。

ii. 受试者［（b）（6）］的［（b）（4）］访视表中第2、3、4周期第1天访视的体重信息。

iii. 受试者［（b）（6）］的［（b）（4）］访视表中第1、2、3、5、6周期第1天访视的体重和/或身高信息。

iv. 试验药物数量记录。

您这种文件管理方式，导致我们不能对您研究场所记录中的信息进行确认。无法知道这些修改的依据和来源。

2. 您未能保存研究中每个受试者的所有观察结果和其他相关数据的足够准确的病历［21 CFR 312.62（b）］

A. FDA审查受试者［（b）（6）］的病历时，发现的不准确填写情况包括但不限于以下：

i. 第13周期第1天访视受试者［（b）（6）］的CRF列出的UPC率为0.21，相应的实验室检测报告显示的UPC率为0.109。

ii. 2006年3月23日基线访视的临床记录，于2006年6月21日补记，信息包括但不限于受试者的［（b）（4）］测试，［（b）（4）］一般状态和受试者入组的知情同意过程。补记的数据来源无法确定。

iii. 第1周期化疗指令表“给药日期栏”显示试验药物给药时间为2006年4月15日。但是，这份表单上方的有一条手写记录“住院患者4月17日化疗给药。”

B. FDA审查受试者［（b）（6）］的病历时，发现的不准确填写情况包括但不限于以下：

i. 基线访视和第1周期第1天访视的病历不一致，我们不能判断这些访视的CRF中的信息的来源在哪里。尤其是第1周期第1天［（b）（4）］访视的原始文件显示，体检、感觉神经评估和生命体征检查于2006年6月19日进行。但第1周期第1天的CRF显示，未进行体检、感觉神经评估，生命体征检查于2006年6月26日进行。另外，基线访视的CRF中显示，体检、感觉神经评估和生命体征检查于2006年6月19日进行，但CRF中生命体征结果与记录在第1周期第1天的［（b）（4）］访视表的不一致。

ii. 第5周期第1天CRF记录的受试者2006年9月15日体重为61.4kg。FDA检查员Keller未能发现支持这个体重数据的原始记录。2006年9月11日的病程记录显示，受试者体重为127磅，但［（b）（4）］访视上记录为58kg。

iii. 第8周期第1天访视CRF记录试验药物给药日期为2006年11月11日。原始记录显示试验药物给药时间为2006年11月20日。

C. FDA审查受试者［（b）（6）］的记录时，发现的不准确填写情况的病历的例子，但不限于以下：

i. 第6周期第1天访视存在两张不同的化疗指令表。研究文件夹中的化疗指令表与试验药房找到的化疗指令表不相同。尤其是研究文件夹中的化疗指令表未签名，记录受试者体重为48kg。试验药房找到的、用来准备试验药物的化疗指令表有签名，记录受试者体重记录为120磅（约54kg）。

ii. 关于第7周期第1天访视的几份原始记录存在不一致的情况。尤其是该次访视存在两份化疗指令表。研究文件夹中的化疗指令表显示受试者体重为45kg。试验药房找到的、用来准备试验药物的化疗指令表，记录受试者体重为55 kg。但第7周期第1天的［（b）（4）］访视工作表上未记录受试者体重的数值。

iii. 受试者［（b）（6）］于［（b）（6）］住院治疗，在FDA对研究场所检查期间，未查见相关文件证实研究场所向伦理委员会提交了SAE报告。

D. 您中心使用申办者的［（b）（4）］工作表作为原始记录。在这一文件的底部，设计了填表人签署名字和日期的地方。但当我们审查这份表格时，我们发现填表人未签名、签日期或未及时签名、签日期是普遍存在的情况。例子包括但不限于以下：

i. 受试者［（b）（6）］第8周期第1天和第12周期第1天两次访视，填表人完成填写后未签名签日期。［（b）（4）］访视工作表记录了受试者［（b）（6）］的感觉神经评估、生命体征、［（b）（4）］一般状态、体格检查、［（b）（4）］检查日期为2006年5月4日，签署日期为2006年8月16日。

ii. 受试者［（b）（6）］第1周期第1天、第2周期第1天、第5周期第1天和第6周期第1天访视，填表人填写表格后未签名、签日期。

iii. 受试者［（b）（6）］第2周期第1天、第3周期第1天、第4周期第1天和第7周期第1天访视，填表人填写表格后未签名、签日期。

研究场所文件上未签名、签日期和/或延迟签名、签日期的情况，让我们对临床研究过程中原始文件的准确性引起关注。

现场检查结束时，您提交给FDA检查员Keller的更新的回复，指出研究场所在临床研究过程中已经对监查员发现的缺陷进行了处理，这导致数据协调员被解雇，更换了全部研究人员。您还提到如果FDA检查员Keller能有时间检查并对记录进行深入审查，会发现方案违背的数量不断下降，因为研究场所对之前发现的缺陷进行了改进，并更换了数据管理团队。

我们认为这一回复是不充分的，尤其是作为临床试验研究者，您有责任确保临床研究依照研究方案进行，并按照适用的FDA法规的要求保持足够和准确的病历。另外，我们发现，您的纠正措施仅仅是解雇、更换了研究人员，没有为保证此类方案违规在当前或未来进行的临床研究中不再发生而准备采取的纠正措施。

本警告信的目的并非是罗列您在试验药物临床研究中存在的所有缺陷。确保遵循法律和FDA相关法规的每一项要求是您的职责。您应当解决这些缺陷，并建立规程，以确保任何正在进行或将来进行的研究均能符合FDA的法规。

自收到这封信的15个工作日内，您应当书面告知本办公室为预防将来发生类似违规情况已经或将要采取的措施。如果不能充分、迅速地解释上述违规问题，可能导致我们在不再通知的情况下采取监管措施。

附：英文原文

Spirtos, Nick M. M.D.

WARNING LETTER

Jan 03, 2009

CERTIFIED MAIL
RETURN RECEIPT REQUESTED

Ref: 09-HFD-45-12-01

Nicola Spirtos, M.D.
Women's Cancer Center of Nevada
3131 La Canada St., Ste 110
Las Vegas, NV 89169

Dear Dr. Spirtos:

Between November 12 and December 1, 2007, CAPT Anthony Keller, representing the U.S. Food and Drug Administration (FDA), conducted an investigation and met with you, to review your conduct of a clinical investigation (Protocol [(b)(4)] entitled "A Pilot Phase Ⅱ Study Evaluating the Combination of [(b)(4)] with [(b)(4)] as First Line Therapy in Patients with [(b)(4)] of the investigational drugs [(b)(4)], performed for [(b)(4)]"

This inspection is a part of the FDA's Bioresearch Monitoring Program, which includes inspections designed to evaluate the conduct of research and to ensure that the rights, safety, and welfare of the human subjects participating in those studies have been protected.

From our review of the establishment inspection report, the documents submitted with that report, and your undated letter provided to FDA investigator Keller at the end of the inspection, we conclude that you did not adhere to the applicable statutory requirements and FDA regulations governing the conduct of clinical investigations. We are aware that at the conclusion of the inspection, FDA investigator Keller presented and discussed with you Form FDA 483, Inspectional Observations. We wish to emphasize the following:

1. You failed to ensure that the investigation was conducted according to the signed investigator statement and investigational plan [21 CFR 312.60].

A. Both the original protocol and Protocol Amendment #1 specified that the study treatment was to be administered in the following concentration and schedule:

[(b)(4)] IV over 30-90 minutes, followed by [(b)(4)] IV as a 1-hour infusion, followed immediately by [(b)(4)] IV over 2 hours.

In addition, both the original protocol and Protocol Amendment #1 specified that all study medications were to be infused on Day 1 every 21 days for 6 Cycles (1 Cycle = 21 days) or until disease progression, and after Cycle 6, [(b)(4)] as a single agent would continue as aninfusion every 3 weeks for a total of 12 months from initiation of therapy. The protocols further stated that the dosing of [(b)(4)] should be adjusted depending upon individual patient tolerance and the dose of [(b)(4)] was to remain fixed at 100% of recommended dose. In addition the protocols stated that if a patient's weight changed by > 10% from screening weight during the study, the study drug dosages were to be recalculated. Examples of protocol violations include but were not limited to the following:

i. For Cycle 2, Subject [(b)(6)] received the investigational drugs in the following incorrect order: [(b)(4)]

ii. With respect to Subject [(b)(6)]

1. For Cycles 1 through 5, your site appears to have reported the values for the weight and height measurements on the chemotherapy order forms based on information from the subject's driver's license (i.e. 190 lbs, 5 foot 3 inches, respectively). We note however, that source documents showed that the subject's weight for these cycles was less than the weight noted on the driver's license:

Cycle	Weight per visit worksheet	Equivalent weight
1	67.3 kg	148.1 lbs
2	67 kg	147.4 lbs
3	61.4 kg	135.1 lbs
4	61.4 kg	135.1 lbs
5	58 kg	127.6 lbs

As the investigational pharmacy prepared the study drugs based on the weight and height values noted per the chemotherapy order forms generated by your site, Subject [(b)(6)] apparently was overdosed with investigational drugs at all of these visits.

2. Between the baseline visit (i.e. June 19, 2006) and the Cycle 5 Day 1 visit the subject's weight had decreased by greater than 10%. However, based on the chemotherapy order forms, you did not adjust the subject's weight, which resulted in a failure to recalculate the dosages.

iii. With respect to Subject [(b)(6)] for Cycles 1 through 6, your site reported the values for the weight and height measurements on the chemotherapy order forms based on the subject's driver's license (i.e. 120 lbs, 4 foot 10 inches, respectively). We note, however, that source documents showed that the subject's weight for these visits was less than the weight noted on the driver's license:

Cycle	Weight per visit worksheet	Equivalent weight
1	45 kg	99 lbs
2	45 kg	99 lbs
3	45 kg	99 lbs
4	45 kg per progress note 49 kg per (b)(4) visit worksheet	99 lbs 107.8 lbs
5	45 kg per progress note 48 kg per (b)(4) visit worksheet	99 lbs 105.6 lbs
6	44.5 kg	97.9 lbs

As the investigational pharmacy prepared the study drugs based on the weight and height values noted per the chemotherapy order forms generated by,your site, Subject [(b)(6)] apparently was overdosed with investigational drugs at all of these visits.

B. The original protocol and Protocol Amendment #1 specified that subjects should be carefully monitored for toxicity and that the dosing of [(b)(4)] were to be adjusted depending on the individual patient tolerance. In addition, the protocols stated that the recommended dose modifications on Day 1 of a new cycle were based on the most severe toxicity observed in the previous cycle and/or upon laboratory values on the scheduled day of treatment in the new cycle. With respect to [(b)(4)], the protocols explicitly detailed the dose modifications needed for Day 1 of the new cycle based on the worst type of toxicity observed in the prior cycle. Specifically, a subject who experiences a Grade 4 neutropenia was to have a delay in the dose, and then a decrease in one dose level when resolved to at least > Absolute Neutrophil Count (ANC) 1200 for neutropenia.

Source documents showed that Subject [(b)(6)] experienced what was identified by your site as a Grade 4 neutropenia on June 8, 2006 at the Cycle 3 Day 8 visit. On June 13, 2006 the ANC rose to $0.6 \times 10^3/\mu L$. Labs showing that the subject's ANC rose above the 1200 mark (i.e. $1.2 \times 10^3/\mu L$) were taken on June 17, 2006. Source records showed that Subject [(b)(6)] had her Cycle 4 Day 1 visit on June 19, and the subject received the standard dosage of investigational drugs on June 20, 2006, without a decrease in dose level as specified in the protocol. We note that the labs showing recovery from the Grade 4 neutropenia were not taken within the 24 hr window specified by the protocol for the hematology tests to be taken on Day 1 of each Cycle (i.e. June 20, 2006). Thus the hematology lab result on June 17, 2006 for the Cycle 4 Day 1 visit is not taken in accordance with the protocol.

C. The original protocol and Protocol Amendment #1 specified that within one working day after a Serious Adverse Event, the investigator was to fill out and submit the SAE notification form. The information on the form was to include an evaluation of the relationship to the study drugs, and the form was also to be signed and dated. Per the written consultation report by Dr. [(b) (6)] dated July 27, 2006, your sub-investigator was aware that Subject [(b) (6)] had been admitted to the hospital with chest pains. During the hospital stay, a left heart catheterization, bilateral selective coronary angiogram and angioplasty were subsequently performed on the subject. You did not submit the initial report of the SAE to the sponsor (signed and dated by you) until December 5, 2006.

D. The original protocol and Protocol Amendment #1 specified that while informed consent could be taken prior to 14 days before study treatment, the baseline study procedures which included but were not limited to a [(b)(4)] performance status evaluation, physical exam, neurosensory assessment, and ECG were to be done within 14 days of study treatment. The following were examples of deviations from protocol requirements:

ⅰ. With respect to Subject [(b)(6)] source documents showed that the baseline study procedures including but not limited to the physical exam, neurological assessment, and [(b) (4)] performance status evaluation were performed on March 23, 2006. The subject did not receive the first dose of investigational drugs until either April 15 or April 17, 2006, which was greater than the 14 days allotted by the protocol.

ⅱ. With respect to Subject [(b)(6)] source documents showed that the baseline study procedures including the physical exam, neurological assessment, vital signs, and [(b)(4)] performance standards were performed on June 16, 2006 and the ECG was performed on June 22, 2006. The subject did not receive the first dose of study treatment until July 21, 2006, which was greater than the 14 days allotted by the protocol.

E. The original protocol and Protocol Amendment #1 specified that at the baseline visit, a urinalysis and urine protein/creatinine (UPC) ratio was to be performed. Source records showed that this was not performed for Subject [(b) (6)] at the baseline visit.

F. The original protocol and Protocol Amendment #1 specified that all study medication will be infused on Day 1 every 21 days for 6 cycles (1 cycle = 21 days) or until disease progression. Thereafter, only [(b)(4)] as a single agent will continue as an infusion every 3 weeks for a total of 12 months from initiation of therapy. With respect to study procedures that were to be performed on the Day 1 visit, the original protocol specified that on Day 1 of each Cycle, specific study procedures including but not limited to a physical exam, vital signs and neurosensory assessment, [(b) (4)] exam, and Peripheral Neurotoxicity Questionnaire were to be administered prior to study drug therapy. Protocol Amendment #1 only changed the requirement that a [(b)(4)] exam was to be performed at least every other cycle. The following protocol deviations included but were not limited to:

ⅰ. With respect to Subject [(b)(6)]:

1. A neurosensory assessment was not performed at the Cycle 1 Day 1 visit.

2. The Cycle 1 Day 1 Peripheral Neurotoxicity Questionnaire was administered on April 11, 2006, which was 6 days prior to the date the subject was dosed with study medication (i.e. April 17, 2006.).

ⅱ. With respect to Subject [(b)(6)]

1. For several cycles where study procedures, including but not limited to the physical exam and neurosensory

assessment were performed on Day 1 of the cycle, the investigational drugs were not administered on Day 1 of the cycle as specified in the protocol:

Cycle	Date of Day 1 visit per visit worksheet and/or CRF	Date of administration of investigational drugs for that cycle
1	June 19, 2006	June 26, 2006
2	July 12, 2006	July 17, 2006
3	August 2, 2006	August 7, 2006
4	August 23, 2006	August 28, 2006
5	September 11, 2006	September 18, 2006
6	October 4, 2006	October 9, 2006

2. The Peripheral Neurotoxicity Questionnaire was not administered at the Day 1 visit of each cycle when the subject was to receive study medication per the protocol requirement. Specifically, source records showed that no questionnaire was administered at the Cycle 1 Day 1 visit. Also, at the Day 1 visit for Cycle 2 and Cycle 5, the questionnaires were done 5 and 7 days, respectively, prior to the date the subject was administered study medication.

iii. With respect to Subject we note that:

1. For several cycles where study procedures, including but not limited to the physical exam and neurosensory assessment were performed on Day 1 of the cycle, the investigational drugs were not administered on Day 1 of the cycle as specified in the protocol.

Examples include:

Cycle	Date of Day 1 visit per visit worksheet and/or CRF	Date of administration of investigational drugs for that cycle
2	August 1, 2006	August 11, 2006
3	August 29, 2006	September 1, 2008
4	September 19, 2006	September 22, 2006
6	October 31, 2006	November 3, 2006

2. The Peripheral Neurotoxicity Questionnaire was not administered at the Day 1 visit of each cycle when the subject was to receive study medication per the protocol requirement. Specifically, a neurotoxicity questionnaire was not completed for the Cycle 6, Day 1 visit. Additionally, for the Day 1 visit for Cycle 2, the questionnaire was completed 10 days prior to the date the subject was administered study medication.

G. The original protocol specified that prior to study medication administration on Day 1 and Day 8 during the cytotoxic chemotherapy and [(b)(4)] treatment, specific laboratory studies were to be performed including hematology (every cycle within a 24 hr window prior to Day 1; except Cycle 1 Day 1 which has a 72 hr window), serum chemistries (every cycle within a 72 hr window, prior to Day 1), coagulation (every cycle within a 72 hr window prior to Day 1), urinalysis and urine protein/creatinine (UPC) determination (every cycle within a 72 hr window) and a [(b)(4)] test (Day 1 each cycle). Protocol Amendment #1, amended some of the requirements for the laboratory studies during the cytotoxic chemotherapy and [(b)(4)] treatment: hematology (72 hr window; required on both Day I and Day 8 of each cycle), serum chemistries (72 hr window; not required on Day 8), coagulation (72 hr window; not required on Day 8), urinalysis and urine protein/creatinine (UPC) determination (72 hr window; at baseline, Day 1 and every cycle prior to chemotherapy treatment; not required on Day 8) and [(b)(4)] test (Day 1 each cycle). In our comparison of the case histories found at your site with the protocol in effect during the time of each visit, protocol deviations were identified. Examples include but are not limited to:

i. With respect to Subject [(b)(4)]

1. Although laboratory samples were taken for certain tests, including the hematology, biochemistry, coagulation and/or the [(b)(4)] test, these laboratory samples were not performed within the protocol specified time periods prior to study drug administration for the Day 1 visits of Cycles 1, 2, 3, 4, 5 and/or 6.

2. Serum chemistries were not performed for the Cycle 1 Day 8 visit or the Cycle 6 Day 8 visit.
3. A urinalysis sample and UPC determination was not performed for the Cycle 1 Day 8, Cycle 2 Day 1, Cycle 3 Day 8, and Cycle 5 Day 1 visits.
4. The partial thromboplastin time (PTT) test was not performed at the Cycle 2 Day 8, Cycle 3 Day 1, Cycle 3 Day 8, Cycle 4 Day 1, and Cycle 6 Day 1 visits.
ii. With respect to Subject [(b)(6)], we note that:
1. The UPC was not performed for the Cycle 4 Day 1 visits.
2. The hematology sample was not performed at the Cycle 2 Day 8 visit.
H. Both the original protocol and Protocol Amendment #1 specified that [(b)(4)] vials were to be refrigerated at [(b)(4)] and should remain refrigerated until just prior to use. Our inspection found that there were no records found prior to January 2007 to confirm that the study medication was stored appropriately per the protocol requirements.
I. The protocol specified that [(b)(4)] was to be stored at temperatures between [(b)(4)] and [(b)(4)] at [(b)(4)] with excursions permitted to [(b)(4)]. Our inspection found that there were no records prior to April 2007 to show that the investigational drugs were stored appropriately per the protocol requirements.
J. Both the original protocol and Protocol Amendment #1 specified that the Investigator was required to ensure compliance with the visit schedule and all procedures required by the protocol and was to provide all information required in the Case Report Form (CRF) in an accurate and legible manner according to the instructions provided and to ensure direct access to source documents to Sponsor Representatives. Both protocols further noted that it was the responsibility of the Investigator to maintain adequate and accurate CRFs designed by the sponsor, to record all observations and other data pertinent to the clinical investigation. All CRFs were to be completed in their entirety in a neat, legible manner to ensure accurate interpretation of the data. In addition, the protocols noted that should a correction be made, the information to be modified must not be overwritten, that the corrected information was to be transcribed by the authorized person next to the previous value, initialed and dated, and that the use of white-out and/or correction fluids was not allowed under any circumstances.
Based on FDA investigator Keller's observations, your site utilized correction fluid and write over corrections in multiple places throughout the source documents that were reviewed during the FDA inspection. Furthermore, these corrections were made without explanation. Examples include but were not limited to:
i. The dose of [(b)(4)] given to the Subject [(b)(6)] as noted on the CRF.
ii. The weight information on the [(b)(4)] visit worksheet for Subject [(b)(6)] at the Day 1 visits of Cycle 2, 3, and 4.
iii. The weight and/or height information on the [(b)(4)] visit worksheet for Subject [(b)(6)] at the Day 1 visit of Cycle 1, 2, 3, 5 and 6.
iv. The investigational agent accountability records.
Your use of these documentation practices leads to the inability to verify the information within the records at your site. The rationale and the source for the corrections could not be determined.

2. You failed to maintain adequate and accurate case histories that record all observations and other data pertinent to the investigation on each individual [21 CFR 312.62(b)].
A. Examples of inaccurate case histories with respect to FDA's review of the records for Subject [(b)(6)] include but were not limited to the following:
i. The Cycle 13 Day 1 visit CRF for Subject [(b)(6)] listed the UPC ratio as 0.21. The corresponding lab report however, showed the UPC ratio as 0.109.
ii. The clinic note for the baseline visit on March 23, 2006 had late entries inputted on June 21, 2006 noting information including but not limited to the subject's [(b)(4)] test, [(b)(4)] performance status and consent process used to enroll the subject into the study. The source for the late entries could not be verified.
iii. The chemotherapy order for the Cycle 1 visit noted in the "date given section" that the investigational drugs were given on April 15, 2006. However, a hand written note written on the top of the order form stated "Chemo Given April 17th In-patient."
B. Examples of inaccurate case histories with respect to FDA's review of the records for Subject [(b)(6)] include but were not limited to the following:

i. The case histories for the Baseline and Day 1 Cycle 1 visits are discrepant and we were unable to determine where information provided in the CFR for these visits was derived. Specifically, the [(b)(4)] visit source document for the Cycle 1 Day 1 visit appears to show that the date the physical exam, neurological assessment and vital signs were taken was on June 19, 2006. The Cycle 1 Day 1 visit CRF, however, notes that the physical exam and neurological assessment were not done and that the vitals signs were taken on June 26, 2006. In addition, the Baseline CRF notes that the physical exam, neurological assessment, and vital signs were done on June 19, 2006, but the vital signs information placed into the CRF does not match the information listed in the [(b)(4)] visit worksheet for the Cycle 1 Day 1 visit.

ii. The Cycle 5 Day 1 CRF listed the subject's weight as 61.4 kg on September 15, 2006. FDA investigator Keller noted that he was unable to find a record to substantiate this weight. The progress note dated September 11, 2006 noted the subject's weight as 127 lbs and the [(b) (4)] visit worksheet noted the subject's weight as 58 kg.

iii. The CRF for the Cycle 8 Day 1 visit noted that the study drug was administered on November 11, 2006. Source records however indicated that the study drug was administered on November 20, 2006.

C. Examples of inaccurate case histories with respect to FDA's review of the records for Subject [(b)(6)] include but were not limited to the following:

i. There were two chemotherapy order forms found for the Cycle 6 Day 1 visit. The chemotherapy order form found in the research file was not similar to the one that was found in the investigational pharmacy. Specifically, the one found in the research file was not signed and noted that the subject weighed 48 kg. The chemotherapy order form found in the investigational pharmacy and used by the pharmacy to prepare the investigational agents, was signed and listed the subject's weight as 120 lbs (approximately 54 kg).

ii. There were discrepancies identified with respect to the source records found for the Cycle 7 Day 1 visit. Specifically, two chemotherapy order forms were found for this visit. The chemotherapy order form found in the research file listed the subject's weight as 45 kg. The chemotherapy order form found in the investigational pharmacy and used by the pharmacy to prepare the investigational agents, listed the subject's weight as 55 kg. The [(b)(4)] visit worksheet for the Cycle 7 Day 1 visit, however, did not note any value for the subject's weight.

iii. During FDA's inspection of your site, no documentation could be found to verify that your site submitted an SAE report to the IRB for Subject [(b)(6)] hospitalization which occurred on [(b)(6)]

D. Your site utilized the sponsor's [(b)(4)] worksheet as a source document. At the bottom of this document, there was a place for the individual who filled out the form to sign and date the form. In our review of this document, we found many instances where the individual who filled out the form either did not sign and date the form or the form was signed and date at a later time. Examples include but were not limited to the following:

i. For the Cycle 8 Day 1 and Cycle 12 Day 1 visits for Subject [(b)(6)], the individual(s) who completed the form did not sign and date when the form was completed. The [(b)(4)] visit worksheet documenting Patient [(b)(6)] neurological assessment, vital signs, [(b)(4)] performance state, physical exam and [(b)(4)] exam performed on May 4, 2006 was signed and dated August 16, 2006.

ii. For the Cycle 1 Day 1, Cycle 2 Day 1, Cycle 5 Day 1 and Cycle 6 Day 1 visits for Subject [(b) (6)], the individual(s) who completed the form did not sign and date when the form was completed.

iii. For the Cycle 2 Day 1, Cycle 3 Day 1, Cycle 4 Day 1, and Cycle 7 Day 1 visits for Subject [(b)(6)] the individual(s) who completed the form did not sign and date when the form was completed.

Your site's lack of signature and date on the forms and/or delayed signature and date of the forms lead to concerns about the accuracy of these source documents during the course of the study.

Per your undated response provided to FDA investigator Keller at the conclusion of the inspection, you noted that your site was responsive to the deficiencies that were identified by the monitors during the course of the study, which led to the termination of the data coordinators and replacement of your entire research staff. You further noted that had FDA investigator Keller had the time to examine and perform a comprehensive review of the records, you believe that he would have found an ever decreasing number of deviations as your site responded to previously noted deficiencies and made changes to the data management team.

We note that this response is inadequate. Specifically, we note that as the clinical investigator, it was your responsibility to ensure that the study was conducted in accordance with the investigational plan and that adequate and accurate case histories were maintained as specified in applicable FDA regulations. In addition, we note that your sole corrective action appears to be the termination and replacement of your staff with no information provided as to corrective actions your site will take to ensure that these violations will not take place in any ongoing or future studies.

This letter is not intended to be an all-inclusive list of deficiencies with your clinical study of an investigational drug. It is your responsibility to ensure adherence to each requirement of the law and relevant FDA regulations. You should address these deficiencies and establish procedures to ensure that any on-going or future studies will be in compliance with FDA regulations.

Within fifteen (15) working days of your receipt of this letter, you should notify this office in writing of the actions you have taken or will be taking to prevent similar violations in the future. Failure to adequately and promptly explain the violations noted above may result in regulatory action without further notice.

If you have any questions, please contact Tejashri Purohit-Sheth, M.D., at 301-796-3402; FAX 301-847-8748. Your written response and any pertinent documentation should be addressed to:

Tejashri Purohit-Sheth, M.D.
Branch Chief
Good Clinical Practice Branch Ⅱ
Division of Scientific Investigations
Office of Compliance
Center for Drug Evaluation and Research
Food and Drug Administration
Bldg 51, Room 5358
10903 New Hampshire Avenue
Silver Spring, MD 20993

Sincerely yours,

{See appended electronic signature page}

Leslie K. Ball, M.D.
Director
Division of Scientific Investigations
Office of Compliance
Center for Drug Evaluation and Research

第139封　给Richard Holub医学博士的警告信

2008年10月1日

参考号：08-HFD-45-09-01

尊敬的Holub博士：

2007年9月4日至10月18日，Denise Terzian女士代表FDA进行了现场检查，与您会面并审查了您实施以下临床研究的情况：

- 试验方案（b）（4）标题为：一个在有轻度至中度阿尔茨海默病患者中以（b）（4）为指标评价试验药物（b）（4）安全性和有效性的双盲，Ⅱ期的临床试验；
- 试验方案（b）（4）标题为：一个在有轻度至中度阿尔茨海默病患者中以（b）（4）为指标评价试验药物（b）（4）有效性的随机、多中心、双盲、安慰剂对照，为期18个月的临床试验；
- 试验方案（b）（4）标题为：一个在有轻度至中度阿尔茨海默病患者中以（b）（4）为指标评价3个剂量组试验药物（b）（4）用药后的安全性、耐受性、有效性的随机、多中心、双盲、安慰剂对照，为期6个月的临床试验。

本次现场检查是FDA的生物研究监查项目的一部分。该项目通过设定的检查方法，对FDA所监管的相关研究的实施情况进行评估，并确保这些研究中受试者的权益、安全和福利得到了保护。

经对FDA现场检查报告、该报告的附件，您在2008年3月15日提交的对FDA 483表的书面回复，我们认为，您没有遵循适用的法律要求和监管临床研究实施及保护受试者的FDA法规。

在现场检查结束时，Terzian女士向您出示并讨论了FDA483表，即现场检查发现的问题。我们希望向您强调如下几点：

1. 您未能亲自进行临床研究或对研究进行监督［21 CFR 312.60］

当您签署上述临床研究的研究者声明（FDA 1572表）时，您同意承担一个临床研究者的责任。特别是您同意在亲自进行或监督研究过程中遇到不能亲自进行的某些方面，应确保所有的助理、同事和员工在协助研究进行时被及时告知他们的义务。

您没有充分监督您所授权的承担研究任务的人。FDA的检查显示，对于试验方案（b）（4）您对接受研究任务的人员的监督不足以确保临床试验按照签署的研究者声明和适用的规定进行。您缺乏足够的监督导致方案违背，药品管理的不足，不充分的知情同意，研究记录（知情同意书）不可用于FDA的检查，不足够和不准确的病历以及以下2~6项中发现的问题。

2. 您未能确保按照签署的研究者声明、研究计划进行研究［21 CFR 312.60］

a. 您没有保证这项研究是按照方案进行的。例子包括，但不限于以下：

关于试验方案（b）（4）

i. 受试者编号并没有按方案要求在该研究点筛选的所有受试者按顺序分配给所有受试者。例子包括，但不限于以下：

（1）受试者（b）（6）于2005年4月22日筛选入组，是这个研究第3个筛选入组的；然而，受试者被分配编号747-004。

（2）受试者（b）（6）于2005年5月12日筛选入组，是这个研究第4个筛选入组的；然而，这个受试者被分配编号747-003。

ⅱ. 方案要求的磁共振成像和计算机断层扫描，简易精神状态检查及改良Hachinski试验受试者747-006、747-007和747-008均没有完成。

ⅲ. 没有按照方案的要求给每个受试者分配一个唯一的六位数编号。具体来说，受试者（b）（6）和（b）（6）的指定编号均为747-005。

ⅳ. 该方案排除在筛选访视前一个月内服用Aleve（萘普生）治疗潜在的受试者。筛选入组时受试者747-004医疗信息表显示该受试者目前正在服用萘普生；然而，该受试者却被随机分组，与方案相违背。此外，方案要求的第43天体格检查和第64天的实验室检测该受试者没有完成。

关于试验方案（b）（4）

ⅴ. 084-009在第2次访视时没有按方案要求进行临床实验室评估和（b）（6）。

ⅵ. 084-002在第7次访视时没有按方案要求进行体格检查。

b. 负责知情同意，确定受试者资格和分发试验药物的研究协调员没有列入FDA1572表，研究者声明和试验方案（b）（4）和（b）（4）中。通过执行这些重要的研究活动，研究协调员应该在FDA表1572s中作为助理研究员。

3. 您未能保存足够准确的试验药物处置记录［21 CFR 312.62（a）］

试验方案（b）（4），研究受试者被分配到原本不是分发给他们的试验药物盒。

具体来说，（b）（4）随机分组确认表显示受试者747-002药盒编号为0495，受试者747-003药盒编号为0655，受试者747-004药盒编号为0582。然而，试验药物标签（吸塑卡标签）显示如下：

a. 发现药包盒编号为0582号的吸塑卡标签对应的是受试者747-002，而非受试者747-004；

b. 发现3张药包盒编号为0495号的试验药物标签对应的是受试者747-003，而非受试者 747-002；

c. 发现12张药包盒编号为0495号的试验药物标签对应的是受试者747-004，而非受试者 747-002。

4. 您未能按照21 CFR 50的要求获得知情同意［21 CFR 312.60］

21 CFR 50.20规定，除50.23和50.24外，FDA法规允许范围内没有研究者可以以人体作为研究对象，除非研究者取得了合法有效的受试者或受试者的合法授权代表的知情同意。此外，FDA规定，知情同意应有文件记录，书面知情同意书是由IRB和签署批准的，经受试者或受试者的合法授权代表签名并签署日期［21 CFR 50.27（a）］。

关于试验方案（b）（4）

a. 受试者2006在2007年2月2日筛选访视时有研究评估和操作；然而，受试者直到2007年5月18日才签署经伦理委员会（IRB）同意的知情同意书。

b. 受试者2005在2007年2月18日筛选访视时根据试验方案（b）（4）进行了研究评估和操作；然而，受试者签署了另外一项研究试验方案（b）（4）的知情同意书，直到2007年3月6日才签署参加试验方案（b）（4）的知情同意书。

关于试验方案（b）（4）

c. 在FDA的检查期间，您不能提供受试者747-007签署的知情同意书。您告诉FDA检查员，这个受试者签署了一份知情同意书，但您找不到这份文件。检查发现，护理员无法回忆起知情同意书被签署。

5. 您未能按要求保留记录，直至研究药物按拟定适应症上市申请获得批准后2年；如果没有提交上市申请或者药物用于适应症的上市申请未被批准，则在研究终止并通知FDA后2年［21 CFR 312.62（c）］

关于试验方案（b）（4），FDA检查时您无法提供受试者747-005和747-006签署的知情同意书。您告诉FDA检查员说，这些受试者签署了知情同意书，但您无法找到这些文件。

6. 您未能保存与研究相关的所有观察结果和其他相关数据的足够及准确的病历［21 CFR 312.62（b）］

例子包括，但不限于以下：

关于试验方案（b）（4）

a. 受试者747-005（b）（6），747-006，747-007和747-008病例报告表没有完成。

b. 受试者（b）（6）被分配的编号为747-005，但2005年7月8日在实验室表中编号为747-007，2005年7月13日在实验室报告中编号为747-008。

在您2008年3月15日对FDA483表的书面回复中您说FDA483表中所列的问题是少数临床研究协调员未能遵遁既定的标准操作规程（SOP）的结果。您提到将采取纠正措施，以确保这样的错误不再重复。这些包括操作过程的选择、培训、研究人员管理，根据SOP的约定研究部门的日常工作操作规程。回复没有解决临床研究者对研究活动监督的过失，并把研究的责任推脱到参加研究人员身上。虽然雇佣合格的员工和提供培训可能有助于与研究相关的活动表现，但不能代替您作为临床研究者的责任，监督您授权给临床研究人员某些研究任务。

本警告信的目的并非是罗列您在试验药物临床研究中存在的所有缺陷。确保遵循法律和相关FDA法规的每一项要求是您的职责。您应当解决这些缺陷，并建立规程，以确保任何正在进行或将来进行的研究均能符合FDA的法规。

自收到这封信的15个工作日内，您应当书面告知本办公室为预防将来发生类似违规行为已经或将要采取的措施。如果不能充分、迅速地解释上述违规问题，可能导致我们在不再通知的情况下采取监管措施。

附：英文原文

Richard Holub, M.D.

WARNING LETTER

OCT 01, 2008

CERTIFIED MAIL
RETURN RECEIPT REQUESTED

Ref: 08-HFD-45-09-01

Richard Holub, M.D.
Neurological Associates of Albany
760 Madison Avenue
Albany, New York 12208

Dear Dr. Holub:

Between September 4 and October 18, 2007, Ms. Denise Terzian, representing the Food and Drug Administration (FDA), conducted an investigation and met with you, to review your conduct of the following clinical investigations:

- Protocol (b)(4) entitled "A Double-Blind, Phase Ⅱ, Safety and Efficacy Evaluation of (b)(4) in Patients with Mild to Moderate Alzheimer's Disease," of the investigational drug (b)(4),performed for (b)(4) ;
- Protocol (b)(4) entitled "A Randomized, Multicenter, Double-blind, Placebo-controlled, 18-month Study of the Efficacy of (b)(4) in Patients with Mild-to-moderate Dementia of the Alzheimer's Type," of the investigational drug (b)(4), performed for (b)(4) ; and
- Protocol (b)(4) entitled "A 6-MONTH, Randomized, Double Blind, Placebo-Controlled, Multicenter, Safety, Tolerability, and Efficacy Study of 3 Doses of (b)(4) in Outpatients With Mild to Moderate Alzheimer's Disease Treated With a (b)(4)," of the investigational drug (b)(4) , performed for (b)(4) .

This inspection is a part of FDA's Bioresearch Monitoring Program, which includes inspections designed to evaluate the conduct of research and to ensure that the rights, safety, and welfare of the human subjects of the study have been protected.

From our review of the establishment inspection report, the documents submitted with that report and your March 15, 2008 letter written in response to the Form FDA 483, Inspectional Observations, we conclude that you did not adhere to the applicable statutory requirements and FDA regulations governing the conduct of clinical investigations and the protection of human subjects.

We are aware that at the conclusion of the inspection Ms. Terzian presented and discussed with you Form FDA 483, Inspectional Observations. We wish to emphasize the following:

1. You failed to personally conduct or supervise the investigation [21 CFR 312.60].

When you signed the investigator statements (Form FDA 1572) for the above-referenced clinical investigations, you agreed to take on the responsibilities of a clinical investigator. You specifically agreed to personally conduct or supervise those aspects of the study you did not personally conduct, and to ensure that all associates, colleagues, and employees assisting in the conduct of the study were informed about their obligations.

You did not adequately supervise individuals to whom you delegated study tasks. The FDA inspection revealed that for protocol (b)(4) your supervision of personnel to whom you delegated study tasks was not adequate to ensure that the clinical trials were conducted according to the signed investigator statement and applicable regulations. Your lack of adequate oversight resulted in protocol violations, inadequate drug accountability, inadequate informed consent, study records (informed consent documents) not being available for the FDA inspection, and inadequate and inaccurate case histories, as noted in items 2-6 below.

2. You failed to ensure that the investigation was conducted according to the signed investigator statement and investigational plan [21 CFR 312.60].

a. You failed to ensure that the study was conducted in accordance with the protocol. Examples include, but are not limited to, the following:

Regarding Protocol (b)(4)

i. The subject numbers were not sequentially assigned to all subjects screened at the site as required by the protocol. Examples include, but are not limited to, the following:

1 Subject (b)(6) screened on April 22, 2005, was the third subject screened for the study; however, the subject was assigned #747-004.

2 Subject (b)(6) screened on May 12, 2005, was the fourth subject screened for the study; however, the subject was assigned #747-003.

ii. Protocol-required magnetic resonance imaging or computer tomography scan, Mini-Mental State Examination, and Modified Hachinski test were not performed for subjects 747-006, 747-007, and 747-008.

iii. A unique six-digit subject number was not assigned to each subject as required by the protocol. Specifically , subject (b)(6) and (b)(6) were both assigned number 747-005.

iv. The protocol excluded potential subjects who were taking Aleve (naproxen) medication one (1) month prior to the screening visit. The Medical Information Sheet for subject 747-004 at screening documents that the subject was currently taking Aleve; however, the subject was randomized in violation of the protocol. In addition, protocol-required physical exams for day 43 and laboratory test for day 64 were not performed for this subject.

Regarding Protocol (b)(4)

v. Protocol-required clinical laboratories assessments and (b)(6) were not performed for subject 084-009 at Visit #2.

vi. Protocol-required physical examination was not performed for subject 084-002 at Visit #7.

b. Study coordinators who administered the informed consent, determined subject eligibility and dispensed study drug were not listed on the Form FDA1572, Statement of Investigator, for protocols (b)(4) and (b)(4). By performing these significant study activities, the study coordinators should have been listed on the Form FDA 1572s as subinvestigators.

3. You failed to maintain adequate and accurate records for disposition of the investigational drug [21 CFR 312.62(a)].

Regarding protocol (b)(4), study subjects were distributed study medication kits not assigned to them. Specifically, the (b)(4) randomization confirmations indicated that subject 747-002 was assigned kit number 0495, subject 747-003 was assigned kit number 0655, and subject 747-004 was assigned kit number 0582. However, study medication labels (blister card labels) revealed the following:

a. A blister card label for kit number 0582 was found identified as distributed to subject 747-002 instead of subject 747-004;

b. Three study medication labels for kit number 0495 was found identified as distributed to subject 747-003 instead of subject 747-002; and

c. Twelve study medication labels for kit number 0495 was found identified as distributed to subject 747-004 instead of subject 747-002.

4. You failed to obtain informed consent in accordance with the provisions of 21 CFR Part 50 [21 CFR 312.60].

21 CFR 50.20 requires that except as provided in sections 50.23 and 50.24, no investigator may involve a human being as a subject in research covered by FDA regulations unless the investigator has obtained the legally effective informed consent of the subject or the subject's legally authorized representative. In addition, the FDA regulations require that informed consent be documented by the use of a written consent form approved by the IRB and signed and dated by the subject or the subject's legally authorized representative at the time of consent [21 CFR 50.27(a)].

Regarding protocol (b)(4)

a. Subject 2006 had study assessments and procedures performed during the screening visit on February 2, 2007; however, the subject did not sign the informed consent form approved by the Institutional Review Board (IRB) until May 18, 2007.

b. Subject 2005 had study assessments and procedures performed for protocol (b)(4) on January 18, 2007 at the screening visit; however, the subject signed a consent form for another study, protocol (b)(4) and did not sign the consent form for participation in protocol (b)(4) until March 6,2007.

Regarding protocol (b)(4)

c. During the FDA inspection you were not able to provide signed informed consent documents for subject 747-007. You told the FDA investigator that this subject signed an informed consent document, but you could not locate the document. Inspection revealed that the caregiver could not recall informed consent document being signed.

5. You failed to retain records required to be maintained by the clinical investigator under 21 CFR part 312 for a period of 2 years following the date a marketing application is approved for the drug for the indication for which it is being investigated; or, if no application is to be filed or if the application is not approved for such indication, until 2 years after the investigation is discontinued and FDA is notified [21 CFR 312.62(c)].

Regarding protocol (b)(4),during the FDA inspection you were not able to provide signed informed consent documents for subjects 747-005 and 747-006. You told the FDA investigator that these subjects signed informed consent documents, but you could not locate the documents.

6. You failed to maintain adequate and accurate case histories that record all observations and data pertinent to the investigation [21 CFR 312.62(b)].

Examples include, but are not limited to, the following:

Regarding protocol (b)(4)

a. No Case Report Forms were completed for subjects 747-005 (b)(6), 747-006, 747-007, and 747-008.

b. Subject (b)(6) was assigned number 747-005, but was identified with number 747-007 on the laboratory form dated July 8, 2005, and number 747-008 on the laboratory report dated July 13, 2005.

In your March 15, 2008 written response to the Form FDA 483 you stated that the Form FDA 483 items were a reflection of the failure of a few clinical research coordinators to adhere to the established Standard Operating Procedures (SOPs). You mentioned correctives actions that will be taken to assure that such errors are not repeated.

These include the process used to select, train, and manage research staff, and SOPs governing the day-to-day work of the research division. The response does not address oversight of the research activities by the clinical investigator and appears to place the burden of responsibility for the research activities on the study staff. Although hiring qualified staff and providing training may help with the performance of study related activities, this does not substitute for your responsibilities as the clinical investigator to supervise those aspects of the studies you delegate to research staff.

This letter is not intended to be an all-inclusive list of deficiencies with your clinical study of an investigational drug. It is your responsibility to ensure adherence to each requirement of the law and relevant FDA regulations. You should address these deficiencies and establish procedures to ensure that any on-going or future studies will be in compliance with FDA regulations.

Within fifteen (15) working days of your receipt of this letter, you should notify this office in writing of the actions you have taken or will be taking to prevent similar violations in the future. Failure to adequately and promptly explain the violations noted above may result in regulatory action without further notice.

If you have any questions, please contact Constance Lewin, M.D., M.P.H., at 301-7963397; FAX 301-847-8748. Your written response and any pertinent documentation should be addressed to:

Constance Lewin, M.D., M.P.H.
Branch Chief, Good Clinical Practice Branch I
Division of Scientific Investigations
Office of Compliance Center for Drug Evaluation and Research
Food and Drug Administration
Bldg 51, Room 5354
10903 New Hampshire Avenue
Silver Spring, MD 20993

Sincerely yours,

{See appended electronic signature page}

Leslie K. Ball, M.D.
Director
Division of Scientific Investigations
Office of Compliance
Center for Drug Evaluation and Research

第140封　给Gardiziola, Gregory, D. O.的警告信

2008年9月3日

参考号：09-HFD-45-0802

尊敬的Gregory博士：

2008年5月9日至30日，Karen Kondas女士代表FDA进行了现场检查，并与您的助理研究员［不公开］医生见面，对您实施的一项临床研究（为［不公开］公司进行的［不公开］临床试验药物［不公开］试验方案［不公开］题目）进行了审查。实施这项研究时，您位于［不公开］，我们注意到您从2003年10月开始负责该项研究，直到2006年5月您离开该诊所，那时起［不公开］医生成为临床研究者。

本次现场检查是FDA的生物研究监查项目的一部分。该项目通过设定的检查方法，对研究的实施情况进行评估，并确保这些研究中受试者的权益、安全和福利得到了保护。

经对FDA现场检查报告（EIR）、该报告的附件，以及［不公开］医生2006年10月19日对FDA483表（现场检查发现的问题）的书面回复进行审查，我们认为，您没有遵循适用的法律要求和监管临床研究实施及保护受试者的FDA法规。我们知道在现场检查结束时，Kondas女士向您的助理研究员出示并讨论了FDA483表。后来，Kondas女士与您讨论了现场检查发现的问题，并向您的办公室传真了一份FDA483表的复印件。我们想强调以下几点：

1. 您未能确保符合适用法规要求的IRB对拟进行的临床研究进行跟踪审查和批准［21 CFR 312.66］

具体而言是，我们的现场检查发现，上面提到的研究的伦理委员会批件于2005年10月7日期满，并且直到2006年10月19日才更新。在这段时间，伦理委员会批准失效时，您筛选、入组或随机化了16名受试者，而且继续进行研究活动（研究的随访和电话联系）。

2. 您未能按照21 CFR 50的要求，获得参加研究的受试者的知情同意［21 CFR 312.60］

21 CFR 50.20要求，除非50.23和50.24提到的情况，没有哪个研究者可以把人类作为研究的受试者，除非研究者得到受试者或受试者合法授权代理人的合法有效的知情同意。此外，FDA法规要求知情同意通过使用书面知情同意书来进行记录，知情同意书由伦理委员会批准，由受试者或受试者的合法授权代理人在同意的时候签署姓名和日期［21 CFR 50.27（a）］。

［不公开］受试者签署了［不公开］研究的同意文件，但是没有签署参加主要研究的知情同意文件。

3. 您未能保留记录到所需的时间段［21 CFR 312.62（c）］

21 CFR 312.62（c）规定，研究者应根据21 CFR 312的规定保存药物相关记录，直至试验药物按拟定适应症上市申请获得批准后2年；如果没有提交上市申请或药物用于该适应症的上市申请未被批准，则保存至研究终止并通知FDA后2年。签署过的知情同意文件，按照21 CFR 312.62（b）规定应当保留，但是［不公开］受试者的找不到了。［不公开］医生2008年6月12日的信函指出，2004年3月5日获得了［不公开］受试者签署了的知情同意文件，并相应地记录在该受试者的病例报告表中。但是，据［不公开］医生所说，该受试者签署过的知情同意文件丢失了。

本警告信的目的并非是罗列您在试验药物临床试验研究中存在的所有缺陷。确保遵循每一项法律和相关FDA法规的要求是您的职责。您应当解决这些缺陷，建立规程，确保任何正在进行的或将来进行的研究都遵循FDA的法规。

自收到这封信的15个工作日内，您应当书面告知本办公室为预防将来发生类似违规行为已经或计划采取的措施。如果不能对上述违规行为进行充分、快速地解释，可能导致我们在不再通知的情况下采取监管措施。

附：英文原文

Gardiziola, Gregory, D.O.

WARNING LETTER

Sep 3, 2008

CERTIFIED MAIL
RETURN RECEIPT REQUESTED
Ref: 08-HFD-45-0802
Gregory Gardziola, D.O.
55 Cross Parks Court
Greenville, SC 29605

Dear Dr. Gardziola:

Between May 9 and 30, 2008, Ms. Karen Kondas, representing the Food and Drug Administration (FDA), conducted an investigation and met with your sub-investigator, Dr. [redacted] to review your conduct of a clinical investigation (protocol [redacted] entitled [redacted] of the investigational drugs [redacted] performed for [redacted]. At the time you performed the study, you were located at [redacted]. We note that you were responsible for the conduct of the study from October 2003 until you left the practice in May 2006, at which time Dr. [redacted] became the clinical investigator.

This inspection is a part of the FDA's Bioresearch Monitoring Program, which includes inspections designed to evaluate the conduct of research and to ensure that the rights, safety, and welfare of the human subjects of those studies have been protected.

From our review of the establishment inspection report and the documents submitted with that report, and Dr. [redacted] June 12, 2008 letter in response to the Form FDA 483, Inspectional Observations, we conclude that you did not adhere to the applicable statutory requirements and FDA regulations governing the conduct of clinical investigations and the protection of human subjects. We are aware that at the conclusion of the inspection, Ms. Kondas presented and discussed with your sub-investigator Form FDA 483. Subsequently, Ms. Kondas discussed the inspection findings with you and faxed a copy of the Form FDA 483 to your office. We wish to emphasize the following:

1. You failed to assure that an Institutional Review Board (IRB) complying with applicable regulatory requirements was responsible for the continuing review and approval of the clinical study 121 CFR 312 .66].

Specifically, our investigation revealed that IRB approval for the above-referenced study expired on October 7, 2005, and was not renewed until October 19, 2006. During this time period, when IRB approval was lapsed you screened, enrolled, or randomized 16 subjects [redacted] and continued to perform research activities (study visits and phone contacts).

2. You failed to obtain informed consent of subjects involved in research in accordance with the provisions of 21 CFR Part 50 [21 CFR 312.60].

21 CFR 50.20 requires that, except as provided in sections 50. 23 and 50. 24, no investigator may involve a human being as a subject in research unless the investigator has obtained the legally effective informed consent of the subject or the subject's legally authorized representative. In addition the FDA regulations require that informed consent be documented by the use of a written consent form approved by the IRB and signed and dated by the subject or the subject's legally authorized representative at the time of consent [21 CFR 50.27(a)] .

Subject [redacted] signed a [redacted] sub-study consent document, but did not sign an informed consent document for participation in the main study.

3. You failed to retain records for the requisite time period [21 CFR 312.62(c)].

21 CFR 312.62(c) requires that an investigator retain records required to be maintained under 21 CFR Part 312 for a period of 2 years following the date a marketing application is approved for the drug for the indication for which it is being investigated; or, if no application is to be filed or if the application is not approved for such indication, until 2 years after the investigation is discontinued and FDA is notified. A signed informed consent document, which was required to be maintained by 21 CFR 312.62(b), could not be located for subject [redacted] Dr. [redacted] letter of June 12, 2008, indicates that a signed informed consent document was obtained from subject [redacted] on March 5, 2004 and was correspondingly documented in the case report for the subject. However, according to Dr. [redacted] the signed informed consent form for this subject was lost.

This letter is not intended to be an all-inclusive list of deficiencies with your clinical study of an investigational drug. It is your responsibility to ensure adherence to each requirement of the law and relevant FDA regulations. You should address these deficiencies and establish procedures to ensure that any on-going or future studies will be in compliance with FDA regulations.

Within fifteen (15) working days of your receipt of this letter, you should notify this office in writing of the actions you have taken or will be taking to prevent similar violations in the future. Failure to adequately and promptly explain the violations noted above may result in regulatory action without further notice.

If you have any questions, please contact Constance Lewin, M.D., M.P.H., at 301-796-3397; FAX 301- 847-8748. Your written response and any pertinent documentation should be addressed to:

Constance Lewin, M.D., M.P.H.
Branch Chief, Good Clinical Practice Branch I
Division of Scientific Investigations
Office of Compliance
Center for Drug Evaluation and Research
Food and Drug Administration
Bldg 51, Room 5354
10903 New Hampshire Avenue
Silver Spring, MD 20993

Sincerely yours,

{See appended electronic signature page}

Leslie K. Ball, M.D.
Director
Division of Scientific Investigations
Office of Compliance
Center for Drug Evaluation and Research

第141封　给Ponugoti, Nagarjuna R.医学博士的警告信

2008年6月6日
参考号：08-HFD-45-0202

尊敬的Ponugoti博士：

2007年9月10日至2007年9月19日，Kimberly Martin女士代表FDA进行了现场检查，与您会面并对您为［不公开］公司所实施的名为“评价中度到重度哮喘［不公开］患者对试验药物［不公开］进行［不公开］临床疗效和长期安全性流行病学研究［不公开］”临床研究［不公开］进行了审查。

本次现场检查是FDA的生物研究监查项目的一部分。该项目通过设定的检查方法，对相关研究的实施情况进行评估，并确保这些研究中受试者的权益、安全和福利得到了保护。

根据对现场检查报告、该报告的附件，以及2007年9月27日对FDA 483表的回复进行审查，我们认为，您没有遵循适用的法律要求和监管临床研究实施的FDA法规。

现场检查结束时，［不公开］女士出示并与您讨论了FDA 483表、即现场检查发现的问题，我们想强调以下几点：

1. 您未能根据21 CFR 50的要求取得并充分记录知情同意［21 CFR 312.60］

知情同意书是由伦理委员会（IRB）批准的、受试者或受试者法定监护人同意并在同意当时签署姓名日期的书面文件证明［21 CFR 50.27，参考21 CFR 312.60］。按照21 CFR 50［参考 21 CFR 312.60］，研究者有义务获得IRB批准的书面形式的知情同意。除了21 CFR 50.23 和 50.24中提到的情况外，不允许研究者以人体作为研究对象，除非研究者获得受试者或者该受试者法定监护人具有法律效力的认可［21 CFR 50.20］。我们的检查发现，参与该项研究的34名受试者中有30名受试者或者该受试者法定监护人没有在知情同意书或者IRB批准认可的书面形式文件签署姓名、日期。直到该试验启动6个月后，IRB才批准终版的知情同意书。另外，没有从受试者、46535、46517和46529获得同意。

2007年9月27日的回复函中，您解释项目申办者在实验开始时没有提供知情同意书，因此您让受试者在入组时签署了“授权书”，以授权使用和披露其健康信息。我们认为您的解释不充分。我们认为授权书中没有提到21 CFR 50.25.中描述的要向受试者解释的构成知情同意书的任何相关要素。当您签署“研究者声明”即FDA1572表时，您同意履行临床研究者的义务，包括确保符合知情同意书相关要求的义务。另外，试验方案规定“患者必须符合参加试验的入选标准：签署知情同意书（有未成年人的情况下，知情同意书必须给孩子父母或法定监护人）”。2004年10月27日的批准函中提到来源于［不公开］人体研究审查委员会的文件规定您作为主要临床研究者对研究的职责。批准函中提到IRB需审查和批准成年人、未成年人和儿童的同意书，所以您应该注意到这些文件对开展临床研究必不可少。确保符合知情同意书的要求是您的职责。

2. 您未能及时向IRB报告给受试者带来风险的所有非预期事件［21 CFR 312.60 和312.66］

研究者有责任确保研究按照研究计划和可适用的规则执行，包括向IRB报告受试者的所有非预期风险［21 CFR 312.60 及 312.66］。我们核查发现受试者46514死于［不公开］。受试者46532死于［不公开］和受试者46505入院。尽管如此，没有文件表明您迅速向IRB报告了这些信息。

在调查期间，您向FDA的核查人员解释虽然您参加了研究者会议，阅读了方案并签署了研究者同意书，但您不知道您需要向IRB报告严重不良事件。在您的回复函中，您陈述您认为申办者会就此跟IRB沟通。我

们认为您的回复不可接受。当您签署“研究者声明”即FDA 1572表时，您同意遵守临床研究者所有职责，包括迅速向IRB报告造成研究受试者或他人风险的不可预测事件。另外，试验方案6.4特别说明“主要研究者必须保证IRB能接收到任何严重不良事件”。

3. 您在IRB的批准已经被撤回的情况下，继续进行与临床研究相关的活动［21 CFR 312.66 和 56.103（a）］

FDA法规要求根据IND（例如，21 CFR 312）开展的临床试验由IRB会议审查、批准及跟踪审查，以达到21 CFR 56的要求（详见 21 CFR 56.103）。临床研究者有责任确保IRB对临床研究开展初始审查及跟踪审查（21 CFR 312.66）。2005年5月12日人体研究审查委员会撤回临床试验的批准后，您继续探视和治疗受试者，违反了这些规定。

尽管您已于2005年5月11日收到IRB撤回批准的通知，但您2005年5月12日后继续取得之前入组的33名受试者中27名受试者知情同意或者受试者父母同意。虽然［不公开］伦理委员会拒绝了您2005年5月22日后提出的关于开展6个月和12个月访视的请求，您仍然在IRB要求临床研究暂停期间完成6名患者的为期6个月研究访视。另外，在您接到该项目临床研究撤回批准通知后，您继续获得15名受试者同意。

在您的回复函中，您陈述您不知道临床试验批准被撤回后您不得执行访视。您的回复不充分。IRB同您联系并明确告知您允许开展试验的批准已被撤回。作为研究者您有责任确保获得IRB对临床试验的后续批准［21 CFR 312.66］。

4. 您未能及时向IRB报告研究活动中的所有变更［21 CFR 312.60 和 312.66］

21 CFR 312.66要求临床研究者确保将研究进行中的所有变更迅速报告给IRB（参考 21 CFR 312.60）。我们发现，2005年9月IRB通知恢复临床试验后，您没有通知IRB您在2006年2月曾中断过研究，且没有递交最终研究报告。我们不接受您解释的您认为这是申办者的责任。您签署的“研究者声明”即FDA1572表，明确规定这是临床研究者的责任，而不是申办者的责任。

5. 您未能保存研究中每个受试者的临床所有研究观察结果和其他相关数据的足够及准确的病历［21 CFR 312.62（b）］

研究者被要求准备和保存足够的、准确的个人病历。该病历需要记录该试验每个接受受试药物或对照药物的受试者所有与研究相关的临床观察结果和数据［21 CFR 312.62（b）］。我们核查发现，您未能按照FDA法规和研究方案对22名受试者的电话随访做出文件记录。

作为临床研究者，您有责任确保研究按照签署的研究者声明、研究计划、适用的规则开展研究，同时保证受试者的权益、安全和福利。

本警告信的目的并非是罗列您在试验药物临床研究中存在的所有缺陷。确保遵循法律和FDA相关法规的每一项要求是您的职责。您应当解决这些缺陷，并建立规程，以确保任何正在进行或将来进行的研究均能符合FDA的法规。

自收到这封信的15个工作日内，您应当书面告知本办公室为预防将来发生类似违规行为已经采取或将要采取的措施。如果不能充分、迅速地解释上述违规问题，可能导致我们在不再通知的情况下采取监管措施。

附：英文原文

Ponugoti, Nagarjuna R., M.D.

WARNING LETTER

Jun 6, 2008

CERTIFIED MAIL
RETURN RECEIPT REQUESTED

Ref: 08-HFD-45-0202

Allergy, Asthma & Immunology
Associates of Terre Haute
4779 S.7th Street
Terre Haute, Indiana 47802

Dear Dr. Ponugoti:

Between September 10,2007 and September 19, 2007, Ms. Kimberly Martin, representing the Food and Drug Administration (FDA), conducted an investigation and met with you to review your conduct of a clinical investigation (protocol) [ ] entitled, "An Epidemiologic Study of [ ] Evaluating Clinical Effectiveness and Long-Term Safety in Patients with Moderate to Severe Asthma [ ] of the investigational drug [ ] performed for [ ]

This inspection is a part of the FDA's Bioresearch Monitoring Program, which includes inspections designed to evaluate the conduct of research and to ensure that the rights, safety and welfare of the human subjects of those studies have been protected.

From our review of the establishment inspection report ,the documents submitted with that report and your September 27, 2007, letter written in response to the Form FDA 483,Inspectional Observations, we conclude that you did not adhere to the applicable statutory requirements and FDA regulations governing the conduct of clinical investigations.

We are aware that at the conclusion of the inspection, Ms. [ ] presented and discussed with you Form FDA 483, Inspectional Observations. We wish to emphasize the following:

1. You failed to obtain and adequately document informed consent in accordance with 21 CFR 50[21 CFR 312.601].

Informed consent must be documented by the use of a written consent form approved by an Institutional Review Board (IRB) and signed and dated by the subject or the subject's legally authorized representative at the time of consent [21 CFR 50.27, see 21 CFR 312.60]. As an investigator, it is your responsibility to obtain informed consent in a written consent form approved by an IRB in compliance with the requirement of 21 CFR Part 50 [see 21 CFR 312.60]. Except as provided in 21 CFR 50.23 and 50.24, no investigator may involve a human being as a subject in research unless the investigator has obtained the legally effective informed consent of the subject or the subject's legally authorized representative [21 CFR 50.20]. Our investigation found that for 30 of the 34 subjects enrolled, informed consent was not obtained or documented by the use of a written consent form approved by the IRB and signed and dated by the subject or the subject's legally authorized representative at the time of consent. The IRB approved consent forms were not completed until six months after the start of the study. In addition, assent was not obtained from subjects 46535, 46517, and 46529.

In your September 27,2007,written response, you explained that the sponsor did not send the consent form in the starter packages for the study, thus you had subjects sign an "Authorization Form" at the time of enrollment, which provided authorization to use and disclose health information. We find your explanation inadequate. Our review of the authorization form reveals that the form does not contain any of the elements required to be provided to subjects to constitute informed consent as described in 21 CFR 50.25. When you signed the "Statement of Investigator", Form FDA 1572, you agreed to fulfill the responsibilities of a clinical investigator that include ensuring that the requirement relating to informed consent are met. In addition, the protocol specified that "patients must meet all the of the following inclusion criteria to be eligible for study entry: signed informed consent document (in the case of a minor, consent must be given by the child's parent or legally authorized representative)…" The approval letter dated October 27,2004, from the [ ] Human Research Review Board documents your role as Principal Investigator with responsibility for the study. The approval letter indicates that the IRB reviewed and approved the Adult Consent Form, Minor Consent Form and Child Assent Form, so you should have been aware that these documents were essential to the conduct of the study. It is your responsibility to ensure compliance with these informed consent requirements.

2. You failed to promptly report to the IRB all unanticipated problems involving risk to human subjects [21 CFR 312.60 and 312.66].

An investigator is responsible for ensuring that the investigation is conducted according to the investigational plan and applicable regulations, including promptly reporting to the IRB all unanticipated problems involving risk to human subjects [21 CFR 312.60 and 312.66]. Our investigation found that Subject 46514 died on [ ]. Subject 46532 died on [ ] and Subject 46505 was hospitalized; however, there is no documentation indicating that you promptly reported this information to the IRB.

During the inspection, you explained to the FDA investigator that you were unaware that you needed to report serious adverse events to the IRB, although you attended the Investigator's Meeting, read the protocol and signed the investigator's agreement. In your written response you state that you were under the impression that the sponsor would communicate with the IRB. We find your response unacceptable. When you signed the "Statement of Investigator", Form FDA 1572, you agreed to comply with all of the responsibilities of a clinical investigator, including promptly reporting to the IRB all unanticipated problems involving risks to human subjects or others. In addition, the protocol specifically states in section 6.4 that "the Principal Investigator must also keep the IRB informed of any significant adverse events."

3. You continued to conduct clinical investigation related activities despite the fact that IRB approval had been withdrawn. [21 CFR 312.66, and 56.103(a)].

FDA regulations require that clinical investigations conducted under an IND (i.e. those subject to 21 CFR Part 312) be reviewed, approved, and under continuing review by an IRB meeting the requirements of 21 CFR part 56 [see 21 CFR 56.103]). Clinical investigators are responsible for assuring that an IRB conducts initial and continuing review of clinical investigations [21 CFR 312.66].You violated these requirements by continuing to see and treat study subjects after [ ] Human Research Review Board withdrew approval of your clinical investigation site on May 12,2005.

Despite your awareness of the withdrawal of IRB approval per the notice you received on May 11, 2005 you continued to obtain informed consent or parental consent from 27 of the 33 subjects previously entered into the study after May 12, 2005. Although [ ] Human Research Board denied the request for you to conduct six-month and twelve-month follow up visits on May 22, 2005, six-month study visits were completed for six study subjects during the period that the clinical investigation was suspended by the IRB. In addition, you pursued obtaining consent from fifteen subjects after you received correspondence withdrawing approval of the clinical investigation.

In your written response, you stated that you did not know you were not permitted to conduct follow up visits after approval had been withdrawn. Your response is inadequate. The IRB correspondence to you clearly documents that approval for the study had been withdrawn, and as the investigator you were responsible for ensuring the continuing approval of the clinical study by the IRB [21 CFR 312.66].

4. You failed to report to the IRB all changes in the research activity [21 CFR 312.60 and 312.66].

Specifically, 21 CFR 312.66 requires clinical investigators to assure that all changes in the research activity are promptly reported to the IRB [see 21 CFR 312.60]. Our investigation found that after having the clinical investigation reinstated by the IRB in September of 2005, you failed to notify the IRB that you were discontinuing the study in February 2006 and failed to submit a final study report. We you're your explanation that you thought this was the sponsor's responsibility to be unacceptable. As noted on the Form FDA 1572 that you signed, this responsibility belongs to the clinical investigator and not to the sponsor.

5. You failed to prepare and maintain adequate and accurate case histories that record all observations and data pertinent to the Investigation on each Individual [21 CFR 312.62(b)].

An investigator is required to prepare and maintain adequate and accurate case histories that record all observations and data pertinent to the investigation on each individual administered the investigational drug or employed as a control in the investigation [21 CFR 312.62(b)]. Our investigation found that you did not document the six-month follow-up that was conducted via telephone in the case histories for 22 subjects as required by FDA regulations and the investigation protocol.

As the clinical investigator, you are responsible for ensuring that the investigation is conducted according to the signed investigator statement, the investigational plan, applicable regulations, and for protecting the rights, safety and welfare of the study subjects.

This letter is not intended to be an all-inclusive list of deficiencies with your clinical study of an investigational drug. It is your responsibility to ensure adherence to each requirement of the law and relevant FDA regulations. You should address these deficiencies and establish procedures to ensure that any on-going or future studies will be in compliance with FDA regulations.

Within fifteen (15) working days of your receipt of this letter, you should notify this office in writing of the actions you have taken or will be taking to prevent similar violations in the future. Failure to adequately and promptly explain the violations noted above may result in regulatory action without further notice.

If you have any questions, please contact Tejashri Purohit-Sheth, M.D. at (301)796-3402 or FAX (301)847-8748. Your written response and any pertinent documentation should be addressed to:

Tejashri Purohit-Sheth. M.D.
Acting Branch Chief
Good Clinical Practice Branch Ⅱ, HFD-47
Page 5 - Nagarjuna R. Ponugoti, M.D.
Division of Scientific Investigations, Bldg 51, Room 5358
Office of Compliance
Center for Drug Evaluation and Research
Food and Drug Administration
10903 New Hampshire Avenue
Silver Spring, MD 20993

Sincerely yours,

{See appended electronic signature page}

Leslie K. Ball, M.D.
Director
Division of Scientific Investigations, HFD-45
Office of Compliance
Center for Drug Evaluation and Research
Food and Drug Administration

第142封　给Corces, Arturo医学博士的警告信

2008年5月28日

参考号：08-HFD-45-050

尊敬的Corces博士：

2007年3月20日至2007年4月26日，Victor Spanioil先生代表FDA进行了现场检查，与您会面并审查了您实施两项临床研究的情况：

- 方案［不公开］IND［不公开］"矫形外科预防凝血防止DVT和PE，选择性接受髋关节置换术的受试者预防VTE延伸进行的［不公开］对照、双盲、随机研究"，为［不公开］执行。
- 方案［不公开］IND［不公开］"临床2B期、随机、多剂量［不公开］在选择性接受全膝关节置换术的受试者预防静脉血栓形成安全性和有效性研究和评估"，为［不公开］执行。

本次现场检查是FDA的生物研究监查项目的一部分。该项目通过设定的检查方法，对相关研究的实施情况进行评估，并确保这些研究中受试者的权益、安全和福利得到了保护。

经过对现场检查报告、该报告附件以及您2007年5月18、24、31日对FDA 483表的书面回复，包括［不公开］准备的展示品的文件夹进行审查，我们认为，您没有遵循适用的法律要求和监管临床研究实施及受试者保护的FDA法规。我们知道，在现场检查结束时，检查员Spanioli向您出示并讨论了FDA 483表，即现场检查发现的问题。我们想强调以下几点：

1. 您未能亲自进行临床研究或对研究进行监督［21 CFR 312.60］

当您为上述临床研究签署临床研究者声明（FDA 1572表）时，您同意承担您机构的临床研究者之职责。您的总体职责（21 CFR 312.60）包括确保研究按照签署的研究者声明、研究计划和适用的法规进行，确保在您的监护下受试者的权益、安全和福利得到保护，确保研究中的试验药物受控。您明确同意亲自开展临床研究或者监督研究中您不能亲自参与的研究。当您需要授权部分研究任务给有资质的其他临床研究者时，您必须对授权的责任人进行充分的监督。我们的现场检查结果表明，您没有对被授权的临床研究责任人进行充分监督，以确保按照签署的研究者声明去保护临床试验中受试者的权益、安全和福利。检查发现，您被授权的研究责任人没有资格承当授权的研究任务。具体如下：

a.对于［不公开］方案中，您授权由［不公开］进行方案规定的临床评估（如体格检查、DVT或肺栓塞信号或症状评估）。根据机构人员授权记录表，［不公开］负责CRFs数据录入。在现场检查期间，［不公开］先生说明他没有进行体格检查和其他检查的培训，或具备相应检查的资格。例如，

i. 受试者［不公开］在2007年3月19日访视期间由［不公开］进行65天体格检查和DVT/PE评估，当时您在英格兰。

ii. 受试者［不公开］在2007年2月27日第13天的评估记录由［不公开］完成，由［不公开］基于受试者问答方式进行DVT/PE评估，而非由有资质的人员进行临床检查。

您在2007年5月18日的答复信中提到［不公开］被列为执行总体研究的授权人。您同时提及［不公开］在PI进行体格检查的现场，并充当抄写员记录PI的检查结果。您还提到［不公开］在PI不在的情况下，无意勾选了受试者［不公开］的其他体格检查项。

我们注意到，研究授权表中［不公开］负责数据录入，而未授权进行受试患者体格检查，而他签署了受试者［不公开］第65天体格检查和评估表及受试者［不公开］第13天评估表，似乎他做了这些检查。

2. 您未能达到知情同意的要求，特别是提供给受试者或其代理人的信息，应使用受试者或其代理人便于理解的语言［21 CFR 50.20］

a. 受试者［不公开］2007年1月3日签署的［不公开］研究的受试者信息和知情同意书共12页，前8页是英语，后4页是西班牙语。没有记录证明该受试者懂英语和西班牙语两种语言。该知情同意书有7处未完成的使用西班牙语、要求用“是”或“不是”来回答的问题。由［不公开］于2007年1月3日签署的研究授权书前3页是英语，最后签字页是西班牙语。由［不公开］签署了日期显示为2007年3月16日的所有英文版知情同意书，但都没有与受试者单独进行讨论并签署姓名、日期的记录，且受试者［不公开］于2007年3月14日完成研究。

b. 受试者［不公开］于2006年10月25日用英语签署［不公开］研究的知情同意书。受试者［不公开］的记录显示，在2006年10月29日手术当天再次签署知情同意，但用西班牙语签署的知情同意书。没有文件证明该受试者懂英语和西班牙语两种语言。

您在2007年5月24日的回复函中提到，不清楚为什么受试者［不公开］在手术当天重新进行了知情同意，虽然该受试者在手术前7天，即2006年10月25日已用英语签订了知情同意书。您的回复未能解释该受试者是否懂双语，也不能解释为什么这个受试者在2006年10月25日被给予了英文版知情同意书，在2006年10月29日被给予了西班牙文版知情同意书。

3. 您未能进行研究或确保按照相关的现行版试验方案进行研究［21 CFR 312.60］

a. 关于这个［不公开］试验方案，受试者［不公开］因为安排冲突未进行第13天的访视，但没有文件说明为什么没有安排其他日期的访视。试验方案要求在第13天需要进行生命体征检查和体格检查，还需要进行血液学和血生化检查的采样。

您在2007年5月18日的回复中提到，您曾多次联系该受试者，但是均没有记录证明。DSI认为您的回复不充分，因为临床研究者有责任确保研究按照正确的流程进行。

b. 试验方案［不公开］4.5.7规定：“研究期间不允许进行气动加压预防血栓形成”。医院的记录表明6名受试者在住院期间接受［不公开］气动加压治疗：［不公开］和［不公开］。

c. 试验方案［不公开］禁止使用气动装置。62名受试者中有5名受试者的记录表明他们在进行全膝关节置换手术住院期间接受过间歇式脚用气动装置的治疗：［不公开］和［不公开］。

您在2007年5月18日的回复函中称，使用间歇式脚用气动装置是［不公开］医疗中心大多数患者的标准治疗，入组该项研究的患者将继续使用该项装置。DSI认为您的回复不可接受，因为试验方案特别规定禁止使用间歇式气动装置。另外，我们检查还发现，2006年9月26日高级研究助理［不公开］和办公室主任［不公开］之间的邮件特别提到治疗期间使用间歇式气动设备是排除标准。

d. 试验方案［不公开］禁止在手术前7天以内和研究治疗期间使用影响血小板功能和凝聚作用的药物，这些药物包括克拉匹多（Peavix）和乙酰水杨酸（Aspirin Ecotrin）。检查发现，受试者［不公开］在参加研究期间接受过克拉匹多和乙酰水杨酸的治疗。

您在2007年5月31日对此的回复是不充分的。受试者［不公开］于2007年1月24日被筛选，2007年1月31日进入活性治疗阶段。您根据药物分发记录说明受试者［不公开］于2007年1月31日中断克拉匹多和乙酰水杨酸的治疗，当天即开始药物治疗，没有按要求在7天前停止给药。

e. 试验方案［不公开］规定为了确保研究盲态，研究者在当地医疗机构不允许测定凝血参数。现场检查发现2006年12月21日对受试者［不公开］进行了凝血参数检测，包括PT INR、PTT和活化部分PTT；2006年10月24日、26日对受试者［不公开］检测了PT、PT INR、APTT。临床研究者均可以对这些受试者的检测结果进行评估。

您于2007年5月18日的答复中称是由于失误所致。

f.［不公开］研究中，受试者［不公开］筛选入组（Day 0）的生化检测样本在2006年12月13日采集。试验室的检测结果显示LDH（乳酸脱氢酶）值为1612 U/L（参考值为100~220 U/L），被标记为“没有临床意义”。该检测项输入时没有责任人签署日期和姓名。相关的血生化“筛查”报告有您的签字，签署日期是2007年1月5日，大约是该受试者髋关节置换手术（2006年12月19日）完成后的三周。没有记录解释LDH值“没有临床意义”的决定过程。

您在2007年5月18日的答复中称，您之所以没有重测是因为血液检测会在受试者手术前作为前期准备工作进行。您也注意到根据NSA钾的结果，筛查时的血样是不可靠的，而且如果LDH值是正确的，将会观察到受试者有慢性或急性组织损伤。您也提到，在手术后采集的血样的检测结果在正常范围内。您的答复是不能接受的。LDH值为1612 U/L是明显超出范围的，临床记录应该说明为什么您认为这是没有临床意义的。另外，您没有解释为什么您在受试者手术后约3周，2007年1月5日才审查入组筛选的实验室检测结果。

g. 试验方案［不公开］要求第6天采两次血样以测定凝血参数。方案规定于给药前及给药后2~4小时各采一次血。受试者［不公开］第6天的给药记录表明，试验药物给药时间是2007年2月19日21:21。给药后采血时间是22:30，约为给药后1小时。受试者［不公开］给药记录表明给药时间为2006年10月30日上午10:19，血样采集记录时间是16:00，约为8小时后。您于2007年5月18日的答复收悉，您称护士录入的时间是错误的，研究协调员在给药期间在现场，坚称血样采集时间符合方案规定的时间要求。DSI认为该回答是不充分的，因为您没有提供相关记录支持您的观点。

h. 试验方案［不公开］规定：“如果治疗期间提前终止，第13天的访视评估必须执行。”记录表明，受试者［不公开］从2007年1月12日至14日接受试验药物（4片和5针），后因康复中心拒绝给药而停止研究。现场检查发现，剩余的试验药物于2007年2月20日返还，第6天及随后的访视及采血均未进行，要求的第13天访视也没有开展。

在您2007年5月18日的回复中提供了2007年4月12日的备忘录，显示您对该患者进行了后续评估。DSI认为这个解释不充分，因为不能解释为什么在受试者结束该项研究后约3个月您对受试者进行随访。

i. 试验方案［不公开］要求在筛选时应排除12导联心电图显示Q-Tc>450毫秒和/或临床体征显示不正常的受试者。记录显示受试者［不公开］2006年9月25日的Q-Tc延迟，值为457毫秒，并于2006年9月25日筛选时签署了知情同意。

您于2007年5月31日的回复中称，ECG结果被送到中心实验室解读。DSI认为您不能解释清楚为什么受试者不符合入组条件而继续入组研究。

j. 试验方案［不公开］要求所有不良事件须全部记录在受试者CRF中。现场检查发现，医疗记录有2006年11月28日受试者［不公开］记忆缺失和右侧股静脉单个血栓，2006年12月7日受试者［不公开］左脚下垂，2007年1月12日、14日受试者［不公开］尿失禁；这些不良事件并没有记录在受试者的CRF中。

您在2007年5月24日的回复中称这些不良事件记录在受试者的病历和体征检查报告中。该答复不充分，因为这些不良事件仍需要记录在受试者的CRF中。

k. 试验方案［不公开］要求排除没有使用适当避孕方法的女性受试者。方案中列出了避孕药物或阻碍法是唯一接受的避孕方法。现场检查发现，年满18周岁的受试者［不公开］完成手术后被“鼓励”节欲至少三个月（2006年12月）。另外，现场检查发现，该受试者之前曾计划进行手术（2006年5月15），但是发现怀孕后实行了流产。

您在2007年5月18日的回复中称，您收到申办者允许该受试者以禁欲的方式避孕。但这种回复不能接受，2007年4月5日来自［不公开］研究助理［不公开］指导员工仅就关于方案规定的避孕事宜与该受试者讨论。

l. 试验方案［不公开］要求每位受试者每天服用4粒受试药物胶囊，治疗期间服用相同剂量，服药时需饮240ml水。现场检查期间发现没有指导性文件，以及已按要求做的记录。

您在2007年5月3日的回复中称方案没有提供怎样确保240ml水被饮用的说明，或者证明该事实。但该回复是不充分的，因为临床研究者有责任确保方案规定的程序被执行并记录。

4. 您未能保存研究中每个受试者的所有观察结果和其他相关数据的足够及准确病历［21 CFR 312.62（b）］ 例如：

a. 关于［不公开］的试验方案，没有按要求将伴随用药记录到伴随用药eCRF，有些原始记录和eCRF中输入的不一致。具体如下：

ⅰ. 原始记录显示受试者［不公开］接受奥美沙坦、对乙酰氨基可待因、马来酸罗格列酮、格列美脲（4mg/2mg）、结合雌激素 1g、奥昔布宁 5mg、美托洛尔，然而CRF记录的只有奥美沙坦、美托洛尔、二甲双胍和奥昔布宁 5mg。另外，服药起始日期不完整，评估医生没有做首字母记录。

ⅱ. 原始记录显示受试者［不公开］服用阿司匹林、叶酸、铁剂、复方对乙酰氨基酚丙氧氨酚、萘普生和维生素。CRF表中只记录了可待因，没有记录开始服药时间。

ⅲ. 受试者［不公开］臀部手术住院时用药小结（2007年2月12~19日）载明服用了阿司匹林和其他几种药物，但这些药物都没有录进eCRF的伴随用药项。eCRF中录入的13种药物有10种没有记录服用药物的开始和结束时间。

我们注意到您在2007年5月24日的回复函中称，这些矛盾的信息是因为信息渠道多样导致的。您准备实施一项标准操作规程的措施收悉，通过建立一套标准程序以确保研究日期的一致性。

b. 研究［不公开］中，受试者［不公开］eCRF结束研究提到，提前结束研究是因为撤回“知情同意”。然而，原始文件表明受试者退出该研究是因为康复中心拒绝该患者继续研究药物。

您于2007年5月24日的回复中解释，该受试者在髋关节置换手术结束后转移到西棕榈滩的康复中心。您的答复没有清楚说明，是因为该受试者撤回知情同意，还是因为康复中心中断了研究。

c. 研究［不公开］中受试者［不公开］的原始记录表明，伴随服药菲诺贝特和卡马西平。该受试者相应的伴随用药eCRF没有记录相应的伴随用药。您于2007年5月31日的答复中称该受试者的这个记录在其eCRF是不经意遗漏的。但您的回复是不充足的，因为您有责任确保试验期间正确完整地进行记录。

5. 您未能保存足够的药物处置记录［21 CFR 312.62］

试验方案［不公开］4.5.8规定，“给药过程应记录（包括日期、时间、剂量和药物分发人的签字）。没有使用的试验药物也应记录”。现场检查发现，2007年3月完成研究的14名受试者的药品分发记录信息不全，没有充分记录受试者的依从性，例如：

a. 受试者［不公开］药物分发记录表显示，药物用量“未知”，并没有解释药物剂量缺失的原因。

b. 受试者［不公开］药物分发记录表显示，片剂和注射剂的数量是未知的，且患者从来没有返还试验药物。

c. 受试者［不公开］药物分发记录表显示，有21片药和16剂注射液分发给该受试者，该受试者返还了19片药的包装，但在“不符的解释”栏未给出任何解释。

d. 受试者［不公开］药物分发记录表显示，用掉的片剂数量是“未知”、注射液数量为16剂，但CRF的记录是所有药物被用掉。

e. 受试者［不公开］药物分发记录表显示，29片药和14剂注射液分配给受试者，11片药和2剂注射剂被退回，“不符和解释”栏是空的。

您于2007年5月18日的回复中提到该项研究复杂，但确保不同护理人员准确给药的指导很有限。该回复不能接受，因为由于不准确的药物分发记录导致我们不能准确评估方案执行的依从性。

本警告信的目的并非是罗列您在试验药物临床研究中存在的所有缺陷。确保遵循法律和相关FDA法规的每一项要求是您的职责。您应当解决这些缺陷，并建立规程，以确保任何正在进行或将来进行的研究均能符合FDA的法规。

自收到这封信的15个工作日内，您应当书面告知本办公室为预防将来发生类似违规情况已经采取或计划采取的措施。如果不能充分、迅速地解释上述违规问题，可能导致我们在不再通知的情况下采取监管措施。

附：英文原文

Corces, Arturo, M.D.

WARNING LETTER

May 28, 2008

CERTIFIED MAIL
RETURN RECEIPT REQUESTED

Ref: 08-HFD-45-050

Arturo Corces, M.D.
7340 SW 79th Street
Miami Institute for Medical Research
Miami, Florida 33186

Dear Dr. Corces:

Between March 20 and April 26, 2007, Mr. Victor Spanioli, representing the Food and Drug Administration(FDA), conducted an investigation and met with you, to review your conduct of two clinical investigations:

- Protocol [redacted] IND [redacted] "Regulation of Coagulation in Orthopedic Surgery to prevent DVT and PE, Controlled,Double-Blind,Randomized Study of [redacted] in the Extended Prevention of VTE in Patients Undergoing Elective Total Hip Replacement,"performed for [redacted] and
- Protocol [redacted] IND [redacted] "A Phase 2B, Randomized, Multicenter Dose-Ranging Study and Assessing the Safety and Efficacy of [redacted] in the Prevention of Venous Thromboembolic Events (VTE) in Subjects Undergoing an Elective, Total Knee Replacement, " performed for [redacted]

This inspection is a part of FDA's Bioresearch Monitoring Program, which includes inspections designed to evaluate the conduct of research and to ensure that the rights, safety, and welfare of the human subjects of the study have been protected.

From our review of the establishment inspection report, the documents submitted with that report,and your May 18, 24 and 31, 2007 letters written in response to the Form FDA 483 including the binders of exhibits prepared by [redacted] we conclude that you did not adhere to the applicable statutory requirements and FDA regulations governing the conduct of clinical investigations and the protection of human subjects.We are aware that at the conclusion of the inspection, Investigator Spanioli presented and discussed with you Form FDA 483,Inspectional Observations. We wish to emphasize the following:

1. You failed to personally conduct or supervise the clinical investigations [21 CFR 312.60]

When you signed the investigator statement (Form FDA 1572) for the above-referenced clinical investigations, you agreed to take on the responsibilities of a clinical investigator at your site. Your general responsibilities (21 CFR 312.60) include ensuring that the investigation is conducted according to the signed investigator statement, the investigational plan and applicable regulations; protecting the rights, safety and welfare of subjects under your care; and ensuring control of drugs under investigation. You specifically agreed to personally conduct the clinical studies or to supervise those aspects of the studies that you did not personally conduct. While you may delegate certain study tasks to individuals qualified to perform them as clinical investigator you must adequately supervise those to whom you delegate authority. Our investigation indicates that your supervision of personnel to whom you delegated study tasks was not adequate to ensure that the clinical trials were conducted according to the signed investigator statement, and in a manner that protected the rights, safety, and welfare of human subjects. The investigation found that you delegated certain tasks to individuals not qualified to perform such tasks. Specifically,

a. For [redacted] protocol, you delegated the performance of protocol-specified clinical evaluations (e.g. physical examinations,and evaluation of signs and symptoms relating to a DVT or pulmonary embolism) to [redacted]. According to the Site Personnel Delegation Log,[redacted] was assigned a role of data entry for CRFs. During the inspection, Mr.[redacted] indicated that he was not trained or qualified to perform physical examinations and other required assessments. For example,

i. For Subject [redacted] the Day 65 physical examination and DVT/PE assessment was performed by [redacted] during a visit date of March 19, 2007, while you were in England.

ii. For Subject [redacted] the Day 13 assessment records dated February 27, 2007, were initialed by [redacted]. The DVT/PE assessment was completed by [redacted] based on the subject's responses to questions instead of a clinical examination by a qualified individual.

We note your response letter dated May 18, 2007 states that [redacted] is listed as the authorized personnel to perform general study procedures. You also state that [redacted] was present at the physical examinations conducted by the PI and acted as a scribe to record results of examinations performed by the PI. You state that [redacted] inadvertently checked all other boxes of the physical evaluation for Subject [redacted] when the PI was not available. We note that [redacted]is listed with the role of data entry on the study delegation log [redacted] is not authorized to conduct physical assessments of study patients,as it appears he did when he signed the Day 65 Physical Exam and Assessments form for Subject [redacted] or the Day 13 Assessment form for Subject [redacted].

2. You failed to meet the requirements for informed consent, specifically therequirement that information given to the subject or the subject's representative shall be in language understandable to thesubject or the representative [21 CFR 50.20].

a. The [redacted] study Research Subject Information and Consent Form signed by Subject [redacted] dated January 3, 2007 is 12 pages long, with the first eight pages written in the English language and the last four pages written in the Spanish language. There was no documentation that this subject is bilingual in both English and Spanish. The section of the consent with seven questions requiring a "yes" or "no"response, appearing in Spanish language text,is not completed. The Research Authorization signed by [redacted] on January 3, 2007 consists of the first three pages in English and the signature last page in Spanish. AII English language versions of these consent forms dated March 16,2007 were signed by [redacted] however, there is no signature or date relating to the individual discussing the consent. Subject [redacted] completed study participation on/or about March 14 2007.

b. The [redacted] study informed consent document signed by Subject [redacted] on October 25, 2006,is in the English language. Records document Subject [redacted] was re-consentedon the day ofsurgery, October 29,2006,using a Spanish language informed consent form. There is no documentation that this subject is bilingual in English and Spanish.

Your May 24, 2007 response letter states that it is unclear why Subject [redacted] was re-consented on the day of surgery, since the subject signed the English informed consent formon October 25, 2006 seven days prior to surgery. Your response does not address whether this subject was bilingual, and does not explain why this subject was given an English consent formon October 25, 2006 and a Spanish consent formon October 29, 2006.

3. You failed to conduct thestudies or ensure they were conducted according to the relevant,current protocols [21 CFR 312.60].

a. For the [redacted] protocol the required 13 day follow up visit for subject[redacted] was not done due to reported scheduling conflicts; however, there is no documentation as to why an alternate date was not scheduled. The protocol required that on day 13,a physical examination with assessment of vital signs be performed, and blood samples be drawn for hematology and clinical chemistry.

Your response letter dated May 18, 2007, states that several attempts were made to contact this subject,but these attempts were not documented. DSI considers your response inadequate, as it is the responsibility of the clinical investigator to ensure that correct study procedures are followed.

b. Section 4.5.7 of the [redacted] protocol states "Thromboprophylaxis with pneumatic compression is not allowed during the study." Hospital records document that the following 6 subjects received [redacted] pneumatic compression therapy during their hospitalization: [redacted] and [redacted]

c. Protocol [redacted] prohibited the use of pneumatic compression devices. Records for 5 of 62 subjects documented that they received intermittent foot pneumatic compression during hospitalization following total knee replacement: [redacted] and [redacted]

Your response letter dated May 18, 2007 states that the use of intermittent pneumatic foot compressiol therapy has been a standard of care for the majority of patients at the [redacted] Medical Center, and that the personnel continued using this device with the patients enrolled in these studies. DSI considers your response to be unacceptable. The protocol specifically prohibited the use of intermittent pneumatic compression devices. Furthermore our investigation found an email exchange of September 26, 2006 between [redacted] Senior Medical Research Associate, [redacted], and Office Manager [redacted] specifically stating that use of planned intermittent pneumatic compression during active treatment period was an exclusion criteria.

d. Protocol [redacted] prohibited the use of drugs known to affect platelet function or coagulation within 7 days prior to surgery and throughout the study treatment period. These included clopidogrel (Plavix) and acetyl salicylicacid (aspirin Ecotrin). The investigation found that Subject [redacted] received both Plavix aspirin,during his/her participation in the study.

Your May 31, 2007 response is insufficient. Subject [redacted] was screened on January 24, 2007, and entered the active treatment phase on January 31,2007. Your letter refers to a Drug Dispensing Record that documents clopidogrel and acetyl salicylicacid for Subject [redacted] were discontinued on January 31, 2007, the same day that active study treatment began, and not seven days before as the protocol required.

e. The [redacted] protocol states that to ensure the blindness of the study the investigator should not measure any coagulation parameter at the local health care facility. The investigation found that coagulation testing for PT INR and PTT, Activated, was performed for Subject [redacted] at the December 21, 2006 visit, and the PT, PT INR and APPT coagulation tests were done for Subject [redacted] on October 24 and 26, 2006. These subject results were available for review by the Clinical Investigator.

In your letter dated May 18, 2007, you state that these tests were ordered in error.

f. For the [redacted] study, the Screening (Day 0) chemistry lab test for Subject [redacted] was collected on December 13, 2006. These lab results documented, among other things, a Lactate Dehydrogenase (LDH) value of 1612 U/L (reference range 100-220 U/L), stamped as “not clinically significant.” This entry did not contain dates or signatures of the responsible person. The associated ‘screening’ hematology report contained your signature and was dated January 5, 2007, approximately three weeks after this subject’s hip replacement surgery on December 19, 2006. No documentation was found explaining the determination that the LDH value was “not clinically significant”.

Your response dated May 18, 2007, states that you chose not to require repeat testing because blood work would be performed prior to the subject’s surgery as part of the pre-operative hospital procedure. You also noted that it appeared that the initial blood sample was unreliable based on the NSA potassium results, and that chronic or acute tissue damage would have been noted in the subject if the initial LDH value was accurate. You also state that blood collection was performed on the day after surgery,and that the lab values were within normal range. This response is unacceptable. An LDH value of 1612 U/L is clearly out of range and clinic records should document why you considered this as “not clinically significant.” Furthermore, you did not explain why you reviewed the screening chemistry lab results on January 5,2007, almost three weeks after the subject’s surgery.

g. The [redacted] Protocol required that blood samples be drawn twice on Day 6to measure coagulation parameters. The protocol specified the times for these blood draws as shortly before intake of the tablet (at trough) and 2-4 hours after intake of tablet (at peak). For Subject [redacted], for the Day 6 sample, the drug administration records document that study drug was administered at 21:21 of February 19,2007. The post-dose blood collection record documents a time of 22:30, or slightly more than 1 hour later. For Subject [redacted] drug administration records document that study drug was administered at10:19 AM on October 30, 2006, and the blood collection records document a time of 16:00, or almost 8 hours later. We acknowledge in your letter dated May 18,2007, you state that the times entered by the nurse were erroneous, and that the Study Coordinator was present during the period of drug administration and firmly recalls the sample collection times as being done within the timeframes specified by the protocol. DSI considers this response to be inadequate because you provided no documentation to support your contention.

h. The [redacted] study protocol states that "in case of premature discontinuation during the treatment phase, all assessments as described for Visit Day 13 have to be performed. Records document that Subject [redacted] received investigational drug from January 12-142007 (four tablets and 5 injections), and was removed from the study because the rehabilitation center declined to administer study medication." The investigation found that remaining doses of study medication were returned on February 20, 2007, and that the Day 6 and other safety follow up visits and blood draws were not performed and the assessments required for the Day 13 follow-up Visit were not done.

We note in your letter dated May 18, 2007 that you include a Note to File, dated April 12, 2007, that documents you contacted this subject for follow-up evaluation. DSI considers this response to be inadequate because it does not explain why your follow-up with this subject occurred approximately 3 months after the subject was discontinued from the study.

i. Protocol [redacted] required the exclusion of subjects with a 12-lead electrocardiogram (ECG) demonstrating QTc >450 msec and/or clinically significant abnormalities at screening. Records document that Subject [redacted] had a prolonged QTc of 457 msec on September 25 2006 and signed an Informed Consent document on September 25, 2006 at screening.

Your May 31, 2007 response letter states that the ECG tracings were sent to a core ECG laboratory for interpretation. DSI considersyour response to be inadequate to explain why you enrolled a subject into the study who did not meet eligibility requirements at study entry.

j. The [redacted] protocol required that all adverse events be fully recorded on the subject's Case Report Form. The investigation found clinic records that documented loss of memory and isolated nonobstructive thrombus in the common femoral vein on the rightside for Subject [redacted] on November28 2006; left foot drop for Subject [redacted] on December 7, 2006; and urinary incontinence for Subject [redacted] on January 12 and 14, 2007. These adverse events were not documented onto the subjects' Case Report Form.

Your May 24, 2007 response states these adverse events were documented in the subject's medical history and physical examination report. This response is insufficient, as these adverse even were required to be documented on the subjects' Case Report Form.

k. The [redacted] protocol excluded female subjects who "are not using adequate birth control method." The protocol lists birth control pills or barrier method as the only acceptable means for birth control. The investigation found that Subject [redacted] who was 18 years of age at the time, was "encouraged" to practice abstinence for at least three months after having the surgical procedure (December 2006). Furthermore, the investigation found that this subject had been previously scheduled to under go surgery (May 15,2006), but was found to have become pregnant and underwent abortion.

Your response letter dated May 18, 2007 states that you received sponsor approval for allowing this subject to use abstinence as a form of birth control.This response is unacceptable. An email dated April 5, 2007 from [redacted] Medical Research Associate [redacted] instructed the staff to discuss only the protocol specified birth control options with this subject.

1. Protocol [redacted] required that each subject be instructed to take 4 capsules of study medication once a day, at the same time of day during the treatment period and that the dose was to be administered with 240 mL of water. The investigation found no documentation that such instructions were given and no record confirming that these requirements were met.

Your May 3, 2007 response states the protocol did not provide instructions of how to ensure that 240 ml of water was consumed, or how to document this fact. This response is unacceptable. It is the responsibility of the clinical investigator to ensure that protocol specified procedures are followed and documented.

4. You failed to maintain adequate and accurate case histories that record all observations and other data pertinent to the investigation on each individual [21 CFR 312.62(b)].For example:

a. For the [redacted] protocol, the concomitant medications required to be entered on the Concomitant Medication eCRF were not entered and some source records were inconsistent with eCRF entries. Specifically,

i. Source records document that Subject [redacted] received Benicar, acetaminophen with codeine, rosiglitazone maleate with glimepiride (4 mg/2mg) , Premarin 1g, oxybutynin 5 mg, and Toprol XL, whereas the Case Report

Form documents only Benicar, Toprol XL, metformin and oxybutynin 5 mg. Furthermore, the Date Started column is not completed, and initials of the reviewing physician are not recorded.

ii. Source records document that Subject [redacted] received concomitant medications aspirin, folic acid, iron, Darvocet, naproxen, and vitamins. The CRF lists codeine as the only concomitant medication, and there are no entries for the Date Started.

iii. For Subject [redacted] the Summary of Medications form for the hip surgery hospitalization(February 12 – 19, 2007) documents the administration of aspirin and several other drugs that are not entered in the Concomitant Medication eCRF. Start and stop dates are not entered for 10 of the 13 drugs listed in this eCRF.

We note that in your response letter dated May 24, 2007, you state that these inconsistencies were due to documentation of information in various sources. We also acknowledge your action to implement a Standard Operating Procedure to establish a standard procedure to ensure consistent documentation of study data.

b. For the [redacted] protocol, for Subject [redacted] The End of Treatment eCRF states that premature termination was due to "consent withdrawn", whereas source records document that the subject was taken off the study because the rehabilitation center refused to continue patient on study drug.

In your letter dated May 24, 2007, you explain the transfer of this subject to a rehabilitation center in West Palm Beach after her hip replacement surgery. Your response does not clarify if the subject with drew consent,or if she was discontinued from the study by the rehabilitation center.

c. For Protocol [redacted] the source records for Subject [redacted] document concomitant medications of fenofirate and carbamazepine. The Concomitant Medication eCRF for this subject does not record these concomitant medications. Your May 31,2007 response letter states this documentation was inadvertently omitted in the eCRF for this subject. Your response is insufficient as it is your responsibility to ensure correct and completed documentation during the conduct of this study.

5. You failed to maintain adequate drug disposition records [21 CFR 312.62].

Protocol [redacted] Section 4.5.8, states "Drug administration will be documented (date,time, dose and signature of dispensing person). Drug account of the unused study medication will be performed." The investigation found that the Drug Dispensing log entries for 14 subjects who completed the study as of March 2007 contained incomplete information and did not adequately account for subject compliance. For example:

a. For Subject [redacted] the Drug Dispensing log document that the amount of drug used was "unknown" with no explanation provided for the lack of drug accountability.

b. For Subject [redacted] the Drug Dispensing log documents the number of tablets and injections administered as unknown and that the patient never returned study medication.

c. For Subject [redacted] the drug Dispensing log documents that 21 tablets and 16 injections were administered to the subject and that the subject returned 19 tablets, with no explanation provided in the "discrepancy" column.

d. For Subject [redacted], the Drug Dispensing Log document that the number of tablets used was "unknown" and that 16 injections were administered whereas the CRF documents that all doses were administered.

e. For Subject [redacted] the Drug Dispensing Log documents that 29 tablets and 14 injections were administered, and 11 tablets and 2 injections were returned, but the "discrepancy explanation" column is left blank.

In your letter dated May 18, 2007, you refer to the complexity of the study with limited instructions regarding assuring administration of investigational drug by various caregivers. This response is unacceptable. Due to the inaccurate drug disposition records, we are unable to accurately assess compliance with the protocol.

This letter is not intended to be an all-inclusive list of deficiencies with your clinical study of an investigational drug. It is your responsibility to-ensure adherence to each requirement of the law and relevant FDA regulations. You must address these deficiencies and establish procedures to ensure that any on-going or future studies will be in compliance with FDA regulations.

Within fifteen(15) working days of your receipt of this letter, you should notify this office in writing of the actions you have taken or will be taking to prevent similar violations in the future. Failure to adequately and promptly explain the violations noted above may result in regulatory action without further notice.

If you have any questions, please contact Tejashri Purohit-Sheth,M.D. at (301)796-3402 or FAX(301)847-8748. Your written response and any pertinent documentation should be addressed to:

Tejashri Purohit-Sheth. M.D.
Branch Chief（Acting）
Good Clinical Practice Branch 2
Division of Scientific Investigations, Bldg 51,Room 5358
Office of Compliance
CDER/FDA
10903 New Hampshire Avenue
Silver Spring, MD 20993

Sincerely yours

{See appended electronic signature page}

Leslie K. Ball M.D.
Director
Division of Scientific Investigations
Bldg 51,Rm.5342
Office of Compliance
Center for Drug Evaluation and Research

第143封　给Nasim, Golzar医学博士的警告信

2008年5月1日

参考号：08-HFD-45-02-04

尊敬的Golzar博士：

2007年7月24日至2007年8月22日，Yvette Lacour-Davis女士代表FDA对您进行了检查，与您会面并审查了您实施的试验药物为［不公开］、申办者为［不公开］的下列临床研究的情况：

- 试验方案［不公开］，题为："一项前瞻、随机、双盲、三臂、多中心、对照研究，评估［不公开］药物每日两次给药7天、［不公开］药物每日两次给药10天与头孢呋新250mg每日两次口服10天相比，治疗急性细菌性鼻窦炎的有效性和安全性"。
- 试验方案［不公开］，题为："一项前瞻、非对照、开放、多中心临床研究，评价［不公开］药物每日两次给药10天治疗社区获得性肺炎有效性和安全性"。
- 试验方案［不公开］，题为："一项前瞻、随机、双盲研究，比较［不公开］药物每日两次给药5天联合阿奇霉素5天（第一天500mg口服，第2至第5天250mg每日一次口服）治疗慢性支气管炎急性发作"。

本次现场检查是FDA的生物研究监查项目的一部分。该项目通过设定的检查方法，评估研究的实施情况，并确保这些研究中受试者的权益、安全和福利得到了保护。

经对现场检查报告、该报告的附件，以及2007年9月8日对FDA 483表即现场检查发现的问题的回复，我们认为，您未能遵循适用的法律要求和监管临床研究实施及受试者保护的FDA法规。

我们知道，在现场检查结束时，Lacour-Davis女士向您出示并讨论了FDA 483表，即现场检查发现的问题，我们想强调以下几点：

1. 您未能按照21 CFR 50的要求获取每位受试者的知情同意［21 CFR 312.60］

具体而言，21 CFR 50.20法规声明：除21 CFR 50.23和21 CFR 50.24所列情况外，在获得受试者或其合法授权代理人的合法有效的知情同意前，研究者不能将人类作为受试者纳入这些法规监管的研究。此外，除21 CFR 56.109（c）所列情况外，知情同意应当使用经IRB批准的书面知情同意书进行记录［21 CFR 50.27（a）］。

在试验方案［不公开］中发现以下违背：

a. 23例受试者中，有4例受试者（4011，4015，4019和4021）在签署知情同意书之前进行了方案规定的基线血样采集。

b. IRB批准的知情同意书要求记录获得受试者合法有效知情同意的实际时间。在受试者4016，4017和4018签署的知情同意书中未记录实际时间。此外，我们无法证实知情同意书的签署时间是否是早于他们接受任何方案规定的程序。

2007年9月18日的书面回复中，您强调所有病例在实施任何研究程序前均已获得受试者的口头同意。但是，口头同意是不够的。21 CFR 50.23和21 CFR 50.24关于免除知情同意要求的情况及21 CFR 56.109（c）关于免除签署IRB批准的书面知情同意书的情况均不适用于本研究。

2. 您未能确保按照批准的研究方案开展研究［21 CFR312.60］

a. 在试验方案［不公开］中发现下列违背：

i. 试验方案规定，纳入研究的必须是根据A）影像学；B）临床标准诊断为急性鼻窦炎的患者，且出现症状和体征时间大于7天，但少于28天。本研究影像学的入选标准包括任何下列表现：出现气-液面、浑浊和/或黏膜增厚大于6mm。入组的30例受试者中有10例（43007，43009，43011，43012，43013，43014，43015，

43019，43021和43030）未达到方案要求的研究入选影像学标准。具体而言，这些受试者的X射线表现未显示出是急性鼻窦炎。

ⅱ. 试验方案规定，入组前7天内接受全身性抗菌药物治疗超过24小时的受试者必须排除。受试者43002尽管在这个排除时间段内一直使用强力霉素，但是于2000年12月12日入组。

ⅲ. 30例受试者中有9例（43001，43002，43003，43004，43005，43006，43009，43013和43014）未按方案要求，在疗效考评访视中进行副鼻窦［不公开］X射线检查。

在2007年9月18日的书面答复中，您强调受试者都具有高度提示急性细菌鼻窦炎的临床体征和症状，无论是否入组研究本来都应该使用抗生素治疗。这个回复是不够的。FDA法规要求，将受试者入组到FDA监管的临床研究的研究者，要遵循研究计划，以帮助确保研究期间采集的数据是可靠的，并且研究参与者的权益、安全和福利得到保护。

b. 试验方案［不公开］规定，提前退出研究的受试者要完成完整的临床评估，采集痰标本进行革兰染色、培养和药敏试验以及方案要求的所有安全性实验室检查。方案进一步强调，若更换抗生素，要在更换前先完成这项检查。此外，方案规定提前退出的受试者要进行临床评估，包括在末次使用替换的抗生素治疗后2~4天进行胸部X射线检查。我们发现受试者17001和17003提前退出该研究，但是既没有按照方案采集痰液，也没有进行替换抗生素后的胸部X射线检查。

c. 在试验方案［不公开］中发现下列违背：

ⅰ. 试验方案版本1和修订版本1（日期：2000年10月15日）规定，为保证一个疗程的微生物学的有效性，研究入选标准要求在适当的治疗前的痰标本应至少确认一种致病菌（即上皮细胞数≤10/低倍视野，WBC≥25/低倍视野）。试验方案版本2和修订版本2（日期：2000年12月8日）进一步说明这项入选标准，即若入组时痰标本WBC＜25/低倍视野，获取另一份WBC≥25/低倍视野的痰样本也是可以接受的，前提是第二份痰样本采集时患者使用研究药物不超过48小时。尽管痰标本不符合试验方案要求的WBC＞25/低倍视野的入选标准，但是受试者4001和4004入组该研究。

ⅱ. 试验方案规定，入组时需获取患者病史，包括呼吸系统既往史、吸烟史、询问相关的基础疾病或状况、总体健康状况等。受试者4001，4002，4003和4004未按方案要求获得足够的病史。

ⅲ. 试验方案规定，入组时需进行基线尿常规检测，受试者4001和4002未按方案要求进行该检测。

ⅳ. 试验方案规定，入组前48小时内，受试者必须通过深咳提供脓性或黏脓性痰标本进行细菌染色、培养及药敏试验。受试者4010未能提供方案要求的用于入组的痰样本，但您仍给其发放了研究药物。

ⅴ. 试验方案规定，在疗效考评访视时，受试者需进行血清妊娠试验。受试者4002，4003和4007未按方案要求进行该试验。

在2007年9月18日的书面答复中，您提到前来就诊的有急性感染的患者需要尽快得到治疗。您进一步声明研究参加者的筛选、入组和随机要以比其他非感染类临床研究明显加快的方式进行；因此在随机前未能拿到所有实验室检查和X射线检查数据进行深入的筛选审查。这个回复是不够的。FDA法规要求，将受试者入组到FDA监管的临床研究的研究者，要遵循研究计划，以帮助确保研究期间采集的数据是可靠的，并且研究参与者的权益、安全和福利得到保护。

3. 您未能准备和保存记录每个个体与研究相关的所有观察结果和其他数据的足够准确的病历［21 CFR 312.62（b）］

a. 在试验方案［不公开］中，入组研究的30例受试者中有17例（43001，43002，43004，43005，43006，43007，43008，43009，43010，43011，43012，43013，43014，43015，43016，43017和43019）电子CRF中报告的疾病的临床症状及体征无法和原始记录的信息相对应。FDA检查时发现了一份日期为2001年2月12日的文件备忘录，记录“目前，对于截至2001年2月12日的研究访视，输入到［不公开］系统的所有规定的鼻窦炎症状以及后续评级，偶尔没有支持性文件。从今以后，输入到［不公开］系统的所有规定的鼻窦炎症状，或任何访视规定的数据都应该要有支持性文件。”FDA在检查期间证实了原始文件的缺失。我们注意到上述的所有

17例受试者都在2001年2月12日前入组。

b. 我们发现对于入组试验方案［不公开］的受试者4001，2001年1月24日治疗前访视的基线疾病临床症状和体征内容，CRF上记录的与原始文件不一致。具体而言，2001年4月12日，您签署修改了受试者4001的CRF，记录受试者有中度而非轻度的喘息。但是，在2001年1月24日治疗前访视完成的P. V. Family & Immediate Medical Care原始文件上，仅记录该受试者在该次访视中有喘息加重，并未记录喘息的程度。

4. 您未能保存足够的关于试验药物数量的处置记录［21 CFR 312.62（a）］

具体而言，入组试验方案［不公开］的受试者17001，其库存药物处置表上记录2000年12月30日归还的药片数量为15片，但是在eCRF上记录受试者当天归还的药片却是12片。

5. 您未能确保伦理委员会对临床研究进行跟踪审查［21 CFR 312.62］

具体而言，21 CFR 312.62要求研究者确保所有研究活动的更改应及时向IRB报告。2000年10月16日对试验方案［不公开］做了修订。然而，在FDA检查期间，您未能提供IRB批准2000年10月16日修订文件的批件复印件。因此，您未能证实已及时向IRB报告了研究活动的这次变动。

本警告信的目的并非是罗列您在试验药物临床研究中的所有缺陷。确保遵循法律和相关FDA法规的每一项要求是您的职责。您必须解决这些缺陷，并建立规程，确保任何正在进行的或未来进行的研究都遵循FDA法规。

自收到这封信的15个工作日内，您必须书面告知本办公室为预防将来类似违规已经采取或将要采取的措施。如果不能充分、迅速地对上述违规作出解释，可能导致我们在不再通知的情况下采取监管措施。

附：英文原文

Nasim, Golzar, M.D.

WARNING LETTER

MAY1, 2008

CERTIFIED MAIL
RETURN RECEIPT REQUESTED

Ref: 08-HFD-45-0204

Nasim Golzar, MD
26516 Crenshaw Blvd
Palos Verdes Peninsula, CA 90274-3970

Dear Dr. Golzar:

Between July 24, 2007 and August 22, 2007, Ms. Yvette Lacour-Davis representing the Food and Drug Administration (FDA), conducted an investigation and met with you to review your conduct of the following clinical investigations of the investigational drug [ ] performed for [ ]

1. Protocol [ ] entitled "Prospective, Randomized, Double-Blind, Three-armed, Multi-Center, Comparative Trial to Evaluate the Efficacy and Safety of [ ] BID for 7 days vs. [ ] BID for 10 days vs. Cefuroxime axetil 250 mg PO BID for 10 days in the Treatment of Acute Bacterial Sinusitis".

2. Protocol [ ] entitled "Prospective, uncontrolled, open label, multi-center clinical trial evaluating the efficacy and safety of [ ] BID for 10 days in the treatment of patients with community acquired pneumonia".

3. Protocol [ ] entitled "Prospective, randomized, double-blind study comparing .[ ] BID for 5 days with Azithromycin for 5 days (500 mg PO day 1, then 250 mg PO OD days 2-5) in the treatment of patients with acute exacerbation of chronic bronchitis".

This inspection is a part of FDA's Bioresearch Monitoring Program, which includes inspections designed to evaluate the conduct of research and to ensure that the rights, safety, and welfare of the human subjects of the study have been protected.

From our review of the establishment inspection report, the documents submitted with that report and your September 18, 2007 letter written in response to the Form FDA 483, "Inspectional Observations", we conclude that you did not adhere to the applicable statutory requirements and FDA regulations governing the conduct of clinical investigations and the protection of human subjects.

We are aware that at the conclusion of the inspection, Ms. Lacour-Davis presented and discussed with you Form FDA 483, Inspectional Observations. We wish to emphasize the following:

1. You failed to obtain informed consent of each human subject in accordance with 21 CFR 50 [21 CFR 312.60].

Specifically, 21 CFR 50.20 states that except as provided in 21 CFR 50.23 and 21 CFR 50.24, no investigator may involve a human being as a subject in research covered by these regulations unless the investigator has obtained the legally effective informed consent of the subject or the subject's legally authorized representative. In addition, except as provided in 21 CFR 56.109(c), informed consent shall be documented by the use of a written consent form approved by the IRB [21 CFR 50.27(a)].

The following violations were noted in reference to Protocol [ ]

a. Four of 23 subjects (4011, 4015, 4019, and 4021) had protocol-specified baseline laboratory blood samples drawn prior to signing and dating the informed consent document.

b. The IRB approved informed consent document required documentation of the actual time in which legally effective informed consent of the subject was obtained. There was no documentation of the actual time in which subjects 4016, 4017 and 4018 signed and dated the consent· forms. In addition, we were unable to verify that these subjects signed and dated the informed consent forms prior to any protocol specified procedures being conducted on them.

In your September 18, 2007 written response, you noted that in all cases the subject had been verbally consented prior to any study procedures being performed. Verbal consent, however, is inadequate. The exceptions in 21 CFR 50.23 and 21 CFR 50.24 to the informed consent requirements, as well as the exception in 21 CFR 56.l09(c) to use of the written consent form approved by the IRB, did not apply to the conduct of this study.

2. You failed to ensure that the studies were conducted according to the approved protocols [21 CFR 312.60].

a. The following violations were noted for Protocol [ ]

i. The protocol specified that to be included in the study the patient must have a clinical diagnosis of acute sinusitis with signs and symptoms present for > 7 days but < 28 days as defined by A) radiographic and B) clinical criteria. The radiographic evidence for inclusion in the study included the presence of any of the following: evidence of air-fluid levels, opacification, and/or >6 mm mucosal thickening. Ten of the 30 enrolled subjects 43007, 43009, 43011, 43012, 43013, 43014, 43015, 43019, 43021, and 43030 failed to meet the protocol required radiographic documentation for inclusion in the study. Specifically, x-rays for these subjects failed to demonstrate acute sinusitis.

ii. The protocol specified that subjects who received systemic antimicrobial agents for more than 24 hours within 7 days prior to enrollment had to be excluded from the study. Subject 43002 was enrolled in the study on 12/12/00 even though the subject had been taking Doxycycline during this exclusionary time period.

iii. For 9 of 30 subjects (43001, 43002, 43003, 43004, 43005, 43006, 43009, 43013, and 43014), a paranasal [ ] view x-ray was not done at the Test of Cure visit, as required by the protocol. In your September 18, 2007, written response, you noted that the patients all had clinical signs and symptoms highly suggestive of acute bacterial sinusitis and would have been treated with antibiotics regardless of enrollment in the study. This answer is inadequate. FDA regulations require that investigators enrolling subjects into FDA regulated clinical research studies follow the investigational plan to help ensure that data collected during the study is reliable and that the rights, safety and welfare of research participants are protected.

b. Protocol [ ] specified that subjects who were prematurely withdrawn from the study were to have a complete clinical assessment, a sputum specimen collected for gram stain, culture and susceptibility testing, and all safety laboratory investigations performed as required by the protocol. The protocol further noted that if an alternate antimicrobial agent was prescribed, this testing should be performed prior to initiation of therapy with the alternate agent. In addition, the protocol specified that these prematurely withdrawn subjects were to have a clinical assessment, including a chest x-ray performed 2 to 4 days after the last dose of therapy with the alternate antibiotic. We note that Subjects 17001 and 17003 were prematurely withdrawn from the study, but did not have their sputum collected, nor did they have post alternate antibiotic chest x-rays taken as required by the protocol.

c. The following violations were noted for Protocol [ ]

ⅰ. Protocol version #1, amendment #1, (dated October 15,2000) specified that for a course of therapy to be microbiologically valid, inclusion in the study required that at least one causative organism be identified in an appropriate pre-treatment sputum specimen (i.e. epithelial cells $<$10/low power field (lpf), WBC $\geqslant$25/lpf). Protocol version #2, amendment #2, (dated December 8, 2000) [hereinafter "the protocol"] further clarified this inclusion criterion noting that if the sputum sample at enrollment had $<$ 25 WBC/lpf, obtaining another sputum sample that demonstrated$>$ 25 WBC/lpf would be acceptable, provided that the patient has received no more than 48 hrs of study medications at the time the second sputum sample was collected. Subjects 4001 and 4004 were enrolled in the study even though their sputum samples did not have the protocol required inclusion criterion of $>$ 25 WBC/lpf.

ⅱ. The protocol specified that at the time of enrollment, a medical history was to be obtained, including past history of respiratory illnesses, smoking history, an inquiry regarding any underlying illness or conditions, and general health status. A complete medical history was not obtained for Subjects 4001, 4002, 4003, and 4004 as required by the protocol.

ⅲ. The protocol specified that at the time of enrollment, a baseline urinalysis test would be performed. Subjects 4001 and 4002 did not have this test as required by the protocol.

ⅳ. The protocol specified that within 48 hrs prior to enrollment, the subject must provide a purulent or muco-purulent sputum by deep expectoration for gram stain, culture, and susceptibility testing. Subject 4010 was unable to produce the protocol required sputum specimen for enrollment; however you still dispensed study medication to this subject.

ⅴ. The protocol specified that at the Test of Cure visit, subjects were to have a serum pregnancy test. Subjects 4002, 4003, and 4007 did not have the test as required by the protocol.

In your September 18, 2007, written response, you noted that patients coming into the office with an acute infection need to be treated quickly. You further stated that study participants had to be screened, enrolled and randomized in a manner that is typically much faster than for other types of non-infectious disease clinical trials; hence there was no in-depth review of screening with all lab and x-ray data in hand before randomization. This answer is inadequate. FDA regulations require that clinical investigators enrolling subjects into FDA regulated clinical studies follow the investigational plan to help ensure the reliability of data collected during the study and that the rights, safety and welfare of research participants are protected.

3. You failed to maintain adequate and accurate case histories that record all observations and other data pertinent to the investigation on each individual [21 CFR 312.62(b)].

a. The clinical signs and symptoms of disease that you reported in the electronic case report form for protocol #[ ] could not be verified against information within the source documents for the 17 of 30 subjects enrolled in the study: 43001, 43002, 43004, 43005, 43006, 43007, 43008, 43009, 43010, 43011, 43012, 43013, 43014, 43015, 43016, 43017, and 43019. A memorandum to file dated 2/12/2001, found during the FDA inspection, noted that "Currently, for all study visits up to 2/12/2001, all specific sinusitis symptoms, and the subsequent ratings entered in the [ ] system, have on occasion no supporting documents. Going forward, all specific sinusitis symptoms, or any visit specific data entered into the [ ] system shall have supporting documents." FDA confirmed the lack of source documents during its inspection. We note that all 17 subjects noted above were enrolled into the study prior to 2/12/2001.

b. We note that there was discrepant information between the case report form and the source documentation for the baseline clinical signs and symptoms of disease at the pre-therapy visit on 1/24/01, for Subject 4001 enrolled in protocol [ ] Specifically, on 4/12/01, you signed and dated a change to the case report form for Subject 4001, which noted that the subject had moderate and not mild wheezing. However, the P.V. Family & Immediate Medical Care source document completed for the pre-therapy visit on 01/24/01 only noted that Subject 4001 had increased wheezing at this visit and did not note the extent of the wheezing.

4. You failed to maintain adequate investigational drug disposition records with respect to quantity [21 CFR 312.62(a)].

Specifically, the Inventory Drug Disposition Log for Subject # 17001 enrolled in protocol # [ ] lists the number of tablets returned as 15 on 12/30/00. However, the electronic Case Report Form, lists the number of tablets returned by the subject 12/30/00 as 12 tabs.

5. You failed to assure Institutional Review Board (IRB) continuing review of clinical investigation [21 CFR 312.66].

Specifically, 21 CFR 312.66 requires clinical investigators to assure that all changes .in the research activity are promptly reported to the IRB. An amendment to Protocol [ ] was made on October 16, 2000. However, during the FDA inspection you failed to provide a copy of the IRB approval of the October 16, 2000 amendment. Thus, you have failed to demonstrate that you promptly reported this change in research activity to the IRB.

This letter is not intended to be an all-inclusive list of deficiencies with your clinical study of an investigational drug. It is your responsibility to ensure adherence to each requirement of the law and relevant FDA regulations. You must address these deficiencies and establish procedures to ensure that any on-going or future studies will be in compliance with FDA regulations.

Within fifteen (15) working days of your receipt of this letter, you must notify this office in writing of the actions you have taken or will be taking to prevent similar violations in the future. Failure to adequately and promptly explain the violations noted above may result in regulatory action without further notice.

If you have any questions, please contact Tejashri Purohit-Sheth, M.D., at 301-796-3402; FAX 301-847-8748. Your written response and any pertinent documentation should be addressed to:

Tejashri Purohit-Sheth, M.D.
Acting Branch Chief
Good Clinical Practice Branch Ⅱ
Division of Scientific Investigations
Office of Compliance
Center for Drug Evaluation and Research
White Oak Bldg 51, Rm 5358
10903 New Hampshire Ave.
Silver Spring, MD 20993

Sincerely yours,

{See appended electronic signature page}

Leslie Ball, MD
Director
Division of Scientific Investigations
Office of Compliance
Center for Drug Evaluation and Research

第144封　给Brar, Saroj医学博士的警告信

2008年3月20日

参考号：08-HFD-45-0301

尊敬的Brar博士：

2007年4月24日至5月18日，Karen Kondas女士代表FDA进行了检查，与您会面并对您开展的两项临床研究进行了审查：

- 试验方案［不公开］题目为"3期临床试验：一项在患有精神分裂症的受试者中进行的随机、双盲、安慰剂对照、平行组临床研究，以评价棕榈酸帕利培酮在防止复发中的作用"，IND［不公开］申办者为强生制药研发有限责任公司。
- 试验方案［不公开］题目为"一项3期随机、安慰剂对照、双盲临床研究：评估［不公开］药物在持续使用锂或丙戊酸/双丙戊酸钠用于治疗急性躁狂或混合性发作的受试者中的安全性和有效性"，申办者为［不公开］公司。

本次现场检查是FDA的生物研究监查项目的一部分。该项目通过设定的检查方法，评估研究的实施情况，并确保这些研究中受试者的权益、安全和福利得到了保护。

经对FDA现场检查报告（EIR）、该报告的附件以及您2006年6月6日（FDA于2007年6月8日收到）对FDA483表书面回复进行审查，我们认为，您没有遵循适用的法律要求和监管临床研究实施及受试者保护的FDA法规。我们知道，在现场检查结束时，检查员Kondas女士向您出示并讨论了FDA483表，即现场检查发现的问题。我们想强调以下几点：

1. 您未能获得使用研究药物的受试者的知情同意［21 CFR 312.60和21 CFR 50.20］

试验方案［不公开］4.2部分要求受试者签署知情同意文件（ICD），以表明他们了解了研究的目的和过程。该方案还要求，不提供本人同意的受试者将被排除。现场检查发现，一名监护人于2006年2月20日为受试者607382签署了ICD。由于知情同意的原因，申办者于2006年4月18日建议该受试者终止临床试验。

您2006年6月6日的信函并没有解释与受试者607382有关的知情同意问题。您的信函并没有解释与受试者607086有关的知情同意问题。该受试者同意当住院并经受妄想期痛苦的时候参加开放标签阶段的研究。您坚持该受试者的知情同意是有效的，部分原因是因为在他首次同意参加临床试验时就被告知进入了研究的开放标签阶段。这种说法是不正确的。对研究阶段的了解并不足以证明对这些阶段进行知情同意。而且，受试者能够在研究的任何时间撤回同意，这强调了实际情况，即按照方案的要求，知情同意必须在每一个研究阶段独立执行［21 CFR 50.25（a）（8）］。

2. 您未能保护在您的监护下受试者的权益、安全和福利［21 CFR 312.60］

a. 试验方案［不公开］6.1.3部分要求，在研究的维持阶段受试者每四周被给予试验药物，而且给药剂量可以在第9、13、17、21周根据受试者的临床需要增加或减少。检查发现，受试者607089在2005年12月27日、研究的维持阶段进行了他的第6次访视，并接受了试验药物。记录证明受试者607089在8天后的2006年1月4日进行了一次非计划的访视，并被给予了另一个剂量的试验药物。

在2006年6月6日的回复中，您表示这个错误当天就被协调者发现，通知了申办者，并写了一个SOP。记录证实申办者建议您每周联系受试者，询问副作用。没有查到2006年1月4日后您联系这名受试者来检查副作用的记录。

b. 检查发现受试者607384入组本研究，2006年2月28日被给予了试验药物，出现代谢失调并于2006年3月10日并被送往医院。直到2006年5月24日，对妄想型精神分裂症症状加重的不良事件记录才被报告给IRB。

3. 您未能进行研究或确保按照研究计划进行研究［21 CFR 312.60］

a. 试验方案［不公开］3.5.1部分，允许受试者在筛选期内接受劳拉西泮治疗，最大剂量4mg/d。基线评估（第1天）之后，方案允许在第一个7天的盲化治疗期间，最大剂量2mg/d。受试者如果不能够减少每日的劳拉西泮摄入量，将被排除出本研究。受试者1006于2006年4月5日参加本研究筛选，2006年5月7日开始接受盲化试验药物。记录显示，这名受试者于2006年4月5日被给予4.5mg劳拉西泮，每日4次；2006年4月6日被给予3.0mg劳拉西泮，每日3次；2006年4月7日被给予5.0mg劳拉西泮，每日4次；2006年4月8日和4月10日被给予3.0mg劳拉西泮，每日3次。这远远超过方案所允许的筛选期和第一个7天的盲化治疗期间的剂量。

在您2006年6月6日的回复中，您表示受试者1006在筛选期和研究的第一个7天内没有给予劳拉西泮。但是，之前和伴随用药表都证实了上述的剂量。

b. 试验方案［不公开］3.1.1部分规定在筛选之前，受试者要用碳酸锂或丙戊酸钠持续治疗至少两周；而且，方案规定，如果筛选时情绪稳定剂的谷期血清浓度不在治疗范围内（0.6~1.2mEq/L），该剂量应重新调整。如果筛选时情绪稳定剂的谷期血清浓度是亚治疗剂量的，情绪稳定剂的剂量必须适当地增加，受试者在重新评估之前应继续用新的剂量治疗7天。记录显示，受试者1012在筛选前接受碳酸锂治疗仅12天，而不是要求的14天。检查还发现受试者1011于2006年8月1日参加本研究筛查。记录显示，该受试者筛选时的碳酸锂水平在亚治疗范围（0.5mEq/L），碳酸锂的剂量由900mg/d上调为1050mg/d，该受试者于4天后的2006年8月4日被随机入组。

您2006年6月6日的回复没有对未能确保受试者1012在筛选前接受满两周的碳酸锂治疗进行解释。您的信函也认可，受试者1011本应该在碳酸锂剂量上调后和接受随机之前等待7天。

c. 试验方案［不公开］3.1.2部分要求，受试者在基线访视后一周（研究第1天和第8天）接受第二个剂量的试验药物。检查员发现，受试者607384于2006年2月28日接受了试验药物的初始注射，于10天之后的2006年3月10日接受了试验药物的第二次注射。

4. 您未能保存对研究中每个受试者的所有研究观察结果和其他相关数据的足够及准确的病历［21 CFR 312.62（b）］

a.具体而言，检查发现对试验方案［不公开］，试验药物工作表记录受试者607084 2006年12月20日接受了编号171466的药物，而访视确认工作表记录该受试者那天接受的药物来自171398研究药盒。试验药物记录又显示受试者607084，2007年1月4日接受了171396研究药盒，而访视确认工作表显示那天171396、171466、171467研究药盒被分发了。一份随后的受试者药物表记录，受试者607084于2007年1月12日接受了编号171466及171467的口服药物，同一天接受了编号132306的注射药物，而访视确认工作表显示仅有编号132306的注射药物。此外，受试者访视记录显示，受试者607084于2007年1月12日14:55分接受了编号132306的注射。

您2006年6月6日的回复信件声称药盒171466于14:55给药，但是并没有提供日期或者对上面描述的多处不一致进行解释。

b. 试验方案［不公开］3.7.3部分要求，在门诊的基础上完成研究的受试者应当至少每周联系一次，以检查他们的情况。

受试者1007于2006年5月1日完成了21天访视，作为门诊患者开始治疗，检查没有发现相关文件可以证实您按照要求联系该受试者检查他/她的情况。受试者1009，2006年5月5日出院，2006年7月18日作为门诊患者完成了该研究，或受试者1012，2006年11月11日作为门诊患者完成了该研究，检查也没有发现文件可以证实他们在门诊期间被联系过。

您2006年6月6日的回复信表示，通常您根据需要“经常地”联系完成了研究的受试者，但是您没有记录这些联系。

c. 试验方案［不公开］4.6部分，提前终止该研究，或者完成了该研究，但是没有进入40周开放标签扩展研究的受试者，要在7天和30天进行一次随访调查，以确定是否发生过不良事件。检查员发现受试者1011于2006年8月17日终止该研究，但是没有文件显示该受试者在7天或30天被联系过。

您2006年6月6日的回复，没有解决这个问题。

d. 试验方案［不公开］原始记录证实，受试者1006由于病情恶化，在2006年5月11日接受了一次计划外的访视，这次访视在病例报告表中没有记录。

您2006年6月6日的回复函表示，通知了申办者，研究协调员被告知在接下来的访视中收集任何数据。您没有提供您联系过的申办者或您在随后的访视中收集了相关数据的记录。

5. 您未能保存足够药物处置记录［21 CFR 312.62（a）］

a. 特别指出的是，检查员发现对于［不公开］试验方案［不公开］记录证实受试者607384在2006年2月28日被随机化到编号132154研究药盒。但是，试验药物工作表和药物计量记录表证实，那天这名受试者接受了编号132165研究药盒。记录显示，编号132154研究药盒被归还给申办者，解释是“没有用过”。这个错误直到2006年3月24日才记录在研究记录中。

您2006年6月6日的回复函表示这个错误被发现，编号132165研究药盒被丢弃了。您的回复没有充分地解释编号132154研究药盒怎样以没有用过而被归还给申办者，以及根据您所回复的编号132165研究药盒如何被丢弃了。

b. 检查员发现［不公开］试验方案［不公开］怎样以受试者1011在2006年8月1日、受试者1009在2006年4月19日和4月21日，关于碳酸锂用药的合并用药工作表和eCRF，与医院记录不一致。

您2006年6月6日的回复函表示这个错误被查到了，通知了申办者，数据被纠正了。但是，您没有提供数据被纠正的任何记录。

本警告信的目的并非是罗列您在试验药物临床试验研究中存在的所有缺陷。确保遵循法律和FDA法规每一项要求是您的职责。您必须解决这些缺陷，并建立规程，确保任何正在进行的或将来进行的研究都符合FDA法规。

自收到本警告信的15个工作日内，您应当书面告知本办公室为防止将来发生类似违规情况您已经或计划采取的措施。如果不能对上述违规行为进行充分、快速地解释，可能导致我们在不再通知的情况下采取监管措施。

附：英文原文

Brar, Saroj M.D.

WARNING LETTER

Mar 20, 2008

CERTIFIED MAIL
RETURN RECEIPT REQUESTED

Ref: 08-HFD-45-0301

Saroj Brar, M.D.
2012 West 25th Street
Cleveland, Ohio 45237

Dear Dr. Brar:

Between April 24 and May 18, 2007, Ms. Karen Kondas, representing the Food and Drug Administration (FDA), conducted an investigation and met with you, to review your conduct of two clinical investigations:

- Protocol [redacted] entitled "Phase 3: A Randomized, Double-Blind, Placebo-Controlled, Parallel-Group Study Evaluating Paliperidone Palmitate in the Prevention of Recurrence in Subjects with Schizophrenia" IND [redacted] sponsored by Johnson & Johnson Pharmaceutical Research & Development LLC., and
- Protocol [redacted] "A Phase 3, Randomized, Placebo-Controlled, Double-Blinded Trial Evaluating the Safety and Efficacy of [redacted] in Subjects Continuing Lithium or Valproic Acid/Divalproex Sodium for the Treatment of an Acute Manic or Mixed Episode," sponsored by [redacted].

This inspection is a part of FDA's Bioresearch Monitoring Program, which includes inspections designed to evaluate the conduct of research and to ensure that the rights, safety, and welfare of the human subjects of the study have been protected.

From our review of the establishment inspection report and the documents submitted with that report, and of your June 6, 2006 [received by FDA on June 8, 2007] letter written in response to the Form FDA 483, we conclude that you did not adhere to the applicable statutory requirements and FDA regulations governing the conduct of clinical investigations and the protection of human subjects. We are aware that at the conclusion of the inspection, Investigator Kondas presented and discussed with you Form FDA 483, Inspectional Observations. We wish to emphasize the following:

1. You failed to obtain informed consent of the subjects to whom the study drug was administered [21 CFR § 312.60; 21 CFR § 50.20].

Section 4.2 of Protocol [redacted] required that subjects sign the informed consent document (ICD) to indicate they understood the purpose of the study and procedures. The protocol also stated that subjects would be excluded if they could not provide their own consent. The investigation found that a guardian signed the ICD for Subject 607382 on February 20, 2006. The sponsor recommended this subject be immediately discontinued from the study for consenting reasons on April 18, 2006.

Your response letter dated June 6, 2006 did not address the issue of consent related to Subject 607382. Your letter did address the issue of informed consent related to Subject 607086. This subject consented to the open-label phase of the study while hospitalized and suffering periods of delusion. You assert that this subject's consent was valid in part because the subject had been informed of the open-label phase of the trial at the time the subject first consented to trial participation. This assertion is improper. Knowledge of trial phases does not suffice to demonstrate informed consent to those phases. Moreover, a subject can withdraw consent at any time during a study, which underscores the fact that informed consent must be established independently at each trial phase required under the protocol [21 CFR § 50.25(a)(8)].

2. You failed to protect the rights, safety, and welfare of subjects under your care [21 CFR § 312.60].

a. Section 6.1.3 of Protocol [redacted] required that subjects be administered study medication every four weeks during the maintenance phase of the study, and that doses may be increased or decreased at Weeks 9, 13, 17 and 21 in response to subject clinical needs. The investigation found that Subject 607089 had his Period 6 Visit during the maintenance phase of the study, on December 27, 2005 and received study medication. Records document that Subject 607089 then presented for an unscheduled visit on January 4, 2006, eight days later, and was administered another dose of study medication.

In your response letter dated June 6, 2006, you state that this mistake was recognized on the same day by the coordinator, that the sponsor was notified, and that an SOP was written. Records document that the sponsor advised you to contact the subject weekly for side effects. There is no documentation that you contacted this subject after January 4, 2006 to check for side effects.

b. The investigation found that Subject 607384, who was enrolled into the study and administered study medication on February 28, 2006, began to decompensate and was admitted to the hospital on March 10, 2006. No record was found for the adverse event of exacerbation of symptoms of paranoid schizophrenia being reported to the IRB until May 24, 2006.

3. You failed to conduct the studies or ensure they were conducted according to the investigational plans [21 CFR § 312.60].

a. Section 3.5.1 of Protocol [redacted] allowed subjects to receive lorazepam during the screening phase at a maximum dose of 4 mg/day. Following baseline (Day 1) assessment, the protocol allowed a maximum of 2 mg/day during the first seven days of blinded therapy. Subjects were to be excluded from the study if unable to reduce their daily lorazepam intake. Subject 1006 was screened for the study on April 5, 2006 and began receiving blinded study medication on April 7, 2006. Records indicate that this subject was administered 4.5 mg lorazepam/four times a day on April 5, 2006; 3.0 mg lorazepam/three times a day on April 6, 2006; 5.0 mg lorazepam/four times a day on April 7, 2006; and 3.0 mg lorazepam/three times a day on April 8 and April 10, 2006. This was more than the doses allowed by the protocol during the screening phase and the first seven days of blinded therapy.

In your response letter dated June 6, 2006, you state that Subject 1006 was not administered lorazepam during the screening phase and first seven days of the study. However, the Prior and Concomitant Medication Worksheet documents the aforementioned doses.

b. Section 3.1.1 of Protocol [redacted] states that subjects be treated continuously with lithium or valproic acid for at least two weeks immediately prior to screening. Furthermore, the protocol states that if the mood stabilizer trough serum concentration was not in the therapeutic range (0.6 - 1.2 mEq/L) at screening, the dose should be re-adjusted. If the mood stabilizer trough serum concentration at screening was sub-therapeutic, the mood stabilizer dose must be increased appropriately and the subject continued on this new dose for seven days prior to reevaluation. The records indicate that Subject 1012 received lithium for only 12 days prior to screening rather than the required 14. The investigation also found that Subject 1011 was screened for the study on August 1, 2006. Records indicate that this subject's lithium level was in the sub-therapeutic range (0.5 mEq/L) at screening. The dose of lithium was adjusted upward to 1050 mg/day from 900 mg/day. This subject was randomized on August 4, 2006, four days later.

Your response letter dated June 6, 2006 does not address the failure to ensure that Subject 1012 received lithium for the full two weeks prior to screening. Your letter agrees that Subject 1011 should have waited seven days after adjusting her lithium dose upwards and before being randomized.

c. Section 3.1.2 of Protocol [redacted] required that subjects receive a second dose of study medication one week after the baseline visit (on Study Days 1 and 8). The investigation found that Subject 607384 received an initial injection of study medication on February 28, 2006 and a second injection of study medication on March 10, 2006, or 10 days later. .

4. You failed to maintain adequate and accurate case histories that record all observations and other data pertinent to the investigation on each individual [21 CFR § 312.62(b)].

Specifically, the investigation found:

a. For Protocol [redacted] the study medication worksheets document Subject 607084 received medication number 171466 on December 20, 2006, whereas the Visit Confirmation worksheet documents that this subject received medication from study kit 171398 on that date. Study medication records next indicate that Subject 607084 received study kit 171396 on January 4, 2007, whereas the Visit Confirmation worksheet shows study kits 171396, 171466, and 171467 were dispensed on that date. A later Subject Medication worksheet documents that Subject 607084 [redacted] received Oral Medication Number 171466 and 171467 on January 12, 2007, and received Injection Medication number 132306 on that date, but the Visit Confirmation worksheet shows only Injection Medication number 132306. In addition, the Subject Visit notes indicated that Subject 607084 received Injection Number 132306 at 14:55 on January 12, 2007.

Your response letter dated June 6, 2006, states that medication kit 171466 was administered at 14:55, but does not provide a date, or explain the multiple discrepancies delineated above.

b. Section 3.7.3 of Protocol [redacted] required that subjects completing the study on an outpatient basis be contacted at least once a week to check on their condition. The investigation found no documentation to verify that Subject 1007, who completed the 21-Day visit on May 1, 2006 and began treatment as an outpatient, was contacted to check on his/her condition, as required. Nor did the investigation find documentation to verify that Subject 1009, who was discharged on May 5, 2006 and completed the trial as an outpatient on July 18, 2006, or Subject 1012, who completed the trial as an outpatient on November 11, 2006, were contacted during the outpatient period.

Your response letter dated June 6, 2006 states generally that you contacted subjects who completed the study "on a regular basis" as required, but that you did not document these contacts.

c. Section 4.6 of Protocol [redacted] required that subjects who discontinued the study early, or completed the study, but did not enter the 40-week open-label extension trial, have a follow-up interview at days 7 and 30, to determine if adverse events had occurred. The investigation found that Subject 1011 discontinued the study on August 17, 2006, but there was no documentation to indicate that this subject was contacted on Days 7 or 30.

Your response letter dated June 6, 2006 does not address this issue.

d. For Protocol [redacted] source records document that Subject 1006 was seen for an unscheduled visit on May 11, 2006 due to exacerbation of their disease. This visit was not documented on a Case Report Form.

Your response letter dated June 6, 2006, states the sponsor was informed, and the study coordinator was told to collect any data on the following visit. You did not provide documentation that you contacted the sponsor or that you gathered any data at the following visit, however.

5. You failed to maintain adequate drug disposition records [21 CFR § 312.62(a)].

a. Specifically, the investigation found that for Protocol [redacted] the [redacted] records document that Subject 607384 was randomized to study kit number 132154 on February 28, 2006. However, the study medication worksheet and the drug accountability records document that this subject received study kit 132165 on that date. Records indicate that study kit 132154 was returned to the sponsor with an explanation of "not used." This error was not documented in the study records until April 24, 2006.

Your response letter dated June 6, 2006 states that the error was recognized and study kit 132165 was discarded. Your response does not adequately explain how study kit 132154 could have been returned to the sponsor as not used, and how study kit 132165 was discarded, as per your response.

b. The investigation found that the concomitant medication worksheets and eCRFs concerning Lithium dosing for Subject 1011 in Protocol [redacted] on August 1, 2006, and for Subject 1009 for April 19, 2006 and April 21, 2006, were inconsistent with hospital records.

Your response letter dated June 6, 2006 states that the error was detected and that the sponsor was informed and the data were rectified. You did not provide any documentation that the records were rectified, however.

This letter is not intended to be an all-inclusive list of deficiencies with your clinical studies of investigational drugs. It is your responsibility to ensure adherence to each requirement of the law and relevant FDA regulations. You must address these deficiencies and establish procedures to ensure that any on-going or future studies will be in compliance with FDA regulations.

Within fifteen (15) working days of your receipt of this letter, you should notify this office in writing of the actions

you have taken or will be taking to prevent similar violations in the future. Failure to adequately and promptly explain the violations noted above may result in regulatory action without further notice.

If you have any questions, please contact Joseph Salewski at (240) 276-3395; FAX (240) 276-8848. Your written response and any pertinent documentation should be addressed to:

Joseph Salewski
Branch Chief (Acting)
Good Clinical Practice Branch Ⅱ,
Division of Scientific Investigations
Office of Compliance
Center for Drug Evaluation and Research
10903 New Hampshire Avenue
Bldg 51, Room 5348
Silver Spring, MD 20993

Sincerely yours,

{See appended electronic signature page}

Leslie Ball, M.D., Director
Division of Scientific Investigations, HFD-45
Office of Compliance
Center for Drug Evaluation and Research

第145封　给Shah, Ashok医学博士的警告信

2008年3月19日

参考号：08-HFD-45-011

尊敬的Shah博士：

2007年4月30日至5月17日，Brunilda Torres女士代表FDA进行了检查，与您会面并审查了您实施的申办者为赛诺菲-安万特制药公司（原安万特制药公司）、试验药物为泰利霉素（Ketek®）的下述临床研究的情况：

- 试验方案［不公开］"一项随机、双盲、平行组、多中心研究，比较泰利霉素与阿奇毒素对社区获得性下呼吸道感染的门诊患者的临床疗效。"
- 试验方案［不公开］"一项随机、开放、多中心试验，评价进行常规治疗的呼吸道感染的门诊患者口服泰利霉素（Ketek®）与阿莫西林/克拉维酸（安灭菌®）治疗的安全性和有效性。"

此次现场检查是FDA的生物研究监查项目的一部分。该项目通过设定的检查方法，评估研究的实施情况，并确保这些研究中受试者的权益、安全和福利得到了保护。

根据现场检查，以及对现场检查报告和相关支持文件的审查，我们认为，您没有遵循适用的法律要求和监管临床研究实施及受试者保护的FDA法规。

在现场检查结束时，Torres女士向您出示并讨论了FDA 483表，即现场检查发现的问题。我们确认收到了您于2007年5月18日对该FDA483表部分条目作出的书面回复。我们想强调以下几点：

1. 您未能确保按照研究计划进行研究［21 CFR 312.60］

试验方案［不公开］

a.在13位入组受试者中有9位未达到肺功能试验合格标准。对于入组试验方案4.2.1部分要求受试者具有记录在案的慢性支气管炎病史且过去12个月内伴有：①基础FEV1为预测值的70%~35%；②FEV1/FVC＜70%的受试者才能入组。您没有确保所有入组受试者都满足肺功能试验（PFT）入选标准，而这一试验标准是诊断AECB不可缺少的。

i. 受试者1和5用以入组受试者的PFT结果缺少受试者的人口学信息和做PFT的日期。FEV1和FEV1/FVC合格标准无法核实，因为肺功能试验存档报告的页面顶部，没有包含写有受试者信息和人口学资料（姓名、检查日期和时间、性别、药物治疗、身高、体重等信息）的页眉。这一顶部部分似乎被移除了，使得我们难以确认受试者的身份及其入选的合格性。您不能提供额外文件来证明这些PFT报告的来源。

ii. 现场检查时，受试者2，4，8和11没有合格PFT存档文件。

iii. 受试者3，7和12的PFT报告显示这些受试者未能满足入选标准，因为他（她）们的FEV1和/或FEV1/FVC测量值未小于70%。

在您2007年5月18日的书面回复中，您声明自己误解了PFT的要求。我们无法接受这一理由，因为作为主要研究者，您必须理解并遵守试验方案中所列出的要求。您不能遵守试验方案制定的入选标准，不仅会令人关注贵研究场所产生的试验数据的有效性，而且会使本来未达到入选标准的受试者暴露于不必要的风险之中。

b. 关于入组，试验方案4.2.1部分要求受试者必须具有记录在案的慢性支气管炎病史且过去12个月内至少有一次慢性支气管炎急性加重（AECB）发作史。您未能确保所有受试者都满足这一试验方案制定的标准。例如，

i. 没有原始文件能够支持受试者1在过去12个月内至少发作过一次AECB。虽然在该受试者2006年1月13

日的口述记录的页面底部手写记录其有过两次AECB发作史，最后一次是2005年6月，但是受试者的医疗记录中没有可以确认以上表述的支持文档。

ii. 没有原始文件能够支持受试者2在过去12个月内至少发作过一次AECB。该受试者2005年11月21日口述的临床访视记录在CRF中被列为能够证明过去12个月内发作过AECB的合格的访视记录，在“评估”的下方记录着该受试者曾患“急性单纯性支气管炎”。但是，有一条未标注日期的手写注释写着“AECB”，但对这一注释没有进一步解释。由于急性单纯性支气管炎与慢性支气管炎急性加重（AECB）截然不同，因此按照这一记录很难支持该受试者在过去12个月内有过AECB发作。

c. 试验方案7.2.1部分要求育龄妇女需做妊娠试验。您没有给受试者4和11进行妊娠试验。

在我们收到的2007年5月18日您的反馈信中，您说受试者4在入选时月经来潮，但是我们认为您的这一回复无法令人接受。试验方案中并没有指出月经来潮时可以不进行妊娠试验。

关于受试者11，您在回复中指出该名受试者过早绝经。但是，没有原始记录可以支持其过早绝经。而且，请注意第一次随访的原始文档工作表第6页，上面写着“自然绝经伴功能失调性子宫出血，”然而这一条被划掉了，且没有给出任何解释，因此不清楚为什么这句话被划掉。

d. 试验方案4.3部分将已知的肾功能不全列为排除标准。但是，根据其在诊所2004年7月27日的门诊记录，您入选的受试者［不公开］患有慢性肾功能不全。

这位受试者应当从研究中排除。考虑到该受试者伴有的肾功能不全，您没有将其排除，而导致其暴露于潜在的危害中。

e. 试验方案6.2.1部分禁止辛伐他汀、洛伐他汀或者阿托伐他汀与泰利霉素同时使用。但是，受试者1和12却被开具了试验方案排除标准中禁止使用的药物。例如，

i. 受试者1既往和伴随治疗的研究总汇总中（CRF的第30页）列出其自2005年6月6日开始持续应用Vytorin（一种依折麦布和辛伐他汀的复方制剂）治疗。表中未标明终止使用时间，而且“持续应用吗？（在治疗终点）”标记框被做了标记。

ii. 受试者12在 2006年2月22日基线随访时相应的口述记录中将复方烟酸洛伐他汀缓释片（一种烟酸和洛伐他汀的复方制剂）列为一种持续应用的药物，但是该受试者的记录中没有证据表明复方烟酸洛伐他汀缓释片被停用。

我们收到您2007年5月18日的回复函，在信中您声明对于进行抗生素治疗的患者，您使其停止使用任何他汀类药物5~7天，所以您认为试验期间该患者没有使用任何他汀类药物。但是，原始文件和CRF文档都不能支持这一说法。

f. 试验方案5.5部分要求试验药物必须锁在限制进出的地方，但是您自己对FDA检查员承认，试验药物是放在一个曾用于储藏医学标本且未上锁的柜子里，而这个柜子放在没有限制进出存放门诊复印机的房间。

试验方案［不公开］

g. 试验方案6.2部分要求“受试者在进入试验时及试验中的任何时间接受的任何治疗都必须如实地记录在病例报告表中。”而以下受试者在最近7天内伴随的药物治疗或抗生素应用却没有在病例报告表中进行报告：

i. 受试者17接受头孢唑啉注射。

ii. 受试者19接受林可霉素注射。

iii. 受试者33接受头孢唑啉注射。

iv. 受试者59接受头孢唑啉注射。

在评价一种抗生素疗效的研究中，合并使用抗生素治疗会对研究结果的解释产生重要的影响，因此，若不对以上伴随治疗进行报告会对研究结果产生潜在的影响。

h. 试验方案8.3部分要求对于8.2部分所指定的观察期内出现的任何不良事件均应当记录于病例报告表中。对于受试者68您没有在病例报告表中记录其两次不良事件。具体而言：

ⅰ. 受试者68在第2次随访时报告出现左手麻刺感4天。

ⅱ. 在2003年2月27日的门诊随访表中记录了受试者68报告“当血糖下降时出现头晕和视物模糊”，在第3次随访的口述记录中写着“头晕和晕倒”。但是在CRF中并未报告。而且，试验方案8.1.4要求视物模糊必须作为特别注意的不良事件进行汇报，但是您并没有在病例报告表中进行报告。

ⅰ. 试验方案7.2.2部分要求初始随访后的17～22天内必须完成治疗后随访。受试者31，61和68的第2次随访没有在试验方案所规定的时间窗内完成。

2. 您未能保存记录研究中每个受试者的与研究相关的所有观察结果和其他相关数据的足够及准确的病历［21 CFR 312.62（b）］

试验方案［不公开］

a. 在几种情况下，研究-随访口述记录进行了回溯性的手写注释修改，但没有标注日期。您在现场检查时承认，口述记录在口述后平均4天才能拿到。这些注释包括但不限于AECB症状和峰流量结果。因为这些手写注释均未标注日期，因此无法确认信息添加上去的时间。以下列举若干，但不仅限于这些：

ⅰ. 受试者5 2005年9月29日的口述记录包括一处未标注日期的手写注释，“AECB”，但是评估报告显示为上呼吸道感染。没有有关为何标注“AECB”和没有标注日期的原因的说明。

ⅱ. 受试者2 2006年1月16日的口述记录的底部记录了峰流量值140，130和120；但是4天后的原始文档中没有可以支持这些添加测量值的证据。

ⅲ. 受试者3 2006年1月17日的口述记录的底部记录了峰流量值100，110和100；但是4天后的原始文档中没有可以支持这些添加测量值的证据。

b. 对于13名受试者中的12名，您对其临床随访表、CRF和/或原始文档工作表做了后期修改，但是并未给出解释。以下列举几个例子，但并不止这些：

ⅰ. 受试者1，2，4和5，第1次随访的CRF中列出了肺功能试验条目，但它们后来又被划掉，没有任何解释。

ⅱ. 受试者1的基线随访CRF中，您初始记录着该受试者满足所有入选和排除标准；然而，在2006年7月25日（受试者入组5个多月后）的记录上注释着该受试者不满足所有合格标准。

ⅲ. 受试者4 2006年1月23日第1次随访的临床随访表中，体温97.9被划掉，又写上了99。对于体温的修改未作出书面解释。

ⅳ. 此外，受试者4的CRF第1次随访的相关药物/手术史部分，有若干条目被划掉，加上“糖尿病”和“无性生活和月经来潮”，但未作出解释。

ⅴ. 受试者8的CRF中2006年2月8日第1次随访记录的“糖尿病”被划掉，但未作出解释。

ⅵ. 受试者11 2006年2月17日的门诊口述记录的底部，手写着“Ketek过敏”，之后又被划掉。请注意该受试者入组日期是2006年2月17日，而修改日期是4月27日。对于这一修改未作出解释。

c. 许多受试者的门诊口述记录、临床随访表、原始文档工作表和/或CRFs记录的信息间存在矛盾。以下列举几个例子，但并不限于此：

ⅰ. 受试者12的CRF上记录的符合资格的AECB发作时间是2005年3月5日，但是根据门诊口述记录，随访时间是2005年3月25日。

ⅱ. 受试者5 2006年1月26日的门诊口述记录中记录着该受试者有水泡音和喘息，但是2006年1月26日的原始文档工作表中却记录无水泡音，无喘息。

ⅲ. 受试者4 第1次随访的原始文档工作表上，在是否是育龄期妇女的方框中勾选了“不是”，但是在第1次随访的CRF中，这个方框勾选了“是”，修改处被圈了出来。

ⅳ. 受试者8 2006年2月8日第1次随访的原始文档工作表中记录着该受试者少量咳痰，但是，在同一天的门诊口述记录或临床随访表中没有当天痰量的原始记录。

3. 您未能在受试者参加临床研究前获得其知情同意［21 CFR 50.20］

试验方案［不公开］

具体而言，受试者1签署知情同意书的时间是2001年11月15日；然而，CRF记录着该受试者进入研究的时间是2001年11月5日。根据这一记录，该受试者在知情同意前便进入了试验。

4. 您未能正确地记录书面的知情同意，因为知情同意文件未经受试者本人或其合法授权代理人签署姓名或日期［21 CFR 50.27（a）］

试验方案［不公开］

具体而言：

a. 受试者1似乎没有在知情同意书上签名。知情同意书签名区中的签名与使用和公开个人健康信息授权书中的签名看起来截然不同。

b. 您在现场检查时承认，并声称当您的所有参与受试者的知情同意书上签署日期时，没有任何受试者在知情同意书上签署日期。

5. 您未能向受试者或受试者合法授权代理人提供经过IRB批准并签署姓名和日期的书面知情同意文件的复印件［21 CFR 50.27（a）］

试验方案［不公开］

a. 没有文件可以表明您向每一位受试者提供了已签上姓名和日期的知情同意书复印件。在现场检查时，您已向FDA区域检查员承认了您没有提供给受试者签名的知情同意书复印件。

试验方案［不公开］

b. 受试者9 2001年12月17日的研究访视记录表明，您2001年12月15日向该受试者提供了知情同意书复印件，然而这一日期是受试者实际同意日期的前两天，也没有文件显示该受试者在2001年12月15日来过诊室。

本警告信的目的并非是罗列您在试验药物临床研究中存在的所有缺陷。确保遵循法律和相关FDA法规的每一项要求是您的职责。您必须解决这些缺陷，并建立规程，以确保任何正在进行或将来进行的研究均能符合FDA的法规。

自收到这封信的15个工作日内，您应当书面告知本办公室为预防将来发生类似违规情况已经采取或计划采取的措施。如果不能充分、迅速地对上述违规问题作出解释，可能导致我们在不再通知的情况下采取监管措施。

附：英文原文

Shah, Ashok M.D.

WARNING LETTER

Mar 19, 2008

CERTIFIED MAIL
RETURN RECEIPT REQUESTED

Ref: 08-HFD-45-011

Ashok Shah, M.D.
3808 South Hopkins Avenue
Titusville, FL 32780

Dear Dr. Shah:

Between April 30,2007 and May 17,2007, Ms. Brunilda Torres, representing the Food and Drug Administration (FDA), conducted an investigation and met with you to review your conduct of the following clinical investigations of the investigational drug Telithromycin (Ketek®), performed for Sanofi-Aventis Pharmaceuticals (formerly Aventis Pharmaceuticals):

1. Protocol [ ] "A Randomized, Double-Blind, Parallel-Group, Multicenter, Study to Compare Clinical Health Outcomes of Telithromycin versus Azithromycin in Outpatients with Community-Acquired Lower Respiratory Tract Infections."

2. Protocol [ ] "A Randomized, Open-Label, Multicenter Trial of the Safety and Effectiveness of Oral Telithromycin (Ketek®) and Amoxicillin/Clavulanic Acid (Augmentin®) in Outpatients with Respiratory Tract Infections in Usual Care Settings."

This inspection is a part of the FDA's Bioresearch Monitoring Program, which includes inspections designed to evaluate the conduct of research and to ensure that the rights, safety, and welfare of the human subjects of those studies have been protected.

Based on this inspection, and from our review of the establishment inspection report and its supporting documents, we conclude that you did not adhere to the applicable statutory requirements and FDA regulations governing the conduct of clinical investigations and the protection of human subjects. At the conclusion of the inspection, Ms. Torres presented and discussed with you the Form FDA 483, Inspectional Observations. We acknowledge receipt of your letter dated May 18, 2007, responding to some items on the Form FDA 483, and wish to emphasize the following:

1. You failed to conduct the study in accordance with the investigational plan [21 CFR 312.601].

Protocol [ ]

a. Nine (9) out of 13 enrolled subjects failed to meet eligibility criteria with respect to pulmonary function testing. For enrollment, Protocol Section 4.2.1 required that subjects have a documented history of chronic bronchitis with 1) a basal FEVl between 70% and 35% predicted and 2) an FEVl/FVC <70% in the past 12 months. You failed to ensure that all enrolled subjects met Pulmonary Function Test (PFT) inclusion criteria, which was integral to the diagnosis of AECB.

i. For Subjects 1 and 5, PFT results used to enroll subjects lack the subject's demographic information, and the date that the test was performed. FEVl and FEVl/FVC eligibility criteria could not be verified as the pulmonary function test on file did not contain the header which includes subject information and demographic data (name, date and time of test, gender, medications, height, weight, etc.), which is printed on the top of the page. It appears that this top section was removed, making it difficult to confirm the subject's identity and therefore subject eligibility for entry. You were unable to provide additional documentation to verify the source of these PFT reports.

ii. For Subjects 2, 4, 8, and 11, there was no qualifying PFT on file at the time of the inspection.

iii. For Subjects 3, 7, and 12, PFT reports reveal that these subjects failed to meet inclusion criteria as their FEVl and/or FEVl /FVC measurements were not < 70%.

In your May 18, 2007 written response, you stated that the PFT requirement was misunderstood by you. This is not an acceptable response. As a principal clinical investigator, you are required to understand and adhere to the requirements set forth in the protocol. Your failure to adhere to inclusion criteria as specified in the protocol has not only raised questions about the validity of the data generated by your site, but also exposed subjects, who may not have been eligible for study entry, to unnecessary risk.

b. For enrollment, Protocol Section 4.2.1 required that subjects have a documented history of chronic bronchitis with at least one episode of an acute exacerbation of chronic bronchitis (AECB) in the past 12 months. You failed to ensure that all subjects met this protocol specified criterion. For example,

i. There is no source documentation to support that Subject #1 had at least one episode of AECB in the past 12 months. Although there is a handwritten note on the bottom of the dictated note dated 1/13/06 stating that the subject had 2 episodes of AECB, the last reported one in June 2005, there are no supporting documents in the subject's medical records to confirm these statements.

ii. There is no source documentation to support-that Subject #2 had at least one episode of AECB in the past 12 months. The dictated clinic visit note dated 11/21/05, which is listed as the qualifying visit for documentation of AECB in the past 12 months in the CRF, states under "Assessment," that the subject had "Acute simple bronchitis." However, there is a handwritten annotation which lists AECB, which is not dated, and there is no explanation for the annotation. As acute simple bronchitis is quite different from acute exacerbation of chronic bronchitis (AECB), it is difficult to support that this subject had an AECB within the past 12 months per this documentation.

c. Protocol Section 7.2.1 required that women of childbearing potential have pregnancy tests conducted. You failed to administer pregnancy tests in Subjects #4 and #ll.

We acknowledge your May 18, 2007 response, in which you stated that Subject #4 was menstruating at the time of enrollment; however, we find your response unacceptable. The protocol did not provide any exceptions with respect to conducting a pregnancy test and concurrent menstruation.

With respect to Subject #11, we acknowledge your response that this subject had early menopause. However, there is no source documentation to support that this subject had early menopause. Furthermore, note that on page 6 of the Source Document Worksheet for Visit 1, it lists "natural menopause with dysfunctional uterine bleeding," however, this has been crossed out without explanation. It is unclear why this was crossed out.

d. Protocol Section 4.3 lists known renal dysfunction as an exclusion criterion. However, you enrolled Subject #8 into this study, when this subject has chronic renal insufficiency, per documentation by a clinic note visit to the [ ] Medical Office, dated 7/27/04.

This subject should have been excluded from study entry. Your failure to exclude this subject from the study exposed the subject to potential harm, given his concomitant renal insufficiency.

e. Protocol section 6.2.1 prohibits the concomitant use of simvastatin, lovastatin, or atorvastatin with telithromycin. However, Subjects #1 and 12 were prescribed medications that were prohibited under the protocol exclusion criteria. For example

i. For Subject #1, the Study Summary Forms for Previous and Concomitant Treatments (page 30 of the CRF) lists Vytorin (a combination of ezetemibe and simvastatin) as ongoing therapy initiated on 06 JUN 2005. There is no end date provided and the tick box for "ongoing? (at end of therapy)" is checked off.

ii.For Subject # 12, the dictated note corresponding to the baseline visit, 2/22/06, lists Advicor (a combination of Niacin and lovastatin) as an ongoing medication. However, there is no evidence in the subject's records that Advicor was discontinued.

We acknowledge your May 18, 2007 response letter that states that it is your practice to stop all statin drugs in patients on antibiotic therapy for 5-7 days and "therefore, this patient didn't take any statins during the trial." However, source and CRF documentation do not support this statement.

f. Protocol Section 5.5 required that study drugs be locked in an area with restricted access; however, per your own admission to the FDA investigator, the study drug was kept inside an unlocked cabinet used to store medical samples and the cabinet was inside an unrestricted access room where the clinic photocopy machine was kept.

Protocol [ ]

g. Protocol section 6.2 required that "all treatments being taken by the subjects on entry to the study or at any time during the study…be documented as such on the case report form." Concomitant medications or antibiotics taken within the last seven days were not reported on the case report form for the following subjects:

i. Subject #17 received a Cefazolin injection

ii. Subject #19 received a Lincocin injection

iii. Subject #33 received a Cefazolin injection

iv. Subject #59 received a Cefazolin injection

The use of concomitant antibiotic treatments in a study evaluating the efficacy of an antibiotic can critically affect the interpretation of results of the study, and therefore the failure to report such concomitant therapies could potentially impact study outcome.

h. Protocol Section 8.3 requires that all adverse events that occur during the observation period set forth in Section 8.2 must be documented on the pages provided in the case report form. For Subject #68, you failed to report two separate adverse events on the case report form. Specifically,

i. Subject #68 reported that she experienced left hand tingling for four days at Visit #2.

ii. Subject #68 reported "lightheadedness and blurry vision when sugar drops" as documented on your clinic visit form dated 2/27/03 and you documented "dizziness and passing out spells" on your dictated note for Visit #3. However, this was not reported on the CRF. Furthermore, Protocol Section 8.1.4 required that blurred vision be reported as an adverse event of special interest; however, you failed to report this on the case report form.

i. Protocol Section 7.2.2 required that post-therapy visits be completed within 17 to 22 days of the initial Visit 1. For Subjects #3 1, #61, and #68, Visit 2 was not conducted within the required protocol window.

2. You failed to maintain adequate and accurate case histories that record all observations and other data pertinent to the investigation on each individual [21 CFR 312.62(b)].

Protocol [ ]

a. In several instances, the study-visit dictated notes were modified by retroactive handwritten annotations on the record, which were not dated. Per your own admission at the time of the inspection, the dictated notes were not available for an average of four days post-dictation. These annotations included, but were not limited to AECB symptoms and peak flow results. Since these handwritten annotations were not dated, the date that the information was added could not be verified. Examples include, but are not limited to the following:

i. For Subject #5, the dictated note dated 9/29/05 includes a handwritten annotation of "AECB" which is not dated. However, the assessment stated upper respiratory tract infection. There is no explanation as to why AECB was annotated on this note nor when this annotation was made.

ii. For Subject #2, the bottom of the dictated note dated 1/16/06 documents peak flow values of 140, 130, and 120; however, there is no source documentation to support the addition of these measurements 4 days later.

iii. For Subject #3, the bottom of the dictated note dated 1/17/06 documents peak flow values of 100, 110, and 100; however, there is no source documentation to support the addition of these measurements 4 days later.

b. For 12 of 13 subjects, you made retroactive corrections to data on the clinic visit form, CRF and /or Source Document Worksheets without explanation. Examples include but are not limited to the following:

i. For Subjects #1, #2, #4, and #5, on the CRF for Visit 1, lung function test entries are listed; however, they are later crossed out without rationale.

ii. For Subject # 1, it is noted that on the CRF for the baseline visit, you had initially noted that the subject met all inclusion and exclusion criteria; however, on 7/25/06 (over 5 months after subject enrolled into the study) the record was annotated to state that the subject did not meet all eligibility criteria.

iii. For Subject #4, a temperature of 97.9 was crossed out and 99 was written on the clinic visit form for Visit 1, dated 1/23/06. There is no written explanation as to why the temperature was changed.

iv. Additionally for Subject #4, there are several entries crossed out on the Visit 1 Relevant Medical/Surgical

History section on the CRF, to include "Diabetes," and "not sexually active and menstruating," without explanation.

v. For Subject #8, on the CRF for Visit 1 dated 2/8/06, "Diabetes Mellitus," is crossed out without explanation.

vi. For Subject #11, on the bottom of the dictated clinic note dated 211 7/06, there is a handwritten annotation that states "allergy to Ketek," which has later been crossed out. Note that the subject was entered into the study on 2/17/06 and the date of the correction is 4/27. No explanation was provided for the correction.

c. Discrepancies were noted between information on your dictated clinic notes, clinic visit forms, source document worksheets and/or CRFs for various subjects. Examples include but are not limited to the following:

i. For Subject # 12, the qualifying episode of AECB was listed as 05 March 2005 on the CRF; however, per the dictated clinic note, the date of the visit was 3/25/05.

ii. For Subject #5, the dictated clinic note dated 1/26/06 documents that the subject had rales and wheezes; however, the Source document Worksheet for 1/26/06 documents rales and wheeze as absent.

iii. For Subject #4, on the Source Document Worksheet for Visit 1, the box in response to whether the female is of childbearing age is checked "No." However, on the CFR for Visit 1, this box is checked as "yes" and circled as a correction.

iv. For Subject #8, the Source Document Worksheet for Visit 1 dated 2/8/06, documents that the subject had mild sputum production; however, the dictated clinic visit note or the clinic visit form for this same date fails to provide source documentation for the sputum production.

3. You failed to obtain informed consent prior to involving a human being as a subject in clinical research. [21 CFR 50.201]

Protocol [ ]

Specifically, Subject #1 signed the Informed Consent Document on 1111 5/01; however, the CRF documents that the subject was entered into the study on 11/5/01. Per this documentation, the subject was enrolled into the study prior to obtaining informed consent.

4. You failed to properly document written informed consent in that the Informed Consent Document was not signed or dated by the subject or the subject's legally authorized representative. [21 CFR 50.27(a)]

Protocol [ ]

Specifically,

a. For Subject #I, it appears that the subject did not sign the Informed Consent Document. The signature in the signature block of the informed consent appears quite distinct from that noted on the signature on the Authorization to Use and Disclose Personal Health Information.

b. None of the subjects dated the Informed Consent Document per your own admission at the time of the inspection, when you stated that you dated the Informed Consent Documents of all participating subjects.

5. You failed to provide a copy of the signed and dated written Informed Consent Document, which had been approved by the IRB to the subject or subject's legally authorized representative [21 CFR 50.27(a)].

Protocol [ ]

a. There is no documentation available to indicate that a copy of the signed and dated Informed Consent Document was provided to each subject. This was confirmed by your own admission to the FDA Field Investigator at the time of the inspection that you did not provide the subjects a copy of the signed Informed Consent Document.

Protocol [ ]

b. For Subject #19, study visit notes dated 12/17/2001 indicate a copy of the Informed Consent Document was provided to the subject on 12/15/2001, two days before the subject was actually consented. There is no documentation to indicate that this subject attended the clinic on 12/15/2001.

This letter is not intended to be an all-inclusive list of deficiencies with your clinical study of an investigational drug. It is your responsibility to ensure adherence to each requirement of the law and relevant FDA regulations. You must address these deficiencies and establish procedures to ensure that any on-going or future studies will be in

compliance with FDA regulations.

Within fifteen (15) working days of your receipt of this letter, you must notify this office in writing of the actions you have taken or will be taking to prevent similar violations in the future. Failure to adequately and promptly explain the violations noted above may result in regulatory action without further notice.

If you have any questions, please contact Joseph Salewski, at (240) 276-8821; FAX (240) 276-8844. Your written response and any pertinent documentation should be addressed to:

Joseph Salewski
Deputy Director
Division of Scientific Investigations IHFD-45
Office of Compliance
Center for Drug Evaluation and Research
7520 Standish Place
Rockville, MD 20855

Sincerely yours,

{See appended electronic signature page]

Leslie Ball, M.D.
Director
Division of Scientific Investigations lHFD-45
Office of Compliance
Center for Drug Evaluation and Research

第146封　给 Whittier, Frederick 医学博士的警告信

2008年3月6日

参考号：08-HFD-45-1201

尊敬的Whittier博士：

2007年8月22日至9月12日，Stephen Kilker先生代表FDA进行了现场检查，与您会面并审查了您实施的申办者为［不公开］、试验药物为［不公开］的下列临床研究的情况：

- 试验方案［不公开］，题为"一项Ⅱ期，多中心、开放、滴定法研究，评估对原来使用一种口服降糖药治疗且血糖控制不佳的2型糖尿病患者，［不公开］剂量上调至一次200mg，每日两次后的有效性、安全性和耐受性的研究"；
- 试验方案［不公开］，题为"一项随机、双盲、安慰剂对照、平行分组的研究，比较［不公开］和安慰剂在合并使用甲氨蝶呤治疗的中、重度活动性风湿性关节炎患者且对既往抗［不公开］治疗反应不佳的患者的安全性和症状体征的改善情况"；
- 试验方案［不公开］，题为"长期扩展研究，评价在完成［不公开］核心研究治疗的患者用［不公开］治疗的安全性"。

本次现场检查是FDA的生物研究监查项目的一部分。该项目通过设定的检查方法，评估由FDA监管的相关研究的实施情况，并帮助确保这些研究中人类受试者的权益、安全和福利得到了保护。

经对现场检查报告、该报告的附件，以及您于2007年10月8日对FDA 483表，即现场检查发现的问题给予的书面回复进行审查，我们认为，您没有遵循适用的法律要求以及监管临床研究实施和受试者保护的FDA法规。我们知道在现场检查结束时，Kilker先生向您出示并讨论了FDA 483表，即现场检查发现的问题。我们想强调以下几点：

1. 您未能按照研究计划进行临床研究［21 CFR 312.60］

关于试验方案［不公开］

a. 在试验方案［不公开］中，被随机的9名受试者中有3名受试者符合排除标准，但并未被排除在本研究之外。这3名受试者的具体情况如下：

i. 受试者5676［不公开］符合排除标准是因为入组前之前曾使用过一种试验性药物进行治疗，所以没有进入本研究的资格。具体而言，这位受试者在2005年8月17日以前一直接受另一种试验性药物治疗，筛选前药物清洗时间小于5个半衰期，符合排除标准。试验方案［不公开］规定，对既往使用任何试验药物治疗的排除标准为：筛选4周（或试验药物的5个半衰期，两个时间中取时间长的）内的治疗。在您之前实施的一项研究［不公开］中，受试者5676［不公开］最后一次接受研究试验药物的时间是2005年8月17日。FDA检查期间在您诊所发现的［不公开］研究的研究者手册（版本日期2005年8月9日）说明［不公开］药物在类风湿关节炎患者的半衰期约为13天。基于该药半衰期为13天，受试者5676要直到2005年8月17日之后5个半衰期或65天后才有资格进行研究筛选。但是该受试者在［不公开］研究的筛选日期为2005年9月28日，距离［不公开］最后一次给药时间仅42天（［不公开］最后一次给药日期2005年8月17日至筛选日2005年9月28日等于42天）。在2007年10月8日的回复中，您指出该受试者入组［不公开］时尚不知道［不公开］药物的半衰期。您提到［不公开］药物的半衰期在研究者手册第12版（版本日期2007年2月26日）提供，但这是该受试者已经入组后才收到。然而如上所述，FDA检查期间在您的诊所中发现了版本日期为2005年8月9日的研究者手册，该版本的研究者手册已经标明［不公开］药物在类风湿关节炎患者中的半衰期约为13天。

ⅱ. 受试者5678［不公开］病历中记录受试者在1998年曾有数月的环磷酰胺（癌得星®）用药史，环磷酰胺是一种被排除的前期治疗药物。试验方案［不公开］规定曾接受过任何烷化剂（例如环磷酰胺）治疗的患者均需被排除。该受试者入组研究［不公开］研究并于2005年10月31日接受第一次试验药物治疗。在2005年11月22日申办者的方案例外、违背/偏离表显示该受试者接受了口服剂量的环磷酰胺（癌得星®），在1998年3月和4月剂量为100mg、每日两次，在1998年5月到9月为100mg、每日一次。在2007年10月8日的回复函中，您声明受试者4578服用癌得星®的时间长度是按周计算，不是按月。受试者的病史与这个声明相矛盾，而且无论如何，方案规定曾使用任何烷化剂都需被排除在外。

ⅲ. 受试者5925［不公开］在2006年1月17日接受过康宁克通®（曲安奈德）注射，违背了方案。试验方案［不公开］规定，受试者在基线前6周内关节内或者肠外使用过糖皮质激素的受试者需要被排除。受试者5925的基线访视是2006年2月23日，2006年1月17日的医疗记录病历记录了该受试者在门诊访视时右肩接受了一次康宁克通®注射。在2006年3月23日备注文件中声明，在例行病历审查中，注意到受试者5925在2006年1月17日接受了一次关节注射，然而，研究护士在筛选时并不知道有这次注射。您2007年10月8日的回复函中声明筛选时研究协调员不知道这次康宁克通®注射。您表示，受试者没有将这一信息告知研究协调员，而且筛选时2006年1月17日的病历口述没有出现在受试者的图表中。然而，在记录了这次康宁克通®注射的2006年1月17日下方，有一张日期为2006年2月6日的手写字条显示“当新的研究组要开始进行筛选时，研究护士会打电话给病人患者，”表明在2006年2月9日筛选之前，患者的病历确实体现了这次康宁克通®注射。作为一名临床研究者，确保遵从方案规定的合格标准是您的职责。

b.在［不公开］方案，被随机的9名受试者中有2名不符合入组标准，但没有被排除在试验之外。这些受试者的详细情况如下：

ⅰ. 受试者5680［不公开］在基线的6周内泼尼松用量大于10mg/d，违背了方案。试验方案［不公开］规定，如果在基线前剂量能稳定至少6周，则允许口服皮质类固醇激素（≤10mg/d的泼尼松或等效的其他激素）。但是，受试者5680的病历记录了在受试者随机日期（即2005年12月7日）之前22天，也就是2005年11月15日泼尼松使用剂量为上午10mg和晚上5mg。同一记录包含了医生建议受试者减少泼尼松用量为5mg、每天两次以有资格参加本研究要求。因此，在基线前该受试者的泼尼松剂量没有稳定足够的时间，也超过了方案允许的剂量（10mg/d）。在2007年12月8日的回复函中您并没有解释这项方案违背。

ⅱ 受试者5924［不公开］的基线前泼尼松剂量稳定没有达到要求的时间。如上所述，试验方案［不公开］规定，如果在基线前剂量能稳定至少6周，则允许口服皮质类固醇激素（≤10mg/d的泼尼松或等效的其他激素）。受试者5924的基线访视时间是2006年2月14日。该受试者2006年1月25日的病历显示“因为缺乏疗效，她中断了泼尼松治疗，但剂量是5mg、每周两次”。病历记录中记录此次随访时医生建议泼尼松用量2.5~5mg早上顿服。该受试者2006年2月6日的“合并用药”表列明泼尼松用量为2.5 mg/d，但该表上所有合并用药的“起始时间”栏均没有时间记录。而且，载明既往和伴随治疗的病例报告表记录泼尼松用量为2.5mg/d，但未记录开始治疗日期。在受试者5924基线后约8个月，日期为2006年10月16日、在2006年10月23日签名的文件备注声明，在2006年1月25日医生的病程记录上泼尼松剂量应该显示的是泼尼松2.5mg/d。该备注文件声明，受试者5924，泼尼松2.5mg/d开始于2005年12月10日。在2007年10月8日的回复函中，您重申：该受试者于2005年12月10日开始泼尼松2.5mg/d、每天一次治疗，至2006年2月14日的基线访视前超过6周。但是，这个在事情发生后数月才记录的信息，显然与该受试者2006年1月25日访视当时或大概的时间由医生写的病程记录相冲突。

关于试验方案［不公开］

c.受试者5679［不公开］在基线前两周内口服过抗生素，违背了方案，但没有被排除在研究外。受试者［不公开］加入2006年5月31日开始的长期扩展研究［不公开］。试验方案［不公开］规定，基线前两周内发生的任何需要口服抗生素治疗的重大感染事件是需要排除的。该研究［不公开］于2006年5月31日开始的第24周的退出访视记录显示，受试者于2006年5月24号开始使用吉速星®（甲磺酸吉米沙星）320mg口服治疗呼吸道感染7天。相应的CRF页记录了抗生素治疗的开始和结束时间，分别为2006年5月23日和2006年5月27日。但在2007年10月8日的回复函中，您并没有解决解释这个问题。

关于试验方案［不公开］

d. 受试者8903［不公开］在2006年11月9日采血检测发现有ALT升高，符合1周内复查的方案标准。但是，在2006年11月14日，重测样本的申请单被错误地标记为“血脂”而不是“肝功能”，从而导致于2006年11月21日重新检测ALT，超过了方案规定的1周的复查时间窗。具体来说，试验方案［不公开］要求，ALT值大于正常上限3倍时必须在1周内重新检测。如果ALT升高被确定，使用试验药物的治疗必须停止，受试者退出试验。中心实验室规定的ALT正常值上限是34，受试者8903于2006年11月9日采血检测的ALT结果为108，符合超过正常值上限3倍的标准。临床研究场所于2006年11月13日收到该结果，2006年11月21日重新检测结果为135。由于药物引起肝酶升高，受试者于2006年11月21日被终止研究，但是该受试者继续服用研究药物直到2006年11月20日。您2007年10月8日的回复函已收到，重测样本的文书错误也提到了。但是，因为没有在方案规定的时间区间内进行复测，将受试者暴露于潜在的危害中。

2.您没有保留记录了每位受试者与研究相关的所有观察发现和其他数据的足够准确的病历［21 CFR 312.62(b)］

关于试验方案［不公开］

a. 在完成最初评估很久以后，研究协调员追溯地对许多病例中评估员做的关节数量做了改变修改。下表提供了最初评估后被更改的肿胀和疼痛的关节数量的例子：

受试者	最初的评估员	初始评估日期	由谁进行更改	对评估更改的日期
5680	某某	2005年12月7日：基线随访访视	某某	2006年1月16日
5680	某某	2006年4月12日：失访18周	某某	2006年4月24日
5924	某某	2006年2月6日：筛查	某某	2006年4月26日
5924	某某	2006年2月14日：基线访视	某某	2006年4月24日
5924	某某	2006年2月28日：2周访视	某某	2006年2月28日和2006年4月24日
5924	某某	2006年3月14日：4周访视	某某	2006年3月30日和2006年4月24日
5924	某某	2006年7月6日：20周访视	某某	2006年7月24日
5925	某某	2006年2月23日：基线访视	某某	2006年3月13日

您在2007年10月8日的回复函中声明，努力修改病例报告表是为了对申办者发出的质疑进行回复。但是，您并没有解释在最初评估很久以后，修改的评估如何被确定。此外，您指出受试者5924有一个无法评估的关节被持续报告，因此做了修正。但是，针对受试者评估所做的额外更改并不涉及无法评估的关节。

关于协议［不公开］

b. 为受试者8901［不公开］制作了一份新的PK（药代动力学）样本制备记录，原始的被废弃，但没有充分的解释。原始记录上的信息一直受到申办者的监查员的质疑，基于2006年11月2日的监查报告，新的记录包含以前在原始记录中未曾显示的信息。具体来说，2006年10月10日申办者监查员的信件声明，eCRF中标记受试者8901第4周的［不公开］样本没做，但原始PK日志却完成了，记录了该样本的离心时间和处理细节。应监查员的请求，访视期间PK日志中的样本处理信息被删除，这个修改有首字母签名并注明日期。但是，下次的监查访视中之后，监查员在2006年11月2日的信件中指出受试者8901的PK日志跟她前次监查访视时看到的不一样。监查员写道，上次随访中她见证的这些修改在新创建的日志中消失了，在新的日志上［不公开］样本被标记为“未做”。新创建的日志也包含所有PK处理信息，而这些信息在上次监查访视时记录为缺失。这些PK处理信息在受试者记录中并未被发现，尽管它是极其重要的原始文件。在2007年10月8日的回复函中，您承认创建了原始日志，并声明原始日志之所以被废弃是因为洒上咖啡导致其“难以辨认”。您也声明已与您的员工一起解决了这个问题。但是，对于在原始记录中没显示的，而在新创建的日志中包含的新的信息，您没有提供足够的解释。

c. 在2006年8月31日受试者8901的［不公开］访视中，原始文件和病程记录似乎是由研究协调员撰写并签署的，但研究协调员那天并不在办公室。在2007年10月8日的回复函中，您承认研究协调员当时在住院，您和另一位员工对受试者进行了访视。此外，您承认研究协调员倒签了访视当日的记录而不是在记录书写的当天签署。您提到您已与您的员工一起解决了这个问题，我们知悉您写了一份说明文件，以澄清病程记录确实是在2006年9月5日撰写的。

d. PK样本处理记录未被完整保存至2006年10月3日。一份2006年11月28日的说明文件指出所有4位受试者（8901，8902，8903和8904）的PK处理信息均未被记录，导致从研究开始至2006年10月3日的信息无法被证实。我们注意到您在2007年10月8日的回复函中承认了这一问题。

本警告信的目的并非是罗列您在试验药物临床研究中存在的所有缺陷。确保遵循法律和相关FDA法规的每一项要求是您的职责。您应当解决这些缺陷，并建立规程，以确保任何正在进行或将来进行的研究均能符合FDA法规。

自收到这封信的15个工作日内，您应当书面告知本办公室为预防将来类似违规情况已经采取或计划采取的措施。如果不能充分、快速地解释上述违规问题，可能导致我们在不再通知的情况下采取监管措施。

附：英文原文

Whittier, Frederick M.D.

WARNING LETTER

Mar 6, 2008

CERTIFIED MAIL
RETURN RECEIPT REQUESTED

Ref: 08-HFD-45-1201

Frederick C. Whittier, M.D.
4565 Dressler Rd. NW, Suite 103
Canton, OH 447 18

Dear Dr. Whitier:

Between August 22 and September 12,2007, Mr. Stephen Kilker, representing the Food and Drug Administration (FDA), conducted an investigation and met with you to review our conduct of the following clinical investigations of the investigational drugs [ ] and [ ] performed for [ ]

• Protocol [ ] entitled “A phase 2, multicenter, open label, titration study to assess the efficacy, safety, and tolerability of [ ] in doses up to 200 mg BID in patients with type 2 diabetes mellitus not optimally controlled with previous treatment with one oral antihyperglycemic agent;”

• Protocol [ ] entitled "A randomized, double-blind, placebo-controlled, parallel group study of the safety and reduction of signs and symptoms during treatment with [ ] versus placebo in combination with methotrexate in patients with moderate to severe active rheumatoid arthritis and an inadequate response to previous anti-[ ] therapy;" and

• Protocol [ ] entitled "Long-term extension study of safety during treatment with [ ] in patients completing treatment in [ ] core studies."

This inspection is a part of the FDA's Bioresearch Monitoring Program, which includes inspections designed to evaluate the conduct of research and to ensure that the rights, safety, and welfare of the human subjects of those studies have been protected.

From our review of the establishment inspection report, the documents submitted with that report, and your October 8, 2007 letter written in response to the Form FDA 483, Inspectional Observations, we conclude that you did not adhere to the applicable statutory requirements and FDA regulations governing the conduct of clinical investigations and the protection of human subjects. We are aware that at the conclusion of the inspection, Mr. Kilker presented and discussed with you Form FDA 483, Inspectional Observations. We wish to emphasize the following:

1. You failed to conduct the clinical investigations according to the investigational plans [21 CFR 312.601].

Regarding Protocol [ ]

a. Of nine subjects randomized in Protocol [ ] three subjects met exclusionary criteria, but were not excluded from the study. The details for these subjects are described below:

i. Subject 5676 [ ] met the exclusionary criterion for previous treatment with an investigational agent, and therefore was not eligible for the study. Specifically, this subject received treatment with another study drug until August 17, 2005, less than 5 half-lives prior to screening, an exclusionary criterion. Protocol [ ]specifies the exclusionary criterion for previous treatment with any investigational agent as treatment within four weeks (or five half-lives of the investigational drug, whichever is longer) of screening. Subject 5676 [ ] was in a prior study under your conduct [ ] in which he received his last study drug dose on August 17, 2005. The investigator brochure (IB)for study [ ] (version date August 9, 2005) found at your clinic during the FDA audit states that the half-life of [ ] in patients with rheumatoid arthritis (RA) is approximately 13 days. Based on a half-life of 13 days, Subject 5676 was not eligible for study screening until 5 half-lives, or 65 days, following the last dose of [ ] on August 17, 2005. However, Subject 5676's screening date for study [ ] was September 28, 2005, only 42 days following his last dose of [ ] last dose of [ ] on 8/17/2005 to screening date of 9/28/2005 = 42 days]. In your October 8, 2007 response letter, you noted that at the time Subject 5676 entered into Study [ ] the half-life of [ ] was not known. You mentioned that the half-life of [ ] was provided in the IB Version 12, dated February 26, 2007, but this was received after the subject was already enrolled. However, the investigator's brochure dated August 9, 2005 was found at your clinic during the FDA audit, as mentioned above. This August 9,2005 version of the IB states that the half-life of [ ] in RA patients is approximately 13 days.

ii. Subject 5678's [ ] medical history documents the use of cyclophosphamide (Cytoxan®), an exclusionary previous treatment, for several months in 1998. Protocol [ ] specifies that any previous treatment with alkylating agents, such as cyclophosphamide, is exclusionary. Subject 5678 was enrolled in study [ ] and received the first dose of study drug on October 31, 2005. The sponsor's Protocol Exception, Violator/Deviator Form dated November 22, 2005 notes that Subject 5678 received twice daily oral doses of cyclophosphamide (Cytoxan®), 100 mg in March and April 1998, and 100 mg once daily from May to September 1998. In your October 8, 2007 response letter, you state that the length of time Subject 4578 was on Cytoxan® was measured in weeks, not months. The subject's medical records contradict this assertion and, in any event, the protocol states that any prior use of alkylating agents is exclusionary.

iii. Subject 5925 [ ] received an injection of Kenalog® (triamcinolone) on January 17, 2006, in violation of the protocol. Protocol [ ] specifies that intra-articular or parenteral corticosteroids administered within six weeks prior to baseline are exclusionary. Subject 5925's baseline visit was February 23, 2006. A January 17, 2006 medical record documents that the subject received an injection of Kenalog® in the right shoulder during a clinic visit. A March 23, 2006 note to file states that during a routine chart review it was noted that Subject 5925 received a joint injection on January 17, 2006, and that the research nurse was not aware of this injection at screening. Your October 8, 2007 response letter states that the Kenalog® injection was not known to the study coordinator at the time of screening. You indicate that the subject did not relay this information to the study coordinator, and at the time of screening, the January 17, 2006 medical record dictation was not present in the subject's chart. However, below the January 17, 2006 progress note documenting the Kenalog® injection, a handwritten note dated February 6, 2006 states that the "study nurse will call patient when new arm of study opens up to be screened," indicating that the patient's medical records did reflect the Kenalog® injection prior to screening on February 9, 2006. As the clinical investigator, it is your responsibility to ensure compliance with protocol-specified eligibility criteria.

b. Of nine subjects randomized in Protocol [ ] two subjects did not meet eligibility requirements. These subjects were not excluded from the study. The details for these subjects are described below:

ⅰ. Subject 5680's[ ] prednisone dose was greater than 10 mg/day within 6 weeks of baseline, in violation of the protocol. Protocol [ ] specifies that oral corticosteroids (≤10 mg/day prednisone or equivalent) are permitted if the dose has been stable for at least 6 weeks prior to baseline. However, Subject 5680's medical records document the subject's prednisone dose as 10 mg in the morning and 5 mg in the evening on November 15, 2005, 22 days prior to the subject's randomization date of December 7, 2005. The same record contains a physician recommendation that the subject decrease his prednisone dose to 5 mg bid to qualify for this study. Accordingly, this subject's prednisone dose was not stable for a sufficient amount of time prior to baseline and exceeded the dose permitted by the protocol (10 mg/day).You did not address this violation in your October 8, 2007 response letter.

ⅱ. Subject 5924's [ ] prednisone dose was not stable for the requisite time prior to baseline. As stated above, Protocol [ ] specifies that oral corticosteroids (≤10 mg/day prednisone or equivalent) are permitted if the dose has been stable for at least 6 weeks prior to baseline. Subject 5924's baseline visit was February 14, 2006. A January 25, 2006 medical record for this subject states that "she discontinued her prednisone for lack of efficacy but the dose was 5 mg twice weekly." The note documents that the physician recommended a prednisone dose of 2.5 mg -5 mg q a.m. at this visit. The"Con Meds" form for this subject dated February 6, 2006 lists the prednisone dose as 2.5 mg per day. None of the medications on the list has a date recorded in the "start date" column. Also, the case report form identifying previous and concomitant treatments documents the prednisone dose as 2.5mg per day, with no start date recorded. A note to file dated October 16, 2006, and signed on October 23, 2006, approximately 8 months after Subject 5924's baseline date, states that the prednisone dose on the January 25, 2006 physician progress note should read prednisone 2.5 mg every day. The note to file states that per Subject 5924, prednisone 2.5 mg daily was started on December 10, 2005. In your October 8, 2007 response letter, you reiterate that the subject began a 2.5 mg daily dose on December 10, 2005, more than 6 weeks before the baseline visit on February 14, 2006. However, this information, recorded months after the fact, is in conflict with the physician›s note apparently written at or about the time of the subject's January 25, 2006 visit.

Regarding Protocol [ ]

c. Subject 5679 [ ] was treated with an oral antibiotic within two weeks prior to baseline, in violation of the protocol, and was not excluded from the study. Subject [ ] rolled over to the long-term extension study, study [ ] May 31, 2006. Protocol [ ] specifies that any major episode of infection requiring treatment with oral antibiotics within two weeks prior to baseline is exclusionary. The May 31, 2006 week 24 withdrawal visit record for Study [ ] documents that the subject was treated for a respiratory infection with Factive® (gemifloxacin mesylate) 320 mg po starting on May 24, 2006 for 7days. The corresponding CFR page documents the start and end dates for this antibiotic as May 23, 2006 and May 27, 2006, respectively. You did not address this observation in your October 8, 2007 response letter.

Regarding Protocol [ ]

d. Subject 8903 [ ] had in an elevated liver enzyme (ALT) result on a sample drawn November 9, 2006 that met the protocol criteria for retesting within one week. However, the requisition for the retest sample on November 14, 2006 was erroneously marked for "lipid panel" instead of a liver panel, which resulted in the ALT retest on November 21, 2006, outside the protocol-specified retesting window of one week. Specifically, Protocol [ ] requires that ALT values greater than three times the upper limit of normal are to be re-measured within one week. If the elevation is confirmed, treatment with the study article must be stopped and the subject withdrawn. The upper limit for ALT as specified by the central study laboratory was 34. Subject 8903's ALT result on a sample from 11/9/2006 was 108, meeting the criterion of greater than three times the upper limit of normal. The ALT result was received by the clinical study site on November 13, 2006. Retesting performed on November 21, 2006 resulted in a value of 135. The subject was discontinued due to medication-induced liver enzyme elevation on November 21, 2006, but had continued to take the study article until November 20, 2006. Your October 8, 2007 response is acknowledged and the clerical error in the retest sample is noted. However, the retesting was not performed within the time frame specified in the protocol, potentially exposing the subject to harm.

2. You failed to maintain adequate and accurate case histories that record all observations and other data pertinent to the investigation on each individual [21CFR 312.62(b)].

Regarding Protocol [ ]

a.A study coordinator retroactively made changes to joint counts performed by assessors in many cases long after the original assessments. Examples of swollen and tender joint counts that were changed after the original dates of assessment are provided in the table below:

Subject	Original Assessor	Date of Original Assessment	Changed by	Date of Change in Assessment
5680	XX	12/7/05: Baseline visit	XX	1/16/06
5680	XX	4/12/06: Escape Week 18	XX	4/24/06
5924	XX	2/6/06: Screening visit	XX	4/26/06
5924	XX	2/14/06: Baseline visit	XX	4/24/06
5924	XX	2/28/06: Week 2 visit	XX	2/28/06 and 4/24/06
5924	XX	3/14/06: Week 4 visit	XX	3/30/06 and 4/24/06
5924	XX	7/6/06: Week 20 visit	XX	7/24/06
5925	XX	2/23/06: Baseline visit	XX	3/13/06

Your October 8, 2007 response letter states that attempts to correct the case report forms were made in response to a query from the sponsor. However, you did not explain how the corrected assessments were determined long after the original assessments were performed. Additionally, you pointed out that subject 5924 had a non-evaluable joint that had consistently been reported, and corrections were made as a result. However, additional changes were made to this subject's assessment that did not pertain to the non-evaluable joint.

Regarding Protocol [ ]

b. A new PK (pharmacokinetic) sample preparation record was made for Subject 8901 [ ] and the original was discarded with no adequate explanation. Information on the original record had been questioned by the sponsor's monitor, and based on a November 2, 2006 monitoring letter, the newly created record contained information that was previously not present on the original record. Specifically, a letter from the sponsor monitor dated October 10, 2006 stated that The [ ]sample at Week 4 for Subject 8901 was marked not done in the eCRF, but the source PK log was completed stating the centrifugation time and processing details for the sample. Per the monitor's request, the sample processing information on the PK log was deleted during the visit, and this change was initialed and dated. However, following the next monitoring visit, the monitor pointed out in a November 2, 2006 letter that the PK log for Subject 8901 was not the same log she saw at the previous monitoring visit. The monitor wrote that the changes she witnessed at the previous visit were missing from the newly created log, and the [ ] sample was labeled as "not done" on the new log. The newly created log also contained all the PK processing information which was noted as missing at the previous monitoring visit. This PK processing information was not found in the subject records, although it is crucial source documentation. In your October 8, 2007 response letter, you acknowledged that the original log was created, and stated that the original was discarded as it was "illegible" due to a coffee spill. You also stated that you have addressed this issue with your staff. However, you did not provide an adequate explanation for the new information contained on the newly created log that had not been present on the original record.

c. For Subject 8901's [ ] visit on August 31, 2006, source and progress notes appear to have been written and signed by a study coordinator, but the study coordinator was not at the office that day. In your October 8, 2007 response letter, you acknowledged that the study coordinator was hospitalized at the time, and you and another staff member performed the subject's visit. Additionally, you acknowledged that the study coordinator back-dated the notes to the day of the visit rather than the day the notes were written. You note that you addressed his issue with your staff, and we acknowledge that you wrote a Note to File to clarify that the progress note was actually written on September 5, 2006.

d. Records of processing of PK samples were not kept adequately through October 3, 2006. A November 28, 2006 Note to File states that PK processing information for all four subjects (8901, 8902, 8903, and 8904) had not been recorded and the information could not be verified from study start through October 3, 2006. We note that you acknowledged this observation in your October 8, 2007 response.

This letter is not intended to be an all-inclusive list of deficiencies with your clinical study of an investigational drug. It is your responsibility to ensure adherence to each requirement of the law and relevant FDA regulations. You should address these deficiencies and establish procedures to ensure that any on-going or future studies will be in compliance with FDA regulations.

Within fifteen (15) working days of your receipt of this letter, you should notify this office in writing of the actions you have taken or will be taking to prevent similar violations in the future. Failure to adequately and promptly explain the violations noted above may result in regulatory action without further notice.

If you have any questions, please contact Constance Lewin, M.D., M.P.H., at (301) 796-3397; FAX (301) 847-8748. Your written response and any pertinent documentation should be addressed to:

Constance Lewin, M.D., M.P.H.
Branch Chief
Good Clinical Practice Branch I
Division of Scientific Investigations, Bldg. 51, Rrn. 5354
Office of Compliance
Center for Drug Evaluation and Research
Food and Drug Administration
10903 New Hampshire Avenue
Silver Spring, MD 20993

Sincerely yours,

{See appended electronic signature page)

Leslie K. Ball, M.D.
Director
Division of Scientific Investigations
Office of Compliance
Center for Drug Evaluation and Research

第147封　给Michael S. Miller，D. O.博士的警告信

2008年2月12日

参考号：CBER-08-02

尊敬的Miller博士：

2007年10月15日至11月5日，FDA对您进行了现场检查，一位FDA检查员与您会面并对您实施临床研究的情况进行了审查，这封信特告知您现场检查的结果。本次现场检查是FDA的生物研究监查项目的一部分，该项目通过设定的检查方法，评估FDA所监管的相关研究的实施情况，现场检查时审查的临床试验包括［不公开］。

现场检查结束时，检查员向您发出并与您讨论了FDA483表，即现场检查发现的问题。

我们已经确认，您违反了发布在美国联邦法规（CFR）第50、312、812部分（可查阅http://www.gpoaccess.gov/cfr/index.html）监管试验药物和医疗器械的临床试验实施的适用法规。对下面列出的每一项违背，都引用了适用的CFR条款。研究1和2与试验药物临床评价有关，受21 CFR 312监管。研究3和4与试验性医疗器械临床评价有关，受21 CFR 812监管。

1. 您未能确保按照21 CFR 50的要求获得知情同意［21 CFR 312.60和812.100］

A. 研究2

i. 在筛选访视时，在研究相关的操作启动时，下列受试者的知情同意书还没有得到受试者签署姓名和日期。

受试者	筛选访视日期	情况
[原文此处被遮蔽]	2006.6.5	2006年7月6日研究协调员记录：该受试者“不经意间漏掉了这张签名页”
[原文此处被遮蔽]	2006.6.19	受试者2006年8月30日签署了知情同意书，但相关记录显示，该名受试者仅在2006年6月16日至6月26日参加了该研究
[原文此处被遮蔽]	2006.7.6	2006年9月7日“解释知情同意的人”在知情同意书上的标注显示，最初签署这份文件时，受试者忽略了这张签名页。应我的请求于2006年8月30日返回，签署了这一页，但签署是最初签署的日期。我也忘了签字，当受试者返回签字的时候我才签的
[原文此处被遮蔽]	2007.2.8	该知情同意书由受试者于2007年5月14日签署，由“解释知情同意的人”于2007年4月30日签署

ii.［不公开］受试者的知情同意书由“解释知情同意的人”签字，日期与受试者在知情同意书上签字的日期不同。因此，并不清楚受试者在知情同意时是否签署了知情同意书。

B. 研究3—某［不公开］受试者的知情同意书没有由受试者签日期。

2. 您未能确保在您的监护下，临床研究按照试验方案、签署的协议、适用法规来进行研究，以保护在您监护下的受试者的权益、安全和福利［21 CFR 312.60和812.100］

A. 研究1

i.［不公开］受试者——尽管该受试者符合筛选失败的标准，但是您还是于2007年3月26日将其随机入组本研究。该受试者的创面于2007年2月19日初始测量为15.1cm^2，2007年3月26日创面减小为7.8cm^2，溃疡面积减少超过30%。试验方案某［不公开］部分描述“如果创面面积改变，相对于筛选时第一次测量，或者a）下降［不公开］……受试者应被考虑为筛选失败，必须退出导入期，转到他们标准的规定治疗。”

此外，试验方案某［不公开］部分要求，在筛选阶段，要进行创面感染评估。但是，根据实验室检查报告，您是在试验第一周采集了该受试者的目标创面拭子。

ii.［不公开］受试者——试验方案［不公开］部分要求"在筛选阶段进行"血液样本的采集和创面感染的评估。23页第0天病例报告表（CFR）显示"没有采集血液样本或创面拭子"。

iii.［不公开］受试者——尽管该受试者符合筛选失败的标准，但是您还是于2007年4月2日将其随机入组本研究。该受试者的创面于2007年3月12日测量为7.8cm^2，2007年4月2日创面增大到8.7cm^2，面积增加超过10%。试验方案［不公开］部分描述"如果创面面积改变，相对于筛选时第一次测量，或者……）增加［不公开］……受试者应被考虑为筛选失败，必须退出导入期，转到他们标准的规定治疗。"

B. 研究2

i.［不公开］受试者——尽管该受试者符合筛选失败的标准，但是您还是继续让该受试者参加本研究。试验方案［不公开］部分要求受试者的体质指数（BMI）小于某值［不公开］，而该受试者2006年6月5日筛选访视时BMI为52.7。

ii.［不公开］受试者——您将该受试者移出本研究，因为他接受了用于［不公开］受试者的供试品创面［不公开］。根据您2007年2月10日签署的文件备忘录，"这是由于研究协调员基于对研究方案关于［不公开］分配的误解而犯的错误。监查员对研究协调员和主要研究者进行了培训，并回顾试验方案与恰当识别正确分配［不公开］。"

试验方案某部分要求，在筛选期间/标准治疗导入期要得到目标［不公开］的X射线结果。该受试者在随机化进入本研究2周内没有进行X射线检查，他于2006年6月19日进入本研究，X射线检查于2006年5月31日进行。

iii.［不公开］受试者——尽管该受试者符合筛选失败的标准，但是您还是继续让该受试者参加本研究。试验方案4.1部分要求合格的受试者年龄在18~85岁，该受试者出生日期为［不公开］，2006年6月19日筛选时年龄为87岁。

C. 研究3

i.［不公开］受试者——您违背了下述方案要求：您未能获取筛选图片或者筛选［不公开］描摹图；您在作为基线访视（治疗访视T1，第0天）的同一天进行了导入期和筛选X射线检查；您在治疗访视T1后超过72小时才进行了T1-A访视（在第0天（基线）治疗访视T1后48 ~ 72小时进行评估）。

ii.［不公开］受试者——CRF"筛选期—访视S1"中记录，该受试者左足或右足都没有明显的脉搏，而您入组了这名不合格的受试者。试验方案［不公开］部分要求每名受试者"足部有充分的血液循环，可以通过试验的目标足有可触及的脉搏来证明。"

iii. 您通过电话收集了研究访视T1A和T2A（在第0天（基线）治疗访视T1后48~72小时进行评估）的信息。试验方案第9部分要求，研究访视T1A和T2A内容包括在您的研究场所更换外部的［不公开］。

D. 研究4

i.［不公开］受试者——尽管该受试者符合多项筛选失败的标准，但是您还是让该受试者入组本研究。试验方案［不公开］部分要求多普勒超声检查，受试者的踝肱指数（ABI）大于等于某值［不公开］、小于等于某值［不公开］，趾肱指数（TBI）大于等于某值［不公开］。试验方案［不公开］部分要求排除筛选血红蛋白低于某值［不公开］的受试者。该受试者的ABI等于1.375，TBI等于0.5，筛选血红蛋白为10.1g/dL。

ii.［不公开］受试者——尽管该受试者筛选血红蛋白为10.8g/dL，符合该研究的排除标准，但是您还是让该受试者入组本研究。试验方案［不公开］部分要求排除筛选血红蛋白低于某值［不公开］的受试者。

3. 您未能准备和保存与研究相关的足够、准确、完整、及时的记录［21 CFR 312.62（b）和812.140（a）（3）］

A．研究1

i.［不公开］受试者——2007年3月26日采集的标本的实验室检查结果"超出参考值结果汇总"显示没

有证据表明您对这些结果的临床意义进行了审查和确定。CRF“第2周第15页［不公开］”某部分［不公开］“血样样本和创面拭子”中提供了指导“返回的实验室检查报告必须由研究者进行审查、签署姓名和日期，任何超出参考值范围的实验室检查结果都要判断临床意义。”

一项实验室检查报告显示该受试者的目标创面拭子采集日期为2007年3月26日，但是那天的CFR表显示没有采集创面拭子。

“初级审核”的CRF不完整，其中第4项的排除标准没有就目标伤口处理暴露骨髓、肌腱、肋膜做标记。

该受试者文件中一份手写的医疗清单显示，没有受试者身份或者信息获取的日期。

CRF第1周第31页中没有显示对研究受试者应用某［不公开］安慰剂治疗的人的姓名首字母，也没有记录对“是否某［不公开］安慰剂运送某［不公开］产品一定不能应用”这一问题的回答。该CRF进一步声明“所有的勾选框都必须打钩后才能向下进行”。

您未签署2007年3月5日、2007年3月12日和2007年3月19日的创面评估进展记录。

该受试者的CRF记录不完整，因为下列CRF页码中没有签署姓名和日期：8、9、12、15、18、22、24、27、32、37。

ii.［不公开］受试者——CRF中没有包括该受试者接受的治疗措施信息。CRF不完整，因为第7、12、18页没有进行要求的对所有项目进行“是”或“否”的勾选。CRF第12和47页没有签署姓名或日期，以确认在访视中记录的数据准确和完整。

iii.［不公开］受试者——该受试者的CRF记录不完整，因为下列CRF页码中没有签署姓名和日期：8、9、15、18、22、24。您未签署2007年3月12日和2007年3月19日的创面评估进展记录。

iv.［不公开］受试者——初始评估CRF显示目标创面在左腿，而下肢静脉评估是在右腿进行，照片也是拍的右腿。

2007年3月26日采集的标本的实验室检查结果“超出参考值结果汇总”显示，没有证据表明您对这些结果的临床意义进行了审查和说明。CRF中关于“血液样本”部分描述“返回的实验室检查报告必须由研究者进行审查、签署姓名和日期，任何超出参考值范围的实验室检查结果都要判断临床意义。”

2007年3月26日采集的创面拭子的实验室检查报告显示，有金黄色葡萄球菌和B 族β溶血性链球菌大量生长，您未在报告上签署姓名或日期。CRF中关于创面拭子采集的部分描述“返回的创面拭子报告必须由研究者进行审查，签署姓名和日期”，但是没有迹象表明您对细菌生长的临床意义进行了评估。

您未对CRF第8、9、12、15、18、22、24、27、32、37和42页签署姓名或日期，以确认CRF内容准确和完整。

2007年4月23日和2007年4月30日的溃疡描摹图未标明实施溃疡描摹的人。

B. 研究2

i.［不公开］受试者——“筛选/标准治疗导入期（第14至11天）”CRF中对排除标准第7项勾选为“否”，这意味着受试者的BMI小于某值［不公开］。这条信息与人口学特征CRF相矛盾，因为该受试者身高5英尺，体重270磅，计算BMI为52.7。这份表格不完整，因为“知情同意”和“生命体征”部分是空白的；“人口学特征”部分的BMI、种族、诊断日期区域没有填写数据；“实验室样本是否采集”没有进行勾选。

ii.［不公开］受试者——研究记录中关于该受试者的死亡相互矛盾。研究文件中一处未签署姓名和日期的标注声称该受试者退出试验，因为该受试者“去世”了。根据2007年6月18日您签署的一份备忘记录，该受试者2006年8月31日还活着，2006年8月30日签署了知情同意书（见本文上述1A项），2006年8月31日后某个时间死亡。FDA现场检查时，可以确定该受试者还活着，被安排2007年10月进行腿部截肢。

iii.［不公开］受试者——该受试者的BMI在“筛选/标准治疗预处理期（第14至11天）”CRF中被错误计算为39。该受试者列为215磅，6英尺1英寸，正确的BMI为28.4。

iv.［不公开］受试者——该受试者文件中一份手写的医疗清单显示，没有受试者身份或者信息获取的日期。

C. 研究3

i.［不公开］受试者——受试者的记录中没有实验室检查结果。试验方案某［不公开］部分规定了筛选期必须进行的实验室检查项目。某［不公开］受试者的原始文件工作表显示，该受试者的实验室检查结果均在正常值范围内。

ii.［不公开］受试者——入组号［不公开］的某［不公开］受试者"治疗阶段-访视T2/第1周"日期为2006年9月8日的CRF显示，获取了目标溃疡的清创后照片。在该受试者文件中没有照片。

受试者的随机记录与受试者总日志不符。受试者随机记录显示该受试者入组号为［不公开］，2006年8月25日进入［不公开］治疗组。受试者总日志显示入组号［不公开］的姓名首字母是［不公开］，入组号［不公开］的姓名首字母是［不公开］。随机化记录显示入组号某［不公开］和某［不公开］的受试者姓名首字母均为［不公开］。

D. 研究4——某［不公开］受试者的文件里没有照片。试验方案某［不公开］部分要求在基线筛选时要拍摄数字照片，CRF显示照片已经拍过。

4. 您未能保存与药物和医疗器械接收、使用、处置相关的准确、完整、及时的记录［21 CFR 312.62（a）和812.140（a）（2）］

A. 研究2——"试验药物数量登记表"中试验药物接收初始日期显示为"未知"。登记表还显示2006年7月13日有一管药被分发，这使［不公开］手头的数量为24，该登记表的下一条项目显示，由于水损害了25个［不公开］被归还给申办者。

B. 研究4——［不公开］数量登记表不完整，因为2005年1月10日至2015年3月14日期间60名受试者条目中有49个批号和保质期限被记录为"未知"。

上述的违背情况并没有打算列出您在进行药物临床研究过程中存在的所有问题。确保遵循法律和适用法规的要求是您作为临床研究者的职责。

自收到这封信的15个工作日内，您需要提供书面材料，关于您已经采取的或将要进行的以纠正这些违规，并在您作为临床研究者的现在或将来的临床研究中，预防将来发生类似违规行为的纠正措施。此外，请提供一份过去5年间您参与的所有的临床试验的完整名单，包括临床研究和供试品的名称、申办者的名称、招募受试者的数量，这些研究的现状。如果不能对本警告信进行回复，并采取适当的纠正措施，有可能导致FDA在不再通知的情况下采取监管措施。此外，FDA有可能按照21 CFR 312.70和812.119对您启动取消资格的程序。

附：英文原文

Michael S. Miller, D.O.

WARNING LETTER

FEB 12, 2008

CERTIFIED MAIL
RETURN RECEIPT REQUESTED

CBER-08-02

Michael S. Miller, D.O.
The Wound Healing Center
1030 South Fourth Street
Terre Haute, Indiana 47807

Dear Dr. Miller:

This letter describes the results of a Food and Drug Administration (FDA) inspection that was conducted from October 15 through November 5, 2007. An FDA investigator met with you to review your conduct of clinical studies. FDA conducted this inspection under the agency's Bioresearch Monitoring Program, which includes inspections designed to review the conduct of research involving investigational products. The studies reviewed at the time of inspection include:

[redacted]

At the end of the inspection, a Form FDA 483, Inspectional Observations, was issued and discussed with you.

We have determined that you violated regulations governing the proper conduct of clinical studies involving investigational drugs and devices, as published in Title 21, Code of Federal Regulations(CFR), Parts 50, 312, and 812 (available at http://www.gpoaccess.gov/cfr/index.html). The applicable provisions of the CFR are cited for each violation listed below. Studies 1 and 2 involve the clinical evaluation of investigational drugs regulated under 21 CFR Part 312. Studies 3 and 4 involve the clinical evaluation of investigational devices regulated under 21 CFR Part 812.

1. You failed to ensure that informed consent was obtained in accordance with 21 CFR Part 50. [21 CFR § 312.60 and 812.100].

A. Study 2:

i. The informed consent forms for the following subjects were not signed and dated by the subjects at the time of the screening visit when study-related procedures were initiated.

Subject	Screening visit date	Comment
[redacted]	6/5/06	On 7/6/06 the study coordinator wrote that the subject "inadvertently left out this signature page."
[redacted]	6/19/06	Subject signed the consent form on 8/30/06, but records indicate the subject participated in the study only from 6/16/06 until 6/26/06.
[redacted]	7/6/06	A notation on the informed consent form entered by the "Person Explaining Consent" on 09/07/06 states "When originally signing this document, the subject overlooked this signature page. He returned at my asking on 8-30-06 and signed the page but signed it for the original date. I also forgot to sign. I signed when the subject returned for signature."
[redacted]	2/8/07	The informed consent form was signed by the subject on 05/14/07 and by the "Person Explaining Consent" on 04/30/07.

ii. The informed consent forms for Subjects [redacted] were signed by the "Person Explaining Consent" on a date different from when the forms were signed by the subjects. Accordingly, it is not clear if the subject signed the consent form at the time of consent.

B. Study 3 —The informed consent form for subject [redacted] was not dated by the subject.

2. You failed to ensure that investigations were conducted according to the investigational plan, the signed agreement, and applicable FDA regulations in order to protect the rights, safety, and welfare of the subjects under your care. [21 CFR § 312.60 and 812.100].

A. Study 1

i. Subject [redacted]-- You randomized Subject [redacted] into the study on 3/26/07 although this subject met a criterion for screen failure. The initial measurement of this subject's wound on 2/19/07 was 15.1 square centimeters (cm^2). On 3/26/07 the subject's wound had decreased to 7.8 cm^2. a greater than 30% reduction in ulcer size. Protocol section [redacted] states "if the wound has changed in size, relative to the first measurement taken in screening, either by a) decreasing by [redacted]..the subject is considered a screen failure and must be discontinued from the run-in period and revert to their standard prescribed therapy."

In addition, protocol section [redacted] requires a wound infection assessment to be performed during the screening phase. Instead, according to the laboratory report, you collected the subject's target wound swab during Week 1.

ii. Subject [redacted]—Protocol section [redacted]requires the collection of blood samples and a wound infection assessment "performed during the screening phase." Page 23 of the Day 0 Case Report Form (CFR) states "did not take blood samples or wound swab."

iii. Subject [redacted]—You randomized Subject [redacted] into the study on 4/2/07 although this subject met a criterion for screen failure. The initial measurement of this subject's wound was 7.8 cm^2 on 3/12/07 and increased to 8.7 cm^2 on 4/2/07, representing a greater than 10% increase in size. Protocol section [redacted] states "if the wound has changed in size, relative to the first measurement taken in screening, either by ...c) has increased by [redacted] ..the subject is considered a screen failure and must be discontinued form the run-in period and revert to their standard prescribed therapy."

B. Study 2

i. Subject [redacted]—You continued this subject in the study although this subject met a criterion for screen failure. Protocol section [redacted] requires subjects have a Body Mass Index (BMI) less than [redacted] This subject's BMI was 52.7 at the screening visit on 6/5/06.

ii. Subject [redacted]—You removed this subject from the study because the subject received the test article wound [redacted] intended for subject [redacted]. According to a Memo to the File you signed on 2/10/07, "this was due to an error on the part of the research coordinator based in a misinterpretation of the study protocol on[redacted] dispensation. Education and review of the protocol and proper identification of the correct [redacted] to be dispensed were reviewed with the research coordinator and the Principal Investigator by the protocol monitor." Protocol section [redacted] requires that an X-ray of the target [redacted]be obtained during the Screening/Standard Care Run-in Period. This subject did not have an X-ray taken within two weeks of randomization into the study. The subject entered the study on6/19/06 and the X-ray was obtained on 5/31/06.

iii. Subject [redacted]—You continued this subject in the study although this subject met a criterion for screen failure. Protocol section 4.1 requires eligible subjects to be between 18 and 85 years of age. The subject's date of birth is [redacted]The subject was 87 years old at the time of screening on 6/19/06.

C. Study 3

i. Subject [redacted]—You violated the following protocol requirements: you did not obtain screening photographs or a screening [redacted] tracing; you performed the run-in phase and screening X-ray on the same day as the Baseline Visit (Treatment Visit T1, Day 0), and you performed the T1-A visit (Evaluation 48-72 hours after Day 0 [Baseline] Treatment Visit T1) more than 72 hours after visit T1.

ii. Subject [redacted]—You enrolled this ineligible subject who had no palpable pulses in either the right or left foot, as documented on the "Screening Period- Visit S1" CRF. Protocol section [redacted] requires each subject "to have adequate circulation to the foot as evidenced by a palpable peripheral pulse on the study target foot."

iii. You collected information for study visits T1A and T2A (Evaluations 48-72 hours after Day 0 [Baseline] Treatment Visit T1) by telephone. Protocol section 9 requires that visits T1A and T2A include changing of the outer [redacted]at your clinical site.

D. Study 4

i. Subject [redacted]—You enrolled this subject into the study although this subject met several criteria for screen failure. Protocol section [redacted] requires a subject's ankle-brachial index (ABI) by Doppler be greater than or equal to [redacted] but less than or equal to [redacted] and a subject's toe-brachial index (TBI) by Doppler be greater than or equal to [redacted] Protocol section [redacted] excludes subjects with screening hemoglobin less than [redacted]. This subject's ABI was equal to 1.375, TBI equal to 0.5, and screening hemoglobin was 10.1 g/dL.

ii. Subject [redacted]—You enrolled this subject into the study although the subject's screening hemoglobin of 10.8 g/dL met the exclusion criterion for the study. Protocol section [redacted] excludes subjects with screening hemoglobin values less than [redacted].

3. You failed to prepare and maintain adequate, accurate, complete, and current records pertinent to the investigations. [21 CFR § 312.62(b) and 812.140(a)(3)].

A. Study 1

i. Subject [redacted]—An "Out of Range Analytes Summary" of laboratory results for a sample collected on 3/26/07 showed no evidence that you reviewed or determined the clinical significance of these results. Section[redacted]"Blood Sampling /Wound Swab" of the "Week-2 Page15 of [redacted] CRF provides the instruction" "Returned Lab reports must be reviewed, signed and dated by the investigator and any out of range lab results assigned clinical significance."

A laboratory report shows the subject's target wound swab was collected on 3/26/07, however, CRFs for that date indicate that a wound swab was not collected.

The "Initial Assessments" CRFs are incomplete in that item 4 of the exclusion criteria is not marked regarding the exposure of visible bone, tendon, or fascia around the target wound.

A hand-written list of medications included in the subject's file showed no subject identification or the date the information was obtained.

Week 1 Page 31 of the CRFs does not show the initials of the individual applying the [redacted] Placebo treatment to the study subject and does not record a response to the question "is the [redacted] Placebo transport [redacted] product must not be applied)." The CRF further states "All boxes must be ticked Yes to proceed."

You failed to sign the Wound Evaluation Progress Notes dated 3/5/07,3/12/07, and 3/19/07.

The CRFs for this subject are incomplete in that the following CRF pages are not signed and dated: 8, 9, 12, 15, 18, 22,24, 27, 32, and 37.

ii. Subject [redacted]—The CRFs do not include information regarding the medications used by the subject. The CRFs are incomplete in that pages 7, 12, and 18 do not have a "Yes" or " No" response required for all of the items. CRF pages 12 and 47 are not signed or dated to confirm the data recorded at the visits are accurate and complete.

iii. Subject [redacted]—CRFs are incomplete in that the following CRF pages are not signed and dated: 8, 9, 15, 18, 22, and 24. You did not sign the Wound Evaluation Progress Notes dated 3/12/07 and 3/19/07.

iv. Subject [redacted]—The Initial Assessments CRF shows the target wound is on the left leg. The Lower Extremity Venous Evaluation was performed on the right leg and photographs were taken of the right leg.

An "Out of Range Analytes Summary" of laboratory results for a sample collected on 3/26/07 showed no evidence of your review or any explanation of the clinical significance of the results. The CRF section regarding "Blood Sampling" states "Returned Lab reports must be reviewed, signed and dated by the investigator and any out of range lab results assigned clinical significance." You did not sign or date the laboratory report for a wound swab collectedon 3/26/07 that showed heavy growth of Staphylococcus aureusand Beta Hemolytic Streptococcus Group B. The CRF section regarding the collection of a wound swab states "Returned swab report must be reviewed, signed, and dated by the Investigator" but there is no indication that you assessed the significance of the microbial growth.

You did not sign or date CRF pages 8, 9, 12, 15, 18, 22, 24, 27, 32, 37 and 42 to verify that the CRF was accurate and complete.

[redacted] tracings of ulcers on 4/23/07 and 4/30/07 did not identify the individual performing the ulcer tracings.

B. Study 2

i. Subject[redacted]—The "Screening/Standard Care Run-In (Day -14 to -11)" CRF shows a response of "No" to exclusion criteria item 7 indicating the subject has a BMI of less than [redacted]This information conflicts with the demographics CRF in that this subject is 5 feet tall and weighs 270 pounds, a calculated BMI of 52.7. This form is incomplete in that the "Informed Consent" and the "Vital Signs" sections are blank; the BMI, Ethnicity, and Date of Diagnosis fields of the "Demographics" section have no data entered; and there is no response to the question "Laboratory samples collected?"

ii. Subject [redacted]—Study records conflict regarding death of this subject. An undated unsigned notation in the study file states this subject was withdrawn because the subject "passed away." According to a Memo of Record that you signed on 6/18/07, this subject was alive as of 8/31/06, signed the consent form on 8/30/06 (see item 1A, above) and died sometime after 8/31/06. At the time of the FDA inspection it was determined the subject was still alive and was scheduled for a leg amputation in October 2007.

iii. Subject [redacted]—This subject's BMI is incorrectly calculated on the "Screening/Standard Care Run-in (Day -14 to -11)" CRF as 39. The subject's weight is listed as 215 pounds and height is 6 feet one inch. The subject's correct BMI is 28.4.

iv. Subject [redacted]—A hand-written list of medications in the subject's file showed no subject identification or the date the information was obtained.

C. Study 3

i. Subject [redacted]—There are no laboratory test results in the subject's records. Protocol section [redacted] specifies the laboratory tests required during the screening period. The Source Document Worksheet for Subject [redacted] shows the subject's laboratory tests were within normal parameters.

ii. Subject [redacted]—The "TREATMENT PHASE - Visit T2/Week 1" CRF for subject [redacted] enrollment number [redacted] dated 9/8/06 indicates post-debridement photographs of the target ulcer were obtained. No photographs were present in the subject's files.

The subject randomization records and the Subject Master Log are discrepant. Subject randomization records show this subject was enrolled as enrollment number [redacted] and [redacted] in the [redacted] treatment group on 8/25/06. The Subject Master Log shows that the initials of enrollment number [redacted] are [redacted] and the initials of enrollment number [redacted] are [redacted] The randomization records show subject initials as [redacted] for both enrollments [redacted] and [redacted].

D. Study 4—No photographs are in the files for subjects [redacted] Section [redacted] of the protocol requires digital photographs to be taken at the time of baseline screening. The CRFs indicate that photos were taken.

4. You failed to maintain accurate, complete and current records relating to the receipt, use, and disposition of drugs and devices. [21 CFR § 312.62(a) and 812.140(a)(2)].

A. Study 2—The "Study Drug Accountability Log" shows "unk" for the initial date of receipt of the study drug. The log also shows one tube dispensed on 7/13/06. The subtraction of this [redacted] makes the number of [redacted] on hand 24. The next entry in the log shows 25 [redacted] were returned to the sponsor due to water damage.

B. Study 4—The [redacted] Accountability Log is incomplete in that "unk" was recorded for the Lot Number and Expiration Date for 49 of 60 subject entries during the period 1/10/05 through 3/14/05.

The violations described above are not intended to be an all inclusive list of problems that may exist with your clinical studies. It is your responsibility as a clinical investigator to ensure compliance with the Act and all applicable regulations.

Within fifteen (15) working days of receiving this letter, please provide written documentation of the additional actions you have taken or will take to correct these violations and prevent the recurrence of similar violations in current or future studies for which you are the clinical investigator. In addition, please provide a complete list of all clinical trials in which you have participated for the last five years, including the name of the study and test article, the name of the sponsor, the number of subjects enrolled, and the current status of the study. Failure to respond to this letter and to take appropriate corrective action could result in the FDA taking regulatory action without further notice to you. In addition, FDA could initiate disqualification proceedings against you in accordance with 21 CFR 312.70 and 812.119.

Please send your written response to:

Christine Drabick, Division of Inspections and Surveillance (HFM-664)
Office of Compliance and Biologics Quality
Center for Biologics Evaluation and Research
Food and Drug Administration
1401 Rockville Pike, Suite 200N
Rockville, Maryland, 20852-1448
Telephone: (301) 827-6221 or (301) 827-6323

We also request that you send a copy of your response to the FDA office listed below.

Sincerely,

/S/

Mary A. Malarkey, Director
Office of Compliance and Biologics Quality
Center for Biologics Evaluation and Research

Cc: Joann Givens, Director
Detroit District Office
Food and Drug Administration
300 River Place, Suite 5900
Detroit, Michigan 48207

第六部分

药物 GLP 警告信

FDA

第148封　给Colorado HistoPrep公司的警告信

2014年3月11日

参考号：14-HFD-45-02-01

尊敬的Bawa博士：

2013年4月10日至5月10日，Theressa Smith女士代表FDA，在贵公司，对您所开展的委托方为（b）（4）[1]，的以下非临床研究：研究（b）（4），“（b）（4）”和研究（b）（4），“（b）（4）”进行了审查。这封警告信特告知您现场检查中发现的违规情况。

本次现场检查是FDA的生物研究监查项目的一部分。该项目通过设定的检查方法，对FDA所监管的相关研究的实施情况进行评估，以确认研究数据符合美国联邦法规21 CFR 58——非临床研究质量管理规范（GLP）的要求，在科学上是有效和准确的。

在现场检查结束时，Smith女士向您出示并讨论了FDA483表，即现场检查发现的问题。您2013年5月27日对该FDA483表的书面回复已收悉。

经对现场检查报告、该报告的附件，以及您2013年5月27日的书面回复进行审查，我们认为，您没有遵循适用的法律要求和监管非临床实验研究的FDA法规。我们想强调以下几点：

1. 您的质量保证部门必须确定，没有适当的授权和记录，不得违背批准的方案或标准操作规程［21 CFR 58.35（b）（5）］

质量保证部门（QAU）必须确定在非临床实验研究实施过程中所有方案和标准操作规程的偏离应经专题负责人授权批准。具体来说，工作人员用“代表性组织”替代丢失的方案特定组织，或收集的组织在出库阶段丢失，以上两种情况未能遵循方案，也未获得专题负责人的授权，您的QAU未能确定这些方案偏离。实例包括如下：

a. 关于研究（b）（4），贵公司使用替代的或非特定组织样本而非方案要求的样本，并未经授权，而您的QAU未能确定，具体如下：

ⅰ）动物 4004 和 4002：贵公司用“采自大块坐骨神经处的肌肉”替代“四头肌”。

ⅱ）动物 1506：贵公司用“采自背部的肌肉”替代“四头肌”。

ⅲ）动物 4506 和 1501：贵公司用“采自耳部的皮肤”替代“乳腺组织皮肤”。

b. 关于研究（b）（4），贵公司使用替代的或非特定组织样本而非方案要求的样本，并未经授权，而您的QAU未能确定。具体情况为，动物1507，贵公司使用“采自肛周的皮肤样本”替代“乳腺组织皮肤”。

c. 关于研究（b）（4），您的QAU未能确定在组织处理过程中发生的未经授权的方案偏离。研究（b）（4）的方案规定，应根据公司内部程序处理福尔马林固定的组织。您的SOP T-3，“修剪大型动物”提供了在组织学处理中修剪每个器官的指导。贵公司填写的“Cororado Histo-Prep 组织表”显示在收集和“修剪”阶段存在的某些特定组织，在出库阶段丢失。例子包括：

ⅰ）动物 1502 和 4004：SOP T-3指出，对于颌下唾液腺，技术员应从每个唾液腺修剪一个横截面，以暴露两种类型的组织。然而，对这两个研究动物，颌下唾液腺已进行横截面修剪和包埋，但在“出库”阶段（如阅片时）未见唾液腺中有次级腺体组织。

ⅱ）动物 1501：SOP T-3规定，对于卵巢，技术员应纵向平分每个卵巢，并提交每个卵巢的一半（共2个）。记录显示修剪了两个卵巢，但在包埋时只收到一个卵巢。

1 (b)(4) 涉及商业秘密，根据法规内容不予公开。

在您2013年5月27日的书面回复中，包括一份关于研究（b）（4）的偏离报告初稿，报告名为“项目差错调查和纠正措施表”，该报告指出您会修订SOP。该回复未包括针对研究（b）（4）的偏离报告，因此不充分；并且针对研究（b）（4）的偏离报告中仅列出丢失或被替换的组织。对研究的影响描述为：“……组织丢失或被替换的情况记录在研究报告的病理学表格中。”您2013年5月27日的书面回复提到已更新研究（b）（4）的病理学表，从而反映所有组织丢失或被替换的情况；然而您的书面回复未提供更新的表格。

对替代或丢失标本的情况缺乏合理解释，以及对这一缺陷缺乏适当的回复，导致我们对研究（b）（4）和研究（b）（4）的病理学数据的科学质量及可靠性的关注。

2. 您的质量保证部门未能完全脱离，并独立于从事研究的人员［21 CFR 58.35（a）］

质量保证部门应完全隔离并独立于实施非临床实验研究操作的人员。这种隔离将允许QAU客观无偏见地评估：每项非临床实验研究是依据经批准的方案和SOP来执行的，并且最终的报告准确反映了原始数据；设施符合GLP要求；现场检查的发现报告给管理层和专题负责人从而允许采取纠正措施。您未能保持质量保证部门完全隔离并独立于实施非临床实验研究操作的人员，从而导致QAU无法达到所需的职能要求。具体来说，您的质量保证部门未能独立于非临床实验研究的实际操作。举例如下：

a. 您的QA经理于2012年8月13日（16只动物）及2012年9月4日（24只动物）接收了研究（b）（4）的组织/标本。根据研究（b）（4）的QA声明，您的QA经理同时稽查了她接收的研究组织/标本。

b. 在研究（b）（4）完成时，您的QA经理于2012年9月6日完成了“切片至封存”的比较，作为“研究后清查”行动的一部分。

c. 您的QA经理于2012年8月30日通过电子邮件联系研究（b）（4）的专题负责人，讨论了组织标本的组织学处理及将来对试验组的评价。

另外，您名为“QAU职责纲要”的SOP将“组织清点/封存计划”列为QA的职责。“切片至封存”的比较被认为是“研究后”行为，也是接受QA经理稽查的研究（b）（4）的一个阶段。由此看来，管理层对允许QAU直接参与实施，同样需接受其稽查的研究行为不以为然。并且，您现行的名为“质量保证职责”的SOP，QAU-4，允许QAU担任专题负责人，参与要求符合GLP研究的计划和实施。这一SOP描述的QAU的某些特定职责被认为是与研究相关的，其中包括帮助检查归还给客户的材料，以及维护客户到达通知。您的SOP，QAU-4，应进行修订，以保证QAU的职责独立于GLP要求符合的研究计划和实施。

在您2013年5月27日的书面回复中，您指出已指示QAU不得参与研究的实施，并且这些任务已指定给其他符合资质的人员。您的回复不充分，因为您未描述改变现有程序的纠正措施。您的书面回复不能保证Cororado Histo-Prep有效纠正这一正在进行的有缺陷的操作，以符合GLP法规的要求。

3. 您的质量保证部门未能确保临床研究总结报告对方法和标准操作规程的描述是准确无误的，并且报告的结果正确反映原始数据［21 CFR 58.35（b）（6）］

QAU应审查最终的研究报告，以保证其报告的结果精确反映了非临床实验研究的原始数据。然而，您的QAU根据SOP QAU-4审查了研究（b）（4）及（b）（4）的总结报告，却未能保证最终的研究报告精确反映了原始数据。例如：

a. 您的QAU稽查了研究（b）（4）及（b）（4）的病理报告，其中有来自10只动物的多个组织的报告为“未见有意义的发现”；然而这些组织从未经过处理，因此无法得出组织病理学结论。

研究编号	动物编号	报告为“未见有意义的发现”或“NSF”
(b)(4)	#1002	垂体
(b)(4)	#1504	胸骨/含骨髓
(b)(4)	#4506	坐骨神经，皮肤/含乳腺组织
(b)(4)	#4006	胸骨/含骨髓
(b)(4)	#1010	垂体
(b)(4)	#4004	甲状腺/甲状旁腺，食管，肺

续表

研究编号	动物编号	报告为“未见有意义的发现”或“NSF”
(b)(4)	#4003	胰腺，十二指肠，空肠，胃，肠系膜，淋巴结，回肠，结肠
(b)(4)	#1508	坐骨神经
(b)(4)	#1502	膀胱
(b)(4)	#4509	皮肤/含乳腺组织

在您2013年5月27日的书面回复中，您解释说，将修订总结报告，以纠正这些错误，包括数据输入错误（例如，更新表格），将由另一QAU独立稽查此修订的总结报告；并且您指出病理表格的所有空白将主动填写，而不会指定为默认值“NSF”。您的回复不充分，因为您未能提供修订的总结报告或其预计完成的日期。尽管您提出病理表在将来不会设置默认值为“NSF”，但未提供书面程序来保证在将来的研究中不会重复出现此缺陷。

b. 在2013年3月28日研究（b）（4）的统计报告中，动物1502的血液学指标（例如，WBC，RBC，HGB，HCT，MCV，MCH，MCHC及PLT）与原始数据不符。

在您2013年5月27日的书面回复中，您指出：“通过修订报告中更新的表已更正此错误。”但您的回复不充分，因为您未能提供修订的总结报告或其预计完成的日期。

c. 对来自研究（b）（4）的临床生化样本的三项临床生化指标（动物1502的ALKP，动物4002的AST和ALT）进行了重复检测，而缺乏合理解释（例如，无错误代码/仪器仪表警告标识的记录）。下列临床生化标本经重复检测，在研究（b）（4）的最终研究报告中报告了第二次检测的结果而无合理解释。

动物/临床生化指标	检测1结果：08/01/12	检测2结果：08/01/12	最终（统计）报告中的结果
#1502/ALKP	289 U/L @ 14:50	266 U/L @ 16:28	266 U/L
#4002/AST	130 U/L @ 15:47	122 U/L @ 16:29	122 U/L
#4002/ALT	140 U/L @ 15:47	137 U/L @ 16:29	137 U/L

Colorado Histo-Prep现行关于重复检测临床生化标本的实际操作常规是：技术员根据对运行的判断和对单个动物数据的审查，返还“看似错误”的标本。

在您2013年5月27日的书面回复中，您指出，您“将找出最好的办法来处理，例如，取两次的平均值等。”您的回复不充分，因为您未能提供书面程序适当描述何时经重复检测的研究标本是可以接受的。您的书面程序还应定义选择记录在最终研究报告中的数据标准（例如是原始值、重测值或平均值）。

在您的书面回复中，您指出，有关人员被告知应“更智慧”地完成他们的工作。您的书面回复不能保证贵公司能有效纠正这一正在进行的操作，以符合GLP法规关于报告非临床安全性数据的要求。因此，FDA担心负责监督Cororado Histo-Prep 的QAU无法有效充分保证数据的可靠性。

4. 并非所有研究中对标准操作规程的偏离都经专题负责人授权并记录在原始数据中［21 CFR 58.81.（a）］

组织必须遵循SOP，以保证非临床实验研究产生数据的质量和可靠性。您的QAU未能遵循SOP，以保证临床病理原始数据的质量，以及研究（b）（4）及（b）（4）中生成的所有报告的质量。例如，您的名为“研究现场检查”的SOP H-20要求对研究特定阶段进行现场检查；名为“质量保证职责”的SOP QAU-4指出，QAU应审查总结报告的准确性。然而，QAU未能对临床病理原始数据进行适当的现场检查，也未对研究（b）（4）及（b）（4）的最终统计报告进行审查，从而未能遵循您的SOP。

在您2013年5月27日的书面回复中，您讨论了贵公司将来会对临床病理数据稽查中发现的问题进行适当处理。然而，您未出具偏离报告来讨论QAU未能现场检查临床病理原始数据，或未能审查研究（b）（4）及（b）（4）最终统计报告的影响。另外，您未能解释将来如何确保QAU稽查所有的临床病理数据和最终的项目报告。因此，FDA担心Colorado Histo-Prep未能采取纠正措施，以确保QAU进行适当的监督。

5. 您的检测部门未能建立关于数据处理、存储、恢复的标准操作规程［21 CFR 58.81.（b）（10）］

一个检测部门应拥有关于非临床实验研究的书面SOP，以确保不同研究之间及不同技术员之间操作程序的一致性。缺乏这样的程序，将无法确保非临床实验研究产生的数据的质量及可靠性。

贵公司未能建立描述电子数据的处理及恢复的SOP。电子数据的处理包括安全（例如，审计追踪）和原始数据的统计分析。处理电子数据的SOP应描述关于将临床病理原始数据的多组统计分析如何与研究记录一并存档的程序。对研究（b）（4），多组统计分析保存在公司的电子服务器上，而未能适当归档。

在现场检查期间，您未能提供FDA检查员关于供统计分析的原始数据的接收程序。并且，您的部门没有关于保存和存档电子数据的明确流程。尽管您提供给FDA检查员SOP H-31，名为“服务器”及“数据存储和灾难恢复”，其描述了电子数据的物理存储在中心文档服务器上，您的SOP缺乏关于如何确保数据安全，以及如何管理和记录信息修改的细节；并且您未能监控对电子统计数据及统计分析的获取及记录修改（通过审计追踪）。因此，无法确保您的数据和数据分析的质量及可靠性。

在您2013年5月27日的书面回复中，您声称将撰写及实施有关SOP，以解决这一问题。您的回复不充分，因为您未能提供新的或修订的SOP，以支持您的纠正措施，也未能提供预计实施SOP的时间计划。

6. 您未能确保所有用于生成、测量及评定数据的设备经过充分测试、校准和标准化［21 CFR 58.63（a）］

用于非临床实验研究中生成原始数据的设备应根据生产商的推荐进行测试、校准和/或标准化。

在处理研究（b）（4）及（b）（4）的组织时，您未能按照生产商的建议更换Tissue Tek 处理器的试剂。根据生产商的Tissue Tek 处理器指南，应在每运行5次后更换用于“清洁周期”的试剂（例如，二甲苯、乙醇和水），以避免石蜡污染。2012年4月至2012年10月，运行超过5次后（例如，运行11，8，6，15及19次后）才更换试剂的情况发生了5次。在非最佳状态的仪器条件下，为非临床实验研究处理组织标本，您未能确保由Tisse Tek 处理器生成的数据的可靠性。

在现场检查期间，您声明该设备未在临床设置下使用，因此不需根据维护指南进行维护。然而，在您2013年5月27日的书面回复中声称，技术员在适当的时间间隔更换了试剂，但未完成相应的记录。另外，您提供了一份用于记录试剂更换的表格，并声称您已修订相应的SOP，以解决此缺陷。您的回复不充分，因为您未能提供一份修订的SOP副本及预计实施该SOP的日期。因此我们无法评估您针对这一违规行为的纠正措施是否适当。

本警告信的目的并非是罗列贵公司在研究中存在的所有缺陷。您2013年5月27日的书面回复考虑非常不充分，确保遵循法律和相关FDA法规的每一项要求是您的职责，您应当解决这些缺陷，并建立规程，以确保任何正在进行或将来进行的研究均符合FDA法规。

自收到这封信的15个工作日内，您应当书面告知本办公室为预防将来再次发生类似违规情况而采取的措施。如果不能充分、迅速地解释上述违规问题，可能导致我们在不再通知的情况下采取监管措施。

附：英文原文

Colorado HistoPrep

WARNING LETTER

MAR 11, 2014

CERTIFIED MAIL
RETURN RECEIPT REQUESTED

Ref: 14-HFD-45-02-01

Rajan S. Bawa, Ph.D.
President
Colorado HistoPrep
702 West Drake Road
Suite G101
Fort Collins, CO 80526

Dear Dr. Bawa:

This Warning Letter informs you of objectionable conditions observed during the U.S. Food and Drug Administration (FDA) inspection conducted at your firm between April 10 and May 10, 2013. Ms. Theressa Smith, representing the FDA, reviewed your conduct of the following nonclinical laboratory studies performed for (b)(4).:

- Study (b)(4), "(b)(4)"; and
- Study (b)(4), "(b)(4)."

This inspection is a part of FDA's Bioresearch Monitoring Program, which includes inspections designed to evaluate the conduct of FDA regulated research to ensure that the data are scientifically valid and accurate, in accordance with Title 21 of the Code of Federal Regulations (CFR), Part 58 – Good Laboratory Practice (GLP) regulations.

At the conclusion of the inspection, Ms. Smith presented and discussed with you Form FDA 483, Inspectional Observations. We acknowledge receipt of your May 27, 2013, written response to the Form FDA 483.

From our review of the FDA establishment inspection report, the documents submitted with that report and your May 27, 2013, written response, we conclude that you did not adhere to the applicable statutory requirements and FDA regulations governing the conduct of nonclinical laboratory studies.

We wish to emphasize the following:

1. Your Quality Assurance Unit must determine that no deviations from approved protocols or Standard Operating Procedures were made without proper authorization and documentation [21 CFR 58.35(b)(5)].

A Quality Assurance Unit (QAU) must determine that all protocol and Standard Operating Procedure (SOP) deviations during the conduct of a nonclinical laboratory study were authorized by the study director. Specifically, your QAU failed to determine that protocol deviations, without authorization by the study director, occurred when personnel failed to follow the protocol and substituted missing protocol defined tissue with "representative tissue," or when collected tissues were missing during the "check out" phase. Examples include the following:

a. For Study (b)(4), your QAU failed to determine that protocol deviations, without authorization, occurred when your firm substituted or used nonspecific tissues samples rather than those required in the protocol for the following:

i) Animals #4004 and #4002: Your firm substituted "quadriceps muscle" with "muscle taken from chunk with sciatic nerve."

ii) Animal #1506: Your firm substituted "quadriceps muscle" with "muscle taken from the back."

iii) Animals #4506 and #1501: Your firm substituted "skin with mammary tissue" with "skin taken from ear."

b. For Study (b)(4), your QAU failed to determine that protocol deviations, without authorization, occurred when your firm substituted or used nonspecific tissue samples rather than those required in the protocol. Specifically, for

Animal #1507, your firm substituted "skin with mammary tissue" with a skin sample from the "perianal region."

c. For Study (b)(4), your QAU failed to determine that protocol deviations, without authorization, occurred during tissue processing. The protocol for Study (b)(4) states that formalin-fixed tissue will be processed in accordance with the firm's internal procedures. Your SOP T3, "TrimmingLarge Animals,"provides instructions for the trimming of each organ during histological processing. During the conduct of Study (b)(4), your firm's written "Colorado HistoPrep Tissue Form" showed that specific tissues were present during tissue collection and the "trimming" phase; however, during the "check out" phase, the specific tissues were noted to be missing. Examples include:

i) Animals #1502 and #4004: SOP T3 states that for submaxillary salivary glands, the technician should trim a cross section from each of the salivary glands to expose both types of tissue. However, for these two study animals, submaxillary salivary glands were trimmed cross sectionally and embedded, and the secondary glandular tissues were not seen on salivary glands at "check out" (i.e., slide review).

ii) Animal #1501: SOP T3 states that for ovaries, the technician should bisect each ovary longitudinally and submit half of each ovary (total of 2). Two ovaries were recorded at "trimming," but only one ovary was received at "embedding."

In your May 27, 2013, written response, you included a draft deviation report for Study (b)(4) titled "Project Error Investigation and Corrective Action Form," which states that you will revise associated SOPs. Your response is inadequate because you did not include a deviation report for Study (b) (4). Further, the deviation report for Study (b)(4) lists only missing and substituted tissue. The description of the study impact says, "... instances of missing tissues or substitutions are present in the pathology tables of the report." Your May 27, 2013, written response states that the pathology tables for Study (b)(4) were updated to reflect all instances of missing or substituted tissues; however, no updated tables were provided with your written response.

Your practice of substituting and omitting tissues without proper justification, and the lack of an appropriate response to this observation, raise concerns regarding the scientific quality and integrity of the pathology data for both Study (b)(4) and Study (b)(4).

2. Your Quality Assurance Unit failed to be entirely separate from and independent of the personnel engaged in the conduct of that study [21 CFR 58.35(a)].

A QAU must remain entirely separate from and independent of the personnel engaged in the conduct of a nonclinical laboratory study. This separation will allow the QAU to provide an objective and unbiased assessment that each nonclinical laboratory study is conducted in accordance with the approved protocol and SOPs; that the final study report accurately reflects the raw data; that the facility is in compliance with GLP requirements; and that the findings from inspections are reported to management and the study director to allow corrective actions. You failed to maintain a QAU that is entirely separated from and independent of the personnel engaged in the conduct of nonclinical laboratory studies, which undermines the QAU from performing its required functions. Specifically, your QAU failed to maintain its independence from the actual conduct of nonclinical laboratory studies. Examples include the following:

a. Your Quality Assurance (QA) Manager received shipments of study tissues/specimens for Study (b)(4) on August 13, 2012 (16 animals), and on September 4, 2012 (24 animals). Your QA Manager also audited the shipments of study tissues/specimens that she received, as noted in the QA Statement for Study (b)(4).

b. At the completion of Study (b)(4), your QA Manager completed the slide-to-block comparison as part of the "Post-study checkout" activities on September 6, 2012.

c. Your QA Manager contacted the study director of Study (b)(4) via e-mail on August 30, 2012, to discuss histological processing of tissues and future evaluations of test groups.

In addition, your SOP titled "QAU Responsibilities Outline" includes "Tissue Counts/Blocking Schemes" as a QAU responsibility. The slide-to-block comparison is considered a "Post-Study" activity, a phase of Study (b)(4) that was also audited by the QA Manager. Therefore, it appears that management is complacent in allowing the QAU to be directly involved in the conduct of a study that is also audited by that QAU. Further, your current SOP QAU-4, "Quality Assurance Responsibilities," allows the QAU to engage the study director in the planning and conduct of GLP-compliant studies. This SOP describes specific QAU responsibilities that are considered study-related activities, including help with the inspection of materials being returned to clients, and the maintenance of client notification of arrival. Your SOP QAU-4 should be revised to ensure that the QAU's responsibilities are independent of the planning and conduct of GLP-compliant studies.

In your May 27, 2013, written response, you indicated that the QAU has been instructed not to conduct any study activities, and that these tasks will be assigned to other qualified personnel. Your response is inadequate because you do not describe specific corrective measures or changes to current procedures. Your written response offers no assurances that Colorado Histo-Prep will correct this ongoing deficient practice effectively and will adhere to GLP regulatory requirements.

3. Your Quality Assurance Unit failed to assure that the final study report accurately described the methods and Standard Operating Procedures, and that the reported results accurately reflect the raw data [21 CFR 58.35(b)(6)].

A QAU is required to review the final study report to ensure that the reported results reflect the raw data of nonclinical laboratory studies accurately. Although your QAU reviewed the final reports of Studies (b)(4) and (b)(4) in accordance with SOP QAU-4, the QAU failed to ensure that the final study reports reflect the raw data accurately. For example:

a. Your QAU audited the pathology reports for Studies (b)(4) and (b)(4), which reported "No Significant Findings" for various tissues from 10 animals; however, those tissues were never processed and could not have been interpreted histopathologically.

Study Number	Animal Number	Tissues Reported as "No Significant Findings" or "NSF"
(b)(4)	#1002	Pituitary
(b)(4)	#1504	Sternum w/marrow
(b)(4)	#4506	Sciatic nerve, skin w/mammary tissue
(b)(4)	#4006	Sternum w/marrow
(b)(4)	#1010	Pituitary
(b)(4)	#4004	Thyroid/parathyroid, esophagus, lungs
(b)(4)	#4003	Pancreas, duodenum, jejunum, stomach, mesenteric, lymph nodes, ileum, colon
(b)(4)	#1508	Sciatic nerve
(b)(4)	#1502	Urinary bladder
(b)(4)	#4509	Skin w/mammary tissue

In your May 27, 2013, written response, you explained that an amended final report will be issued with corrections, including data-entry errors (e.g., updated tables), and that the amended final report will be independently audited by another QAU. In addition, you stated that all fields in the pathology tables will be made proactive and will not have default values of "NSF" assigned. Your response is inadequate because you failed to provide either a final amended report or an estimated date by which an amended report will be issued. Although you stated that the default setting for the construction of future pathology tables will no longer be "NSF," no written procedure was provided to ensure that this observation will not be repeated in future studies.

b. Hematology parameters (i.e., WBC, RBC, HGB, HCT, MCV, MCH, MCHC, and PLT) do not correspond to the raw data for Animal #1502 in the statistical report of Study (b)(4), dated March 28, 2013.

In your May 27, 2013, written response, you stated that "this error has been fixed and new tables will reflect the corrections in the amended report." However, your response is inadequate because you did not provide either the final amended report for Study (b)(4) or an estimated date by which an amended report will be issued.

c. Clinical chemistry serum samples from Study (b)(4) for three different clinical chemistry parameters (ALKP from Animal #1502, and AST and ALT from Animal #4002) were reanalyzed without any justification (i.e., no documented error codes/instrumentation flags). The following clinical chemistry samples were repeated, and the second result was reported without justification in the final report of Study (b)(4):

Animal & Clinical Chemistry Parameter	Test 1 Result: 08/01/12	Test 2 Result: 08/01/12	Reported Resultin Final (Statistical) Report
#1502/ALKP	289 U/L @ 14:50	266 U/L @ 16:28	266 U/L
#4002/AST	130 U/L @ 15:47	122 U/L @ 16:29	122 U/L
#4002/ALT	140 U/L @ 15:47	137 U/L @ 16:29	137 U/L

Colorado Histo-Prep's current practice of reanalyzing clinical chemistry samples is to rerun samples that "appear in error," based on the technician's knowledge of the run and review of individual animal data.

In your May 27, 2013, written response, you indicated that you "will figure out the best way to deal with this, e.g. average of 2 values, etc." Your response is inadequate because you failed to provide a written procedure that adequately describes when it is acceptable to reanalyze study samples. Your written procedure should also define the criteria for selecting the data (i.e., original, retest, or average) that should be reported in the final study report.

In your written response, you stated that personnel have been told to perform their jobs "more diligently." However, your response offered no assurance that your firm will correct this ongoing practice effectively and will adhere to GLP regulatory requirements for reporting nonclinical safety data. Thus, the FDA is concerned that the QAU oversight at Colorado HistoPrep is neither effective nor adequate to ensure data integrity.

4. Not all deviations from standard operating procedures in a study were authorized by the study director and documented in the raw data [21 CFR 58.81(a)].

A facility must follow SOPs in order to ensure the quality and integrity of the data generated in a nonclinical laboratory study. Your QAU failed to follow SOPs to ensure the quality of clinical pathology raw data, and the quality of all reports generated during the conduct of Studies (b)(4) and (b)(4). For example, your SOP H-20, "Inspection of Studies," states that the QAU is required to inspect study specific phases; and SOP QAU-4, "Quality Assurance Responsibilities," states that final project reports are reviewed by the QAU for accuracy. However, the QAU failed to follow your SOPs by not inspecting the clinical pathology raw data appropriately and by not reviewing the statistics final reports for Studies (b)(4) and (b)(4).

In your May 27, 2013, written response, you discussed how your firm will implement the findings from audits of clinical pathology data in the future. However, you did not issue a deviation report discussing the impact of the QAU's failure to inspect the clinical pathology raw data, or their failure to review the statistics final reports for Studies (b)(4) and (b)(4). Additionally, you failed to explain how you will ensure that the QAU will audit all clinical pathology data and final project reports in the future. As a consequence, FDA is concerned that Colorado Histo-Prep has not instituted corrective procedures to ensure proper QAU oversight.

5. Your testing facility failed to establish standard operating procedures for data handling storage, and retrieval [21 CFR 58.81(b)(10)].

A testing facility is required to have written SOPs for nonclinical laboratory studies that ensure consistency of procedures from study to study and from technician to technician. Without such procedures, the quality and integrity of data generated in nonclinical laboratory studies cannot be ensured.

Your firm failed to establish SOPs describing the handling and retrieval of electronic data. Handling of electronic data includes the security (e.g., audit trails) and statistical analysis of raw data.

Specifically, the SOP for handling electronic data should describe a procedure for the archiving of multiple statistical analyses of the clinical pathology raw data with the study records. For Study (b)(4) multiple sets of statistical analyses were maintained on the firm's electronic server, and were not archived appropriately.

During the inspection, you failed to provide the FDA Investigator with any procedures related to raw data received for statistical analysis. Furthermore, your facility does not have a defined process for saving and archiving electronic data. Although you provided the FDA Investigator with SOP H-31, "Server" and "Data Storage and Disaster Recovery," which describes the physical storage of electronic data in a central file server, your SOP lacks details concerning how you ensure the security of data, and how changes to the files are managed and documented. Furthermore, you failed to monitor access and record changes (via an audit trail) of electronic statistical data and statistical analyses. Thus, the quality and integrity of your data and analyses cannot be ensured.

In your May 27, 2013, written response, you stated that SOPs will be written and implemented to address the issue. Your response is inadequate, however, because you failed to provide the new or revised SOPs to support your corrective actions, and a timeline for their anticipated implementation.

6. You failed to ensure that all equipment used in the generation, measurement, or assessment of data is adequately tested, calibrated, and/or standardized [21 CFR 58.63(a)]

Equipment used to generate raw data in a nonclinical laboratory study is required to be tested, calibrated and/or standardized, based on the manufacturer's recommendations.

You failed to replace reagents in the Tissue Tek processor in accordance with the manufacturer's recommendations when you processed tissues for Studies (b)(4) and (b)(4). According to the manufacturer's guide for the Tissue Tek processor, reagents (i.e., xylene, alcohol and water) used in the "Clean Cycle" should be replaced after every five runs to avoid paraffin contamination. Between April 2012 and October 2012, there were five instances when the reagents were changed after more than 5 runs (i.e., after 11, 8, 6, 15, and 19 runs). By using suboptimal instrumentation conditions to process tissues for nonclinical laboratory studies, you failed to ensure the integrity of the data generated by the Tissue Tek processor.

During the inspection, you stated that this equipment is not used in a clinical setting, and therefore, there is no need to perform the maintenance as described in the maintenance guide. However, in your May 27, 2013, written response, you stated that the technician had changed the reagents at appropiate intervals, but neglected to properly document the reagent changes. In addition, you provided a form used to record reagent changes and stated that you revised the corresponding SOP to address this deficiency. Your response is inadequate, however, because you failed to provide a copy of the revised SOP and an anticipated date for its implementation. Thus, we are unable to assess the adequacy of your response and corrective action for this violation.

This letter is not intended to be an all-inclusive list of deficiencies at your facility. Your written responses, dated May 27, 2013, are severely inadequate, and it is your responsibility to ensure adherence to each requirement of the law and relevant FDA regulations. You should address these deficiencies and establish procedures to ensure that any ongoing or future studies will be in compliance with FDA regulations.

Within fifteen (15) business days of your receipt of this letter, you should notify OSI in writing of the actions you have taken or will take to prevent similar violations in the future. Your written response should include any documentation necessary to show that full and adequate correction has been or will be achieved. Please include the projected completion dates for each action to be accomplished. Failure to address the violations noted above adequately and promptly may result in regulatory action without further notice.

If you have any questions, please contact Charles R. Bonapace, Pharm.D., at 3017961507; FAX 301 8478748. Your written response and any pertinent documentation should be addressed to:

Charles R. Bonapace, Pharm.D.
Acting Branch Chief, Good Laboratory Practice Branch
Division of Bioequivalence and Good Laboratory Practice Compliance
Office of Scientific Investigations
Office of Compliance
Center for Drug Evaluation and Research Office of Medical Products and Tobacco Food and Drug Administration
Building 51, Room 5228
10903 New Hampshire Avenue
Silver Spring, MD 20993

Sincerely yours,

{See appended electronic signature page}

Sean Y. Kassim, Ph.D. Acting Director

Office of Scientific Investigations
Office of Compliance
Center for Drug Evaluation and Research
Food and Drug Administration

第 149 封　给 SNBL 美国有限公司的警告信

2010年8月9日

参考号：10-HFD-45-08-01

尊敬的Tsusaki博士：

2008年7月21日至8月1日及2009年11月16日至20日，FDA的代表在位于Everett，WA的SNBL USA，Ltd.（SNBL），对您所开展的研究进行了现场检查。本次现场检查是FDA的生物研究监查项目的一部分。该项目通过设定的检查方法，评估所开展的研究是否符合美国联邦法规第21篇第58部分——药物非临床研究质量管理规范（GLP）文件的要求，该法规适用于FDA所监管产品的非临床研究。两次现场检查结束时，检查员分别就2008年和2009年的检查向Steven L. Meyer和James K. Klaassen出示并讨论了FDA483表，即现场检查发现的问题。

经对现场检查报告和该报告的附件，以及您2008年8月20日、2008年10月2日和2009年12月9日的书面回复进行审查，我们认为，SNBL没有遵循适用的法律要求和监管非临床研究的FDA法规。我们想强调以下几点：

1. 试验机构负责人未能确保试验人员清楚地理解其将履行的职责［21 CFR 58.31（f）］

具体而言，试验机构负责人并未向工作人员提供有关总结报告撰写的适当说明，导致专题负责人例行撰写了总结报告，该报告部分基于参与此项研究的研究人员的报告草案，且QAU（质量保证部门）对该总结报告进行了稽查。于2008年（研究SNBL. 118.06、SNBL.210.07和SNBL.053.06）和2009年（研究SNBL.258.10、SNBL.010.27、SNBL.289.03、SNBL.293.01和SNBL.010.22）的现场检查期间，FDA发现大量此类重大缺陷。我们注意到，1978年最终法案（1978 Final Rule）的前言中强调了试验人员的报告需个人签署并注明日期，对明确试验人员对报告准确性负责而言是非常重要的[1]。

此外，1987年最终法案的前言中声明“……经病理学家签署和注明日期包含对组织样本进行组织病理学评估的相关原始数据的病理学总结报告。”[2]由于SNBL专题负责人使用试验人员未经签署姓名和日期的报告草案撰写总结报告并递交给申办者，故此，缺乏同意和确定，不能确认试验人员的原始数据的准确性。此外，鉴于SNBL专题负责人邀请申办者对试验人员的报告和总结报告均进行修订和编辑，因此，无法排除对数据诠释和报告存在的偏倚。

您于2009年12月9日的书面回复中声明，SNBL对2008年8月1日的FDA 483表提及的上述问题有所误解。基于如下原因，我们认为您的申诉并无依据：

- 现场检查结果第7条明确地记录了2008年现场检查期间发现的缺陷，即：“专题负责人使用试验人员未经签署的报告草案撰写总结报告。”
- SNBL2008年8月20日及2008年10月2日的书面回复声明“专题负责人将被要求确保总结报告撰写时使用的是最终版的试验人员的报告。”

因此，您对此问题误解的申诉并不合理且缺乏依据。自然，SNBL并未作出保证：将有效地纠正该持续发生的缺陷，并将遵守非临床安全性数据报告的GLP法规要求。

2. 试验机构负责人未能确保供试品混合物的稳定性经过适当检测［21 CFR 58.31（d）］

2009年现场检查时，研究SNBL.284.01的总结报告声明，供试品混合物在使用条件（即室温）下稳定，尽管试验方法并未证实其稳定性。因此，SNBL未能确保试验系统接受方案规定剂量的供试品。

在2009年12月9日的回复中，您指出SNBL将对与研究SNBL.284.01使用相同供试品的所有研究开展适当的稳定性试验，并修订总结报告。然而，由于标准操作规程（SOP）并未要求使用适当的方法验证稳定性，导致受该缺陷影响的研究不仅仅是SNBL.284.01一项研究。尽管您声明SNBL已开始对使用不当方法评估稳定性的其他研究进行审查，但FDA认为试验机构负责人并没有认识到之前的不足或并未指派合格人员解决此问题，进而导致该问题对多家申办者的多项安全性研究造成不良影响。

3. 试验机构负责人未能执行非临床研究方法相关的书面标准操作规程，该规程应足以确保研究过程中生成数据的质量和完整性［21 CFR 58.81（a）］

2008年现场检查时，FDA发现试验机构负责人未制定无菌制备给药溶液的SOP，但SNBL进行的研究已包括需要无菌制备的项目（如侧脑室用药的供试品混合物）。2009年现场检查时，FDA仍发现存在无菌制备的问题。具体而言，供试品部仍有过期的生物安全柜的复核和维护SOP，并未使用现版SOP进行替换；工作人员未能完成所需的生物安全柜使用培训，而且生物安全柜的性能验证和复核并不充分。

由于试验机构负责人未能专注于持续遵守关键职责，以确保GLP合规性，故引起FDA对SNBL得到的非临床安全性数据有效性的关注。2008年现场检查后的回复函中声明，SNBL将就已发现的缺陷采取纠正措施。2009年现场检查发现，多项已发现的缺陷尚未纠正，事实上还多次重蹈覆辙，与SNBL所声明的截然相反。由于试验机构负责人在一年多时间内未能采取适当的纠正措施，故不能说明SNBL具备有效管理符合GLP规范的试验机构的能力。

4. 专题负责人未能确保遵守所有适用的GLP法规，且所有试验数据（包括对试验系统非预期反应的观察结果）得到准确的记录和复核［21 CFR 58.33（e）和58.33（b）］

举例如下：

a. 如上文1. 所述，FDA在两次现场检查中发现，专题负责人多次撰写不含试验人员必要原始数据的总结报告草案。

b. 在2008年现场检查时，FDA发现专题负责人在其复核过程中未能查出研究SNBL.118.06的终版毒代动力学报告中存在的错误，即使用了给药溶液的药物浓度，而非脑脊液药物浓度。

c. FDA发现专题负责人未能确保非临床研究中所用的生物分析方法的准确性。

ⅰ. 2008年现场检查时，FDA发现SNBL在毒代动力学检测中未使用质控样品，来确保生物分析方法的定量准确性，以及决定是否接受/拒绝各分析批（如研究SNBL.210.07）。

ⅱ. 2008年现场检查时，FDA发现SNBL并未拒绝超过预定接受限度的生物分析批（如研究SNBL.195.01.BA.1）。

ⅲ. 2009年现场检查时，FDA发现尚未解决研究SNBL.200.13中检测样品去甲肾上腺素浓度的生物分析方法所存在的重大缺陷（如检测精密度差及经过长期储存后的稳定性未获证实）。在您2009年12月9日的回复函中，您同意该方法未经验证，而贵机构使用了未经验证的方法。

ⅳ.2009年现场检查时，FDA发现一个精密度异常结果被选择性地从支持研究SNBL.289.03的方法验证SNBL.289.05中剔除了。

尽管SNBL在其2008年8月20日和2008年10月2日的回复函中声明，其将会修订规程，并提供额外的人员培训，以纠正生物分析研究过程中存在的缺陷，然而，2009年现场检查发现缺陷仍然存在。对此，无法保证SNBL有能力实施适当的控制和纠正措施确保专题负责人对非临床安全性研究所用生物分析方法的准确性进行记录和确认。

5. 质量保证部门未能就该试验机构开展所有非临床研究制定准确的主计划表，该表以供试品为索引，包括试验系统、研究性质、研究开始日期、每个研究的现状、申办者识别号和专题负责人的姓名［21 CFR 58.35（b）（1）］

具体而言，2008年现场检查时，发现有多项研究的专题负责人身份信息并未列出。2009年现场检查时，FDA发现检查开始时提供的初始主计划表中多项已归档研究的目前状态有误。

6. 质量保证部门没有合适的授权和记录，未能确定没有发生标准操作规程偏离［21 CFR 58.35（b）（5）］

具体而言，下面列举发生了违反SNBL规程的未批准和未记录的偏离：

a. 21个涉及GLP工作的部门中有14个并未于指定的时间内进行2008~2009年稽查计划中的现场检查。

b. 机构存档和生物安全柜相关的旧版SOP复印件未撤出工作场所，且未使用新版本进行替换。

c. 工作人员未能完成规定的机构存档和生物安全柜相关的SOP培训。

d. 工作人员未能在要求的时间内按照规定对档案室中借阅物品的状态进行跟踪和记录。

e. 如下述项7. b. 条所述，未按照规定的时间对移液器进行校准。

根据2008年8月20日、2008年10月2日及2009年12月9日的回复函，SNBL承认这些缺陷，并已提出纠正措施。然而，您并未提供充足的信息评估相关措施的充分性。例如，在您2009年12月9日的回复中，您声明SNBL QAU在日后将密切管理机构设施现场检查，但并未说明如何及时取得成效。此外，鉴于研究机构负责人整体缺乏实施GLP基本要素的责任心，FDA认为SNBL QAU的监管既无效且不足以确保数据的完整性。

7. 您未能充分地检查、清洁和维护设备，对产生、测量或评估数据所用的仪器设备未进行充分的测试、校准和标准化［21 CFR 58.63（a）］

2009年现场检查时，FDA发现有大量设备并未根据SNBL规程的规定进行校准。例如：

a. 色谱柱柱温箱的温度校准已于2008年8月过期，然而，直至2009年9月，研究SNBL.990.40 两项生物分析方法验证和样品分析试验一直使用该仪器。

b. 一年以来，生物分析部门对多个移液器的性能未做充分评估，尽管SNBL规程要求每个月对在用的移液器进行校验。此外，多个移液器的季度校正已过期，违反了SNBL规定的规程。

8. 专题负责人未在研究总结报告上签署姓名和日期［21 CFR 58.185（b）］

例如，2008年FDA现场检查时，发现研究SNBL.223.07、SNBL.109.01和SNBL.053.04的报告草案未经签署，持续了3~5年。

SNBL在其2008年8月20日和2008年10月2日的回复中声明，将会完成这些报告的最终版。与该声明截然相反的是，2009年现场检查时发现，研究SNBL.053.04仍然缺少最终版本，在该版报告中，专题负责人已签署试验总结报告并注明日期，但信息并不充分。具体而言，专题负责人依赖同行审评的病理学声明（日期为2005年6月1日），其比研究病理学家的实际报告（日期为2009年4月25日）早约4年。

9. 您未能使专题负责人以修订案的形式对试验总结报告作出修改或补充［21 CFR 58.185（c）］

在2008年现场检查时，FDA发现研究SNBL.210.07的毒代动力学测试中缺乏质控样品，以确定含量测定方法的性能，且ECG报告并未包含相关数据表。您2008年8月20日和2008年10月2日的回复中声明，SNBL将采取适当的措施解决这些缺陷。然而，2009年FDA现场检查时发现，专题负责人未以修订案形式对试验总结报告作出必要的修正或补充。

本警告信的目的并非是罗列您在试验药物非临床研究中存在的所有缺陷。根据FDA现场检查发现的问题证实，SNBL试验机构负责人未能履行其主要职责，建立适当的制度和规程确保向FDA提交的非临床安全性数据的质量和可靠性。此外，专题负责人和QAU部门对研究监管的严重缺陷可能是由于试验机构负责人缺乏实施GLP关键要素的责任心所致。2008年现场检查后，SNBL于2008年8月20日及2008年10月2日承诺将采取纠正措施。然而，2009年的跟踪现场检查，FDA发现试验机构负责人未能纠正SNBL于2008年现场检查后认可的缺陷，因此，导致近期的现场检查中再次发现此类问题，持续不遵守GLP规定。鉴于此，SNBL于2009年12月9日的书面回复无法令人信服，也未提供充足的可信证据证明其能够遵守GLP。确保SNBL的运行和程序完全遵守适用的法律和法规是您的职责。

自收到这封信的15个工作日内，您应当书面告知本办公室为预防将来发生类似违规情况而采取的措施。书面回复中应包括必要文件来说明全面及充分的纠正措施能得以实施。同时请说明将采取的各项措施的预计完成日期。如果对本警告信的回复不能令人满意，未能采取适当的纠正措施，FDA将根据21 CFR 58.204采取监管措施，包括取消资格。

您2010年1月25日、2010年4月15日及2010年7月20日对FDA 483表的回复函收悉，但这些回复函是在现场检查结束15个工作日后才收到的。根据2009年8月11日发布的局长执行倡议（Commissioner's Enforcement Initiative），尽管我们已对这些回复进行审查，但在本警告信中并未对这些回复函进行讨论。如您认为这些对FDA 483表的书面回复已全面说明了您为预防将来发生类似违规情况而采取的措施，请于15个工作日内以书面形式联系我们。对本信的回复，您可参考2010年1月25日、2010年4月15日及2010年7月20日的书面回复。

附：英文原文

SNBL USA LTD.

WARNING LETTER

Aug 9, 2010

CERTIFIED MAIL
RETURN RECEIPT REQUESTED

Ref: 10-HFD-45-08-01

Hideshi Tsusaki, D.V.M., Ph.D.
President, COO
SNBL USA, Ltd.
6605 Merrill Creek Parkway
Everett, WA 98203

Dear Dr. Tsusaki:

Between July 21 and August 1, 2008, and between November 16 and 20, 2009, representatives of Food and Drug Administration (FDA) inspected SNBL USA, Ltd. (SBLN) in Everett, WA. These inspections are part of FDA's Bioresearch Monitoring Program, which includes inspections designed to verify compliance with Title 21 of the Code of Federal Regulations (CFR), Part 58-Good Laboratory Practices (GLP) regulations.The regulations at 21 CFR 58 apply to nonclinical laboratory studies of products regulated by FDA. We are aware that at the conclusion of both inspections, our investigators presented and discussed with Steven L. Meyer and James K. Klaassen, DVM, Ph.D., Form FDA 483, Inspectional Observations for the respective inspection in 2008 and 2009.

From our review of the establishment inspection reports and the documents submitted with those reports, and your firm's written responses dated August 20, 2008, October 2, 2008, and December 9, 2009, we conclude that SNBL did not adhere to the applicable statutory requirements and FDA regulations governing the conduct of nonclinical laboratory studies. We wish to emphasize the following:

1. Testing Facility Management failed to ensure that personnel clearly understand the functions they are to perform [21 CFR 58.31(f)].

Specifically, Testing Facility Management did not provide personnel with proper instructions on the preparation of final reports. As a result, Study Directors routinely prepared, and the Quality Assurance Unitaudited, final reports based in part on unsigned draft reports of contributing scientists. FDA found numerous examples of this significant deficiency during the inspections Conducted in both 2008 (Studies SNBL.118.06, SNBL.210.07, and SNBL.053.06) and 2009 (Studies SNBL. 258.10, SNBL. 010.27,SNBL.289.03,SNBL.293.01, and SNBL.010.22).We note that the preamble to the 1978 Final Rule emphasized the importance of individually signed and dated contributing scientist reports in establishing the contributing scientists' individual accountability for accurate reporting.[1] Furthermore, the preamble to the 1987 Final Rule stated that "...only the signed and dated final report of the pathologist comprises raw data respecting histopathological evaluation of tissue specimens."[2] Because SNBL Study Directors prepared and submitted final report to sponsors with draft contributing scientist reports that were not signed and dated, they lacked accountability and confirmation that the contributing scientists' raw data was accurate. Furthermore, given that SNBLStudy Directors invite the study sponsors to comment on and edit both the contributing scientist reports and the final report, bias in data interpretation and reporting cannot be ruled out.

Your December 9, 2009, written response claimed that SNBL misunderstood this issue as it was cited on the Form FDA 483, lnspectional Observations, dated August 1, 2008. Your claim has no basis for the following reasons:

- lnspectional Observation Item7 clearly documented the deficiency found during the 2008 inspection thus:"The Study Director prepared the final report using unsigned draft reports of Contributing Scientists."
- The SNBL written responses dated August 20, 2008, and October 2,2008, stated that "Study Directors will be instructed to ensure that the final versions of contributing scientist reports are utilized during final report preparation."

Consequently, your claim of misunderstanding the issue is not justified and lacks merit. In this regard, SNBL offers no assurance that SNBL will effectively correct this ongoing deficient practice and will adhere to GLP regulatory requirements for reporting nonclinical safety data.

2. Testing Facility Management failed to ensure that test article mixtures were appropriately tested for stability [21 CFR 58.31(d)].

At the 2009 inspection, for Study SNBL.284.01, the final report stated that the test article mixture was considered stable under the conditions of use (i.e., ambient temperature) even though the testing method did not demonstrate stability. Thus, SNBL failed to ensure that test systems were administered with the protocol-required dose of test article.

In your response dated December 9, 2009, you indicated that SNBL will conduct appropriate stability testing and amend the final reports for all studies that used the same test article as Study SNBL.284.01. However, because your standard operating procedures (SOPs) failed to require the use of methods appropriate for demonstrating stability, the impact of this deficiency extends beyond the test article used in Study SNBL.284.01. Although you stated that SNBL initiated a review of other studies in which inappropriate methods were used to assess stability, FDA is concerned that Testing Facility Management did not recognize this failure previously or assign qualified staff to address this issue, and that as a result, this deficiency adversely affected multiple safety studies for multiple sponsors.

3. Testing Facility Management failed to implement standard operating procedures (SOPs)in writing setting forth nonclinical laboratory study methods that are adequate to ensure the quality and integrity of the data generated in the course of a study [21 CFR 58.81(a)].

In the 2008 inspection, FDA found that Testing Facility Management failed to maintain an SOP for sterile preparation of dosing solutions, even though SNBL's workload included studies requiring aseptic preparation (e.g., test article mixtures for intracerebro-ventricular administration). In the 2009 inspection, FDA found continued failure in aseptic preparation. Specifically, an outdated SOP for verification and maintenance of biological safety cabinets in the test article department was not removed and replaced with the current SOP; staff failed to complete required training in biological safety cabinet use; and validation and verification performance of biological safety cabinets was inadequate.

Because Testing Facility Management failed to attend to its core responsibilities to remain GLP-compliant, FDA is concerned about the validity of nonclinical safety data generated by SNBL. Your responses following the 2008 inspection stated that SNBL would initiate corrective actions for the identified deficiencies. The 2009 inspection found that, in direct contrast with SNBL's statement, some of the identified deficiencies had not been corrected, and indeed many had been repeated. Because Testing Facility Management failed for over a year to implement appropriate corrective actions, SNBL's ability to effectively manage a GLP-compliant testing facility has not been demonstrated.

4. The Study Director failed to ensure that all applicable GLP regulations were followed and all experimental data, including observations of unanticipated responses of the test system, were accurately recorded and verified [21 CFR 58.33(e) and 58.33(b)].

The following examples are provided:

a. As described above under Item 1, FDA found in both inspections that Study Directors repeatedly prepared draft final reports without the necessary raw data from contributing scientists.

b. At the 2008 inspection, FDA found that the Study Directory failed to verify the final toxicokinetics report for Study SNBL.118.06 in that it erroneously contained drug concentrations in dosing solutions, instead of drug concentrations in cerebrospinal fluid.

c. FDA found that Study Directors failed to ensure that bioanalytical methods used in nonclinical laboratory studies were accurate.

i. At the 2008 inspection, FDA found that SNBL failed to use quality control samples in toxicokinetic assays to ensure quantitative accuracy of the bioanalytical method, and to decide acceptance/rejection of individual runs (e.g., Study SNBL.210.07).

ii. At the 2008 inspection, FDA found that SNBL failed to reject bioanalytical runs that exceeded the a *priori* acceptance limit (e.g., Study SNBL.195.01.BA.1).

iii. At the 2009 inspection, FDA found that significant deficiencies in the bioanalytical method for measuring noradrenaline concentrations samples from Study SNBL.200. 13 were not addressed (e.g., large degree of assay imprecision, stability following long-term storage was not demonstrated). In your response dated December 9, 2009, you agreed that the method was not valid for use, yet your facility used the invalid method. iv. At the 2009 inspection, FDA found that an aberrant precision result was selectively excluded from method validation SNBL.289.05 in support of Study SNBL.289.03.

Although the SNBL responses, dated August 20, 2008 and October 2, 2008, stated that procedures would be revised and additional staff training would be provided to correct deficiencies in bioanalytical study conduct, the 2009 inspection found continuing deficiencies. In this regard, there is no assurance that SNBL is capable of instituting appropriate controls and correcting procedures to ensure that the Study Director records and verifies the accuracy of bioanalytical methods used in nonclinical safety studies.

5. The Quality Assurance Unit failed to maintain an accurate master schedule sheet of all nonclinical laboratory studies conducted at the testing facility indexed by test article and containing the test system, nature of study, date study was initiated, current status of each study identity of the sponsor, and name of the study director [21 CFR 58.35(b)(1)].

Specifically, at the 2008 inspection, the identity of the Study Director was not listed for several studies. At the 2009 inspection, FDA found that the initial master schedule provided at the start of the inspection contained incorrect entries regarding the current status of several studies which had been archived.

6. The Quality Assurance Unit failed to determine that no deviations from SOPs were made without proper authorization and documentation [21 CFR 58.35(b)(5)].

Specifically, unapproved and undocumented deviations occurred against procedures established by SNBL in the following examples:

a. Facility inspections in the 2008-2009 audit plan were not conducted within the required time frame in 14 of the 21 departments involved in GLP work.

b. Outdated copies of SOPs related to the facility archive and biological safety cabinets were not removed from workspaces and replaced with the new versions.

c. Staff failed to complete required training on SOPs related to the facility archive and biological safety cabinets.

d. Staff failed to follow up on and to document the status of materials checked out of the archive in accordance with the required time frame.

e. Pipettes' calibrations were not made in accordance with required time frames, as described in Item 7b below.

In your responses dated August 20, 2008, October 2, 2008, and December 9, 2009, SNBL acknowledged these deficiencies and proposed corrective actions. However, you did not provide sufficient information to assess the adequacy of such actions. For example, in your response dated December 9, 2009, you stated that SNBL QAU would closely manage facility inspections in the future without describing how you would achieve timeliness. Furthermore, in light of the overall lack of responsibility of Testing Facility Management to implement basic elements of GLP compliance, FDA is concerned that QAU oversight at SNBL is neither effective nor adequate to ensure data integrity.

7. You failed to adequately inspect, clean, and maintain equipment. Equipment used for the generation, measurement, or assessment of data was not adequately tested, calibrated, and standardized [21 CFR 58.63(a)].

In the 2009 inspection, FDA found that numerous pieces of equipment were not calibrated according to the schedule defined by SNBL procedures. For example:

a. The temperature verification for a chromatography column heater had expired in August 2008, yet the apparatus was used through September 2009 in two bioanalytical method validations and sample analyses for Study SNBL.990.40.

b. The adequate performance of multiple pipettes in the analytical biology area was not assessed for up to one year, even though SNBL procedures required monthly verification of such active pipettes. Furthermore, multiple pipettes had expired quarterly calibrations, in violation of required SNBL procedures.

8. Study Directors failed to sign and date final reports [21 CFR 58.185(b)].

For example, in the 2008 inspection, FDA found that draft reports for Studies SNBL.223.07, SNBL.109.01, and SNBL.053.04 were unsigned for three to five years. The SNBL responses dated August 20, 2008 and October 2, 2008 stated that these reports would be finalized. In contrast to those statements, FDA found during the 2009 inspection that Study SNBL.053.04 still lacked appropriate finalization, in that the Study Director signed and dated the final report without adequate information. Specifically, the Study Director relied on a peer review pathology statement (dated June 1, 2005) that preceded the study pathologist's actual report (dated April 25, 2009) by about four years.

9. You failed to make corrections or additions to a final report in the form of an amendment by the Study Director [21 CFR 58.185(c)].

In the 2008 inspection, FDA found that toxicokinetic assays in Study SNBL.210.07 lacked quality control samples to determine assay performance,and that the ECG report failed to include relevant data tables. Your responses dated August 20, 2008 and October 2, 2008 stated that SNBL would establish appropriate procedures to address these deficiencies. However, FDA found during the 2009 inspection that the Study Director had not made the necessary corrections or additions to the final report in the form of an amendment.

This letter is not intended to be an all-inclusive list of deficiencies at your facility. As evidenced by FDA's inspectional findings, SNBL Testing Facility Management failed to fulfill its primary responsibility to establish appropriate policies and procedures intended to ensure the quality and integrity of nonclinical safety data for FDA submission. Furthermore, the serious deficiencies found in oversight by the Study Director and the Quality Assurance Unit can be contributed to the lack of responsibility of Testing Facility Management to establish core elements necessary for GLP compliance. SNBL responses, dated August 20, 2008 and October 2, 2008, promised corrective action following the 2008 inspection. However, during the 2009 follow-up inspection, FDA found that Testing Facility Management failed to correct the deficiencies that SNBL had agreed upon after the 2008 inspection, thus leading to the problems found during the recent inspection and resulting in a continued lack of GLP compliance. For this reason, SNBL's written response, dated December 9, 2009, does not inspire confidence or provide sufficient convincing evidence that compliance will be achieved. It is your responsibility to ensure that SNBL's practices and procedures comply fully with all applicable statutes and regulations.

Within fifteen (15) business days of your receipt of this letter, you should notify this office in writing of the actions you have taken to prevent similar violations in the future. Your written response should include any documentation necessary to show that full and adequate correction will be achieved. Please include the projected completion dates for each action to be accomplished. Failure to respond satisfactorily to this letter and take appropriate corrective action could result in FDA taking regulatory action including disqualification in accordance with 21 CFR 58.204.

We acknowledge receipt of your written responses dated January 25, 2010, April 15, 2010, and July 20, 2010, to Form FDA 483, but note that these responses were received more than fifteen (15) business days from close of the inspection. Thus, while we have reviewed these responses, we have not included a discussion of them in this letter as per the Commissioner's Enforcement Initiative announced August 11, 2009. If you believe these written responses to the Form FDA 483 fully explain the actions you have taken to prevent similar violations in the future, please communicate that to us in writing within fifteen (15) business days. You may reference the written responses dated January 25, 2010, April 15, 2010, and July 20, 2010, in your response to this letter.

We appreciate the cooperation shown to the FDA Investigators during the inspections. If you have any questions, please contact Sam H. Haidar, Ph.D., R.Ph., at 301-796-4777; FAX 301-847-8748. Your written response and any pertinent documentation should be addressed to:

Sam H. Haidar, Ph.D.,R.Ph.
Acting Branch Chief
GLP and Bioequivalence Investigations Branch
Division of Scientific Investigations
Office of Compliance
Center for Drug Evaluation and Research
Food and Drug Administration
Bldg 51, Room 5210
10903 New Hampshire Avenue
Silver Spring, MD 20993

Sincerely

/S/

LeslieK.Ball, M.D.
Director
Division of Scientific Investigations
Office of Compliance
Venter for Drug Evaluation and Research
Food and Drug Administration

---

1 43Fed.Reg. 60009(December 22, 1978)
2 52Fed.Reg.33770(September 4, 1987)

第150封　给Continuum健康伙伴有限公司的警告信

2009年8月17日

参考号：CBER-09-07

尊敬的Sadiq博士：

这封信特告知您2009年4月29日结束的FDA进行现场检查的结果。来自纽约区办公室的FDA检查员，与您和员工中的其他委员会面，并对您公司依据非临床研究质量管理规范（GLP）的法规［美国联邦法规（CFR）第21篇第58部分］实施的非临床研究（b）（4）和（b）（4）进行了审查。本次现场检查是FDA的生物研究监查项目的一部分。该项目通过设定的检查方法，审查试验药物相关研究的实施情况。

现场检查结束时，检查员出示并与您和其他人员讨论了FDA 483表，即现场检查发现的问题。我们已经审查了您寄给纽约区办公室，日期为2009年7月17日，对FDA 483表的回复函。

根据在现场检查中获得的信息，我们得出这样的结论：纽约多发性硬化症研究中心（MSRCNY）违反了发表在21 CFR 58用于监管非临床研究合规实施的GLP法规，在每项违规下均引用了CFR的适用规定。

1. 试验机构负责人未能设立负责监督每项研究的质量保证部门［21 CFR 58.31（c）和58.35（a），（b），（c）］

在现场检测期间，贵公司还没有设立质量保证部门（QAU）负责监督每一项研究，以确保符合法规，包括但不仅限于以下内容：

a. 保存一份所有非临床试验研究的主计划表的复印件，该表以供试品为索引，还包括试验系统、研究性质、研究开始的日期、每项研究当前状态、申办者的识别号和专题负责人的名字。

b. 保存质量保证部门负责的所有非临床试验研究相关的所有方案的复印件。

c. 以适当的时间定期，检查每一项非临床试验室研究，确保研究的完整性，并对每一个周期性检查，留存有书面的、正确签署姓名、日期的记录。

d. 给机构负责人和专题负责人提交定期的状态报告，提示在研究过程中出现的任何问题以及采取的纠正措施。

e. 确定没有未经合适特权和记录的方案和标准操作规程偏离。

f. 审查研究总结报告，以确保报告准确描述方法和标准操作规程，报告结果准确地反映了非临床试验研究的原始数据。

g. 撰写和签署一份声明包含在总结报告中，声明中详细报告检查的日期和报告给管理者和专题负责人检查中发现的问题。

h. 保持覆盖质量保证部门的职责书面程序。

在您7月17日的回复函中，您声明已设立一个独立的质量保证部门，将遵循GLP“指南”进行检查。质保人员清楚地理解自己履行的职责和功能，是很重要的。上述列出的职能不仅仅是“指南”，也不局限于检查。它们是为了保证在联邦食品药品和化妆品法案21 CFR 58.1的监管下，产品申请批准的安全性数据的质量和完整性而设立的监管要求。

在您的来信中，您仅解决了少数职责和职能。文件名为“质量保证服务”的文件，提供了一个涉及检查的清单，如设施、设备、储存、方法和操作，但并未说明质保部门会实际检查哪些内容，他们将会采用什么标准，当发现错误或问题时会采取什么措施，以及他们将如何记录和报告他们发现的问题，所有这一切都是法规要求的。

您声明，在每（b）（4）个月将进行研究项目检查，这将在质量保证部门SOP中描述，同时包含检查日期，执行检查的人员以及被检查的研究所处的阶段或环节。您也说明质保人员不会参与目前新药申报相关的申请事项。QAU书面程序将描述您将如何确保QA人员不会参与任何将由他们检查的非临床研究。

请为QAU准备书面的SOP，并在您对这封信的回复中提供一份复印件。

2. 专题负责人未能确保遵守所有适用的GLP法规［21 CFR 58.33（2）］

在贵机构非临床试验研究过程中，专题负责人未能遵守非临床研究质量管理规范（GLP）。

这项违规行为没有写入 FDA-483，然而，所有写入这封警告信内的缺陷都是违反GLP。

专题负责人有责任确保遵守所有适用的GLP法规。

3. 未能确保有一个与试验系统安置区域相隔离，用于动物饲料的专用存储区域［21 CFR 58.45］

法规规定试验系统为“任何动物……研究中给予供试品或对照品”。21 CFR 58.3（i）FDA的现场检查发现，动物饲料储存在动物房内。

在您7月17日的来信中声明，这一违规行为已经在检查过程中被纠正。FDA检查员并没有被告知该纠正措施。您在信中没有说明该违规行为是被如何纠正的。在您的书面程序中，应详细介绍动物饲料、垫料、物料和设备的储存情况。作为您回复这封信的一部分请提供修订过的SOP。

回复函中您声称，确保符合这一项GLP要求主要是动物设施工作人员的责任。然而，GLP法规规定，专题负责人是研究项目的首要责任人，应在非临床试验研究过程中承担全部责任。

4. 未能对用于产生、测量或评估数据的仪器设备进行充分测试、校准和标准化的标准检验设备［21 CFR 58.63］

a. 未保存维护所有设备的检查、维护、测试、校准和/或标准化操作适当的书面记录。具体而言，在检查的非临床试验研究中使用的组织病理学实验室或细胞培养实验室设备没有维护记录。

在您7月17日的回复函中说明，一个活页夹已被放置在实验室中，存放所有的设备检查、维护、测试和校准记录。您声称冰箱的温度将被手动记录，而每个研究人员将负责检查他或她的工作台附近的冰箱温度。细胞培养管理人员将记录细胞培养室的温度，一个研究助理将进行检查，以确保所有的实验室人员都记录每天的温度。您声称这些变更将确保有足够的维护记录。

您提出的纠正措施是不充分的。这项缺陷并不仅仅是关于低温冰箱和冷藏冰箱的温度记录。它涉及设备维修保养文件，校准，标准化和清洁的记录，以及维护保养是否是例行执行，并遵循标准操作规程等。

在您对这封信的回复中，请解释您们充分的纠正措施，并提供修改后的书面程序。

b. 动物护理设施的动物笼具清洗机被认为在（b）（4）华氏度运行。审查这个笼具清洗机的时间温度记录图表发现图表日期记录为9 / 2 / 2002。检查发现时间温度记录装置已坏，数字显示不显示温度。您正在使用的（b）（4）有一个温度范围（b）（4）华氏度，但笼具清洗机SOP并未列出笼具清洁机适于运行的温度。

您7月17日的来信包括修订笼具清洗机SOP，增加了温度需求（b）（4）“验证温度（b）（4）华氏度已经达到了。”您没有提及的事实是，时间温度记录装置已经损坏，数字显示器不显示温度，文件最后记录表的日期是9 / 2 / 2002。

SOP列明（b）（4）不同的物品，将会通过笼具清洗机，再加上1个维护保养周期；SOP列明了使用（b）（4）未详细说明的不同配方用于清洗笼子和瓶子，（b）（4）不同洗涤时间周期，但未要求应满足的温度阀值。SOP规定了温度（b）（4）仅适用于每天的（b）（4）负荷，这并不能保证该负荷或任何后续批次达到未具体要求的温度。

请提供一个更全面的回复和提交修订后的SOP。作为温度（B）（4）一种替代的选择，贵公司应该考虑修复或更换已损坏的时间温度记录仪和数字显示设备，由外部厂商进行笼具清洗机上的时间/温度验证，并把它放入常规的维护/校准计划。

5. 未能建立所需的书面标准操作规程（SOPs）［21 CFR 58.81（b）（11）］

在组织病理学实验室或细胞培养实验室没有设备维护SOP。

在7月17日回复函中您声称，活页夹已经到位用于存放所有的SOP。这不足以确保需要的SOP已经建立。

您7月17日与回复函一同提交的SOP是不充分的。描述设备维护保养SOP应包括其他方面；校准，标准化，维护和清洁时间表，执行这些职能的人员，是日常维护还是设备故障维护，SOP应提出记录设备缺陷的性质，缺陷如何被发现、什么时候被发现和任何纠正缺陷采取的补救措施。

例如，对于（b）（4）培养箱的SOP，只是写明维持清洁的要求，并未写明怎么清洁它们，用什么清洁它们，多长时间清洁，谁执行清洁。移液器和天平SOP存在同样的问题。实验室冷藏冰箱和低温冰箱的SOP写明设备将定期或必要时除霜，而不是设定一个除霜的计划表或标准。SOP还指出，冷藏冰箱和低温冰箱没有数显温度，将使用温度计读取温度，但不需要使用校准的温度计。这些只是SOP中少数应提出的问题，并不是一份详尽清单。

请修改现行SOP，并在您对这封警告信的书面回复中一并提交。

6. 未能确保研究进行中所有试剂和溶液都适合使用［21 CFR 58.83］

通过对存放在组织病理学实验室的试剂和溶液的现场检查，发现了许多试剂和溶液，已经过了有效期1~4年。

您7月17日信中指出，实验室助理研究员将检查到期日期，任何过期的试剂将被处理。您信中所附的SOP仅仅声明："检查化学品的到期日期，如果过期，丢弃化学品并再订购。"这是不充分的，因为您的SOP并没有明确如何记录执行的检查。例如，使用一个"使用日志"，其中记录批号和有效期。SOP也没有规定谁将负责进行检查或处理过期的试剂和溶液。试剂和溶液的检查也应涵盖在质量保证部门的SOP中。

请修改现行SOP并在您对这封警告信的书面回复中一并提交。

7. 未能遵循方案进行非临床试验研究［21 CFR 58.130（a），（c）和（d）］

a.（b）（4）研究的（b）（4）天的（b）（4）组的（b）（4）和（b）（4）动物的体重和临床评分被记录在了不正确的来源的动物名下。

您7月17日的来信中，承认在（b）（4）天的实验中，以上所述动物的EAE评分记录不正确。

b. 试验方案（b）（4）要求动物在等级（b）（4）上进行评估。然而，我们审阅（b）（4）组的数据发现，等级（b）（4）和增量（b）（4）一起使用。另一份记录显示，有另一个含+/−评分（b）（4），（b）（4）增量和（b）（4）值的评分系统。

在您7月17日的信中，您承认在没有适当的授权和记录的情况下您修改了方案，并说明，将来您在修改方案时会提前获得授权，并在将来的试验中充分记录修改过程。

c.（b）（4）组（b）（4）研究（b）（4）组的（b）（4）在实验期间发生死亡，随后，所有其他动物被重新分配新的号码来填补这个空白，结果导致（b）（4）变成（b）（4）等。

在您7月17日的来信中，您承认（b）（4）动物死亡后，重新分配了动物ID号码，您声明以后不会再重新分配ID号码。

您们宣称，上述项目7a~7c存在误差，并没有减弱研究数据的完整性。我们不同意。法规规定非临床实验研究应当按照试验方案进行。您没有按照方案进行研究。您没有提交或获得方案的批准，就改变了在方案中列出的分级量表。数据被错误地记录下来，动物被重新分配了新的识别号。这些行为和违规，直接影响研究的完整性。

8. 未能定期分析试验动物用的饲料和水［21 CFR 58.90（g）］

现场检查动物护理设施时发现，在动物房内，给予试验方案（b）（4）中使用的实验系统的饲料和水，都没有被分析以确认已知的会干扰研究的污染物，或存在的干扰物在方案要求的检测限度之下。

在您7月17日的信中，您指出所有的饲料厂家都遵照GMP标准。在检查结束时，您说您会要求饲料制造商提供饲料的分析证书。请修改您公司的SOP，明确您将如何采取行动确保符合法规要求。

在您7月17日的信中，您提供的用于（b）（4）的水的分析数据似乎是足够了。请修改您的SOP说明多久会对水进行检查，也就是说每月、每季度等。SOP还应该列出应检查哪些污染物。

您还说您已经送了一些文件到纽约区办公室，包括：①IACUC SOP；②对员工的培训记录；③（b）（4）和（b）（4）的活动日志；④微生物培养箱的报告；⑤5/15/2007，9/1720/07，2/20/2008和 9/9/2008 IACUC关于（b）（4）和（b）（4）的备忘录；⑥对啮齿动物用饲料污染物检测报告。无论是纽约区办公室，还是我们的办公室，都没有收到这些参考文件。请在对这封警告信回复中提供这些文件的复印件。

本警告信的目的并非是罗列贵机构存在的所有缺陷。确保遵循法律和相关FDA法规的每一项要求是您的职责。您有责任进行调查、确定原因并改正FDA证实的违规情况，有责任对贵公司整体上的操作进行审查，以确保符合适用于非临床试验研究的监管要求。您应该立即采取行动，纠正这些违规情况并防止再次发生。如果不能做到，可能导致FDA在不再通知的情况下采取监管措施。

自收到本警告信的15个工作日内，请提交书面的文件，告知本办公室为了防止再次发生类似的违规情况，您已经采取的具体步骤。如果在回复前您不能完成所有的纠正措施，请说明延迟的原因和完成纠正措施的时间范围。

附：英文原文

Continuum Health Partners , Inc.

WARNING LETTER

August 17, 2009

By Certified Mail - Return Receipt Requested
And By Facsimile Transmission

CBER-09-07

Saud A. Sadiq, M.D., Director
Multiple Sclerosis Research Center of New York
521 West 5ih Street, 4th Floor
New York, New York 10019

Dear Dr. Sadiq:

This letter describes the results of a Food and Drug Administration (FDA) inspection that concluded on April 29, 2009. The FDA investigators from the New York District Office met with you and members of your staff to review your firm's conduct of studies (b)(4) and (b)(4) performed under the Good Laboratory Practice (GLP) regulations [Title 21, Code of Federal Regulations, (CFR) Part 58]. The inspection was conducted as part of FDA's Bioresearch Monitoring Program, which includes inspections designed to review research involving investigational products.

At the conclusion of the inspection, a Form FDA 483, Inspectional Observations, was issued to and discussed with you and members of your staff. We have reviewed your letter dated July 17, 2009, sent to the New York District Office, written in response to the Form FDA 483.

Based upon the information obtained during the inspection, we conclude that the Multiple Sclerosis Research Center of New York (MSRCNY) has violated GLP regulations governing the proper conduct of nonclinical studies as published under 21 CFR Part 58. The applicable provisions of the CFR are cited for each violation.

1. Failure of the testing facility management to establish a Quality Assurance Unit responsible for monitoring each study. [21 CFR § 58.31 (c) and 58.35 (a), (b), (c)].

At the time of the inspection, your firm had not established a quality assurance unit (QAU) responsible for

monitoring each study to assure conformance with the regulations, including but not limited to the following:
a. Maintaining a copy of the master schedule sheet of all nonclinical laboratory studies conducted at the testing facility indexed by test article and containing the test system, nature of the study, date study was initiated, current status of each study, identity of the sponsor, and name of the study director.
b. Maintaining copies of all protocols pertaining to all nonclinical laboratory studies for which the unit is responsible.
c. Inspecting each nonclinical laboratory study at intervals adequate to assure the integrity of the study and maintaining written and properly signed records of each periodic inspection.
d. Submitting periodic status reports to the testing facility management and study director, noting any problems and the corrective action taken.
e. Determining that no deviations from approved protocols or standard operating procedures (SOPs) were made without proper authorization and documentation.
f. Reviewing the final study report to assure that the report accurately describes the methods and standard operating procedures, and that the reported results accurately reflect the raw data of the nonclinical laboratory study.
g. Preparing and signing a statement to be included with the final study report that specifies the dates of inspection and findings reported to management and to the study director.
h. Maintaining written procedures covering the responsibilities of the QAU.

In your July 17th letter you state that you have formed an independent QAU that will follow GLP "guidelines" in its inspections. It is important that the QAU staff clearly understand their responsibilities and the functions they are required to perform. The functions listed above are more than just "guidelines," and are not limited to inspections. They are regulatory requirements designed to assure the quality and integrity of the safety data filed in applications for approval of products regulated under the Federal Food, Drug, and Cosmetic Act. 21 CFR 58.1

In your letter you addressed only a few of these responsibilities and functions. The document titled "Quality Assurance Services" provides a list of things to be inspected, such as facilities, equipment, storage, and methods and practices, but does not state what the QAU will actually look at, what criteria they will use to ascertain compliance, what actions they will take when errors or problems are found, and how they will document and report their findings, all of which are required by the regulations. You state that studies will be inspected every (b)(4)months, which should be described in the QAU SOPs, along with the dates of inspection, who performed the inspection, and the phase or segment of the study that was inspected. You also state that QAU personnel will not be involved with the current IND related application. The QAU written procedures should describe how you will ensure that QAU staff will not be otherwise involved in any nonclinical study that they will inspect.

Please prepare written SOPs for the QAU, and provide a copy with your response to this letter.

2. Failure of the study director to ensure that all applicable good laboratory practice regulations are followed. [21 CFR § 58.33(e)].

The study director failed to follow all good laboratory practice regulations (GLPs) for the nonclinical laboratory study being conducted at your facility.

This violation was not cited on the Form FDA-483. However, the failures cited in this Warning Letter are all violations of the GLP regulations.

The study director is responsible for assuring that all applicable GLP regulations are followed.

3. Failure to ensure that there is a dedicated storage area for animal feed that is separate from areas housing the test systems. [21 CFR § 58.45].

The regulations define test system as "any animal ... to which the test or control is administered or added for study." 21 CFR 58.3(i). The FDA inspection found that animal feed was stored in the animal housing area.

In your July 17th letter, you state this violation was corrected during the inspection. The FDA investigators were not apprised of this correction. You do not state in your letter how this violation was corrected. The storage of animal feed, bedding, supplies and equipment should be covered in detail in your written procedures. Please provide the revised SOP as part of your response to this letter.

In your letter you state that the responsibility for ensuring compliance for this GLP requirement is primarily with the animal facility staff. However, the GLP regulations require that the study director be the single point of study control, who maintains overall responsibility for the nonclinical laboratory study.

4. Failure to adequately test, calibrate and standardize equipment used for the generation, measurement, or assessment of data. [21 CFR § 58.63].

a. Adequate written records are not maintained of all equipment inspection, maintenance, testing, calibration and/or standardization operations. Specifically, there are no maintenance records for the equipment in the Histopathology - Pathology Laboratory or the Cell Culture Laboratory that were used for the inspected nonclinical laboratory study.

You state in your July 17th letter that a binder has been placed in the laboratory to hold all written records of equipment inspection, maintenance, testing, and calibration. You state that temperatures of freezers and refrigerators will be manually recorded, and that each researcher will be responsible for checking the temperature on the refrigerator near his or her bench. The cell culture manager will record temperatures in the cell culture room, and a research assistant will check to ensure that all laboratory personnel are recording daily temperatures. You state these changes will ensure that there are adequate maintenance records.

Your proposed corrective actions are incomplete. This violation does not concern only the recording of temperatures of freezers and refrigerators. It concerns maintaining records that document equipment maintenance, calibration, standardization, and cleaning, and whether maintenance is routine and follows standard operating procedures.

In your response to this letter, please explain your complete corrective actions and provide revised written procedures.

b. The animal cage washer in the Animal Care Facility is rated to be run at (b)(4)°F. A review of the time-temperature recording chart for this cage washer found the chart to be dated 9/2/2002. The time-temperature recording device was found to be broken, and the digital display does not display the temperature. The (b)(4) you are using has a range of (b)(4)°F, but the SOPs for the cage washer do not list the temperature at which the cage washer is to be run.

Your July 17th letter includes a revised cage washer SOP that adds a requirement for temperature (b)(4) "to validate that a temperature of (b)(4) degrees Fahrenheit has been reached." You did not address the fact that the time-temperature recording device was found broken, that the digital display does not display the temperature, and that the last recording chart on file was dated 9/2/2002.

The SOP lists (b)(4) different items that are run through the cage washer, plus a maintenance cycle; the SOP lists the use of (b)(4) different unspecified formulas used to clean the cages and bottles,(b)(4) different wash-time cycles, but no required temperature threshold that must be met. The SOP states that a temperature (b)(4) is to be used only on the (b)(4) load of each day, which does not ensure that the load or any subsequent runs achieved the unspecified required temperature.

Please provide a more complete response and submit a revised SOP. As an alternative to the temperature (b)(4) your firm should consider repairing or replacing the broken time-temperature recording and the digital display devices, having an outside firm perform a time/temperature validation on the cage washer and putting it on a routine maintenance/calibration schedule.

5. Failure to establish required written standard operating procedures (SOPs). [21 CFR § 58.81(b)(11)].

There are no SOPs for the maintenance of equipment in the Histo-Pathology Laboratory or the Cell Culture Laboratory.

You state in your July 17th letter that a binder has been put in place to hold all SOPs.This is inadequate to ensure that required SOPs are actually established.

The SOPs that were submitted with your July 17th response are inadequate. The SOPs that describe equipment maintenance should include among other things; calibration, standardization, maintenance and cleaning schedules, who performs these functions, and whether maintenance is routine or a result of equipment defect. The SOPs should address documenting the nature of an equipment defect, how and when the defect was discovered, and any remedial action taken to correct the defect.

For example, the SOP for the (b)(4) incubators only states the requirement to maintain clean incubators, but does not state how they are to be cleaned, what to clean them with, how often, and who performs the cleaning. The same is true for the pipettes and balance scales. The SOP for the laboratory refrigerators and freezers states the equipment will be defrosted periodically or when deemed necessary, instead of setting a defrosting schedule or criteria for determining such a schedule. The SOP also states that refrigerators and freezers without a digital temperature read-out will use a thermometer, but it does not require the use of a calibrated thermometer. These are just a few of the things the SOPs should address It is not an exhaustive list.

Please revise the current SOPs and submit them with your written response to this Warning Letter.

6. Failure to ensure that all reagents and solutions used in the conduct of the study are suitable for use. [21 CFR § 58.83].

The inspection of the reagents and solutions stored in the Histopathology Pathology Laboratory found numerous reagents and solutions to have passed their expiration dates for periods of between one and four years.

Your July 17th letter states that laboratory research assistants will check the expiration dates and any outdated reagents will be disposed of. The SOP provided with your letter only states: "Check expiration dates of chemicals. Discard and reorder if expired." This is insufficient, because your SOP does not address how you will document that these checks are being done. For example, implementing a "use log" where lot numbers and expiration dates are recorded. The SOP also does not state who will be responsible for conducting this check or for the disposal of out of date reagents and solutions. The inspection of reagents and solutions should also be covered in the QAU's SOPs.

Please revise the current SOPs and submit them with your written response to this Warning Letter.

7. Failure to conduct nonclinical laboratory studies in accordance with the protocol. [21 CFR § 58.130(a), (c), and (d)].

a. The weight and clinical scoring data for animals identified as (b)(4) and (b)(4) in Group (b)(4) of study (b)(4) for days (b)(4) were attributed to the incorrect source animals.

In your letter of July 17th, you admitted that the EAE scores for the above referenced animals were incorrectly transcribed during days (b)(4) of the experiment.

b. Protocol (b)(4) required that the animals be evaluated on a scale of (b)(4). However, our review of the data for Group (b)(4) found that a scale of (b)(4) was used with increments of (b)(4). Another document showed an additional scoring system of (b)(4) with plus/minus scoring, (b)(4) increments and one (b)(4) value.

In your July 17th letter you acknowledge that you modified the protocol without proper authorization and documentation, and state that, in the future, you will obtain prior authorization for any amendments to a protocol, and fully document the amendment process in all future experiments.

c. Animal (b)(4) from the Group (b)(4) animals in study (b)(4) died during the experiment. Subsequently all other animals reassigned new numbers to fill the void, resulting in (b)(4) becoming (b)(4), and so on.

In your July 17th letter you acknowledged that the animal IDs were reassigned upon the death of animal (b)(4) and you state that you will not reassign identification numbers in the future.

You claim that the errors cited in items 7a to 7c, above, did not compromise the integrity of the study data. We disagree. The regulations state the nonclinical laboratory study shall be conducted in accordance with the protocol. You did not conduct the study in accordance with the protocol. You changed the grading scale that was listed in the protocol without submitting or obtaining approval for a protocol amendment. Data were incorrectly recorded, and animals were assigned new identification numbers. These actions and regulatory violations directly affect the integrity of the study.

8. Failure to periodically analyze feed and water used for test animals. [21 CFR § 58.90(g)].

Inspection of the Animal Care Facility found that neither feed nor water for the test systems used for Protocol (b)(4) housed in Animal Room (b)(4) are analyzed to ensure that contaminants known to be capable of interfering with the study and reasonably expected to be present in such feed and water are not present at levels above those specified in the protocol.

You indicate in your July 17th letter that all feed manufacturers are GMP compliant. At the end of the inspection you stated that you will request certificates of analysis from the feed manufacturers. Please revise your firm's SOPs to specify how you will ensure compliance with these regulatory requirements.

The analytical data you provided in your July 17th letter for the water used for the (b)(4) appears to be adequate. Please revise your SOP to define how often the water will be checked, i.e., monthly, quarterly, etc. The procedures should also list the contaminants which are to be checked.

You also state that you had sent a number of documents to the New York District Office, including: (1) the IACUC SOP; (2) training records for one staff member; (3) activity logs for (b)(4) and (b)(4); (4) microbiology swabs of cages report; (5) IACUC minutes in reference to (b)(4) and (b)(4) dated 5/15/07, 9/17/07, 2/20/08 and 9/9/08; and (6) a report on rodent diet contamination check. Neither the New York District Office nor our office received these referenced documents. Please provide a copy of these documents with your response to this Warning Letter.

The deviations listed above are not intended to be an all-inclusive list of deficiencies at your facility. It is your responsibility to ensure that your establishment is in compliance with all requirements of the law and applicable federal regulations. You are responsible for investigating, determining causes of, and correcting violations identified by the FDA, and for reviewing your firm's operations as a whole to ensure that you are in compliance with the regulatory requirements applicable to nonclinical laboratory studies. You should take prompt action to correct these deviations and prevent their recurrence. Failure to do so may result in FDA initiating regulatory action without further notice.

We request that you notify this office in writing, within fifteen (15) working days of receipt of this letter, of the specific steps you have taken to correct the noted violations and to prevent their recurrence. If you cannot complete all of the corrections before you respond, please state the reason for your delay and the time frame within which the corrections will be completed.

Please send your response and the requested documentation to:

Robert L. Wesley
Division of Inspections and Surveillance (HFM-664)
Office of Compliance and Biologics Quality
Center for Biologics Evaluation and Research
1401 Rockville Pike, Suite 200N
Rockville, Maryland 20852-1448
Telephone (301) 827-6338

We also request that you send a copy of your response to the FDA District Office listed below.

Sincerely,

/S/

Mary A. Malarkey
Director
Office of Compliance and Biologics Quality
Center for Biologics Evaluation and Research

第151封　给华盛顿生物技术股份有限公司的警告信

2009年2月17日

参考号：CBER-09-04

尊敬的O'Neill博士：

2008年10月3日，FDA Baltimore地区办公室的一名检查员和生物制品评价研究中心（CBER）的一名毒理学家，对您公司按照非临床研究质量管理规范（GLP）方面的法规［美国联邦法规（CFR）第21篇第58部分］所开展的研究TOX［（b）（4）[1]］、TOX［（b）（4）］和［（b）（4）］进行了现场检查。这封警告信特告知您现场检查中发现的违规情况。本次现场检查是FDA的生物研究监查项目的一部分。该项目通过设定的检查方法，审查试验药物研究的实施情况。

在现场检查结束时，检查人员向您出示并讨论了FDA483表，即现场检查发现的问题。

根据我们现场检查获得的信息，我们的结论是：华盛顿生物技术股份有限公司（WBI）违反了21 CFR 58非临床研究相关的GLP规定和要求。以下逐条列出违规情况和相应的CFR条款：

1. 未能确保参与或负责监督非临床研究的每位人员具备教育、培训和相关经验，或上述几项的综合能力，能够执行所分配的职责［21 CFR 58.29（a），58.33］

a. 所检查的3项研究的专题负责人缺乏教育、培训和经验，或上述某几项的综合能力，无法承担GLP专题负责人的职责。

b. TOX［（b）（4）］的项目经理进行了一次尸检，但缺乏尸检相关的教育、培训、经验，或上述几项的综合能力。

2. 未能确保为每个参与或监督非临床研究的人员保存一份关于培训、工作经验和工作描述的现况摘要［21 CFR 58.29（b）］

您未保存以下员工的上述文件：

a. 试验 TOX［（b）（4）］、TOX［（b）（4）］和［（b）（4）］的专题负责人。

b. 试验 TOX［（b）（4）］替任的专题负责人。

c. 负责监督试验 TOX［（b）（4）］数据统计分析的高级科学家。

d. 负责进行试验 TOX［（b）（4）］统计分析的统计师。

e. 试验 TOX［（b）（4）］的项目经理。

f. 负责试验 TOX［（b）（4）］尸检的实验室技术人员。

3. 试验机构负责人未能履行其职责［21 CFR 58.31（a）和（g）］

a. 试验机构未按照 21 CFR 58.33 的要求指派合格的专题负责人。

b. 试验机构未确保质量保证部门报告任何违规情况，并与专题负责人沟通，且未确保执行和记录纠正措施。

4. 未确保专题负责人履行其职责［21 CFR 58.33（a），（b），（c）和（f）］

a. 研究主任未能确保遵循所有试验方案或记录和批准方案变更。

b. 研究主任未能确保根据试验方案要求准确记录和验证实验数据。

c. 当发生不可预见的、可能影响非临床研究质量和完整性的情形时，专题负责人未能确保将其记录，并采取和/或记录纠正措施。其中，试验方案 TOX［（b）（4）］对尸检有特定要求，但并未执行。专题负责人

1 (b)(4) 涉及商业秘密，根据法规内容不予披露的标注。

未发现该方案偏离，也未采取纠正措施。

d. 试验TOX［（b）（4）］和［（b）（4）］的专题负责人未确保对所有原始数据、记录、方案、样本和总结报告在试验期间或试验结束时进行归档。

5. 质量保证部门未能履行职责［21 CFR 58.35（a）；58.35（b）（1）（3）和（7）；58.35（c）］

a. QAU未完全独立于研究的参与和主管人员。试验TOX［（b）（4）］的QAU经理直接汇报给专题负责人。

b. QAU未保存一份在该机构所有非临床研究的总计划表。此外，总计划表未列出供试品、检验系统、试验起始日期、申办者，以及专题负责人的名字。

c. QAU未对试验进行定期检查，以保证试验的真实性。此外，QAU未保存试验TOX［（b）（4）］和［（b）（4）］定期检查的书面、经签字的记录。

d. QAU未在TOX［（b）（4）］最终试验报告中准备和签署一项声明，其内容包括将检查与发现问题报告给管理者及专题负责人的日期。

e. 无有关QAU职责和流程的书面文件、QAU更新维护的记录，以及记录索引的方法。

6. 未能对设备进行充分检查、清洁和维护［21 CFR 58.63］

没有对［（b）（4）］检查、清洁、维护、测试、标定或标准化的书面记录，包括试验TOX［（b）（4）］供试品的贮存，试验 TOX［（b）（4）］和TOX［（b）（4）］所用的离心机，以及试验TOX［（b）（4）］所用的［（b）（4）］。

7. 未能建立和遵守满足管理需要的、并足以保证研究过程中生成数据的质量与完整性的非临床研究方法的书面标准操作规程 ［21 CFR 58.81（a）和（b）（6）、（b）（7）和（b）（11）］

a. SOP的重大偏离未经专题负责人确认，也未记录在相应试验的原始数据中。如：

ⅰ. 规程 1661.3 要求采血前麻醉，且要求记录所用的麻醉剂。试验TOX［（b）（4）］的总结报告中无2007年10月18日和2007年11月12日进行眼眶采血所用麻醉剂的记录。

ⅱ. 规程 1686.3 要求大鼠在放血前进行麻醉，并记录所用麻醉剂。［（b）（4）］试验TOX［（b）（4）］未记录动物编号2～10和动物编号12放血前所用的麻醉剂。

ⅲ. 规程 8060.4要求在［（b）（4）］基础上对机构设施进行稽查。

2006年1月至2008年9月没有任何设施稽查的记录。

ⅳ. 规程420.11要求饲养大鼠的鼠笼相对湿度维持在［（b）（4）］下。“室温/湿度的日志记录”显示试验TOX［（b）（4）］中湿度偏离了规定的范围。

ⅴ. 规程400.8要求稽查“室温/湿度的日志记录”“动物检查记录”“饲养笼/设备状态报告”和“动物活动记录”。没有记录显示在2007年8月至2007年11月间对试验 TOX［（b）（4）］的上述记录进行稽查。

b. 未对以下工作制定书面SOP：

ⅰ. 试验中濒死或死亡动物的处理。

ⅱ. 动物尸检或尸检后的检查。

ⅲ. 设备的维护和校准。

具体来说，未对试验 TOX［（b）（4）］和 TOX［（b）（4）］所用−80°C冰箱、离心机和分光光度计的维护和校准建立SOP。

8. 未能确认并记录每批供试品或对照品的特征、含量、纯度和组分［21 CFR 58.105（a）］

专题负责人未从申办者处获得试验TOX［（b）（4）］所用供试品的检验报告，其应记录供试品的批号、规格、纯度和组分。

9. 未能确保每个研究均有一个经过批准的书面方案，其中清楚地表明实施该研究的目的和所有方法［21 CFR 58.120（a）］

a. 试验TOX［（b）（4）］的方案未显示该试验在第［（b）（4）］天进行实验室检测和数据分析所用的统

计方法。

b. 试验 TOX［（b）（4）］TOX［（b）（4）］和［（b）（4）］无申办者对试验方案批准的记录。

10. 未能按照方案进行非临床研究［21 CFR 58.130（a）（c）和（d）］

a. 试验 TOX［（b）（4）］中出现以下方案违背。

i. 方案要求对试验中所有死亡的动物进行尸检，所有出现异常的器官进行摘除、保存并送至组织学检查。编号11的动物尸检显示脾脏增大，但未有该器官保存并送至组织学检查的记录。

ii. 未遵循方案进行实验室分析。如：

（1）编号33的动物肾和编号35的动物肺送至组织病理学检查，但方案并未要求这些检查。

（2）编号28的动物在尸检中抽取的肾积液送至分析实验室进行检测，但方案并未要求这项检测。该样品的这项分析结果未记录在总结报告中。

iii. 在最初的［（b）（4）］动物完成最终给药后，该试验加入了额外的动物，其并未遵循方案的规定。

iv. "放血血清样本"在2007年11月13日运送至申办者，其并未遵循方案的规定。

v. 方案要求在试验的第［（b）（4）］天进行放血，但试验［（b）（4）］只中的35只动物直至试验第［（b）（4）］天才进行放血。

vi. 方案要求在放血后立即进行尸检，但放血30分钟后才进行尸检。

b. 试验 TOX［（b）（4）］的样本未标明测试系统、试验编号、类型和收集日期。

c. 试验 TOX［（b）（4）］样本进行肉眼尸检观察的所有发现未提供给病理学家进行组织病理学评估。

11. 未能建立非临床研究结果的完整报告［21 CFR 58.185（a）（2）～（4），（6）（9）～（10）（13），（b）和（c）］

a. 试验 TOX［（b）（4）］的总结报告未记录原始试验方案的所有变更，以及专题负责人对这些变更的批准。

b. 试验 TOX［（b）（4）］的总结报告未标明数据分析所用的统计学方法。

c. 试验 TOX［（b）（4）］的总结报告未标明供试品和对照品的名称、化学文摘号或编号、规格、纯度，以及组分或其他相关特性。

d. 试验 TOX［（b）（4）］的最终报告未包括对所用方法的准确描述。如：

i. 总结报告提到，动物随机入组；但未有动物随机化的记录，且贵公司无动物随机化相关的书面程序。

ii. 总结报告与试验动物实施安乐死所用方法的实验室记录不一致。

e. 总结报告未说明可能影响数据质量或可靠性的所有情形。如：

i. 试验 TOX［（b）（4）］的总结报告将［（b）（4）］治疗组作为［（b）（4）］，但方案和原始数据文件将［（b）（4）］治疗组作为［（b）（4）］

ii. 试验 TOX［（b）（4）］的总结报告未说明用于样品贮存或进行［（b）（4）］扫描分析的单独实验室的环境条件。在2008年7月22日样品制备和2008年8月7日样品分析期间，未有样品的贮存记录。

f. 最终试验报告无专题负责人的名字、其他科学家或专业人员的名字、试验中涉及的所有监督人员的名字。具体来说，

i. 试验［（b）（4）］的总结报告无专题负责人的名字，且未经专题负责人签署名字和日期。

ii. 试验 TOX［（b）（4）］将 Sean P. O'Neill 博士列为专题负责人；但试验 TOX［（b）（4）］的总结报告将［（b）（6）］列为研究主任。期间无专题负责人变更的记录。

iii. 试验 TOX［（b）（4）］的总结报告无试验中涉及所有科学家和专业人员的名字。

g. 试验 TOX［（b）（4）］的总结报告未记录所有样本的贮存地点。

h. 专题负责人未按照修订的格式提交总结报告的更正或增补。具体来说，试验［（b）（4）］有两个版本的总结报告，其中一份由专题负责人于2008年1月18日签署，另一份于2008年6月18日签署。2008年6月的总结报告未标示为总结报告的修订版。

12.未能储存并保留生成的、作为非临床研究结果的所有原始数据、文件记录、方案、总结报告和标本［21 CFR 58.190（a）和58.195（b）］

试验 TOX［（b）（4）］和［（b）（4）］的专题负责人未保证所有原始数据、记录、方案、样本和最终报告在试验期间或试验终止时进行存档。如：

a. 试验 TOX［（b）（4）］中指定收集的动物器官在试验结束时未进行归档。

b. 试验［（b）（4）］的方案在试验结束时未进行归档。

本警告信的目的并非是罗列贵公司中存在的所有违规和缺陷。确保贵公司遵循法律法规的要求是您的职责。您有责任对FDA提出的违规情况进行调查、确定原因和纠正，并对整个机构进行全面审查，以确保遵循所有非临床研究相关的法律法规。您应尽快采取措施纠正这些违规问题，并防止其再次发生。如未采取措施，可能导致我们在不再通知的情况下采取监管措施。

自收到这封信的15个工作日内，我们要求您书面告知本办公室您为纠正违规行为、预防将来发生类似违规行为采取的具体步骤。如果您不能在回复日期前完成所有的纠正措施，请陈述延迟理由和可以完成所有措施的时限。

请告知本次检查所涉及的3项研究TOX［（b）（4）］、TOX［（b）（4）］和［（b）（4）］的申办者，贵公司未遵循21 CFR 58开展GLP研究。您在回复时请附上一份贵公司通知上述申办者的书面说明。

附：英文原文

Washington Biotechnology, Inc

Warning Letter

FEB 17, 2009

By Certified Mail - Return Receipt Requested
And By Facsimile Transmission

CBER-09-04

Sean P. O'Neill, Ph.D., President
Washington Biotechnology, Inc.
9075 Guilford Road
Columbia, Maryland 21046

Dear Dr. O'Neill:

This letter describes the results of a Food and Drug Administration (FDA) inspection that concluded on October 3, 2008. An FDA investigator from the Baltimore District Office and a toxicologist from the FDA Center for Biologics Evaluation and Research met with you and members of your staff to review your firm's conduct of studies TOX-[(b)(4)] TOX-[(b)(4)] and [(b) (4)] performed under the Good Laboratory Practices (GLP) regulations [Title 21, Code of Federal Regulations, (CFR) Part 58]. The inspection was conducted as part of FDA's Bioresearch Monitoring Program, which includes inspections designed to review research involving investigational products.

At the conclusion of the inspection, a Form FDA 483, Inspectional Observations, was issued to and discussed with you.

Based upon the information obtained during the inspection, we conclude that Washington Biotechnology Inc. (WBI) has violated GLP regulations governing the proper conduct of nonclinical studies as published under 21 CFR Part 58. The applicable provisions of the CFR are cited for each violation.

1. Failure to ensure that each individual engaged in the conduct of or responsible for the supervision of a nonclinical laboratory study has the education, training, and experience, or combination thereof, to enable that individual to perform the assigned functions. [21 CFR § 58.29(a), 58.33].

a. The study director for the three studies reviewed during the inspection lacks the education, training, and experience, or combination thereof, to perform his functions as GLP study director.

b. The project manager for study TOX-[(b)(4)] performed a necropsy despite lacking the education, training, and experience; or combination thereof, to perform necropsies.

2. Failure to ensure that the testing facility maintains a current summary of training and experience and job description for each individual engaged in or supervising the conduct of a nonclinical laboratory study. [21 CFR § 58.29(b)].

You failed to maintain such documentation for the following individuals:

a. The study director for studies TOX-[(b)(4)] TOX-[(b)(4)] and [(b) (4)].

b. The replacement study director for study TOX [(b)(4)].

c. The senior scientist responsible for overseeing the statistical analysis of data for study TOX-[(b)(4)].

d. The statistician responsible for performing statistical analysis for study TOX-[(b)(4)].

e. The project manager for study TOX-[(b)(4)].

f. The laboratory technician responsible for performing necropsies for study TOX[(b)(4)].

3. Failure of testing facility management to fulfill its responsibilities. [21 CFR § 58.31(a) and (g)].

a. The testing facility management failed to designate a qualified study director as described in 21 CFR 58.33.

b. The testing facility management failed to assure that deviations from the regulations were reported by the quality assurance unit and communicated to the study director, and that corrective actions were taken and documented.

4. Failure to ensure that the study director fulfills his or her responsibilities. [21 CFR § 58.33(a), (b), (c), and (f)].

a. The study director failed to assure that the protocols for each study were followed or that changes to the protocol were documented and approved.

b. The study director failed to assure that experimental data was accurately recorded and verified as required by each study protocol.

c. The study director failed to assure that unforeseen circumstances that may affect the quality and integrity of the nonclinical laboratory study were noted when they occurred, and that corrective action was taken and/or documented. Specifically, the TOX[(b)(4)] protocol contained specific requirements about conducting necropsies but these requirements were not followed. The study director failed to note this deviation from protocol and to take corrective actions.

d. The study director for studies TOX [(b)(4)] and [(b)(4)] failed to assure that all raw data, documentation, protocols, specimens, and final reports were transferred to the archives during or at the close of the studies.

5. Failure of the Quality Assurance Unit (QAU) to fulfill its responsibilities. [21 CFR § 58.35(a); 58.35(b)(1), (3), and (7); 58.35(c)].

a. The QAU was not entirely separate from and independent of the personnel engaged in the direction and conduct of that study. The QAU manager for study TOX [(b)(4)] reported directly to the study director.

b. The QAU failed to maintain a complete copy of the master schedule sheet of all nonclinical laboratory studies conducted at the testing facility. Specifically, the master schedule failed to identify the test article, test system, the dates studies were initiated, the sponsor, and the name of the study director.

c. The QAU failed to inspect studies at intervals adequate to assure the integrity of the studies. Specifically, the QAU failed to maintain written and properly signed records of each periodic inspection of studies TOX [(b)(4)] and [(b)(4)]

d. The QAU failed to prepare and sign a statement to be included with the final report for study TOX [(b)(4)] which specified the dates of inspection and findings reported to management and the study director.

e. There is no written documentation of the responsibilities and procedures applicable to the QAU, the records maintained by the QAU, and the method for indexing records.

6. Failure to adequately inspect, clean, and maintain equipment. [21 CFR § 58.63].

There is no written documentation of the inspection, cleaning, maintenance, testing, calibration, or standardization of the [(b)(4)] in which the test article for study TOX [(b)(4)] was stored, the centrifuges used for studies TOX-[(b)(4)] and TOX [(b)(4)] and the [(b)(4)] used in study TOX-[(b)(4)].

7. Failure to establish and follow standard operating procedures (SOPs) setting forth nonclinical laboratory study methods that management is satisfied are adequate to insure the quality and integrity of the data generated in the course of a study. [21 CFR § 58.81 (a) and (b)(6), (b)(7), and (b)(11)].

a. Significant deviations from the SOPs were neither authorized by the study director nor documented in the raw data of the applicable studies. For example:

i. Procedure 1661.3 requires that anesthesia be used for blood draws, and that the anesthetic used be documented. The final report for study TOX-[(b)(4)] contains no documentation of the anesthesia used for orbital bleeds conducted on October 18, 2007 and November 12, 2007.

ii. Procedure 1686.3 requires that rats be anesthetized prior to exsanguination, and the anesthetic used be documented. There is no documentation that anesthesia was used prior to the exsanguinations of animals 2 through 10 and animals 12 through [(b)(4)] in study TOX [(b)(4)].

iii. Procedure 8060.4 requires facility audits to be conducted on a [(b)(4)] basis. There is no documentation of any facility audits between January 2006 and September 2008.

iv. Procedure 420.11 requires that rooms housing rats be maintained at [(b)(4)] relative humidity. The "Room Temperature/Humidity Daily Record," documents deviations from the required humidity range for rats included in study TOX-[(b)(4)].

v. Procedure 400.8 requires that "Room Temperature/Humidity Daily Record," "Animal Inspection Record," " Room/Equipment Status Report," and "Census Activity Record," be audited. There is no documentation that these records were audited for study TOX-[(b)(4)] from August 2007 through November 2007.

b. Written SOPs have not been established for the following:

i. The handling of animals found moribund or dead during a study.

ii. Necropsy or post-mortem examination of animals.

iii. The maintenance and calibration of equipment. Specifically, SOPs have not been established for the maintenance and calibration of the -80℃ freezer, the centrifuges, and the spectrophotometer used for studies TOX [(b)(4)] and TOX[(b)(4)].

8. Failure to determine and document the identity, strength, purity, and composition of each batch of the test or control article. [21 CFR § 58.105(a)].

The study director failed to procure a certificate of analysis from the sponsor that documented the identity, strength, purity, and composition for the test article used for study TOX-[(b)(4)].

9. Failure to assure that each study has an approved written protocol that clearly indicates the objectives and all methods for the conduct of the study. [21 CFR § 58.120(a)].

a. The protocol for the TOX [(b)(4)] study failed to identify the statistical methods to be used for data analysis and the laboratory assays to be performed on day [(b)(4)] of the study.

b. The protocols for studies TOX [(b)(4)] TOX [(b)(4)] and [(b)(4)] failed to document sponsor approval of the protocols.

10. Failure to conduct nonclinical laboratory studies in accordance with the protocol. [21 CFR § 58.130(a), (c), and (d)].

a. The following protocol violations occurred in study TOX [(b)(4)]

i. The protocol required that any animal found dead during the study be necropsied, and any organ displaying abnormalities be removed, preserved, and sent for histological examination. The necropsy of animal 11 indicated an enlarged spleen, however, there is no documentation that this organ was preserved and sent for histological examination.

ii. Laboratory analyses were conducted that were not authorized by the protocol. For example,

1. The kidneys from animal 33 and the lungs from animal 35 were sent for histopathological examination, even though these examinations were not required by the protocol.

2. Fluid extracted from the kidney of animal 28 during necropsy was sent to an analytical laboratory for testing, even though this testing was not required by the protocol. The results of the analysis of this sample are not documented in the final report.

iii. Additional animals were added to the study after the final dosing of the [(b)(4)] original animals, which was not authorized by the protocol.

iv. "Exsanguination Serum Samples" were shipped to the study sponsor on November 13, 2007, which was not authorized by the protocol.

v. The protocol required exsanguination to be performed on day [(b)(4)] of the study. However, 35 of the [(b)(4)] animals included in the study were not exsanguinated until day [(b) (4)] the study.

vi. The protocol required necropsies to be performed immediately following exsanguination. However, necropsies were not performed until 30 minutes after the exsanguinations.

b. Specimens for study TOX [(b)(4)] ere not identified by test system, study, nature, and date of collection.

c. Records of gross findings for all specimens from postmortem observations conducted in study TOX [(b)(4)] were not provided to the pathologist performing the histopathological evaluations.

11. Failure to prepare complete reports of nonclinical laboratory study results. [21 CFR § 58.185(a)(2)-(4), (6), (9)-(10), (13); (b); and (c)].

a. The final study report for TOX [(b)(4)] does not document all changes to the original study protocol, or the study director's approval of the changes.

b. The final study report for study TOX [(b)(4)] fails to identify the statistical methods employed for data analysis.

c. The final study report for study TOX [(b)(4)] fails to identify the test and control articles by name, chemical abstracts number or code number, strength, purity, and composition or other appropriate characteristics.

d. The final study report for study TOX [(b)(4)] does not include an accurate description of the methods used. For example,

i. The final report states that the animals were randomly assigned to study groups; however, there is no documentation that animals were randomized and the firm does not have a written procedure for randomization of animals.

ii. The final report conflicts with the laboratory notebook regarding the method employed to euthanize the study animals.

e. Final study reports fail to describe all circumstances that may have affected the quality or integrity of the data. For example:

i. The final report for study TOX [(b)(4)] refers to the [(b)(4)] treatment groups as [(b)(4)] but the protocol and raw data document the [(b)(4)] treatment groups as [(b)(4)].

ii. The final report for study TOX [(b)(4)] does not describe the circumstances under which a separate research laboratory was used to store samples or analyze [(b)(4)] scans. There is no documentation of the storage of the samples between preparation on July 22, 2008, and analysis on August 7, 2008.

f. Final study reports do not include the name of the study director, the names of other scientists or professionals, and the names of all supervisory personnel involved in the studies. Specifically,

i. The final report for study [(b(4)] does not include the name of the study director, and was not signed and dated by the study director.

ii. The protocol for study TOX [(b)(4)] lists Dr. Sean P. O'Neill as the study director; however, the final report for study TOX [(b)(4)] lists [(b) (6)] as the study director. There is no documentation of the change in study directors.

iii. The final report for study TOX [(b(4)] does not include the names of all of the scientists or professionals involved in the study.

g. The final report for study TOX [(b)(4)] does not document the location where all specimens were stored.

h. Corrections or additions to the final reports were not submitted by the study director in the form of an amendment. Specifically, there are two versions of the final report for study TOX [(b)(4)], one of which was signed by the study director on January 18, 2008 and the other on June 18, 2008. The June 2008 final report is not identified as an amended final report.

12. Failure to store and retain all raw data, documentation, protocols, final reports and specimens generated as a result of nonclinical laboratory studies. [21 CFR § 58.190(a) and 58.195(b)].

The study director for studies TOX [(b)(4)] and [(b)(4)] failed to assure that all raw data, documentation, protocols, specimens, and final reports were transferred to the archives during or at the close of the study. For example:

a. The animal organs directed for collection in study TOX[(b)(4)] were not transferred to the archives at the close of the study.

b. The protocal for [(b)(4)] was not transterred to the archivces at the close of the study.

The deviations listed above are not intended to be an all-inclusive list of deficiencies at your facility. It is your responsibility to ensure that your establishment is in compliance with all requirements of the law and applicable federal regulations. You are responsible for investigating, determining causes of, and correcting violations identified by the FDA, and for reviewing your firm's operations as a whole to ensure that you are in compliance with the regulatory requirements applicable to nonclinical laboratory studies. You should take prompt action to correct these deviations and prevent their recurrence. Failure to do so may result in FDA initiating regulatory action without further notice.

We request that you notify this office in writing, within fifteen (15) working days of receipt of this letter, of the specific steps you have taken to correct the noted violations and to prevent their recurrence. If you cannot complete all of the corrections before you respond, please state the reason for your delay and the time frame within which the corrections will be completed.

Please notify the sponsors of the three studies that were the subjects of the inspection, TOX-[(b) (4)], TOX-[(b)(4)] and [(b)(4)] advising them that your firm failed to conduct the corresponding GLP studies in compliance with Federal regulations under Part 58 of the CFR. As part of your response to this letter, please include a copy of your written notification to these sponsors.

Please send your response and the requested documentation to:

Robert L. Wesley, CSO
Division of Inspections and Surveillance (HFM-664)
Office of Compliance and Biologics Quality
Center for Biologics Evaluation and Research
1401 Rockville Pike, Suite 200N
Rockville, Maryland 20852-1448
Telephone (301) 827-6338

We also request that you send a copy of your response to the FDA District Office listed below.

Sincerely,

/S/

Mary A. Malarkey
Director
Office of Compliance and Biologics Quality
Center for Biologics Evaluation and Research

第152封　给BioReliance公司的警告信

2009年1月5日

参考号：CBER-09-01

尊敬的Kramer博士：

这封信特告知您2008年9月29日结束的，FDA对BioReliance 公司进行现场检查的结果。FDA检查员们与您和员工中的其他人员会面，并对BioReliance公司按照非临床研究质量管理规范（GLP）的法规［美国联邦法规（CFR）第21篇58部分］实施的非临床研究（b）（4）［（b）（4）涉及商业秘密，根据法规内容不予披露的标注］和（b）（4）进行了审查。本次现场检查是FDA的生物研究监查项目的一部分。该项目通过设定的检查方法，审查试验药物相关研究的实施情况。

现场检查结束时，检查员出示并与您和其他BioReliance人员讨论了FDA 483表，即现场检查发现的问题。我们收到并审查了您10月28日给FDA Baltimore地区办公室主任对FDA 483表的回复函。

根据在现场检查中和您10月28日回复函中获得的信息，我们的结论是BioReliance违反了21 CFR58非临床研究相关的GLP法规和要求。以下逐条列出违规情况和相应的CFR条款。

1. 专题负责人未能确保当发生那些可能会影响非临床研究质量和完整性的情况时要进行记录，要采取纠正措施并记录［21 CFR 58.33（c）］质量保证部门未经授权和记录未能确定没有标准操作规程偏离［21 CFR 58.35（b）（5）］。未能按照方案进行非临床研究［21 CFR 58.130（a）］

贵公司没有每日检查所有动物笼内的饲料和饮水情况，或者未隔12天清理一次研究（b）（4）用动物笼。方案规定的笼清理间隔时间为（b）（4）。即没有按照“动物护理时间表”SOP OPBT0206.R06的规定（b）（4）检查所有动物。BioReliance动物饲养人员在“体内生物制剂活性测定研究的临床观察记录”中注明：四只动物死亡，且其他动物“因笼中缺少饲料而蜷缩”。又发现其他动物死亡，并对部分动物进行肢解，或者发现死亡并送去尸检。（b）（4）体重表显示，从2006年11月17日至2006年11月28日，38%的试验动物体重平均下降超过10%；另外15%的动物体重平均下降5%~10%。动物房记录显示，动物有饲料和饮水，但笼变更日志显示，未对笼进行清理。这一问题增加了缺少饲料和饮水之外的原因而导致体重下降的可能性。没有对试验动物进行动物房间号的追踪记录，因此，无法确定发现动物死亡或蜷缩的动物室中是否开展了其他GLP研究。

A.（b）（4）的专题负责人未调查上述情况。没有偏离报告记录未进行动物笼消毒的情况，并且也未向申办者报告。在FDA现场检查期间，“事件详情报告”重新打开，并在现场检查其间制定“纠正/预防措施”文件。

B. QAU未能编制偏离报告或未能着手调查这些事件的相关情况。贵公司在事件发生一年后才进行调查。以回复对FDA关于最终研究报告方面的疑问。

您10月28日的回复函中说明，BioReliance认为这些偏离是独立事件，没有显著影响研究完整性或有效性。该回复函进一步说明，您对最终研究报告进行了最后修订，纳入通过调查后所得到的结果和结论。您报告称，对FDA通过（2007年11月至2008年6月）研究主计划表进行现场检查时提出疑问的（b）（4）GLP研究，BioReliance进行了所要求的笼具更换。因缺少记录，且该事件信息存在矛盾，我们无法确定您所认为的“独立事件”的准确性。事件发生一年内，专题负责人和QAU既未调查该事件，又未形成偏离报告。这些表明，未将动物体重不可预见性下降事件通知专题负责人，也未进行任何调查。本研究的动物饲养记录中关于完成动物喂食和笼清理的信息不一致。因此，无法确定本研究中发生了什么，且无法评估问题的程度。

2005年10月20日结束的FDA既往检查期间也发现笼清理和消毒存在缺陷。此外，您还说明，重新对BioReliance实验室工作人员进行了特定表格和SOP的使用培训，包括“动物房日志”“笼具变更日志”“数据记录”SOP、“支持GxP操作的记录错误纠正中所用的缩略语”SOP以及“动物护理计划表”SOP。修订FMDC0332表，要求在最少（b）（4）时进行笼变更的确认。

2. 未能确保参与或负责监督非临床研究的每位人员具备相关教育、培训和经验，或上述几项的综合能力，能够执行所分配的职责［21 CFR 58.29（a）］

QAU未发现和报告专题负责人没有按BioReliance SOP OPBT0290GLP第5.3节和ODTD2001第5.4节的规定及时完成GLP培训。研究（b）（4）和（b）（4）的负责人未按照BioReliance SOP OpDL0052第5.3节的规定至少每（b）（4）参加一次GLP培训。在本警告信涉及的研究期间，专题负责人的GLP培训存在问题。

10月28日的回复函称，该专题负责人具有超过20年的GLP 专题负责人经验，5个月未参加GLP的再培训不会影响研究（b）（4）和（b）（4）的GLP符合性。现场检查期间，BioReliance向FDA研究者提供了当前正在开发的培训通知系统的流程图。

3. 未能准备一份非临床研究总结报告，其中包含了对所有会影响质量和数据可靠性的情况描述［21 CFR 58.185（a）（9）］

A.（b）（4）的最终版研究报告中没有上述第1项所列的BioReliance在动物饲养中存在问题。这些问题导致试验系统发生变化，无法确定该系统对GLP研究结局造成的潜在影响。

您在回复函中称，在研究实施期间以及研究报告中，BioReliance向申办者报告了关于缺少饲料的不可预见情况，包括研究动物临床观察结果和体重数据。没有记录证明BioReliance向申办者报告其未消毒鼠笼。FDA检查员提供的一封电子邮件显示，申办者曾要求BioReliance提供研究动物死亡的相关信息。FDA检查员要求提交可以证明BioReliance向申办者报告了其未在适当间隔内消毒鼠笼的文件，但至今您尚未向FDA提交该证明文件。

B. 没有记录可以溯源（b）（4）和（b）（4）研究动物所用的研究室位置。因缺少该类证明文件，无法对环境、动物饲养情况、动物室消毒情况进行明确的评价。

现场检查期间，贵公司修改了“笼变更日志”，添加了研究动物饲养室的相关记录。

C.（b）（4）高剂量组23/（b）（4）只小鼠“触诊记录”中有可触及的病变，而解剖员在肉眼检查时发现该组仅有一只动物的接种部位出现结节，BioReliance未能按方案要求报告这一差异情况。方案规定“病理学家应总结供试品组和对照品组的所有结果（临床、肉眼检查和显微镜观察结果），并在研究结束时提供给申办者”这一差异情况也未包含在最终的病理报告中。

您的回复函中未就现场检查发现的上述问题予以说明。

此外，我们还关注现场检查结束时FDA检查员与贵方讨论的以下问题：

A. BioReliance未能记录体内生物制剂试验区域中试验动物在动物室中的具体位置。

B. 关于对被检查的某研究用供试品和对照品（b）（4）的说明，研究记录和口头声明不一致。BioReliance质量体系负责人和QA经理都表示，（b）（4）是“（b）（4）”，而不是整个检查所提及的及方案中所确定的（b）（4）。在供试品制备记录和终版研究报告中，（b）（4）均未被作为一个组分或（b）（4）。

C. BioReliance 的（b）（4）和（b）（4）小鼠均属于被检查方案的范围。方案或BioReliance SOP均不要求（b）（4）。现场检查期间，BioReliance向FDA检查员提供了一个其他涉及（b）（4）其他GLP研究的（b）（4）列表，其中，（b）（4）试验未按照BioReliance的规定进行。现场检查期间，BioReliance向FDA检查员提供了一个纳入（b）（4）测定数据的修订版SOP。现场检查结束时，FDA检查员要求提交（b）（4）研究的任何（b）（4）特征性质的文件。

以上所列举的偏离情况，并非是罗列贵公司存在的所有GLP缺陷。作为GLP试验机构，您应负责确保按照FDA的法规开展非临床研究。

给您下发本警告信是因为现场检查时发现的问题的性质非常严重。请注意，未能实施有效的纠正措施和/

或进一步发生违规情况，可能导致FDA在不再通知的情况下采取监管措施。

自收到本警告信的15个工作日内，请提交书面的文件，说明为了纠正上述违规情况并预防当前或将来的非临床研究中再次发生类似的违规情况，您已经采取或将要采取的额外措施。

附：英文原文

BioReliance Corporation

WARNING LETTER

JAN 5, 2009

By Certified Mail - Return Receipt Requested
And By Facsimile Transmission

CBER-09-01

James J. Kramer, Ph.D.
Vice President of Operations
BioReliance Corporation
14920 Broschart Road
Rockville, Maryland 20850

Dear Dr. Kramer:

This letter describes the results of a Food and Drug Administration (FDA) inspection that concluded on September 29, 2008. The FDA investigators met with you and other members of your staff to review BioReliance Corporation's conduct of nonclinical laboratory studies (b)(4) and (b)(4) performed under the Good Laboratory Practice (GLP) for Nonclinical Laboratory Studies regulations [Title 21, Code of Federal Regulations, (CFR) Part 58]. The inspection was conducted as part of FDA's Bioresearch Monitoring Program, which includes inspections designed to review research involving investigational products.

At the end of the inspection a Form FDA 483, Inspectional Observations, was issued and discussed with you and other BioReliance staff. We received and reviewed your October 28 Letter responding to the Form FDA 483, addressed to the FDA Baltimore District Director.

Based upon the information obtained during the inspection and your October 28 Letter, we conclude that BioReliance has violated GLP regulations governing the proper conduct of nonclinical studies as published under 21 CFR Part 58. The applicable provisions of the CFR are cited for each violation.

1. Failure of the study director to assure that unforeseen circumstances that may affect the quality and integrity of the nonclinical laboratory study were noted when they occurred and corrective action was taken and documented. [21 CFR § 58.33(c)]. Failure of the quality assurance unit (QAU) to determine that no deviations from approved standard operating procedures (SOPs) were made without proper authorization and documentation. [21 CFR § 58.35(b)(5)]. Failure to conduct nonclinical laboratory studies in accordance with the protocol. [21 CFR § 58.130(a)].

Your firm did not check every animal cage for feed and water each day, or clean the animal cages for study (b)(4) for twelve days. The protocol-specified interval for cleaning cages is (b)(4). As a result, the animals were not checked (b)(4) as required in the "Animal Care Schedule" SOP OPBT0206.R06. BioReliance animal care staff noted on the "Clinical Observation Record for In Vivo Biologics Assays" that four animals were found dead and others "hunched, possibly due to lack of food in cage." Other animals were found dead and partially cannibalized, or found dead and sent to necropsy. The (b)(4) body weight charts showed 38% of the study animals lost an average of more than of 10% of their body weight during the period from November 17 to November 28, 2006; another 15% of the animals lost an average of 5% to 10% of body weight. The Animal Room Logs showed the animals had food and water, but the Cage Changing Log shows that cleaning had not been performed. This discrepancy raises the possibility that causes other than the absence of food and water could have contributed to the weight loss. There was no documented tracking of study animals to specific animal rooms, and it is not possible to determine what other GLP studies took place in the room where dead and hunched animals were found.

A. The (b)(4) Study Director did not investigate these circumstances. There was no deviation report to document the lack of animal cage sanitation, and no report was made to the study sponsor. The "Event Details Report" was re-opened during the FDA inspection and a document entitled "Corrective/Preventative Actions" was prepared during the inspection.

B. The QAU failed to generate a deviation report or to initiate an investigation into the circumstances of these events. Your firm's investigation took place more than one year after these events occurred, in response to an FDA inquiry regarding the final study report.

Your October 28 Letter explains that BioReliance considers these deviations to be an isolated event with no significant impact on integrity of the study or study validity criteria. The Letter further explains that the final study report was eventually amended to include results and conclusions from your investigation of these events. You report that BioReliance performed required cage changes for (b)(4) GLP studies that were queried during the FDA inspection using a master schedule for studies that took place from November 2007 to June 2008. It is not possible to determine the accuracy of your statement that this was an isolated event because of the lack of documentation and also conflicting information regarding this incident at BioReliance. No study director or QAU investigations took place and no deviation report was generated within a year of the incident. These events demonstrate that the study director was either not informed about the unforeseen loss of animal weight, or did not act to investigate. Animal husbandry records for this study are in disagreement concerning the accomplishment of animal feeding and cage cleaning. As a result it is not possible to determine what happened in this study or to assess the extent of the problems.

Cage cleaning and sanitizing deficiencies were also noted during your previous FDA inspection which ended on October 20, 2005. You also report that the BioReliance laboratory staff was retrained concerning use of specific forms and SOPs, including the "Animal Room Log," "Cage Changing Log," "Recording of Data" SOP, "Abbreviations Used in Error Corrections on Documents Supporting GxP Operations" SOP, and the "Animal Care Schedule" SOP. Form FMDC0332 was revised to require confirmation of cage change performance at a minimum of (b)(4).

2. Failure to ensure that each individual engaged in the conduct of, or responsible for the supervision of a nonclinical laboratory study has the education, training, and experience or combination thereof to enable that individual to perform their assigned functions. [21 CFR § 58.29(a)].

The QAU failed to detect and report that the study director was overdue for GLP training, as required by BioReliance SOPs OPBT0290 section 5.3 and ODTD 2001 section 5.4. The study director for studies (b)(4) and (b)(4) did not participate in GLP training at least every (b)(4), as required in BioReliance SOP OPDL0052 section 5.3. The Director's GLP training deficiency occurred during the same period as the deficiencies for the studies noted in this letter.

The October 28 Letter states that this individual has more than 20 years of experience as a GLP study director, and your firm does not believe a GLP refresher-training gap of 5 months compromised GLP compliance for studies (b)(4) and (b)(4). During the inspection BioReliance gave the FDA investigators a flow chart showing a training notification system currently under development.

3. Failure to prepare a final nonclinical laboratory study report that included a description of all circumstances that may have affected the quality or integrity of the data. [21 CFR § 58.185 (a)(9)].

A. There is no description in the (b)(4) final study report of BioReliance's animal husbandry lapses described in item 1, above. These deficiencies introduced a variable into the test system whose potential effects on the outcome of the GLP study cannot not be determined.

Your letter explains that BioReliance reported to the sponsor unforeseen circumstances relating to lack of food, including study animal clinical observations and weight data, during the conduct of the study as well as within the study report. There is no documentation showing BioReliance reported its failure to sanitize mouse cages to the sponsor. The FDA investigators were furnished an e-mail that shows the sponsor asked BioReliance for information concerning deaths of study animals. The FDA investigators requested documentation showing that BioReliance reported its failure to sanitize mouse cages at appropriate intervals to the sponsor, but you have not provided the documentation to FDA.

B. There was no documentation to track specific study room locations for (b)(4) and (b)(4) study animals. The lack of such documentation makes a definitive evaluation of the environmental, animal husbandry, and room sanitation conditions impossible.

During the inspection your firm revised the "Cage Changing Log" to document the room where the study animals are housed.

C. BioReliance did not report discrepant clinical observations involving palpable lesions noted on the "Palpation Records" for 23 of the (b)(4) mice in the (b)(4) high dose group. Prosectors found only one animal in this group with a nodule at the site of inoculation on gross examination. This discrepancy was not included in the final pathology report, as required by the study protocol in which "the pathologist is required to summarize all the findings (clinical, gross and microscopic) for the test and control groups and present them to the study sponsor at the end of the study."

Your letter does not address this inspectional observation.

We are also concerned about the following issues, which the FDA investigators discussed with you at the close of the inspection:

A. BioReliance does not track specific room locations of test animals in the in vivobiologics testing area.

B. Study documents and verbal statements conflict regarding the (b)(4) for the inspected studies' test and control articles. The BioReliance Director of Quality Systems and Quality Assurance Manager both stated that the (b)(4) was "(b)(4)," not (b)(4) as noted throughout the inspection and specified in the protocols. (b)(4) is not listed as a component or an (b)(4) in the test article preparation documentation or the corresponding final study reports for the protocols.

C. BioReliance (b)(4) under the inspected protocols, and the (b)(4) mice. Neither the protocols nor the BioReliance SOPs required (b)(4). During the inspection, BioReliance furnished the FDA investigators a listing of (b)(4) other GLP studies involving the (b)(4), in which, according to BioReliance, (b)(4) testing were not performed. During the inspection, BioReliance furnished the FDA investigators with a revised SOP to include measurement of (b)(4). At the close of the inspection, the FDA investigators requested documentation for any (b)(4) characterization for the (b)(4) studies.

The deviations listed above are not intended to be an all-inclusive list of GLP deficiencies that may exist at your testing facility. As a GLP-testing facility, you are responsible for ensuring that you conduct nonclinical studies according to FDA regulations.

This Warning Letter is issued to you because of the serious nature of the observations noted at the time of the FDA inspection. Please be advised that failure to implement effective corrective actions and/or commission of further violations may result in the FDA taking regulatory action without further notice.

Within fifteen (15) working days of receiving this letter, please provide written documentation of the additional actions you have taken or will take, to correct the above violations and prevent the recurrence of similar violations in current or future nonclinical studies.

Please send your written documentation to:

Anthony D. Hawkins
Division of Inspections and Surveillance (HFM-664)
Office of Compliance and Biologics Quality
Center for Biologics Evaluation and Research
1401 Rockville Pike, Suite 200N
Rockville, Maryland 20852-1448

Telephone (301) 827-6338

We request that you send a copy of your response to the FDA District Office listed below.

Sincerely,

Mary A. Malarkey
Director
Office of Compliance and Biologics Quality
Center for Biologics Evaluation and Research

Cc: Evelyn Bonnin, District Director
Food and Drug Administration
6000 Metro Drive, Suite 101
Baltimore, Maryland 21215

附 录

FDA

专业术语及缩略语英汉对照表

英文	中文	缩略语
abbreviate new drug application	仿制药申请	ANDA
active controlled	阳性对照	
adverse drug reaction	药物不良反应	ADR
adverse event	不良事件	AE
applicable regulatory requirement(s)	适用的法规要求	
audit	稽查	
audit certificate	稽查证明	
audit report	稽查报告	
audit trail	审计追踪/稽查轨迹	
bioavailability	生物利用度	BA
bioequivalence	生物等效性	BE
Bioresearch Monitoring Program	生物研究监查项目	BIMO
blinding/masking	设盲	
case histories	病历	
Case Report Form	病例报告表	CFR
Center for Biologics Evaluation and Research	生物制品审评研究中心	CBER
Center for Drug Evaluation and Research	药品审评研究中心	CDER
certified copy	核准的复印件	
checkin	登记	
clinical investigator	临床研究者	CI
clinical trial/study	临床试验/研究	
clinical trial/study report	临床试验/研究报告	CSR
comparator /or product	对照药物	
comparative trial	对照研究	
compliance in relation to trials	试验的依从性	
confidentiality	保密性	
conflict of interest	利益冲突	
continuing review	跟踪审查	
contract research organization	合同研究组织	CRO
contract/agreement	合同/协议	
convened meetings	召集会议	
coordinating investigator	协调研究者	
corrective action plan	纠正措施计划	
Data Monitoring Committee	数据监查委员会	
Data and Safety Monitoring Board	数据与安全监查委员会	DSMB
deliberation or voting on IRB	伦理委员会的审查或投票	

direct access	直接访问权限	
documentation	文件/文件化	
dose adjustments	剂量调整	
double blind	双盲	
eligibility criteria	合格标准	
essential documents	核心文件	
Establishment Inspection Report	现场检查报告	EIR
fiscal quarter	财务季度	
Form FDA 483	FDA 483表	
Good Clinical Practice	临床试验质量管理规范	GCP
Good Laboratory Practice	非临床研究质量管理规范	GLP
imparitial witness	独立见证人	
inclusion/exclusion criteria	入选/排除标准	
Independent Data-Monitoring Committee	独立的数据监查委员会/数据监查委员会	IDMC
Independent Ethics Committee	伦理委员会	IEC
informed consent	知情同意	IC
informed evaluation	知情评价	
initial review	初始审查	
inspection	现场检查	
inspectional observations	现场检查发现的问题	
inspection report	现场检查报告	IR
institution（medical）	医疗机构	
Institutional Review Board	伦理委员会	IRB
integrity of the data/data integrity	数据可靠性	DI
Interim clinical study report	临床研究中期报告	
investigational product	试验药物	IP
investigational medicinal product	试验药物	IMP
investigational new drug application	新药临床试验申请	IND
investigator	研究者	
investigator's brochure	研究者手册	IB
legally acceptable representative	法律认可的代理人	
Marketing Authorisation Application	上市许可申请	MAA
Marketing Authorisation Holder	上市许可持有人	MAH
meeting minutes	会议记录	
memos-to-file	备忘录文件	
monitoring	监查	
monitoring plan	监查计划	
monitoring report	监查报告	
multicentre trial	多中心试验	
New Drug Application	新药上市申请	NDA
nonclinical study	非临床研究	
office of compliance	合规办公室	

open label	开放的（非盲法的）	
opinion in relation to IEC	伦理委员会意见	
original medical record	原始医疗记录	
parallel group	平行组	
physical exam worksheets	体检表	
physical examinations	体格检查	PE
placebo	安慰剂	
principal investigator	主要研究者	PI
protocol	试验方案	
protocol amendment	试验方案的修正案	
quality assurance	质量保证	QA
quality control	质量控制	QC
randomization	随机化	
regulatory authorities	监管部门	RA
rescreening	复筛	
screening	筛选	
screening eligibility checklist	筛查合格表	
serious adverse drug reaction	严重药物不良反应	SADR
serious adverse event	严重不良事件	SAE
single-blind	单盲	
source data	原始数据	
source documents	原始文件	
sponsor	申办者	
sponsor-investigator	申办–研究者	
standard operating procedures	标准操作规程	SOP
subinvestigator	授权研究者	
subject identification code	受试者识别代码	
subject/trial subject	受试者/试验受试者	
trial site	试验场所	
unexpected adverse drug reaction	非预期的药物不良反应	
validation of computerized systems	计算机化系统验证	CSV
vulnerable subjects	弱势受试者	
well-being of the trial subjects	受试者的健康	